Emergency Nursing
CORE CURRICULUM

Emergency Nursing
CORE CURRICULUM
SEVENTH EDITION

Edited by

Vicki Sweet, MSN, RN, MICN, CEN, FAEN
ALS/CQI Coordinator
Orange County Emergency Medical Services
Santa Ana, California
Associate Faculty, Health Sciences & Human Services
Saddleback College
Mission Viejo, California

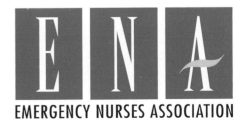

ELSEVIER

ELSEVIER

3251 Riverport Lane
St. Louis, Missouri 63043

EMERGENCY NURSING CORE CURRICULUM ISBN: 978-0-323-44374-6
Copyright © 2018, Elsevier Inc. All Rights Reserved.

Notices

Previous editions copyrighted 2007, 2000, 1994, and 1987.

Senior Content Strategist: Sandra Clark
Content Development Manager: Billie Sharp, Lisa Newton
Associate Content Development Specialist: Samantha Dalton
Publishing Services Manager: Julie Eddy
Project Manager: Mike Sheets
Design Direction: Brian Salisbury

Printed in India

Last digit is the print number: 9 8 7 6 5 4

Working together
to grow libraries in
developing countries

www.elsevier.com • www.bookaid.org

CONTRIBUTORS

Anne C. Albers, MSN, RN, CPNP-PC
Pediatric Nurse Practitioner
Washington University St. Louis
St. Louis Children's Hospital
St. Louis, MO, US

Teri Arruda, DNP, FNP-BC, CEN
Nurse Practitioner

Cynthia Baxter, RN, DNP, ACNS-BC, NEA-BC, VHA-CM
Chief Nurse, Ambulatory Care
College of Nursing
University of Kentucky
Lexington VA Medical Center
Lexington, KY, US

Denise Bayer, MSN, RN, CEN, FAEN
CEO/Consultant
Bayer Healthcare Consulting
Riverside, CA, US

Sue Anne Bell, PhD, FNP-BC
Clinical Associate Professor
School of Nursing
University of Michigan
Ann Arbor, MI, US

Nancy M. Bonalumi, DNP, RN, CEN, FAEN
President
NMB Global Leadership, LLC
Lancaster, PA, US

Karen Cameron, RN, BSN, CPTC, CTBS
Call Center, Manager
Gift of Hope Organ & Tissue Donor Network
Itasca, IL, US

Melody R. Campbell, DNP, RN, CEN, TCRN, CCRN, CCNS
Trauma Program Manager & Critical Care Clinical Nurse
    Specialist
Kettering Medical Center
Kettering, OH, US

Mary Jo Cerepani, DNP, FNP-BC, CEN
Assistant Professor & Director of Advanced Practitioner Services
University of Pittsburgh
Pittsburgh, PA, US

Garrett K. Chan, PhD, APRN, FAEN, FPCN, FNAP, FAAN
Director of Advanced Practice
Stanford Health Care
Stanford, CA, US

Joni Hentzen Daniels, MSN, RN, CEN, CCRN, CNS
Clinical Nurse Specialist – Emergency Care, Regional Director,
    Clinical Services
EmCare, Inc, Southwest Division
Houston, TX, US

Michael De Laby, MSN, RN, CCRN, CFRN, TCRN, NRP
EMS Systems & Standards Chief
Orange County Emergency Medical Services
Santa Ana, CA, US

Nancy J. Denke, DNP, ACNP-BC, FNP-BC, CEN, CCRN, FAEN
Ortho/Neuro Nurse Practitioner
HonorHealth Scottsdale Osborn Medical Center
Scottsdale, AZ, US

Jennifer Denno, MSN, RN, CEN
Clinical Educator, Emergency Services
Sutter Medical Center, Sacramento
Sacramento, CA, US

Margaret Flanagan, MSN, FNP-BC, RN
Adjunct Faculty, Retired
California State University, Long Beach
Long Beach, CA, US

Kathleen Flarity, DNP, PhD, CEN, CFRN, FAEN
Mobilization Assistant to the Chief
Air Force Nurse Corps
Office of the Surgeon General
Headquarters United States Air Force
Washington, DC, US
Nurse Scientist
University of Colorado Health
Colorado Springs, CO, US

Joyce Foresman-Capuzzi, MSN, APRN, RN-BC, CCNS, CEN, CPN, CTRN, CCRN, CPEN, AFN-BC, SANE-A, EMT-P, FAEN
Clinical Nurse Educator
Lankenau Medical Center
Wynnewood, PA, US

Reneé Semonin Holleran, FNP-BC, PhD, CEN, CCRN (Emeritus), CFRN and CTRN (Retired), FAEN
Family Nurse Practitioner
Alta View Senior Clinic
Hope Free Clinic
Salt Lake City, UT, US

Kathleen Sanders Jordan, DNP, MS, RN, FNP-BC, ENP-BC, SANE-P
Clinical Assistant Professor
School of Nursing
University of North Carolina at Charlotte
Nurse Practitioner
Mid-Atlantic Emergency Medicine Associates
Charlotte, NC, US

Betty L. Kuiper, PhDc, MSN, APRN, ACNS-BC, CEN
Nursing and Institutional Research Coordinator
Baptist Health Paducah
Paducah, KY, US

Arnitha Lim, BSN, MBA, RN, CNOR, CTBS
Director, Tissue Program
Gift of Hope Organ & Tissue Donor Network
Itasca, IL, US

Kyle Madigan, RN, MSN, CMTE, CFRN, CTRN, CEN, CCRN
Director – Dartmouth-Hitchcock Advanced Response Team
(DHART)
Dartmouth-Hitchcock Medical Center
Lebanon, NH, US

Tamara C. McConnell, RN, MSN, LNC, PHN
Emergency Medical Services Administrator, Orange County
Emergency Medical Services
Orange County Health Care Agency
Santa Ana, CA, US

Justin J. Milici, MSN, RN, CEN, CPEN, CFRN, CCRN
RN III – Emergency Services
Parkland Health and Hospital System
Dallas, TX, US

Joanne E. Navarroli, MSN RN CEN
Staff/Trauma Nurse
Chandler Regional Medical Center – Dignity Health
Chandler, AZ, US

Mary Hugo Nielson, DNP, APRN, ANP-BC, ANP
Assistant Professor
Western Connecticut State University
Danbury, CT, US

Karen M. O'Connell, Lt Col, USAF, NC, PhD, RN, CEN, NEA-BC
Nurse Scientist/Director, Clinical Investigations
Wright-Patterson Medical Center
Wright-Patterson Air Force Base, OH, US

Walter A. Perez, MSN, CEN, CCRN
Staff Nurse
VA Greater Los Angeles Healthcare System
Los Angeles, CA, US

Jaime V. Pitner, MSN, RN, MICP, CEN, RHC
Administrative Director of Nursing
RWJ Barnabas Health
Toms River, NJ, US

Kristine Kenney Powell, MSN, RN, CEN, NEA-BC, FAEN
Director of Emergency Services-North Texas
Baylor Scott & White Health
Dallas, TX, US

Elda G. Ramirez, PhD, RN, FNP-BC, FAANP, FAEN
Professor – Clinical Nursing
School of Nursing
University of Texas Health Science Center at Houston
Houston, TX, US

Rebecca L. Reilly, BS, CTBS
Donor Services Field Representative
AlloSource
Centennial, CO, US

Nancy Zeller Smith, MS, RN, OCN
Director, Education Department; Director, Charles A. Sammons
Center
Baylor Scott and White Regional Medical Center at Grapevine
Grapevine, TX, US

Jeff Solheim, MSN, RN, CEN, CFRN, FAEN
Founder/Executive Director
Project Helping Hands
Grants Pass, OR, US

Stephen J. Stapleton, PhD, MS, RN, CEN, FAEN
Assistant Professor
Mennonite College of Nursing
Illinois State University
Normal, IL, US

Rebecca A. Steinmann, MS, APN, CPEN, CEN, TCRN, CCRN, CCNS, FAEN
Clinical Nurse Specialist, Emergency Care Center
Ann & Robert H. Lurie Children's Hospital of Chicago
Chicago, IL, US

Debbie Travers, PhD, RN, FAEN, CEN
Associate Professor
University of North Carolina at Chapel Hill
Chapel Hill, NC, US

Christine Trotter, CCRN, ACNP
Abdominal Transplant Surgery Nurse Practitioner
Critical Care Nurse Practitioner
University of Chicago
Chicago, IL, US

Anna M. Valdez, PhD, RN, CEN, CFRN, CNE, FAEN
Faculty
Walden University
Minneapolis, MN, US

Sharon Vanairsdale, MS, APRN, ACNS-BC, NP-C, CEN
Program Director for Serious Communicable Diseases
Emory University
Atlanta, GA, US

Barbara Weintraub, RN, MSN, MPH, CEN, CPEN, APN, FAEN
Manager, Emergency Department
Community First Medical Center
Chicago, IL, US

Lisa Adams Wolf, PhD, RN, CEN, FAEN
Director, Institute for Emergency Nursing Research
Emergency Nurses Association
Des Plaines, IL, US

LaToria Woods, MSN, RN, APN, CCNS
Senior Associate – Nursing Education, Institute for Emergency
Nursing Research
Emergency Nurses Association
Des Plaines, IL, US

Cheryl Wraa, MSN, RN, FAEN
Director, TCAR Programs
Laurelwood Education Programs
Sacramento, CA, US

REVIEWERS

Sharon Saunderson Coffey, DNP, FNP-C, ACNS-BC, CEN, CCRN, CHEP
Adjunct Faculty
Barry University
Miami Shores, FL, US

Yvette Cole, DNP-C, MSN-Ed, FNP-C, CCRN, CEN, PCCN, CPEN
Family Nurse Practitioner
Lake City Medical Center
Lake City, FL, US

Candy M. Corral, RN, CNS-BC, MSN, CEN, SCRN
Director of Clinical Partnerships
Huntington Hospital
Pasadena, CA, US

Anthony John Cruz, RN, MSN
ER Director
Anaheim Global Medical Center
Anaheim, CA, US

Denise L. Garee, MSN, RN, CEN, CHSE, PhD(c)
Owner and President
Nurse D Cares
Deerfield Beach, FL, US

Stacie Hunsaker, RN, MSN, CEN, CPEN
RN – Emergency Department
Intermountain Healthcare
Salt Lake City, Utah,
Assistant Teaching Professor
College of Nursing
Brigham Young University
Provo, UT, US

Diane Phillips Irwin, RN, MSN-HCSM, BS
Consultant

Lori Kelty, MSN-Ed, CCRN, CEN, NE
Assistant Professor of Nursing
Mercer County Community College
West Windsor, NJ, US

Kent Lee, RN, MSN, CPEN, CNS
Clinical Nurse Specialist
Children's Hospital of Orange County
Orange, CA, US

Lisa Matamoros, DNP, RN-BC, CEN, CHSE, CPEN
Advanced Education Specialist
Johns Hopkins All Children's Hospital
St. Petersburg, FL, US

Tamara C. McConnell, RN, MSN, LNC, PHN
Emergency Medical Services Administrator, Orange County
    Emergency Medical Services
Orange County Health Care Agency
Santa Ana, CA, US

Stacy Merritt, DNP, APRN, ACNP-BC, FNP-BC, CEN
Nurse Practitioner
Faster Care Urgent Care
Sumter, SC, US

Brittany M. Newberry, PhD, MSN, MPH, APRN, ENP-BC, FNP-BC
Nurse Practitioner
Piedmont Mountainside
Jasper, GA, US
VP Education and Professional Development
HospitalMD
Peachtree City, GA, US

Laurie Nolan-Kelley, DNP(c), MSN, RN CNL, CEN, TCRN, EMT-P
Registered Nurse
Western Connecticut Health Network
Norwalk, CT, US

Mary E. O'Sheilds, MS, RN
Interim Director – Emergency Services
BE Smith Interim Services
Lenexa, KS, US

Ruthie Robinson, PhD, RN, CNS, FAEN, CEN, NEA-BC
Director, Graduate Nursing Studies
Lamar University
Beaumont, TX, US

Mary Russell, EdD, MSN, RN, RPT, CEN
Registered Nurse, Emergency Services
Boca Raton Regional Hospital
Boca Raton, FL, US

Susan F. Sanders, PhD, APRN, ACNS-BC, CEN
Assistant Professor of Nursing
Georgia Southern University
Statesboro, GA, US

Carla E. Schneider, MSN, CEN, MICN
Director, Emergency Department
Hoag Memorial Hospital Presbyterian
Newport Beach, CA, US

Karen L. Sharp, MSN, RN
Director, Emergency Services
Memorial Care Health System–Saddleback Memorial
Laguna Hills, CA, US

Dustin Spencer, DNP, RN, NRP, NP-C, ENP-BC
Assistant Professor
Saginaw Valley State University
University Center, MI, US

Noel Stevens, CRNP, AGACNP-BC, MS, BSN, BA, CEN, CCRN
Nurse Practitioner
Baltimore County Detention Center
Towson, MD, US

Diane Fuller Switzer, DNP, ARNP, FNP-BC, ENP-BC, CEN, CCRN
Emergency Nurse Practitioner
Harborview Medical Center
Assistant Clinical Faculty
College of Nursing
Seattle University
Adjunct Clinical Faculty
School of Nursing
University of Washington
Seattle, WA, US

Stephanie B. Turner, EdD, MSN, RN
Assistant Professor
Capstone College of Nursing
University of Alabama
Tuscaloosa, AL, US

We would like to dedicate this edition of the *Emergency Nursing Core Curriculum* to emergency nurses worldwide. Your commitment to safe practice and safe care is a tribute to the nursing profession.

PREFACE

Emergency Nursing Core Curriculum, seventh edition, represents a body of knowledge in the specialty of emergency nursing. The practice of emergency nursing has changed significantly in 40-plus years and with that practice comes a change in our core knowledge and skills. Today's emergency nurse practices in a variety of arenas and must be prepared to face a dynamic and rapidly changing health care environment.

The goal of *Emergency Nursing Core Curriculum,* seventh edition, is to provide today's emergency nurse with current, evidence-based information in a concise format. Individual chapters have been revised and updated in order to provide the most current information available. Some chapters have been combined and others have been added.

The seventh edition includes the usual clinical topics as well as many that affect today's emergency nurse on a daily basis. These topics include emerging diseases and personal protective procedures, end-of-life issues, hemodynamic monitoring concepts, complementary and alternative therapies, as well as forensic evidence collection. The goal of this revision is to provide both current clinical practice and current trends in practice settings and research.

Emergency Nursing Core Curriculum, seventh edition, would not have been possible without the expertise of each contributor and reviewer. The willingness to meet tight deadlines was crucial to this project's success. The support from the Emergency Nurses Association and the editors from Elsevier, Inc. was invaluable. I am deeply indebted to all who contributed to this revision.

Vicki Sweet, MSN, RN, MICN, CEN, FAEN

ACKNOWLEDGMENTS

This revision would not have been possible without the contributions of expert authors and reviewers. Thank you for your commitment to emergency nursing excellence.

The expertise of the publishing staff at Elsevier cannot be overlooked. Their attention to detail and constant communication with the project editor and with ENA staff kept the project on track.

Thank you also to the Emergency Nurses Association. Having the support of the ENA Board of Directors, the Executive Directors, as well as professional staff liaisons contributed significantly to the success of this revision. I could not have done it without you.

Vicki Sweet, MSN, RN, MICN, CEN, FAEN
Editor, Seventh Edition

Nancy MacRae, MS
ENA Executive Director
Matthew F. Powers, MS, BSN, RN MICP, CEN
ENA Interim Executive Director/ Past President

2018 ENA Board of Directors
Jeff Solheim, MSN, RN, CEN, CFRN, FAEN
President

2017 ENA Board of Directors
Karen K. Wiley, MSN, RN, CEN
President

2016 ENA Board of Directors
Kathleen E. Carlson, MSN, RN, CEN, FAEN
President
Josie Howard-Ruben, PhD, APN-CNS, AOCN, CHPN
ENA Chief Nursing Officer
Marilyn Noettl, MS, RN
ENA Senior Associate

CONTENTS

PART 2
Clinical Emergencies

PART 3
Trauma Emergencies

PART 4
Professional Components

CHAPTER 1

Nursing Assessment and Resuscitation

Nancy J. Denke, DNP, ACNP-BC, FNP-BC, CEN, CCRN, FAEN

Safe Care, Safe Practice

No matter the reason for the patient's presentation to the emergency department (ED), the care team's responsibilities are to be prepared to receive any patient while protecting themselves. This means the team must comply with universal precautions, perform hand hygiene, and don personal protective equipment.

I. Primary Assessment

Even though the reasons for presenting to the ED can vary, forming a general impression of the patient is important (e.g., sick, sicker, sickest). The goal then of the primary assessment is to rapidly but systematically obtain essential subjective and objective** information, interpret this information, identify potential life-threatening states, and immediately intervene when indicated. The ABCDE mnemonic can facilitate this process using a systematic

** NOTE: Subjective data is information that is communicated either by patients themselves or others. Objective data is information obtained through observations during the physical examination or through test results.

approach. If a potential life-threatening state is identified at any time during this process, the assessment is stopped momentarily until appropriate stabilizing interventions are initiated and priorities of care achieved. It must be noted at this time if uncontrolled bleeding is present on arrival of this patient to the ED, and if so, the priorities of assessment must be reorganized to **C-ABCDE**. Evidence has proven that under certain circumstances, such as external peripheral hemorrhage, the priorities must be reorganized to address and control hemorrhage prior to proceeding with the assessment.[1]

A. OVERVIEW OF MAJOR COMPONENTS

1. Subjective data collection
   a. Brief one-line statement
      1) Chief complaint
      2) Precipitating event/onset of symptoms
      3) Mechanism of injury (see Chapter 31)
   b. Progression of condition from first symptom or injury to initiation of care
      1) History of present illness/injury/chief complaint
         a) Location of problem
         b) Duration of symptoms

c) Characteristics
d) Aggravating factors
e) Relieving factors
f) Treatment prior to arrival

2. Objective data collection
   a. Airway patency with simultaneous cervical spine protection for all or suspected trauma patients
   b. Breathing effectiveness
   c. Circulation effectiveness
   d. Disability (brief neurologic assessment)
   e. Exposure/environmental controls

B. INDIVIDUAL COMPONENTS OF PRIMARY ASSESSMENT

1. Assessment of airway, with simultaneous cervical spine (C-spine) protection if indicated
   a. Subjective data collection
      1) No history related to airway problem
      2) No dyspnea, dysphagia, or dysarthria
   b. Objective data collection
      1) Patient able to open mouth widely, and mouth is clear
      2) Patient able to speak or appropriately vocalize for age without dysphonia or muffled speech (this indicates a protected airway)
      3) No foreign material, drooling, or obstruction visible in upper airway (e.g., blood, vomitus, loose teeth, foreign bodies, debris, angioedema)
      4) Equal rise and fall of chest with ventilations
      5) Absence of adventitious upper airway noises (e.g., stridor, grunting)
      6) Use of the mnemonic AVPU—a quick assessment of alertness and if patient will be able to protect his or her airway[1]
         a) **A** = alert
         b) **V** = responds to verbal stimuli
         c) **P** = responds only to painful stimuli
         d) **U** = unresponsive
   c. Action/intervention
      1) If mechanism of injury, symptoms, or physical findings suggest a spinal cord injury, alignment and protection of the cervical spine must be achieved
         a) This can be achieved with manual stabilization or with the use of a rigid collar
      2) Verify that airway is open, clear, and patency is maintained
      3) Maintain a position that will facilitate adequate patency
      4) Continue to monitor
   d. Assessment of partially obstructed or obstructed/unacceptable finding requiring immediate intervention
      1) Subjective data collection
         a) Trauma to face, mouth, pharynx, neck, or chest
         b) Patient eating or drinking when difficulty began
         c) Recent vomiting

d) Contact with allergen
e) Patient discovered putting objects into mouth

2) Objective data collection
   a) Absence of breathing
   b) Panic behavior, hands on throat, waving arms, grabbing at clothing
   c) Patient unable to speak or vocalize appropriate for age
   d) Substernal, intercostal retractions
   e) Drooling in patient other than infant
   f) Nasal flaring, especially in infant
   g) Facial weakness or paralysis
   h) Facial engorgement: ruddy/bright purple skin color
   i) Violent coughing with lacrimation
   j) Sitting up and leaning forward; tripod position
   k) Decreased level of consciousness
   l) Inspiratory and/or expiratory stridor
   m) Pale, cyanotic, dusky gray skin color, especially mucous membranes and nail beds
   n) Singed nasal/facial hair
   o) Carbonaceous sputum

e. Possible etiologies of total airway obstruction
   1) Current or preexisting diseases/illness
   2) Trauma: blunt or penetrating forces (stab to neck with risk of expanding hematoma), inhalation injury (singed nasal/facial hair, carbonaceous sputum)
   3) Tongue, occluding upper airway in unconscious patient
   4) Saliva/sputum
   5) Vomitus
   6) Blood
   7) Dislodged teeth/dentures (may be loose or knocked out as a result of facial injury)
   8) Food (e.g., meat, fish, hot dogs, hard candy, marshmallows, nuts)
   9) Any item small enough to fit into mouth or nose (e.g., marbles, small toy parts, coins, latex balloons, plastic bags, beanbag foam balls)
   10) Airway edema secondary to allergen exposure

f. Analysis: differential nursing diagnoses/collaborative problems
   1) Ineffective airway clearance
   2) Impaired gas exchange
   3) Impaired airway patency
   4) Anxiety/fear

g. Planning and implementation/interventions (Interventions for ineffective airway clearance must be implemented before proceeding in the primary assessment [see Section II, Resuscitation])

h. Evaluation and ongoing monitoring
   1) Airway patency

2. Cervical spine
   a. Assessment (should occur simultaneously with airway assessment)

1) Acceptable/stable
   a) Subjective data collection
      (1) No history of injury and no injury is suspected
      (2) No history of degenerative bone disease (e.g., ankylosing spondylitis, osteoporosis)
      (3) No complaints of pain on movement (flexion/extension or side/side) or with palpation of neck
   b) Objective data collection
      (1) Movement in all extremities without limitation, weakness, or sensory changes
      (2) Breathing effective: no intercostal retractions or abdominal breathing
      (3) If mechanism of injury suggests potential for injury, stabilize or immobilize patient's cervical spine
2) Unacceptable or requiring immediate intervention/unstable
   a) Subjective data collection
      (1) Mechanism of injury with potential for cervical trauma (e.g., direct injury to head or neck; trauma involving sudden deceleration as in motor vehicle crash or fall; high-voltage electrical shock [see Chapter 30])
3) Symptoms: inability to move extremities, C-spine pain or tenderness, palpable deformity or sensory loss
   a) Objective data collection: possibility of no objective findings as nondisplaced fractures of cervical spine may not compromise neurologic system
      (1) Paralysis, paresthesia, or hypersensitivity
      (2) Abdominal breathing indicating possible diaphragm paralysis
      (3) Decreased or absent movement/sensation below level of injury
      (4) Weakness
      (5) Bowel or bladder incontinence or retention
      (6) Loss of sympathetic outflow
         (a) Hypotension
         (b) Bradycardia
      (7) Flaccid paralysis
      (8) Loss of sphincter tone
      (9) Priapism
      (10) Warm, dry skin
      (11) Bounding peripheral pulses
      (12) Hypothermia; poikilothermy (loss of temperature regulation and patient's body assumes temperature of external environment)
      (13) Inability to shiver or sweat
b. Possible etiologies of C-spine injury
   1) Current or preexisting diseases/illness
   2) Trauma: blunt or penetrating forces
      3) Flexion or flexion/rotation injuries
      4) Compression injury
      5) Head or facial injury
   c. Analysis: differential nursing diagnoses/collaborative problems
      1) Ineffective airway clearance
      2) Ineffective breathing pattern
      3) Impaired gas exchange
      4) Ineffective tissue perfusion: renal, cerebral, cardiopulmonary, spinal cord, gastrointestinal, peripheral
      5) Risk for injury
      6) Ineffective thermoregulation
   d. Planning and implementation/interventions (Interventions to stabilize and protect the cervical spine must be implemented before proceeding in the primary assessment [see Section II, Resuscitation])
   e. Evaluation and ongoing monitoring
      1) C-spine stabilization and protection
3. Breathing
   a. Assessment (be sure to expose chest)
      1) Effective
         a) Subjective data collection
            (1) No distress
            (2) No history of injury to head, chest, or abdomen
            (3) No deviation from patient's usual breathing pattern
         b) Objective data collection
            (1) Chest rises and falls spontaneously
            (2) Exhaled air may be felt or heard escaping from nose, mouth, or stoma
            (3) Respiration quality smooth, even
            (4) Chest expansion equal bilaterally
            (5) Possible mild tachypnea, retracting, wheezing, and accessory muscle use
            (6) Oxygen saturation measured by pulse oximetry (SpO_2) 94–98% (or patient's normal baseline)
      2) Compromised or absent/unacceptable finding requiring immediate intervention that differs depending on whether breathing is compromised or absent
         a) Subjective data collection
            (1) Blunt or penetrating injury to neck, chest, back, or abdomen
            (2) Severe asthma, emphysema, cardiovascular disease
            (3) Dyspnea
            (4) History of respiratory arrest
         b) Objective data collection
            (1) Apnea or agonal breathing (slower than 10 breaths/minute in adults)
            (2) Work of breathing: use of accessory muscles, abdominal breathing, nasal flaring, grunting (in pediatrics)

      (3) Marked tachypnea

      (4) Shallow, weak, gasping respirations

      (5) Skin color: pallor, dusky, cyanotic

      (6) Marked increase in respiratory effort

      (7) Kussmaul respirations: regular, rapid, deep, labored

      (8) Cheyne-Stokes respirations: alternating periods of hyperventilation and apnea

      (9) Decreased/absent breath sounds, unilaterally or bilaterally

      (10) Inability to converse in phrases or complete sentences

      (11) Severe retractions

      (12) Open or sucking chest wounds

      (13) Paradoxical chest wall movement

      (14) Pulse oximeter SpO_2 less than 94% (or patient's baseline)

      (15) Arterial blood gas acutely abnormal/uncompensated

      (16) Decreased rate of respirations

      (17) Contusions/abrasions or deformities to chest wall

      (18) Jugular venous distention (JVD) or tracheal deviation

      (19) Signs of inhalation injury: singed nares, facial burns

      (20) Unable to lay flat

      (21) Decreasing level of consciousness

      (22) Tracheal deviation

  b. Possible etiologies

    1) Current or preexisting diseases/illness

    2) Trauma: blunt or penetrating forces, brain injury, C-spine injury, or burns

    3) Aspiration

    4) Chemical/drug exposure

    5) Allergen or dust exposure

  c. Analysis: differential nursing diagnoses/collaborative problems

    1) Ineffective breathing pattern

    2) Impaired gas exchange

    3) Anxiety/fear

  d. Planning and implementation/interventions (Interventions for compromised or absence of breathing must be implemented before proceeding in the primary assessment [see Section II, Resuscitation])

  e. Evaluation and ongoing monitoring

    1) Respiratory rate and effort

    2) Oxygen saturation

    3) Level of consciousness

4. Circulation

  a. Pulse

    1) Assessment

      a) Acceptable or adequate

        (1) Subjective data collection

          (a) No report of cardiac arrest prior to arrival

          (b) No report of life-threatening dysrhythmia

          (c) No report or suspicion of significant blood loss

        (2) Objective data collection

          (a) Central and peripheral pulse palpable

          (b) Heart rate: approximately 60 to 100 beats/minute in uncompromised adults

          (c) Heart rate: approximately 100 to 180 beats/minute in uncompromised infants, approximately 80 to 120 beats/minute in uncompromised small children

          (d) Rhythm regular

          (e) Skin color, temperature, moisture: pink, warm, dry

      b) Compromised or absent/unacceptable requiring immediate intervention

        (1) Subjective data collection

          (a) Unconsciousness or significantly altered level of consciousness

          (b) Reported cardiac arrest

          (c) Reported or suspected significant blood loss

          (d) Weak or absent peripheral or central pulses

          (e) Skin color: pale, dusky, cyanotic

          (f) Skin temperature and moisture: cool, clammy

        (2) Objective data collection

          (a) Heart rate: less than 60 beats/minute or greater than 100 beats/minute and weak in adults

          (b) Heart rate: less than 100 beats/minute or greater than 220 beats/minute in infants, less than 80 beats/minute or greater than 180 beats/minute in small children

          (c) Unresponsive or significantly altered level of consciousness

          (d) Nonpalpable central (carotid and/or femoral) or peripheral pulse: 100

          (e) Uncontrolled bleeding

    2) Possible etiologies of pulse abnormalities

      a) Current or preexisting diseases/illness

      b) Trauma: blunt or penetrating forces—swollen deformed extremities, rigid abdomen

      c) Chemical/drug exposure

      d) Hypothermia/hyperthermia

      e) Uncontrolled bleeding

      f) Arrhythmia

    3) Analysis: differential nursing diagnoses/collaborative problems

      a) Decreased cardiac output

b) Ineffective tissue perfusion: renal, cerebral, cardiopulmonary, gastrointestinal, peripheral

4) Interventions (Interventions for inadequate circulation must be implemented before proceeding in the primary assessment [see Section II, Resuscitation])

5) Evaluation and ongoing monitoring
   a) Central or peripheral pulses: quality, rate
   b) Bleeding controlled
   c) Level of consciousness
   d) Skin color, temperature, moisture

b. Bleeding
   1) Assessment
      a) Acceptable or adequate
         (1) Subjective data collection
            (a) No history of disease or injury that could result in significant bleeding
            (b) Active external bleeding easily controlled prior to arrival
         (2) Objective collection
            (a) No visible active bleeding
            (b) Any visible bleeding is limited to oozing, low volume, dark red color
      b) Unacceptable finding requiring immediate intervention
         (1) Subjective data collection
            (a) Reported or suspected significant blood loss prior to arrival
            (b) Inability to control external bleeding enroute
         (2) Objective data collection
            (a) Uncontrolled, pulsating, or high-flow bleeding
            (b) Marked pallor of skin, lip margins, or nail beds
            (c) Large amount of bleeding or clots in emesis, nares or oral cavity, stool, or vagina
            (d) Gross swelling of injured extremities (e.g., thigh)
            (e) Distended, rigid abdomen
            (f) Systolic blood pressure less than 90 mm Hg in adults, rapid heart rate, thready, weak pulse
   2) Possible etiologies
      a) Current or preexisting diseases/illness
      b) Trauma: blunt or penetrating forces
   3) Analysis: differential nursing diagnoses/collaborative problems
      a) Impaired gas exchange
      b) Deficient fluid volume
      c) Decreased cardiac output
      d) Ineffective tissue perfusion: renal, cerebral, cardiopulmonary, gastrointestinal, peripheral
      e) Anxiety/fear

4) Planning and implementation/interventions (Interventions for bleeding must be implemented before proceeding in the primary assessment [see Section II, Resuscitation])

5) Evaluation and ongoing monitoring
   a) Blood loss controlled

c. Perfusion
   1) Assessment
      a) Acceptable
         (1) Subjective data collection
            (a) No history of injury or disease that could result in decreased perfusion
         (2) Objective data collection
            (a) Patient alert and oriented to person, place, time, and event
            (b) Skin warm and dry
            (c) Capillary refill brisk, less than 2 to 3 seconds (reliable in children only)
            (d) Pulse rate within normal limits; palpable in all extremities
            (e) Blood pressure within normal limits for age/weight
      b) Unacceptable/requiring immediate intervention
         (1) Subjective data collection
            (a) Patient weak, lightheaded, nauseated, experiencing visual dimming
            (b) Patient verbalizes sense of impending doom
            (c) Patient verbalizes feeling short of breath
            (d) Complaints suggestive of acute, inadequate organ perfusion (e.g., sudden onset of painless visual loss [retinal artery occlusion], sudden onset of testicular pain [testicular torsion])
         (2) Objective data collection
            (a) Alerted level of consciousness: restlessness, anxiety, confusion, disorientation, obtundation
            (b) Increased respiratory effort or work of breathing
            (c) Skin moisture/temperature: diaphoretic, cool
            (d) Skin color: pale, dusky, cyanosis
            (e) Pallor or cyanosis of nail beds or lip margins
            (f) Central or peripheral pulses: weak, thready, rapid
            (g) Vomiting, retching
            (h) Capillary refill delayed >2 seconds (reliable in children only)
            (i) Hypotension (systolic <90 mm Hg in adults)

(j) Extremity injury with diminished/absent pulse

(k) Other indicators of acute, organ-specific, diminished perfusion (may be identified during more in-depth secondary or focused assessment—i.e., retinal artery occlusion [see Chapter 23], testicular torsion [see Chapter 17])

2) Possible etiologies
   a) Current or preexisting diseases/illness
   b) Trauma: blunt or penetrating forces

3) Analysis: differential nursing diagnoses/collaborative problems
   a) Deficient fluid volume
   b) Decreased cardiac output
   c) Ineffective tissue perfusion: cardiopulmonary, renal, gastrointestinal, peripheral
   d) Anxiety/fear

4) Planning and implementation/interventions (Interventions for inadequate perfusion must be implemented before proceeding in the primary assessment [see Section II, Resuscitation])

5) Evaluation and ongoing monitoring
   a) Peripheral and/or organ-specific tissue perfusion

5. Disability (brief neurologic assessment)
  a. Assessment
    1) Acceptable
      a) Subjective data collection
        (1) No history of loss of consciousness
        (2) No history of neurologic trauma
        (3) No sudden onset of severe headache
      b) Objective data collection
        (1) Determine gross level of consciousness using AVPU scale
        (2) Pupil assessment—equality/reactivity: pupils equal, round, briskly reactive to light, and accommodate
        (3) Glasgow Coma Scale or Pediatric Coma Scale scores 15 (see Appendix A)
        (4) Motor/movement
          (a) Ability to respond to commands (avoid commands such as hand grasping, which may be reflexive)
          (b) Moves all four extremities
        (5) Sensory
          (a) Pain
          (b) Fine touch
    2) Unacceptable/requiring immediate intervention
      a) Subjective data collection
        (1) History of loss of consciousness or unconscious/coma
        (2) Head or traumatic brain injury
        (3) Sudden onset of severe headache
        (4) History of diabetes or alcohol abuse

      b) Objective data collection
        (1) Altered level of consciousness: restless, stupor, coma
        (2) Pupillary assessment; equality/reactivity: unequal, "blown," slow, or absent reaction to light
        (3) Abnormal flexion/extension positioning
        (4) Hypoglycemia
        (5) Elevated blood alcohol or positive drug screen
        (6) Loss of pain or fine touch sensation

  b. Possible etiologies
    1) Current or preexisting diseases/illness
    2) Trauma: blunt or penetrating forces
    3) Substance and/or alcohol use/abuse
    4) Medication toxicity
    5) Toxic environmental exposure
    6) Hyperthermia/hypothermia
    7) Electrolyte/acid-base balance disturbance

  c. Analysis: differential nursing diagnoses/collaborative problems
    1) Risk for ineffective airway clearance
    2) Ineffective breathing pattern
    3) Impaired gas exchange
    4) Ineffective tissue perfusion: cerebral
    5) Risk for aspiration
    6) Risk for injury
    7) Ineffective temperature control

  d. Planning and implementation/interventions (Interventions for acute neurologic disability must be implemented before proceeding in the primary assessment [see Section II, Resuscitation])

  e. Evaluation and ongoing monitoring
    1) Level of consciousness

6. Exposure/environmental controls
  a. Assessment
    1) Acceptable/stable
      a) Subjective data collection
        (1) No history of unexposed injury
        (2) No history of prolonged environmental exposure
        (3) No history of thermoregulatory disease
        (4) No history of critical infectious illness exposure
        (5) No history of head injury
        (6) No history of spinal cord injury
      b) Objective data collection
        (1) No injuries noted
        (2) No petechial/purpura rash
    2) Unacceptable/requiring immediate interventions/unstable
      a) Subjective data collection
        (1) Complaint of chest, abdominal, extremity, spinal or head injury or pain
        (2) Recent exposure to critical infectious illness
        (3) Prolonged exposure to environmental elements

b) Objective data collection
  (1) Observable head, spinal, chest, abdominal, extremity injury
  (2) Petechial rash
  (3) Tachycardia/bradycardia
  (4) Subnormal/elevated temperature
b. Possible etiologies
  1) Current or preexisting diseases/illness
  2) Trauma: blunt or penetrating forces
  3) Substance and/or alcohol use/abuse
  4) Medication toxicity
  5) Environmental exposure
c. Analysis: differential nursing diagnoses/collaborative problems
  1) Risk for injury
  2) Ineffective thermoregulation: hyperthermia or hypothermia
d. Planning and implementation/interventions (Interventions to expose hidden injuries, petechiae, purpura, etc., and maintain patient's body temperature must be implemented before proceeding in the primary assessment [see Section II, Resuscitation])
e. Evaluation and ongoing monitoring
  1) Body temperature
  2) Change in obvious injury or rashes to the body

II. Resuscitation

The goal of the resuscitation in the primary assessment is to correct all life-threatening deviations from normal. Resuscitation priorities follow the same ABCDE mnemonic, because interventions occur simultaneously during the primary assessment.

A. AIRWAY/CERVICAL SPINE PROTECTION

1. Open airway
  a. Basic airway management
    1) If patients are alert or respond to verbal stimuli, ask them to open their mouth
    2) Jaw-thrust maneuver or chin lift: use on any patient who is unresponsive and may have a C-spine injury; performed without tilting the head
      a) If C-spine injury is suspected, manually stabilize the cervical spine with two hands holding the head and neck in alignment until a semirigid collar can be applied
    3) Inspect and auscultate for:
      a) Loose objects or foreign debris: remove without blindly finger sweeping the mouth; remove only visualized material
      b) Tongue
      c) Blood, vomitus, secretions
      d) Edema
      e) Evidence of inhalation injury: burns, soot
      f) Abnormal sounds: snoring, gurgling, stridor
    4) Clear airway:
      a) Suction gently, as deep suctioning may stimulate the gag reflex or vagal nerve leading to bradycardia
      b) Chest or abdominal thrusts: use to remove foreign objects obstructing the airway
      c) If foreign body is observed it may be removed carefully with forceps
    5) Maintain patent airway
      a) Airway adjuncts
        (1) Oropharyngeal airway
          (a) Use only in unconscious patients
          (b) Insertion will stimulate the gag reflex and may cause vomiting, aspiration, or laryngospasm in conscious patients
          (c) Insert in the mouth behind the tongue
          (d) If patients tolerate the oral airway, they are likely to require a definitive airway
        (2) Nasopharyngeal airway
          (a) Use in conscious or semiconscious patients
          (b) Useful when unable to place oropharyngeal airway (i.e., trismus, massive trauma)
          (c) Inserted into one nostril and gently passed into the posterior oropharynx; should be lubricated
          (d) Should not be used in the presence of significant head or facial trauma
  b. Predicting a difficult airway
    1) Important to assess airway prior to attempting intubation
    2) Factors may predict difficulties with airway maneuvers
      a) C-spine injury
      b) Mandible or maxillofacial trauma
      c) Limited mouth opening
      d) Anatomical variations: short, muscular neck; receding chin
2. C-spine protection
  a. Maintain/provide immobilization/stabilization protection
    1) If the patient arrives immobilized/stabilized on a backboard: leave the board in place until the primary and secondary assessments are completed and resuscitative measures for airway, breathing, and circulation have been initiated
    2) If the patient is at risk for C-spine injury and is not immobilized/stabilized: maintain the head in a neutral position (manually or with head blocks), place a semirigid cervical collar around the neck, and keep the bed flat; logroll the patient in the event of copious vomiting and when inspecting posterior surfaces

b. Remove the backboard as soon as possible to prevent skin breakdown; however, spinal precautions (semirigid cervical collar, head in neutral position, logrolling, and flat bed) should be followed until the cervical spine is cleared per institutional protocols

c. Continually maintain and monitor airway patency and breathing effectiveness, especially when patients are immobilized/stabilized on a backboard

d. **REMEMBER**: The cervical spine is determined to be stable only if:
  1) There is no posterior midline cervical tenderness
  2) The patient is alert and oriented to person, place, time, and event, and able to follow commands with no signs of intoxication
  3) There is no focal neurological deficit
  4) There are no distracting injuries

B. BREATHING

1. Positioning
   a. High Fowler's position
   b. Orthopneic position (seated propped up in bed with pillows or sitting bent forward with the arms supported on a table or chair arms)
2. O_2: devices used to administer O_2 to patients with adequate respiratory effort
   a. Low-flow system
      1) Nasal cannula
      2) Simple face mask
      3) Partial rebreather
   b. High-flow system
      1) Venturi mask
      2) Aerosol mask
      3) Tracheal collar
      4) Nonrebreather mask with reservoir bag
3. Noninvasive ventilation (NIV)
   a. Method of delivering oxygen by positive pressure mask that allows the provider to postpone or prevent invasive tracheal intubation in patients with acute respiratory failure
   b. Ventilation through a tight-fitting face or nasal mask for short-term ventilatory support for respiratory failure without intubation, usually as a result of pulmonary edema, heart failure, or chronic obstructive pulmonary disease; requires an alert and cooperative patient
   c. Should not exceed 25 cm H_2O at any point regardless of the mode of NIV being used
   d. Two primary modalities
      1) Continuous positive airway pressure (CPAP)
         a) Fixed positive pressure throughout the respiratory cycle
         b) Start at 10 cm H_2O
         c) Titrate based on PCO_2, PaO_2, and bedside SpO_2
      2) Bilevel positive pressure ventilation (BiPAP)

         a) When the ventilator delivers different levels of pressure during inspiration (IPAP) and expiration (EPAP)
         b) Start with IPAP of between 12 and 15 cm H_2O, and EPAP of between 4 and 7 cm H_2O
         c) Titrated up or down depending on the clinical effect and patient comfort
   e. Absolute contraindications
      1) Need for urgent endotracheal intubation
      2) Decreased level of consciousness
      3) Excess respiratory secretions and risk of vomiting and aspiration
      4) Past facial surgery precluding mask fitting
   f. Relative contraindications
      1) Hemodynamic instability
      2) Severe hypoxia and/or hypercapnia, PaO_2/FiO_2 ratio of <200 mm Hg, $PaCO_2$ >60 mm Hg
4. Positive pressure ventilation
   a. Mouth-to-mask ventilation: used for apneic patient if bag-mask ventilation device is not available or effective
   b. Bag-mask ventilation: provides oxygenation and ventilatory support in apneic patient or patient with inadequate respirations: may be used with mask and bag-valve or LMA and bag-valve device
   c. Mechanical ventilator: provides oxygenation and ventilatory support in an intubated patient who is apneic or has inadequate respirations due to respiratory fatigue, respiratory arrest, tachypnea/bradypnea, clinical deterioration
5. Advanced airway management
   a. Definitive airway (endotracheal intubation)
      1) Nasal or oral intubation
         a) Use to establish and maintain airway patency, reduce risk of aspiration, and provide a mechanism to deliver high concentrations of O_2
            (1) Nasal tracheal intubation (NTI) performed blindly and patient must be breathing on own with a high failure rate
            (2) Contraindications for NTI
               (a) Patient is apneic
               (b) Midface fracture: LeFort II or III
               (c) Basilar skull fracture
               (d) Fractures of the cribiform plate or frontal sinus
               (e) Pregnant trauma patient due to fragile nasal mucosa
         b) Use of rapid-sequence induction protocols may be required before intubation
            (1) 7 Ps
               (a) Preparation: assemble suction and all needed equipment/medications
               (b) Preoxygenate with 100% O_2
               (c) Pretreatment
                  (i) LOAD (lidocaine, opioids, atropine, defasciculating agent)

(ii) Sedative: ketamine, midazolam, or etomidate

(d) Paralysis: succinylcholine or vecuronium/rocuronium

(e) Protection and positioning: pass the tube

(f) Placement with proof: use esophageal intubation detector, check breath sounds, CO_2 detector

(g) Postintubation management: sedation and analgesia

c) Gum elastic bougie may be used when the vocal cords are not visible with direct laryngoscopy

(1) Can be placed blindly beyond the epiglottis with tip pointing anteriorly

(2) Tracheal positioning is confirmed when either the tracheal rings are felt or "clicks" are heard

d) Use of a flexible fiberoptic laryngoscope may be technically demanding but is considered the safest and the most effective method to intubate a patient who has a known or suspected difficult intubation

(1) Permits direct visual control of the intubation procedure

e) Retrograde intubation

(1) Useful for patients who are breathing and have an anatomic problem that makes orotracheal intubation impossible or dangerous when no fiberoptic laryngoscope is available

(2) Can take up to 4 minutes to perform, so may not be useful in a critical situation

(3) Done on an awake patient while using a BVM to keep the patient oxygenated

(4) Performed under local anesthesia; cannula is inserted through the cricothyroid membrane into the trachea and a guidewire is passed through the needle upward through the vocal cords into the pharynx or mouth

b. Supraglottic airways

1) Laryngeal mask airway (LMA) is not a definitive airway

a) Supraglottic airway device with an elliptical mask at the distal end, which is inserted into the posterior pharynx covering the supraglottic structures

b) Once mask is inflated it will form a seal over the larynx

c) Not typically used in nonfasting patients but may be used as a rescue airway when intubation fails; but risk of aspiration is not eliminated

2) Combitube airway (used in emergency situations and difficult airways)

a) A dual-lumen tube inserted blindly into the posterior pharynx, usually into the esophagus; placed to a depth that lines up the teeth between the two proximal markings on the tube

b) It has a low-volume inflatable distal cuff and a much larger proximal cuff designed to occlude the oro- and nasopharynx

c) Ventilation can be accomplished with the tube in either the trachea or the esophagus through the lumen that produces chest rise

d) May be used by providers without intubation skills or as a rescue method for difficult airway

e) Possible increased incidence of sore throat, dysphagia, and upper airway hematoma with this device

f) Contraindications for its use

(1) Conscious patient

(2) Intact gag

(3) Pediatric patient (under 16 years of age)

(4) Ingestion of caustic substances

(5) Latex-sensitive individuals

3) King laryngeal tube

a) Single lumen tube with a distal and proximal balloon that occludes the esophagus and oropharynx and quickly establishes a secure airway with a blind insertion

b) Latex free

c) Prevents gastric inflation and aspiration

d) Cannot be used with an intact gag reflex

e) Should not be used on patients with known esophageal disease or patients who have ingested caustic substances

c. Surgical airway

1) Needle cricothyrotomy or percutaneous transtracheal jet insufflation (transtracheal needle ventilation)

a) Indicated when intubation fails and other airway options are not appropriate or available

b) Insertion of a needle or over-the-needle catheter into the cricothyroid membrane into the trachea

(1) Complications

(a) Aspiration of blood

(b) Esophageal laceration

(c) Hematoma

(d) Subcutaneous emphysema

c) Jet insufflation

(1) Performed by placing a large-caliber cannula 12–14 G (adults) and 16–18 G (children) through the cricothyroid membrane into the trachea below an obstruction as a temporary measure

(2) Connected to high-pressure O_2 delivery device

(3) Can cause barotrauma (i.e., pneumothorax, pulmonary rupture)

(4) Indicated infants and children younger than 12 years because they have a smaller cricothyroid membrane and a more funnel-shaped, compliant larynx

(5) Can be used for approximately 40 minutes, after which time carbon dioxide accumulates and can be devastating in patients with head trauma

2) Cricothyroidotomy

a) Indicated when intubation tube cannot be passed through the cords because of edema, trauma, or fracture

b) Small endotracheal or tracheostomy tube is inserted through the cricothyroid membrane (midneck) after a small incision is made

c) May be accomplished surgically or percutaneously

d) Care with children—absolute contraindication to surgical cricothyroidotomy is age (<12 years)

e) Permanent tracheostomy should be placed within 24 hours

f) Complications

(1) Aspiration

(2) False passage into the tissue

(3) Laceration of the esophagus

(4) Tracheal laceration

(5) Mediastinal emphysema

3) Tracheostomy

a) Surgical airway placed low in the neck

b) Difficult and prone to complications when performed on an emergency basis; rarely indicated outside the controlled setting of the operating room

6. Epinephrine: administer for allergic reaction with compromise of airway/breathing

a. Usual route of administration is subcutaneous injection, intravenous administration only for patients with profound hypotension or cardiac arrest

7. Needle thoracentesis

a. Indicated when immediate decompression of a tension pneumothorax is required because of severe respiratory or cardiac compromise; a temporary measure

b. Second intercostal space midclavicular line

8. Chest tube insertion

a. Indicated for pneumothorax greater than 10% or hemothorax

9. Mobile chest drain

a. Use with patient breathing spontaneously and who require a chest tube without the need for suction to reexpand the lung or drain the pleural space

10. Metered-dose inhaler (MDI) or nebulizer: medication inhalation therapy for bronchospasm

C. CIRCULATION/BLEEDING

1. Interventions for inadequate or absent pulse

a. Initiate or continue chest compressions per basic life support (BLS) standards

1) Pulseless patients

2) Chest compressions may also be indicated in the presence of an inadequate pulse rate, especially in a child (pulse <60 in child <8 years of age)

b. Place on cardiac monitor and attach pulse oximetry and end tidal CO_2 detector

c. Defibrillation per advanced life support (ALS) protocols for ventricular fibrillation/pulseless ventricular tachycardia

d. Cardioversion per ALS protocols for tachycardia (infant >220, child >180) with hemodynamic compromise

e. External cardiac pacing for hemodynamically significant heart block

f. Administer medications per ALS protocols

g. Pericardiocentesis: to relieve pericardial tamponade

1) Beck triad: muffled heart tones, distended neck veins, hypotension

h. FAST exam to inspect for pericardial tamponade

i. Prepare and assist with emergency thoracotomy as indicated (blunt trauma only)

2. Control significant bleeding

a. Apply direct pressure to external bleeding

b. Elevate the bleeding extremity if possible

c. Bleeding vessels may be clamped or ligated by a physician

d. Consider the use of a tourniquet

e. Splint fractures

1) Pelvic binder/sheeting or stabilizer for unstable pelvic fractures

2) Consider traction splint for midshaft femur fractures

f. Interventions to control copious epistaxis (see Chapters 13 and 36), gastrointestinal bleeding (see Chapter 11), vaginal hemorrhaging (see Chapters 23 and 37), and clotting abnormalities (see Chapters 19 and 33)

3. Interventions to improve perfusion

a. Administer high-flow supplemental O_2

b. Obtain vascular access

1) Cannulate two large-caliber intravenous (IV) catheters (14–16 caliber for adult; 18–20 caliber for children)

a) If venous access is difficult in a critically ill or injured patient, intraosseous access may be accomplished in children and adults

2) Vascular access is used

a) Collect blood samples

(1) Type and crossmatch

(2) Hemoglobin and hematocrit

(3) Lactate/base excess

(4) ABG

(5) Other specimens as indicated by clinical situation

b) Administer fluid replacement to restore organ perfusion
  (1) Warmed isotonic crystalloid solutions: 1–2 liters or 20 mL/kg for pediatric patients
  (2) Hypoallergenic colloids/plasma expanders
  (3) Blood products: fresh frozen plasma (FFP), platelets, cryoprecipitate, packed RBCs
    (a) 10 mL/kg for pediatric patients
    (b) Use blood tubing
  (4) Tranexamic acid (TXA)
c) Administer pharmacologic therapy as ordered
c. Position patient to optimize perfusion to the brain
  1) Head of bed flat or elevated as per institution protocol or as ordered
  2) Legs elevated if possible (modified Trendelenburg's position)
    a) Do not use Trendelenburg's position (head lower than body) because it has not been shown to be superior to leg elevation alone and may lead to respiratory distress and increased intracranial pressure
d. Definitive intervention
  1) Damage control resuscitation—permissive hypotension, control coagulopathies (keep patient warm; administer factor VII or protein complex concentrate [PCC])
  2) Damage control surgery
  3) Consider embolization/angioembolization
e. Pneumatic antishock garment (PASG) or medical antishock trousers (MAST)
  1) No longer used to improve systemic perfusion because no evidence exists to demonstrate their effectiveness

D. DISABILITY (NEUROLOGIC STATUS)

1. Identify possible etiologies of decreased level of consciousness
   a. Medications, substance abuse, alcohol toxicity, or withdrawal
   b. Current or preexisting diseases/illness
   c. Trauma: blunt or penetrating forces
   d. Psychological dysfunction
2. Interventions for altered neurologic status
   a. Ensure adequate oxygenation and perfusion (see Sections IIB, Breathing, and IIC, Circulation/Bleeding)
   b. Maintain head midline, position head of bed flat or elevated per institutional policy or as prescribed; do not place head lower than body because this may increase intracranial pressure
   c. Administer pharmacologic therapy as ordered
     1) Narcotic or benzodiazepine overdose
       a) Naloxone (Narcan™)
       b) Flumazenil (Romazicon™)
     2) Hypoglycemia

a) Bedside glucose
b) Consider concomitant administration of thiamine in severely malnourished patients, especially those with history of chronic alcohol abuse
3) Head trauma
  a) Glasgow Coma Scale (GCS) and pupillary reaction
    (1) Consider intubation with GCS <8
  b) Mannitol (Osmitrol™)
  c) Neuromuscular blockers
  d) Sedatives/barbiturates
  e) Anticonvulsants
  f) Consider CT head scan

E. EXPOSURE/ENVIRONMENTAL CONTROLS

1. Exposure: remove all the patient's clothing to allow adequate examination
   a. Cut clothing, without destroying physical or forensic evidence (see Chapter 44), if necessary to prevent further injury or pain
   b. Exercise caution for possible sharp objects (e.g., needles) or weapons in pockets
2. Environmental controls: prevent heat loss and increase in coagulopathies
   a. Dry the patient, if necessary, to prevent additional heat loss by evaporation
   b. Cover the patient for privacy and warmth; use warm blankets or forced air warmers as indicated
     1) Keep patient's head warm and dry
   c. Administer warm oxygen or warm intravenous fluids and blood products
   d. Use heating lights or increase ambient temperature as indicated
   e. Patients at increased risk for iatrogenic hypothermia include children, the elderly, and patients with poor systemic perfusion

III. Secondary Assessment

The secondary assessment is a brief/focused exam performed after the primary assessment and resuscitation. The goal of this assessment is to discover all other abnormalities or injuries that are not life threatening. It is also valuable for discovering occult problems in patients with a poor or confusing history. Once additional abnormalities or injuries have been identified, a more focused, detailed assessment is performed. A useful mnemonic to assist in completion of the secondary assessment is

F = full set of vital signs/facilitate family presence
G = get resuscitation adjuncts (LMNOP; see upcoming discussion)
H = history and head-to-toe assessment
I = inspect posterior surfaces/remove spine board

A. FULL SET OF VITAL SIGNS/ FACILITATE FAMILY PRESENCE

1. Full set of vital signs (see Appendix B for age-specific normal ranges)
   a. Blood pressure
      1) Not a reliable indicator of perfusion in children because they are able to maintain "normal" blood pressure until severely compromised
      2) May not be a reliable indicator in the elderly because of increased systolic blood pressure with age, making hypotension less obvious
      3) Frequent and serial blood pressure measurements
      4) Mean arterial pressure (MAP): automatically calculated on monitor (MAP = [(2 × diastolic) + systolic] / 3)
   b. Pulse: rate, rhythm, quality
      1) Central pulse: more accurate than peripheral pulse
         a) Apical
         b) Carotid
         c) Femoral
      2) Peripheral pulse
         a) Radial
         b) Brachial
         c) Posterior tibialis
         d) Dorsalis pedis
   c. Temperature
      1) Oral
      2) Rectal
      3) Axillary
      4) Bladder through a catheter with a thermistor probe
      5) Tympanic: accuracy highly subject to operator technique
      6) Temporal artery scanning
   d. Respirations: rate, depth, quality, work of breathing
2. Facilitate family presence (see Chapter 5)
   a. Family presence may reduce anxiety
   b. Assess family's desire to be present at bedside
   c. Assign someone to support family members while in the room
      1) Explain procedures and events to family using an honest, sensitive, and caring approach
      2) Escort family out if events are such that they cannot remain in the room

B. GET RESUSCITATION ADJUNCTS (LMNOP MNEMONIC)

1. **L**: Laboratory studies
   a. Type and crossmatch
   b. Arterial blood gas (ABG)
   c. Lactate
2. **M**: Monitor cardiac rate and rhythm
   a. Monitor for dysrhythmias
   b. Pulseless electrical activity (PEA): consider cardiac tamponade, tension pneumothorax, or profuse hypovolemia

3. **N**: Consider placement of naso- or orogastric tube to prevent vomiting and aspiration, relief of gastric distension
4. **O**: Oxygenation and ventilation
   a. Pulse oximetry
      1) Normal value: 92–98%
   b. $ETCO_2$ monitoring (capnography)
      1) Normal value 35–45 mm Hg
5. **P**: Assess pain (see Chapter 8)
   a. PQRST mnemonic
      1) Provocation/precipitating factors
      2) Quality and character
      3) Region/radiation
      4) Severity: use age-appropriate tool
      5) Temporal factors: time of onset, constant versus intermittent (see Appendix C)
   b. Assess pain using an appropriate pain scale
      1) FACES pain rating scale for patients approximately 3 years of age and older
      2) Visual analog scale for school-age children and adolescents
      3) FLACC (Faces, Legs, Arms, Cry, Consolability) Scale for infants and preverbal children
      4) Numeric rating scale for older school-age children and adolescents
   c. Management of pain
      1) Nonpharmacologic measures
         a) Reposition if not contraindicated
         b) Splint, elevate ice-injured extremities
         c) Use age-appropriate distraction techniques (see Chapter 8)
         d) Padding over bony prominences
      2) Administer pharmacologic therapy as ordered
         a) Nonnarcotic analgesics
         b) Nonsteroidal antiinflammatory drugs (NSAIDs)
         c) Narcotics

C. HISTORY AND HEAD-TO-TOE ASSESSMENT

1. History of present illness/injury/chief complaint
   a. MIST mnemonic—prehospital assessment
      1) **M** = mechanism of injury (MOI)
      2) **I** = injuries/illness sustained
      3) **S** = signs and symptoms (found in the field)
      4) **T** = treatment (in the field)
   b. CIAMPEDS (chief complaint; immunizations, isolation; allergies; medications; past medical history, parent's/caregiver's impression; events surrounding the condition; diet, diapers; symptoms): components of pediatric history (see Chapter 2)
   c. Patient's own history using SAMPLE mnemonic
      1) **S** = symptoms associated with the injury
      2) **A** = allergies and tetanus status
      3) **M** = medications currently used including over-the-counter (OTC) and anticoagulants

4) **P** = past medical history (PMH), to include hospitalization/surgeries
5) **L** = last oral intake
6) **E** = events and environmental factors related to injury/illness

d. CLIENT OUTCOMES mnemonic—integrates ethnocultural considerations into "data" gathering and provides culturally consistent care
   1) **C** = character of the symptoms (intensity and severity)
   2) **L** = location (radiation if present)
   3) **I** = impact of the symptoms/illness on patient's activities of daily living (ADLs) and quality of life
   4) **E** = expectations of the caregiving process
   5) **N** = neglect or abuse, to include signs of physical and emotional neglect or abuse which may play a role in the patient's condition; does the injury match the mechanism?
   6) **T** = timing, to include onset, duration, frequency of symptoms
   7) **O** = other symptoms that occur in association with the major presenting symptom
   8) **U** = understanding/beliefs about the possible causes of the illness (patient, family, caretaker)
   9) **T** = treatment (medications, therapies that patient has tried to alleviate symptoms)
   10) **C** = complementary alternative medicine (CAM)
   11) **O** = options for care that are important to the patient (advance directives)
   12) **M** = modulating factors that precipitate, aggravate, or alleviate symptoms
   13) **E** = exposure to infectious agents, toxic materials, etc.
   14) **S** = spirituality, to include spiritual beliefs, values, needs

e. Content and time of most recently ingested food, alcohol/drugs
f. Comorbid factors
   1) Pregnancy >20 weeks
   2) Obesity
   3) Elderly/geriatric patient
g. Efforts to relieve symptoms
   1) Home remedies
   2) Complementary Alternative Medicine—(CAM) therapies
   3) Medications
      a) Prescription
      b) OTC/herbal
   4) Physician visits
h. Prehospital emergency medical services (EMS) care
i. Mechanism of injury/illness (see Chapter 31)
   1) MIVT, if not previously obtained
      a) **M** = mechanism of injury/events leading up to illness
      b) **I** = injuries sustained/symptoms

c) **V** = vital signs prior to arrival/presentation on arrival of EMS
      d) **T** = treatment prior to arrival/first aid/remedy started
j. Source of data collection/gathering
   1) Patient
   2) Family or significant other
   3) Caregiver
   4) EMS personnel
   5) Bystander
   6) Use of translator

2. Past medical history
   a. Check for presence of medical information in wallet, medical alert jewelry, medical records, etc.
   b. General health status
      1) Patient's definition of own health
      2) Current or preexisting diseases/illness/injuries/surgeries
         a) Respiratory disease
         b) Cardiovascular disease; risk factors
         c) Neurologic disease
         d) Endocrine disease
         e) Hepatic disease
         f) Infectious disease
         g) Hematologic disease
         h) Immunosuppression
         i) Autoimmune disease
         j) Psychological disorders—psychiatric or mental health
      3) Recent trauma: blunt or penetrating forces
      4) Substance and/or alcohol use/abuse—past and present use
      5) Detoxification history
      6) Smoking history
      7) Sexual history
         a) Last normal menstrual period: female patients of childbearing age
         b) Contraception
         c) Number of children, pregnancies, and live births
      8) Environmental exposures
      9) Morbid obesity, malnourishment, or eating disorder history
   c. Related to present problem or current event
      1) Previous episodes: number, duration, date, treatment
      2) Previous injury to same area and treatment
      3) Previous therapy, complementary/alternative therapy
   d. Current medications
      1) Prescription
      2) OTC/herbal
      3) Use of another person's medications
   e. Complementary Alternative Medicine—(CAM) therapies
   f. Allergies
      1) Medication—prescription, OTC

2) Food/beverages
3) Latex
4) Iodine
5) Environmental

g. Immunization status
   1) Tetanus
   2) Childhood illnesses
   3) Pneumococci
   4) Influenza

3. Psychological/social/environmental factors: collection of a complete social and psychological history may be limited; however, in some situations this information is essential in order to make appropriate treatment and realistic follow-up plans

a. Risk factors
   1) Smoking in the home
   2) Substance and/or alcohol use/abuse in the home
   3) Safety
      a) Possible/actual assault, abuse, or intimate partner violence situations (see Chapters 3 and 40)
      b) Use of seat belts
      c) Texting while driving
      d) Drinking and driving
   4) Psychiatric history (personal or family members)
   5) Literacy

b. Behavior appropriate for age and developmental stage
c. Occupation/profession
d. Hobbies/avocations
e. Meaning of illness, injury, or event to patient/family
f. Patient's/family's expectations of care
g. Support system
   1) Family structure
   2) Significant others
   3) Social agencies
   4) Religious affiliation
   5) Caregivers
h. Responsibilities
   1) Self
   2) Family
   3) Business
   4) Community
i. Cultural beliefs and practices
j. Spirituality
k. Living accommodations
   1) House
   2) Apartment
   3) Accessibility (e.g., stairs)
   4) Homeless, shelters
l. Affordability and accessibility to care—socioeconomic status

4. Head-to-toe assessment (Review of systems): a complete/comprehensive head-to-toe assessment is necessary for all critically ill or injured patients; a more focused head-to-toe assessment may be completed

when a patient presents with a specific minor injury or symptoms limited to one body system

a. General appearance
   1) Behavior, affect, mental alertness, facial expressions, eye contact
   2) Odors
      a) Ethanol
      b) Acetone, indicative of ketosis
      c) Gasoline, indicative of spilled fuel
      d) Urine
      e) Feces
      f) Metallic, indicative of blood loss
      g) Chemicals
      h) Other
   3) Gait/mobility/posture
   4) Speech pattern/hearing
   5) Hygiene: dishevelled appearance, appropriateness of patient's attire
   6) Level of distress/discomfort
   7) Weight loss or gain
   8) Changes in appetite

b. Technique sequence
   1) Inspect, palpate, auscultate (look, listen, feel), except in abdomen, where auscultation should precede palpation; palpation prior to auscultation of the abdomen may stimulate peristalsis leading to bowel sounds being heard and altering the findings
   2) Percussion rarely used in emergent settings, but can be performed once the patient is stabilized

c. Skin/mucous membranes/nail beds
   1) Inspection
      a) Integrity: lacerations, ecchymosis, abrasions, avulsions, puncture wounds, burns, foreign objects
      b) Color
         (1) Pink
         (2) Pallor
         (3) Erythema, flushed
         (4) Jaundice
         (5) Cyanosis
      c) Rash/lesions
      d) Abscess formation
      e) Cellulitis, lymphangitis
   2) Palpation
      a) Moisture/turgor
         (1) Dry
         (2) Moist
         (3) Diaphoresis
         (4) Tenting
         (5) Edema
         (6) Pitting
      b) Temperature
         (1) Cool
         (2) Cold

(3) Warm

(4) Hot

d. Head and face

1) Inspection

a) Skin integrity: lacerations, abrasions, avulsions, lesions, puncture wounds, burns, foreign objects, color

b) Ecchymosis: bilateral periorbital ecchymosis (raccoon eyes) or "black eyes" may indicate basilar skull fracture

c) Edema

d) Presence of pink or gray tissue (possible brain tissue)

e) Facial symmetry—features and structures

(1) Unilateral facial droop—think Bell palsy vs. stroke

f) Malocclusion of teeth

g) Trismus

h) Ability to raise eyebrows, smile

2) Palpation

a) Bony deformity, depression, tenderness

b) Angulation

c) Open fracture

d) Loose teeth

e) Sensation of forehead, and each side of face

e. Eyes

1) Inspection

a) Skin integrity of lids: lacerations, ecchymosis, abrasions, avulsions, puncture wounds, burns, foreign objects

b) Gross visual acuity/peripheral vision—use of Snellen chart

c) Pupillary size, equality, reaction to light—PERRLA, miosis

(1) Brisk vs. sluggish

(2) Round vs. irregular shaped

(3) Unequal—anisocoria (physiological in about 20% of population)

(4) Cloudy cornea—glaucoma

(5) Photophobia/excessive tearing/pain—may indicate foreign body

d) Iris/sclera/conjunctiva

(1) Color

(2) Bleeding (subconjunctival hemorrhage)

(3) Excessive tearing

(4) Discharge

(5) Foreign object/body (FB)

(6) Ulcerations

(7) Hyphema—accumulation of red blood cells within the anterior chamber

e) Globe integrity

f) Lid edema/lesions—evert upper lid and assess for FB

g) Ptosis—drooping of eyelid

h) Excessive blinking or inability to open eyes (blepharospasm)

i) Nystagmus

j) Extraocular movements: ability to move eyes in all directions—smoothness of movements

k) Exophthalmos/proptosis—bulging of the eye anteriorly out of the orbit

l) Contact lenses (remove if present), corrective eyewear

2) Palpation

a) Tenderness or step-off may indicate fracture

(1) Supraorbital/infraorbital ridges

(2) Zygoma

f. Ears

1) Inspection

a) Skin integrity: lacerations, ecchymosis, abrasions, avulsions, puncture wounds, burns, foreign objects

b) Blood

(1) External pinna or canal

(2) Behind tympanic membrane (hemotympanium)

c) Clear fluid: may be cerebrospinal fluid (CSF), which indicates an open skull fracture; do not pack ears

d) Ecchymosis behind ear, over the mastoid bone (Battle sign); may be indicative of basilar skull fracture (not evident immediately after injury, but 6–8 hours later)

e) Exposed cartilage

f) Purulent drainage/crusting: may be indicative of external canal infection or otitis media with ruptured tympanic membrane

g) External hematoma

h) Symmetry

2) Palpation

a) Preauricular and postauricular lymph nodes

b) External ear

g. Nose

1) Inspection

a) Skin integrity: lacerations, ecchymosis, abrasions, avulsions, puncture wounds, burns, foreign objects (especially in the pediatric population)

b) Bleeding/discharge

c) Deformity, swelling

d) Septal hematoma

e) Rhinorrhea: may be CSF, which indicates an open skull fracture; do not pack nose

f) Symmetry

2) Palpation

a) Bony tenderness—bridge and soft tissue

b) Deformity

h. Mouth

1) Inspection

a) Skin integrity: lacerations, ecchymosis, abrasions, avulsions, puncture wounds, burns, foreign objects

b) Symmetry

c) Number of teeth

d) Inspect mucosa/gums for color, ulcerations, lesions, trauma

e) Tongue color and movement/deviation

f) Drooling

g) Malodorous breath

  (1) Fruity sweet—ketones: diabetic ketoacidosis

  (2) Foul (fecal) smelling: intestinal obstruction

  (3) Halitosis: tonsillitis, respiratory infection, gingivitis

  (4) Ethanol: alcohol intoxication

i. Neck

1) Inspection

a) Skin integrity: lacerations, ecchymosis, abrasions, avulsions, puncture wounds, burns, foreign objects

b) Edema

2) Auscultation

a) Carotid bruits—use bell of stethoscope and light pressure

  (1) Blowing or swishing sounds reflect turbulent blood flow

3) Palpation

a) Tracheal position

  (1) Deviation: may indicate tension pneumothorax

    (a) Not easily visualized except on chest radiograph

    (b) May be palpable above sternal notch

b) Neck veins

  (1) Distended (jugular venous distention [JVD]): may indicate heart failure, tension pneumothorax, or cardiac tamponade

  (2) Flat: may indicate hypovolemia

c) Subcutaneous emphysema

  (1) May indicate disruption of trachea or bronchial tree

d) Step-off or deformity along cervical spine

  (1) Maintain manual immobilization/stabilization of the head during palpation of the posterior neck

  (2) Tenderness or muscle spasm

4) Geriatric

a) Limited range of motion due to degenerative changes

j. Chest

1) Inspection—symmetry and integrity of the chest wall

a) Spontaneous breathing and accessory muscle use

  (1) Rate, depth, effort—expansion and excursion during ventilation

    (a) Expansion may be decreased in the geriatric population

  (2) Accessory or abdominal muscle usage

  (3) Paradoxical movements or respiratory pattern

  (4) Tire quickly—may see this in the geriatric population

b) Bony deformities

  (1) Paradoxical chest wall movement indicates a flail chest

    (a) Pulmonary contusion frequently present in the lung beneath the flail segment

  (2) Barrel chest—think COPD

  (3) Kyphosis especially in the geriatric population

c) Skin integrity—anterior, posterior, axilla

  (1) Lacerations, abrasions, avulsions, puncture wounds, burns, foreign objects, color, scars

  (2) Burns may result from airbag deployment

  (3) Loss of subcutaneous tissue in the geriatric population

d) Ecchymosis

  (1) Round abrasion may indicate steering wheel impact

  (2) Ecchymosis diagonally across chest/neck may indicate safety belt injury

e) Sputum—color, acute/chronic

2) Palpation

a) Tenderness, crepitus (a crinkly-like sensation)

b) Subcutaneous emphysema (a gentle bubbly-like feeling)

  (1) May indicate disruption of trachea or bronchial tree

  (2) Always requires attention

c) Bulges, depressions

3) Auscultation—DO NOT PERFORM OVER THE GOWN OR CLOTHING—CHEST SHOULD BE EXPOSED!

a) Breath sounds—pitch, quality, duration of inspiratory/expiratory phases

  (1) Presence, bilaterally

  (2) Adventitious sounds

    (a) Wheezes—musical, squeaks; high pitched (asthma)

    (b) Crackles—bubbly sound heard on inspiration and not cleared with cough; discontinuous sounds

    (c) Rhonchi—coarse rumbling sounds

  (3) Depth and equality bilaterally

  (4) Cough—dry/moist; spasmodic

  (5) Stridor

  (6) Snoring/gurgling

  (7) Sudden onset of stridor or wheezes in pediatric population—consider foreign body

  (8) Grunting in infants and small children

b) Heart sounds
   (1) S₁, S₂
      (a) S₁ heard best at apex of the heart
      (b) S₂ heard best at base of the heart
      (c) Splitting of S₂ (a "stutter") may indicate left bundle branch block
   (2) S₃, S₄—low pitched and best heard with bell of stethoscope
      (a) Presence of S₃ (follows S₂) indicates left ventricular (systolic) dysfunction; CHF
      (b) S₃ normal in children and young adults
      (c) Presence of S₄ (precedes S₁) indicates diastolic dysfunction due to noncompliant ventricle; hypertension
      (d) S₄ common in older individuals
   (3) Muffled, distant: may indicate pericardial tamponade
   (4) Murmurs or rubs—what is the quality (how loud)?
      (a) Sounds that occur during systole or diastole as a result of turbulent blood flow
      (b) May indicate mitral valve regurgitation
      (c) Friction rub
         (i) Creaky-scratchy noise
         (ii) Due to inflammation
         (iii) May occur after myocardial infarction or with pericarditis
4) Percussion
   a) Resonance: normal lung tissue
   b) Hyperresonance: hyperinflated lung tissue (emphysema or asthma), or air-filled thoracic cavity (pneumothorax)
   c) Dullness/flatness: fluid-filled or consolidated lung tissue (pneumonia, pneumothorax) or fluid-filled thoracic cavity (hemothorax)
5) Apgar score in newborns
6) Children
   a) Respiratory effort
   b) Work of breathing—nasal flaring, grunting, head bobbing, intercostal/abdominal muscle use (retraction at xiphoid process or suprasternal notch)
k. Abdomen/flanks—think anatomically where organs live
   1) Inspection
      a) Divided into four quadrants
      b) Patient movement (or lack of)
         (1) Peritonitis—prefer to lie very still
         (2) Renal or biliary colic—unable to find a comfortable position; writhing
         (3) Legs flexed at the knees

c) Skin integrity: lacerations, abrasions, avulsions, puncture wounds, burns, foreign objects/bodies, evisceration, scars, striae, spider angiomas, color, drainage
d) Contour
   (1) Flat
   (2) Distention
      (a) Trauma, acute distention is most likely caused by air or intraabdominal blood accumulation
      (b) Children—mouth breather
      (c) Girth
   (3) Pregnant—outline of the fetus (rupture amniotic sac)
   (4) Obese
   (5) Hernia (umbilical)
   (6) Peristalsis/movement of the abdominal wall
   (7) Newborn: umbilical cord stump (color, drainage)
e) Ecchymosis
   (1) Flank (Grey Turner sign): late finding suggestive of retroperitoneal bleeding
      (a) Flank discoloration
   (2) Periumbilical (Cullen sign): late finding suggestive of intraperitoneal bleeding
      (a) Bluish discoloration of the umbilicus
   (3) Other possible causes of Grey Turner or Cullen sign
      (a) Ruptured ectopic pregnancy
      (b) Coagulopathy
2) Auscultation
   a) Bowel sounds in all quadrants
      (1) Present
      (2) Absent
         (a) Indicative of paralytic ileus or diminished perfusion, listen for at least 1 minute in each quadrant to determine true absence
      (3) Hypoactive
         (a) Diminished perfusion
      (4) Hyperactive (high pitched)
         (a) Intestinal obstruction
   b) Bruit: indicates turbulent flow through arteries
      (1) Vascular sounds similar to heart murmurs
      (2) May see with renal stenosis
   c) Friction rubs—vascular disease
      (1) Hepatic or splenic disorder—heard in upper quadrants
   d) Sounds heard in the chest—diaphragmatic injury
3) Palpation—warm hands and stethoscope; ask if patient is ticklish
   a) All quadrants: ask patient to indicate area of pain—palpate area known to be painful last
      (1) Light then deep

b) Soft
c) Tenderness, guarding
  (1) Tenderness over McBurney point—appendicitis
  (2) Psoas sign—flexion of the right hip against resistance
  (3) Murphy sign—palpate below right costal margin, pain with deep breath; seen with acute cholecystitis, hepatitis, or hepatomegaly
  (4) Rovsing sign—palpate left lower quadrant and it elicits pain in the right lower quadrant indicates appendicitis
d) Rigid, boardlike, indicating peritoneal irritation
e) Masses
  (1) Pulsatile: possible aortic aneurysm or dissection
  (2) Solid: possible tumor or stool
f) Referred pain—pain to left shoulder (Kehr sign) due to presence of blood or other irritants in the peritoneal cavity
4) Percussion: rarely performed
  a) Tympany, a hollow sound indicating presence of air or gas
  b) Dullness, a heavy sound indicating fluid (e.g., blood) or a mass
    (1) Shifting dullness (waves)—ascites
5) Neonate
  a) Abdomen of the neonate is protuberant
  b) Inspect umbilical cord
  c) Inspect for umbilical hernia—common in African-Americans
  d) Inspect for jaundice
  e) Olive-shaped mass palpated in right upper quadrant—pyloric stenosis
6) Pediatric
  a) Intussusception—present with tense abdomen, vomiting, and colicky pain
    (1) Red, currant jelly stool
    (2) Peak 3–12 months
  b) Aortic pulsation common in lean children
  c) Flex hips and knees to palpate abdomen
  d) Peristaltic waves—pyloric stenosis
  e) If ticklish have child place a hand over yours during palpation
l. Pelvis/perineum
  1) Inspection
    a) Skin integrity: lacerations, ecchymosis, abrasions, avulsions, puncture wounds, burns, foreign objects
    b) Bleeding
      (1) Urethral (blood at the meatus): trauma to urethra, bladder
      (2) Genital: trauma to vagina, uterus; open pelvic fracture; pregnancy related; trauma to penis, scrotum (scrotal or labial hematoma)

(3) Rectal: injury to rectum, anus, large bowel; open pelvic fracture; lower gastrointestinal bleeding secondary to disease process; lower GI bleed; hemorrhoids
c) Priapism
d) Genital lesions, masses/edema or discharge (color, odor)
e) Symmetry
  (1) Asymmetrical testicle may be a torsion
  (2) Symmetry of iliac crests and size of buttock
  (3) Shortening and external rotation—hip fracture
f) Gait and posture
g) Pain and/or urge but unable to void
2) Palpation
  a) Pelvic stability/tenderness
    (1) Gentle pressure over the iliac wings downward and medially
    (2) Press gently with heel of hand on the symphysis pubis
  b) Genital examination
    (1) Prostate exam
    (2) Inguinal hernia exam
    (3) Testes for masses or tenderness
      (a) Firm tender mass—testicular cancer
  c) Pelvic exam
    (1) Speculum
    (2) Bimanual
  d) Rectal examination
    (1) Loss of sphincter tone: spinal cord injury above S1
    (2) Stool for occult blood
    (3) Should be performed on all males and females who present with abdominal pain
m. Extremities
  1) Inspection
    a) Symmetry
    b) Soft tissue injury
      (1) Skin integrity: lacerations, abrasions, avulsions, puncture wounds, burns, impaled objects, color
      (2) Closed fracture: not associated with an open wound
      (3) Open fracture: open wounds associated with a fracture; high risk for infection; prophylactic antibiotics will be prescribed
    c) Deformity—angulation, protruding bony fragments
    d) Ecchymosis
    e) Edema
    f) Gait
    g) Splints—previously applied for correct placement
    h) Dialysis catheter, peripherally inserted central catheters (PICC)

2) Palpation
   a) Tenderness/pain (PQRST)
   b) Instability, deformity, step-off
   c) Crepitus
3) Motor function—onset, quality, associated symptoms, mechanism of injury
   a) Spontaneous movement
   b) Motor strength against resistance (flexion and extension)
   c) Symmetry of strength
   d) Range of motion (ROM)—flexion, extension, supination, pronation
4) Sensory function—onset, quality, associated symptoms; sense touch in all four extremities
   a) Sharp-dull
   b) Two-point discrimination
5) Circulatory status
   a) Color, skin temperature
   b) Pulses distal to injury
      (1) Compare one side with the other
      (2) Femoral popliteal, dorsalis pedis, posterior tibialis
   c) Capillary refill
   d) Skin moisture
6) Neonatal
   a) To inspect the hip, need to place infant frog legged; if groin crease below the anus, think hip dislocation
7) Children
   a) Compare to opposite extremity
   b) Bones are pliable
8) Geriatric
   a) Osteoporosis can cause brittle bones and increase risk of fractures
   b) Limited mobility due to arthritic changes
   c) Pain restriction to ROM is different from mechanical restrictions
   d) Always assess pain that is caused by decreased ROM and change in sensation

D. INSPECT POSTERIOR SURFACES

1. Logroll the patient, with ample assistance to maintain spinal alignment if there is any potential for spinal injury
   a. If patient is on a spinal board, promote timely removal
2. Splint/support injured extremities and attempt not to roll the patient onto an injured extremity
3. Inspection
   a. Skin integrity: lacerations, ecchymosis, avulsions, abrasions, puncture wounds, foreign bodies, impaled objects, color, scars
   b. All posterior surfaces of back, flanks, buttocks, thighs
   c. Blood in or around the rectum
4. Palpation

a. Tenderness, step-off, deformity, muscle spasms along the vertebral column and flanks
b. Tenderness of costovertebral angle
c. May assist with performance of rectal examination if not previously done
   1) Presence or absence of rectal tone
   2) Presence of high-riding prostate

IV. Focused Assessment

The focused assessment is a detailed assessment of any area or system that has an abnormality or injury. Refer to specific chapters for details of focused assessment.

V. Diagnostic Procedures

Laboratory, imaging, and other studies such as ECGs are obtained in conjunction with the primary, secondary, and focused assessments. Appropriate diagnostic tests are discussed in more detail within each clinical chapter. Point-of-care testing for glucose, arterial blood gas, hemoglobin, pregnancy, urine, and occult blood in stool or emesis is commonly performed in the emergency department setting.

VI. Analysis: Differential Nursing Diagnoses/Collaborative Problems

Nursing diagnosis is a clinical judgment about the individual, family, or community responses to and risk for actual health problems and life processes. It provides the basis for selection of nursing interventions to achieve outcomes for which the nurse is accountable. A nursing diagnosis made by professional nurses describes actual or potential health problems that nurses, by virtue of their education and experience, are able and licensed to treat.

Collaborative problems are those that nurses cannot treat independently and require involvement of other members of the health care team.

VII. Planning and Implementation/Interventions

Planning involves selecting appropriate interventions to manage identified health care problems and needs. These nursing actions include both collaborative and independent interventions. All interventions are patient oriented and goal directed. General interventions appropriate for all patients include:
1. Determine priorities of care
2. Relieve anxiety/apprehension

3. Allow significant others to remain with the patient if they are supportive
4. Educate the patient and significant others
5. Relieve pain

VIII. Evaluation and Ongoing Monitoring

This is the determination of whether the desired responses to interventions have been achieved. If positive outcomes are not demonstrated, further assessment is indicated, along with reevaluation of the plan of care and specific interventions.

1. Continuously monitor primary and secondary assessment along with vital signs, pain, and any procedures; and treat as indicated
2. Monitor the patient's responses/outcomes, and modify the nursing care plan as appropriate
3. If positive patient outcomes are not demonstrated, reevaluate the assessment and/or plan of care

IX. Documentation of Nursing Assessments and Resuscitation

A. SUBJECTIVE DATA COLLECTION

B. OBJECTIVE DATA COLLECTION

C. ANALYSIS: DIFFERENTIAL NURSING DIAGNOSES/ COLLABORATIVE PROBLEMS

D. PLANNING AND IMPLEMENTATION/ INTERVENTIONS

E. EVALUATION AND ONGOING MONITORING

X. Age-Related Considerations

A. PEDIATRIC

Children are not small adults. They have unique anatomic and physiologic differences that affect assessment and intervention.

1. Airway
   a. Neonates are obligate nose breathers until 6–8 months of age
   b. Small airway diameter, more easily occluded by secretions
   c. Greater amounts of soft tissue surrounding airway, prone to edema, which may compromise airway
   d. Large tongue
   e. Cricoid cartilage: narrowest part of airway
   f. Soft laryngeal cartilage

2. Cervical spine
   a. Head large in relation to body; therefore, at greater risk for injury
   b. Prominent occiput in children up to 8 years may result in flexion of the neck when the patient is supine on a backboard; pad upper back to maintain neutral alignment (external auditory meatus in line with shoulders) on a backboard
   c. If possible, place a parent or caregiver in the patient's direct line of vision to decrease struggling when the patient is immobilized on a backboard

3. Breathing
   a. Poorly developed intercostal accessory muscles
   b. Thin chest wall, breath sounds easily transmitted from one area to another
   c. Decreased pulmonary reserve
   d. Higher O_2 requirements owing to higher metabolic rate
   e. Respiratory rates are faster
   f. Use abdominal muscles for breathing

4. Circulation
   a. Myocardium: infants have less contractile mass and less compliant ventricles and therefore are unable to increase stroke volume to accommodate large increase in preload (e.g., intravenous fluids)
   b. Primarily maintain cardiac output with increased heart rate and vasoconstriction
   c. Able to maintain cardiac output for long periods of time: strong compensatory mechanisms
   d. Less total circulatory blood volume than adults: approximately 80 mL/kg

5. Disability (neurologic status)
   a. Use a modified coma scale for preverbal children (see Appendix A)
   b. Infants: muscle tone (slightly flexed), fontanels, recognition of caregivers
   c. Age-appropriate behavior
   d. Positive Babinski normal in infant until walking stage
   e. Bedside glucose testing

6. Exposure/environmental controls
   a. May lose heat rapidly (due to less body fat); keep covered (especially head in small infants)
   b. Thinner skin and higher rate of insensible water loss

7. Full set of vitals/focused adjuncts/facilitate family presence
   a. Vital signs
      1) Normal ranges vary with age (see Appendix B)
      2) Hypotension is a late sign of shock; may not appear until circulating volume is decreased by 50%; capillary refill (central) is a better indicator of perfusion than blood pressure in small children
      3) Use appropriately sized cuff for blood pressure and other equipment
      4) Use brachial or apical site for pulse rates in infants

5) Obtain an actual weight whenever possible in kilograms; use length-based resuscitation tape to estimate weight in a critically ill or injured child

6) Use toy or bright object to distract infant during assessment

b. Resuscitation adjuncts
   1) Use appropriately sized supplies and equipment; length-based resuscitation tape contains this information
   2) Avoid nasal gastric tubes in small infants because they are obligate nose breathers
   3) Consider decompression with a gastric tube especially if child was crying or bag-mask ventilation
   4) Apply pulse oximeter probe to a warm extremity
   5) Children may have difficulty localizing source of pain

c. Facilitate family presence—promote family-centered care at all times
   1) Parents/primary caregivers provide emotional support to the child
   2) Parents/primary caregivers usually prefer to be present during all aspects of care, including invasive or resuscitative procedures
   3) Valuable source of information about what is "normal" or baseline for the child

8. Growth and development
   a. Infants
      1) Trust development
      2) Attachment to parents; minimize separation from parents; stranger anxiety onset at 7–9 months
      3) Older infants may localize pain
      4) Health care providers should focus on establishing trust and rapport with parents
   b. Toddlers
      1) Developing autonomy
      2) Increased safety concerns
      3) Fear of pain, separation from parents
   c. Preschoolers
      1) Learning to do things for self
      2) Magical thinking
   d. School-age children
      1) Able to understand body anatomy and function
      2) Maintaining control is important; want to cooperate
      3) Modesty and privacy needs
   e. Adolescents
      1) Peer relationships are important
      2) Sensitive to being different from peer group
      3) Privacy is critical
      4) High-risk behaviors: unprotected sexual activity, careless driving, substance use/abuse

9. "Pearls"
   a. Differences in illness in children and adults are anatomic, physiologic, and psychological
   b. Treat child and parent as one unit: avoid separation

c. Give simple instructions or one choice to increase the child's sense of control
d. Use play therapy, if time permits; allow the child to have a favorite toy for security
e. Avoid threatening behavior such as sudden movement or loud noises
f. Be honest with the child; if the procedure will hurt, say so
g. Protect modesty, respect privacy
h. Explain procedures to the extent possible, according to the child's developmental level
i. Examine the painful area last, if possible
j. Do painful or intrusive procedures (e.g., rectal temperature) last

B. GERIATRIC

1. Airway
   a. Diminished airway compliance
   b. Increased airway resistance
   c. Decreased ciliary action
   d. Decreased gag
   e. Presence of dentures or partials
2. Cervical spine
   a. Degenerative bony changes increase risk for fracture
   b. May require padding under head to achieve neutral head alignment in the presence of kyphosis
3. Breathing
   a. Loss of thoracic muscle mass
   b. Diminished lung compliance
   c. Decreased vital capacity
   d. May be unable to tolerate supine position
   e. Labored breathing causes rapid exhaustion, predisposing elderly patients to respiratory arrest
   f. Degenerative bony changes limit visualization of vocal cords with intubation
4. Circulation
   a. History of cardiac disease; decreased cardiac output
   b. Decreased peripheral blood flow
   c. Atherosclerosis may impair ability to vasoconstrict
   d. Decreased baroreceptor sensitivity, less able to mount a tachycardic response to hypotension
   e. Anemia may be caused by chronic disease and malnutrition
   f. Elevated systolic blood pressure may mask hypotension
5. Disability (neurologic status)
   a. Decreased cerebral blood flow
   b. Loss of functioning neurons and cerebral atrophy are normal with aging and increased in Alzheimer's disease and alcohol abuse
   c. Slowed nerve transmission, slowed reflexes increase risk for injury
   d. Do not assume that dementia or confusion is the patient's normal baseline

e. Patients who are hearing impaired may appear confused when they answer questions inappropriately

f. Confusion is a common sign of illness in the elderly; do not assume it is dementia

g. Higher incidence of chronic subdural hematoma—use of anticoagulants, antiplatelets, alcohol abuse

h. Brain tissue atrophy

6. Exposure/environmental controls

a. Prone to hypothermia secondary to decreased metabolic rate and loss of subcutaneous fat

b. Thinner skin

7. "Pearls"

a. Older adults may dismiss significant symptoms as "normal for age": investigate each complaint

b. Decreased pain sensation is common with advanced age

c. Keep manipulation of body to a minimum to avoid fatigue

d. Poor elasticity of skin can mimic dehydration; examine lateral cheeks for turgor

e. Skin more friable and prone to injury, especially from prolonged backboard time

f. Do not assume that patient is hearing impaired; it may offend the patient

g. Treat patients with respect; use first name only with the patient's permission; do not use terms such as "honey" or "dear"

h. Increased risk of skin breakdown

i. Predisposed to medication toxicities and adverse reactions

1) Reduced renal excretory function

2) Polypharmacy increases risk of drug interactions

j. Less able to manage multiple stimuli simultaneously and divide attention

1) Slow pace of history gathering

2) Avoid simultaneous interventions and questions when possible

C. BARIATRIC PATIENT

1. Use appropriate sized equipment

a. Cuff that is too small can produce false high reading

b. Forearm may be used to assess BP but results may be higher than those taken in upper arm

c. Know weight capacity of conventional equipment—be familiar with bariatric equipment available in the department

2. Anatomy and physiology

a. Respiratory insufficiency due to chest wall weight, decreased chest wall compliance

b. Nocturnal gastric reflux

c. Left ventricular hypertrophy—pulmonary hypertension

d. Elevated blood viscosity—venous stasis/pulmonary embolus

1) Thromboembolism prevention should be initiated—antiembolism stockings, compression

devices, prophylactic anticoagulant therapy, early mobilization

e. Osteoarthritis—weight-bearing joint deterioration

f. Abdominal wall weakness

3. Airway

a. High risk for gastric reflux or aspiration

b. Use a two-handed bilateral jaw thrust

c. Reverse Trendelenburg position will benefit airway and work of breathing

4. Breathing

a. Higher respiratory rate

b. Positional dyspnea—weakened respiratory muscles may quickly lead to fatigue and respiratory failure

c. Anticipate potential use of bilevel positive airway pressure (BiPAP)

5. Resuscitative adjuncts

a. If patient has had recent bariatric surgery, blind insertion of gastric tube is contraindicated

b. Pain medications based on IBW not on actual weight—lipophilic medications are taken up by adipose tissue and slowly released; therefore, they should be titrated according to patient responses

6. Treat patient with dignity—protect patient privacy

Reference

1. Emergency Nurses Association: *Geriatric emergency nursing education course (GENE)*, Des Plaines, IL, 2014, Emergency Nurses Association.

Bibliography

American College of Surgeons: *ATLS student manual*, ed 9, Chicago, 2014, American College of Surgeons.

Emergency Nurses Association: *Presenting the option for family presence*, ed 3, Des Plaines, IL, 2010, Emergency Nurses Association.

Emergency Nurses Association: *Emergency nursing pediatric provider manual*, ed 4, Des Plaines, IL, 2012, Emergency Nurses Association.

Emergency Nurses Association: *Geriatric emergency nursing education course (GENE)*, Des Plaines, IL, 2014, Emergency Nurses Association.

Emergency Nurses Association: *Trauma nursing core course provider manual*, ed 7, Des Plaines, IL, 2014, Emergency Nurses Association.

Hammond BB, Gerber-Zimmermann P: *Sheehy's manual of emergency care*, ed 7, St. Louis, MO, 2013, Mosby/Elsevier.

Howard PK, Steinmann RA: *Sheehy's emergency nursing: Principles and practice*, ed 6, St. Louis, MO, 2010, Mosby/Elsevier.

Kleinman ME, et al.: Part 5: Adult basic life support and cardiopulmonary resuscitation quality: 2015 American Heart Association guidelines for cardiopulmonary resuscitation and emergency cardiovascular care, *Circulation* 132(18 Suppl. 2):S414–S435, 2015. Retrieved from http://circ.ahajournals.org/content/132/18_suppl_2/S414.full (Level VII or D).

Proehl JA: *Emergency nursing procedures*, ed 4, Philadelphia, 2009, Saunders/Elsevier.

Debbie Travers, PHD, RN, FAEN, CEN

Triage is an information-collecting and decision-making process. It is performed in order to sort injured and ill patients into categories of acuity and prioritization based on the urgency of their medical or psychological needs. Triage begins when the patient enters the emergency department and is performed either in a specified triage location or at the patient's bedside. The practice of triage is changing, with many EDs implementing immediate bedding of patients when there are open ED beds. Triage has become more of an assessment process that can take place anywhere in the ED, rather than triage always being a place (the triage area) where the triage nurse performs the triage assessment. Patients' priorities may change as their conditions stabilize or deteriorate after triage. Thus triage is an assessment process in which the triage nurse documents a snapshot of the patient's status at the time of initial presentation to the ED, and determines the prioritization for treatment. Triage assessment and assignment of an acuity rating do not fulfill the legal requirement of the patient's receiving a medical screening examination (MSE) under the United States Emergency Medical Treatment and Active Labor Act (EMTALA [see Chapter 45]).

I. Triage Overview

A. OBJECTIVES

1. Identify patients who need immediate care and treatment
2. Perform a brief assessment on all incoming patients
3. Assign an appropriate acuity level
4. Assign location of care if applicable

B. NURSING QUALIFICATIONS

1. Emergency Nurses Association (ENA) recommendations
   a. Registered nurse with a minimum 6 months of emergency nursing experience
   b. Completion of triage education course involving
      1) Didactic component
      2) Clinical orientation with a preceptor
   c. Current certification in Basic Life Support (BLS) and Advanced Cardiac Life Support (ACLS)
   d. Successful completion of Trauma Nursing Core Course Provider (TNCC-P)
   e. Successful completion of Emergency Nursing Pediatric Course Provider (ENPC-P)
   f. Certified Emergency Nurse (CEN) credential (preferred)
2. Additional qualifications
   a. Strong interpersonal skills
   b. Ability to conduct a brief, focused interview
   c. Strong physical assessment skills
   d. Ability to make rapid, accurate decisions
   e. Ability to work collaboratively with other members of the health care team
   f. Ability to adjust to workload fluctuations
   g. Ability to effectively communicate understanding of patient and family expectations

h. Understand cultural and religious concerns that could arise at triage
i. Possess knowledge of specific institutional policies affecting triage

C. ASSESSMENT

1. Purpose
   a. Perform a rapid assessment in order to
      1) Determine the urgency of a patient's need for emergency care
      2) Gather pertinent assessment data to determine an accurate acuity rating
      3) Identify patients with life-threatening and potentially life-threatening conditions to ensure they receive immediate treatment
      4) Identify patients without apparent life-threatening conditions
2. "Across-the-room" assessment
   a. Triage nurse's first contact with patient, using sense of sight, hearing, and smell
   b. Purpose: identify obvious life-threatening conditions
      1) The triage assessment should not be completed in the triage area on patients who are clearly in need of immediate, lifesaving interventions or on those who are at high risk for serious illness
      2) Immediately place patient in treatment area once a life-threatening or high-risk condition is identified
   c. Brief primary assessment (see Chapters 1 and 32)
      1) Airway and cervical spine
      2) Breathing
      3) Circulation
      4) Disability
      5) Exposure/environmental controls
3. Subjective data collection
   a. If English is a second language, use a hospital interpreter or, if necessary, a family member to obtain information
   b. Information gathered from appropriate sources
      1) Patients: if able to speak for self
      2) Family, other historian, such as a caretaker, guardian, friend, caseworker
      3) Emergency medical services (EMS) personnel
   c. Chief complaint
      1) Determine patient's primary reason for seeking ED care
      2) Document chief complaint as accurately as possible in words used by the patient, family member, or other historian
      3) Patients with multiple complaints or history/long duration of illness
         a) Focus on problem requiring treatment today
   d. Brief history of present illness/injury
      1) Elicit and document a focused history of present illness/injury

a) Description of symptoms
b) Any precipitating events, illnesses
   (1) Possible/actual victim of assault, abuse, or intimate partner violence situations (see Chapter 3)
c) Duration and progression of symptoms
d) Pain assessment (see Chapter 8)
e) Mechanism of injury and related information (see Chapter 31)
f) Efforts to relieve symptoms and response, prior to arrival at emergency department
   e. Significant past medical history
      1) Current or preexisting diseases/illness
      2) Last normal menstrual period: female patients of childbearing age
      3) Smoking/tobacco history
      4) Current medications
         a) Include prescription, over-the-counter medications, and alternative therapies (e.g., herbals, acupuncture)
      5) Allergies
      6) Immunization status when indicated
4. Objective data collection (see Chapters 1 and 32)
   a. Secondary and focused assessments related to chief complaint

D. ACUITY RATING SYSTEMS

Combining the information collected from the "across-the-room" assessment and subjective and objective data, a triage acuity rating is assigned to the patient.
1. Five-level triage rating systems
   a. Currently recommended as the standard by the ENA and American College of Emergency Physicians (ACEP)[1]
   b. Examples and comparisons (Tables 2.1 and 2.2)
      1) Canadian Triage and Acuity Scale (CTAS): utilizes lists of clinical descriptors for each level of acuity
      2) Emergency Severity Index (ESI): integrates acuity levels and utilization of resources
      3) Australasian Triage Scale (ATS): utilizes lists of clinical descriptors for each level of acuity
      4) Manchester: combines subjective and objective data collection based on flowcharts
         a) Triage nurse selects a presentational flowchart (e.g., chest pain)
         b) Flowchart questions are followed until a positive answer is given; corresponding color level is then assigned

E. LOCATION OF CARE ASSIGNMENT

Triage nurses are typically responsible for addressing the initial logistical considerations related to each patient's ED visit. The logistical decision as to where continuing treatment will be provided is *distinct from* the triage acuity rating decision.

1. Logistical considerations
   a. Treatment areas within the emergency department
      1) Acute versus urgent care, fast-track area
      2) Pediatric versus adult area
      3) Surgical versus medical area
      4) Specialty area needs, such as
         a) Gynecology
         b) Ocular, ear, nose, throat area
         c) Trauma/medical resuscitation

   d) Chest pain area
   e) Behavioral health (psychiatric)
   f) Isolation needs
   b. Treatment areas outside the emergency department
      1) Using institutional-approved policies or protocols and in compliance with EMTALA, triage nurses may send a patient to areas outside the emergency department but within the hospital
         a) Fast-track or urgent care
         b) Mental health services
         c) Labor and delivery

F. TREATMENT AND DIAGNOSTIC TESTING

1. Triage treatments
   a. Basic first aid
      1) Nursing interventions
         a) Wound care, bleeding control
         b) Application of ice and elevation of injured extremities
         c) Providing rest and comfort (e.g., slings, wheelchairs)
   b. Written policies for initiating treatment
      1) Administering antipyretic medications for fever control
      2) Obtaining glucose level by point-of-care testing
      3) Administering analgesic medications for mild pain (e.g., acetaminophen, ibuprofen)
      4) Instilling topical anesthetic medication for eye injuries

Table 2.1

Five-Level Acuity Rating Systems

CTAS	ESI	ATS	Manchester
Categories			
Resuscitation	Level 1	Resuscitation	Immediate (red)
Emergent	Level 2	Emergent	Very urgent (orange)
Urgent	Level 3	Urgent	Urgent (yellow)
Less urgent	Level 4	Semi urgent	Standard (green)
Nonurgent	Level 5	Nonurgent	Nonurgent (blue)
Time Frame			
Resuscitation	Level 1	Resuscitation	Immediate

CTAS, Canadian Triage and Acuity Scale; *ESI,* Emergency Severity Index; *ATS,* Australasian Triage Scale.

Data from Gilboy, N., Tanabe, P., Travers, D. A., Rosenau, A. M., & Eitel, D. R. (2013). *Emergency severity index, version 4: Implementation handbook, 2012 edition.* Retrieved from http://www.ahrq.gov/professionals/systems/hospital/esi/index.html.

Table 2.2

Comparisons of Five-Level Triage Systems

Criteria	CTAS	ESI	ATS	Manchester
Pain scale incorporation	Uses 10-point scale	Uses 10-point scale. If rating is greater than 7/10, consider triage level 2	Not specified	Major factor for each flowchart
Incorporates pediatric patients	Yes	Vital sign criteria included	Not specifically, but generally recognized	Not addressed in flowcharts
Uses sentinel diagnosis	Yes	No	Yes	52 chief complaints versus sentinel diagnoses
Educational material available	Web-based training	Published manual and training video	Training video	Published manual
Additional comments		Has four major decision points: A: Is patient dying? B: Should patient wait? C: Resource prediction (incorporated into levels 3–5) D: Patient's vital signs		Algorithmic flowchart based on 52 chief complaints

CTAS, Canadian Triage and Acuity Scale; *ESI,* Emergency Severity Index; *ATS,* Australasian Triage Scale.

Modified from Fernandes, C., Tanabe, P., Gilboy, N., Johnson, L. A., McNair, R. S., Rosenau, A. M., Sawchuk, P., Thompson, D. A., Travers, D. A., Bonalumi, N., & Suter, R. E. (2005). Five-level triage: A report from the ACEP/ENA five-level triage task force. *Journal of Emergency Nursing, 31*(1), 39–50.

2. Initiating diagnostic tests at triage
   a. Institutional-approved policies or protocols must be in place and followed
   b. Competency-based education of policy/protocol use is recommended
   c. Often utilized when department is overcrowded and wait times are longer
   d. Examples
      1) Ordering radiographs of injured extremities
      2) Obtaining 12- to 15-lead electrocardiograms on patients with the potential for having acute coronary syndromes
      3) Obtaining urine and ordering/performing urinalysis on patients with suspected urinary tract infection
      4) Obtaining urine and ordering/performing pregnancy tests when appropriate
      5) Obtaining blood and ordering specific diagnostic tests

G. DECISION-MAKING PROCESS

1. Scientific evidence is lacking that demonstrates how triage nurses make acuity rating decisions. It is believed to be based on
   a. Knowledge of human anatomy, physiology, pathophysiology, pharmacology, and other related disciplines
   b. Clinical portraits: through experience, emergency nurses accumulate memories or pictures of what certain conditions look like
   c. Rules of thumb, such as all women of childbearing age are pregnant until proven otherwise
   d. *Gestalt,* instinct, or intuition
   e. Knowledge and use of specific hospital triage guidelines

H. INTERFACILITY TRANSFERS

1. Emergency departments may receive transfers from health centers, other hospital emergency departments, nursing homes, and other long-term care facilities as a result of
   a. Specific transfer agreements between facilities
   b. Capabilities of the accepting facility such as a regional referral center
2. Transfer patients should have triage assessment performed on arrival to the emergency department
3. Other considerations of transfer patients
   a. Obtain patient information from
      1) Transferring facility
      2) Transport personnel
      3) Patient and/or family
   b. Additional information
      1) Medications, treatment, course of care at transferring facility
      2) Medications, treatment, course of care while enroute to receiving facility

3) Name and contact information of patient's primary care physician

II. Additional Triage Responsibilities

A. WAITING ROOM MANAGEMENT

1. Triage nurse is clinically and legally responsible for patients in waiting room
   a. Must be accessible to patients/others in waiting room
   b. Must be able to view the waiting room and periodically perform a minimal "across-the-room" assessment of waiting patients
2. Safety
   a. Waiting room must remain a safe environment for patients and others
   b. Triage personnel must work closely with other hospital personnel to identify unsafe conditions/situations
      1) Patients who are potentially a danger to self or others
         a) Notify hospital security/law enforcement personnel to
            (1) Stay with patient
            (2) Screen/search for weapons or other items (e.g., medications) that the patient may use to harm self or others
         b) Relocate persons from waiting room to more secure location as soon as possible
3. Reassessment
   a. Consider a triage reassessment policy that may include
      1) Reassessment time frames based on patient acuity level
         a) More frequent assessments for more acute patients
      2) Components of patient reassessment
         a) Vital signs, pain rating
         b) General appearance, mental status
         c) Information relevant to chief complaint (e.g., wound status for lacerations, respiratory status for asthma exacerbation)
      3) Reassessment documentation
4. Initiation of patient teaching
   a. Injury prevention (e.g., helmet, car seat, seat belt use)
   b. Providing written patient/family education information (e.g., department operations, triage process)

B. COMMUNICATION ISSUES

1. Customer service—patient satisfaction
   a. The patient's and family's first impression of emergency clinical staff is the triage nurse

b. Be courteous, respectful, empathetic, calm, and practice active listening

c. Explain to the patient and others expectations regarding wait times

　　1) Patients frequently are not treated on a "first come, first served" basis but instead by acuity

　　2) Wait times may vary and are influenced by many factors

　　　　a) Patient acuity ratings

　　　　b) Location of care (e.g., acute, nonacute areas of emergency department)

　　　　c) Specialty area needs

　　　　d) Volume and criticality of other patients in the emergency department

　　　　e) Staffing for nurses, physicians, ancillary personnel

　　3) Attempt to provide accurate estimates of wait time

　　　　a) When in doubt, overestimate wait times

　　4) If available, patient pagers may be provided if prolonged wait time is expected

2. Visitors

　a. Department visitation policy should include

　　1) Process for identification of visitors

　　2) Number of visitors in treatment area at a time

　　3) Minimum age limits (e.g., no children under specified age)

　b. Triage nurse may be responsible for communicating and/or enforcing policy

　c. Triage nurse may serve as liaison between family in waiting room and primary (bedside) nurse and/or treating provider

　d. Ensure patient confidentiality

3. Dealing with upset patients, families, visitors (service recovery)

　a. Determine nature of problem

　b. Attempt to address problem in real time

　　1) Provide information

　　2) Allow person to vent, but not become hostile or violent

　c. Identification of violent/potentially violent patients and/or visitors

　　1) Objective signs: increasing agitation including pacing, clenched fists, yelling, verbal threats, signs of alcohol or drug use

　　2) Subjective information from the patient, family, police, or others

　d. Deescalating actions

　　1) Verbal escalation

　　　　a) Manage with verbal interventions

　　　　b) Anxiety: provide support and explanations, answer questions

　　　　c) Agitation: be directive and address specific needs, set appropriate limits

　　2) Verbally threatening

　　　　a) Take threat seriously

　　　　b) Involve hospital security and/or police

　　3) Physically acting out

　　　　a) Initiate immediate security response

　　　　b) Take actions to protect others

　e. Solicit help if needed

　　1) Involve patient advocate/relations personnel if available

　　2) Involve supervising personnel as needed

4. Public and media relations

　a. Notify public and media relations of any high-profile patient or unusual incident per institutional policy

　b. Transfer all telephone calls and inquiries about the incident or patient(s) per institutional policy

5. Arrival of families of critically ill or deceased patients

　a. Anticipate family arrival

　b. Escort family to a private waiting area

　c. Contact hospital chaplain, social worker, or other support personnel if available

　d. Notify treating emergency personnel of family arrival

III. Administrative Responsibilities

A. SAFETY

1. Implementation of safety measures

　a. Security and/or police presence

　b. Security monitoring with cameras in specific locations

　c. Panic buttons

　d. Restricted access doors

　e. Employee identification badges

　f. Metal detectors

B. INFECTION CONTROL

1. Enforcement of universal precautions and good handwashing between patients

2. Policy implementation concerning respiratory hygiene and cough etiquette

　a. Application of appropriate masks for patients with suspected droplet infection or tuberculosis

3. Screening policy for all incoming patients with signs and symptoms of infection

　a. Presence of fever, chills, rash, cough, recent exposure to infection

　b. History of immunosuppression

　c. Recent foreign travel (see Chapters 9 and 20)

4. Other infection control policies

　a. If possible, provide physical separation of patients with suspected infections

　　1) Post signage outside bay or room to alert all ED personnel of isolation precautions and glove, gown, or mask requirements

　b. Notification of appropriate personnel of need for a positive- or negative-pressure room

C. TRIAGE LEGALITIES

1. EMTALA
   a. All patients presenting to an emergency department for care, regardless of the hospital's capabilities, must have an MSE performed to determine whether a medical emergency condition exists (see Chapter 45)
      1) Triage is not an MSE
      2) An MSE is performed by a physician or an independent licensed practitioner (i.e., nurse practitioner, physician assistant) as identified by hospital bylaws
      3) All hospitals receiving federal funding in the United States must comply with EMTALA
      4) If an emergency medical condition exists, the patient must be stabilized prior to transfer
2. Left without being seen (LWBS), left without treatment (LWOT), or left without notification (elopement)
   a. A competent, registered ED patient may elect to leave the department prior to receiving an MSE
   b. If triage nurse is aware that the patient is leaving or considering leaving
      1) Notify the supervising nurse or attending physician of patient's intent per institutional policy
      2) Provide information to the patient about risks of leaving prior to being seen
      3) If possible, have patient sign a medical release
      4) Document
         a) Patient's mental capacity
         b) Notification of appropriate personnel
         c) Explanation of risks of leaving and patient's understanding of risks
         d) Attempts made to locate or contact patients who have eloped
   c. Rates of LWBS, LWOT, or elopements should be tracked
      1) National rate 1.7%[1]
3. Consent for treatment (see Chapter 45)
   a. All physically able and mentally competent adult patients must provide consent for emergency treatment
   b. Age of majority for providing emergency treatment consent varies from state to state
   c. Minor patients (under the age of majority)
      1) State laws vary regarding minors seeking care for pregnancy-related problems, sexually transmitted diseases, sexual assault, abuse, drug and alcohol treatment, and life- or limb-threatening conditions
      2) Consent obtained from parent or guardian
      3) Emancipated minors
         a) Individuals below the age of majority who are self-supporting and recognized by the legal system as an adult
         b) Individuals below the age of majority who are in the military, married, or pregnant
   d. Implied consent
      1) Allows for lifesaving treatment in an emergency situation when the patient is unable or incapable of giving consent
4. Patient confidentiality and privacy (see Chapter 45)
   a. Privacy and confidentiality must be maintained in triage area
5. Providing telephone advice
   a. Written departmental/institutional policy and protocols must be followed
   b. Instruct callers to dial 911, or emergency phone number appropriate for the area, if medical emergency exists

D. TRIAGE PERFORMANCE IMPROVEMENT

1. Triage process should be part of overall ED quality improvement plan
   a. Monitoring indicators
      1) Rates of under- or overtriage
      2) Adverse events associated with triage
      3) Time intervals
         a) Time of arrival to triage time
         b) Time of triage to first physician/practitioner interaction
         c) Length of stay by triage acuity category
      4) Measurement of admission rates by triage acuity level
      5) Specific patient populations such as trauma or pediatrics
      6) Frequency and appropriateness of reassessment of patients remaining in the waiting area
   b. Share results with staff
   c. Restaff as needed
   d. If process/practice changes are made, then remonitor

E. TRIAGE DATA UTILIZATION

1. Benchmarking
   a. ED case mix examples
      1) Number of patients in each triage acuity category
      2) Most common chief complaints
      3) Pediatric versus adult patients
   b. Performance measure examples
      1) Wait times by triage acuity category
      2) Length of stay by triage acuity category
      3) Description of patients who leave ED without being seen: acuity levels, chief complaints
      4) Time intervals (e.g., door to admit time)
2. Surveillance: the collection and interpretation of routinely collected health data
   a. Syndromic surveillance
      1) Aggregation of electronic symptom data that are captured early in the course of illness, and analyzed for signals that could indicate a disease

outbreak requiring investigation and response by the public health system

    2) Data (chief complaints, triage notes, assessment findings) frequently used for syndromic surveillance because the data are timely, increasingly available in electronic form, and population based

  b. Injury surveillance

  c. National ED surveillance

    1) National Hospital Ambulatory Medical Care Survey (NCHS, 2010)

      a) Annual national survey of emergency departments in the United States

      b) Conducted by the National Center for Health Statistics

3. Research (see Chapter 47)

  a. Triage data used for a variety of research studies

    1) Clinical research examples

      a) Stratification of patients by acuity

      b) Grouping of patients by chief complaint category

  b. Administrative research examples

    1) Evaluation of department overcrowding using triage acuity data

    2) Nurse staffing ratios by triage acuity case mix

    3) Patient flow, throughput to inpatient units

IV. Selected Considerations

A. POPULATIONS

1. Pediatrics

  a. Incidence of illness/injury in children

    1) Children less than 15 years of age account for 19% of all ED visits[2]

    2) About one-fifth of children less than 15 years of age are seen in pediatric emergency departments[2]

    3) National ED visit rate for infants under 12 months of age was 9.5 visits per 100 persons in 2007[2]

  b. Infants and children decompensate rapidly

  c. Additional knowledge required

    1) Pediatric growth and development including milestones

    2) Communication with the patient and caregiver

    3) Response to pain

    4) Assessment

    5) Common pediatric illness or injuries

    6) Injury prevention

  d. Care is family centered

    1) Meeting the physiologic, psychosocial, and emotional needs of the pediatric patient and family

  e. Pediatric assessment

    1) Pediatric assessment triangle[3]

Box 2.1

CIAMPEDS

C: Chief complaint

I: Immunizations, isolation

A: Allergies

M: Medications

P: Past medical history, parent's/caregiver's impression of the child's condition

E: Events surrounding the illness or injury

D: Diet; diapers

S: Symptoms associated with the illness or injury

From Emergency Nurses Association. (2012). *Emergency nursing pediatric course provider manual* (4th ed.). Des Plaines, IL: Emergency Nurses Association.

---

      a) Begins with "across-the-room" assessment

      b) Before touching the child, the registered nurse performs a visual or observational assessment

        (1) Appearance

        (2) Work of breathing

        (3) Circulation to skin

    2) Followed by completion of the primary and secondary assessments (see Chapters 1 and 32)

      a) Vital signs: normal ranges of heart rate, respiratory rate, blood pressure for each age group (see Appendix B), oxygen saturation, temperature

      b) Pain level (see Chapter 8)

      c) Accurate weight (in kilograms)

      d) History

        (1) Mechanism of injury (see Chapter 31)

        (2) CIAMPEDS (Box 2.1) from parent/caregiver

        (3) Tailor questions to patient's developmental level and ability to communicate

  f. Triage red flags (Table 2.3)

2. Geriatrics

  a. In 2009-10, 15% of patients seen in emergency departments in the United States were age 65 or older[4]

  b. More likely to have chronic medical problems and take multiple medications

  c. Physiologic effects of aging on each system must be considered

  d. Triage considerations

    1) Past medical and medication histories are more complex

    2) Triage interview frequently takes longer

    3) Atypical presentations must be considered

    4) There may be a delay in seeking care

    5) Pain perception may be altered

    6) Confusion is a common sign of illness

    7) Minor problems are often more complicated

    8) Consider elder abuse and neglect

Table 2.3

Triage Red Flags

Airway
Apnea
Choking
Drooling
Audible airway sounds
Positioning

Breathing
Grunting
Sternal retractions, increased work of breathing
Irregular respiratory patterns
Respiratory rate >60 breaths/min
Respiratory rate <20 breaths/min for children less than 6 yr
Respiratory rate less than 15 breaths/min for children less than 15 yr
Absence of breath sounds
Cyanosis

Circulation
Cool or clammy skin
Tachycardia, bradycardia
Heart rate >200 beats/min
Heart rate <60 beats/min
Hypotension
Diminished or absent peripheral pulses
Decreased tearing, sunken eyes

Disability
Altered level of consciousness
Inconsolability
Sunken or bulging fontanel

Exposure
Petechiae
Purpura
Signs and symptoms of maltreatment/abuse

Full set of vital signs
Hypothermia
Temperature >100.4°F (38°C) in infant age 3 mo or less
Temperature >104–105°F (40.0–40.6°C) at any age

Give comfort
Severe pain

History
History of chronic illness
History of family crisis
Return visit to emergency department within 24 hr

9) Assess compliance with medications and treatments
10) Consider asking about a health care proxy or advance directive

B. ILLNESS/INJURY

1. Behavioral health (psychiatric) conditions
   a. Patients frequently seek care in the emergency department when their coping mechanisms fail
   b. Conditions requiring immediate safety measures and treatment (including continuous monitoring) to protect the patient and others include[5,6]
      1) Active suicidal or homicidal ideation
      2) Physically or verbally acting out

   c. Subjective data collection
      1) History of present illness/injury/chief complaint
      2) Past psychiatric history including hospitalizations, medications
         a) Obtain from patient and/or family/friends
      3) Safety assessment: threats or actions indicating a potential for violence toward self or others
         a) Suicidal (Table 2.4) or homicidal
            (1) Thoughts
            (2) Does the patient have a plan?
            (3) Does the patient have the means to carry out the plan?
            (4) History of attempts: number and method
      4) Substance abuse
         a) Alcohol
            (1) History of alcohol abuse and treatment
            (2) Amount consumed in the last 24 hours
            (3) Time and amount of last drink
            (4) History of seizures related to alcohol withdrawal
         b) Drugs
            (1) History of substance abuse and treatment
            (2) Drugs used recently and route of use
            (3) Timing of last use
      5) Presence of visual, auditory, tactile hallucinations
      6) Presence of paranoid statements
      7) Patient's mood
   d. Objective data collection
      1) Affect
      2) Speech and content of speech
      3) Current behavior or activity
      4) Personal appearance including hygiene and dress
      5) Eye contact
      6) Orientation
2. Cognitive impairments
   a. Determine baseline mental status from parent/caregiver
   b. Causes of chronic cognitive impairment
      1) Dementia
      2) Alzheimer's disease
      3) Developmental disability
      4) Previous stroke or head trauma
      5) Psychiatric conditions
      6) Children with developmental delays
      7) Adults with conditions such as Down syndrome
   c. Dealing with cognitively impaired patient at triage
      1) Obtain history and assessment information from family/caregiver
      2) Determine from parent/caregiver deviations from baseline
      3) From parent/caregiver obtain information on how best to communicate with patient
      4) Allow parent/caregiver to stay with patient at all times
      5) Minimize stimulation

Table 2.4	
Triage-Based Management for Patients with Suicidal or Homicidal Ideation or Behavior	
Risk Level	**Interventions**
High-risk patients include those who:	One-to-one constant staff observations and/or security
Have made a moderately to nearly lethal suicide attempt	Locked door preventing elopement from area
Have suicide ideations	Rapid evaluation by licensed medical provider and/or mental health provider
Have command hallucinations	Inpatient admission
Are psychotic	Sedation and/or restraints as necessary
Express other signs of acute risk	
Have recent onset of major psychiatric syndromes	
Have been recently discharged from psychiatric inpatient unit	
Have history of acts/threats of aggression	
Moderate-risk patients include those who:	Locked door preventing elopement from area
Have suicide ideation with some level of suicide intents, but who have taken no action	At least 15-min checks by personnel
Have no other acute risk factors	Psychiatric/psychological evaluation soon/when sober
Have psychomotor retardation	May be monitored by family if locked door prevents elopement
Are currently in treatment with confirmed good therapeutic alliance	
Lower-risk patients include those who:	May wait in waiting room, especially if accompanied by family/friend and in view of personnel
Have some mild or passive suicide ideation, with no plan or intent	May wait for psychiatric/psychological evaluation
Have no history of suicide attempt	
Have a good and available support system	

3. Pregnancy
   a. Conditions requiring immediate treatment
      1) Hemorrhage: internal or external
         a) Ruptured ectopic pregnancy
         b) Abruptio placentae
         c) Placenta previa
      2) Imminent delivery (crowning)
      3) Eclampsia
   b. Consider pregnancy in any woman of childbearing age (11 to 55 or more years of age)
   c. Triage history should include last normal menstrual period
   d. Subjective data collection
      1) History of present illness/injury/chief complaint
      2) Reproductive history: gravida, para, abortion (spontaneous or therapeutic), ectopic
      3) Expected date of confinement (EDC)
      4) Number of fetuses
      5) Known pregnancy complication such as hypertension or pregnancy-induced diabetes
      6) Common chief complaints
         a) Bleeding or discharge
         b) Pain
   e. Objective data collection
      1) Fetal heart tones: normal is 120–160 beats/minute
      2) Fetal activity

3) Presence of contractions
4) Signs of imminent delivery (e.g., crowning, umbilical cord exposure)

4. Chronic illness
   a. Patients with serious chronic illness
      1) Likely to have acute complications and illnesses
      2) May require higher triage acuity rating
   b. Examples
      1) Immunocompromised patients at risk of occult infection
      2) Patients on anticoagulants at higher risk of bleeding
      3) Patients with chronic respiratory disease are vulnerable to acute respiratory infections

5. Trauma
   a. Conditions requiring immediate treatment
      1) Obstructed or partially obstructed airway
      2) Mechanism of injury (see Chapter 31) and signs or symptoms of a potential C-spine injury
      3) Breathing difficulties
      4) Signs and/or symptoms of internal or external bleeding
      5) Change in level of consciousness
   b. In 2007, one third of all ED visits were attributable to injury[2]

c. Primary assessment is completed first with life-threatening injuries identified and treated (see Chapter 32)

d. Subjective data collection
   1) Obtain history from prehospital providers
   2) History of events from patient
      a) Date and time of injury
      b) Mechanism of injury (see Chapter 31)
      c) Protective devices used (e.g., seat belt, helmet)
      d) Current complaints/injuries

6. Wounds
   a. Subjective data collection
      1) History of injury/chief complaint
         a) How did the injury occur?
         b) Date and time of injury
         c) Type of injury: blunt or penetrating forces
         d) What has the patient done to relieve pain, bleeding, or other symptoms?
      2) Tetanus immunization history
   b. Objective data collection
      1) Unwrap and expose all injuries for adequate evaluation
      2) Assess for active bleeding
      3) Assess for circulatory compromise
      4) Evaluate size, extent of tissue damage or loss, and location of injury
      5) Assess for gross wound contamination
   c. Provide first aid
      1) Apply dressing to protect the injury from further contamination
      2) Control bleeding with application of direct pressure or pressure dressing and elevation; tourniquet use is a last resort
      3) Stabilize any impaled foreign body
   d. Specific injuries
      1) Burns
         a) Conditions requiring immediate treatment
            (1) Inhalation injury
            (2) Partial-thickness burns greater than 20% of body surface area (BSA)
            (3) Full-thickness burns greater than 10% BSA
            (4) Significant electrical burn
         b) Subjective data collection
            (1) Type of burn
            (2) Circumstances surrounding the burn
            (3) Assess for other injuries
         c) Objective data collection
            (1) Signs of airway involvement
            (2) Location and extent of burns
            (3) Depth of burn
         d) First aid
            (1) Burns less than 5% of BSA: apply moist sterile compresses over burned tissue
            (2) Chemical burns: identify agent and verify appropriateness of saline dressing application

2) Bites and stings
   a) Conditions requiring immediate treatment
      (1) Signs of anaphylaxis
      (2) Bites associated with systemic reaction
      (3) Bites with potential for significant envenomation
   b) Subjective data collection
      (1) History of present injury/chief complaint
      (2) Description of animal, reptile, insect causing the injury or bite
      (3) Location of the bite/injury
      (4) Additional complaints
      (5) Past or familial history of allergies or reactions to bites or stings
   c) Objective data collection
      (1) Type and location of wound
      (2) Wound description
      (3) Systemic symptoms
3) Amputations
   a) Preserve amputated part by wrapping it in moist sterile gauze and placing it in a sealed plastic bag on ice
4) High-pressure injuries from paint or grease guns are serious and should be seen rapidly

7. Musculoskeletal injuries
   a. Conditions requiring immediate treatment
      1) Pulseless extremity
      2) Hemorrhage
      3) Open fracture
      4) Compartment syndrome
   b. Subjective data collection
      1) History of present injury/chief complaint
      2) Description of event resulting in injury
         a) Date and time of the injury
         b) How patient landed when injury occurred and the position of extremity
         c) Sounds heard at the time of injury (e.g., a pop or snap)
         d) Symptoms present directly after the injury
         e) Ability to walk, bear weight, or use the affected extremity
         f) Cause of injury
      3) History of previous orthopedic injuries or surgeries, bone disease
   c. Objective data collection
      1) Obvious deformity: compare side to side
      2) Assessment of presence/absence of the five Ps distal to injury
         a) Pain
         b) Pallor or skin color and temperature
         c) Pulses and capillary refill
         d) Paresthesias or abnormal sensation
         e) Paralysis: assess motor function
   d. Provide first aid
      1) Splint affected extremity including joint above and below injury
      2) Apply ice

    3) Elevate extremity

    4) Educate and encourage the patient to rest the injured extremity

    5) Remove constricting clothing or jewelry in the area of and distal to injury

8. Respiratory illness

  a. Conditions requiring immediate treatment

    1) Oxygen saturation <90% (small children, <95%)

    2) Adult respiratory rate <10 or >30

    3) Cyanosis

    4) Labored breathing

    5) Inability to talk in full sentences

    6) Abnormal airway sounds such as stridor

  b. Remove extra layers of clothing to accurately count respirations

  c. Subjective data collection

    1) History of present illness/injury/chief complaint

    2) Prior intubations or intensive care unit (ICU) admission for respiratory problems

    3) Chronic respiratory or cardiovascular disease

    4) Smoking history

  d. Objective data collection

    1) Inspection

      a) Assess work of breathing

      b) Nasal flaring

      c) Use of accessory muscles

      d) Retractions

      e) Patient's ability to simultaneously breathe and speak in full sentences

    2) Listen and auscultate for audible abnormal breathing

      a) Wheezing

      b) Stridor

      c) Crackles or rhonchi

      d) Breath sound equality

  e. Initiate respiratory isolation if patient at risk for acute communicable respiratory infection

    1) Apply appropriate mask

    2) Arrange appropriate isolation

9. Altered mental status

  a. Conditions requiring immediate treatment

    1) Unresponsiveness

    2) Acute decrease in level of consciousness

      a) Responsive only to pain

      b) Minimally responsive to verbal stimuli

      c) Fluctuating level of consciousness

    3) Acute confusion

    4) "Worst headache of my life" complaint

    5) Signs and symptoms of stroke

  b. Subjective data collection

    1) History of present illness/injury/chief complaint

    2) Important to determine baseline: Is altered mental status acute or chronic?

    3) Onset, duration

    4) Substance abuse or ingestion

    5) Acute visual or balance changes

  c. Objective data collection

    1) Orientation to time, place, person

    2) Glasgow Coma Scale score (see Appendix A)

    3) Speech; ability to articulate clearly and respond appropriately to questions

    4) Unilateral weakness such as facial droop, pronator drift

  d. Identify potential candidates for fibrinolytic therapy or clot-specific fibrinolysis and facilitate rapid assessment and treatment

    1) Move patient to treatment area (if bed available)

10. Cardiovascular illness

  a. Conditions requiring immediate treatment

    1) Crushing substernal chest pain or other symptoms indicating an acute coronary syndrome, with unstable vital signs, severe diaphoresis, and/or pallor

    2) Symptomatic bradycardia or tachycardia (e.g., with accompanying hypotension, chest pain, altered mental status, diaphoresis)

    3) Syncopal episode

    4) Heart failure with oxygen saturation <90%

  b. Subjective data collection

    1) History of present illness/injury/chief complaint

    2) PQRST of pain (see Chapter 8)

    3) Cardiac risk factors

    4) Previous history of respiratory or cardiovascular problems

  c. Objective data collection

    1) Presence of diaphoresis, emesis, shortness of breath

    2) Pain location: midsternal area; may present with pain in other areas such as jaw, left arm, shoulder, abdomen, back

    3) Abnormal vital signs

  d. Identify potential candidates for fibrinolytic therapy or cardiac catheterization and facilitate rapid assessment and treatment

    1) Move patient to treatment area (if bed available)

  e. For possible acute myocardial infarction, perform electrocardiogram immediately at triage or if treatment bed not immediately available per institutional policy

11. Abdominal illnesses

  a. Conditions requiring immediate treatment

    1) Expanding or acute aortic abdominal aneurysm

    2) Suspected mesenteric ischemia

    3) Ruptured appendix/peritonitis

  b. Subjective data collection

    1) History of present illness/injury/chief complaint

    2) Have patient point with one finger to most painful location

    3) Consider conditions related to gastrointestinal, genitourinary, reproductive systems

      a) Female: determine last normal menstrual period

      b) Male: assess for possible testicular torsion

4) History of abdominal surgeries/illnesses
5) History of diarrhea, constipation, nausea, vomiting
6) Pain description
   c. Objective data collection
   1) Signs of hypovolemia
   2) Signs of peritoneal irritation
   3) Ability to ambulate or sit
   4) Color of skin/sclera
   5) Odors
   6) Objective signs of pain
12. Ocular, ear, nose, throat conditions
    a. Ocular complaints
    1) Conditions requiring immediate treatment
       a) Sudden loss of vision
       b) Chemical (acid or alkali) exposure
       c) Diminished loss of vision with pain
       d) Significant eye injury
       e) Sudden onset of severe eye pain
    2) Subjective data collection
       a) History of present illness/injury/chief complaint: one or both eyes
          (1) Mechanism, date, time of injury, if applicable
          (2) Changes in vision
              (a) Loss of vision in one or both eyes, decreased acuity/blurred vision
              (b) Diplopia
              (c) Complaints of flashes of light or floaters
          (3) Pain
          (4) Drainage
          (5) Use of eye protective equipment
          (6) Treatments prior to arrival
       b) History of previous eye problems, surgery
       c) Use of glasses or contact lenses
    3) Objective data collection
       a) Brief inspection of eye for drainage, blood, swelling, redness, foreign body
       b) Test visual acuity
       c) Gross visual field testing
    b. Ear conditions
    1) Subjective data collection
       a) History of present illness/injury/chief complaint: one or both ears
          (1) Pain
          (2) Discharge
          (3) Changes in hearing
          (4) Fever and chills
          (5) Dizziness or ringing in the ears
          (6) Other symptoms such as cold or change in behavior
       b) History of ear infections, problems, trauma
       c) Treatments prior to arrival
    2) Objective data collection
       a) Obvious drainage

b) Patient's behavior such as infant pulling on the ear or crying
   c. Nasal conditions
   1) Conditions requiring immediate treatment
      a) Hemorrhages
   2) Subjective data collection
      a) History of present illness/injury/chief complaint
         (1) Time of onset
         (2) Bleeding: cause if known
         (3) Amount of bleeding, presence of clots, duration of bleeding, unilateral or bilateral nares
         (4) Nasal discharge: color, amount, odor, unilateral or bilateral nares
         (5) Treatment prior to arrival
         (6) Associated symptoms of dizziness, vomiting
      b) History of nosebleeds, trauma, foreign bodies, nose picking, or intranasal administration of drugs such as cocaine
   3) Objective data collection
      a) Nasal or postnasal bleeding or discharge
   4) Provide first aid for anterior bleeding
      a) Have patient gently blow clots from nose
      b) Assist patient in applying direct pressure to nostrils for 5–10 minutes
   d. Throat conditions
   1) Conditions requiring immediate treatment include any patient with difficulty maintaining a patent airway or having significant respiratory distress
      a) Stridor or other abnormal sounds
      b) Muffled voice
      c) Inability to swallow secretions
      d) Drooling in an age group that should not drool
   2) Subjective data collection
      a) History of present illness/injury/chief complaint
         (1) Onset of symptoms
         (2) Presence of fever, chills, sore throat
         (3) Unilateral or bilateral facial, oral, throat swelling
      b) History of similar episodes
   3) Objective data collection
      a) Ability to cough and swallow
      b) Obvious neck swelling
   e. Dental complaints
   1) Subjective data collection
      a) History of present illness/injury/chief complaint
         (1) Mechanism, date, time of injury, if applicable
         (2) Time of onset
      b) Recent dental procedures or oral surgery

      c) Last dental examination
      d) Consider whether the pain/discomfort could
         be cardiac pain
   2) Objective data collection
      a) General oral hygiene and general condition
         of the teeth and gums
         (1) Broken or missing teeth: intact tooth
             with root may be reimplanted within 30
             minutes of injury
         (2) Obvious caries
         (3) Dentures or partial plates
      b) Presence of swelling, redness, pus
   3) First aid
      a) Place missing permanent tooth in a com-
         mercial tooth preservative or saliva, milk, or
         saline if preservative not available
13. Environmental-related complaints
   a. Conditions requiring immediate treatment
      1) Cold exposure
         a) With shivering, lethargy, and/or confusion
         b) Frozen digits
      2) Heat exposure
         a) Syncope or near syncope
         b) Muscle cramps
         c) Lethargy and/or confusion
         d) Temperature >102°F (38.8°C)
   b. Pediatric and geriatric patients especially vulner-
      able to heat- and cold-related emergencies

References

1. American College of Emergency Physicians: Triage scale standardization. Retrieved from http://www.acep.org/Clinical-Practice-Management/Triage-Scale-Standardization/, 2010.
2. Niska R, Bhuiya F, Xu J: *National Hospital Ambulatory Medical Care Survey: 2007 emergency department summary*, Advance data from Vital and Health Statistics No. 26. Hyattsville, MD, 2010, National Center for Health Statistics.
3. Emergency Nurses Association: *Emergency nursing pediatric course provider manual*, ed 4, Des Plaines, IL, 2012, Emergency Nurses Association.
4. Albert M, McCaig LF, Ashman JJ: *Emergency department visits by persons aged 65 and over: United States, 2009-2010*, NCHS Data Brief No. 230. Hyattsville, MD, 2013, National Center for Health Statistics.
5. The Joint Commission: *Behavioural Health Accreditation Program*, National patient safety goals effective, 2015. January 1, 2015. Retrieved from http://www.jointcommission.org/bhc_2015_npsgs/.
6. American Psychiatric Association Task Force on Psychiatric Emergency Services: Report and recommendations regarding psychiatric emergency and crisis services: a review and model program descriptions. Retrieved from http://www.emergencypsychiatry.org/data/tfr200201.pdf, 2002.

Bibliography

Australasian College of Emergency Medicine. (n.d.): Australasian triage scale. Retrieved from http://www.enw.org/AustralianTriageScales%20Guidelines.pdf.
Canadian Association of Emergency Physicians. (n.d.): Canadian triage and acuity scale. Retrieved from http://www.caep.ca/resources/ctas.
Emergency Nurses Association: *Making the right decision: a triage curriculum*, ed 2, Des Plaines, IL, 2001, Emergency Nurses Association.
Emergency Nurses Association and the American College of Emergency Physicians. (n.d.): Standardized ED triage scale and acuity categorization: joint ENA/ACEP statement. Retrieved from https://www.ena.org/SiteCollectionDocuments/Position%20Statements/Joint/StandardizedEDTriageScaleandAcuityCategorization.pdf.
Fernandes C, Tanabe P, Gilboy N, Johnson LA, McNair RS, Rosenau AM, Sawchuk P, Thompson DA, Travers DA, Bonalumi N, Suter RE. Five-level triage: a report from the ACEP/ENA five-level triage task force, *J Emerg Nurs* 31(1):39–50, 2005.
Gilboy N, Tanabe P, Travers DA, Rosenau AM, Eitel DR: *Emergency severity index, version 4: Implementation handbook, 2012 edition*, AHRQ Publication No. 12-0014. Rockville, MD, 2013, Agency for Healthcare Research and Quality. Retrieved from http://www.ahrq.gov/professionals/systems/hospital/esi/index.html.

CHAPTER 3

Abuse and Neglect

Mary Hugo Nielson, DNP, APRN, ANP-BC, ANP

MAJOR TOPICS
General Strategy
Assessment
Analysis: Differential Nursing Diagnoses/
  Collaborative Problems
Planning and Implementation/Interventions
Evaluation and Ongoing Monitoring

Documentation of Interventions and Patient Response
Age-Related Considerations
Specific Abuse/Assault Emergencies
Child Maltreatment
Elder Abuse/Neglect
Intimate Partner Violence (Domestic Violence)
Sexual Assault

I. General Strategy

A. ASSESSMENT

1. Primary and secondary assessment/resuscitation (see Chapters 1 and 32)
2. Focused assessment
   a. Subjective data collection
      1) History of present illness/injury/chief complaint
         a) "Red flags" of history
            (1) Inconsistent history: injuries/illness do not appear to have logically been caused by the stated history
            (2) Changing or adding explanatory history when patient or caregiver is questioned
            (3) Mechanism of injury unlikely in view of patient's age, physical development, or condition
            (4) Delay by caregiver in seeking treatment
            (5) Overbearing individual who intimidates individual family members by body positions, facial expressions, or verbal threats and/or speaks for the victim of injury
         b) Somatic complaints (e.g., headache, abdominal pain, weakness)
         c) Recent injury
         d) Stated assault
         e) Efforts to relieve symptoms
            (1) Home remedies
            (2) Alternative therapies
            (3) Medications
               (a) Prescription
               (b) Over-the-counter/herbal
      2) Past medical history
         a) Current or preexisting diseases/illness
         b) Previous history of abuse/neglect
         c) Previous housing at shelter
         d) Substance and/or alcohol use/abuse
         e) Last normal menstrual period: female patients of childbearing age
         f) Medications
            (1) Prescription
            (2) Allergies to medications
            (3) Allergies to other
            (4) Immunization status
      3) Psychological/social/environmental factors
         a) Fear of reporting abuse
         b) Caregivers contributing factors (Table 3.1)
         c) Fear of retaliation
         d) Physical, financial, or social isolation of patient
         e) Munchausen syndrome by proxy
   b. Objective data
      1) General appearance
         a) Level of consciousness, behavior, affect
         b) Vital signs
         c) Odors
         d) Gait
         e) Hygiene
         f) Level of distress/discomfort
      2) Inspection
         a) Soft tissue injuries: ecchymotic areas, different stages of healing
         b) Burns
         c) Patterned injuries

TABLE 3.1

Contributing Caregiver Factors for
Maltreatment of:

Older Adults	Children
Alcohol or substance abuse	Parental history of child maltreatment in family of origin
Inability to cope with stress	Substance abuse
Lack of training in caring for elder	Mental health issues, including depression
Lack of social support from other potential caregivers	Nonbiological, transient caregivers in the home
High emotional or financial dependence on the older adult	Parental thoughts and emotions that tend to support or justify maltreatment behaviors
Depression	Social isolation
	Parental stress, poor parent-child relationships
	Parental characteristics such as young age, low education, single parenthood, large number of dependent children, low income

From "Understanding Elder Abuse Fact Sheet 2016." Centers for Disease Control and Prevention, https://www.cdc.gov/violenceprevention/pdf/em-factsheet-a.pdf. Accessed April 5, 2017. "Child Abuse and Neglect: Risk and Protective Factors." Centers for Disease Control and Prevention, www.cdc.gov/violenceprevention/childmaltreatment/riskprotectivefactors.html. Accessed April 5, 2017.

    3) Auscultation
        a) Breath sounds
        b) Heart sounds
        c) Bowel sounds
        d) Fetal heart tones if pregnant
    4) Palpation
        a) Skin temperature, moisture
        b) Areas of tenderness, deformity
    5) Percussion
        a) Abdominal tympany versus dullness
3. Diagnostic procedures
    a. Laboratory studies
        1) Complete blood count (CBC) with differential
        2) Serum chemistries including glucose, blood urea nitrogen (BUN), creatinine
        3) Serum and urine toxicology screens
        4) Type and crossmatch
        5) Urinalysis; pregnancy test in female patients of childbearing age
        6) Baseline human immunodeficiency virus (HIV), and hepatitis B and C
        7) Rapid plasma reagin (RPR)
        8) Cultures for sexually transmitted diseases unless prophylactically treated
        9) Evidence collection swabs (e.g., anogenital and oral areas)
        10) Forensic testing: DNA, ABO blood groups

    b. Imaging studies
        1) Radiograph of injured/tender area
        2) Battered-child (full body) radiographs
        3) Head or abdominal computed tomography (CT) scan, as indicated by injuries
    c. Other
        1) 12- to 15-lead electrocardiogram (ECG)
        2) Physical evidence collection (e.g., fingernail scrapings, clothing)
        3) Alternate lighting source

B. ANALYSIS: DIFFERENTIAL NURSING DIAGNOSES/COLLABORATIVE PROBLEMS

1. Risk for injury
2. Risk for ineffective coping
3. Risk for impaired skin integrity
4. Anxiety/fear
5. Pain
6. Risk for self-directed violence
7. Rape-trauma syndrome
8. Posttraumatic stress syndrome

C. PLANNING AND IMPLEMENTATION/INTERVENTIONS

1. Determine priorities of care
    a. Maintain airway, breathing, and circulation (see Chapters 1 and 32)
    b. Provide supplemental oxygen as indicated
    c. Establish intravenous (IV) access for administration of crystalloid fluids/blood products/medications
    d. Obtain and set up equipment and supplies
    e. Prepare for/assist with medical interventions
    f. Administer pharmacologic therapy as ordered
    g. Expose patient
        1) Assess for any other deformities or injuries
    h. Obtain a full set of vital signs including pain scale
2. Relieve anxiety/apprehension
    a. If the person accompanying the patient is suspected to be involved, allow for privacy to interview patient
3. Allow significant others to remain with patient if supportive
4. Educate patient and significant others

D. EVALUATION AND ONGOING MONITORING

1. Continuously monitor and treat as indicated
2. Monitor patient response/outcomes, and modify nursing care plan as appropriate
3. If positive patient outcomes are not demonstrated, reevaluate assessment and/or plan of care
4. Provide resources
    a. Rape crisis
    b. Women's shelters

E. DOCUMENTATION OF INTERVENTIONS AND PATIENT RESPONSE

F. AGE-RELATED CONSIDERATIONS

1. Pediatrics
   a. Growth or development related
      1) Dependent on caregiver to meet physical and emotional needs
      2) If an experienced pediatric examiner is not available and the assault is not acute (recent), the examination may be postponed until a time when an examiner is available
      3) Determine local policy or state law regarding consent when preparing to examine an adolescent. Patient may not want parents contacted, so determine whether parental consent is required
      4) Determine the adolescent's knowledge base of sexual function and terminology
   b. "Pearls"
      1) The uncooperative pediatric patient should not be restrained in order to complete an examination, to avoid further traumatization for the child
      2) Risk factors for abuse
         a) Infant separation at birth as a result of prematurity or illness
         b) Congenital anomalies or chronic medical conditions
         c) Behavior problems, fussy infants
         d) Developmental disabilities
      3) Assess for possibility of long-term molestation in the pediatric age group
2. Geriatrics
   a. Aging related
      1) Each year an estimated 1 in 10 persons over the age of 60 is the victim of abuse or neglect
      2) Increased incidence of soft tissue injury resulting from force
         a) Soft tissue is more friable and may lead to increased bleeding
      3) Consider patient comfort when performing pelvic examination
      4) Dependent on caregivers to meet physical and emotional needs
   b. "Pearls"
      1) Women are more often victims because they make up a larger proportion of the older population
      2) Determine patient's degree of comfort when discussing sexual function and terminology

II. Specific Abuse/Assault Emergencies

A. CHILD MALTREATMENT

Child maltreatment can be described as physical, sexual, or psychological abuse and neglect that is committed by a parent or other caregiver. Each has unique characteristics and requires individual approaches. Annually, more than 3.3 million cases are investigated by authorities in the United States. Approximately 2,000 children die each year from injury or neglect. Many of these seriously injured and murdered children have previously presented to the emergency department for initial care.

Children who have been sexually assaulted or molested should be referred to a child abuse medical specialist or specialized program. The most important treatment priority is ensuring the health and safety of the child. It is estimated that over 200,000 American minors are at risk for human trafficking and sexual exploitation. Children who are trafficked often experience mental health problems and suffer physical and sexual assaults. The emergency care provider's ability to maintain a nonjudgmental approach aids in his or her ability to communicate therapeutically with the patient and family.

Emergency care of the maltreated child includes a number of important steps. These steps include a suspicion of abuse, history taking, establishing the diagnosis, treating injuries, reporting to appropriate child protective agencies and/or law enforcement, documenting findings, discussing safety, and recommending follow-up physical/psychological care.

1. Assessment
   a. Subjective data collection
      1) History of present illness/injury/chief complaint (Table 3.2)
         a) Injury
            (1) Bruises, fractures, tissue disruption
            (2) Burns
            (3) Mechanism of injury
         b) Lethargy, new-onset seizure, coma
         c) Feeding problems; failure to thrive
         d) Persistent vomiting, hemoptysis
         e) Genital bleeding, discharge
         f) Regressive or "acting out" behaviors
         g) Recurring vague physical illness: Munchausen syndrome by proxy
      2) Past medical history
         a) Current or preexisting diseases/illness
            (1) Leukemia, hemophilia, other blood dyscrasias
            (2) Glutaricaciduria type 1: amino acid metabolism disorder resulting in retinal hemorrhages and subdural hematomas

Table 3.2
History Questioning
Use Open-Ended Questions:
Does any place on your body hurt?
What happens when you do something that your parents may not like?
Have people ever hit you?
What happens at (home, school, day care) when people get angry?
Are you afraid of anyone?
Where do you sleep?

      (3) Osteogenesis imperfecta
      (4) Mental, physical, or behavioral difficulties
    b) Medications
    c) Allergies to medications
    d) Allergies to other
    e) Immunization status
  b. Objective data collection
    1) Physical examination
      a) General appearance
        (1) Level of consciousness, behavior, affect: awake to comatose, behavior normal to quiet and subdued, or "acting out"
        (2) Vital signs: normal to hypotension, tachycardia, tachypnea
        (3) Hygiene: clean to unkempt, malnourished
        (4) Moderate to severe distress/discomfort
      b) Inspection
        (1) Injuries in various stages of healing (e.g., fractures) (Table 3.3)
        (2) Injuries that do not match the given history
        (3) Injuries with identifiable pattern (e.g., hand, object)
        (4) Multiple bruising of soft tissues in various stages
        (5) Burns
          (a) Identifiable pattern (e.g., cigarette, heater, hot water immersion)
      c) Auscultation
        (1) Lung sounds
        (2) Heart sounds
        (3) Bowel sounds
      d) Palpation
        (1) Skin and mucous membranes
        (2) Areas of tenderness
    2) Diagnostic procedures
      a) CBC with differential
      b) Complete chemistry profile including BUN and creatinine
      c) Coagulation profile in any child with suspicious bruising
      d) Urinalysis; pregnancy test in female patients of childbearing age
      e) Liver transaminases and amylase
      f) Stool guaiac
      g) Radiographic bone survey
        (1) Full radiographic abuse survey (skeletal survey) indicated in any child age 2 years or younger
      h) Head CT scan
        (1) Noncontrast CT scan indicated in any child with head trauma
      i) Abdominal CT scan
        (1) Indicated in unconscious child or the child with signs of abdominal trauma
2. Analysis: differential nursing diagnoses/collaborative problems
  a. Risk for caregiver role strain
  b. Impaired parenting
  c. Risk for impaired parent-infant/child attachment
  d. Risk for injury
  e. Ineffective individual and/or family coping
  f. Risk for impaired skin integrity
  g. Anxiety/fear
3. Planning and implementation/interventions
  a. Maintain airway, breathing, and circulation (see Chapters 1 and 32)
  b. Provide supplemental oxygen as indicated
  c. Establish IV access for administration of crystalloid fluids/blood products/medications as needed
  d. Prepare for/assist with medical interventions
    1) Initiate or continue Basic Life Support (BLS) and Advanced Life Support (ALS) per protocols if respiratory or cardiac arrest is present
    2) Institute cardiac and pulse oximetry monitoring as indicated
    3) Photograph all injuries when possible
      a) Identify photograph with child's name
      b) Identify date of photograph
      c) Identify body location of photograph; ruler or colorimetric chart may be added to aid in identifying size and type of injury
      d) Take three photographs of injuries
        (1) One photo of the injury at a distance to place the injury and body part in perspective to the whole body
        (2) One close-up photo of the injury
        (3) One of the injury with a ruler for size perspective
    4) Assist with collection and maintenance of physical and forensic evidence as indicated (see Chapter 40)
    5) Assist with treatment of injuries associated with abuse
    6) Insert gastric tube and attach to suction as indicated

Table 3.3

Inflicted Injury Fractures

Low Specificity Fractures
Clavicle fractures
Long-bone shaft fractures (unless child is not yet ambulatory)
Linear skull fractures

Moderate Specificity Fractures
Multiple fractures
Fractures of different ages
Epiphyseal separation
Digital fractures
Complete skull fractures
Spinal fractures

High Specificity Fractures
Rib fractures
Scapular fractures
Sternal fractures
Infants with unexplained fractures

7) Insert indwelling urinary catheter as indicated
8) Notify appropriate reporting agency
9) Assist with possible hospital admission or placement in another safe environment
10) Expose patient
    a) Assess for any other deformities or injuries
11) Obtain a full set of vital signs using appropriate pain scale
   e. Administer pharmacologic therapy as ordered
     1) ALS medications per protocols as indicated
     2) Nonnarcotic analgesics as indicated
     3) Narcotics as indicated
     4) Antibiotics
     5) Tetanus immunization
4. Evaluation and ongoing monitoring
   a. Level of consciousness
   b. Hemodynamic status
   c. Breath sounds and pulse oximetry
   d. Cardiac rate and rhythm
   e. Pain relief
   f. Intake and output

B. ELDER ABUSE/NEGLECT

The elder adult who has been abused may present to the emergency department for care. Emergency care professionals need to be aware of subtle signs of abuse. Elder abuse, which is any act or omission that results in psychological, emotional, physical, or financial harm to a person at least 60 years of age, is categorized into several types (Table 3.4) that may stem from various risk factors (Table 3.5). Available statistics for cases of sexual abuse and assault are underestimated, and it is common for intimate partners and family members to be the offender.

It is an American Medical Association recommendation to routinely ask older adults about abuse, even if signs are absent. Questions should be nonjudgmental and asked in a direct, nonthreatening manner. Multiple factors are involved in the management of older persons who have been abused, including immediate care, long-term assessment and care, education, and prevention. Intervention can be a lengthy process.

Multidisciplinary teams (i.e., social workers, physicians, nurses, administrators) can assist in these situations. The goal is to provide the older adult with a more fulfilling and enjoyable life. Immediate care focuses on treating the physical manifestations of abuse and ensuring the safety of the patient.

1. Assessment
   a. Subjective data collection
     1) History of present illness/injury/chief complaint (Table 3.6)
       a) May report history of abuse
         (1) Date and time of abuse/injury
         (2) Location of where abuse took place
         (3) Use of penetrating foreign objects in the abuse
       b) Bruises, welts, lacerations, rope marks, burns

c) Venereal disease or genital infections
d) Several injuries in various stages of healing
e) Unexplained injuries or injuries inconsistent with history
f) Delay in seeking treatment
g) Contradictory explanations given by the patient and caregiver
h) Changes in behavior

Table 3.4

Types of Elder Abuse

Neglect
Failure or refusal of the caregiver to provide necessities such as shelter, food, water, clothing, personal hygiene, medicine, access to medical care, or a safe environment

Self-Neglect
Behavior of an elder person that threatens his or her own health or safety
Emotional or psychological
Purposeful interaction with the intent to inflict anguish, distress, or pain, including verbal assaults, insults, threats, or humiliation

Physical Abuse
Use of physical force that results in pain or injury: slapping, hitting, biting, kicking, pushing, shoving, shaking, pinching, burning, striking with an object; also includes inappropriate use of drugs and physical restraints, force feeding, or using physical punishment

Sexual Abuse
Consists of nonconsensual sexual contact with an elderly individual or sexual contact with any elderly individual who is incapable of giving consent, including but not limited to sexual assault, rape, sodomy, or coerced nudity

Financial Abuse
Also known as material exploitation or financial exploitation, which involves illegal or improper use of an elderly person's money, funds, assets, or property; includes actions such as deceiving or forcing an elder to sign legal documents (e.g., wills), forging an elder's signature on legal documents, misusing or stealing an elder's possessions or money

Abandonment
Willful desertion of an elderly person by a caregiver

Department of Health and Human Services. National Center on Elder Abuse. (2015). Types of abuse. Retrieved from http://ncea.aoa.gov/FAQ/Type_Abuse/.

Table 3.5

Risk Factors for Abuse

Neglect: low income, poor health, poor social support
Emotional: low social support, physical dependence
Physical: substance abuse, mental illness, social isolation, low social support
Sexual: low social support, prior traumatic events
Financial: disability
Risk factors of a nursing facility: no abuse prevention policies, poor staffing and screening, high staff turnover, resident overcrowding

Table 3.6

Older Adult Abuse History Questions

Physical abuse: Do you feel safe where you live? Does anyone at home hurt you?

Psychological abuse: Does someone help you with your medications? Are you afraid of anyone at home?

Sexual abuse: Does someone touch you without your consent? Are you made to do things you don't want to?

Neglect: Who prepares your food? Are you alone a lot?

Financial abuse: Who takes care of your checkbook? Had you signed documents that you did not understand?

2) Past medical history
   a) Current or preexisting diseases/illness
   b) Substance or alcohol use/abuse in the home
   c) Medications and adherence to medications
   d) Allergies to medications
   e) Allergies to other
   f) Immunization status
   b. Objective data collection
   1) Physical examination
      a) General appearance
         (1) Level of consciousness, behavior, affect: alert, confused, comatose, fearful
         (2) Unkempt, poor hygiene
         (3) Malnourished: excluding physical condition of failure to thrive at the end of life
         (4) Moderate to severe distress/discomfort
      b) Inspection
         (1) Abrasions, ecchymosis, or lacerations in differing stages of healing
         (2) Skin breakdown
         (3) Dry mucous membranes
         (4) Decubitus ulcers
      c) Auscultation
         (1) Lung sounds
         (2) Heart sounds
         (3) Bowel sounds
      d) Palpation
         (1) Areas of tenderness
      e) Percussion
         (1) Tympany versus dullness of abdominal organs
   2) Diagnostic procedures
      a) CBC with differential
      b) Serum chemistries including glucose, BUN, and creatinine
      c) Serum and urine toxicology screens
      d) Urinalysis
      e) Radiographs as identified by physical examination findings
      f) Head CT scan
      g) ECG
2. Analysis: differential nursing diagnoses/collaborative problems
   a. Ineffective denial
   b. Ineffective individual and family coping
   c. Hopelessness
   d. Powerlessness
3. Planning and implementation/interventions
   a. Maintain airway, breathing, and circulation (see Chapters 1 and 32)
   b. Provide supplemental oxygen as indicated
   c. Establish IV access for administration of crystalloid fluids/blood products/medications as needed
   d. Prepare for/assist with medical interventions
      1) Initiate or continue BLS and ALS per protocols if respiratory or cardiac arrest is present
      2) Institute cardiac and pulse oximetry monitoring as indicated
      3) Photograph all injuries when possible
         a) Identify photograph with patient's name
         b) Identify date of photograph
         c) Identify body location of photograph; ruler or colorimetric chart may be added to aid in identifying size and type of injury
         d) Take three photographs of injuries
            (1) One photo of the injury at a distance to place the injury and body part in perspective to the whole body
            (2) One close-up photo of the injury
            (3) One photo of the injury with a ruler for size perspective
      4) Assist with collection and maintenance of physical and forensic evidence as indicated (see Chapter 43)
      5) Assist with treatment of injuries associated with abuse
      6) Insert gastric tube and attach to suction as indicated
      7) Insert indwelling urinary catheter as indicated
      8) Expose the patient
         a) Assess for any other deformity or injury
      9) Obtain a full set of vital signs including pain scale
      10) Notify appropriate reporting agency
      11) Assist with possible hospital admission or placement in another safe environment
   e. Administer pharmacologic therapy as ordered
      1) ALS medications per protocols as indicated
      2) Nonnarcotic analgesics
      3) Narcotics
      4) Antibiotics
      5) Tetanus immunization
   f. Educate patient
      1) Determine patient's safety if returning to home
      2) Allow patient to return home if patient is mentally competent and refuses further interventions
      3) Discuss obtaining a protective court order
4. Evaluation and ongoing monitoring
   a. Level of consciousness
   b. Hemodynamic status

Table 3.7

Aspects of History Taking

History Taking Considerations

Batterers may accompany patient to the emergency department.

Batterer may refuse to leave patient alone or to answer questions.

Translator (if required) should not be a member of the patient's or suspected abuser's family.

History Taking Questions to Ask

Have you been hit, kicked, or punched by someone in the past year?

Is a partner from a previous relationship making you feel unsafe?

Do you feel safe in your current relationship?

Does your partner ever force you to engage in sexual activity?

c. Breath sounds and pulse oximetry
d. Cardiac rate and rhythm
e. Pain relief
f. Intake and output

C. INTIMATE PARTNER VIOLENCE (DOMESTIC VIOLENCE)

Intimate partner violence is the victimization of a person with whom the abuser has had an intimate, romantic, or spousal relationship, which may or may not have involved a sexual relationship. Intimate partner violence can be sexual, psychological, or physical harm, which can occur between heterosexual or same-sex couples. This type of violence occurs in both younger and older men and women, and occurs in all socioeconomic groups. It has been estimated that 27.3% of women and 11.5% of men have experienced some form of intimate partner violence.

Intimate partner violence consists of a pattern of behaviors including physical violence, psychological abuse, and nonconsensual sexual behavior. It may also be associated with physical or social isolation.

Since 1992, The Joint Commission (TJC) has required hospitals seeking accreditation to develop and implement intimate partner violence protocols and training guidelines. This includes the requirement that hospitals and clinics routinely screen for intimate partner violence. Recognition of abuse requires a high index of suspicion. It is estimated that an accurate diagnosis of intimate partner violence is present in 1 of 25 cases.

1. Assessment
   a. Subjective data collection
      1) History of present illness/injury/chief complaint (Table 3.7)
         a) Date and time of assault
         b) Location of assault
         c) Use of penetrating foreign objects or other weapons in assault
         d) Palpitations, chest pain
         e) Dyspnea
         f) Abdominal pain
         g) Unexplained injury, or inconsistent with history
         h) Genital discharge, bleeding
         i) Substance or alcohol abuse in home
         j) Depression, suicide ideation
      2) Past medical history
         a) Current or preexisting diseases/illness
         b) Previous episodes of abuse
         c) Self-mutilation
         d) Medications
         e) Allergies to medications
         f) Allergies to other
         g) Immunization status
   b. Objective data collection
      1) Physical examination
         a) General appearance
            (1) Level of consciousness, behavior, affect: alert to comatose, angry, fearful, agitated
            (2) Moderate to severe distress/discomfort
         b) Inspection
            (1) Injuries
               (a) Ecchymosis, petechiae
               (b) Bilateral extremity injury
               (c) Multiple injuries
               (d) Fingernail scratches, cigarette burns, rope burns, bite marks, slap marks, patterned imprints
               (e) Subconjunctival hemorrhage
               (f) Upper extremity defensive wounds or injuries
         c) Auscultation
            (1) Lung sounds
            (2) Heart sounds
            (3) Bowel sounds
         d) Palpation
            (1) Areas of tenderness
         e) Percussion
            (1) Tympany versus dullness of abdominal organs
      2) Diagnostic procedures
         a) CBC with differential
         b) Complete metabolic profile
         c) Urinalysis; pregnancy test in female patients of childbearing age
         d) Radiographs as determined by physical examination findings
2. Analysis: differential nursing diagnoses/collaborative problems
   a. Ineffective denial
   b. Ineffective individual and family coping
   c. Hopelessness
   d. Powerlessness
   e. Self-mutilation
   f. Suicidal thoughts
3. Planning and implementation/interventions
   a. Maintain airway, breathing, and circulation (see Chapters 1 and 32)

b. Provide supplemental oxygen as indicated
c. Establish IV access for administration of crystalloid fluids/blood products/medications as needed
d. Prepare for/assist with medical interventions
  1) Initiate or continue BLS and ALS per protocols if respiratory or cardiac arrest is present
  2) Institute cardiac and pulse oximetry monitoring as indicated
  3) Photograph all injuries when possible
    a) Identify photograph with patient's name
    b) Identify date of photograph
    c) Identify body location of photograph; ruler or colorimetric chart may be added to aid in identifying size and type of injury
    d) Take three photographs of injuries
      (1) One photo of the injury at a distance to place the injury and body part in perspective to the whole body
      (2) One close-up photo of the injury
      (3) One photo of the injury with a ruler for size perspective
  4) Assist with collection and maintenance of physical and forensic evidence as indicated (see Chapter 43)
  5) Assist with treatment of injuries associated with assault
  6) Insert gastric tube and attach to suction as indicated
  7) Insert indwelling urinary catheter as indicated
  8) Expose the patient
    a) Assess for other deformity or injury
  9) Obtain a full set of vital signs including pain
  10) Notify appropriate reporting agency
  11) Assist with possible hospital admission or other safe environment
e. Administer pharmacologic therapy as ordered
  1) ALS medications per protocols as indicated
  2) Nonnarcotic analgesics
  3) Narcotics
  4) Antibiotics
  5) Tetanus immunization
f. Educate patient
  1) Identify risks to patient and children
  2) Discuss patient safety, safety escape plan, and available options
  3) Reassure patient that no one deserves to be abused
  4) Offer services of an agency advocate
    a) Frequently a volunteer from a shelter or domestic violence response agency
    b) Depending on agency procedures, the advocate may respond to the emergency department or be reached by a hotline number: National Domestic Violence Hotline (1-800-799-7233) or TTY (1-800-787-3224)
  5) Inform patient that violence at home may escalate
  6) Offer referral to shelter, legal services, and counseling
4. Evaluation and ongoing monitoring
  a. Level of consciousness
  b. Hemodynamic status
  c. Lung sounds and pulse oximetry
  d. Cardiac rate and rhythm
  e. Pain relief
  f. Intake and output

D. SEXUAL ASSAULT

Sexual assault is any type of sexual activity in which one person does not agree to engage but is forced to comply. Both psychological coercion and physical force can be parts of sexual assault. Rape is the means by which the abuser dominates and controls his or her victim. Girls and women and boys and men of all ages have been victims of sexual assault. It is estimated that more than 23 million women and 2 million men in the United States have experienced rape during their lifetimes.

Human trafficking is modern-day slavery that affects 17,500 to 20,000 victims in the United States annually. Human sex trafficking includes victims of all ages and both sexes. Both the sexual assault victims and the human trafficking victim may present to emergency departments with a myriad of complaints. Not all patients will readily admit to being either sexually assaulted or victims of human trafficking; therefore, the nurse has a responsibility to assess the patient and ask sensitive questions to determine whether the patient has been sexually assaulted. The entire emergency team must communicate with the patient in a nonjudgmental manner. The positive hospital experience can have an important impact on the patient's physical and psychological recovery from the assault. Every sexual assault victim requires a complete and in-depth physical examination and the opportunity to consent to a sexual assault forensic examination.

Many hospitals and counties have developed Sexual Assault Response Teams (SARTs). The SART consists of a victim advocate, a police officer, and most often a Sexual Assault Nurse/Forensic Examiner (SANE/SAFE). SART programs provide one-on-one comprehensive and compassionate medical care. The goal of the SART examination is to ensure that the patient's medical and psychological needs are attended to along with obtaining an appropriate forensic examination.

The SANE is a registered nurse who has received additional forensic nursing training. Law enforcement should be present at the hospital at the adult patient's request. This allows for sharing of vital information and aids in the maintenance of the legal chain of evidence. Officers should not be in the room during the patient examinations. The victim advocate supports the patient's emotional needs. These specialized teams have demonstrated improved care delivery to victims of sexual assault.

It is imperative that the patient be made aware of the medical team's mandatory reporter status (as required by law) even though the patient may choose not to speak with law enforcement officers. Requirements for the forensic examination of minors must also be determined.

1. Assessment
   a. Subjective data collection
      1) History of present assault/injury/chief complaint
         a) Date and time of assault
         b) Location of assault
         c) Use of penetrating foreign objects or other weapons in assault
         d) Consensual intercourse within last 5 days (vaginal, oral, rectal)
         e) Postassault hygiene
            (1) Bathed, showered, douched
         f) Loss of memory/consciousness
         g) Voluntary substance or alcohol use
         h) Involuntary drug use
            (1) "Date rape" drugs such as flunitrazepam (Rohypnol), ketamine, and gamma-hydroxybutyric acid (GHB): follow local protocols for drug testing
            (2) Other common date rape drug use such as alcohol, benzodiazepines, and diphenhydramine
         i) Injuries that the patient may have inflicted on the perpetrator
         j) Contraceptive/lubricant use by the perpetrator
      2) Past medical history
         a) Current or preexisting diseases/illness
         b) Recent gynecologic/obstetric/urologic illness/injury
            (1) Last normal menstrual period
         c) Medications (including contraceptives)
         d) Allergies to medications
         e) Allergies to other
         f) Immunization status
   b. Objective data collection
      1) Physical examination
         a) General appearance
            (1) Level of consciousness, behavior, affect: alert to comatose, crying, fearful, calm
            (2) Moderate to severe distress/discomfort
         b) Inspection
            (1) Abrasions
            (2) Lacerations
            (3) Ecchymotic areas: suction injury (commonly known as a "hickey")
            (4) Bite marks
            (5) Finger (nail) marks
            (6) Genital/perineal lacerations, abrasions, ecchymosis
            (7) Buttocks area: lacerations, abrasions, ecchymosis
         c) Auscultation
            (1) Lung sounds
            (2) Heart sounds
            (3) Bowel sounds
         d) Palpation
            (1) Areas of tenderness
         e) Percussion
            (1) Tympany
            (2) Dullness
      2) Diagnostic procedures
         a) CBC with differential
         b) Urinalysis; pregnancy test in female patients of childbearing age
         c) RPR test
         d) Serum and urine toxicology screen
         e) Other studies as indicated by local policy
            (1) Blood sample for forensic laboratory evaluation (DNA, ABO groups)
            (2) Baseline gonorrhea and chlamydia testing
            (3) Prophylactic treatment of sexually transmitted diseases may be substituted as appropriate
            (4) Baseline human immunodeficiency virus (HIV) and/or hepatitis testing
         f) Alternate light source: scan the body with ultraviolet light
            (1) Fluorescent areas may be seminal fluid
            (2) Swab fluorescent areas
         g) Evidence collection (see Chapter 43)
            (1) Patient's clothing: place in paper bags, not plastic
            (2) Swabs/slides, during an oral, vaginal (pelvic), penile, and/or rectal examination
            (3) Photography (35 mm and/or colposcopy)
2. Analysis: differential nursing diagnoses/collaborative problems
   a. Rape trauma syndrome
   b. PTSD
   c. Impaired skin integrity
   d. Ineffective coping
   e. Anxiety
3. Planning and implementation/interventions
   a. Maintain airway, breathing, and circulation (see Chapters 1 and 32)
   b. Provide supplemental oxygen as indicated
   c. Establish IV access for administration of crystalloid fluids/blood products/medications as needed
   d. Prepare for/assist with medical interventions
      1) Provide privacy for patients promptly on arrival and during all aspects of care
      2) Assist with treatment of injuries associated with assault
      3) Assist with forensic examination (see Chapter 40)
         a) All evidence is collected and labeled according to local or state policies with
            (1) Patient's name

(2) Medical record number

(3) Date, time

(4) Sample source

(5) Registered nurse's initials

b) Local or state policy may dictate that all swabs and slides be air dried prior to packaging. Swab boxes, slides carriers, and envelopes should be used to house the evidence. All evidence is kept in the custody of the nurse until it is passed to the law enforcement officer

(1) Label outside of evidence kit if moist swabs are present inside the kit

c) Have patient remove clothing while standing on a paper sheet if possible. Place each piece of clothing in a separate paper bag, labeled, and sealed

d) Obtain photographs per local policy (35 mm and/or colposcopy)

e) Fingernail scrapings evidence

(1) Use a cotton-tipped applicator, clean toothpick, or manicure stick to collect material under each fingernail. Place used applicator and material from each hand into a different envelope

f) Oral evidence

(1) Examine for injury or the presence of trace evidence

(2) Per local policy, collect swabs for seminal fluid if the patient was made to orally copulate the perpetrator. Prepare dry mount slides using the swabs and label to indicate which swab was used to make which slide

(3) Buccal swabs may also be taken for a reference sample. Place swabs in patient's buccal mucosa until saturated

g) Pubic hair evidence

(1) Place a paper sheet under the buttock. Using a comb or soft brush, comb downward to remove foreign hairs/material. Evidence tape may be used if area has been previously shaved. Fold the paper sheet, comb or brush, and collected hairs and place in an envelope

(2) Reference sample: pluck/pull or cut close to the skin (approximately 20 to 30 hairs) from a minimum of two different areas in the pubic region

h) Pelvic examination evidence

(1) Collect any foreign material or matted hairs

(2) Vaginal swabs per local policy. Swabs may be used to make dry mount slides. If more than 48 hours has elapsed from the time of the assault, consider also collecting cervical swabs

(3) Prepare wet mount slide for examination under microscope for presence of motile or nonmotile sperm

i) Anal/rectal examination evidence

(1) Collect any foreign material or matted hairs

(2) Cleanse perianal area after vaginal or penile specimens have been taken and foreign material has been collected

(3) Anal swabs: prepare slides as indicated by local policy

j) External genitalia (male)

(1) Collect penile swabs: evidence collected by holding the swabs together and swabbing the glans, shaft, and base of the penis with a rotating motion to ensure a uniform sample

e. Offer patient a shower after the examination

f. Administer pharmacologic therapy as ordered

1) Antibiotics: sexually transmitted disease prophylaxis per Centers for Disease Control and Prevention guidelines including HIV medications if high-risk exposure

2) Pregnancy-prevention medication within 72 hours of the assault. Plan B package instructions:

a) Take one white pill after unprotected sexual contact and an additional white pill 12 hours later

b) Each dose contains 0.75 mg of levonorgestrel

c) Must have a documented negative pregnancy test at the time of the examination before pregnancy-prevention medication can be administered

d) Ensure antiemetic is prescribed along with Plan B

g. Ensure chain of custody

1) Deliver packaged clothing directly to law enforcement officer

2) Place all collected evidence together in a carrier/box and deliver evidence box directly to law enforcement officer. The box itself and/or accompanying documentation must indicate the date/time the evidence was obtained by the nurse and the date/time the evidence box was given to the law enforcement officer. The officer will sign/date and time the evidence box

h. Educate patient and significant others

1) Support patient recovery

2) Dispel myths and misconceptions

a) No one has the right to violate another person

b) The patient did not cause the attack

(1) The victim did not ask for the assault by something he or she did or did not do

3) Follow up with primary health care provider in 1 to 2 weeks

Part 1

    4) Offer information regarding testing for HIV and hepatitis

    5) Telephone follow-up with victim advocate

4. Evaluation and ongoing monitoring

    a. Hemodynamic status

    b. Emotional status

    c. Pain relief

Bibliography

Anetzbeerger G, Dayton C: *Elder abuse risk factors podcast*, Washington, DC, 2015, Department of Health and Human Services. National Center on Elder Abuse. Retrieved from http://www.ncea.aoa.gov/Resources/Webinar/docs/Elder_Abuse_Risk_Factors.Podcast_Key_Points.2013.pdf.

Blodget B: *Sexual assault—A guide for primary care providers*, The Clinical Advisor, 2015, September.

Burnett LB: *Medscape: domestic violence clinical presentations.* Retrieved from http://emedicine.medscape.com/article/805546-clinical, 2015.

Burnett LB: *Emedicine: domestic violence.* Retrieved from http://www.emedicine.com/emerg/topic153.htm, 2006.

Centers for Disease Control and Prevention: *Child maltreatment: definitions.* Retrieved from http://www.cdc.gov/violenceprevention/childmaltreatment/definitions.html, 2015.

Centers for Disease Control and Prevention: *Elder abuse prevention.* Retrieved from http://www.cdc.gov/features/elderabuse/, 2015.

Centers for Disease Control and Prevention: *Injury prevention and control: division of violence prevention, elder abuse: definitions.* Retrieved from http://www.cdc.gov/violenceprevention/elderabuse/definitions.html, 2015.

Centers for Disease Control and Prevention: *Injury prevention and control: division of violence prevention, intimate partner violence.* Retrieved from http://www.cdc.gov/violenceprevention/intimatepartnerviolence/, 2015.

Centers for Disease Control and Prevention: *Sexually transmitted disease guidelines.* Retrieved from http://www.cdc.gov/mmwr/preview/mmwrhtml/rr6403a1.htm, 2015.

Choi NG, Mayer J: Elder abuse, neglect, and exploitation: risk factors and prevention strategies, *J Gerontol Soc Work* 33:5–25, 2000.

Department of Health and Human Services. National Center on Elder Abuse: *Types of abuse.* Retrieved from http://ncea.aoa.gov/FAQ/Typese/, 2015.

Emergency Nurses Association: *Emergency nursing pediatric course*, Des Plaines, IL, 2013, Emergency Nurses Association p. 346.

Ernewein C, Nieves R: Human sex trafficking; recognition, treatment, and referral of pediatric victims, *J Nurse Pract* 11:8, 2015.

International Association of Forensic Nurses: *Sexual assault nurse examiner educational guidelines*, Elkridge, MD 2015.

National Sexual Violence Resource Center (NSVRC): *Sexual violence in later life. A technical assistance guide for health care providers*, Enola, PA, 2013, NSVRC Publications.

Stanford Medicine: *Child abuse. Fractures.* Retrieved from http://childabuse.stanford.edu/screening/fractures.html, 2015.

Stanford Medicine: *Child abuse. Screening children.* Retrieved from http://childabuse.stanford.edu/screening/children.html, 2015.

Stanford Medicine: *Elder abuse, how to screen.* Retrieved from http://elderabuse.stanford.edu/screening/how_screen.html, 2015.

Taylor RB: *Preventing violence against women and children.* Retrieved from http://www.milbank.org/reports/violence.html, 1998.

U.S. Department of Justice Office of Justice Programs: *Recognizing when a child's injury or illness is caused by abuse*, Washington, DC, 2014, Office of Justice Programs. Office of Juvenile Justice and Delinquency Prevention.

U.S. Department of Justice Office on Violence Against Women: *A national protocol for sexual assault medical forensic examinations*, ed 2, NCJ 228119. Rockville, MD, 2013, NCJRS.

CHAPTER 4

Complementary/Alternative Therapies

Vicki Sweet, MSN, RN, MICN, CEN, FAEN

I. Introduction

Although not necessarily new, the use of complementary and alternative medicine (CAM) therapies continues to increase throughout the United States. Some patients fully ascribe to "alternative" therapies and turn away from conventional Western medicine, and other patients use alternative or dietary remedies to complement the medical regimens prescribed by their health care practitioners. This approach is sometimes referred to as "integrative" or "holistic" medicine. The term holistic, familiar to nursing, is often incorrectly used by patients in describing the complementary therapies they may be using. "Homeopathic" is also another term often used to describe CAM; however, as will be shown, homeopathy is a unique practice.

Unfortunately, information on complementary, integrative, or alternative therapy use is not always shared with health care providers. In some cases, certain remedies may potentiate the effects of prescription medications; in others, the effects may be contradictory. It is essential, then, for the emergency nurse to be knowledgeable about therapies and to address the use of CAM in all emergency patients. Some therapies are quite safe; others, if used improperly, may have dangerous interactions with prescribed treatments, and patients may present to the emergency department because of these reactions.

II. Types of Complementary/ Alternative Therapies

A. ACUPUNCTURE

1. An ancient therapy of using thin needles to correct imbalances in the flow of the body's energy, or "chi"

2. The World Health Organization considers acupuncture to be appropriate treatment for such disorders as anxiety, back pain, migraines, infertility, blood pressure regulation, smoking cessation, among others
3. Considered relatively safe when performed by a trained practitioner. Licensure for use of acupuncture is required in some states in order to provide for adherence to infection control and safety guidelines
4. Complications
   a. Minor
      1) Bruising
      2) Local bleeding
   b. Serious
      1) Nerve damage
      2) Pneumothorax (very low risk)

B. AROMATHERAPY

1. Use of essential oils for healing
2. Therapy based on belief that sense of smell is connected with memory and emotion and that this connection affects health
3. Proponents believe it reduces stress and alleviates minor conditions
4. Complications
   a. Accidental ingestion or inhalation of potentially toxic essential oils
   b. Topical reaction including contact dermatitis, rash, pruritus

C. HERBOLOGY/NUTRITIONAL SUPPLEMENTS

1. Often recognized as safe
2. Complications

a. Frequently taken without appropriate guidance from health care providers
b. Labeling vague and nonspecific
c. No U.S. government regulation of quality or standardization of preparations
d. Unexpected outcomes such as stroke and liver failure have occurred
e. Multiple herb–drug interactions (Table 4.1)

D. HOMEOPATHY

1. Belief that "like cures like"; a system of medical practice that treats a disease through the administration of minute doses of a remedy that would, in healthy persons, produce symptoms similar to those of the disease
2. Prepared through series of dilutions and successions (vigorous shaking). The more dilute the preparation, the stronger it is considered to be
3. Considered safe and nontoxic

E. HYPNOTHERAPY/GUIDED IMAGERY

1. Belief that the mind influences body health and well-being
2. Assists person into state of relaxation
3. Useful in pain management, anxiety, and stress-related disorders

F. NATUROPATHY

1. Based on concept that the body can heal itself: a system of treatment of disease that avoids drugs and surgery and emphasizes the use of natural agents (e.g., air, water, sunshine) and physical means (e.g., manipulation, electrical treatment)
2. Emphasis on prevention and healthy living

III. General Strategy

A. ASSESSMENT

1. Subjective data collection
   a. History of present illness/chief complaint
      1) Relationship to use of alternative therapy
         a) Use of over-the-counter herbs, dietary supplements, vitamins
            (1) Reason for use
            (2) Dosage
            (3) Name of substance
         b) Recent reactions from alternative therapies use
      2) Receiving care from herbalist, acupuncturist, naturopathic practitioner, nutritionist, or natural healer
   b. Past medical history
      1) Current or preexisting diseases/illness
         a) Cardiovascular
         b) Diabetes

         c) Acute viral illness
         d) Chronic respiratory disease
         e) Chronic renal disease
         f) Chronic fatigue syndrome
         g) Fibromyalgia
         h) Chronic pain
         i) Osteoarthritis
         j) Immunosuppression disorders
      2) Substance and/or alcohol use/abuse
      3) Smoking history
      4) Last normal menstrual period: female patients of childbearing age
      5) Current medications
         a) Prescription
         b) Over-the-counter/herbal/dietary supplements
      6) Allergies
2. Objective data collection
   a. General appearance
      1) Level of consciousness, behavior, affect
      2) Vital signs
      3) Odors
      4) Gait
      5) Hygiene
      6) Level of distress/discomfort
   b. Inspection
      1) Cutaneous reactions
      2) Localized bleeding
      3) Cardiac dysrhythmias on monitor
   c. Auscultation
      1) Breath sounds
      2) Heart sounds
      3) Bowel sounds
   d. Palpation
      1) Areas of tenderness
3. Diagnostic procedures: frequently none
   a. Complete blood count (CBC) with differential
   b. Coagulation profile if active bleeding
   c. Serum chemistries including glucose, blood urea nitrogen (BUN), and creatinine
   d. Liver function panel
   e. Serum and urine toxicology screen
   f. Urinalysis; pregnancy test in female patients of childbearing age
   g. 12-lead ECG, in cases of cardiac complaints (e.g., palpitations, syncope)

B. PLANNING AND IMPLEMENTATION/ INTERVENTIONS

1. Determine priorities of care
   a. Provide supplemental oxygen as indicated
   b. Establish IV access for administration of crystalloid fluid/medications as needed
   c. Obtain and set up equipment and supplies
   d. Prepare for/assist with medical interventions
   e. Administer pharmacologic therapy as ordered

Table 4.1

Common Herbs: Usage, Actions, Reactions, and Interactions*

Herb: Common Name	Scientific Name	Common Usage	Actions	Possible Side Effects	Drug Interactions
Aloe	*Aloe barbadensis; A. vera*	Topical: Wound healing Burns Oral: Laxative	Topical gel: Antiinflammatory Antimicrobial Antiparasitic Oral juice: Irritation of large intestine	Topical gel: Allergic or hypersensitivity reaction Oral juice: Bloody diarrhea Red urine Fluid/electrolyte imbalance	Topical gel: None Oral juice: May potentiate antidysrhythmics, cardiac glycosides, diuretics, and steroids
Bilberry	*Vaccinium myrtillus*	Arthritis Diabetes Vascular problems Visual disorders "Antiaging"	Antioxidant Decreased platelet activity Decreased vascular permeability May decrease blood glucose	Mild GI upset More than 1.5 g/kg/day could be fatal	Anticoagulants Antiplatelets
Capsicum	*Capsicum sp.*	Topical: Arthritis Pain Oral: GI problems Joint pain	Topical: Stimulates local nerve fibers to decrease pain	Blepharospasm Lacrimation Burning sensation	Topical: None Oral: Antiplatelet Decreased effect of antihypertensives and MAO inhibitors
Chamomile (German)	*Matricaria recutita*	Topical: Skin inflammation Wounds Burns Oral: Cough, URI GI disturbances Insomnia Anxiety	Antiinflammatory Antispasmodic Antibacterial Anxiolytic	Allergic reaction	Anticoagulants Benzodiazepines
Dong quai	*Angelica sinensis*	Gynecologic disorders Circulation Menopausal symptoms PMS	Antispasmodic Vasodilation May affect uterine activity	Bleeding Photosensitivity	Anticoagulants
Echinacea	*Echinacea angustifolia; E. pallida; E. purpurea*	Topical: Wounds Burns Oral: URI	Topical: Antibacterial Oral: Stimulates immune system Antiinflammatory	Allergic reaction	Immunosuppressants
Evening primrose	*Oenothera biennis*	Topical: Psoriasis Oral: Menopausal symptoms PMS Rheumatoid arthritis	Contains rich source of omega-6 fatty acid Decreases platelet aggregation	Topical: Rash Oral: GI upset Headache May decrease seizure threshold	Antiinflammatories Beta-blockers Antipsychotics Anticoagulants Phenothiazines
Fenugreek	*Trigonella foenum-graecum*	Constipation Diabetes mellitus Elevated cholesterol GI problems	May decrease cholesterol and blood glucose May decrease calcium oxalate deposits in kidney	GI upset Allergic reaction	Anticoagulants Diabetic agents

Continued

Table 4.1

Common Herbs: Usage, Actions, Reactions, and Interactions*—cont'd

Herb: Common Name	Scientific Name	Common Usage	Actions	Possible Side Effects	Drug Interactions
Feverfew	*Tanacetum parthenium*	Colds Fevers Body aches Migraine prophylaxis	Spasmolytic Antiinflammatory Possible inhibition of prostaglandin synthesis	Contact dermatitis Anxiety Insomnia Tachycardia	Anticoagulants Nonsteroidal antiinflammatory drugs
Garlic	*Allium sativum*	Topical: Infections Oral: Elevated cholesterol	Topical: Antimicrobial Oral: May inhibit hepatic cholesterol synthesis May decrease cellular lipid concentration	Topical: Contact dermatitis Oral: Breath odor Allergic reaction Nausea	Anticoagulants Antiplatelets Diabetic agents Protease inhibitors
Ginger	*Zingiber officinale*	Arthritis Dyspepsia Nausea/vomiting	Antiemetic (stimulates gastric secretions) Antiinflammatory Inhibits platelet aggregation Positive inotropic	Heartburn Possible dysrhythmia with overdosage	Anticoagulants Diabetic agents
Ginkgo biloba	*Ginkgo biloba*	Memory impairment Intermittent claudication	Arterial and venous vasoactive changes Increased microvascular blood flow Inhibition of platelet activating factor	GI upset Allergic reaction Headache	Anticoagulants Anticonvulsants Antiplatelets May alter insulin requirements
Ginseng (American)	*Panax quinquefolius*	Energy Adaptogen* Stamina	Has both CNS depressant and stimulant effects	Headache Hypertension Insomnia	Anticoagulants Diabetic agents MAO inhibitors
Ginseng (Asian)	*Panax ginseng*	Decreased susceptibility to illness Promotion of health Stamina	Antiinflammatory Decreases serum glucose Stimulant Smooth muscle relaxation	Headache Hypoglycemia Insomnia Mastalgia Diarrhea	Anticoagulants Diabetic agents MAO inhibitors
Ginseng (Siberian)	*Eleutherococcus senticosus*	Adaptogen* Diabetes	Immune system stimulation May decrease serum glucose levels	Diarrhea Euphoria Insomnia	Anticoagulants Antihypertensives Digoxin (may increase serum levels) Diabetic agents
Kava kava	*Piper methysticum*	Anxiety Insomnia Muscle spasms	Analgesic CNS effects Muscle relaxant Psychotropic	GI upset Mydriasis Hepatitis Liver injury Altered reflexes	Potentiates benzodiazepines and barbiturates May decrease effect of levodopa
Licorice	*Glycyrrhiza glabra*	Antiinflammatory Cough GI disturbances	Aldosterone-like effects Antiinflammatory Expectorant May mimic endogenous steroids	Hypertension Hypernatremia Hypokalemia	Antihypertensives Anticoagulants Digoxin Diabetic agents Procainamide
Ma huang	*Ephedra sinica*	Asthma Bronchospasm Nasal congestion	Ephedrine-like effects	Anxiety Insomnia Stroke Tachycardia Urinary retention	Beta-blockers MAO inhibitors Phenothiazines Sympathomimetics
St. John's wort	*Hypericum perforatum*	Wound healing Depression, mild Diuretic Melancholy	Possible inhibition of serotonin reuptake	GI upset Allergic reaction	Selective serotonin reuptake inhibitors (SSRIs) Cyclosporine Over-the-counter cold and flu preparations

Table 4.1

Common Herbs: Usage, Actions, Reactions, and Interactions*—cont'd

Herb: Common Name	Scientific Name	Common Usage	Actions	Possible Side Effects	Drug Interactions
Valerian	*Valeriana officinalis*	Anxiety Insomnia	Anxiolytic CNS depression	Blurred vision Hangover effect Headache	Potentiates sedatives and hypnotics
Yohimbe	*Pausinystalia yohimbe*	Aphrodisiac Erectile dysfunction	$Alpha_2$-adrenergic blocker	Anxiety Hypertension Insomnia Tachycardia	Potentiates CNS stimulants Potentiates $alpha_2$-blockers Decreases effects of antihypertensives

*Not intended to be all-inclusive. Consult an evidence-based herbal resource for complete information.

Data from Ernst, E. (2001). The desktop guide to complementary and alternative medicine: An evidence-based approach. London: Harcourt; Fetrow, C. W., & Avila, J. R. (1999). Professional's handbook of complementary and alternative medicines. Springhouse, PA: Springhouse; LaGow, B. (Ed.). (2004). PDR for herbal medicines (3rd ed.). Montvale, NJ: Thomson PDR; and Rotblatt, M., & Ziment, I. (2002). Evidence-based herbal medicine. Philadelphia, PA: Hanley & Belfus.

*Adaptogen is term used by herbalists to refer to an herb that helps the body adapt to physiologic stressors.

CNS, central nervous system; GI, gastrointestinal; MAO, monoamine oxidase; PMS, premenstrual syndrome; URI, upper respiratory infection.

2. Relieve anxiety/apprehension
3. Allow significant others to remain with patient if they are supportive
4. Educate patient and significant others
   a. Uses of alternatives therapies to control symptoms
   b. Interactions of herbs, supplements, vitamins, other medications

C. EVALUATION AND ONGOING MONITORING

1. Continuously monitor and treat as indicated
   a. Hemodynamic status
   b. Cardiac rate and rhythm
   c. Resolution of presenting symptoms
2. Monitor patient response/outcomes, and modify nursing care plan as appropriate
3. If positive patient outcomes are not demonstrated, reevaluate assessment and/or plan of care

D. DOCUMENTATION OF INTERVENTIONS AND PATIENT RESPONSE

Bibliography

Antoniades J, Jones K, Hassed C, Piterman L: Sleep…naturally, *Altern Complement Ther* 18(3):136–139, 2012.

Eisenberg DM: The Institute of Medicine report on complementary and alternative medicine in the United States: personal reflections on its content and implications, *Altern Ther Health Med* 11(3):10–15, 2005.

Ekor M: The growing use of herbal medicines: issues relating to adverse reactions and challenges in monitoring safety, *Front Pharmacol* 4(177):1–10, 2013.

Ernst E: *The desktop guide to complementary and alternative medicine: An evidence-based approach*, London, 2001, Harcourt.

Gurley BJ: Pharmacokinetic herb-drug interactions (part 1): origins, mechanisms, and the impact of botanical dietary supplements, *Planta Medica* 78(13):1478–1489, 2012. Retrieved from http//www.ncbi.nlm.nih.gov/pubmed/22322396.

Gurley BJ, Fifer EK, Gardner Z: Pharmacokinetic herb-drug interactions (part 2): drug interactions involving popular botanical dietary supplements and their clinical relevance, *Planta Medica* 78(13):1490–1514, 2012. Retrieved from http://www.ncbi.nlm.nih.gov/pubmed/22565299.

Hebert PR, Barice J, Hennekens CH: Treatment of low back pain: The potential clinical and public health benefits of topical herbal remedies, *J Altern Complement Med* 20(4):219–220, 2014.

Karch AM: *Focus on nursing pharmacology*, ed 6, Philadelphia, PA, 2013, Wolters Kluwer/Lippincott Williams & Wilkins.

LaGow B, editor: *PDR for herbal medicines*, ed 3, Montvale, NJ, 2004, Thomson PDR.

Lao L, Hamilton GR, Fu J, Berman BM: Is acupuncture safe? A systematic review of case reports, *Altern Ther Health Med* 9(1):72–82, 2003.

National Institutes of Health: National Center for Complementary and Integrative Health website, https://nccih.nih.gov/health/providers/digest/herb-drug.

National Institutes of Health: Office of Dietary Supplements website, http://www.ods.od.nih.gov.

PDR Network, LLC: *PDR® for non-prescription drugs, dietary supplements, and herbs*, Montvale, NJ, 2011, PDR.

Rogers EA, Gough JE, Brewer KL: Are emergency department patients at risk for herb-drug interactions? *Acad Emerg Med* 8(9):932–934, 2001.

Woodrow R, Colbert BJ, Smith DM: *Essentials of pharmacology for health occupations*, ed 6, Clifton Park, NY, 2011, Delmar/Cengage Learning.

CHAPTER 5
Palliative and End-of-Life Care

Garrett K. Chan, PHD, APRN, FAEN, FPCN, FNAP, FAAN

I. Overview

According to the Centers for Disease Control and Prevention, approximately 183,000 persons died in emergency departments in the United States in 2011 and approximately 286,000 persons who were admitted to the hospital from the emergency department died during that hospital stay.[1] Because the emergency department is a fast-paced and frequently high-stress, high-anxiety department, end-of-life issues are often given a lower priority. Clinical personnel may make decisions regarding patient care with suboptimal levels of information.[2–4] Relationships among personnel, patients, and families are limited during a time of crisis.[5, 6] Additionally, the emergency department is usually a place of transition where patients receive stabilizing treatment and then are either transferred out or discharged. Patients usually do not remain in the emergency department for the duration of their hospital stay.[7]

The United States is a rescue-oriented culture.[7] Cardiopulmonary resuscitation and other advanced life support measures are routinely employed in end-of-life scenarios. However, some patients do not require or want basic or advanced life support measures performed, and they may request only care-and-comfort measures at the end of their life.[7] It is important to recognize that some patients have

a poor prognosis, and although staff members have many interventions available (e.g., intubation equipment, chest compressions), these interventions are not appropriate for all patients at or near the end of life. Careful exploration with patients and families regarding their life goals and expectations for care can help determine what interventions are appropriate.[8] For example, patients in severe respiratory distress may be brought to the emergency department by ambulance not necessarily for mechanical ventilation but because it became frightening for the family to have the patient die at home.

The interval referred to as the "end of life" is not well defined and is used inconsistently,[9] but the term frequently applies to any interval when a patient is approaching the finality of cardiopulmonary or brain death. Emergency department staff members have a pivotal role in providing care that may be most beneficial to the patient and family. Planning that care requires engagement with the patient and family in order to explore goals and to determine which interventions are and are not appropriate. It is also important to determine, from the patient if possible, who should receive information and who should be allowed in the treatment area at this end stage.[10]

Emergency nurses encounter death frequently in their clinical practice, and caring for dying patients may become routine,[11] sometimes leading nurses to become desensitized to the suffering around them.[6] Conversely, patients and families are often unfamiliar with death and dying. They come to the emergency department with unexpected injuries or illnesses, with chronic disease exacerbations, or with terminal illnesses seeking symptom management and lifesaving or life-prolonging treatment.[7] Patients and families are often in crisis and seek help and answers from emergency personnel.[6]

There are seven trajectories of approaching death in the emergency department: (1) dead on arrival; (2) resuscitation in the field, resuscitative efforts in the emergency department, died in the emergency department; (3) resuscitation in the field, resuscitative efforts in the emergency department, resuscitated, and admitted to the hospital; (4) terminally ill, coming to the emergency department; (5) frail, hovering near death; (6) arriving at the emergency department alive and then suffering cardiac arrest or sudden death in the emergency department; and (7) potentially preventable death by acts of omission or commission.[12] Although emergency health care providers are masters at resuscitation, there are dying trajectories that require care interventions other than resuscitative measures. Some dying trajectories benefit from aggressive symptom management and humanistic care, whereas others call for more aggressive interventions.

Recognition of poor prognoses and framing beneficial interventions with the patient and family will help determine the plan of care. Although resuscitative measures are the standard of care in the emergency department, they may not be appropriate for all patients near the end of life. Fear of liability may be a concern of emergency personnel.[7, 8] However, expanding the definition of "success" from the traditional concept of resuscitation to include aggressive palliative care management can ease emergency personnel's feelings of abandoning the patient.[8]

II. Palliative Care Symptom Management

Palliative care is patient and family centered and multidisciplinary; it includes symptom management, emotional/psychological care, social care, spiritual/existential care, advanced care planning, and bereavement care for survivors.[13–15] Palliative care can be given concurrently in every situation in the emergency department, in situations where there may be a simple extremity fracture or if the patient is near the end of life. In end-stage disease, treatment to relieve symptoms may be more appropriate than treatment of the underlying cause, such as infection or tumor progression. The patient must be assessed and reassessed for the presence, improvement, or reduction of symptoms before and after any intervention. Many interventions may be seen as palliative as well as therapeutic.

In patients who are near the end of life, careful consideration should be made when ordering diagnostic tests. Each test ordered should help determine an intervention. However, if the results will not change the management of the patient's condition, the test should be questioned for its appropriateness.[16]

A. ADVANCED PREPARATION BEFORE DECIDING ON A PLAN OF CARE[17]

1. Identify the diagnosis and prognosis
   a. Use a model of trajectories of approaching death such as the following trajectories[12] to understand what the potential outcome of the patient may be:
      1) Dead on arrival
      2) Resuscitation in the field, resuscitative efforts in the emergency department, could die in the emergency department
      3) Resuscitation in the field, resuscitative efforts in the emergency department, resuscitated, and admitted to the hospital
      4) Terminally ill, but still coming to the emergency department
      5) Frail, hovering near death
      6) Arrives at the emergency department alive and then suffering cardiac arrest or sudden death in the emergency department
      7) Potentially preventable death by acts of omission or commission
2. Determine what the patient or surrogate already knows
3. Ask whether the patient has an advance directive and/or a Physician's Order for Life Sustaining Treatment, which clearly states the patient's wishes. If it is not readily available, ask the surrogate decision maker what the advance directive states, and request a written copy as soon as possible. Document in the medical record what the surrogate decision maker states is in the advance directive
4. Seek assistance from other members of the health care team (e.g., social worker, chaplain, patient care advocate) or ask the patient or family whether they want help in contacting someone to be with them in the emergency department
5. Establish a therapeutic milieu[17]
   a. Identify a private and quiet place in the emergency department where all family members and significant others can be seen and heard
   b. Minimize interruptions
6. Seek patient and surrogate knowledge about diagnosis and prognosis[17]
   a. Correct inaccuracies and misconceptions
   b. Provide additional information
   c. Communicate effectively[17]
      1) Avoid jargon, slang, acronyms
      2) Assess whether statements have shared definitions—for example, the question "Do you want us to do 'everything' for your loved one?" may have a different meaning to each person

3) Demonstrate empathy
4) Be honest and direct
5) Patients and families may not be able to understand fully what is trying to be communicated to them. It is possible and permissible to help ground the family by telling them what could be done in this situation. One approach can be, "I understand that this is a very difficult time and we are providing you with a lot of choices. May I tell you what I might consider if this was my loved one?" If the answer is yes, then proceed. If the answer is no, then tell them that you will be available to provide more information and help initiate the plan of care based on their decisions

7. Make a palliative care treatment recommendation[17]
   a. Provide rationale for recommendations
   b. Answer all questions
   c. Explore the possibility of a "do not resuscitate (DNR)," "do not attempt resuscitation (DNAR)," or "allow natural death (AND)" order that will avoid heroic interventions such as chest compressions, defibrillation, intubation/mechanical ventilation, and/or vasopressors as these interventions have a low probability of success

8. Seek patient or surrogate agreement with recommendations[17]

B. COMMON SYMPTOMS (TABLE 5.1)

1. Pain (see Chapter 8)
   a. Pain and discomfort are common in patients near the end of life
   b. Inadequate pain relief
      1) Hastens death
      2) Increases physiologic stress
      3) Potentially diminishes immunocompetency
      4) Decreases mobility
      5) Worsens risk of developing pneumonia and thromboembolism
      6) Increases work of breathing and myocardial oxygen requirements
      7) Impairs the individual's quality of life
      8) Relief of pain at end of life may allow the patient to "let go"
   c. Pain versus suffering at end of life
      1) Existential distress, fear of the dying process, and grief may alter expressions of pain
      2) Pain in the terminally ill is complex and includes dimensions of psychological, social, and spiritual distress along with physical pain
      3) Management of pain at end of life must be based on an interdisciplinary approach
   d. Nonpharmacologic interventions
      1) Warm packs
      2) Cold packs
      3) Distraction/music therapy
      4) Massage
      5) Radiation therapy
      6) Position of comfort
   e. Pharmacologic interventions
      1) Narcotics
      2) Nonnarcotic analgesics
      3) Acetaminophen
      4) Nonsteroidal antiinflammatory drugs (NSAIDs)
      5) Adjuvant agents
         a) Tricyclic antidepressants
         b) Anticonvulsants
         c) Local anesthetics
         d) Corticosteroids
         e) Baclofen (Lioresal)
         f) Bisphosphonate medications (e.g., alendronate [Fosamax])

2. Dyspnea[16]
   a. Defined as distressing shortness of breath and is frequently called breathlessness. The experience of dyspnea can be very frightening
   b. Diseases most commonly associated with this symptom include lung disease, heart disease, stroke, dementia, end-stage renal disease, and metastatic cancer
   c. Planning and implementation/interventions
      1) Determine priorities of care
      2) Provide position of comfort
      3) Provide supplemental oxygen as indicated
         a) Oxygen use in nonhypoxemic patients may have limited benefit. A trial of oxygen should always be considered
      4) Establish IV access for administration of crystalloid fluids/blood products/medications as needed
         a) Blood transfusions to increase oxygenation in the anemic patient
      5) Prepare for/assist with medical interventions
         a) Institute cardiac and pulse oximetry monitoring as indicated
         b) Thoracentesis to promote better lung inflation by removing fluid from the pleural space
         c) Stent placement to open an occluded airway
         d) Paracentesis, when dyspnea is secondary to ascites, may improve ability to breathe
         e) Nonpharmacologic treatment techniques
            (1) Counseling may include the use of cognitive-behavioral, interpersonal, and complementary strategies
            (2) Pursed-lip breathing slows respiratory rate and decreases small airway collapse
            (3) Energy conservation techniques can save energy, reduce fatigue, and allow the patient to maintain control of lifestyle changes
            (4) Fans, open windows, and air conditioners that circulate air, especially across a

Table 5.1

Common Symptoms at the End of Life

Body System	Symptoms
Pulmonary	Dyspnea
	Cough
	Head/nasal congestion
	"Death rattle"
	Respiratory distress/respiratory depression
Neurologic/functional	Pain
	Spinal cord compression
	Weakness
	Fatigue
	Immobility
	Insomnia
	Confusion/dementia/delirium
	Memory changes
Gastrointestinal	Nausea/vomiting
	Dysphagia
	Anorexia
	Weight loss
	Unpleasant taste
	Ascites
	Constipation/obstipation/bowel obstruction
	Diarrhea
	Incontinence of bowel
	Hiccups
Urinary	Incontinence of bladder
	Bladder spasms
	Changes in function or control
Integumentary	Decubitus
	Mucositis
	Candidiasis
	Pruritus
	Edema
	Hemorrhage
	Infection (e.g., herpes zoster)
	Diaphoresis
Psychiatric	Depression
	Anxiety
Other	Fever

Modified from Ferrell, B. R. (1998). HOPE: Home Care Outreach for Palliative Care Education Project. Duarte, CA: City of Hope.

person's cheek (not directly into the nasal/oral mucosa), can reduce dyspnea

    (5) Elevation of the head of the bed and the ability of the patient to sit in a forward and upright position reduce choking sensations and promote expansion of the lungs. Placing the patient's arms on pillows may promote air exchange

    (6) Spiritual support can promote comfort and relaxation

    (7) Education of patient and family reduces anxiety

    (8) Music can promote relaxation and distraction

    (9) Calm room environment by reducing stimuli and encouraging a smoke- and allergen-free atmosphere

  6) Administer pharmacologic therapy as ordered (Table 5.2)

3. Cough[16]

  a. Of palliative care patients, 39% to 80% will experience cough-related problems

  b. Cough, like dyspnea, can be frustrating and debilitating for the patient and can cause pain, fatigue, vomiting, and insomnia. An ongoing cough is also a constant reminder of the evolving disease process. Cough is frequently present in advanced diseases such as bronchitis, heart failure, acquired immunodeficiency syndrome (AIDS), and various cancers; however, patients with lung cancer most commonly experience this symptom

  c. Planning and implementation/interventions

    1) Determine priorities of care

    2) Provide supplemental oxygen as indicated

      a) Oxygen use in nonhypoxemic patients may have limited benefit. A trial of oxygen should always be considered

    3) Prepare for/assist with medical interventions

      a) Institute cardiac and pulse oximetry monitoring as indicated

      b) Nonpharmacologic treatment techniques

        (1) Chest physiotherapy has ability to help a frail patient mobilize secretions

        (2) Humidifier, typically cool, can help comfort a rapid breathing state and thin secretions

        (3) Elevate the head of the bed/position the patient to allow the patient to clear or manage secretions more effectively

        (4) Caffeinated beverages have been reported to have an effect in dilating pulmonary vessels

        (5) Radiation may be utilized, especially with hemoptysis

    4) Administer pharmacologic therapy as ordered (Table 5.3)

4. Nausea/vomiting[16]

  a. The incidence of nausea is quite common in advanced disease; it occurs in up to 60% of terminally ill patients;[18] vomiting occurs in approximately 30% of patients, but unfortunately, this symptom has not been well researched in patients with advanced disease

  b. The pathophysiology of nausea and vomiting is extremely complex, requiring careful assessment of the cause, which should lead to an appropriate treatment

Table 5.2

Pharmacologic Treatment for Dyspnea

Class of Drug	Examples	Mechanism of Action	Dosages/Routes/Comments
Opioids	Morphine	Exact mechanism for dyspnea not completely understood	IV: 1–4 mg every 15 min to 4 hr PRN Subcutaneous: 1–4 mg every 30 min to 4 hr PRN PO: 5–15 mg, pill or liquid form every 1–4 hr PRN Rectal: 5–15 mg every 1–4 hr PRN suppository; may need to be compounded
	Fentanyl (Sublimaze)		IV: 25–40 mcg every 15 min PRN SL: 25–40 mcg every 15 min PRN
Bronchodilators (used frequently in airway obstruction, COPD, and asthma conditions)	Albuterol (Proventil, Ventolin)	Relax smooth muscles of respiratory tract thus relieving bronchospasm	Dosages highly variable and dependent on patient's overall health status, smoking history, age, and presence of comorbid factors May cause anxiety and cough while worsening dyspnea
		Stimulate beta$_2$-agonist, adrenergic receptors of sympathetic nervous sympathetic nervous system Relax smooth muscles of bronchial tree	Drugs available in metered-dose inhalers, nebulizers, or orally
Diuretics (used in heart failure, reduce fluid overload)	Furosemide (Lasix)	Inhibits reabsorption of electrolytes in ascending limb of the loop of Henle, thus enhancing excretion of sodium chloride, potassium, calcium, and other electrolytes	PO: 20–80 mg IV: 20–40 mg Dosage varies widely and should be adjusted to patient's requirement and response
Benzodiazepines	Lorazepam (Ativan) Conflicting reports about the efficacy in the treatment of dyspnea Therefore, should not be considered a first-line treatment	Appear to act on thalamic/hypothalamic areas of the CNS to produce anxiolytic, sedative, hypnotic effects and skeletal muscle relaxation	IV: 0.5–2 mg every 8–12 hr PO: 0.5–2 mg every 8–12 hr IM: 0.5–2 mg every 6–12 hr All routes every 8–12 hr for anxiety Dosages may vary significantly and should be adjusted to patient's requirements and responses
Nonbenzodiazepine anxiolytic	Buspirone (BuSpar)	No effect on pulmonary function tests or arterial blood gases, but improves exercise tolerance and decreases sensation of breathlessness in patients with COPD	
Steroids (used in asthma and COPD)	Dexamethasone (Decadron)	Mechanism not fully understood Affects antibody systems Appears to decrease inflammation (especially associated with vena cava syndrome) and suppresses immune response	Aerosol: 0.25–20 mg IV: 0.25–20 mg PO: 0.25–20 mg IM: 0.25–20 mg
Antibiotics	Beta-Lactam agents	Varies by agent	Varies according to antibiotic given
Antifungals (used to treat pulmonary infections)	Fluconazole (Diflucan)	Varies by agent	Dose varies, typically 200 mg PO day 1 then 100 mg daily
Anticoagulants	Heparin Warfarin (Coumadin)	Prevents clot formation and thus may prevent future incidence of pulmonary emboli	Varies according to laboratory results

Permission to use materials from the End-of-Life Nursing Education Consortium (ELNEC) curriculum was granted by the American Association of Colleges of Nursing (AACN) and the City of Hope National Medical Center (COH). The ELNEC Project is a national end-of-life educational program administered by COH and the AACN designed to enhance palliative care in nursing. The ELNEC Project was originally funded by a grant from the Robert Wood Johnson Foundation with additional support from funding organizations (the National Cancer Institute, Aetna Foundation, and Archstone Foundation). Materials are copyrighted by the COH and AACN and are used with permission. Further information about the ELNEC Project can be found at http://www.aacn.nche.edu/ELNEC.
CNS, central nervous system; *COPD,* chronic obstructive pulmonary disease; *IM,* intramuscular; *IV,* intravenous; *PO,* oral; *PRN,* as needed; *SL,* sublingual.

Table 5.3

Pharmacologic Treatment for Cough

Class of Drug	Examples	Mechanism of Action	Comments
Bronchodilators	Terbutaline (Brethine)	Relax smooth muscles and decrease cough in airway disease	Dosages vary widely
Cough suppressants Opiates	Morphine sulfate, codeine	Central CNS action, suppresses cough	Dosages vary
Local anesthetics	Benzonatate (Tessalon Perles) Benzonatate (Tessalon)	Suppresses cough stimulus (anecdotal reports) Inhibits cough by anesthetizing stretch receptors that mediate cough reflex	5 mL of 2% lidocaine via nebulizer every 4 hr PRN 100 mg PO 3 times a day; may be administered every 4 hr up to 600 mg daily Should not be chewed or dissolved in mouth
Cough expectorants	Guaifenesin	Increases production of respiratory tract fluids; decreases secretion viscosity	
Antibiotics	Penicillin	Treat pneumonias or infections of the airway passages	Infrequently used in palliative care but may prove useful in an infectious process
Steroids	Dexamethasone (Decadron)	Decrease inflammation of airways or compression of an airway by tumor	
Anticholinergics	Atropine Hyoscine Hydrobromide (Scopolamine)	Decrease secretion production; decrease cough	
Nebulized saline or humidifier		Used to thin secretions	

Permission to use materials from the End-of-Life Nursing Education Consortium (ELNEC) curriculum was granted by the American Association of Colleges of Nursing (AACN) and the City of Hope National Medical Center (COH). The ELNEC Project is a national end-of-life educational program administered by COH and the AACN designed to enhance palliative care in nursing. The ELNEC Project was originally funded by a grant from the Robert Wood Johnson Foundation with additional support from funding organizations (the National Cancer Institute, Aetna Foundation, and Archstone Foundation). Materials are copyrighted by the COH and AACN and are used with permission. Further information about the ELNEC Project can be found at http://www.aacn.nche.edu/ELNEC.
CNS, central nervous system; *PO,* orally; *PRN,* as needed.

1) Nausea and vomiting can be acute, anticipatory, or delayed
c. Planning and implementation/interventions
  1) Determine priorities of care
  2) Provide supplemental oxygen as indicated
  3) Establish IV access for administration of crystalloid fluids/medications as needed
    a) Intravenous hydration for severe nausea/vomiting must be carefully considered. Total parental nutrition (TPN) and peripheral nutrition have limited roles in palliative care. Some may argue that they have no role in end-stage disease
  4) Prepare for/assist with medical interventions
    a) Insert gastric tube and attach to suction as indicated
      (1) Nasogastric tube may relieve pressure and provide comfort
    b) In rare cases, such as unresectable obstruction, a draining percutaneous endoscopic gastrostomy (PEG) tube may be placed
    c) Anticipatory nausea can be treated by the use of distraction or relaxation techniques, acupuncture, music therapy, or hypnosis
    d) Serving meals at room temperature with clear fluids while avoiding strong smells may be beneficial
    e) Encourage the patient to eat slowly; avoid large, high-bulk meals
    f) Patients who are weak should be positioned to avoid aspiration
  5) Administer pharmacologic therapy as ordered
    a) Anticholinergics (e.g., hyoscine hydrobromide [Scopolamine]) may be helpful in treating motion sickness, intractable vomiting, or small bowel obstruction
    b) Antihistamines are commonly used in intestinal obstruction, increased intracranial pressure, or peritoneal irritation, and when vestibular causes exist (e.g., meclizine [Antivert] or cyclizine [Marezine])
    c) Octreotide (Sandostatin) may be administered for unresectable intestinal obstruction
    d) Phenothiazines (e.g., prochlorperazine [Compazine]) used for general nausea and vomiting are not highly recommended for routine use in palliative care

e) Steroids (e.g., dexamethasone [Decadron]), administered alone or with other agents for nausea and vomiting, are appropriate for cytotoxic-induced emesis

f) Prokinetic agents (e.g., metoclopramide [Reglan]) can treat gastric stasis or ileus

g) Antibiotics can decrease the impact of infectious processes

h) Antifungals (e.g., nystatin) can decrease the impact of fungal infections such as candidiasis

i) Butyrophenones (e.g., haloperidol [Haldol]) are used to treat nausea that is induced chemically, mechanically, or by opioids

j) Cannabinoids are a second-line antiemetic and typically more effective in young adults

k) Benzodiazepines (e.g., lorazepam [Ativan]) are most effective in treating nausea exacerbated by anxiety

l) Serotonin receptor agonists are used for postoperative nausea and vomiting and chemotherapy-related emesis. These include ondansetron hydrochloride (Zofran) and granisetron hydrochloride (Kytril)

5. Diarrhea[16]

a. Diarrhea is the frequent passage of loose, non-formed stool resulting in three or more bowel movements in 1 day.[19] Although much less common than constipation in the palliative care setting, diarrhea remains a common symptom

b. It may be especially problematic in patients with human immunodeficiency virus (HIV) infection. It can dramatically affect a person's quality of life.[19]

c. Continuous diarrhea produces fatigue, electrolyte abnormalities, and depression and may cause a person to become homebound. Ongoing diarrhea can exhaust both patients and family. This situation can be embarrassing and time consuming and can lead to problems such as skin breakdown and dehydration

d. Planning and implementation/interventions

1) Determine priorities of care

2) Establish IV access for administration of crystalloid fluids/medications

a) Infuse normal saline solutions as appropriate

3) Prepare for/assist with medical interventions

a) Treat the underlying cause as appropriate

4) Administer pharmacologic therapy as ordered (Table 5.4)

a) Pancreatic enzymes

5) Educate patient and significant others

a) Dietary modifications

(1) Initiate a clear liquid diet. Avoid milk, proteins, fats, alcohol, hot spices, and gas-forming foods, such as broccoli, cauliflower, cabbage, sauerkraut, corn, or beans

(2) Promote hydration by suggesting fluids that may improve electrolyte status (e.g., sports drinks, juices)

6. Constipation/obstipation[16]

Table 5.4

Pharmacologic Treatment for Diarrhea

Class of Drug	Examples	Mechanism of Action	Comments
Opioids	Diphenoxylate hydrochloride (Lomotil)	Suppress forward peristalsis and increase sphincter tone	5 mg PO every 6 hours
	Loperamide hydrochloride (Imodium)		Start at 4 mg PO, then 2 mg after each loose stool, not to exceed 16 mg daily
Bulk-forming agents	Psyllium (Metamucil)	Promote absorption of liquid and increase thickness of stool	Give 1–3 times daily; many preparations available. Patient must be able to drink at least 8 glasses of water daily
Antibiotics	Metronidazole (Flagyl)	Eliminate infectious processes	Antibiotic choice based on cause
Steroids	Dexamethasone (Decadron)	Decrease inflammation in the gut and provide some relief in partial bowel obstruction and ulcerative colitis	
Somatostatin	Octreotide (Sandostatin)	Slows transit time by decreasing secretions	Suppresses diarrhea associated with carcinoid tumors and AIDS

Permission to use materials from the End-of-Life Nursing Education Consortium (ELNEC) curriculum was granted by the American Association of Colleges of Nursing and the City of Hope. The End-of-Life Nursing Education Consortium (ELNEC) Project is a national end-of-life educational program administered by City of Hope National Medical Center (COH) and the American Association of Colleges of Nursing (AACN) designed to enhance palliative care in nursing. The ELNEC Project was originally funded by a grant from the Robert Wood Johnson Foundation with additional support from funding organizations (the National Cancer Institute, Aetna Foundation, and Archstone Foundation). Materials are copyrighted by COH and AACN and are used with permission. Further information about the ELNEC Project can be found at http://www.aacn.nche.edu/ELNEC.

AIDS, acquired immunodeficiency syndrome; *PO,* orally.

a. Constipation is the infrequent passage of stool

b. Obstipation is severe constipation or intestinal obstruction

c. Associated symptoms may include rectal pressure, straining, cramps, distention, and/or the sensation of bloating

d. Constipation is a frequent symptom in patients at the end of life

e. Although constipation occurs in approximately 10% of the general population, its incidence can be as high as 50% to 78% in the ill adult

f. Constipation may be a highly embarrassing issue for the patient, and this situation can frequently evolve to a severe problem. Talking frankly and openly regarding this symptom and encouraging discussion help prevent significant distress. Discuss with the patient how to address this issue. Prevention is the key.

g. Planning and implementation/interventions

1) Determine priorities of care

2) Prepare for/assist with medical interventions

a) Assist with possible hospital admission

(1) There may be an indication for palliative surgery to resect the bowel or place an intraluminal stent to allow passage of flatus or fecal material through the obstruction[20, 21]

3) Administer pharmacologic therapy as ordered (Table 5.5)

a) Prophylactic stool softener

b) Naloxone hydrochloride (Narcan) in small amounts if opioid-induced constipation is suspected. Caution must be taken to not reverse the analgesic effects of the opioids (Fig. 5.1)

4) Educate patient and significant others

a) Encourage patient to drink plenty of fluids as tolerated while increasing activity as appropriate

b) Encourage patient's own bowel regimens as long as they are effective and not contraindicated

c) Consider using oral agents before rectal agents

d) High-fiber foods are useful if adequate fluid intake is maintained

e) Suppositories and/or enemas should be considered when the patient is no longer able to tolerate oral medications or they have become ineffective. Enemas should be avoided as part of a routine bowel regime but may be necessary in some cases

f) Metoclopramide (Reglan), when given parenterally, has been shown to be effective

Table 5.5

Pharmacologic Treatment for Constipation*

Class of Drug	Examples	Mechanism of Action	Comments
Stimulant	Senna or senna combinations	Stimulates bowel	Should be used with caution when liver disease is present
Laxatives Bulk	Psyllium (Metamucil)	Increase intestinal transit time	Not recommended if bowel obstruction is impending or patient has limited fluid intake (less than 8 glasses/day), may not be appropriate in end-of-life care
Lubricant	Mineral oil	Lubricates and softens stool	Decreases absorption of vitamins and minerals. Associated with aspiration pneumonia in the frail elderly
Detergent/softener	Docusate (Colace)	Softens stool, may stimulate colon	
Combination	Casanthrol and docusate	Combines mild stimulant with softener	
Osmotic	Sorbitol, lactulose	Nonabsorbable sugars pull fluid into gastrointestinal tract	Typically used in patients with chronic constipation, especially in opiate use
Magnesium salts	Milk of Magnesia	Osmotic	Prolonged use or overdosage of saline laxative may lead to life-threatening electrolyte disturbances

*Note: Multiple over-the-counter preparations are available; see individual dosing guidelines.

Permission to use materials from the End-of-Life Nursing Education Consortium (ELNEC) curriculum was granted by the American Association of Colleges of Nursing (AACN) and the City of Hope National Medical Center (COH). The ELNEC Project is a national end-of-life educational program administered by COH and the AACN designed to enhance palliative care in nursing. The ELNEC Project was originally funded by a grant from the Robert Wood Johnson Foundation with additional support from funding organizations (the National Cancer Institute, Aetna Foundation, and Archstone Foundation). Materials are copyrighted by the COH and AACN and are used with permission. Further information about the ELNEC Project can be found at http://www.aacn.nche.edu/ELNEC.

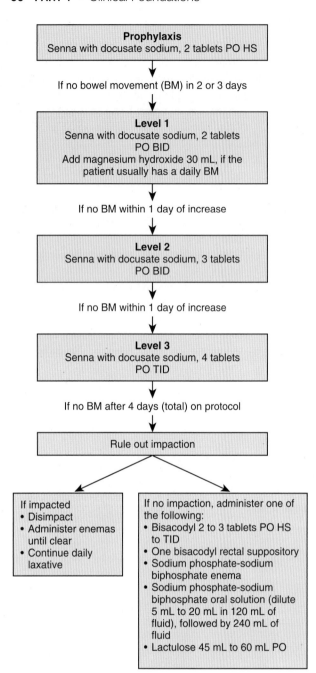

FIG. 5.1 Algorithm to prevent and manage opioid-induced constipation. *BID*, twice daily; *BM*, bowel movement; *PO*, orally; *TID*, three times daily. (*Permission to use materials from the End-of-Life Nursing Education Consortium [ELNEC] curriculum was granted by the American Association of Colleges of Nursing [AACN] and the City of Hope National Medical Center [COH]. The ELNEC Project is a national end-of-life educational program administered by the COH and the AACN designed to enhance palliative care in nursing. The ELNEC Project was originally funded by a grant from the Robert Wood Johnson Foundation with additional support from funding organizations [the National Cancer Institute, Aetna Foundation, and Archstone Foundation]. Materials are copyrighted by the COH and AACN and are used with permission. Further information about the ELNEC Project can be found at* http://www.aacn.nche.edu/ELNEC.)

by increasing gastric motility and intestinal transit time

7. Delirium/agitation/confusion[16]
   a. Delirium is an acute change in cognition or awareness and may be related to a variety of causes (Table 5.6)
   b. Terminal delirium is common in patients near death. Early detection and assessment may lead to resolution of delirium if the cause is reversible, but in all cases, patient and family support is essential[22]
   c. Agitation is a common symptom accompanying delirium (hyperactive delirium), although withdrawn behaviors (hypoactive delirium) can also occur
   d. Confusion refers to disorientation, inappropriate behavior or communication, and/or hallucinations
   e. Delirium, agitation, or confusion may be associated with a reversible cause, or it can be a very late symptom indicating that a patient is close to death. Treatment may be limited to identifying the reversible cause and treating that cause. Careful consideration of the benefits versus the risks of treatment should be considered, as with all other symptoms.
   f. Planning and implementation/interventions
      1) Determine priorities of care
      2) Prepare for/assist with medical intervention
         a) Minimize external stimulation, family intervention regarding treatment options
         b) Institute nonpharmacologic treatments such as relaxation/distraction therapy, massage
         c) Hydration may be indicated based on assessment of potential benefits or burdens
      3) Administer pharmacologic therapy as ordered
         a) Neuroleptics (e.g., haloperidol [Haldol], chlorpromazine [Thorazine]) or benzodiazepines for acute agitation; monitor closely for potential side effects of these agents
         b) Midazolam (Versed) for neuromuscular symptoms (e.g., tremors, twitching)

8. Depression[16] (see Chapter 27)
   a. Depression can be described as a broad spectrum of responses that range from "expected, transient, and nonclinical sadness to extremes of major clinical depressive disorders and suicidality"[23]
   b. Depression and anxiety are frequent comorbid factors in chronic medical illness; unfortunately, the symptoms are frequently unrecognized and undertreated. Symptoms usually respond to treatment; therefore, recognition of their existence is extremely important
   c. Depression occurs in about 25% to 77% of the terminally ill population.
   d. Early diagnosis can improve outcomes and allow individuals to feel better while having more energy to achieve their goals
   e. Persistent feelings of helplessness, hopelessness, inadequacy, depression, and suicidal ideation are not normal at the end of life. These symptoms should be aggressively evaluated and treated

f. Planning and implementation/interventions
  1) Determine priorities of care
    a) Patients with immediate, lethal, and precise suicide plans and resources to carry out the plan should be immediately evaluated by psychiatric professionals, hospitalized, or placed under appropriate close and continuous supervision

2) Prepare for/assist with medical interventions
  a) Promote and facilitate autonomy and control
  b) Increase patient and family participation in care, thus promoting a sense of control and reducing feelings of helplessness
  c) Reminiscence and life review can assist terminally ill patients to focus on life accomplishments and to promote closure and resolution of life events for the patient and family
  d) Grief counseling can assist patients and families to deal with past, present, and future losses
  e) Maximize symptom management to decrease physical stressors that can exacerbate depression and anxiety symptoms
  f) Psychiatric counseling may be needed for those experiencing significant inability to cope with the experience of their medical illness
  g) Assist the patient to draw on previous sources of strength, such as faith and other belief systems
  h) Assist the patient to reframe negative thoughts into positive thoughts
  i) Seek further assistance from a mental health or palliative care professional
3) Administer pharmacologic therapy as ordered (Table 5.7)

Table 5.6
Causes of Delirium

D	Drug use (e.g., new dose adjustment, psychotropics, recreational, illicit)
E	Electrolyte (e.g., hyponatremia, hypoxemia, hypoglycemia/hyperglycemia)
L	Lack of drugs (i.e., withdrawal) or liver failure
I	Infection or ischemia (e.g., myocardial)
R	Renal failure or reduced sensory input (e.g., blindness, deafness, darkness, change in surroundings)
I	Intracranial problems (e.g., stroke, bleeding, meningitis, postictal state) or impaction of stool
U	Urinary retention, urinary infection
M	Metastases to the brain or myocardial problems

Data from Storey, P. (1994). Symptom control in advanced cancer. *Seminars in Oncology, 21,* 748–753; and Merck Manual. (2006). Delirium. Retrieved from http://www.merck.com/mrkshared/mmg/sec5/ch39/ch39a.jsp.

Table 5.7
Pharmacologic Treatments for Depression

Class of Drug	Examples	Mechanism of Action	Comments
Antidepressants	SSRIs: Fluoxetine (Prozac), Paroxetine (Paxil), Sertraline (Zoloft)	Block serotonin reuptake	Some SSRIs have long half-lives and thus may have limited use for the terminally ill
	Tricyclic: Amitriptyline (Elavil), Nortriptyline	Block reuptake of various neurotransmitters at the neuronal membrane Improve sleep	
Stimulants	Methylphenidate (Concerta)	Stimulates CNS and respiratory centers, increases appetite and energy levels, improves mood, reduces sedation	Starting dose 5–10 mg every morning and at noon, titrate to effect; acts quickly
Nonbenzodiazepines	Buspirone hydrochloride (BuSpar)	Mechanism of action complex: acts on multiple CNS sites to produce anxiolytic activity	Useful in patients with mixed anxiety and depressive symptoms
			Starting dose 10–15 mg PO daily in divided doses, then titrated up to no higher than 60 mg PO daily
			Slow onset; duration of effect may be limited
Steroids	Dexamethasone (Decadron)	Improves appetite and elevates mood, thus enhancing a sense of well-being	

CNS, central nervous system; *PO,* orally; *SSRI,* selective serotonin reuptake inhibitor.

Permission to use materials from the End-of-Life Nursing Education Consortium (ELNEC) curriculum was granted by the American Association of Colleges of Nursing (AACN) and the City of Hope National Medical Center (COH). The ELNEC Project is a national end-of-life educational program administered by COH and the AACN designed to enhance palliative care in nursing. The ELNEC Project was originally funded by a grant from the Robert Wood Johnson Foundation with additional support from funding organizations (the National Cancer Institute, Aetna Foundation, and Archstone Foundation). Materials are copyrighted by the COH and AACN and are used with permission. Further information about the ELNEC Project can be found at http://www.aacn.nche.edu/ELNEC.

Table 5.8

Pharmacologic Treatment for Anxiety

Class of Drug	Examples	Mechanism of Action	Comments
Antidepressants	SSRIs: Fluoxetine (Prozac), Paroxetine (Paxil), Sertraline (Zoloft)	Block serotonin reuptake	Useful in treating transient anxiety and panic attacks; use cautiously in terminally ill
Benzodiazepines/anticonvulsants	Alprazolam (Xanax) Lorazepam (Ativan) Clonazepam (Klonopin) Temazepam (Restoril) Midazolam (Versed)	Appear to act on limbic-thalamic-hypothalamic areas of the CNS to produce anxiolytic, sedative, hypnotic effects and skeletal muscle relaxation	Dose varies Midazolam and lorazepam used parenterally in terminal restlessness/agitation
Neuroleptics	Haloperidol (Haldol)	Precise mechanism unclear, depresses the CNS at level of brain, midbrain, brainstem reticular formation	Used in severe agitation when benzodiazepines are not effective; especially useful when treating delusions and hallucinations that accompany anxiety and in demented patients
Nonbenzodiazepines	Buspirone (BuSpar)	Mechanism of action complex: acts on multiple CNS sites to produce anxiolytic activity	Useful in patients with mixed anxiety and depressive symptoms

CNS, central nervous system; *SSRI,* selective serotonin reuptake inhibitor.

Permission to use materials from the End-of-Life Nursing Education Consortium (ELNEC) curriculum was granted by the American Association of Colleges of Nursing (AACN) and the City of Hope National Medical Center (COH). The ELNEC Project is a national end-of-life educational program administered by COH and the AACN designed to enhance palliative care in nursing. The ELNEC Project was originally funded by a grant from the Robert Wood Johnson Foundation with additional support from funding organizations (the National Cancer Institute, Aetna Foundation, and Archstone Foundation). Materials are copyrighted by the COH and AACN and are used with permission. Further information about the ELNEC Project can be found at http://www.aacn.nche.edu/ELNEC.

9. Anxiety (see Chapter 27)
   a. Anxiety is a subjective feeling of apprehension, tension, insecurity, and uneasiness, usually without a known cause
   b. Signs and symptoms that accompany anxiety occur along a continuum that can be assessed as mild, moderate, or severe. The greater the threat perceived by the patient, the greater the anxiety response
   c. Planning and implementation/intervention
      1) Determine priorities of care
      2) Prepare for/assist with medical interventions
         a) Acknowledge patient fears, using open-ended questions, reflecting, clarifying, and using empathetic listening and remarks to help the patient identify effective coping strategies used in the past and to learn new coping skills
         b) Allow patient to articulate anger and provide appropriate reassurance and support
         c) Provide concrete information to eliminate fear of the unknown, and in appropriate situations, provide stressful event warning
         d) Encourage use of a stress diary, to help the patient understand relationships among situation, thoughts, and feelings
         e) Explore patient experiences with "near-miss" events
         f) Maximize symptom management to decrease physical stressors that can exacerbate depression and anxiety symptoms
         g) Promote use of relaxation and guided imagery techniques through the use of audiotapes, breathing exercises, progressive muscle relaxation
         h) Psychiatric counseling may be needed for those experiencing significant inability to cope with the experience of their medical illness
      3) Administer pharmacologic therapy as ordered (Table 5.8)

III. Possible Triggers for Obtaining a Palliative Care Consult

Recent research in emergency and palliative care has focused on identifying situations when a palliative care consult may be beneficial in the emergency department.[24] From the research, these situations involve much suffering, complex psychosocial issues, and a high probability of death. These situations could trigger a palliative care consult. Getting help from another specialty that can dedicate time and expertise is beneficial for the patients, families, and emergency department staff. The literature suggests that there be a quick (1- to 2-minute) initial screening process by the triage nurse.[24] Following are recommendations for the initial screening to determine if a palliative care consult should be initiated by emergency department clinicians (e.g., treatment RN, social worker, physician, nurse practitioner, physician assistant).

1. Age>65 years and/or chronic life-limiting illness
   a. Each emergency department should identify high-volume illnesses (e.g., metastatic cancer, end-stage congestive heart failure, end-stage COPD) based on the population served by the institution
2. Functional status of the patient (e.g., bed-bound)
3. Low caregiver or social support
4. Frequent emergency department admissions or hospitalizations
   a. Set the time and definition such as more than three admissions to the emergency department and/or hospital within a 3-month period
5. The "would you be surprised" question is used to help with a prognosis of the patient
   a. For example, if you were to ask yourself, "Would I be surprised that the patient would live for another 12 months?" and the answer is, "Yes, I would be surprised that the patient would live for another 12 months," then that is a fairly good prognostic tool to say that the patient is nearing the end of life

IV. Family Presence During Resuscitation

Since 1993, the Emergency Nurses Association (ENA) has been involved in research and policy development for allowing the option for family presence during resuscitation and invasive procedures.[25–29] There has been a move away from the traditional paternalistic approach of health care toward a more collaborative practice with family involvement.[24] Increasingly, other professional organizations have incorporated the option for family presence during resuscitation and invasive procedures and have developed guidelines and position statements in support of this practice.[30] Core curricula designed for resuscitation such as the American Heart Association's Advanced Life Support (ALS) and Pediatric Advanced Life Support (PALS), the Advanced Pediatric Life Support (APLS)—the Pediatric Emergency Medicine Resource, the Trauma Nursing Core Course (TNCC), and the Emergency Nursing Pediatric Course (ENPC)—have included guidelines for the option for family presence.[31]

A. BENEFITS OF FAMILY PRESENCE

1. Facilitates family grieving and provides closure for survivors[25]
2. Allows for an open process to reduce questioning whether personnel adequately attempted to resuscitate the patient[29, 32]
3. Resuscitation efforts may be terminated at the request of the family[33]

B. POTENTIAL RISKS OF FAMILY PRESENCE[25]

Although the following potential risks have been cited in the literature, there is no evidence that they have occurred, with the exception of the increased level of psychological stress on medical personnel. The potential risks are presented to give a balanced perspective on this issue.

1. A negative effect on family member for witnessing the event's survivors[24]
2. Increased level of psychological stress on the medical staff
3. Family interference with the resuscitation process
4. Lack of support for family members
5. Increased risk of medicolegal litigation

C. CORE ELEMENTS OF FAMILY PRESENCE PROGRAMS[30,34,35]

1. Appropriate personnel and facilities, along with education survivors[25]
2. Preparation of the family for the experience
3. Provision of a dedicated person to accompany the family
4. Safety of the health care team at all times

V. Death Notification

A. BEREAVEMENT CARE

1. Delivering news of death is complicated and difficult. Nurses often state they feel unprepared to notify survivors about death[36]
2. Simple interventions can be helpful to survivors in their grief during bereavement
   a. Death notification
      1) Death notification can be in person or over the telephone, or it may include the assistance from other agencies such as police departments
      2) The manner used to deliver the news has a significant impact on how survivors remember the last moments of the patient's life. It is important to be clear in the verbiage to include the words that the person has died
      3) Repetition is very helpful because it is difficult for survivors to comprehend all the information given to them[37]
   b. Be present[37]
      1) Bereaved survivors may feel abandoned and may need someone to answer questions and review the events in an effort to understand and cope with the situation
      2) Some nurses feel unprepared and uncomfortable in working with grieving survivors
      3) Allow the survivors time and space for their grief reactions but do not move away from them.[6, 36, 38] Grief reactions can range from anger, disbelief, sadness, helplessness, chest pain, headache, agitation, crying, and social withdrawal.[37] Only intervene if the survivors are at risk of hurting themselves or others

c. Encourage survivors to view the deceased person[36,37]
1) Use the patient's real name and avoid using the term "the body." This allows the patient to remain a socially alive person until survivors can come to terms with the patient's death.[36] Viewing or touching the body may help the grieving process[6, 39]
2) Describe to the survivors what they will see before they enter the room[33]
3) Assist the survivors to follow particular cultural, religious, or spiritual rituals that are important to them
4) If there is suspicion of an unexpected, unnatural, suspicious, or violent death, ensure evidence preservation (see Chapter 44).[40] Postmortem care is important to increase the possibility that the crime suspect is successfully prosecuted.[7] Involvement with the medical examiner's or coroner's office is crucial and often mandatory. Procedures developed in conjunction with the medical examiner's or coroner's office regarding survivor presence during pronouncement of death may help ease anxiety and bereavement[7, 36]

d. Follow-up[37]
1) Provide survivors with written information about what to do next[39]
2) Telephone follow-up calls are also helpful to survivors. They provide an opportunity to ask questions and demonstrate that the emergency staff remembers the survivors.[6, 36, 38] This is an important humanistic aspect of clinical practice

VI. End-of-Life Legalities/Ethics

A. ADVANCE DIRECTIVES[16] (SEE CHAPTER 45)

The Patient Self-Determination Act requires providers to inform patients what their state provides in the form of advance directives and requires hospitals to inform patients of their right to accept or refuse medical treatment and to make advance directives. The act is intended to protect patients' views and choices when they become incapacitated and unable to make decisions about their care.

1. Decision-making capacity[16]
a. The informed consent process requires that a patient have the mental ability to comprehend information, contemplate options, evaluate risks and consequences, and communicate decisions
b. Every adult is presumed to have decisional capacity and authority unless proven differently
c. Decision-making capacity can be permanent, temporary, intermittent, or situational depending on current medications, disease process, or level of communication with patients and families. For example, if language is not used at a level that a patient or family can understand, then the capacity to make

decisions is impaired. Additionally, patients who do not speak English may not be able to make informed decisions if an appropriate translator/interpreter is not available
d. Although frequently used interchangeably, "capacity" is different from "competence." Competence is a legal status determined by a court, whereas decisional capacity within health care is an assessment provided by physicians
e. When a patient lacks the capacity to choose, mechanisms and laws dictate who is appropriate to choose for the patient. Some of these mechanisms are living wills, health care proxy/surrogate, and power of attorney for health care decisions
f. The two most common forms of advance directives are living wills (a form of instructional directive to limit life-sustaining medical treatment in the event of a life-threatening illness) and durable power of attorney for health care (an appointment of a health care agent or proxy to make decisions according to the incapacitated patient's preference)
g. Other types of instructional directives include personal letters, a values history, and a medical directive[41,42]

2. Advance directives[16]
a. An advance directive is a written method for patients to plan and communicate their care and treatment choices when they no longer are able to speak for themselves, and are based on the individual's self-determination
b. Nurses need to be aware of their state laws regarding advance directives. Advance directive forms and state statutes may differ, but a sensible, clear, documented plan is generally persuasive to caregivers and courts
c. Nurses advocate for respecting a patient's advance directive. Advance directives should be utilized to promote continuity of care across settings
d. Social workers and hospices are resources for patients and families to obtain information and/or counseling on advance directives and be guided through decision making at the end of life
e. Advance directive documents offer legal protection for patient rights. Courts and legislatures have recognized these as valid indicators of a patient's previously expressed desires. Advance directives give immunity to health care professionals who, in good faith, follow the directive
f. Living wills[16]
1) Prepared while the patient has decisional capacity
2) Describe the patient's preferences in the event that he or she becomes incapable of making decisions or communicating decisions
3) Usually describes what type of life-prolonging procedures the patient would or would not want and circumstances under which these procedures would be carried out, withheld, or withdrawn

4) Documentation of living will: copies should be in patient's home, physician's record, hospital record, and outpatient record and with surrogate/proxy
5) Variations exist by state, so professionals must be familiar with state laws
g. Durable power of attorney for health care[16]
1) This advance directive allows for the appointment of a decision maker (i.e., surrogate or proxy) in the case of future incapacity
2) The patient must choose a durable power of attorney while capacitated
3) Durable power of attorney for health care document specifies which powers the patient gives to the person holding the power of attorney
4) May include arrangements for consent to medical, therapeutic, and surgical procedures, including administration of medications
5) The patient has the right to choose anyone to be the surrogate/proxy and can change that person at any time
6) The health care surrogate/proxy must agree to become the decision maker when the patient is no longer capable
7) Responsibilities and rights of the health care surrogate/proxy
   a) Reviewing the patient's medical records to become informed of patient status and prognosis
   b) Consulting with health care providers
   c) Giving consent
   d) Applying for medical benefits on the patient's behalf
   e) Making life-prolonging/terminating decisions if the surrogate form meets requirements of the living will statute
3. DNR[16]/ DNAR/No Code/AND[43–45]
   a. These are physician orders found in prehospital and inpatient settings
   b. DNR, DNAR, No Code, and AND share the common meaning of prohibiting life-sustaining/life-extending interventions such as chest compressions, defibrillation, intubation, and vasopressor use
   c. Health care professionals should be familiar with their local institution's definitions of these orders and which are used in the institution
   d. The presence of this type of order does not exclude the health care professional's moral obligation to provide care to patients.[35] Examples of continued care in the presence of a DNR/DNAR/No Code/AND order include symptom management and emotional/psychosocial/spiritual care
   e. The DNAR form confirms and expresses that if cardiopulmonary arrest occurs, no resuscitative measures will be initiated[16]

1) A written order from a physician is required. This is the only intervention that requires an order prohibiting it[16]
2) Not required by standards or law for admission to hospice programs[16]
3) A decision not to resuscitate is an opportunity to clarify the benefit, necessity, and desirability of other interventions[16]

B. ORGAN AND TISSUE DONATION (SEE CHAPTER 7)

Federal law (Public Law 99-5-9; Section 9318) and Medicare regulations require that hospitals give the surviving family members the chance to authorize donation of their family member's tissues and organs.[8] Initiating the conversation about organ and tissue procurement may be difficult; however, some families have initiated the conversation with health care providers. An important aspect surrounding organ or tissue procurement is respecting the family's grieving process and giving them all the information they need to make a decision with which they will be comfortable. Organs and tissues can be procured after cardiac death or brain death. The following guidelines by Kelly[34] are helpful in working with families and organ/tissue procurement organizations.
1. Follow hospital protocols for organ procurement. Hospital protocols will identify who is to serve as a liaison between the family and the transplant program staff
2. Recent guidelines by the Centers for Medicare/Medicaid Services (CMS) require that hospitals inform their organ procurement office of all deaths that occur and that trained staff members discuss organ donation and obtain consent
3. Arrange for the regional transplant program (RTP) personnel to provide annual updates on organ donation. Doing so will ensure that clinical staff members have current information on caring for the potential donor and updated information on legislation in the state
4. Respect each person's individual beliefs. Identify which staff members support organ donation and work with them to enhance the skills needed to speak with families and provide care to the donor
5. Be knowledgeable about state and federal regulations; post guidelines in a conspicuous place

C. POSTMORTEM PROCEDURES

The ENA and the American College of Emergency Physicians (ACEP) have developed position statements regarding use of the newly deceased patient for procedural practice.[46, 47] The ENA and ACEP agree that there is a need to teach and practice many lifesaving skills in order to provide those same skills in emergency situations. However, there are many ethical concerns regarding the use of a newly deceased person to teach and practice needed skills.

Therefore, the ENA's and ACEP's position is that consent must be obtained from family for the performance of these invasive procedures.

D. AUTOPSY

1. The decision to perform an autopsy is usually made by the medical examiner or coroner's office in the county in which the patient died
2. Emergency departments should develop policies and procedures delineating when to contact the medical examiner or coroner
3. Several factors are taken in account to determine whether an autopsy is warranted
   a. Any death associated with a known or suspected criminal activity is cause for an autopsy
   b. Autopsies are performed to determine the cause of any sudden, traumatic, or unexpected death
   c. Family members may request an autopsy. The autopsy may be performed by any pathologist rather than by the medical examiner
   d. Regulations vary from state to state and even within states
   e. Emergency department personnel should consult with their local medical examiner, coroner, and other agencies to determine local regulations and preferences[34]

E. WITHHOLDING/WITHDRAWING LIFE-SUSTAINING MEASURES

Withholding or withdrawing treatments is challenging to emergency personnel because they are trained and called on to institute resuscitation interventions; however, withholding or withdrawing of treatments may be morally and legally justified and has strong roots in common law. Patients and surrogate decision makers may be allowed to refuse or withdraw a treatment at any time, according to hospital's patient's bill of rights. Withholding treatment is considered morally equivalent to withdrawing treatment; the end result is the patient is without the treatment. However, at times it may be more difficult for personnel to withhold, rather than withdraw, treatment.

The End-of-Life Nursing Education Consortium (ELNEC)[16] makes the following points about withholding or withdrawing treatments.

1. Common reasons for considering withholding/withdrawing therapy
   a. Patient choice
   b. Undesirable quality of life
   c. Burdens outweigh benefits
   d. Prolonging dying
2. When a capacitated patient or designated surrogate decides that a proposed treatment will impose undue burdens, the patient or the surrogate should be entitled to refuse initiation of the treatments, based on the patient's right to self-determination

3. Similarly, when a patient or surrogate in collaboration with the responsible health care professional decides that a treatment has become more burdensome than beneficial to the patient, it is appropriate to withdraw that care
4. Common treatments that may be withheld or withdrawn include
   a. Medically provided hydration and nutrition
   b. Ventilation
   c. Cardiopulmonary resuscitation
   d. Dialysis
   e. Antibiotic use
   f. Automatic implantable cardioverter defibrillators (AICDs)
5. Health care professionals may find it difficult to discontinue life-sustaining treatment because they have been trained to do everything possible to support life
6. Withdrawal or withholding treatment is a decision/action that allows the disease to progress on its natural course. It is not a decision/action intended to cause death

F. PRINCIPLE OF DOUBLE EFFECT

The ethical principle of double effect distinguishes between the consequences a person intends and those that are unintended but foreseen. It may be applicable in various situations in which an action has two effects, one good and one bad.[48] In other words, a single action may have two foreseen effects, one good and one bad. The agent (or person) performing the action intends the good effect to occur, yet if the bad effect were to occur, the action would still be permissible.

The principle of double effect is most commonly applied in the administration of pain-relieving medication to patients who are dying. Opioids are used to relieve pain and other symptoms of suffering (i.e., the good effect). However, opioids also have the potential side effect of causing respiratory and cardiovascular depression that may, if left untreated, lead to death (i.e., the bad effect). If the clinician's intention is to relieve pain and suffering yet incidentally foresees that the patient may die, it is morally and legally permissible to administer the opioid if the intention is to relieve suffering. If the primary intention is to have the patient die, then it is not morally or legally permissible to administer the opioid.

G. PARTICULARLY SIGNIFICANT DEATHS

1. Some deaths affect individuals on a significant level because the death of the patient may remind them of the death of someone close to them
   a. Death of children
   b. Fetal demise
   c. Mass casualty
   d. Death of someone the clinician knows
   e. Particularly horrific, traumatic death

2. It is important for the clinician to recognize that the death was meaningful in order to manage the stress of the event
3. Colleagues must discover ways to support each other rather than dismissing the impact the death has on a clinician
4. Some strategies can be used immediately after the incident; other strategies are more long term.[49, 50] Examples of strategies include
   a. Ask to be relieved from care responsibilities and take a break, if possible
   b. Ask for reassignment to another part of the emergency department, if possible[48]
   c. Find a colleague or friend with whom the event can be discussed. Consider speaking with the department manager about stress debriefing
   d. Self-reflection: Take a moment to reflect on feelings after exposure to the event. What do you think? How do you behave? Pay attention to any physical symptoms and to thoughts and feelings[49]
   e. Self-monitoring: Assess responses to traumatic situations and compare them with normal responses[49]
   f. Minimize the impact of negative thoughts[49]
   g. Focus on what was done right[48]
   h. Include therapies that follow basic health principles[49, 50]
      1) Physical exercise
      2) Meditation
      3) Humor
      4) Music
      5) Relaxation (e.g., acupressure, reflexology, therapeutic massage)
      6) Guided imagery
      7) Eat properly
      8) Get adequate rest

H. BURNOUT AND POSTTRAUMATIC STRESS

1. Symptoms may include[49]
   a. Increase in the number of sick days
   b. Indecision
   c. Difficulty with problem solving
   d. Isolation or withdrawal
   e. Behavioral outbursts
   f. Denial and shock
   g. Fixation on a single detail
   h. Immobilization
   i. Feeling of extreme serenity
   j. Emotionally numbing responses
   k. Intrusive responses
2. Signs of burnout or posttraumatic stress may include[49]
   a. Tachycardia
   b. Increased respiration rate
   c. Elevated blood pressure

References

1. Centers for Disease Control and Prevention. (n.d.). National Hospital Ambulatory Medical Care Survey: 2011 Emergency Department Summary Tables. Retrieved from http://www.cdc.gov/nchs/data/ahcd/nhamcs_emergency/2011_ed_web_tables.pdf.
2. Iserson KV: Withholding and withdrawing medical treatment: an emergency medicine perspective, *Ann Emerg Med* 28:51–54, 1996.
3. Emergency Nurses Association: Resuscitative decisions. Retrieved from http://www.ena.org/about/position/resuscitativedecision.asp, 1998.
4. Marco CA: Ethical issues of resuscitation, *Emerg Med Clin North Am* 17:527–538, 1999. xiii–xiv.
5. Sanders AB: Unique aspects of ethics in emergency medicine. In Iserson KV, Sanders AB, Mathieu D, editors: *Ethics in emergency medicine*, ed 2., Tuscon, AZ, 1995, Galen Press, pp 7–10.
6. Walters DT, Tupin JP: Family grief in the emergency department, *Emerg Med Clin North Am* 9:189–207, 1991.
7. Chan GK: End-of-life care models and emergency department care, *Acad Emerg Med* 11:79–86, 2004.
8. Campbell M, Zalenski R: The emergency department. In Ferrell BR, Coyle N, editors: *Textbook of palliative care,* ed 2, New York, 2006, Oxford University Press, pp 861–869.
9. National Institutes of Health: National Institutes of Health state-of-the-science conference statement. Retrieved from http://consensus.nih.gov/ta/024/024EndOfLifepostconfINTRO.htm, 2004.
10. Kamienski MC: Family-centered care in the ED, *Am J Nurs* 104:59–62, 2004.
11. Chan GK: Understanding end-of-life caring practices in the emergency department: developing Merleau-Ponty's notions of intentional arc and maximum grip through praxis and phronesis, *Nurs Philos* 6:19–32, 2005.
12. Chan GK: Trajectories of approaching death in the emergency department: clinician narratives of patient transitions to the end of life, *J Pain Symptom Manage* 42(6):864–881, 2011.
13. Lasts Acts: Means to a better end: a report on dying in America today. Retrieved from http://www.rwjf.org/files/ publications/other/meansbetterend.pdf, 2002.
14. Field MJ, Cassel CK: *Approaching death: improving care at the end of life*, Washington, DC, 1997, Institute of Medicine, p 437.
15. World Health Organization: *Cancer pain relief and palliative care*, Geneva, 1990, World Health Organization.
16. Ferrell BR, Grant M, editors: *End-of-Life Nursing Education Consortium (ELNEC) Curriculum.* © The ELNEC Project, Washington, DC, 2001, American Association of Colleges of Nursing.
17. Campbell M: *Foregoing life-sustaining therapy: how to care for the patient who is near death*, Aliso Viejo, CA, 1998, American Association of Critical-Care Nurses.
18. King C: Nausea and vomiting. In Ferrell BR, Coyle N, editors: *Textbook of palliative nursing*, ed 2, New York, 2006, Oxford University Press, pp 177–194.
19. Economou DC: Bowel management: constipation, diarrhea, obstruction, and ascites. In Ferrell BR, Coyle N, editors: *Textbook of palliative nursing*, ed 2, New York, 2006, Oxford University Press, pp 219–248.

20. Ferrell BR, Juarez G, Borneman T: The role of nursing in caring for patients undergoing surgery for advanced disease. In Ferrell BR, Coyle N, editors: *Textbook of palliative nursing*, ed 2, New York, 2006, Oxford University Press, pp 871–879.

21. Vrazas JI, Ferris S, Bau S, Faragher I: Stenting for obstructing colorectal malignancy: an interim or definitive procedure, *Australia and New Zealand Journal of Surgery* 72:392–396, 2002.

22. Kuebler KK, Heidrich DE, Vena C, English N: Delirium, confusion, agitation. In Ferrell BR, Coyle N, editors: *Textbook of palliative nursing*, ed 2, New York, 2006, Oxford University Press, pp 401–120.

23. Pasacreta JV, Minarik PA, Nield-Anderson L: Anxiety and depression. In Ferrell BR, Coyle N, editors: *Textbook of palliative nursing*, ed 2, New York, 2006, Oxford University Press, pp 375–400.

24. Lamba S, DeSandre PL, Todd KH, et al.: Integration of palliative care into emergency medicine: the Improving Palliative Care in Emergency Medicine (IPAL-EM) collaboration, *J Emerg Med* 46(2):264–270, 2014.

25. Moreland P: Family presence during invasive procedures and resuscitation in the emergency department: a review of the literature, *J Emerg Nurs* 31:58–72, 2005. quiz 119.

26. Emergency Nurses Association: *Presenting the option for family presence*, ed 2, Des Plaines, IL, 2001, Emergency Nurses Association.

27. Eichhorn DJ, Meyers TA, Guzzetta CE, Clark AP, Klein JD, Taliaferro E: Family presence during invasive procedures and resuscitation: hearing the voice of the patient, *Am J Nurs* 101:48–55, 2001.

28. Hanson C, Strawser D: Family presence during cardiopulmonary resuscitation: foote Hospital emergency department's nine-year perspective, *J Emerg Nurs* 18:104–106, 1992.

29. Meyers TA, Eichhorn DJ, Guzzetta CE, Clark AP, Klein JD, Taliaferro E, Calvin A: Family presence during invasive procedures and resuscitation, *Am J Nurs* 100:32–42, 2000.

30. Henderson DP, Knapp JF: Report of the National Consensus Conference on Family Presence During Pediatric Cardiopulmonary Resuscitation and Procedures, *J Emerg Nurs* 32:23–29, 2006.

31. Emergency Nurses Association: Family presence at the bedside during invasive procedures and cardiopulmonary resuscitation. Retrieved from http://www.ena.org/about/position/PDFs/4E6C256B26994E319F66C65748BFBDBF.pdf, 2005.

32. Tsai E: Should family members be present during cardiopulmonary resuscitation? *N Eng J Med* 346:1019–1021, 2002.

33. Doyle CJ, Post H, Burney RE, Maino J, Keefe M, Rhee KJ: Family participation during resuscitation: an option, *Ann Emerg Med* 16:673–675, 1987.

34. Kelly CT: Death and dying in the emergency department. In Oman KS, Koziol-McLain J, Scheetz LJ, editors: *Emergency nursing secrets*, Philadelphia, PA, 2001, Hanley & Belfus, pp 27–32.

35. Iserson KV: The gravest words: sudden-death notifications and emergency care, *Ann Emerg Med* 36:75–77, 2000.

36. Denke NJ: End of life in the emergency department. In Newberry L, editor: *Sheey's emergency nursing: principles and practice*, ed 5, St. Louis, MO, 2003, Mosby, pp 183–188.

37. Davies J: Grieving after a sudden death: the impact of the initial intervention, *Accid Emerg Nurs* 8:181–184, 1997.

38. Kent H, McDowell J: Sudden bereavement in acute care settings, *Nurs Stand* 19:38–42, 2004.

39. Li SP, Chan CW, Lee DT: Helpfulness of nursing actions to suddenly bereaved family members in an accident and emergency setting in Hong Kong, *J Adv Nurs* 40:170–180, 2002.

40. Lynch VA: Clinical forensic nursing: a new perspective in the management of crime victims from trauma to trial, *Crit Care Nurs Clin North Am* 7:489–507, 1995.

41. Emanuel L, von Gunten C, Ferris F, editors: *The Education for Physicians on End-of-life Care (EPEC) Curriculum.* © *The EPEC Project.* Princeton, NJ, 1999, Robert Wood Johnson Foundation.

42. Patient Self-Determination Act: *In Ominbus Budget Reconciliation Act of 1990. PL 101–508*, 1990.

43. Meyer C: Allow natural death: an alternative to DNR? Retrieved from http://hospicepatients.org/and.html, 2006.

44. Knox C, Vereb JA: Allow natural death: a more humane approach to discussing end-of-life directives, *J Emerg Nurs* 31:560–561, 2005.

45. Cohen RW: A tale of two conversations, *Hastings Cent Rep* 34:49, 2004.

46. Emergency Nurses Association: The use of the newly deceased patient for procedural practice. Retrieved from http://www.ena.org/about/position/PDFs/Use-of-NewlyDeceased.PDF, 2002.

47. American College of Emergency Physicians (ACEP): Ethical issues in emergency department care at the end of life. Retrieved from http://www.acep.org/webportal/PracticeResources/PolicyStatements/ethics/ethicalissuesendlife.htm, 2006.

48. Williams G: The principle of double effect and terminal sedation, *Medical Law Review* 9:41–53, 2001.

49. Badger JM: Understanding secondary traumatic stress, *Am J Nurs* 101:26–32, 2001.

50. Campbell PM: Self-care for the caregiver. In Oman KS, Koziol-McLain J, Scheetz LJ, editors: *Emergency nursing secrets*, Philadelphia, PA, 2001, Hanley & Belfus, pp 33–36.

Bibliography

American Geriatrics Society Panel on Chronic Pain in Older Persons: the management of chronic pain in older persons, *J Am Geriatr Soc* 46:635–651, 1998.

Burkle Jr FM: Mass casualty management of a large-scale bioterrorist event: an epidemiological approach that shapes triage decisions, *Emerg Med Clin North Am* 20:409–436, 2002.

Chochinov HM, Wilson KG, Enns M, Lander S: Depression, hopelessness, and suicidal ideation in the terminally ill, *Psychosomatics* 39:366–370, 1998.

Emergency Nurses Association: End-of-life care in the emergency department. Retrieved from http://www.ena.org/about/position/endoflife.asp, 2002.

Ersek M: Enhancing effective pain management by addressing patient barriers to analgesic use, *J Hosp Palliat Nurs* 1:87–96, 1999.

Ferrell BR, Borneman T: Pain and suffering at the end of life for older patients and their families, *Generations* 23:12–17, 1999.

Ferrell BR, Ferrell BA: *Pain in the elderly: A report of the Task Force on Pain in the Elderly of the International Association for the Study of Pain*, Seattle, WA, 1996, IASP Press.

Green WG: Mass casualty incident management: The Virginia model. Retrieved from http://www.richmond.edu/~wgreen/conf7.pdf, 2000.

Hott C: Caring for the survivors, *Ann Emerg Med* 39:570–572, 2002.

Jacox A, Carr DB, Payne R, Berde CB, Bereitbart W, Cain JM, … Weissman DE: *Management of cancer pain: adults*, Rockville, MD, 1994, Agency for Health Care Policy and Research.

Kendrick KR, Baxi SC, Smith RM: Usefulness of the modified 0-10 Borg scale in assessing the degree of dyspnea in patients with COPD and asthma, *J Emerg Nurs* 26:216–222, 2000.

Luce JM, Alpers A: End-of-life care: what do the American courts say? *Crit Care Med* 29:N40–N45, 2001.

Malone RE: Dimensions of vulnerability in emergency nurses' narratives, *Adv Nurs Sci* 23:1–11, 2000.

McCaffery M, Pasero C: *Pain clinical manual*, ed 2, St. Louis, MO, 1999, Mosby.

McClain K, Perkins P: Terminally ill patients in the emergency department: a practical overview of end-of-life issues, *J Adv Nurs* 28:515–522, 2002.

Mitty EL: Ethnicity and end of life decision-making, *Reflect Nurs Leadersh* 27:28–31, 2001. 46.

Morrison RS, Wallenstein S, Natale DK, Senzel RS, Huang LL: "We don't carry that": failure of pharmacies in predominantly nonwhite neighborhoods to stock opioid analgesics, *N Engl J Med* 58:125–129, 2000.

Ng B, Dimsdale JE, Shragg P, Deutsch R: Ethnic differences in analgesic consumption for post operative pain, *Psychometric Medicine* 58:125–129, 1996.

Payne SA, Dean SJ, Kalus C: A comparative study of death anxiety in hospice and emergency nurses, *J Adv Nurs* 28:700–706, 1998.

Roth AJ, Breitbart W: Psychiatric emergencies in terminally ill cancer patients, *Hematol Oncol Clin North Am* 10:235–259, 1996.

Sulmasy DP: Commentary: double effect—intention is the solution, not the problem, *J Law, Med Ethics* 28:26–29, 2000.

MAJOR TOPICS
Invasive Hemodynamic Monitoring Basics
Concepts
Types of Monitoring Systems
Pressure Monitoring System Components
Obtain Accurate Data
Setting Up Pressure Monitoring System with
Transducer

Leveling the Transducer and Zeroing the Monitor
Complications
Specific Pressure Monitoring Systems
Central Venous Pressure Monitoring
Arterial Pressure Monitoring
$SCVO_2$, SVO_2 Monitoring
Passive Leg Raise Monitoring
Intracranial Pressure Monitoring

I. Invasive Hemodynamic Monitoring Basics

Critically ill patients have dynamic and rapidly changing profiles that require monitoring parameters beyond the physical examination, imaging, and laboratory results. The practice of placing devices into the vascular system or the brain allows the bedside clinician to rapidly and accurately identify and manage changes as they occur in the patient. Hemodynamic monitoring is the process by which the interrelationship of blood pressure, heart rate, vascular volumes, ventricular function, and other physical properties of blood are measured. Analysis of the hemodynamic parameters assists the nurse in assessing the accuracy of circulation, perfusion, and oxygenation of the body. Whenever possible, consent should be obtained prior to performing these invasive procedures.

A. CONCEPTS

1. Cardiac output
   a. Cardiac output (CO) is the amount of blood pumped by the ventricles each minute. This value is based on body size; cardiac index is the value that has been adjusted for a person's body surface area (BSA). Factors affecting CO include diastolic filling, heart rate, stroke volume, contractility, fiber stretch, preload, afterload, ventricle pressure, and ventricular size and wall thickness.
   b. The calculation for CO is stroke volume (SV) × heart rate.
2. Frank-Starling law of the heart (see Fig. 6.1)

   a. The force of heart contractions is related to the myocardial fiber stretch prior to contraction. The contractile force increases as the fibers are stretched, but only to a certain point. After that, there is ventricular failure as the fibers are unable to stretch any further
3. Pascal's law
   a. A pressure change at any given point in a confined fluid space results in a similar pressure change to the entire fluid volume
   b. In a fluid-filled tube, pressure at both ends of the tube is equal
4. Preload and afterload
   a. Preload is determined by venous return to the heart. It is affected by venous constriction and dilation, and total blood volume
   b. Preload can decrease during hypovolemia, trauma, hemorrhage, diuresis, vomiting and diarrhea, third spacing (ascites, sepsis, congestive heart failure), and diaphoresis. Preload increases with administration of fluids and venous constriction
   c. Afterload is the resistance to ventricular emptying during systole where the ventricle must overcome the pressure to open the aortic and pulmonary valves to pump blood into the vasculature. This is affected by the length of the vessel, the viscosity of the blood, vasoconstriction of the vasculature, and any obstructions to the outflow tract
   d. Increased afterload causes include aortic/pulmonic stenosis, hypothermia, hypertension, and the presence of vasoconstrictors. Decreased afterload can

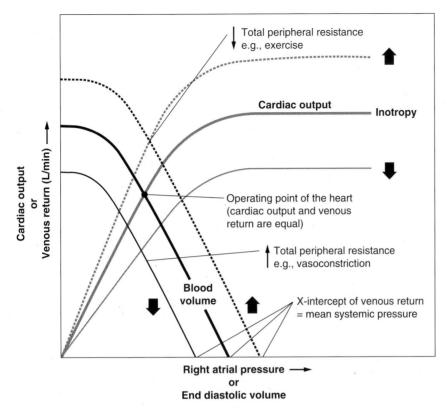

FIG. 6.1 Frank Starling curve. Cardiac output is dependent upon the interrelationship of venous return and cardiac function (Starling curve) so that blood entering the right heart (venous return) will equal blood leaving the left heart (cardiac output). The intersection point of these curves will vary according to the quantity of venous return and cardiac output. For example, in hypovolemia, reduced venous return places the patient on the steep rising part of the Starling curve. In hypervolemia, a patient will be on the flatter part of the Starling curve. Other factors such as vasodilation, change in contractility, and increased sympathetic stimulation or exercise will also shift the intersection point of the curves. *(From Lough, M. E. [2016].Hemodynamic monitoring: Evolving technology and clinical practice. St. Louis, MO: Elsevier.)*

occur during shock states, hypovolemia, and in the presence of vasodilatory medications
5. Pressure signal transmission
    a. Pressure changes in a vessel can be sent through fluid-filled tubing to a monitor and displayed as a numeric value, waveform, or both

B. TYPES OF MONITORING SYSTEMS

1. Fluid system with transducer, amplifier, and monitor
    a. The transducer receives pressure signals and converts to electronic signals
    b. The amplifier enhances transducer-generated signals and filters out unwanted artifact
    c. The monitor displays amplifier-enhanced signals on an oscilloscope
        1) Vertical axis represents pressure
        2) Horizontal axis moves with time
    d. Used for central venous pressure (CVP), arterial, pulmonary artery (PA), and intracranial pressure (ICP) monitoring (Fig. 6.2)
    e. Newer models have an integrated digital display and do not require a pressure bag system
2. Bioreactance monitoring system: Uses alternating current to measure phase shift to determine fluid responsiveness. This measurement translates to stroke volume; along with heart rate, the system can provide cardiac output readings
3. Fiberoptic monitoring systems (Fig. 6.3)
    a. Pressure signal is sent by fragile fiberoptics to monitor

b. Increased accuracy and decreased complexity compared with transducer system
c. Currently used primarily for ICP monitoring

C. PRESSURE MONITORING SYSTEM COMPONENTS

1. Catheter: provides access to patient's vessels/brain for monitoring pressure
2. Stopcock(s) (Fig. 6.4)
    a. Allows clinician to isolate infusing fluid and transmit pressure signals directly from vessel to transducer
    b. Allows flush solution to flow continuously and reduces the risk of clot formation at catheter tip
    c. Allows clinician to open system to atmospheric pressure for zeroing
    d. Allows blood to be withdrawn from vessel without dilution from flush solution
        Note: Review the directions of stopcocks to open/close because they vary among manufacturers.
    e. Allows the clinician to close the ICP system during transport to stop any overdrainage while the patient is being moved
3. Rigid pressure tubing (for fluid-filled transducer system): optimizes physiologic signal transmission
    a. Compliant tubing distorts pressure signals and causes overdamped tracings
    b. Long tubing also distorts tracing; allow no greater than 4 feet of tubing between catheter and transducer

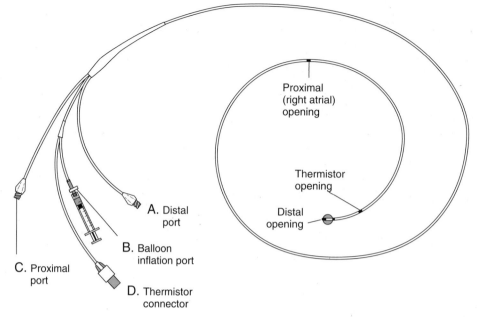

FIG. 6.2 **The 7-French quad-ruple-lumen, thermodilution pulmonary artery catheter.** *(From Darovic, G. O. [2004]. Handbook of hemodynamic monitoring [2nd ed.]. Philadel-phia, PA: Saunders.)*

A. Distal port

B. Balloon inflation port

C. Proximal port

D. Thermistor connector

Proximal (right atrial) opening

Thermistor opening

Distal opening

4. Flush device with capillary restrictors: keeps system patent by allowing a continuous flow of solutions through line
   a. Capillary restrictor limits flow of solution
   b. An activator (fast flush device) can bypass the re-strictor to allow rapid flow of flush solution through line (e.g., while priming the line and to clear line after blood draws)
5. Dead-end caps (nonvented): maintain sterility of stop-cock ports
6. Transducer: senses physiologic pressure signals and converts them to an electrical signal with proportion-ate changes
7. Monitor and amplifier: creates readable signals, filters out unwanted artifact and displays waveform on oscil-loscope
8. Flush solution: keeps line patent
   a. Transducer system
      1) 300 mm Hg pressure overcomes resistance of pressure tubing and allows a continuous flush at 1 to 5 mL per hour and prevents backflow
      2) Normal saline used for pressurized fluid
9. Pressure-infuser bag or cuff: capable of providing 300 mm Hg pressure

D. OBTAIN ACCURATE DATA

The clinician must take measures to ensure that the data obtained from invasive monitoring systems are accurate and reflective of the patient's physiologic status. Box 6.1 identifies the characteristics of a reliable monitoring system. Other variables to consider are patient position, height of the transducer, zero referencing, and dynamic response testing.

1. Dynamic response testing: a means to assess the trans-ducer's ability to accurately reproduce variations in the patient's vascular pressures

   a. Activate the fast flush device and observe the char-acteristics of the waveform produced on the monitor
   b. Resulting waveform (Box 6.2) described as
      1) Optimally damped
      2) Overdamped
      3) Underdamped

E. SETTING UP PRESSURE MONITORING SYSTEM WITH TRANSDUCER

(See CVP section for water manometer setup and ICP sec-tion for fiberoptic setup.)

Note: Individual systems may have specific require-ments. Always review manufacturer's guidelines to ensure that all requirements are met.

1. Turn monitor on; some monitors require time to warm up
2. Gather supplies specific to type of system being used and physician request
3. Exchange vented caps on stopcocks with dead-end caps to ensure sterility
4. Close roller clamp on tubing and turn stopcocks OFF to side ports of system
5. Insert tubing spike into bag of flush solution. Fill drip chamber halfway. Open roller clamp and slowly flush solution through soft (pliable) portion of tubing up to transducer. Close roller clamp (or per institutional policy)
6. Attach pressure bag and inflate to 300 mm Hg to allow the line to be "primed" when the fast flush device is activated (or per institutional policy)
7. Open roller clamp. Activate fast flush device with a slow, steady squeeze or pull, depending on model. Flush entire line until all air is removed. Flushing too quickly can cause air to collect in system

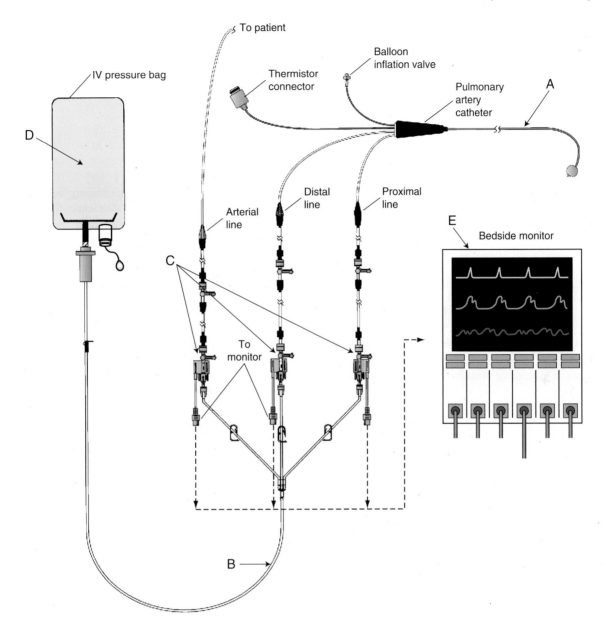

FIG. 6.3 Components of an invasive monitoring system (pulmonary artery catheter and designated arterial line) connected to one flush solution. **A,** Invasive catheter. **B,** Noncompliant pressure tubing. **C,** Transducer and zeroing stopcock. **D,** Pressurized flush system. **E,** Bedside monitoring system. (Not to scale.) *(From Sole, M. L. [2013]. Introduction to critical care nursing [6th ed.]. St. Louis, MO: Elsevier.)*

8. Flush each stopcock. At each stopcock
   a. Turn arrow OFF to distal portion (patient end) of line
   b. Open stopcock to air and point port upward (air rises)
   c. Activate fast flush device to flush stopcock port
   d. Replace cap, maintaining sterility
   e. Turn stopcock OFF to side port
9. Inspect entire line, transducer, and stopcock ports for air bubbles. If one is located, flush air out of closest port distal to bubble. Occasionally, the bubble will adhere to side of tubing. It can be released by slightly tapping the tubing

10. Set scale on monitor appropriate to device being used. Generally, the scale for CVP monitoring is 0–30 mm Hg and for arterial monitoring can be 0–200 mm Hg. Patients with lower blood pressures should have the scale set as close as possible to their range to ensure accurate measurement. This might warrant the scale be set as low as 0–100 mm Hg. Both scales should show the waveform clearly to ensure that the reading is being done closest to the patient's values. Also, the clinician will be able to view waveform characteristics if the range is set closely

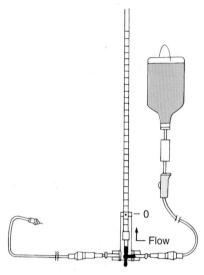

FIG. 6.4 The stopcock is turned to fill the manometer to 25 cm H$_2$O. *(From Roberts, J., & Hedges, J. [2004].* Clinical procedures in emergency medicine *[4th ed.]. Philadelphia, PA: Saunders.)*

Box 6.1

Characteristics of a Reliable Monitoring System

The system should be as simple as possible. Extra stopcocks and manifolds decrease the fidelity of the monitoring system and increase the risk of fluid leak, microbial line contamination, and air bubble collection.

All connecting tubing should be of low compliance (stiff) and no longer than 3–4 feet. Low-compliance tubing is identified on packaging as "monitoring tubing."

Tubing connectors should be tight. Use Luer-Lok connections, and inspect frequently for fluid leaks.

The catheter and connection tubing must be patent. Use a continuous flush device for cardiovascular pressure monitoring, and inspect frequently to see that the pressure bag is inflated to 300 mm Hg.

The system must be free of air bubbles or clots. Even pinpoint air bubbles decrease the fidelity of monitoring systems.

Keep the connecting tubing away from areas of patient movement. Jostling of tubing results in an externally induced whip artifact.

From Davoric, G. O. (2004). *Handbook of hemodynamic monitoring* (2nd ed.). Philadelphia, PA: Saunders.

Box 6.2

Dynamic Response Testing (Square Wave, Frequency Response Testing) Using the Fast Flush System

Optimally Damped System

When the fast flush of the continuous flush system is activated and quickly released, a sharp upstroke terminates in a flat line at the maximal indicator on the monitor and hard copy. This is then followed by an immediate rapid downstroke extending below baseline with just one or two oscillations within 0.12 second (minimal ringing) and a quick return to baseline. The patient's pressure waveform is also clearly defined, with all components of the waveform, such as the dicrotic notch on an arterial waveform, clearly visible.

Intervention: There is no adjustment in the monitoring system required.

Overdamped System

The upstroke of the square wave appears somewhat slurred, the waveform does not extend below the baseline after the fast flush, and there is no ringing after the flush. The patient's waveform displays a falsely decreased systolic pressure and false high diastolic pressure as well as poorly defined components of the pressure tracing, such as a diminished or absent dicrotic notch on arterial waveforms.

Intervention: To correct for the problem:

1. Check for the presence of blood clots, blood left in the catheter after blood sampling, or air bubbles at any point from the catheter tip to the transducer diaphragm and eliminate these as necessary.
2. Use low-compliance (rigid), short (less than 3–4 feet) monitoring tubing.
3. Connect all line components securely.
4. Check for kinks in the line.

Underdamped System

The waveform is characterized by numerous amplified oscillations above and below the baseline after the fast flush. The monitored pressure wave displays false high systolic pressure (overshoot), possibly false low diastolic pressure, and "ringing" artifacts on the waveform.

Intervention: To correct the problem, remove all air bubbles (particularly pinpoint air bubbles) in the fluid system; use large-bore, shorter tubing; or use a damping device.

From Davoric, G. O. (2004). *Handbook of hemodynamic monitoring* (2nd ed.). Philadelphia, PA: Saunders.

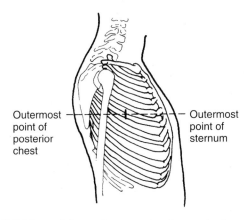

FIG. 6.5 The midchest reference point for monitoring circulatory pressures. This is a point midway between the outermost portion of the anterior and posterior surfaces of the chest and under the sternal angle of Louis. *(From Darovic, G. O. [2004]. Handbook of hemodynamic monitoring [2nd ed.]. St. Louis, MO: Mosby.)*

In the figure: "Outermost point of posterior chest", "Outermost point of sternum"

F. LEVELING THE TRANSDUCER AND ZEROING THE MONITOR

1. Ensure accurate pressure readings by aligning the pressure transducer on the same vertical plane as the catheter tip
   a. The phlebostatic axis is the reference point used to estimate the level of the in situ catheter. It is identified as the point midway between the anteroposterior chest wall at the fourth intercostal space (Fig. 6.5)
   b. Use a level device to ensure that the transducer is in line with the phlebostatic axis. The leveling point should be communicated during clinician hand-off to minimize changes in measurements
   c. When the level of the transducer is at the phlebostatic axis, the hydrostatic pressure effects are nil
2. Zeroing. Physiologic pressures are interpreted relative to atmospheric pressure (Note: for water manometer zeroing, see CVP section; for fiberoptic system, see ICP section.)
   a. To zero the transducer system to atmospheric pressure, accurately align the transducer with the reference point identifying the phlebostatic axis
      1) For every inch the transducer is below the correct reference point, the pressure reading will be 2 mm Hg greater
      2) For every inch the transducer is above the correct reference point, the pressure reading will be 2 mm Hg less
   b. Turn the stopcock next to the transducer OFF to the patient and open to the sideport
   c. Remove the sterile cap to open the sideport to air (atmospheric pressure)
   d. Follow the manufacturer's guidelines to zero the monitor
   e. Replace the cap on the sideport, maintaining sterility
   f. Turn the stopcock OFF to the sideport and open to the patient

G. COMPLICATIONS

There are many potential risks associated with invasive hemodynamic monitoring. The clinician is responsible for using appropriate techniques to prevent complications as well as for continuously monitoring for the development of these adverse consequences.

1. Local and systemic infectious complications
   a. Sterile technique during insertion is mandatory
   b. The Centers for Disease Control and Prevention has issued Guidelines for the Prevention of Central Line Associated Blood Stream Infections[1] with recommendations for catheter type, entry site, catheter length, and replacement of catheters, tubing systems, and dressings
2. Bleeding back into the system
   a. Prevented by maintaining a forward flow within the system and ensuring that there are no leaks in the setup (e.g., loose connections or stopcocks in the wrong position)
3. Thrombus formation
   a. Catheters can form a thrombus after insertion due to platelet adherence. Clearing catheter obstructions such as a fibrin sheath that can form within 5–7 days of insertion can be done with thrombolytic agents per institution protocol
   b. Troubleshooting
      1) Table 6.1 summarizes possible solutions to common problems associated with pressure monitoring systems

II. Specific Pressure Monitoring Systems

A. CENTRAL VENOUS PRESSURE MONITORING

1. Basic function
   a. CVP represents the pressure in the vena cava and right atrium (RA)
   b. Represents RA filling pressures (preload) and reflects right ventricular (RV) function in the absence of tricuspid disorder
2. Indications and contraindications
   a. Monitor volume status
   b. Assess RV function
   c. No specific contraindications
3. Parameters measured
   a. CVP; normal 6–10 mm Hg. Patients on ventilators will have higher CVP values due to positive pressure in the intrathoracic cavity. Septic patients may have a goal of 8–12 mm Hg for their CVP depending on institution protocol and patient tolerance. High CVP values in the absence of hypervolemia may be caused by cardiomegaly, left-sided heart failure, pulmonary hypertension, and cardiac tamponade

Table 6.1

Troubleshooting Pressure Monitoring Systems

**Always check patient first for signs of acute distress before troubleshooting the device.

Problem	Possible Causes or Solutions
No waveform	Check the power supply. Check the pressure range setting on the monitoring equipment. Check zero reference and calibration of the equipment. Check for loose connection in the pressure-monitoring line. Check to be certain that stopcocks are not turned off to the patient. Be certain that the connecting tubing is not kinked or compressed. It is possible that the catheter is occluded or has moved out of the vessel. If this is suspected, try to aspirate blood from the line. Blood clot has occluded the vessel. Note: Fast flushing the line may dislodge a loose clot and cause distal embolization. *Never use a syringe to aggressively flush any hemodynamic monitoring line.*
Artifact	Check for electrical interference. Check for patient movement. Catheter whip may be the problem (pulmonary artery catheters). Perform the dynamic response test to determine underdamping. Use an alternative method of measurement when possible, such as cuff arterial blood pressure monitoring.
Waveform drifting	Check to see whether a temperature change of intravenous solution (new flush bag hung) or environmental temperature change has occurred. Rezero the system.
Unable to flush line with the continuous flushing system	Check the stopcocks and tubing for kinks. Check to see that the pressure bag is inflated to the appropriate level. Reposition the catheter to move it away from the vessel walls or to remove catheter kinks. Gently aspirate with a syringe (do not apply excessive force to aspirate).
Reading too high	Check zero calibration. Check to see whether the transducer is located at the midchest level. Check the stopcocks and make certain they are open to the patient. Check the flow rate of the automatic flush device (flow too fast). The standard flush device delivers 3 microdrops per minute. Check for underdamping of the system. If it is caused by overshoot or undershoot artifact, track mean pressures.
Reading too low	Check to see whether the transducer is located at the midchest level. Check for loose connections and leaks. Check for air bubbles. Rezero and calibrate. Quickly evaluate the patient for shock.
Overdamped waveform	Check for air bubbles in the system. Check for kinks in the tubing. Check for blood in the system. Suspect possible occlusion at the catheter tip (i.e., thrombus), or the catheter tip may be resting against the vessel wall. Note: A term sometimes used for this phenomenon is high-pressure damping. This refers to a baseline that elevates and remains elevated, usually at the upper limit of the pressure monitoring range. This is invariably caused either by an electrical failure of the monitor amplifier or by total occlusion at some point in the fluid-filled line. Check the stopcocks, tubing, and catheter patency.

From Davoric, G. O. (2004). *Handbook of hemodynamic monitoring* (2nd ed.). Philadelphia, PA: Saunders.

4. Ongoing management
   a. Obtain and document CVP measurements as ordered by physician
   b. Trends in CVP values are often more indicative of a patient's condition than a single absolute value
   c. Administer medication, fluid, and other interventions as ordered in relation to CVP values

5. Complications
   a. Inaccurate CVP readings may be caused by
      1) Increased intrathoracic pressure (e.g., ventilator, coughing)
      2) Inconsistent use of appropriate reference point
      3) Malposition of central venous catheter
      4) Presence of air bubbles within system

B. ARTERIAL PRESSURE MONITORING

1. Basic function
   a. Insertion of catheter directly into an artery allows for continuous monitoring of arterial pressures as well as access to blood samples from the arterial system
   b. Theoretically, any artery can be utilized. Considerations in selection of site include
      1) Ease of access
      2) Presence of auxiliary circulation
      3) Presence of trauma or infection at desired site
      4) Need to immobilize site
      5) Size of catheter selected
      6) Risk for complications associated with selected site
2. Indications and contraindications
   a. Indications
      1) Continuous monitoring of arterial pressure in critically ill or injured patients or those with rapidly changing conditions
      2) Patients whose condition requires frequent access for blood samples, particularly from the arterial system
      3) Need for continuous mean arterial pressure (MAP) values (e.g., to calculate cerebral perfusion pressure or titrate vasoactive medications)
   b. Relative contraindications
      1) Patients with peripheral vascular disease
      2) Patients with bleeding disorders or those receiving anticoagulants or fibrinolytic agents
      3) Presence of infection over or near selected arterial site
   c. Absolute contraindications: clinicians must perform the Allen test to check for collateral circulation before inserting an arterial catheter
3. Parameters measured
   a. Systolic blood pressure (SBP); normal adult values 100–120 mm Hg
      1) Pressure increases with increasing distance from the aortic root
   b. Diastolic blood pressure (DBP); normal adult values 60–90 mm Hg
   c. MAP
      1) Can be calculated with the following formula: MAP = [(2 x diastolic)+systolic] / 3
      2) Calculated automatically by most monitors
      3) MAP remains consistent throughout the arterial circulation
   d. Because indirect (cuff) blood pressures and direct (arterial line) blood pressures are based on different variables (pressure versus flow), it is useful to obtain baseline correlations when the arterial line is first inserted
4. Waveforms
   a. Arterial waveforms have a sharp upstroke with a dicrotic notch representing the cardiac cycle transitioning from systole to diastole (Fig. 6.6)

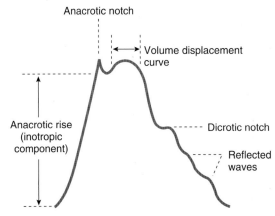

FIG. 6.6 The arterial waveform. Creation of the arterial pressure wave and acceleration of blood flow correlate with the inotropic upstroke. The rounded shoulder represents blood volume displacement and distention of the arterial walls. Normally, the peak of both the inotropic and volume displacement phases are equal in amplitude. The descending limb represents diastolic runoff of blood; the dicrotic notch separates systole from diastole. Additional humps on the downslope relate to pulse waves reflected from the periphery. *(From Darovic, G. O. [2004]. Handbook of hemodynamic monitoring [2nd ed.]. Philadelphia, PA: Saunders.)*

   b. Conditions that may affect the morphology of the arterial waveform are
      1) Dysrhythmias: premature beats have lower SBPs because of incomplete ventricular filling
      2) Hypertension: a rapid anacrotic rise and significantly enlarged phases throughout
      3) Hypotension: waveform appears damped, and dicrotic notch may not be appreciated
5. Ongoing management
   a. Obtain pressure readings as ordered
   b. Withdraw blood specimens as ordered for laboratory testing
      1) Select appropriate size syringe(s) for volume of blood to be withdrawn
      2) Gather appropriate size waste syringe per institutional protocol
      3) Follow institutional policy and procedure for blood withdrawal and blood gas retrieval
6. Complications
   a. Tissue ischemia or necrosis
   b. Infection
   c. Hemorrhage
   d. Accidental intraarterial drug injection

C. SCVO$_2$, SVO$_2$ MONITORING

1. Basic function
   a. Measures tissue perfusion at the cellular level. Other vital signs such as blood pressure and pulse oximetry do not reflect the actual gas exchange at organ and internal tissue levels
   b. Reflects values of oxygen demand (DO$_2$) and oxygen consumption (VO$_2$)

Part 1

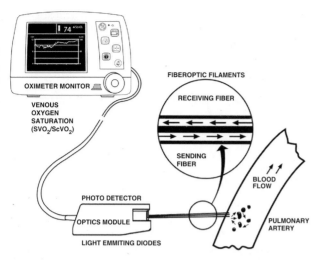

FIG. 6.7 Oximetry system with reflectance spectrophotometry. *(From Edwards Lifesciences LLC. [2002].* Understanding mixed venous oxygen saturation [SVO₂] monitoring using the Swan Ganz TD System *[2nd ed.]. Irvine, CA: Edwards Lifesciences.)*

c. SVO$_2$ is a true value obtained with a pulmonary catheter and reflects central venous oxygen saturation. ScVO$_2$ is a value of mixed venous oxygen saturation that is reflected from blood in the superior vena cava by a central line

d. Normal range values for SVO$_2$ are 60–80% and 70% for ScVO$_2$. ScVO$_2$ usually runs 7% higher than SVO$_2$ due to the blood mixing as it enters the right atrium

e. Low ScVO$_2$ values can indicate alterations in cardiac output, oxygen consumption, oxygenation, hemoglobin

2. Indications and contraindications
   a. Indications
      1) Assessment of end organ and tissue perfusion in septic patients
      2) Assessment of response to fluid resuscitation in septic patients
   b. Relative contraindications
      1) Coagulopathy
      2) Aortic dissection/aneurysm

3. Waveform measured
   a. ScVO$_2$: continuous waveform measurements available on commercial monitors (Fig. 6.7)

4. Ongoing management
   a. Assessment of values as fluid resuscitation and blood products are administered

5. Complications
   a. Complications are related to the central catheter and include but are not limited to infection, thrombus, pneumothorax, hemothorax, and coagulopathy

D. PASSIVE LEG RAISE MONITORING

1. Basic function
   a. Passive leg raise testing indicates whether cardiac output will increase with volume expansion. This

reversible maneuver mimics rapid volume expansion by shifting approximately 300 mL venous blood from lower limbs toward intrathoracic compartment

2. Indications and contraindications
   a. Indications: assessment of whether fluid expansion will help patients in hypovolemic shock and give indications as to the ability of the heart to respond
   b. Contraindications: patients with neurological injuries

3. Parameters measured
   a. If patient is fluid responsive, stroke volume index (SVI) will increase by 10% or greater as compared to its baseline. Specific monitor and devices are used for this procedure. Follow all hospital policies and equipment instructions
   b. Test is positive: SVI rises ≥10%: patient is fluid responsive
   c. Test is negative: SVI rises <10%; patient is not fluid responsive

4. Ongoing management
   a. Assessments will determine fluid resuscitation orders

5. Complications
   a. Due to nature of the procedure, no fluid is added and is therefore considered a reversible and safe test without complications in most critically ill patients

E. INTRACRANIAL PRESSURE MONITORING

1. Basic function
   a. ICP monitoring may be employed to calculate the cerebral perfusion pressure (CPP), an indicator of cerebral blood flow
   b. Various ICP monitors are available (Table 6.2)
   c. Use of extraventricular devices (EVDs) also allows for withdrawal of cerebral spinal fluid (CSF) as a means to control elevated ICP

2. Indications and contraindications
   a. Indications
      1) Severe head injury or ischemic cerebral event
      2) Anoxic event that may contribute to secondary cerebral injury
      3) To monitor interventions directed at managing patient's ICP/CPP
   b. Contraindications
      1) Severe coagulopathy
      2) Infections or open wound near planned insertion site

3. Parameters measured
   a. ICP: pressure exerted by intracranial contents; measured directly. Normal: 1–15 mm Hg
   b. CPP: pressure by which the brain is perfused; derived (CPP = MAP–ICP). Normal 60–85 mm Hg depending on treatment goals; 50 mm Hg minimum required to perfuse brain

4. Waveforms (Fig. 6.8)
   a. Waveforms produced by various devices are visually similar

Table 6.2

Comparison of Intracranial Pressure Monitors

Type	Site	Advantages	Disadvantages
Subarachnoid bolt	Subarachnoid space	Can be used with small or collapsed ventricles; does not penetrate brain parenchyma; low infection rates; low cost; ease and safety of insertion	Does not allow CSF drainage or withdrawal; becomes occluded; may dampen to give unreliable readings after a few days; brain tissue may herniate into bolt
Intraventricular catheter	Ventricles	Ventricular site provides more accuracy; CSF cultures can be collected; CSF can be withdrawn to control ICP; contrast materials can be injected for radiologic studies	Risk of hemorrhage; increased risk of infection; risk of CSF leak at site; artifacts may cause dampening of recordings; more difficult to insert
Epidural sensor	Epidural space	Ease of insertion; least invasive; recommended in case of meningitis and CNS infection; less risk of infection; does not require recalibration	Slower response time; fragile; can become wedged against skull; affected by heat or febrile patient; expensive; diaphragm can rupture; less accurate; unable to drain CSF

CNS, central nervous system; *CSF,* cerebrospinal fluid; *ICP,* intracranial pressure.
From Barker, E. (2002). *Neuroscience nursing: A spectrum of care* (2nd ed.). St. Louis, MO: Mosby.

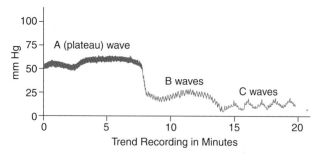

FIG. 6.8 Intracranial pressure waves. Composite diagram of A (plateau) waves, B (sawtooth) waves, and C (small, rhythmic) waves. *(From Barker, E. [2007]. Neuroscience nursing [3rd ed.]. St. Louis, MO: Mosby.)*

    b. Fluctuations with respirations and heartbeats are normal
5. Ongoing management
    a. Measure pressure and calculate CPP at intervals ordered by physician
    b. Drain excess cerebrospinal fluid and/or blood as ordered by physician; check ICP level at regular intervals per institution protocol to minimize the risk of overdrainage
    c. Maintain strict aseptic technique when accessing system
    d. Monitor for signs and symptoms of infection
6. Complications
    a. Infection
    b. Iatrogenic epidural hematoma
    c. Occlusion of ventricular catheter
    d. Fracture of fiberoptic catheter

Bibliography

American Association of Critical Care Nurses, Chulay M, Burns SM: *AACN essentials of critical care nursing,* New York, NY, 2006, McGraw-Hill, Medical Publication Division, pp 65–109.

Centers for Disease Control: Guidelines for the prevention of intravascular catheter-related infections. Retrieved from http://www.cdc.gov/hicpac/pdf/guidelines/bsi-guidelines-2011.pdf, 2011.

Cheetah Medical: How it works. Retrieved from http://www.cheetah-medical.com/how-it-works, 2013.

Cheetah Medical: Passive leg raise protocol with the Cheetah Nicom system. Retrieved from http://files.cheetahmedical.net dna-/JADXGHEm_jezvAwdq2-xuNWCvnJCk6jZ0dE3flB6kb I/mtime:1398868310/sites/default/files/PLR_Challenge_F.pdf, 2013.

Lifesciences Edwards: Quick guide to cardiopulmonary care. Retrieved from http://ht.edwards.com/scin/edwards/sitecollecti onimages/products/mininvasive/ewquickguide2ed.pdf, 2010.

Marschall J, Mermel LA, Fakih M, Hadaway L, Kallen A, O'Grady NP, Yokoe DS. Strategies to prevent central line–associated bloodstream infections in acute care hospitals: 2014 update, *Infect Control Hosp Epidemiol* 35(7):753–771, 2014. Retrieved from http://doi.org/10.1086/676533.

Medscape: Intracranial pressure monitoring. Retrieved from http://emedicine.medscape.com/article/1829950-overview, 2015.

Pittman JAL, Ping JS, Mark JB: Arterial and central venous pressure monitoring, *Int Anesthesiol Clin* 42(1):13–30, 2004, Winter. Retrieved from http://journals.lww.com/anesthesiaclinics/Citation/2004/04210/Arterial_and_Central_Venous_Pressure_Monitoring.4.aspx.

Prabhakar H, Sandhu K, Bhagat H, Durga P, Chawla R: Current concepts of optimal cerebral perfusion pressure in traumatic brain injury, *J Anaesthesiol Clin Pharmacol* 30(3): 318–327, 2014, July-September. http://dx.doi.org/10.4103/0970-9185.137260.

CHAPTER 7
Organ and Tissue Donation

Arnitha Lim, BSN, MBA, RN, CNOR, CTBS
Karen Cameron, RN, BSN, CPTC, CTBS
Rebecca Reilly, BS, CTBS

I. Overview

Each year in the United States, approximately 1 million tissue transplants are performed.[1] In 2014, according to statistics from the U.S. Department of Health and Human Services, there were 29,532 organs transplanted with 123,851 people on the waiting list for organs.[2] However, an average of 22 people die each day waiting for transplants that cannot take place because of the shortage of donated organs.[3] More than 1 million tissue transplants are done each year and the surgical need for tissue has been steadily rising. Each year, approximately 30,000 tissue donors save and heal lives. Although health care

advancements, medicine, and preservation techniques for organ and tissues have improved along with public education and awareness, there remains a critical shortage of lifesaving organs and tissue. Fig. 7.1 shows the widening gap between organs needed and those on the waiting list. Tables 7.1 and 7.2 describe organs transplanted by age group. For organ donation, there are two primary sources of transplantable organs: deceased (cadaveric) donors and living donors. Deceased donors account for most of the organs transplanted. The limiting factor in the provision of successful transplantation remains donor availability. Waiting time for an organ can vary by region and organ type. Recipient wait time may range from months to years.

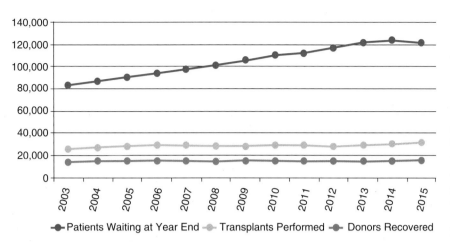

FIG. 7.1 Gap between organ donors, organ transplants, and organ waiting list. *(From U.S. Department of Health and Human Services. [2016]. Organ Procurement and Transplantation Network: Liver allocation and distribution policy. Available at* https://optn.trans plant.hrsa.gov/.)

Table 7.1

Organ Donors, Transplants, and Waiting List

Year	Organ Donors*	Organ Transplant	Organ Waiting List
1991	6,953	15,756	23,198
2001	12,702	24,239	79,524
2011	14,149	28,539	112,816
2012	14,011	28,054	117,040
2013	14,257	28,954	121,272
2014	14,412	29,532	123,851

*Including living and deceased donors
Data retrieved from http://organdonor.gov/about/data.html.

Table 7.2

Eye Donors and Transplants

Year	2013	2014
Total number eye and cornea donors	62,274	65,558
Corneas transplanted*	68,526	72,013

*Intermediate-term preserved corneas
From Eye Bank Association of America Statistics, http://restoresight.org/who-we-are/statistics/.

Changes in medical technology as well as in governmental legislation are making donation a more common occurrence in the emergency department. Emergency nurses are positioned to play an influential role in helping to support families through the donation decision-making process. A health care provider's personal perspective on organ and tissue donation does influence his or her professional practice.[4] Because of this, it is imperative that emergency department nurses not impose their own beliefs surrounding organ and tissue donation onto the organ and tissue donation process. A patient who is a candidate for organ donation may arrive to the emergency department with a catastrophic brain injury secondary to trauma, stroke, or anoxia. The role of the emergency team is to stabilize the patient hemodynamically as well as maintain perfusion and oxygenation, thus preserving the life of the patient and the opportunity for donation. Often the emergency staff may not realize that, in providing the highest quality of care in the presence of a devastating brain injury, the life of the patient may be lost, thus creating an opportunity for a family to choose donation and possibly saving the lives of seven organ recipients and countless numbers of tissue recipients and restoring sight to two cornea recipients.

II. Legislation and Regulation

A. UNIFORM ANATOMICAL GIFT ACT (UAGA)

1. The first legislation passed to affect transplantation
2. Established donor cards and designated a hierarchy of next of kin that provided consent for organ, tissue, and eye donation
3. The most recent revision (2013) changed the language from "consent" to "authorization" and
   a. Identifies who can give authorization for donation
      1) Recognizes the rights of individuals to choose the disposition of their body without requiring agreement or consultation with family members
      2) Identifies the rights of donor families
      3) Identifies that disposition is not limited to the purpose of transplantation
      4) Allows a person to donate his or her body or any part of the body for transplantation, medical education, or medical research
   b. Provides instruction as to how authorization should be obtained
   c. Allows for directed donation, meaning the family has the right to request that an organ or tissue be made available to a specific person
      1) Further legislative support at the state and federal levels followed the UAGA, which vary from state to state. Each state has the ability to amend their respective UAGAs

B. UNIFORM DETERMINATION OF DEATH ACT (UDDA)

1. Proposed in 1980 by the American Bar Association, the American Medical Association, the National Conference of Commissioners on Uniform State Laws, and the President's Commission for the Study of Ethical Problems in Medicine and Biomedical and Behavioral Research
2. Defined death as
   a. Irreversible cessation of circulatory and respiratory function, or
   b. Irreversible cessation of all functions of the brain, including the brainstem
3. Allows individual states or specific hospital policy to determine practice

C. OMNIBUS RECONCILIATION ACT OF 1986

1. Referred to as "Required Request," this act was created to support the rights of survivors to have an opportunity to choose organ/tissue and/or eye donation
2. The goal of this legislation was to increase the awareness of hospital personnel regarding their responsibility concerning the rights of individuals to either donate any part of their body, or to decline such donation
3. For a hospital to participate in Medicare reimbursement programs it must
   a. Develop and implement policies that identify potential donors
   b. Inform patients and families about donation
4. This particular aspect of the law caused a great deal of stress on hospital personnel, many of whom were reluctant to engage in such conversations with a bereaved family sensing it would be perceived as cruel or insensitive
5. The expectation of an increase in donor numbers as a result of this law was not realized because many health care workers were reluctant to have this conversation
6. Some hospitals instituted policies that required that all patients be asked about donation upon admission to the hospital
7. This approach also had a negative effect on donation rates leading to fear and mistrust of medical institutions across the country

D. NATIONAL ORGAN TRANSPLANT ACT (NOTA)

1. Passed in 1984 and established a national task force on organ transplantation to deal with the medical, legal, ethical, and financial issues surrounding organ donation and transplantation
2. NOTA required the formation of a national Organ Procurement and Transplantation Network (OPTN)
   a. The OPTN is responsible for maintaining the following through a federal contract holder
      1) Waiting list
      2) National system of sharing/matching
      3) Registry for transplant recipients
      4) Registry for bone marrow donors
3. NOTA is also responsible for
   a. Prohibiting the sale of human organs for transplantation
   b. Authorizing financial assistance for organ procurement organizations (OPOs)
   c. Requiring that OPOs be nonprofit entities
   d. Defining the service area of the OPO
   e. Requiring that OPOs be part of the OPTN
   f. Providing assistance for financial coverage of immunosuppressive drug therapy for transplant recipients during the first year following transplantation.

E. HEALTH CARE FINANCING ADMINISTRATION (HCFA)

1. HCFA founded in 1998
2. After implementation of the Omnibus Reconciliation Act, there was no significant increase in referral rates or donation rates
3. In an effort to make improvements in this area, it focused on increasing the number of referrals made to OPOs
4. This ruling required hospitals that receive Medicare funding to
   a. Notify the OPO when a patient has died or death is imminent
   b. Allow the OPO to determine medical suitability for donation
   c. Work with the OPO to initiate a discussion of donation with family of the potential donor
   d. Allow the OPO to have the donation discussion with family
   e. Allow the OPO to provide education to medical staff on donation-related issues
   f. Allow for a medical record review of all deaths to help improve identification and referral process for the hospital
5. Regulatory agencies[5]
   a. Federal oversight is managed under umbrella of the U.S. Department of Health Resources and Services Administration (HRSA) with collaboration from
      1) Centers for Medicare and Medicaid Service (CMS)
      2) Centers for Disease Control and Prevention (CDC)
      3) National Institutes of Health (NIH)
      4) Agency for Healthcare Research and Quality (AHRQ)
      5) Food and Drug Administration (FDA)
   b. Organ donation has further oversight from these regulatory agencies
      1) United Network for Organ Sharing (UNOS)
      2) Association of Organ Procurement Organizations (AOPO)
      3) Additional state, county, local oversight

   c. Tissue donation has additional oversight from these regulatory agencies
    1) American Association of Tissue Banks (AATB)
    2) Eye Bank Association of America (EBAA)
    3) Additional state, county, local oversight
  6. Donor designation
    a. Since the inception of the UAGA, the donor card has been available and was the equivalent to permission for donation for transplantation, medical education, and research of organs, tissues, and eyes
    b. Many times the survivors were caught up in the emotions of grief and pain, they overturned their loved one's desire to help others through the act of donation, and said no to the request of donation
    c. The majority of OPOs chose not to act on the information provided by the card and pursued permission from survivors of the decedent
    d. Since that time, each state has implemented donor designation laws that support the rights of individuals to make the choice of donation which cannot be overturned by their next of kin
    e. Much like a do not resuscitate (DNR) status, donor designation is defined by Donate Life America as a documented, legally authorized commitment by an individual to make an anatomical gift that cannot be revoked by anyone other than the registered donor

F. ROLE OF THE LOCAL OPO

1. Assist hospitals in creating policies and procedures for declaration of death
2. May advise on interventions consistent with maintaining a patient's organ function
3. Determines patients' eligibility and/or suitability for donation
4. Determines if the patient is on donor registry
    a. If the patient is not on the registry, an OPO representative has authorization for conversation with the family
    b. If the patient is on the registry, an OPO representative has informative conversation with family about donation
5. Manages the recovery, preservation, and transportation related to the donation
6. Reviews and arranges for
    a. Reimbursement of all hospital charges associated with the donation
    b. Recovery of all donated organs and/or tissue

III. Donation Opportunities

A. LIVING DONATION

1. The kidney is the most commonly transplanted organ from a living donor
2. Living liver donation, where a segment of the donor's liver is transplanted, occurs less often, and the donor is usually related to the recipient

3. Also, in rare cases, a segment of organs such as lung, intestine, or pancreas can be transplanted from a living donor[6]

B. DECEASED DONATION

1. Organ
    a. Heart beating: patient taken to OR on ventilator and ventilation continues until circulatory cessation (cross clamp)
    1) Death is declared by neurological criteria
    2) Patient remains on ventilator
    3) Patient requires hemodynamic support
    4) Organs that can be donated: heart, lungs, liver, pancreas, kidneys, intestine
    5) Can also donate tissue and eyes
    b. Donation after circulatory death (also referred to as non-heart-beating/asystolic)
    1) Patient is removed from vent support with an expectation that cardiac arrest will happen shortly thereafter
    2) Death is declared by cardio/pulmonary criteria
    3) Recovery of organs begins after declaration of death
    4) Organs that may be donated: kidneys, liver, lungs, pancreas
    5) Can also donate tissue and eyes
2. Tissue
    a. Tissue can be donated through both living donation and after circulatory death
    b. According to U.S. Department of Health and Human Services, examples of tissue donation by living donors are[5]
    1) Amnion
    2) Skin for autotransplant
    3) Bone after hip or knee replacements
    4) Blood
    5) Marrow
    6) Blood stem cells
    7) Umbilical cord blood
    c. Types of tissue donation after circulatory death that can be utilized for transplantation include but are not limited to
    1) Bone: can be used for repair of fractures, spine fusions, osteosarcoma, joint degradation
    2) Ligaments and tendons: can be used for tendon repairs such as anterior cruciate ligament repair
    3) Fascia: can be used for repair of bladder incontinence
    4) Cartilage: can be used to repair cartilage defects
    5) Ocular tissues (corneas and sclera): can be used to restore sight
    6) Skin: can be used on burn patients (split thickness skin) or post mastectomy and wound repairs (full thickness skin)

Part 1

7) Vascular grafts (veins and arteries): can be used on AV fistulas, open heart surgery with bypass grafts (CABG), and leg bypass surgeries to improve circulation
8) Pericardium: can be used for pericardial patches and open heart surgery reinforcement of anastomosis sites
9) Amniotic membrane: when used alone and without added cells, can help with ocular repair
10) Dura mater: can be used for dura repair
11) Heart valve allografts: can be used for HV replacement
12) Hematopoietic stem cells derived from peripheral or umbilical cord blood: can be used for stimulation of stem cell replacement for disease systems
13) Semen: can be used in vitro
14) Oocytes
15) Embryos

3. Ocular tissue
   a. Restoring sight to patients suffering from corneal blindness is made possible through cornea donation
   b. Eye bank facilitates this process
      1) U.S. eye banks provided 72,013 corneas for transplant in 2014 and provided a further 28,000 corneas for international transplant[7]
      2) The need remains large with 10 million cornea-blind individuals worldwide[7]

C. IMPACT OF DONATION ON MEDICAL RESEARCH

1. Organ and tissue
   a. Organ tissue, bones, tendons, skin, and other structural tissues are used in research studies and clinical trials (see Table 7.3)
   b. Authorization is required in same manner as for transplant
   c. Clinical studies are typically evaluated by a scientific advisory committee consisting of physicians, PhDs, and donor family representatives
   d. Most important criteria for studies is whether they will have a significant, positive impact and further the field of work
   e. Researchers at many prestigious learning institutions rely on donor tissue
   f. Before donor tissue was available for research, clinicians had access to nonhuman tissue only, which does not mimic the human body in how it behaves and reacts to stimuli
   g. Human tissue has a different structure which animal tissue cannot replicate
   h. Human tissue for modeling and testing allows for more accuracy in predicting how that tissue will respond to therapeutic and pharmacologic treatments

2. Eye
   a. Donated eye tissue can be used for research on many causes of blindness such as glaucoma, retinal disease, diabetes complications, and other sight disorders[7]
   b. Research can help lead to understanding the causes and disease progression and thus to cures and new treatments[7]

IV. Safety in Donation

A. INFECTIOUS DISEASE TESTING

1. All donors undergo testing prior to transplant
2. Infectious disease testing is performed in accordance with AOPO, FDA, and AATB guidelines at a CLIA-approved laboratory
3. Examples of testing performed
   a. HIV 1/HIV 2 antibody
   b. HIV-1 NAT
   c. HBc antibody (total, IgM, IgG)
   d. HBsAg
   e. HCV antibody
   f. HCV NAT
   g. Syphilis (*Treponema pallidum*)
   h. CMV
   i. EBV
   j. The presence of an infectious disease does not prevent donation; however, it can prevent transplantation[8]
4. Microbiological testing for tissue donation
   a. Presterilization cultures are established to represent all recovered tissues on a donor
   b. Results must be documented in donor record

B. TISSUES

1. Some OPOs maintain "tissue bio-repositories" with tissue samples
2. Tissues uses
   a. Evaluate effectiveness of screening kits
   b. Test donor matching methodologies
   c. Perform clinical trials

C. DONOR/RECIPIENT MATCHING

1. Polymerase chain reaction (PCR)
   a. PCR is used to match donor and recipient human leukocyte antigen (HLA)
   b. Donor and recipient HLA must match or the immune system will attack the tissue and/or organ and cause rejection
2. Virtual crossmatching
   a. Virtual crossmatching uses a computer to predict compatibility based on PCR results in fewer than 6 hours
3. Both technologies improve safety of match and speed up the process, thus saving lives of recipients on organ waiting lists

Table 7.3

Clinical Study/Research Using Donor Tissue

Study Title	Purpose	Tissue Type
Lung Tissue Repository	Evaluate the molecular and physiological mechanisms that cause a range of lung diseases, including asthma, COPD, and cystic fibrosis, with the ultimate goal of prevention.	Lung
Alcohol and Lung Transplantation: Understanding Donor and Recipient Consequences	Determine the effects of long-term alcohol use by donors on lung allograft recipients.	Lung and trachea
Ex-Vivo Lung Perfusion	Determine the effectiveness of ex-vivo lung perfusion on donor lungs with the goal of increasing lung tissue donation.	Lung
Calcium Cycling in the Human Heart	Understand normal heart functionality at the cellular level, what factors impact the pumping function of the heart and how changes in calcium cycling could increase vulnerability to arrhythmias in heart disease. Ultimate goal is to develop new treatments to prevent cardiac arrhythmias.	Heart
JNK Suppression of Connexin 43 Enhances A-fib in Aged Atria	Identify the pivotal role of a specific enzyme that helps lead to atrial fibrillation in aged atria, which will be used to understand how cardiovascular disease impacts older patients differently than younger patients.	Heart
Develop Competencies for Isolating Human Islet Cells for Eventual Transplantation	Test the hypothesis that islet transplantation in patients with established kidney transplants leads to a reduced risk of diabetes-related complications.	Pancreatic-islet cells
Pancreas and Islet Repository	Study the efficacy of islet cell transplantation to treat type 1 diabetes.	Pancreatic-islet cells
Protection Against Oxidative Stress in Islet Isolation	Better understand islet isolation techniques for transplantation.	Pancreatic-islet cells
Isolation of Human Facilitating Cells from Deceased Donor Bone Marrow	Develop methods to identify people who may not need immunosuppressive agents to prevent rejection of transplanted organs, thus eliminating the lifelong expense associated with taking antirejection medications.	Vertebrae
Normothermic Preservation in Deceased Donor Kidneys	Determine if normothermic preservation is a viable option for the "rescue and repair" of damaged donor kidneys. Goal is to increase the number of kidney transplantations using deceased donor kidneys.	Kidney
Studies of Pediatric Angiogenesis	Compare normal lymphatic tissues to lymphatic malformations to better understand the origins of vascular anomalies that develop in utero or shortly after birth.	Lymph Node
Peptide Therapy for Intervertebral Disc Degeneration and Low Back Pain	Determine if a specific treatment will be beneficial in decreasing inflammation and pain.	Lumbar Spine
Bone and Joint Tissue Repository	Evaluate the physiological structure of the joint system, how load and injury lead to osteoarthritis and other orthopedic conditions, and develop new treatments and medications for rheumatoid arthritis and other conditions.	Various Joint
Human Abdominal Wall Fascia for Validation of a Fine Element Model of a Novel Suture Design	Investigate an alternative suture design that may increase the strength of the surgical closure and decrease the incidence of postsurgical hernia formation.	Abdominal

From Gift of Hope Organ & Tissue Donor Network Connections Newsletter, Q3 2015.

V. Donation Referrals

A. DONATION REFERRAL CRITERIA

1. A living donation referral can be made based on
   a. Potential donor medical/social history
   b. Significant hypertension or hypotension or cardiac arrest
   c. Insulin-dependent diabetes
   d. Serum creatinine level greater than 1.5 mg; patients may have renal failure, which must be closely monitored for evaluation
   e. Alcohol and/or substance use/abuse
   f. Presence of infectious disease
   g. HIV and hepatitis are relative contraindicators to organ donation

 h. Screen for malignancy
 i. Previous surgical procedures
 j. Organ-specific function
2. A nonliving donation referral can be made based on
 a. No active cancer outside the central nervous system
 b. No HIV-positive result
 c. Age limit is dependent upon the local OPO, but typically there is none
3. In the case of impending death, the following strategies should be considered
 a. Plan to declare using neurological criteria
 b. Plan to remove life-sustaining therapies (DCD donor)
 c. Triggers as specified by the local OPO
4. In the case of cardiac death, a referral should be made as soon as possible after death is declared
5. When referring a donation, the following information should be shared
 a. Caller information
  1) Name of the hospital
  2) Unit name
  3) Caller contact information
 b. Patient demographics
  1) Reason for hospitalization
  2) Past medical history
  3) Summary of treatment modalities
 c. Family member and/or decision maker
  1) Contact information
  2) Level of engagement
  3) Describe their understanding of the situation
 d. In the case of cardiac death, note
  1) Time declared
  2) Current location of the body
6. The OPO should provide the following information
 a. Referral number
 b. Suitability for donation
 c. Donor designation
 d. Instructions of next steps

VI. OPO Donor Evaluation

A. ORGAN/TISSUE (SEE FIG. 7.2)

1. Role of emergency department personnel
 a. Frequently first to identify potential donor
 b. Immediate notification of OPO
 c. Support family through the organ donation process

B. EYE[7]

1. The eye bank has a short time frame within which to contact the donor family, obtain consent, and recover ocular tissue (typically, within 12 hours of death)
2. Of critical importance is obtaining contact information for the donor family

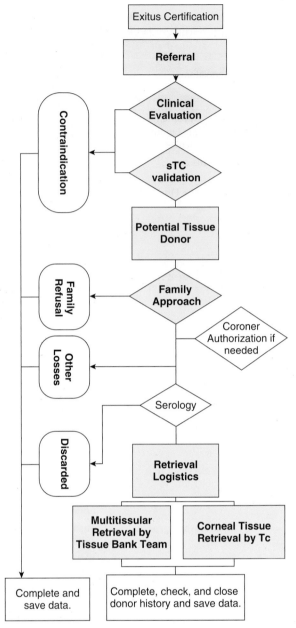

FIG. 7.2 Tissue Evaluation Process (*From Rodríguez, A., Sandiumenge, A., Masnou, N., … Pont, T. [2015]. Medical students for tissue procurement, a 10-year experience in a large university hospital: An exportable model? Transplantation Proceedings, 47[8], 2314–2317.*)

VII. Determination of Brain Death

A. GUIDELINES

1. Irreversible cessation of circulatory and respiratory functions (2% of all donors)
2. Irreversible cessation of all brain functions, including brainstem (98% of all donors)
3. Diagnosis of death requires both cessation of function and irreversibility

4. Confirmatory testing: potential donor must be on ventilator and have cause for underlying neurologic injury
5. Table 7.4 shows American Academy of Neurology's brain death declaration guidelines
6. See Table 7.5 for complicating conditions

Table 7.4

American Academy of Neurology Brain Death Declaration Guidelines

Phase	Activity
I	Clinical Evaluation Establish irreversible and proximate cause of coma Achieve normal core temperature Achieve normal systolic blood pressure Perform one neurological examination

II	Neurologic Assessment
	Coma
	    Must lack all evidence of responsiveness
	Absence of brainstem reflexes
	    Absence of pupillary response to bright light in both eyes
	    Absence of ocular movements using oculocephalic testing and oculovestibular reflex testing
	    Absence of corneal reflex
	    Absence of facial muscle movement to a noxious stimuli
	    Absence of the pharyngeal and tracheal reflexes
	Apnea
	    Absence of a breathing drive

III	Ancillary Tests Used in the case of uncertainty in the neurologic assessment or when apnea cannot be performed Preferred ancillary tests include EEG, cerebral angiography, nuclear scan, transcranial Doppler

IV	Documentation
	The documented time of death is either:
	    When the PCO_2 reached the targeted value, or
	    When ancillary test results are officially interpreted

From American Academy of Neurology Clinician Guideline Supplement, Update: Determining Brain Death in Adults, 2010.

Table 7.5

Conditions Complicating Determination of Brain Death*

Drug or metabolic intoxication	Barbiturates, alcohol, sedatives, neuromuscular blockade
Hypothermia	Core temperature less than 32°C or 90°F
Medical conditions	Severe electrolyte, acid-base, or endocrine instability

*Complicating conditions may mimic brain death. These conditions must be corrected before determination of brain death can be made.

VIII. Donor Family Authorization

The recommended practice is to separate the death notice conversation from the donation conversation. Donation should not be discussed unless the family understands that the patient is not going to survive or is dead.

A. CORE ELEMENTS FOR AUTHORIZATION

1. Name of the donor
2. Name, address, and telephone number of the authorizing person and his/her relationship to the donor
3. Explanation that the organ and/or tissue is a gift and that neither the donor's estate nor the authorizing person will receive monetary compensation or valuable consideration for said gift
4. Description of the general types of tissue to be recovered
5. Description of the permitted use(s) of the recovered tissues
   a. Transplant
   b. Therapy
   c. Research
   d. Education
6. Explanation that recovery of tissue requires the following actions and the Document of Gift/Authorization thus specifically authorizes
   a. Access to, and required disclosure of, the donor's medical and other relevant records
   b. Testing and reporting for transmissible diseases
   c. Removal of specimens for the purpose of determining suitability and/or compatibility of donor and recipient, which may include, but are not limited to
      1) Spleen
      2) Lymph nodes
      3) Blood samples
   d. Release to the tissue bank of any and all records and reports of a medical examiner, coroner, or pathologist
   e. Other requirements as may be applicable for the specific donation or tissue bank, such as transport of body, archiving of samples
   f. Contact information for the organization represented by the donation coordinator
   g. Any additional information required by laws or regulations

B. AUTHORIZING PERSON

1. Provide information to the authorizing person
   a. General description of the recovery such as timing, relocation of donor if applicable, contact information
   b. Explanation that costs directly related to the evaluation, recovery, preservation, and placement of tissues will not be charged to family
   c. Explanation regarding the impact the donation process may have on burial arrangements and appearance of the body

d. Explanation that a document of authorization is available
e. Any explanation required by law (e.g., multiple organizations [nonprofit and/or for profit] may be involved in facilitating the gift(s), reference to the possibility that tissue may be transplanted abroad) must be included
2. Qualifications for an authorizing person
  a. Health care agent or power of attorney (POA)[9]
  b. Spouse
  c. Adult children
  d. Parents
  e. Adult siblings
  f. Adult grandchildren
  g. Grandparents
  h. Adults who exhibited special care or concern
  i. Legal guardian
  j. Whomever the responsibility would lie with to dispose of the body
    1) Support family's decision whether or not they accept donation

IX. Interacting with and Supporting Donor's Family

A. ASSESS

1. Family's understanding of death
2. Family's cultural and religious belief systems
3. Role(s) of prospective donor in family
4. Meaning of death of loved one to family
5. Family's understanding of and feelings about organ or tissue donation
6. Meaning of donation to family
7. Wishes of prospective donor, if known

B. ADDITIONAL ANALYSIS

1. Additional analysis may be necessary and require differential nursing diagnoses and collaborative problem solving
  a. Dysfunctional family processes
  b. Anticipatory grieving
  c. Deficient knowledge
  d. Ineffective family coping

C. NEXT OF KIN

1. In the event the next of kin is unable to make a decision
  a. Support the decision, no matter what is decided
  b. Offer to make a referral to social worker, chaplain, and/or crisis intervention nurse
  c. Make referral to appropriate community agency
2. Donor's family will either meet a representative from the OPO in person at the hospital or receive a call from the OPO representative to explain donation options

X. Maintaining Viability of Potential Organ Donors

Once brain death is declared and authorization obtained, the emphasis shifts to supporting the viability of the organs being donated.

A. MAINTAIN ADEQUATE INTRAVASCULAR VOLUME

B. MAINTAIN NORMAL BLOOD PRESSURE (BP) AND NORMOTHERMIA

C. ESTABLISH DIURESIS

D. OPTIMIZE OXYGENATION AND ACID-BASE BALANCE

XI. Maintaining Viability of Potential Tissue/Ocular Donor

A. COOLING OF THE BODY

1. Through the morgue or by using ice bags

B. DOCUMENTATION

1. Document admission and course history with specific attention to
  a. Fluids and blood products administered
  b. Both actual IV sites and IV access (location) attempts
  c. Blood draw sites

C. COORDINATION

1. Coordinate with medical examiner and funeral homes

D. OCULAR TISSUE DONATION

1. Take actions to help preserve eye donation opportunity
  a. Elevate the head with bed or rolled towel
  b. Moisten eyes and close eyelids
  c. Cool eye area (not directly on the eyelids)
    1) Example: ice in glove on forehead

XII. Pre- and Posttransplantation Emergencies (see Chapter 25)

A. REJECTION AND INFECTION

1. Two major posttransplant emergencies for which patients seek treatment in an emergency department: rejection and infection
2. Rejection is the recognition and response to foreign donor antigens by the recipient's immune system

Table 7.6

Classification and Characteristics of Rejection Responses

	Hyperacute	Acute	Chronic
Time frame	Occurs within minutes to hours after graft	Occurs 1 week to 1 year after transplantation	Occurs over months to years after transplantation
Outcome	Rapid loss of organ function in vascular supply to graft	Accelerated deterioration in organ function	Gradual decrease in organ function resulting from progressive fibrotic changes
Immune response	Preformed antibodies react quickly to class I HLA (ABO) antigens from donor tissue; more prevalent in those with history of multiple transfusions or pregnancies	T-cell response (cellular immunity) and antibody system activated, producing inflammatory and immune responses to transfusions or pregnancies	Actual cause unknown; response may be T-cell action and immune system mediators, such as interleukins and lymphokines or prior transplant
Confirmation of Rejection	Tissue necrosis demonstrated by laboratory studies	Laboratory studies indicating loss of organ function; organ biopsy; symptoms may not appear until process is well advanced	Presence of infiltrates of inflammatory cells and vascular and tissue damage leading to organ failure; nonspecific inflammatory changes; specific changes related to graft type
Treatment	None; improved crossmatching and careful screening to reduce incidence	Immunosuppressive therapy; regular follow-up; extent of rejection determined by recipient's response to therapy	Retransplantation

a. Antigens can be part of the ABO system, HLA antigens, or antigens to which humans are exposed in daily life

b. Three classifications of rejection: hyperacute, acute, chronic (Table 7.6)

3. Infection can be bacterial, fungal, or viral

   a. Bacterial: usually seen during first 6 months

     1) Meningitis

     2) Pneumonia

   b. Fungal

     1) Candida

     2) Aspergillus

   c. Viral: usually seen 6 months after transplantation

     1) Cytomegalovirus (CMV)

     2) Herpes simplex or zoster

References

1. Donate Life America: Organ donation statistics. Retrieved from http://donatelife.net/statistics/, 2016.

2. U.S. Department of Health and Human Services: The gap continues to widen. Retrieved from http://www.organdonor.gov/about/graphdescription.html, 2016.

3. U.S. Department of Health and Human Services: The need is real: Data. Retrieved from http://organdonor.gov/about/data.html, 2016.

4. Marck CH, Weiland TJ, Neate SL, et al.: Personal attitudes and beliefs regarding organ and tissue donation: a cross-sectional survey of Australian emergency department clinicians, *Prog Transplant* 22(3), 2012, September. Retrieved from http://pit.sagepub.com/content/22/3/317.refs.

5. U.S. Department of Health and Human Services: Organ and tissue donation from living donors. Retrieved from http://www.organdonor.gov/about/livedonation.html, 2016.

6. United Network for Organ Sharing: Living donation. Retrieved from https://www.unos.org/donation/living-donation/, 2015.

7. Eye Bank Association of America: Facts & statistics. Retrieved from http://www.restoresight.org, 2016.

8. The American Association of Tissue Banks: Overview and updates; 13th edition of AATB. *Standards for Tissue Banking*. Retrieved from http://aatb.org/aatb/files/ccLibraryFiles/Filename/000000001206/AATB%20Standards%20for%20Tissue%20Banking%2013th%20edition%202-17-16.pdf, 2015.

9. Uniform Law Commission: The National Conference of Commissioners on Uniform State Laws: Anatomical Gift Act of 2006. Retrieved from http://www.uniformlaws.org/Act.aspx?title=Anatomical%20Gift%20Act%20(2006), 2016.

Bibliography

Illinois Anatomical Gift Act. (2014). 755 ILCS 50/.

Rodgers SG: Legal framework for organ donation and transplantation, *Nurs Clin North Am* 24(4), 1989, December.

Uniform Anatomical Gift Act: Retrieved from http://www.uniformlaws.org/shared/docs/anatomical_gift/uaga_final_aug09, 2009.

United Network for Organ Sharing: Retrieved from http://www.unos.org, 2016.

U.S. Department of Health and Human Services: Health Care Financing Act, *Federal Register* 63, 1998.

CHAPTER 8

Pain Management

Stephen J. Stapleton, PHD, MS, RN, CEN, FAEN

I. Pain Overview

Pain is a complex, subjective phenomenon often viewed as a warning sign indicating something is wrong. The International Association for the Study of Pain (IASP) defines pain as "an unpleasant sensory and emotional experience associated with actual or potential tissue damage, or described in terms of such damage."[1] Pain is one of the most common reasons people seek medical attention. Many patients present to the emergency department with moderate to severe pain and expect their pain to be relieved. Clinical findings often do not correlate well with the severity of the pain a patient perceives. Recognizing the subjectivity of the pain experience, emergency nurses play a critical role in the assessment and management of patients' pain.

II. Definitions

These definitions originate from the International Association for the Study of Pain.[1]

A. PAIN

1. An unpleasant sensory and emotional experience
2. Associated with actual or potential tissue damage or described in terms of such damage
   a. Acute pain: usually has a short duration and an identifiable cause such as trauma, injury, or a surgical procedure; tissue is damaged and the pain sensation serves as a warning to the body of an injury
   b. Chronic pain: lasts longer than the normal healing period (3–6 months); has no purpose and can exist without injury
   c. Cancer pain: a result of cancer, the spread of cancer, tumor growth, or side effects of cancer treatment (chemotherapy)
   d. Neuropathic pain: a type of chronic pain that is caused by an injury to a peripheral nerve or the CNS
3. Personal and subjective experience
   a. Can only be described by person experiencing pain
   b. Exists whenever the person says it does

B. ADDICTION

1. Behavioral pattern characterized by compulsively obtaining and using a substance
2. Results in physical, social, and psychological harm to user

C. ALLODYNIA

1. Pain caused by a stimulus not normally eliciting pain

D. CO-ANALGESICS

1. Medications with pain-relieving properties that are not primarily identified as an analgesic but in clinical practice demonstrate either independent or additive analgesic properties[2]

E. DEPENDENCE

1. Reliance on a substance
2. Abrupt discontinuance would cause impairment of function

F. PAIN MANAGEMENT

1. Comprehensive approach to needs of a patient who is experiencing problems associated with acute or chronic pain

G. PAIN THRESHOLD

1. Least level of stimulus intensity perceived as painful

H. TOLERANCE

1. Greatest level of discomfort a person is prepared to endure
2. Person requires increased amount of substance to achieve desired effect

I. SUFFERING

1. Physical or emotional reaction to pain
2. Feeling of helplessness, hopelessness, or uncontrollability

J. OLIGOANALGESIA[3-5]

1. A term used to describe the phenomenon of poorly managed or inadequate pain management
2. The undertreatment of pain

III. Pain Physiology

Emergency nurses need an understanding of basic physiology of pain to effectively assess, intervene, and evaluate patient outcomes.

A. NEUROANATOMY[6]

1. Afferent pathway
   a. Nociceptors (pain receptors) in the tissues respond to pleasant and painful stimuli
      1) Stimulation of nociceptors produces impulse transmission through fibers
         a) Small C fibers: unmyelinated; transmit burning and aching sensations; relatively slow. Often called *slow pain-wave* or *second pain*, due to the slower onset and longer duration, is typically caused by chemical stimuli or persistent mechanical or thermal stimulation
         b) Larger A-delta fibers: myelinated; transmit sharp and well-localized sensations; relatively fast. Often called *fast pain* or *first pain*, typically caused by mechanical or thermal stimulation
      2) Terminate in the dorsal horn of the spinal cord
         a) Transmission of impulses between peripheral nociceptive neurons and dorsal horn neurons in the spinal cord is mediated by neurotransmitters
            (1) Amino acids (e.g., glutamate)
            (2) Amino acid derivatives (e.g., norepinephrine)
      3) Modulate pain patterns in the dorsal horn
      4) Transmit impulses to midbrain via the neospinothalamic tract (acute pain) and to limbic system via the paleospinothalamic tract (dull and burning pain)
   b. Nociceptors translate noxious stimuli into signals that are transmitted by a dorsal root ganglion to the dorsal horn of the spinal cord
   c. Nociceptors respond to mechanical, thermal, chemical stimulation
      1) Mechanical stimuli are caused by intense pressure applied to the skin or from an extreme muscle stretch
      2) Extreme heat and cold stimulate nociceptors
      3) Chemical stimuli arise from chemical mediators released from injured and inflamed tissues, which either stimulate or sensitize nociceptors
      4) Chemical agents such as bradykinin, histamine, serotonin, and potassium, which act to sensitize nociceptors and the lowering of the activation threshold causing the transmission of afferent signals to the dorsal horn causing neurogenic inflammation, are released as a result of the inflammatory response
      5) Prostaglandins are other chemical mediators that may act alone or in concert with other mediators
2. Central nervous system
   a. Includes limbic system, reticular formation, thalamus, hypothalamus, medulla, cortex
   b. Arousal, discrimination, and localization of pain; coping response; release of corticosteroids; cardiovascular responses; modulation of spinal pain transmission
3. Efferent pathway
   a. Fibers connecting the reticular formation, midbrain, and substantia gelatinosa in the dorsal horn of the spinal cord

b. Afferent fibers stimulate the periaqueductal gray matter in the midbrain, which then stimulates the efferent pathway

c. Modulates or inhibits pain impulses

4. Neuromodulation

   a. Endorphins: a group of neuropeptides that inhibit pain transmission in the brain and spinal cord

     1) Beta-lipotropin: responsible for feeling of well-being

     2) Enkephalin: weaker than other endorphins but longer lasting and more potent than morphine

     3) Dynorphin: generally impedes pain impulse

     4) Endomorphin: very antinociceptive

     5) Opiate receptors

   b. Mu (μ) receptors on the membrane of afferent neurons inhibit the release of excitatory neurotransmitters

   c. Beta (β) receptors react with enkephalins to modulate pain transmission

   d. Kappa (κ) receptors produce sedation and some analgesia

   e. Sigma (σ) receptors cause pupil dilation and dysphoria

B. EFFECT OF MEDICATIONS ON MODULATING PAIN[7]

1. Stimulation of afferent pathways results in activation of circuits in supraspinal and spinal cord levels; each synaptic link is subject to modulation

2. Mechanisms of drug action

   a. Acetaminophen, effective analgesic without antiinflammatory or coagulation effects

     1) Inhibit prostaglandin synthesis in CNS

     2) Mechanism of action is not fully understood

     3) Caution when 2 g/day; consider acetaminophen in combination with OTC cold and fever medications and opioid analgesics such as codeine, hydrocodone, oxycodone

     4) When combined with NSAIDs, analgesic efficacy increases

   b. Aspirin

     1) Inhibits prostaglandin production, decreases platelet aggregation

     2) Produces analgesia and decreased inflammation

   c. NSAID: synthesized at the site of injury; inhibits prostaglandin synthesis, which reduces hyperalgesia

     1) Useful for nociceptive pain

     2) COX-2 selectivity reduces bleeding and GI effects

     3) May increase BP and cardiovascular risks

     4) Risks increase with age

   d. Opiates: interact with mu and kappa receptors; powerful effect on brainstem and periphery

     1) Recommended and effective for management of moderate to severe pain

   e. Corticosteroids

     1) Limited role in pain management

     2) Effectiveness found in acute and subacute pain related to tendon and synovial injuries and inflammatory processes

   f. Antidepressants (norepinephrine, serotonin, dopamine reuptake inhibitors) are shown to increase availability of norepinephrine and serotonin in the CNS

     1) Used in chronic pain conditions; role in acute pain is unclear

     2) Antidepressants that increase synaptic norepinephrine levels (tricyclic antidepressants, or TCAs) may be effective analgesics

     3) Anticholinergic side effects are common

     4) Dose-related QT prolongation occurs with TCAs

     5) An increased risk of suicide and mania may occur

   g. Anticonvulsants (sodium channel blockers)

     1) Lidocaine, carbamazepine, oxcarbazepine, and lamotrigine are effective in trigeminal neuropathy, diabetic peripheral neuropathy, HIV-related neuropathy, and MS

   h. Calcium channel blockers

     1) Gabapentin and pregabalin are effective for diabetic peripheral neuropathy and fibromyalgia

   i. Local anesthetics: block sodium channels and thus prevent transmission of nerve impulses

C. PAIN THEORIES[6,8]

1. Specificity theory

   a. Refers to presence of dedicated pathways for each somatosensory modality

   b. Specific sensation that is independent of other sensations

2. Intensity theory

   a. Defines pain as an emotion that occurs when a stimulus is stronger than usual, not as a unique sensory experience

3. Pattern theory

   a. Proposes that pain receptors share endings or pathways with other sensory modalities

   b. Different patterns of activity of the same neurons can be used to signal painful or nonpainful stimuli

4. Gate control theory[9]

   a. Nociceptors and touch fibers synapse in two different regions within dorsal horn of the spinal cord

   b. Modulations of inputs in the spinal dorsal horns and brain act as gating mechanism

   c. With a stimulus, a sequence of events occurs

     1) Pain impulse is transmitted via nociceptor fibers in the periphery to the substantia gelatinosa through large A-delta and small C fibers

     2) At the terminus of the nociceptive fibers, neurotransmitters such as substance P, adenosine triphosphate, and glutamate carry the impulse across the synapse to the dorsal horn

     3) A gating mechanism regulates transmission from the spinal cord to the brain, where pain is perceived

4) Stimulation of large fibers closes the gate and thus decreases transmission of impulses unless persistent
5) Stimulation of small fibers opens the gate and enhances pain perception
d. The spinal gating mechanism is also influenced by fibers descending from the brain
1) The conducting fibers carry precise information about the nature and location of the stimulus
2) Through efferent pathways, the CNS may close, partially close, or open the gate
3) Descending fibers release endogenous opioids that bind to opioid receptor sites and thereby prevent release of neurotransmitters such as substance P, thus inhibiting transmission of pain impulses and producing analgesia
4) Cognitive function can also modulate pain perception and individual's pain response
5. Neuromatrix theory[10]
a. A widespread network of neurons consists of loops between the thalamus and cortex and between the cortex and limbic systems; neural processes are modulated by stimuli from the body but can also act in the absence of stimuli
1) Stimuli trigger neural patterns but do not produce them
2) Cyclic processing of impulses produces characteristic pattern in the entire matrix that leaves a neurosignature
3) Signature patterns are converted to awareness of the experience and activation of spinal cord neurons to produce muscle patterns for action
b. Neural inputs modulate continuous output of the neuromatrix to produce a wide variety of experiences felt by the individual
1) Awareness of the experience involves multiple dimensions (e.g., sensory, affective, evaluative) simultaneously
2) Pain qualities are not learned but may be innately produced by neurosignature and interpreted by the brain

D. TYPES OF PAIN[6]

1. Acute pain (Table 8.1)

Table 8.1

Comparison of the Characteristics of Acute and Chronic Pain

Characteristic	Acute Pain	Chronic Pain
Experience	An event	A state of existence
Source	External agent or internal disease	Unknown or treatment unsuccessful
Onset	Usually sudden	Sudden or develops insidiously
Duration	Transient (up to 6 months)	Prolonged (months to years)
Pain identification	Painful and nonpainful areas generally well identified	Painful and nonpainful areas less easily differentiated; change in sensation becomes more difficult to evaluate
Clinical signs	Consistent with sympathetic fight-or-flight response • Increased heart rate • Increased stroke volume • Increased blood pressure • Increased pupillary dilation • Increased muscle tension • Decreased gastric motility • Decreased salivary flow	Absence of autonomic responses
Psychological component	Associated anxiety	• Increased irritability • Associated depression • Somatic preoccupation • Withdrawal from outside interests • Decreased strength of relationships
Significance	Informs person something is wrong	Person looks for significance
Pattern	Self-limiting or readily corrected	Continuous or intermittent; intensity may vary or remain constant
Course	Suffering usually decreases over time	Suffering usually increases over time
Actions	Leads to actions to relieve pain	Leads to actions to modify pain
Prognosis	Likelihood of complete relief	Complete relief usually not possible
Other types of responses		• Decreased sleep • Decreased libido • Appetite changes

Modified from Heuther, S., Rodway, G., & DeFriez, C. (2014). Pain, temperature, sleep, and sensory function. In S. Heuther & K. McCance (Eds.), *Understanding pathophysiology* (7th ed., pp. 485–495). St. Louis, MO: Elsevier: Mosby; Porth, C. M. (2015). Somatosensory function, pain, and headache. In C. M. Porth (Ed.), *Essentials of pathophysiology: Concepts of altered health states* (4th ed., pp. 854–879). Philadelphia, PA: Wolters Kluwer.

a. Elicited by injury to body tissues

b. Generally associated with trauma, acute illness, surgery, burns, or other conditions that are of limited duration; generally relieved when healing takes place

c. Diagnostic clues include the pain's location, radiation, intensity, and duration, along with factors that aggravate or relieve pain

2. Chronic pain (Table 8.1)

a. Pain is highly variable and persists longer than might be expected

b. May be perpetuated by factors remote from the original cause and extend beyond the expected healing time; generally lasts longer than 3 months

c. Biological factors contributing to chronic pain

1) Peripheral mechanisms result from persistent stimulation of nociceptors; for example, the inflammatory process where inflammatory mediators are released from injured tissue increase sensitivity of the C fibers leading to an increased duration of pain. Chronic musculoskeletal, visceral, and vascular disorders are examples.

2) Peripheral-central mechanisms caused by an abnormal functioning of the peripheral and central portions of the somatosensory system result from a partial or complete loss of descending inhibitory pathways or spontaneous firing of regenerate nerve fibers. Examples include causalgia, phantom limb pain, and postherpetic neuralgia.

3) Central mechanisms associated with disease or injury to the CNS and characterized by burning, aching, hyperalgesia, dysesthesia; may be superficial (skin) or deep (bone or muscle) pain.

3. Nociceptive pain

a. Represents the normal response to noxious insult or injury of tissues such as skin, muscles, visceral organs, joints, tendons, or bones

1) Somatic pain: arises from skin, muscle, joint, connective tissue, or bone; generally well localized and described as aching or throbbing

2) Visceral pain: arises from internal organs such as the bladder or intestine; poorly localized and described as cramping

4. Neuropathic pain

a. Caused by damage to peripheral or central nerve cells

1) Peripheral

a) Arises from injury to either single or multiple peripheral nerves

b) Felt along nerve distributions

c) Described as burning, shooting, stabbing, or like an electric shock

d) Examples include diabetic neuropathy, herpetic neuralgia, radiculopathy, trigeminal neuralgia

2) Central

a) Arises from injury to either peripheral or central nerves or is associated with ANS dysregulation

b) Examples include phantom limb pain (peripheral) or complex regional pain syndromes (central)

5. Inflammatory pain

a. Caused by the activation and sensitization of the nociceptive pain pathway when a variety of mediators are released at a site of tissue inflammation

1) Examples include appendicitis, rheumatoid arthritis, inflammatory bowel disease

6. Cancer pain

a. Pain caused by the disease itself or by treatments for the disease, and is usually classified as chronic pain

1) Pharmacologic and nonpharmacologic interventions are utilized

2) Palliative radiation, antineoplastic therapies, and palliative surgery often aid to alleviate cancer pain

IV. General Strategy

A. ASSESSMENT

1. Primary and secondary assessment/resuscitation (see Chapters 1 and 32)

2. Focused assessment

a. Subjective data collection

1) History of present illness/injury/chief complaint

a) Patient's self-report of pain

b) History of pain related to current illness or injury (PQRST)

P: Provoking or palliating factors: What makes the pain better or worse?

Q: Quality: Have patient describe what the pain feels like in own words

R: Region/radiation: Have patient point to where the pain is located and tell whether it spreads to other areas of the body

S: Severity/intensity: Offer a rating scale

T: Timing: Have patient tell when pain began, and if pain is better, worse, or the same now

c) Efforts to relieve symptoms

(1) Home remedies

(2) Alternative therapies

(3) Medications

(a) Prescription

(b) OTC/herbal

2) Past medical history

a) Current or preexisting diseases/illness

b) Previous pain history

3) Chronic painful conditions

a) New or recurring problem

b) Substance and/or alcohol use/abuse

c) Last normal menstrual period: female patients of childbearing age

d) Current medications

(1) Prescription

(2) OTC/herbal

e) Nonpharmacologic interventions: massage, ice, heat, splinting, aroma therapy, rest, sleep
f) Food or drink: type, amount, last full meal
g) Coping mechanisms
h) Allergies
4) Psychological/social/environmental factors
a) Anxiety/depression
b) Aggravating or alleviating factors
(1) Effect of pain on function
(2) Family support
(3) Possible/actual victim of assault, abuse, or intimate partner violence situations (see Chapters 3 and 40)
c) Expressions of pain
(1) Response to pain is learned and can be influenced by demographics
(a) Age[11,12]
(b) Gender[13,14]
(c) Ethnicity[15,16]
(d) Culture[17-20]
(i) Culture refers to lifestyle, the learned and shared believes, values, knowledge, rules, symbols that guide behavior of a particular group of people[21]
(ii) Must be aware of individual bias and treat each individual as unique[22]
(e) Religion[23,24]
d) Pain behavior is also learned, yet adaptive, and is related to pain threshold and pain tolerance
e) Pain expressions can be verbal, behavioral, emotional, and physical[25] (Table 8.2)

Table 8.2

Behavioral Responses to Pain

Age Group	Vocalizations	Facial Expressions	Body Movements	Coping Strategies
Infants	Crying Fussy Irritable	Lowered brows drawn together Eyes closed (young infant) Eyes open (older infant) Mouth open	Generalized body responses; rigid or thrashing (young infant) Localized body response; withdraws stimulated area (older infant)	Oral stimulation (sucking) Crying Fetal position
Toddlers Preschoolers	Crying Screaming Asking to stop painful stimulus Pointing to area of pain	Eyes closed or open Furrowed brow	Physical resistance Uncooperative Restless Clinging	Oral stimulation Crying while sleeping (toddlers) Rocking Lying still or being active (preschoolers)
School Age	Crying Verbalizing pain quality Location Duration	Withdrawn facial expression Furrowed brow	Muscle rigidity Gritted teeth Clenched fists Squinting/guarding Lying still	Verbal stalling Being active or lying still Talking about the pain Using distraction techniques Playing or watching television Sleeping
Adolescents	Verbalizing Crying	Withdrawn Eyes closed Furrowed brow	Muscle tension and body control Splinting/guarding Lying still	Verbalizing pain Taking medication or initiating actions to relieve pain Sleeping Lying still
Adults	Groaning Moaning Sobbing Grunting Shouting Praying Crying out for help	Frowning Staring Furrowed brow Teeth clenching	Thrashing Tossing Rocking Muscle rigidity	Protective behaviors Posturing Massaging
Elderly	Sighing Moaning Grunting Chanting Praying Crying for help	Eyes squeezed closed Withdrawn look Furrowed brow Staring	Rocking Clutching side rails Muscle rigidity	Wandering Rubbing Guarding

Modified from Bernardo, L., & Conway, A. (1998). Pain assessment and management. In T. Sond & J. Rogers (Eds.), *Manual of pediatric emergency nursing* (pp. 686–711). St. Louis, MO: Mosby-Year Book; Katz, E., Kellerman, K., & Siegel, S. (1980). Behavioral distress in children with cancer undergoing medical procedures: Developmental considerations. *Journal of Consulting and Clinical Psychology, 48*(3), 356–365. Copyright © (1980) by the American Psychological Association.

b. Objective data collection
  1) General appearance
    a) Psychological
      (1) Change in level of consciousness
      (2) Change in emotional state
    b) Observations of behavior and vital signs should not be used solely in place of self-report
      (1) Crying, moaning, grimacing, frowning
      (2) Rubbing or splinting a body part, limping
    c) Positioning and movement
    d) Physiologic
      (1) Elevated blood pressure
      (2) Elevated heart rate
      (3) Change in respiratory rate and pattern
    e) Level of distress/discomfort
  2) Obtain a pain rating
    a) Adult
      (1) Visual analogue scale
      (2) Numeric rating scale
      (3) Graphic rating scale: number and word
      (4) Thermometer-like scale
    b) Infant/pediatric[25] (Table 8.3)
      (1) N-Pass
      (2) r-FLACC
      (3) FACES
      (4) VAS
  3) Inspection
    a) Position
    b) Skin color
    c) External bleeding
    d) Skin integrity
    e) Obvious deformity
    f) Edema
  4) Auscultation
    a) Lung sounds
    b) Bowel sounds
  5) Palpation
    a) Areas of tenderness: light, deep (as appropriate)
    b) Save painful part until last
3. Diagnostic procedures
  a. Laboratory studies: determined by possible cause of pain

Table 8.3

Sample Pediatric Pain Emergency Department Assessment Protocol

Pain assessment frequency	• Assess for presence of pain in triage; may defer due to critical condition • Pain reassessment within 1 hour of pain-relieving nonpharmacologic and/or pharmacologic intervention • Patients determined to have pain during ED visit will be assessed for pain within 30 minutes of discharge
Utilize appropriate standardized pediatric pain scale with each pain assessment	• N-PASS will be used to assess pain in infants less than 3 months • r-FLACC scale will be used to assess pain in children ages 3 months to 3 years, cognitively impaired children, and those unable to utilize a subjective scale due to clinical condition • Wong-Baker FACES will be used to assess pain in children age 3 and older • Visual analogue scale will be used to assess pain in children ages 8 and older

Ask patient to identify location (all assessments) and characteristics (triage only) of pain	• Ask toddler and preschool patients if they "hurt" or have an "owie" and ask them to point or tell you where it hurts
	• Ask the school age and adolescent patient if they have pain
	If they report pain ask about additional pain descriptors including:
	  • Location
	  • Onset ("When did the pain begin?")
	  • Progression ("What makes the pain worse and what makes the pain better?")
	  • Quality ("Are there words to describe your pain?")
	  • Effect on daily activities ("Does the pain stop you from doing things you normally do?")

Documentation	• Type of pain assessment scale used with each assessment and pain score • Location of pain and additional pain characteristics such as onset, progression quality, and effect on daily activities as appropriate
N-PASS	It is important to observe the infant for approximately 5 minutes before scoring each category. Score each category and add each score to determine pain score. Sedation-specific criteria will not be scored. Total from 0 to 10.
r-FLACC	Observe the patient for at least 1–3 minutes (5 minutes if asleep). Score each category and add each score to determine pain score. Total from 0 to 10. Includes common pain expressive behaviors seen in cognitively impaired. Can be individualized.
FACES	Explain that each face is for a person who has no pain (hurt) or some, or a lot of pain (0 to 10). Ask the patient to point to the face that best describes own pain.
VAS	On a scale from 0 to 10 where 0 is "no pain" and 10 is the "worst pain" ask the patient to point or state the number that best describes own pain.

Data from Hummel, Puchalski, Greech, & Weiss, 2008; Illinois Emergency Medical Services for Children (EMSC), 2013; Malviya, Voepel-Lewis, Burke, Merkel, & Tait, 2006; Stinton, Kavanagh, Yamada, Gill, & Stevens, 2006; Wong & Baker, 1998; Habich & Letizia, 2015.

b. Imaging studies: determined by possible cause of pain

c. Electrocardiogram: determined by possible cause of pain

B. ANALYSIS: DIFFERENTIAL NURSING DIAGNOSES/COLLABORATIVE PROBLEMS

1. Acute pain
   a. Somatic pain is superficial, from the skin or close to body surface
      1) Characteristics
         a) Sharp and well localized
         b) Dull, aching, poorly localized; often accompanied by nausea and vomiting
   b. Visceral pain locates in internal organs, abdomen, or skeleton
      1) Characteristics
         a) Poorly localized
         b) Associated with nausea and vomiting, hypotension, restlessness, sometimes shock
         c) Often radiates or is referred (i.e., present in an area that is away from its origin)
   c. Chronic pain is prolonged pain for more than 6 months
      1) Characteristics
         a) Persistent (e.g., back pain)
         b) Intermittent (e.g., migraines)
      2) May be caused or aggravated by a decreased level of endorphins or an increased amount of C-neuron stimulation
         a) Central pain is caused by a lesion or dysfunction in the CNS
         b) Neuropathic pain results from trauma or disease of the peripheral nerves
            (1) Tingling
            (2) Burning
            (3) Shooting

C. PLANNING AND IMPLEMENTATION/INTERVENTIONS

1. Determine priorities of care
   a. Maintain airway, breathing, circulation (see Chapters 1 and 32)
   b. Provide supplemental oxygen as indicated
   c. Establish IV access for administration of crystalloid fluid/blood products/medications as needed
   d. Obtain and set up equipment and supplies
   e. Prepare for/assist with medical interventions
      1) Treat underlying conditions related to disease or injury
      2) Institute cardiac and pulse oximetry monitoring
      3) Assist with hospital admission as indicated
   f. Provide measures for pain relief
      1) Use therapeutic communication; accept patient's report of pain

2) Provide culturally competent care by considering patient's and family's cultural, social, psychological needs
3) Elicit participation by patient and family in the management of patient's pain
4) Involve patient and family in pain management decisions
5) Consider nonpharmacologic interventions to reduce pain
   a) Positioning
      (1) Place in position of comfort that reduces or relieves pain
      (2) Apply sling, swathe, or splint to injured extremities
      (3) Support positioning with pillows, towel rolls, foam wedges
   b) Cutaneous stimulation
      (1) Ice for sprains, fractures, bleeding
      (2) Heat for muscle spasms/cramps or IV infiltration; avoid heat to the abdomen if patient is a surgical candidate
      (3) Massage for tense muscles; avoid if inflammation is present
      (4) Pressure with or without massage
      (5) Vibration may cause numbness and/or anesthesia in the area stimulated and, if continued for 30 minutes or more, can provide pain relief for several hours
   c) Relaxation/distraction
      (1) Directs attention away from pain
      (2) Breathe slowly and regularly
      (3) Slowly contract and release muscle groups
      (4) Guided imagery to imagine a pleasant place or event
      (5) Soothing music, allow patient preference; can be a sleep aid
      (6) Visiting with family and friends
      (7) A negative consequence of the use of relaxation or distraction techniques is that patients may not "look like" they are in pain
   g. Administer pharmacologic therapy as ordered (Table 8.4)
      1) Diagnosis-based overview of pharmacologic treatments[7]
         a) Nociceptive pain
            (1) Rest
            (2) Ice
            (3) NSAIDs
            (4) Opioids
         b) Neuropathic pain
            (1) Tricyclic antidepressants
            (2) Serotonin-norepinephrine reuptake inhibitors
            (3) Antiepileptics
            (4) Opioids

Table 8.4

Common Medications Used for Pain Relief

Classification						
Nonopioid Analgesics	Nonopioid analgesics are used to control mild to moderate pain and fever					
	Medication	**Indication**	**Contraindications**	**Side Effects**	**Pregnancy Category**	**Route(s)**
	Acetaminophen	Mild to moderate pain	Hypersensitivity; active liver disease or severe dysfunction; alcoholism	Generally safe and well tolerated	B—PO, rectal C—IV	PO, rectal, IV
	Salicylates (aspirin)	Mild to moderate pain; TIA and MI prophylaxis	Hypersensitivity; bleeding disorders; vitamin K deficiency; peptic ulcer disease; do not administer to children with flulike symptoms because of its risk of Reye's syndrome	Gastric upset; bleeding, prolonged prothrombin time; CNS and metabolic toxicity at high dosages or with prolonged use	D—first trimester	PO, rectal
NSAIDs	NSAIDs are used to control mild to moderate pain, fever, and inflammatory conditions					
	Medication	**Indication**	**Contraindications**	**Side Effects**	**Pregnancy Category**	**Route(s)**
	Ibuprofen	Mild to moderate pain; inflammatory disorders	Hypersensitivity; GI bleed; use cautiously in cardiovascular, renal or hepatic disease	Headache, dizziness, drowsiness, tinnitus; arrhythmias, hypertension	C—up to 30 weeks D—>30 weeks	PO, IV
	Indomethacin	Inflammatory disorders	Hypersensitivity; alcohol intolerance; active GI bleed	Dizziness, headache, tinnitus	B—First trimester	PO, IV
	Ketorolac	Short-term management of pain; antipyretic; antiinflammatory	Hypersensitivity; preoperative use; peptic ulcer; GI bleed	Stroke, drowsiness, dizziness, euphoria, headache, MI; GI bleed	C	PO, IM, IV, IN
	Naproxen	Mild to moderate pain, dysmenorrhea, fever, inflammatory disorders	Hypersensitivity; active GI bleed, ulcers, lactation	Dizziness, drowsiness, headache	B—First trimester	PO

Classification

Opioid analgesics are used for the management of moderate to severe pain.

Opioid Analgesics						
Buprenorphine Schedule III	Moderate to severe pain	Hypersensitivity; respiratory depression, asthma, paralytic ileus	Confusion, dysphoria, hallucinations, sedation, dizziness, euphoria floating feeling, headache, unusual dreams	C	IM, IV, transdermal
Codeine Schedule II, III, IV	Mild to moderate pain, cough suppression	Hypersensitivity; head trauma, increased ICP, renal, hepatic, pulmonary disease	Confusion, sedation, dysphoria, euphoria, hallucinations, headache, unusual dreams	C	PO
Fentanyl (Sublimaze) Schedule II	Analgesic supplement, Induction-maintenance of anesthesia, severe pain	Hypersensitivity; use cautiously in geriatric, debilitated, critically ill, diabetes, renal, pulmonary, or hepatic disease	Confusion, paradoxical excitation-delirium, depression, drowsiness	C	IM, IV, IN, transdermal
Hydrocodone Schedule II, III	Moderate to severe pain, antitussive	Hypersensitivity; respiratory depression, paralytic ileus, asthma	Confusion, dizziness, sedation, euphoria, hallucinations, headache, unusual dreams	C	PO
Hydromorphone (Dilaudid) Schedule II	Moderate to severe pain	Hypersensitivity; respiratory depression, asthma, head trauma, renal, hepatic, or pulmonary disease	Confusion, sedation, dizziness, dysphoria, euphoria, floating feeling, hallucinations, headache	C	PO, rectal, SQ, IM
Methadone Schedule II	Moderate to severe pain. Detoxification and maintenance therapy for opioid use disorder	Hypersensitivity; significant respiratory depression, asthma, paralytic ileus, ETOH intolerance	Confusion, sedation, dizziness, dysphoria, euphoria, floating feeling, hallucinations, headache, unusual dreams. Hypotension, bradycardia, constipation	C	IV, IM, PO, subcutaneous
Morphine sulfate Schedule II	Severe pain, pulmonary edema, MI pain	Hypersensitivity; respiratory depression, asthma, paralytic ileus	Confusion, sedation, dizziness, dysphoria, euphoria floating feeling, hallucinations, headache, unusual dreams, respiratory depression, hypotension, bradycardia, constipation, nausea, vomiting	C	PO, IM, SQ, rectal, IV, epidural, IT, IN
Oxycodone (Oxycontin) Schedule II	Moderate to severe pain	Hypersensitivity; respiratory depression, paralytic ileus, asthma	Confusion, sedation, dizziness, dysphoria, euphoria floating feeling, hallucinations, headache, unusual dreams, respiratory depression, orthostatic hypotension, constipation	B	PO, rectal
Tramadol Schedule II	Moderate to severe pain	Hypersensitivity; cross sensitivity with other opioids	Seizures, dizziness, headache, somnolence, anxiety, CNS stimulation, confusion, coordination disturbance, euphoria, malaise, nervousness, sleep disorder, weakness	C	PO

Continued

Table 8.4

Common Medications Used for Pain Relief—cont'd

Classification

Classification						
Skeletal Muscle Relaxants	Diazepam (Valium) Schedule IV	Antianxiety, anticonvulsant, sedative/hypnotic, skeletal muscle relaxants	Hypersensitivity; cross sensitivity with other benzodiazepines, comatose patients, myasthenia gravis, severe pulmonary impairment, sleep apnea, hepatic dysfunction, CNS depression	Dizziness, drowsiness, lethargy, depression, hangover, ataxia, slurred speech, headache, paradoxical excitation. Respiratory depression, hypotension	D	PO, IM, IV, rectal,
	Lorazepam (Ativan) Schedule IV	Anxiety disorder, sedation, decreased seizures	Hypersensitivity; cross sensitivity with other benzodiazepines, CNS depression, uncontrolled severe pain, hypotension, sleep apnea	Dizziness, drowsiness, lethargy, hangover, headache, ataxia, slurred speech, forgetfulness, confusion, mental depression, rhythmic myoclonic jerking paradoxical excitation, respiratory depression	D	PO, IM, IV, SL
Local anesthetics	Lidocaine Mepivacaine Procaine Tetracaine	Local anesthesia prior to painful procedures	Hypersensitivity	Blanching, redness, alteration in temperature sensation, edema, itching, rash, hyperpigmentation	B	Locally
	LET (Lidocaine, Epinephrine, Tetracaine)	Local anesthesia prior to painful procedures	Hypersensitivity	Blanching, redness, alteration in temperature sensation, edema, itching, rash, hyperpigmentation	B	Topically
	EMLA cream	Local anesthesia prior to painful procedures	Hypersensitivity	Blanching, redness, alteration in temperature sensation, edema, itching, rash, hyperpigmentation	B	Topically

Pregnancy Category:

A – Studies have not shown an increased risk to the fetus.

B – Animal studies have demonstrated no harm to the fetus but well-controlled human studies have failed to demonstrate a risk to the fetus.

C – Animal studies have shown an adverse effect to the fetus and there are no well-controlled studies in pregnant women.

D – Studies in pregnant women have demonstrated a risk to the fetus. Benefits may outweigh the risks.

X – Studies have demonstrated positive evidence of fetal abnormalities. The use in pregnant women is contraindicated.

   c) Co-occurring pain syndromes (functional or central sensitization)
     (1) Tricyclic antidepressants
     (2) Serotonin-norepinephrine reuptake inhibitors
     (3) Antiepileptics
   d) Opioid use disorder
     (1) Substance abuse treatment
     (2) Abstinence or medication-assisted treatments (e.g., methadone maintenance)
 2) Administer analgesics and/or adjuvant medications to augment analgesics as prescribed. The World Health Organization (WHO) recommends the use of the analgesic ladder as a systematic plan for the use of analgesic medications.[26] The three steps of the analgesic ladder suggest the types of medications appropriate for different pain intensities (Fig. 8.1).
   a) Step 1 uses nonopioid analgesics and possibly other adjuvant analgesics for mild pain.
   b) Step 2 adds a mild opioid when the pain is moderate.
   c) Step 3 includes the use of stronger opioids when pain is moderate to severe (Fig. 8.1)
 3) Patient-controlled analgesia (PCA)
   a) Indications: used in patients with acute or chronic pain who are able to communicate, understand explanations, and follow directions
   b) Assess vital signs and pain level
   c) Explain use of pump to patient and family members

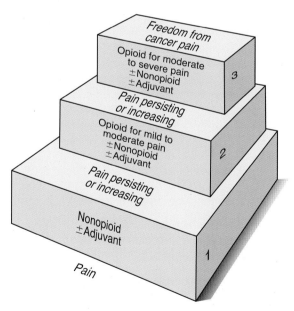

Fig. 8.1 WHO analgesic ladder. *(From World Health Organization. [1996]. Cancer pain relief [2nd ed.]. Geneva: World Health Organization. Retrieved from http://apps.who.int/iris/bitstream/10665/37896/1/9241544821.pdf. Reproduced with permission of the World Health Organization.)*

   d) Collaborate with physician, patient, and family about dosage, lockout interval, basal rate, and amount of dosage on demand
   e) Assist patient to use PCA pump
 4) Procedural sedation medications (Table 8.5)
2. Relieve anxiety/apprehension
3. Allow significant others to remain with patient if supportive
4. Educate patient and significant others
  a. Inform patient and family about efficacy and safety of opioid analgesia

D. EVALUATION AND ONGOING MONITORING

1. Continuously monitor and treat as indicated
  a. Level of consciousness
  b. Hemodynamic status
  c. Breath sounds, respiratory rate, and pulse oximetry
  d. Cardiac rate and rhythm
  e. Pain relief
2. Monitor patient response/outcomes, and modify nursing care plan as appropriate
3. If positive patient outcomes are not demonstrated, reevaluate assessment and/or plan of care

E. DOCUMENTATION OF INTERVENTIONS AND PATIENT RESPONSE

F. AGE-RELATED CONSIDERATIONS

1. Pediatrics
  a. Growth or development related
   1) Children's pain tolerance increases with age
   2) Children's developmental level influences pain behavior
   3) Localization of pain begins during infancy
   4) Preschoolers can anticipate pain
   5) School-age children can verbalize pain and describe location and intensity
  b. "Pearls"
   1) Children may not admit to pain to avoid injection
   2) Distraction techniques can aid in keeping the child's mind occupied and away from pain
   3) Opioids are no more dangerous for children than for adults
2. Geriatrics
  a. Aging related
   1) Pain is not a normal aging consequence
   2) Chronic pain alters the person's quality of life
   3) Chronic pain may be caused by a myriad of conditions
  b. "Pearls"
   1) Adequate treatment may require deviation from clinical pathways
   2) Administer pain-relieving medications at lower dose and increase slowly

TABLE 8.5

Medications Commonly Used in Procedural Sedation

(Note: Nursing practice may vary from state to state in terms of authorization to administer certain sedation medications. Consult your agency/facility practice guidelines for indications, contraindications, administration and monitoring)

Medication	Initial Dose/Route	Onset	Duration	Repeat Dose	Nursing Considerations
Dexmedetomidine (Precedex)	Adult: • 1 mcg/kg IV loading dose (over 10 minutes) followed by 0.6 mg/kg per hour Pediatric: • 1–3 mcg/kg loading dose (over 10 minutes) followed by 0.5–2 mcg/kg per hour continuous infusion if intubated	Adult: • Rapid Pediatric: • 5–10 minutes	Adult: Pediatric: • 30–75 minutes	Adult: Pediatric: • N/A for continuous infusion • Titrate infusing rate PRN	Adult: For newly-intubated patients, usually in intensive care settings. Generally, only used for up to 24 hours May be used for procedural sedation Pediatric: • Sedation and modest analgesia without respiratory depression. • Commonly used for diagnostic imaging (CT, MRI). • Common adverse events: bradycardia, hypertension, or, especially with loading dose, hypotension. General Cautions: children who are debilitated, inadequately hydrated, or have reduced cardiac output. • Absolute contraindication: patients receiving digoxin or other medications acting on sinus node or with sinus node dysfunction.
Etomidate (Amidate®)	Adult: • 0.1–0.15 mg/kg Pediatric: • 0.1–0.3 mg/kg IV • Lower dose in children with renal or hepatic insufficiency	Adult: • 5–15 seconds Pediatric: • <0.5	Adult: • 5–15minutes Pediatric: • 5–15	Adult: • 0.05 mg/kg every 3–5 minutes Pediatric: • 0.05 mg/kg every 3–5 minutes titrate up to 0.6 mg/kg total dose to desired sedation	Adult: • Sedative. No analgesia.Rapid recovery • Generally maintains cardio-respiratory stability. • Elderly or renal/hepatic insufficiency: use loser dose range. • Myoclonus, injection site pain, nausea/vomiting may occur. Pediatric: • Rapid onset and recovery. Commonly used for brief diagnostic imaging (e.g., head CT). • Reduces intracranial pressure. Hemodynamic and respiratory stability maintained in most patients making it a good choice if cardiovascular status is unknown or compromised (e.g., trauma patient). • Common adverse effects: pain at the injection site, transient non-epileptiform myoclonus, vomiting. Myoclonus and vomiting reduced by premedication with midazolam. • Relatively contraindicated in children with severe illness such as suspected sepsis. • Absolute contraindications: children with congenital or acquired adrenal insufficiency.

Medication	Initial Dose/Route	Onset	Duration	Repeat Dose	Nursing Considerations
Ketamine (Ketalar®)	Adult: • 1–2 mg/kg IV over 1–2 minutes Pediatric: • 1–1.5 mg/kg IV over 1–2 minutes • 4-5mg/kg IM • When given with propofol, reduce initial dose to 0.5 mg/kg	Adult: • 0.5 -1 minutes Pediatric: • 1–2 minutes	Adult: • 5–45 minutes Pediatric: • 15–30 minutes	Adult: • 0.25–0.5 mg/kg every 5–10 minutes Pediatric: • 0.5–1 mg/kg every 10 minutes titrating to desired level of sedation	Adult: • Dissociative and amnestic. • Minimal respiratory depression. • Does not inhibit protective reflexes. Pediatric: • Provides sedation AND analgesia for moderately to severely painful procedures. Minimal respiratory depression and. General Cautions Common adverse events • Vomiting, emergence phenomenon; vomiting may be reduced by premedication with Anti-emetics • Laryngospasm or apnea is rare and may be more common with intramuscular administration. General Cautions: age younger than 12 months, active pulmonary infections (including URI), known or suspected cardiac disease, suspected increased intracranial pressure (e.g., head trauma with signs or symptoms, intracranial mass, or hydrocephalus), glaucoma or acute eye injury (open globe). General Cautions: age younger than 3 months or patients with known or suspected psychosis.
Methohexital (Brevital®)	Adult: • 0.75–1 mg/kg Pediatric: • 0.5–1 mg/kg IV	Adult: • 10-30 seconds Pediatric: • 30-60 seconds	Adult: • 10–40 minutes Pediatric: • 5–10 minutes	Adult: • 0.5 mg/kg every 2–5 minutes Pediatric: • 0.5 mg/kg IV (maximum 40 mg per dose) every 2–5 minutes, titrate up to 2 mg/kg (160 mg total dose)	Cannot come in contact with silicone, as might be used in vial stoppers or syringes. May cause immediate breakdown of the silicone. Adult: • Sedative and amnestic. No analgesia. • Cardio-respiratory depression, hypotension, tachycardia can occur. Emergency airway equipment must be immediately available. • Can precipitate or worsen seizures. Pediatric: • Short-acting barbiturate option for noninvasive diagnostic procedures. • More adverse events than pentobarbital. • All patients:Common adverse effects: respiratory depression, hypotension, and myocardial depression. • Caution patients with cardiac, liver, or renal insufficiency. • Absolute contraindications: porphyria or partial seizure disorder (may precipitate seizures).

Continued

TABLE 8.5

Medications Commonly Used in Procedural Sedation—cont'd

(Note: Nursing practice may vary from state to state in terms of authorization to administer certain sedation medications. Consult your agency/facility practice guidelines for indications, contraindications, administration and monitoring)

Medication	Initial Dose/Route	Onset	Duration	Repeat Dose	Nursing Considerations
Midazolam (Versed®)	Adult: • 1–2.5mg slow IV • Maximum 2.5 mg per dose • Maximum if elderly 1.5 mg Pediatric: • 6 months to 5 years: 0.05–0.1 mg/kg IV. Maximum single dose = 2 mg. • 6–12 years: 0.025–0.05 mg/kg IV. May be given IM, but slower onset- Maximum single dose = 2 mg.	Adult: • 1–2.5 minutes Pediatric: • 1–3 minutes	Adult: • 10–60 minutes Pediatric: • 10–15 minutes, depending upon total dose administered	Adult: • May repeat after 2–5 minutes Pediatric: • After initial IV dose, repeat after 2–5 minutes titrating to desired level of sedation • 6 months to 5 years: up to 0.2 mg/kg per dose. Maximum total dose 6 mg. • 6–12 years; 0.1 mg/kg. Maximum total dose 10 mg.	Adult: • Sedative and anxiolytic. No analgesia. • Relatively slow onset; requires more cautious titration. • Prolonged effect or delayed recovery in elderly, obese, or impaired hepatic function. • Use reduced dose in combination with other agents. Pediatric: • Provides sedation but NO analgesia. For painful procedures, consider adding analgesia General Cautions: • When combined with fentanyl can produce moderate or deep sedation, but less effective and more adverse respiratory events reported when compared to sedation with ketamine alone or combined with propofol. • Flumazenil can reverse effects but should be avoided in patients with seizure disorder or who are chronically maintained on benzodiazepines. General Cautions: Common adverse effects: respiratory depression, and apnea, especially when combined with opioid medications (e.g., fentanyl); paradoxical reactions, including hyperactivity, aggressive behavior, and inconsolable crying. • Close monitoring of respiratory status is required.
Phenobarbital (Luminal®)	Adult: • 1–3 mg/kg IV Pediatric: • 1–2 mg/kg IV • Maximum 100 mg per dose	Adult: • 5–10 minutes Pediatric: • 1–5 minutes	Adult: • Dose-dependent Pediatric: • 15–90 minutes	Adult: Pediatric:	Adult: • Caution in patients with cardiac disease or hepatic insufficiency Pediatric: • Short-acting barbiturate option for noninvasive diagnostic procedures. • Better efficacy seen in children <8 years old. General Cautions Common adverse effects all ages: respiratory depression, hypotension, and increased heart rate, especially with intravenous use or in combination with opioid or benzodiazepine, emergence reactions. • Absolute contraindications all ages: porphyria.

Medication	Initial Dose/Route	Onset	Duration	Repeat Dose	Nursing Considerations
Propofol (Diprivan®)	Adult: • 0.5–1 mg/kg Pediatric: • Initiate infusion at 25 mcg/kg per minute and titrate gradually to response (range 50–200 mcg/kg per minute)^OR • 0.5–1 mg/kg IV bolus dose (children 2 years of age and older) • 1–2 mg/kg IV bolus dose (infants 6 months to 2 years of age) • Significant dose reduction necessary for patients who are debilitated or with reduced cardiac output	Adult: • 0.5–1 minute Pediatric: • <0.5 minutes	Adult: • 5 minutes Pediatric: 5–15 minutes after single bolus dose, longer after prolonged infusion or when repeated bolus doses are given.	Adult: 0.5 mg/kg every 3–5 minutes Pediatric: • Not applicable for continuous IV infusion, titrate infusion rate as needed. • Additional IV bolus dose 0.5 mg/kg every 3–5 minutes titrating as needed up to 3 mg/kg. Wait at least 3–5 minutes between doses to assess effect.	Adult: • Sedative and amnestic. No analgesia. • Rapid onset • Respiratory depression, hypotension, injection site pain may occur. Airway management must be immediately available. • Elderly: reduce dose by 20%, slower administration. • Screen for allergies to egg lecithin, soybean oil (potential allergens). Pediatric: • Provides sedation but NO analgesia. For painful procedures, consider an analgesic agent • Rapid onset of sedation with good neurologic recovery. • Peripheral injection site pain. General Cautions • Common adverse events all ages: Respiratory depression, oxygen desaturation, apnea, hypotension, and/or rapid transition to deeper levels of sedation, especially with overly rapid administration of bolus injection. • Absolute contraindications: egg or soy allergy, porphyria.

• Doses are given as a suggested range for the initial dose.
• Children may differ markedly with respect to efficacy of any single dose and careful titration to effect by using repetitive dosing to achieve the desired depth; and duration of sedation is necessary for any individual patient.
• Suggested initial doses should be reduced approximately 50% for patients who are debilitated or with reduced cardiac output.
• Elderly patients are at increased risk of adverse events with these agents and dosing should be adjusted accordingly.
(Data from http://www.uptodate.com/contents/search?sp=0&source=USER_PREF&search=procedural+sedation+in+the+emergency+department&searchType=PLAIN_TEXT); Karch AM (2013). Focus on Nursing Pharmacology (6th Ed). Philadelphia, PA: Wolters Kluwer Health/Lippincott Williams & Wilkins; Woodrow R, Colbert BJ & Smith DM (2011). Essentials of Pharmacology for Health Occupations (6th Ed.) . Clifton Park, NY: Delmar Publishing)

V. Pain Management Practice

A. BARRIERS TO EFFECTIVE PAIN MANAGEMENT[27-29]

1. Attitudes of emergency health care providers
2. Hidden biases, misconceptions, and knowledge deficits regarding pain
   a. Race
   b. Age
      1) Pediatric-specific pain management protocols
      2) Geriatric-specific pain management protocols
   c. Gender
   d. Insurance status
   e. Cultural competency
   f. Psychological condition
   g. Behavioral issues
   h. Cognitive ability
   i. Level of consciousness
   j. Nonverbal patients
3. Inadequate initial pain assessment and reassessment of pain relief
4. Lack of time to adequately assess and control pain
5. Failure to accept patients' reports of pain
6. Withholding pain-relieving medication
7. Exaggerated fears of addiction
8. Poor communication (language barriers)
9. Patients' reluctance to report pain
10. Patients' reluctance to take opioids
11. Reluctance to administer opioids
12. ED crowding
13. Patient-centered pain management outcomes

B. ACUTE PAIN MANAGEMENT MYTHS[30]

1. Administering an opioid to a patient with abdominal pain will interfere with an accurate diagnosis
2. Neonates and infants do not require analgesic medications
3. Geriatric patients do not require analgesic medications as often as other adults because they complain of pain less frequently
4. Antiemetic medications are required prior to administering an opioid
5. Opioid-dependent patients do not require more pain medications than opioid naïve patients

C. ENABLERS TO EFFECTIVE PAIN MANAGEMENT [27-29]

1. Nurse-initiated analgesia protocols
2. Use of a pain management champion
3. Attending pain management education courses
4. Protocols for assessing patients' pain
5. Performance improvement initiatives aimed at improving pain management outcomes and patient satisfaction
6. Use of a validated pain assessment scale

D. IMPROVING PAIN MANAGEMENT PRACTICE

1. Changing attitudes
2. Continuing education related to realities and myths of pain management
3. Evidence-based practice and research initiatives
4. Cultural sensitivity
5. Age-specific pain management protocols
6. Use of validated pain assessment scales for initial assessment and reassessment
7. Addressing documentation issues
8. Recognizing the cognitive and emotional experience of pain[31]
9. Engaging interdisciplinary, team approaches to pain management[31]

VI. Procedural Sedation

Procedural sedation represents a dynamic continuum where patients are moving from one level of consciousness to another without a clear point of transition.[32] The goal of procedural sedation is to effectively alleviate patient anxiety, pain, and discomfort while allowing for the safe performance of painful and nonpainful procedures.[32] Responses to medications used in procedural sedation vary from patient to patient; therefore, it is the responsibility of the emergency nurse to recognize and manage potential complications. The Joint Commission (TJC) has standard definitions for four levels of sedation and anesthesia:

- Minimal sedation, in which the patient responds normally
- Moderate sedation/analgesia (conscious sedation), in which an airway and cardiovascular function is maintained
- Deep sedation/analgesia, in which the patient is not easily aroused
- Anesthesia, in which patients require assisted ventilation

Sedating a patient prior to performing a procedure is useful in controlling excessive movements and minimizing pain and anxiety during the procedure. The goal of procedural sedation is to induce a state of depressed level of consciousness, but allow the patient to maintain his or her own protective airway reflexes and oxygenation.

The Emergency Nurses Association supports the routine use of procedural sedation by appropriately trained and credentialed emergency nurses and physicians.[33] Medications used in procedural sedation include, but are not limited to, etomidate, propofol, ketamine, fentanyl, and midazolam, which may be administered by emergency nurses in the presence of a physician, APN, or other health care professional credentialed and privileged for procedural sedation. Emergency nurses should be trained and competent in the following:

- Principles of oxygen delivery, transport and uptake, and respiratory physiology
- Age-appropriate airway management including the monitoring of patient's oxygenation and ventilation
- Knowledge of anatomy, physiology, pharmacology, cardiac dysrhythmia recognition, and complications related to procedural sedation and analgesia
- Initiation of cardiac resuscitation procedures
- Identification of various levels of sedation
- Pre- and postprocedural nursing care of the patient undergoing procedural sedation
- Recognition of legal/liability ramifications associated with administering procedural sedation[33]

Institutional policies, procedures, clinical guidelines, and protocols for procedural sedation that are age specific must be in place prior to performing these procedures. These include:

- Equipment and supplies
- Mandatory education and competency validation
- Risk management
- Quality monitoring, patient outcomes
- Required documentation[33]

A. INDICATIONS FOR PROCEDURAL SEDATION: DIAGNOSTIC AND THERAPEUTIC PROCEDURES

1. Abscess incision and drainage
2. Suturing
3. Fracture reduction and orthopedic procedures
4. Burn and wound debridement
5. Laceration repair (especially in pediatrics)
6. Foreign body removal
7. Elective and nonelective cardioversion
8. Thoracostomy tube insertion
9. Intubation and mechanical ventilation
10. Radiologic studies in agitated or uncooperative patient[32]

B. ASSESSMENT

1. General considerations
   a. Past medical history
   b. Past anesthesia history
   c. Medication history
   d. Last meal
      1) No evidence supports fasting in the ED
      2) No evidence supports gastric emptying
2. Physical considerations
   a. Vital signs
   b. Pulse oximetry, capnography
   c. Cardiac monitoring

C. PROCEDURE

1. Obtain baseline vital signs and level of consciousness
2. Explain procedure to patient and family
3. Facilitate obtaining informed consent
4. Obtain venous access
5. Bring appropriate equipment to bedside
   a. Cardiac monitor
   b. Blood pressure monitor
   c. Pulse oximeter (capnography)
   d. Suction and oxygen equipment
   e. Airway management equipment (ET tube[s] and bag-valve mask)
   f. IV supplies
   g. Reversal agents
   h. Crash cart
6. Assist with administration and titration of prescribed medications and reversal medications as indicated
7. Maintain continuous pulse oximetry, capnography, blood pressure, heart rate monitoring during procedure
8. Document vital signs, level of consciousness, and cardiopulmonary status every 5–15 minutes during procedure, per hospital protocol

D. POSTPROCEDURE DISCHARGE CRITERIA

1. Continuous monitoring of patient until responsive to voice or gentle stimulation
2. Assess patient for readiness for discharge: awake, able to swallow, able to ambulate
3. Mental status and physical function should have returned to a point where the patient can care for self with minimal to no assistance
4. Symptoms such as pain, light-headedness, and nausea should be well controlled
5. Determine vital signs: should be within 15% of admission readings
6. Document patient condition and to whom patient is released at discharge. A reliable person who can provide support and supervision should be present at the patient's home for at least a few hours
7. Clear written discharge instructions should be given and explained to the patient and family member or friend who will be assisting with patient's care following procedural sedation. The clinician should explain what was done, the expected course, potential problems, what to do if problems arise, when and where to follow up, and when to return to normal activities

E. INSTITUTIONAL RESPONSIBILITIES

1. Provide and maintain competency-based education for nursing personnel
2. Supply appropriate equipment for monitoring patient's oxygenation, ventilation, circulation during procedure
3. During procedure, ensure physical supervision is provided by personnel capable of initiating advanced emergency airway management and hemodynamic stabilization

References

1. International Association for the Study of Pain (IASP). Retrieved from http://www.iasp-pain.org/.

2. Malec M, Shega JW: Pain management in the elderly, *Med Clin North Am* 99:337–350, 2015.

3. Vlahaki D, Milne W: Oligoanalgesia in a rural emergency department, *Can J Rural Med* 13:62–67, 2008.

4. Todd KH, Ducharme J, Choiniere M, et al.: Pain in the emergency department: results of the pain and emergency medicine initiative (PEMI) multicenter study, *J Pain* 8:460–466, 2007.

5. Pollack CV, Viscusi ER: Improving acute pain management in emergency medicine, *Hosp Pract* 43:36–45, 2015.

6. Porth CM: *Essentials of pathophysiology: concepts of altered health states*, Philadelphia, PA, 2015, Wolters Kluwer.

7. Tauben D: Nonopioid medications for pain, *Phys Med Rehabil Clin N Am* 26:219–248, 2015.

8. Moayedi M, Davis KD: Theories of pain: from specificity to gate control, *J Neurophysiol* 109:5–12, 2012.

9. Melzack R, Wall PD: Pain mechanisms: a new theory, *Science* 150:971–979, 1965.

10. Melzack R: Pain and the neuromatrix in the brain, *J Dent Educ* 65:1378–1382, 2001.

11. Anderson L, FitzGerald M, Luck L: An integrative literature review of interventions to reduce violence against emergency department nurses, *J Clin Nurs* 19:2520–2530, 2010.

12. Brown D: A literature review exploring how healthcare professionals contribute to the assessment and control of postoperative pain in older people, *J Clin Nurs* 13:74–90, 2004.

13. Ely B: Pediatric nurses' pain management practice: barriers to change, *Pediatr Nurs* 27:473–480, 2001.

14. Greenberger P: Women, men, and pain, *J Womens Health Gend Based Med* 10:309–310, 2001.

15. Jackson R, Iezzi T, Gunderson J, Nagasaka T, Fitch A: Gender differences in pain perception: the mediating role of self-efficacy beliefs, *Sex Roles* 47:561–568, 2002.

16. Bonham V: Race, ethnicity, and pain treatment: striving to understand the causes and solutions to the disparities in pain management, *J Law Med Ethics* 29:52–68, 2001.

17. Green C, Baker T, Sato Y, et al.: Race and chronic pain: a comparative study of young black and white Americans presenting for management, *J Pain* 4:176–183, 2003.

18. Tamayo-Sarver J, Hinz S, Cydulka R, et al.: Racial and ethnic disparities in emergency department analgesic prescription, *Am J Public Health* 93:1067–1073, 2003.

19. Lasch KE: Culture, pain, and culturally sensitive pain care, *Pain Manag Nurs* 1:16–22, 2000.

20. Lee A, Gink T, Ho T: Opioid requirements and responses in Asians, *Anaesth Intensive Care* 25:665–670, 1997.

21. Racher F, Annis R: Respecting culture and honoring diversity in community practice, *Res Theory Nurs Pract* 21:255–270, 2007.

22. Spencer C, Burke P: The impact of culture on pain management, *Med Surg Matters* 20:12–15, 2011.

23. Ludwig-Beymer P: Transcultural aspects of pain. In *Transcultural concepts in nursing care*, ed 4, Philadelphia, PA, 2003, JB Lippincott.

24. Rippentropp E, Altmaier E, Chen J, et al.: The relationship between religion/spirituality and physical health, mental health, and pain in a chronic pain population, *Pain* 116:227–288, 2001.

25. Habich M, Letizia M: Pediatric pain assessment in the emergency department: a nursing evidence-based practice protocol, *Pediatr Nurs* 41:198–202, 2015.

26. IOM (Institute of Medicine): *Relieving pain in America: a blueprint for transforming prevention, care, education, and research*, Washington, DC, 2011, The National Academies Press.

27. Pretorius A, Searle J, Marshall B: Barriers and enablers to emergency department nurses' management of patients' pain, *Pain Manag Nurs* 16:372–379, 2015.

28. Stang AS, Hartling L, Fera C, et al.: Quality indicators for the assessment and management of pain in the emergency department: a systematic review, *Pain Res Manag* 19:e179–e190, 2014.

29. Ucuzal M, Dogan R, Dogan R: Emergency nurses' knowledge, attitude and clinical decision making skills about pain, *Int Emerg Nurs* 23:75–80, 2015.

30. Olszewski A, Kennedy K, Kary A, et al.: The painful truth: five acute pain management myths in the ED, *Can J Emerg Nurs* 37:22–24, 2014.

31. Institute of Medicine: Relieving pain in America: a blueprint for transforming prevention, care, education, and research. Retrieved from http://www.nationalacademies.org/hmd/Reports/2011/Relieving-Pain-in-America-A-Blueprint-for-Transforming-Prevention-Care-Education-Research.aspx, 2011.

32. Godwin A, Whisenant B: Procedural sedation. In Adams JG, editor: *Emergency medicine*, Philadelphia, PA, 2008, Saunders: Elsevier, p 111.

33. ENA: Procedural sedation consensus statement. Retrieved from https://www.ena.org/SiteCollectionDocuments/Position%20Statements/Archived/Procedural_Sedation_Consensus_Statement.pdf, 2008.

Bibliography

Barton ED, Collings J, DeBlieux PMC, Gisondi MA, Nadel ES: *Emergency medicine*, Philadelphia, PA, 2008, Saunders-Elsevier.

D'Arcy Y: *How to manage pain in the elderly*, Indianapolis, IN, 2010, Sigma Theta Tau International.

D'Arcy Y: *Acute pain management: an evidence-based approach for nurses*, New York, NY, 2011, Springer Publishing Company.

Heuther S, McCance K, editors: Understanding pathophysiology, ed 7, St. Louis, MO: Elsevier: Mosby.

IOM (Institute of Medicine): *Relieving pain in America: a blueprint for transforming prevention, care, education, and research*, Washington, DC, 2011, The National Academies Press.

Parson G, Preece W: *Principles and practice of managing pain: a guide for nurses and allied health professionals*, New York, NY, 2010, McGaw-Hill.

Porth CM: *Essentials of pathophysiology*, ed 4, Philadelphia, PA, 2015, Wolters Kluwer.

Turk DC, Melzack R: *Handbook of pain assessment*, New York, NY, 2011, The Guilford Press.

Vallerand AH, Sanoski C, Deglin JH: *Drug guide for nurses*, ed 14, Philadelphia, PA, 2015, F. A. Davis Company.

CHAPTER 9

Isolation and Personal Protective Equipment

Anna M. Valdez, PHD, RN, CEN, CFRN, CNE, FAEN

I. General Strategy

Identification of patients with potential communicable disease begins upon initial patient contact. Early identification of infectious illness, proper and timely use of personal protective equipment (PPE), appropriate use of isolation, and effective communication are critical elements in the management of patients with a known or potential infectious illness.[1,2]

A. DETECTION OF INFECTIOUS ILLNESS AND RELATED SIGNS AND SYMPTOMS

1. Primary and secondary assessment/resuscitation (see Chapter 1)
2. Focused assessment (see Chapter 20)

B. HAND HYGIENE[1,3-5]

1. Health care workers' hands are the most common source of infection transmission in clinical environments
2. Hand hygiene is the single most effective practice for reducing the spread of infection yet hand hygiene compliance remains low in health care workers
3. Hand hygiene should occur before and after any patient contact or contact with potentially contaminated surfaces, prior to and following clinical procedures, and after removing and discarding PPE

4. Wash hands with soap and water or an alcohol-based product before and after patient contact or contact with patient's environment
   a. Wash hands with soap and water when visibly soiled or in potential contact with *Clostridium difficile* contaminate
      1) Routine handwashing should take 15–60 seconds (Fig. 9.1)
      2) Wet hands
      3) Apply enough soap to cover all hand surfaces
      4) Vigorously rub all hand surfaces including the palm, dorsum, and in between fingers
      5) Rinse hands with water
      6) Dry hands thoroughly
      7) Turn off water using hands-free approach or by using a paper towel if necessary
   b. Use alcohol-based products before and after any patient contact or contact with surfaces touched by patients (exception is exposure or potential exposure to *Clostridium difficile* contaminate, then wash hands with soap and water)
      1) Apply alcohol-based product to palm of hand
      2) Rub over all hand surfaces including the palm, dorsum, and in between fingers for 15–30 seconds
      3) Allow hands to dry
5. Keep nails trimmed low and do not wear nail extenders

How to Handwash?

WASH HANDS WHEN VISIBLY SOILED! OTHERWISE, USE HANDRUB

🕐 **Duration of the entire procedure:** 40-60 seconds

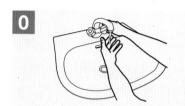

0

Wet hands with water;

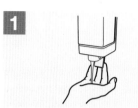

1

Apply enough soap to cover
all hand surfaces;

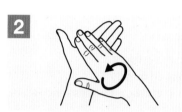

2

Rub hands palm to palm;

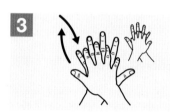

3

Right palm over left dorsum with
interlaced fingers and vice versa;

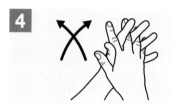

4

Palm to palm with fingers interlaced;

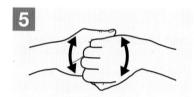

5

Backs of fingers to opposing palms
with fingers interlocked;

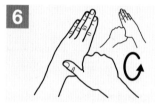

6

Rotational rubbing of left thumb
clasped in right palm and vice versa;

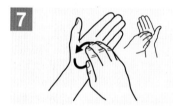

7

Rotational rubbing, backwards and
forwards with clasped fingers of right
hand in left palm and vice versa;

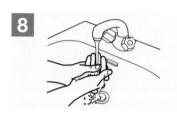

8

Rinse hands with water;

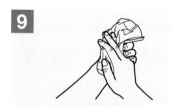

9

Dry hands thoroughly
with a single use towel;

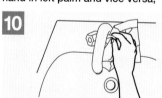

10

Use towel to turn off faucet;

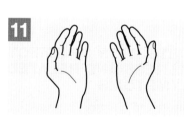

11

Your hands are now safe.

FIG. 9.1 How to handwash *(From World Health Organization. [2014].* Interim Infection Prevention and Control Guidance for Care of Patients with Suspected or Confirmed Filovirus Haemorrhagic Fever in Health-Care Settings, with Focus on Ebola. How to handwash. *Available at* http://www.who.int/csr/resources/publications/who-ipc-guidance-ebolafinal-09082014.pdf?ua=1*)*

C. USE OF PERSONAL PROTECTIVE EQUIPMENT

1. Determine potential mode of transmission
2. Select appropriate PPE as indicated based on
   a. Type of exposure anticipated: splash, spray, touch, category of isolation precautions
   b. Durability and appropriateness for the task
   c. Personnel fitness/medical hardiness
   d. Training/competency in needed PPE equipment
3. Provide masks for patients who present with a cough if patient is able to tolerate a mask and per hospital policy (may not be appropriate for smaller pediatrics without supervision)

D. ISOLATE PATIENT IF INDICATED

1. Place patient in appropriate isolation area
2. Maintain isolation until discontinued according to facility policy or diagnostic testing results indicate it is not necessary

E. NOTIFICATION, DOCUMENTATION, AND COMMUNICATION

1. Notify other health care workers of findings
   a. Verbally report high-risk findings to other health care personnel involved in patient care
   b. Use signage for transmission-based precaution levels as per policy
2. Document care, isolation level, and use of standard or transmission-based precautions
3. Notify infection control department or personnel in hospital and/or local public health department or other relevant agencies as indicated

II. Personal Protective Equipment[1,6-13]

The Occupational Health and Safety Administration (OSHA) defined personal protective equipment as "specialized clothing or equipment, worn by an employee for protection against infectious materials." PPE is designed to protect the skin, airways, mucous membranes, and clothing. Emergency nurses must be knowledgeable about where to access PPE and how to select appropriate PPE based on type of precautions needed. It is important to follow organization-specific policies and procedures related to PPE selection, use, removal, and disposal. Emergency nurses also need to practice using PPE including donning and doffing procedures and working in complex care situations while wearing a wide range of personal protective equipment. The CDC states the overall goal is to improve personnel safety in the health care environment through appropriate use of PPE.

Appropriate use of PPE is based on a risk assessment of the anticipated level of exposure and protection needed. There is a wide variety of PPE, including but not limited to gloves, masks, respirators, protective gowns, eye protectors, face shields, and foot coverings, which may be worn alone or in combination based on the level of risk.

A. GLOVES

1. Gloves are used to protect both the health care provider and patient
   a. Follow facility policy regarding open wounds on any part of the health care worker's body
2. Use gloves when anticipating contact with blood, body fluids, nonintact skin, mucous membranes, patient sweat, and other potentially infectious materials including potentially contaminated or visibly soiled equipment and surfaces
3. Gloves should also be worn when having direct contact with patients that are infected or colonized with pathogens that are spread through the contact route (see transmission-based precautions)
4. A single pair of properly fitting gloves provides an adequate barrier for routine patient care situations
5. Double gloving may be needed for high-risk patient encounters
6. Gloves are single use and should be removed immediately following patient contact
   a. Do not use the same gloves to provide care for more than one patient or to perform more than one procedure with the same patient
   b. Hand hygiene should not occur while gloves are on, except to decontaminate gloves during the doffing procedure or to disinfect gloves during patient care while in full PPE (see Ebola donning and doffing procedure guidance)
   c. Immediately replace gloves with tears, punctures, or other damage; based on contamination risk, wash hands with either alcohol-based hand sanitizer or soap and water before replacing gloves
7. Glove use
   a. Select the correct glove type (Note: Follow institutional policy and procedure on glove selection and use.)
      1) Nonsterile disposable
         a) Used for routine care and contact that does not require a sterile approach
         b) Made from variety of materials including nitrile, latex, and vinyl
         c) When selecting the type of nonsterile glove consider type of protection needed (e.g., microbiological, chemical, and/or cytotoxic substances) and whether or not a latex sensitivity exists
         d) Know the organizational policy regarding glove selection and latex-free requirements
      2) Sterile gloves
         a) Use when maintenance of a sterile environment is required
      3) Glove material
         a) Vinyl
         b) Latex

c) Nitrile

d) Other

b. Utility gloves

   1) Used for nonpatient care activities only

      a) Select correct glove size

         (1) Gloves should fit properly to allow for dexterity needed to provide safe care and not be too loose or too tight

         (2) Gloves should be of a quality not to rip or tear too easily as gloves can be worn for up to several hours and need to stand up to the task

      b) Put on (don) gloves. Do: work from "clean to dirty"

         (1) Apply (don) gloves by holding the wrist portion of the glove to allow the other hand to enter the glove with ease

         (2) When gloves are worn in combination with other PPE they are often applied last and should be applied over the protective gown or coverall

      c) Remove (doff) gloves immediately after use and before contact with clean areas or other people (see doffing procedures)

         (1) Carefully remove gloves to avoid contamination of hands and clothing or making any contaminate on gloves airborne

         (2) Using a gloved hand, pinch the other glove near the wrist and gently pull it over the hand while turning the contaminated side of the glove inward (the glove should be pulled off so it is inside out)

         (3) Hold the removed glove in the remaining gloved hand

         (4) Slide the fingers of the ungloved hand between the glove and gloved wrist

         (5) Remove the second glove by rolling it down the hand while folding the first glove inside

         (6) Discard both gloves according to facility policy

      d) Perform hand hygiene

   2) Once gloves are donned, limit opportunities for "touch contamination" by not touching self—including face or other exposed skin surfaces, other parts of PPE, or any environmental surfaces except as necessary

B. PROTECTIVE COVERS/GOWNS/ COVERALLS

1. Protective covers, aprons, and gowns are disposable and used to protect clothing and skin when close patient contact is expected, potential for splashing or spraying of bodily fluids is present, and/or when indicated according to Standard and Transmission-based Precautions

2. Intended for single use only

3. Selection of gown or apron or coverall

   a. The purpose of a gown is to protect the body and arms; if only body needs protection, use gown or apron

   b. Material properties of gown: cotton versus synthetic material and the need for fluid resistance

   c. Clean versus sterile: Selection is based on the need to remain within either a sterile or a clean environment

4. Protective covers or gowns are always worn in combination with gloves and may also be combined with other PPE including face shields, mask, and/or respirators

5. Protective cover/gown/coverall use

   a. Donning the gown or protective garment

      1) Select an appropriate cover or gown that is large enough to allow freedom of movement

      2) Check to ensure that there are no tears or holes in the protective gown or cover before donning the garment

      3) Don the protective cover or gown (refer to facility policy) by fully covering the front of the body and arms

      4) If using a protective gown tie it on the side snuggly but not tight enough to be restrictive or difficult to remove

   b. Doffing the gown/cover (or follow institutional policy)

      1) Remove protective cover/gown before leaving patient room or in a designated doffing area to prevent contamination of clean areas

      2) Protective garments should be removed in a manner that prevents contamination of the skin or clothing

      3) First remove contaminated gloves

         a) If wearing inner gloves, move to next step

         b) If only wearing single gloves, then apply clean gloves

            (1) Untie gown or cover; a properly protected doffing partner can assist with untying the gown being careful to avoid contamination or cross contamination

         c) Carefully remove the gown by rolling it forward over the shoulders; contaminated surfaces should be rolled inward so there is no contact with the noncontaminated side of the garment

         d) Discard the protective cover or gown according to facility policy

C. SURGICAL AND PROCEDURE MASKS

1. Masks are used to protect health care providers and patients from direct contact with infectious materials

   a. Intended to be worn by health care personnel to prevent exposure to potentially infectious material, such as respiratory secretions or splashed/sprayed blood and body fluid

b. Also worn by health care personnel during sterile procedures to prevent contamination of sterile area; selection of facial PPE is determined by the isolation precautions required for patient and/or the nature of patient contact

c. Can be placed on patients to prevent potential exposure to infectious respiratory secretions through coughing and sneezing

2. Surgical masks do not provide a tight seal and do not provide a barrier to aerosolized particles; therefore, they do not provide respiratory protection from airborne pathogens

3. There are a wide variety of surgical, procedure, and isolation masks available; it is important to understand the type of protection provided by the various masks available and how they are expected to be used per facility policy

4. Using masks for personal protection
   a. Masks may tie, use elastic, or have ear loops
   b. For specific donning and doffing procedures consult the manufacturer instructions and/or facility policy
   c. Surgical and procedure masks should always fit comfortably and cover the mouth and nose completely
   d. Change the mask if it becomes soiled, wet, torn, or damaged

D. FACE AND EYE PROTECTION

1. Face and eye protection including goggles and shields are used to protect the eyes and skin from contact with potentially infectious materials

2. Must be worn when splashing or spraying of blood, body fluids, or other infectious materials is anticipated

3. Personal eyeglasses and contact lenses are not considered adequate eye protection

4. Face shields are general single-use disposable items; however, eye protection may be reusable
   a. Reusable items must be decontaminated or sterilized after use

5. Using face and/or eye protection
   a. Apply the equipment per manufacturer instructions
   b. Face shields and eye protection should not be touched while in use and need to be removed immediately following use and disposed of properly or cleaned according to manufacturer recommendations
   c. When removing eye and face protection remember that the front surface is considered contaminated and should not be touched with ungloved hands. Care should be taken when removing face protection with a contaminated gloved hand

E. RESPIRATORY PROTECTION[1,7-14]

1. Respirators are used to prevent infection from airborne infectious agents such as *Myobacterium tuberculosis* and *Neisseria meningitis*

2. Respirators must be worn during contact with patients with known or possible airborne illness and should also be worn as PPE during procedures where respiratory secretions may be aerosolized, including intubation, suctioning, and bronchoscopies

3. Respiratory protection requires the use of a respirator with 95% or higher filtration such as the N-95, N-99, and/or P-100 respirator

4. In the United States, respiratory protection is regulated by the Occupational Health and Safety Administration under 29 CFR 1910.134[7]
   a. Properly fitted respirators, medical evaluation, and training must be made available by the employer at no cost when needed to protect employee health
   b. Employers must have a respiratory protection plan and provide fit testing for employees prior to using a respirator in the clinical setting. Fit testing must occur before using the brand and type of respiratory protection available to health care staff in the area they are working

5. Respirators must be properly fitted and emergency nurses must be trained on how to use them correctly to prevent unintentional exposure to pathogens

6. There are three common types of respirators used in health care. Respirators vary by manufacturer. Follow institutional policy on respirator selection and use
   a. Filtering face piece respirators (most common)
      1) Must be rated 95% or higher at filtering out airborne particulates. Different respirator ratings include N if they are not resistant to oil, R if somewhat resistant to oil, and P if strongly resistant to oil (See http://www.ede.gov/niosh/nppti/topics/respirators/factsheets/respsars.html for PPE ratings.)
      2) Filters droplets and aerosol-size particles from the air
      3) Must be properly fitted to the face to provide a tight seal around mouth and nose
         a) Facial hair prevents a proper seal
         b) Recommended guidance for extended used can be found at http://www.cdc.gov/niosh/topics/hcwcontrols/recommendedguidanceextuse.html
      4) These are disposable, single-use respirators
      5) Advantages include being easily accessible, disposable, nonpowered, noiseless, and easy to use with minimal training
      6) Disadvantages include common issues with face seal leaks, increased resistance to breathing, discomfort for wearer, requires fit testing, and impaired efficacy when wet, damaged, or creased
      7) When using a filtering face piece respirator (e.g., N-95), always follow the manufacturer's donning and doffing procedures, which vary by type of mask used
         a) Select an appropriately sized respirator based on fit testing results and medical evaluation
         b) Hold the respirator in the palm of your hand with straps facing the floor

Part 1

c) Place the respirator over your nose and mouth
d) Pull the bottom strap up and over your head so it sits below your ears
e) Pull the second strap over the head so it sits at the crown of the head
f) Mold the nosepiece over the ridge of the nose to ensure a tight seal
g) Perform a positive and negative pressure face seal check

b. Air purifying respirators
  1) Nonpowered
    a) Air is drawn through cartridges or filters by the wearer's respiratory effort
  2) Powered air purifying respirator (PAPR)
    a) A blower draws air through one or more filters and it is delivered to the person wearing the respirator
    3) When used, advantages of a HEPA filter include a high level of respiratory protection, no fit testing requirement, hood provides face and eye protection, more comfortable for wearer, and can be safely used with facial hair
    4) Disadvantages include storage needs, increased training requirements, must be able to maintain charged batteries to supply power, can impede clinical performance, increased risk for trips and falls, impaired communication due to noise, and speech is muffled by hood
    5) Donning a PAPR includes many steps and requires detailed training

c. Air supplying respirators include self-contained breathing apparatus (SCBA) and supplied air respirators
  1) Both deliver the air that the wearer will breathe resulting in highest level of respiratory protection
  2) Requires extensive initial and ongoing training

7. Always follow manufacturer's instructions and facility policy for the use of any type of respirators
8. Do not attempt to use a respirator without appropriate training, medical evaluation, and practice using the equipment

F. DONNING PERSONAL PROTECTIVE EQUIPMENT

1. Always don equipment prior to patient contact; preferably this should occur before entering the patient room in a designated donning area
2. PPE must be donned correctly to provide protection from infectious agents
  a. When possible have a trained observer monitor the donning process
  b. Because the sequence and actions involved in each donning and doffing step are critical to avoid exposure, a trained observer should read aloud to the health care worker each step in the procedure checklist and visually confirm and document that the step

has been completed correctly. The trained observer has the sole responsibility of ensuring that personnel adhere to donning and doffing processes. The trained observer must be knowledgeable about all PPE recommended in the facility's protocol and the correct donning and doffing procedures, including how to dispose of used PPE, and must be qualified to provide guidance and recommendations to the health care worker[11]

3. Predonning activities
  a. Complete training and competency validation on use of PPE, including practice donning, doffing, and working in PPE
    1) Detailed training guidance is available on the CDC webpage at http://www.cdc.gov/vhf/ebola/hcp/ppe-training/index.html
  b. Review relevant policies and procedures
  c. Gather equipment in appropriate sizes
  d. Visually inspect PPE for tears, holes, or damage
  e. Remove jewelry and personal items
  f. Perform hand hygiene
  g. Take temperature and prehydrate if using protective clothing and/or respirator

4. The order for donning PPE depends upon the combination of equipment being used and facility policies and procedures
5. When using a combination of gown/coverall and N95 respirator, the equipment should be donned in the following order
  a. Boot or shoe covers
  b. Inner gloves
  c. Gown or coverall
  d. N95 respirator
  e. Surgical hood
  f. Outer apron (if indicated)
  g. Outer gloves
  h. Face shield
6. When using a combination of gown/coverall and PAPR in a high-risk environment (e.g., caring for a patient with Ebola virus disease, or EVD) the PPE should be donned in the following order
  a. Boot or shoe covers
  b. Inner gloves
  c. Gown or coverall
  d. PAPR
  e. Outer gloves
  f. PAPR hood
  g. Outer apron (if indicated)

G. SAFE USE OF PPE DURING PATIENT CARE

1. Verify correct application of PPE following the donning procedure and prior to patient contact or entering a contaminated area
  a. When possible have a trained observer monitor the donning process using a standardized checklist

b. Have another health care provider or trained observer check to ensure that PPE is covering all body surfaces prior to entering the care environment
2. Wear PPE at all times while working in a potentially contaminated area and during patient contact
3. Disinfect soiled gloves with an alcohol-based hand rub (ABHR) after contact with body fluids
4. Do not adjust PPE during patient care
5. Immediately move to the doffing area if a breach in PPE or significant splash occurs

H. DOFFING PERSONAL PROTECTIVE EQUIPMENT

1. During PPE removal, the risk of contamination is high
2. PPE should be removed inside the patient room or in a designated doffing area when indicated (e.g., airborne illness, EVD)
3. In high-risk doffing procedures such as following EVD patient care, a trained observer should monitor the doffing procedure
4. A trained assistant dressed in appropriate PPE may be needed to ensure safe removal of PPE during the doffing process
5. PPE must be removed carefully in the correct order to prevent self-contamination or exposure to pathogens
6. When using a combination of gown/coverall and N95 respirator the equipment should be doffed in the following order
   a. Disinfect outer gloves with an ABHR
   b. Remove outer apron (if worn)
   c. Disinfect outer gloves with an ABHR
   d. Remove and discard outer gloves
   e. Inspect and disinfect inner gloves
   f. Remove the face shield
   g. Disinfect inner gloves with an ABHR
   h. Remove the surgical hood
   i. Disinfect inner gloves with an ABHR
   j. Remove the gown or coverall
   k. Disinfect inner gloves with an ABHR
   l. Remove boot or shoe covers
   m. Change inner gloves
   n. Remove the N95 respirator
   o. Disinfect the new inner gloves
   p. Disinfect shoes
   q. Disinfect the inner gloves
   r. Remove and discard inner gloves
   s. Perform hand hygiene
   t. Check body for contaminants
   u. Exit the doffing area
7. When using a combination of gown/coverall and PAPR, the equipment should be doffed in the following order:
   a. Disinfect outer gloves with an ABHR
   b. Remove outer apron (if worn)
   c. Disinfect outer gloves with an ABHR
   d. Remove boot or shoe covers
   e. Disinfect outer gloves with an ABHR

f. Remove and discard outer gloves
g. Inspect inner gloves
h. Remove the respirator
i. Remove the gown or coverall
j. Disinfect inner gloves with an ABHR
k. Disinfect shoes
l. Disinfect inner gloves with an ABHR
m. Remove and discard inner gloves
n. Perform hand hygiene
o. Check body for contaminants
p. Exit the doffing area

III. Precautions to Prevent Transmission of Infectious Agents[1]

A. STANDARD PRECAUTIONS

1. Emergency personnel should observe standard precautions for *all* patients as part of routine infection control measures in the health care setting
2. Standard precautions are based on the principle that all blood, body fluids, secretions, excretions (except sweat), and mucous membranes are potentially infected with a variety of pathogens
3. Must be implemented whenever contact with nonintact skin, body fluids, or mucous membranes is anticipated
4. Standard precautions always include hand hygiene and may include any of the previously outlined PPE based on the type of exposure that is anticipated
   a. Hand hygiene
      1) Wash hands before and after patient contact and procedures
      2) Wash or disinfect hands with an ABHR before leaving patient's room or care environment, or use soap and water for potential exposure to *Clostridium difficile*
   b. Gloves are routinely used in standard precautions and must be worn when
      1) Contact with blood or body fluids is anticipated
      2) Touching mucous membranes like inside the mouth, rectum, and vagina
      3) Touching nonintact skin or when your hands have nonintact skin
      4) Contact with surfaces, supplies, or equipment that may be contaminated
   c. Masks and protective eye wear or face shields are used to protect the eyes, mouth, and nose when splashing or spraying of body fluids is possible (i.e., intubation, wound irrigation)
   d. Gowns and other protective covers must be used when splashing or spraying of body fluids is expected
   e. Equipment that is contaminated with body fluids or has come in contact with mucous membranes must be discarded, sterilized, or disinfected after use

5. Respiratory hygiene[1,15]
   a. Aimed at preventing the spread of undiagnosed respiratory illnesses
   b. Applies to any patient who presents with a cough, congestion, rhinorrhea, or increased respiratory secretions
   c. Includes several actions in the emergency setting
      1) Posting signs asking patients to cover their mouth and nose when coughing or sneezing
      2) Providing patient education about respiratory hygiene including how to cover the mouth and nose when coughing
      3) Immediately discarding tissues used to cover the mouth and nose during coughing
      4) Wearing a mask if tolerated based on patient's age and condition
      5) Keeping a distance of 3 feet or more from others while waiting in common areas
      6) Washing hands frequently and following any contact with respiratory secretions
6. Safe injection practices[1]
   a. An important element of standard precautions and infection control practices
   b. Use a sterile, single-use, disposable needle and syringe for each injection given
   c. Never reuse needles or syringes on the same patient or with multiple patients
   d. When possible use single-dose vials for medication administration
   e. Always use aseptic technique, including a sterile needle and syringe, when accessing single-dose or multidose medication vials

B. TRANSMISSION-BASED PRECAUTIONS AND ISOLATION[1]

1. Used in addition to standard precautions
2. Based on type of known or suspected infection and mode of transmission
3. Some illnesses have multiple routes of transmission that require health care personnel to use a combination of transmission-based precautions
   a. Examples of diseases that require a combination of transmission-based precautions include viral hemorrhagic fever (Ebola virus disease, Marburg) and severe acute respiratory syndrome (SARS)
4. There are three categories of transmission-based precautions
   a. Contact precautions
      1) Used to prevent the spread of infection when the known or suspected infectious agent is spread by direct or indirect contact with a patient or the patient's environment
      2) Examples of infections requiring contact precautions include but are not limited to noroviruses, *Clostridium difficile*, vancomycin-resistant enterococci (VRE), and respiratory syncytial virus (RSV)

3) Also used when there is a significant amount of wound drainage, fecal incontinence, or other uncontrolled secretions that have the potential to create extensive environmental contamination
4) Contact precautions consist of the following
   a) Private patient room if possible; if not possible keep at least 3 feet spatial separation between patients and consult an infection control specialist for rooming guidance
   b) Post appropriate signage alerting staff and visitors to precautions required
   c) Perform hand hygiene before and after patient contact or contact with the patient's environment
   d) Use soap and water for hand hygiene if hands are visibly soiled or after caring for a patient with diarrhea
   e) Gloves and gowns should be worn for any patient contact or contact with the patient's environment
   f) Don PPE prior to entering the patient's care environment and discard prior to exiting the room or in the designated doffing area
   g) Disinfect the patient's room before allowing a new patient to be placed in the room
   h) Have patient use a private bathroom if possible; if not, disinfect the bathroom after use if the patient has diarrhea
b. Droplet precautions
   1) Used to prevent the spread of infection when the known or suspected infectious agent is spread by close respiratory or mucous membrane contact with respiratory secretions
   2) Examples of infections requiring droplet precautions include but are not limited to influenza viruses, *Bordetella pertussis* (whooping cough), *Neisseria meningitides*, and group A streptococcus (during first 24 hours of antibiotic treatment)
   3) Special air handling and ventilation is not required for droplet precautions because the pathogens involved do not remain infectious for prolonged periods or over long distances suspended in air
   4) Droplet precautions consist of the following
      a) Private patient room if possible; if not possible keep at least 3 feet spatial separation between patients and consult with an infection control specialist for guidance on rooming patients
      b) Post appropriate signage alerting staff and visitors to precautions required
      c) Perform hand hygiene before and after patient contact or contact with the patient's environment
      d) Health care personnel must don a surgical or procedure mask before patient contact or upon entering the patient's room

e) Patients should be wearing a mask (if tolerated) and follow respiratory hygiene standards when outside of their room

f) Use standard precautions as indicated in addition to wearing a mask

c. Airborne precautions

1) Used to prevent the spread of infection when the known or suspected infectious agents remain infectious over long distances when suspended in air

a) Examples of infections requiring airborne precautions include but are not limited to varicella virus (chickenpox), *Mycobacterium tuberculosis* (TB), severe acute respiratory syndrome (SARS), and rubeola virus (measles)

2) Special air handling and ventilation is required and the patient must be placed in an airborne infection isolation room (AIIR)

3) In settings where an AIIR is not available (e.g., exam rooms, ground and air transport) place the patient in a private area with the door closed, ask the patient to wear a mask (if tolerated), and all personnel must wear an N95 or higher respirator while in the care environment

4) If possible, nonimmune health care personnel should not care for patients on airborne precautions with vaccine-preventable airborne illnesses (e.g., measles and chickenpox)

5) Airborne precautions consist of the following

a) Immediately place patient in an airborne infection isolation room (e.g., negative pressure)

b) Post appropriate signage alerting staff and visitors to precautions required

c) Perform hand hygiene before and after patient contact or contact with the patient's environment

d) Health care personnel must don a properly fitted respirator before patient contact or upon entering the patient's room

e) Patients should be wearing a mask (if tolerated) and follow respiratory hygiene standards when outside of their room

f) Use standard precautions as indicated in addition to wearing a respirator

d. When transmission-based precautions are used, health care providers should consider the psychosocial impact on the patient and provide supportive measures to counteract adverse effects

C. PROTECTIVE PRECAUTIONS

1. A protective environment is required for patients who are significantly immunosuppressed to minimize the risk of acquiring a fungal infection

2. Patients requiring protective precautions should be placed in a private positive-pressure room

3. Do not allow live plants or flowers in the patient's room

4. All visitors and health care personnel must perform hand hygiene before entering the patient room and after patient contact

5. Visitors and health care personnel must don a surgical or procedure mask before entering the patient's room

6. Gloves and gowns should also be worn if indicated (Table 9.1)

IV. Organizational Infection Control Recommendations[1,2,16-18]

Preventing the spread of infection and communicable diseases is a priority for emergency nurses and their employers. Health care settings and emergency nurses must be prepared to protect patients and health care providers from a wide range of infectious agents. Additionally, health care settings must be proactive in planning for and managing communicable diseases and preventing the transmission of infection.

A. ADMINISTRATIVE MEASURES

1. Development of infection prevention plans, policies, procedures

2. Provision of human and fiscal resources to manage infection prevention and employee health

3. Infection prevention planning

a. Organizational risk assessment

b. Compliance with regulatory standards and professional organization recommendations

1) Occupational Health and Safety Administration

2) National Institute for Occupational Safety and Health

3) Centers for Disease Control and Prevention

4) Centers for Medicare and Medicaid Services

5) World Health Organization

6) The Joint Commission

7) Emergency Nurses Association

c. Collaborative planning with local public health agencies and community health care partners

d. Development of a safety culture

4. Environmental controls and processes

a. Isolation rooms

b. Filtration devices

c. Limiting visitors when appropriate

d. Use of safety devices

5. Surveillance plan

a. Early identification of communicable disease or illness

b. Monitor for signs and symptoms of outbreaks

c. Collaborate with local, state, and federal partners on surveillance programs (e.g., Biowatch, EpiX, ESSENCE)

Table 9.1

Standard and Transmission-Based Precautions Chart

Precaution Type	Patient type	Patient Placement	Gloves	Gown or Cover	Eye Protection/ Face Shield	Mask	Respirator	Other Considerations
Standard Precautions	All patients	Private room not required	Yes, if contact with blood, body fluids, or mucous membranes	Yes, if splashing or spraying of body fluids	Yes, if splashing or spraying of body fluids	Yes, if splashing or spraying of body fluids	Not required	None
Transmission-Based Precautions								
Contact Precautions	Patients with rash, stool incontinence, diarrhea, uncontrolled secretions or known infection spread by direct or indirect contact	Private room	Yes	Yes	Yes, if splashing or spraying of body fluids	Yes, if splashing or spraying of body fluids	Not required	Provide dedicated medical equipment (preferably disposable)
Droplet Precautions	Patients with known or suspected illness that is spread through contact with respiratory secretions	Private room	Yes, if contact with blood, body fluids, or mucous membranes	Yes, if contact with blood, body fluids, or respiratory secretions	Yes, if splashing or spraying of body fluids and/or secretions	Yes	No, except during aerosol generating procedures like intubation	Reinforce respiratory hygiene practices and have patient wear a mask during transport
Airborne Precautions	Patients with known or suspected illness that remains infectious for long distances when suspended in air	Private airborne infection isolation room	Yes, if contact with blood, body fluids, mucous membranes, or respiratory secretions	Yes, if contact with blood, body fluids, or respiratory secretions	Yes, if splashing or spraying of body fluids and/or secretions	No, does not provide respiratory protection	Yes, N95 or higher	Reinforce respiratory hygiene practices and have patient wear a mask if tolerated during transport
Protective Precautions	Patients with significant immunosuppression	Private positive-pressure room with HEPA filtration	Yes, for direct patient contact	Yes, for direct patient contact	Yes, if splashing or spraying of body fluids/ secretions	Yes, to protect the patient	No	No live flowers or plants in patient room

6. Standardized treatment protocols
   a. Use standardized treatment protocols based on current evidence
7. Medication, supplies, and equipment
   a. Ensure availability of medications to treat patients in a large-scale communicable illness event
   b. Health care organizations must have appropriate PPE and supplies on hand in multiple sizes and readily accessible to health care personnel
8. Vaccinations
   a. Ensure that health care personnel are properly educated on the benefits and risks associated with immunizations
   b. Lack of knowledge and understanding of vaccine efficacy is associated with low health care worker vaccination rates
   c. Include immunization status in employee health interactions
   d. Avoid assigning nonimmune health care personnel to care for patients with vaccine preventable illnesses
   e. Ensure annual influenza vaccination availability for patients and health care workers
9. Education and training should be provided for all health care personnel
   a. Infection control and prevention measures, policies, procedures
   b. Standard and transmission-based precautions
   c. Safe and appropriate use of personal protective equipment
   d. Entering and exiting isolation areas
   e. Disease-specific treatment protocols
   f. Importance of health care personnel vaccinations
10. Practice and drills
    a. Plan for and practice large-scale infectious disease/illness events
       1) Participate in local, regional, state exercises
       2) Utilize practice events to strengthen infection prevention and emergency response plans
    b. Plan for and practice small-scale high-risk events, including but not limited to presentation of a patient with suspected EVD or SARS
       1) Practice team approach including high-risk procedures while wearing appropriate personal protective equipment
       2) Simulation within the ED is an effective strategy for practicing infectious illness events
          a) Provides hands-on experience in the emergency practice setting using available equipment and supplies
          b) Facilitates interprofessional training to simulate real-life team interactions
          c) Identifies gaps in training, communication, resources
          d) Prepares health care workers for complexities of providing care in PPE without risk of disease transmission

References

1. Siegel JD, Rhineheart E, Jackson M, Chiarello L, the Healthcare Infection Control Practices Committee: 2007 Guideline for isolation precautions: preventing transmission of infectious agents in healthcare settings. Retrieved from http://www.cdc.gov/hicpac/pdf/isolation/Isolation2007.pdf, 2007.
2. Emergency Nurses Association: Position statement. Communicable diseases in the emergency department. Retrieved from https://www.ena.org/SiteCollectionDocuments/Position%20Statements/CommDisease.pdf, 2010.
3. World Health Organization: How to wash your hands. Retrieved from http://www.who.int/gpsc/5may/How_To_Hand Wash_Poster.pdf, 2009, May.
4. World Health Organization: How to rub your hands. Retrieved from http://www.who.int/gpsc/5may/How_To_Hand Rub_Poster.pdf, 2009, May.
5. Allegranzi B, Pittet D: Role of hand hygiene in healthcare-associated infection prevention, *J Hosp Infect* 73(4):305–315, 2009.
6. World Health Organization: Glove use information leaflet. Retrieved from http://www.who.int/gpsc/5may/Glove_Use_Information_Leaflet.pdf, 2009, August.
7. Occupational Safety & Health Administration: Major requirements of OSHA's respiratory protection standard 29 CFR 1910.134. Retrieved from https://www.osha.gov/dte/library/respirators/major_requirements.pdf, 2006.
8. Centers for Disease Control and Prevention: Ebola (Ebola Virus Disease). Information for healthcare workers and settings. Retrieved from http://www.cdc.gov/vhf/ebola/hcp/index.html, 2015.
9. Centers for Disease Control and Prevention: Guidance for donning and doffing personal protective equipment (PPE) during management of patients with Ebola virus disease in U.S. hospitals. Retrieved from http://www.cdc.gov/vhf/ebola/hcp/ppe-training/index.html, 2014, Oct. 29.
10. Centers for Disease Control and Prevention: Guidance for the use and selection of personal protective equipment (PPE) in healthcare settings. Retrieved from http://www.cdc.gov/hai/pdfs/ppe/ppeslides6-29-04.pdf, 2004.
11. Centers for Disease Control and Prevention: Guidance on personal protective equipment to be used by healthcare workers during management of patients with Ebola virus disease in U.S. hospitals, including procedures for putting on (donning) and removing (doffing). Retrieved from http://www.cdc.gov/vhf/ebola/hcp/procedures-for-ppe.html, 2015, Aug. 17.
12. United States Department of Health and Human Services: Personal protective equipment. Retrieved from http://chemm.nlm.nih.gov/ppe.htm#medical, 2014, Oct. 31.
13. Bunyan D, Ritchie L, Jenkins D, Coia JE: Respiratory and facial protection: a critical review of recent literature, *J Hosp Infect* 85(3):165–169, 2013, http://dx.doi.org/10.1016/j.hin.2013.07.011.
14. Tompkins BM, Kerchberger JP: Personal protective equipment for care of pandemic influenza patients: a training workshop for the powered air purifying respirator, *Anesth Analg* 111(4):933–945, 2010, http://dx.doi.org/10.1213/ANE.0b013e3181e780f8.
15. Rothman RE, Irvin CB, Moran GJ, et al.: Respiratory hygiene in the emergency department, *J Emerg Nurs* 33(2):119–134, 2007.

16. Gammon J, Morgan-Samuel H, Gould D: A review of the evidence for suboptimal compliance of healthcare practitioners to standard/universal infection control precautions, *J Clin Nurs* 17(2):157–167, 2008.

17. Patterson MD, Geis GL, Falcone RA, LeMaster T, Wears RL: In situ simulation: detection of safety threats and teamwork training in a high risk emergency department, *BMJ Qual Saf* 22(6): 468–477, 2013, http://dx.doi.org/10.1136/bmjqs-2012-000942.

18. Wheeler DS, Geis G, Mack EH, LeMaster T, Patterson MD: High-reliability emergency response teams in the hospital: improving quality and safety using in situ simulation training, *BMJ Qual Saf* 22(6):507–514, 2013, http://dx.doi.org/10.1136/bmjqs-2012-000931.

CHAPTER 10

Children with Special Health Needs (CSHN)

Barbara Weintraub, ARNP, MSN, MPH, CEN, CPEN, FAEN

I. Legislation

A. INDIVIDUALS WITH DISABILITIES EDUCATION IMPROVEMENT ACT OF 2004

1. The Individuals with Disabilities Education Improvement Act (IDEA) is a law ensuring services to children with disabilities throughout the nation. IDEA governs how states and public agencies provide early intervention, special education, and related services to more than 6.5 million eligible infants, toddlers, children, and youth with disabilities

B. AMERICANS WITH DISABILITIES ACT OF 1990[1]

1. The Americans with Disabilities Act (ADA) is a civil rights law which ensures that areas of school buildings such as classrooms, washrooms, playgrounds, and buses be modified to be accessible to students with disabilities

C. REHABILITATION ACT OF 1973, SECTION 504

1. The Rehabilitation Act of 1973 is a civil rights law which prohibits discrimination against individuals who have disabilities. Section 504 of the Rehabilitation Act addresses many disabilities that are not covered under IDEA. Section 504 prohibits discrimination to service availability, accessibility, delivery, employment, and the administrative activities and responsibilities of organizations receiving federal financial assistance. A recipient of federal financial assistance may not, on the basis of disability:[1]
   a. Be denied, as qualified individuals, the opportunity to participate in or benefit from federally funded programs, services, or other benefits
   b. Be denied access to programs, services, benefits, or opportunities to participate as a result of physical barriers

D. PATIENT PROTECTION AND AFFORDABLE CARE ACT (PPACA) OF 2010

1. The Patient Protection and Affordable Care Act (PPACA) was signed into law on March 23, 2010. It offers the opportunity to close gaps in insurance coverage. Cost of health insurance and the affordability of this coverage is a serious issue for families, because CSHN utilize services at a higher rate than the typical

child. Expenditures by payers for the care of CSHN are almost three times higher than for other children, and account for about 42% of all medical care costs for all children. While 18% of all CSHN families report that taking care of their child has created financial hardship, the burden can be even higher for children with specific conditions[2]

E. TITLE V MATERNAL AND CHILD HEALTH SERVICES BLOCK GRANT PROGRAM

1. The Title V Maternal and Child Health Services Block Grant aims to improve the health and well-being of women, particularly mothers, and children. Its funds, dispersed to grantees from 59 states and jurisdictions, seek to provide
   a. Access to preventive and child care services as well as rehabilitative services for certain children
   b. Family-centered, community-based systems of coordinated care for children with special health care needs[3]

II. Demographics

A. DEFINITION

1. The Maternal and Child Health Bureau has defined children with special health needs (CSHN)[4] as, "Those who have one or more chronic physical, developmental, behavioral, or emotional conditions and who also require health and related services of a type or amount beyond that required by children generally"

B. PREVALENCE

1. In 2009, 15.1% of all children in the United States were considered to have special health care needs[5]
2. One of every five households in the United States has at least one child with special health care needs[5]
3. Approximately 14.6 million children ages 0–17 years in the United States (19.8%) have special health care needs[5]
4. Prevalence of CSHN ranges from 14.4% to 26.4% across the 50 states and the District of Columbia[5]
5. About 65% of CSHN experience more complex service needs that go beyond a primary need for prescription medications to manage their health condition[5]
6. Compared to children not meeting CSHN criteria (non-CSHN), CSHN are more likely to be male (58.1% vs. 49.4%) and older (12–17 years) (43.2% vs. 31.8%)[6]

III. General Strategy

A. HEALTH HISTORY CONSIDERATIONS IN CSHN

In general, assessment follows the same priorities as for non-CSHN—utilize CIAMPEDS.
1. Chief complaint

   a. Relationship of chief complaint to underlying disability
   b. Parental concerns as they are this child's expert
   c. CSHN present with both disability-related and non-disability, normal childhood illnesses
2. Immunization status; vaccination history: may not be up to date r/t disability considerations
3. Allergies
   a. Substance
   b. Reaction experienced
   c. How treated
4. Medications
5. Past medical history
   a. Normal childhood illnesses
   b. Disability-related illnesses
      1) Problems encountered
      2) Hospitalizations
      3) Intensive care admissions
6. Parents' impression
   a. Particularly important as parents are experts on child's condition and treatments
7. Events: proceed as for non-CSHN
8. Diet/diapers: establish change from baseline
9. Symptoms: consider parent's analysis of symptoms' importance

B. PRIMARY ASSESSMENT CONSIDERATIONS IN CSHN

1. Consider child's developmental level, rather than anatomic age, in ability to cooperate
2. Possible assessment findings in CSHN
   a. Airway
      1) Decreased ability to handle secretions (e.g., cerebral palsy, esophageal atresia)
      2) Increased size of tongue (e.g., Down syndrome)
      3) Decreased level of consciousness
      4) Abnormal size, placement, or openings of/into airway structures (e.g., Pierre Robin, tracheomalacia, tracheoesophageal fistula)
      5) Presence of airway adjuncts (e.g., tracheostomy)
   b. Breathing
      1) Alterations in immunological system predisposing to pneumonia (e.g., HIV, sickle cell disease, severe combined immunodeficiency)
      2) Abnormality of ribcage, diaphragm, or intercostal muscles (e.g., kyphoscoliosis, spinal muscular atrophy, congenital diaphragmatic hernia)
      3) Alteration in pulmonary-alveolar surface or other lung structures (e.g., cystic fibrosis, pulmonary hypoplasia)[7]
      4) Disorders of oxygen-carrying capacity of blood (e.g., thalassemia, hereditary spherocytosis)
      5) Disorders of neurologic stimulus or pathways for breathing (e.g., Ondine curse [central hypoventilation syndrome])

c. Circulation
   1) Congenital heart abnormalities (e.g., hypoplastic left heart, aortic valve stenosis)
   2) Rhythm disturbances (e.g., congenital third degree heart block, Wolff Parkinson White)
   3) Abnormal peripheral vasculature (e.g., Sturge-Weber, cystic hygroma)
   4) Abnormalities of blood affecting circulation (e.g., hemophilia, ITP)
   5) Abnormalities affecting circulatory volume (e.g., congenital adrenal hyperplasia)
d. Disability
   1) Must be compared to child's own baseline
   2) Decreased level of consciousness (e.g., infantile spasms, Dandy-Walker syndrome)

C. SECONDARY/FOCUSED ASSESSMENT CONSIDERATIONS IN CSHN

1. Exposure and environmental control
   a. Abnormalities of central thermoregulation (e.g., hypothyroidism, Riley Day syndrome)
   b. Abnormalities of skin affecting heat loss (e.g., epidermolysis bullosa, major burns)
   c. Examine for signs of abuse or neglect. Children with special health care needs are 2–3.6 times more likely to experience increased risk of all forms of child maltreatment when compared to children without such needs[8,9]
2. Full set of vital signs
   a. Evaluate vital signs against patient's normal, rather than against normal for age
   b. Obtain parental advice regarding preferred route of temperature measurement
3. Family presence
   a. Utilize family input to compare child's condition to baseline. Family's expertise in child's condition is paramount
   b. Caregivers may be more directive in your care of the patient
      1) Loss of control
      2) Perceive child as more vulnerable than reality
      3) Unrealistic perception as to level of care needed[10]
4. Give comfort measures
   a. Decreased sensitivity to pain (congenital analgesia)
   b. Increased sensitivity to pain (e.g., complex regional pain syndrome)
5. History of present illness
   a. Obtain from child if age appropriate. Do not assume the child cannot communicate regardless of appearance
   b. Factors specific to child's special needs
      1) Previous similar episodes
      2) Previous successful treatments
      3) Change from patient's baseline
   c. Smoking, substance, and/or alcohol use: research suggests some adolescents with special needs may engage more frequently in some risk-taking behaviors[11]

d. Last menstrual period/sexual history
   1) Sexual development can be delayed or come early (Turner syndrome, McCune-Albright syndrome)[12]
   2) Menstrual manipulation sometimes implemented by parents to eliminate menstrual cycle[13]
   3) Menses may affect or be affected by child's disability (e.g., seizures, clotting disorders)[13]
   4) Most CSHN experience interest in learning about approaching potential partners, dating, and having sexual experiences[14]

D. DIFFERENCES IN HEAD TO TOE ASSESSMENT

1. Obtain parental suggestion on order of exam
2. Enlist help of family if needed to examine child

E. AGE-RELATED CONSIDERATIONS

1. Due to advances in medicine, children with some chronic illnesses may now live into adulthood, surviving diseases that had in the past been considered "pediatric diseases"[15]
2. Need to consider plans to accommodate transition from pediatrician-based care to internist-based care[16]

IV. Specific Special Health Care Needs

A. AUTISM SPECTRUM DISORDERS (ASD)[17]

1. Range of neurodevelopmental disorders
   a. Autism
   b. Asperger syndrome
   c. Childhood disintegrative disorder
   d. Pervasive developmental disability
2. Defining characteristics
   a. Impairment in use of nonverbal behaviors/communication
   b. Restricted, repetitive, and stereotyped patterns of behavior interest and activities
   c. Sensory dysfunctions (visual auditory, tactile) are common
3. Common comorbid conditions
   a. Anxiety disorder (43–84% of those with ASD)
   b. Depression (30%)
   c. Obsessive-compulsive disorders (37%)
   d. Seizure disorder (5–49%)
   e. Motor delays (9–19%)
   f. Hypotonia (50%)
4. Emergency department considerations
   a. Presenting conditions
      1) Common childhood illnesses and injuries
      2) Injuries attributable to autistic behaviors (head banging, lack of danger awareness)
      3) Comorbid conditions

b. Treatment considerations
   1) Auditory defensiveness: place in quiet area of ED to decrease auditory stimuli; speak in low, slow, calm voice; set alarms to sound only outside of room
   2) Visual defensiveness: dim lights, converse with child even if he or she avoids eye contact, limit machine settings to avoid flashing lights
   3) Tactile defensiveness: limit amount and duration of touching; approach child gradually and enlist help of parents
   4) Resistance to change: allow child to keep clothes on to the extent possible, try to limit movement from room, utilize portable x-rays; keep family within child's sight

B. CONGENITAL HEART DISEASE

1. Most common birth defect
   a. Occurs in approximately 8 of every 1,000 births
   b. Congenital heart disease accounts for nearly one third of all major congenital anomalies[18]
   c. Mortality has decreased by 31% between 1987 and 2005[19]
2. Defining characteristics
   a. Classified according to patterns of blood flow; cyanotic or acyanotic
   b. Range from single anomalies to complex, multiple anomalies
   c. 8% occur with a syndrome and are genetic, 2% due to environment, 90% multifactorial[20]
3. Common comorbid conditions[19]
   a. Chromosomal abnormalities (DiGeorge syndrome, trisomy 21)
   b. Developmental delays
   c. Impaired immunity (DiGeorge, posttransplant)
4. Emergency department considerations
   a. Presenting conditions
      1) May present undiagnosed in extremis as previously patent ductus arteriosus closes
      2) Congestive heart failure
      3) Cyanosis or tiring during feeding
      4) Syncope
      5) Common childhood illnesses and injuries
   b. Treatment considerations
      1) If undiagnosed and presenting within first weeks of life, consider possibility of ductal-dependent lesion; consider prostaglandin E_1 to keep ductus open until definitive surgery available
      2) Administer oxygen cautiously; oxygen is a vasodilator and can lead to development of pulmonary edema[20]

C. SPINA BIFIDA

1. Definition[21]
   a. Neural tube defect with familial tendency. Defect occurs during development of the spinal cord in the first trimester of pregnancy

b. Myelomeningocele is the most complex congenital abnormality compatible with long-term survival[22]
c. Each year, about 1,500 babies are born with spina bifida
d. At least 75% of children born with this birth defect can be expected to reach their early twenties[21]
2. Defining characteristics
   a. Three main types
      1) Spina bifida occulta: usually without disability. Small gap exists in the spine, without opening or sac on the back. Spinal cord and nerves are usually normal. May not be discovered until late childhood or adulthood
      2) Meningocele: may have minor disabilities. Sac of fluid extrudes through opening in the back; spinal cord is not involved. There is usually little or no nerve damage
      3) Myelomeningocele: causes moderate to severe disability. Sac of fluid extrudes through opening in the back; a portion of the spinal cord and nerves are in this sac and are damaged
3. Common comorbid conditions
   a. Hydrocephalus: 90% of the people with myelomeningocele
   b. Tethered spinal cord: abnormal attachment of distal end of spinal cord to spinal canal; can cause spinal nerve damage due to stretching as child grows
   c. Arnold Chiari II malformation: occurs when the lower part of the brain is displaced from the back of the skull down into the upper neck; may partially obstruct flow of cerebrospinal fluid and lead to hydrocephalus[23]
   d. Orthopedic anomalies such as club foot, hip dislocation, scoliosis
4. Emergency department considerations
   a. Presenting conditions[24]
      1) Fever
      2) Vomiting
      3) Headache
      4) Abdominal pain
      5) Genitourinary symptoms
      6) Urinary tract infection
      7) Cellulitis
      8) Seizure
      9) Headache
      10) Dehydration
      11) Shunt failure
      12) Common childhood illnesses and injuries
   b. Treatment considerations
      1) Latex allergy: possibly three quarters of those with the condition are allergic to latex, or natural rubber[25]
      2) Depressive symptoms among those with spina bifida (48%) were higher than the frequency estimated for people aged 18–34 years from the general population (10%)[21]
      3) Examine for pressure ulcers in areas with decreased/absent sensation

V. Special Considerations

A. EMERGENCY INFORMATION FORM

1. Assists in prompt and appropriate care for CSHN by concisely summarizing crucial information in a standardized format. Available at http://www.acep.org and http://www.aap.org

B. DISASTER PLANNING

1. Anticipate loss of medical home, possible loss of utilities needed for the technologically dependent, challenges in compliance with evacuation orders

References

1. Illinois Emergency Medical Services for Children: Planning for students with special needs. In Zonia L, editor: *School nurse emergency care course*, ed 5, Maywood, IL, 2015, Loyola University Medical Center, pp 339–352.
2. Farrell KH: The Affordable Care Act and children with special health care needs: an analysis and steps for state policymakers. Retrieved from http://hdwg.org/sites/default/files/ACAandCSHCNpaper.pdf, 2011, January.
3. Health Resources and Services Administration Maternal and Child Health. (n.d.): Title V Maternal and Child Health Services Block Grant Program. Retrieved from http://mchb.hrsa.gov/programs/titlevgrants/.
4. McPherson AP: A new definition of children with special health care needs, *Pediatr* 137–140, 1998.
5. Child and Adolescent Health Measurement Initiative: Who are children with special health care needs? Retrieved from http://www.cahmi.org/wp-content/uploads/2014/06/CSHCNSwhoarecshcn_revised_07b-pdf.pdf, 2013.
6. Data Resource Center for Child & Adolescent Health: National Survey of Children with Special Health Care Needs. Retrieved from http://www.childhealthdata.org/learn/NS-CSHCN, 2009/2010.
7. Snow S: *Initial assessment. Emergency nursing pediatric course*, ed 4, Des Plaines, IL, 2013, Emergency Nurses Association, pp 63–82. chapter 5.
8. Giardino AP: Providing medical evaluations for possible child maltreatment to children with special health care needs, *Child Abuse Negl* 1083–1222, 2003.
9. Behar S: Best practices in the emergency department management of children with special needs, *Pediatr Emerg Med Pract* 12(6), 2015.
10. Evans E: Children and youth with special health care needs. In Thomas DB, editor: *Core curriculum for pediatric emergency nursing*, ed 2, Des Plaines, IL, 2009, Emergency Nurses Association, pp 77–81.
11. McNamara J: Learning disabilities and risk-taking behavior in adolescents: A comparison of those with and without co-morbid attention-deficit/hyperactivity disorder, *J Learn Disabil* 561–574, 2008.
12. Fladera ML-B: *A severe LHRH-independent precocious puberty in a 26-month-old girl with a clinical diagnosis of McCune-Albright syndrome*, European Society for Paediatric Endocrinology, 2014.
13. Quint E: Menstrual and reproductive issues in adolescents with physician and developmental disabilities, *Obstet Gynecol* 367–375, 2014.
14. Chivers JM: Training in sexuality and relationships: an Australian model, *Sex Disabil* 73–80, 2000.
15. Cravero J: Caring for adults with pediatric diseases, *ASA Refresher Courses in Anesthesiology* 25–36, 2009.
16. Flume P: Smoothing the transition from pediatric to adult care: Lessons learned, *Curr Opin Pulm Med* 611–614, 2009.
17. Giarelli EN: Sensory stimuli as obstacles to emergency care for children with autism spectrum disorder, *Advanced Emergency Nursing Journal* 145–163, 2014.
18. van der Linde D: Birth prevalence of congenital heart disease worldwide: a systematic review and meta-analysis, *J Am Coll Cardiol* 2241–2247, 2011.
19. Boyle L: The school age child with congenital heart disease, *Matern Child Nurs* 16–23, 2015.
20. Redfearn S: Cardiovascular system. In Soud TR, editor: *Manual of pediatric emergency nursing*, St. Louis, MO, 1998, Mosby-Year Book, pp 233–265.
21. Centers for Disease Control and Prevention: Spina bifida. Retrieved from Centers for Disease Control and Prevention website, at http://www.cdc.gov/ncbddd/spinabifida/facts.html, 2015, September 29.
22. Bowman RM: Spina bifida outcome: a 25-year prospective, *Pediatr Neurosurg* 114–120, 2001.
23. National Institute of Neurological Disorders and Stroke: Chiari malformation fact sheet: National Institute of Neurological Disorders and Stroke (NINDS). Retrieved from http://www.ninds.nih.gov/disorders/chiari/detail_chiari.htm#186143087, 2015, August 27.
24. Caterino JM: Descriptive analysis of 258 emergency department visits by spina bifida patients, *J Emerg Med* 17–22, 2006.
25. National Institute of Health: Eunice Kennedy Shriver National Institute of Child Health and Human Development. Retrieved from https://www.nichd.nih.gov/health/topics/spina bifida/conditioninfo/Pages/disorders-conditions.aspx, 2012, November 30.

CHAPTER 11
Abdominal Emergencies

Margaret A. Flanagan, MSN, FNP-BC, RN

I. General Strategy

A. ASSESSMENT

1. Primary and secondary assessment/resuscitation (see Chapter 1)
2. Focused assessment
   a. Subjective data collection
      1) History of present illness/chief complaint
         a) Pain: PQRST (see Chapter 8)
         b) Vomiting
            (1) Timing of pain in relation to onset of vomiting/diarrhea
            (2) Blood (color—e.g., dark brown, bright red)
            (3) Bile
            (4) Fecal matter
            (5) Onset
            (6) Frequency
            (7) Duration
         c) Diarrhea
         d) Gastrointestinal (GI) bleeding
         e) Recent changes in weight
         f) Changes in bowel habits
         g) Changes in appetite
         h) Efforts to relieve symptoms
            (1) Home remedies
            (2) Alternative therapies
            (3) Medications
               (a) Prescription
               (b) OTC/herbal
         i) Aggravating factors
         j) Recent trauma
      2) Past medical history
         a) Current and preexisting diseases/illness
         b) Previous surgical procedures
         c) Recent foreign travel
         d) Substance and/or alcohol use/abuse
         e) Smoking history
         f) Last normal menstrual period: female patients of childbearing age
         g) Current medications
            (1) Prescription
            (2) OTC/herbal
         h) Allergies
         i) Immunization status
      3) Psychological/social/environmental factors
         a) Lifestyle
         b) Coping patterns
         c) Precipitating events
         d) Possible/actual assault, abuse, or intimate partner violence situations (see Chapters 3 and 40)
   b. Objective data collection
      1) General appearance
         a) Level of consciousness, behavior, affect
         b) Vital signs

c) Odors

d) Gait

e) Hygiene

f) Level of distress/discomfort

2) Inspection

   a) Contour (flat, distended, rounded, herniation)

   b) Obvious pulsating mass

   c) Symmetry

   d) Umbilicus (contour, location, herniation)

   e) Striae

   f) Diastasis rectus

   g) Lesions

   h) Scars

   i) Discolorations

   j) Signs of trauma

3) Auscultation

   a) Bowel sounds: present or absent; character

   b) Bruit

4) Palpation/percussion

   a) Abdominal tenderness

   b) Rigidity/guarding

   c) Masses

   d) Rebound tenderness with deep palpation: indicating peritoneal irritation

   e) Percussion sounds: tympanic, dullness

   f) Spleen or liver enlargement

5) Rectal examination: check stool for occult blood

3. Diagnostic procedures

   a. Laboratory studies

   1) Complete blood count (CBC) with differential

   2) Serum chemistries including glucose, blood urea nitrogen (BUN), and creatinine

   3) Liver function tests (aspartate aminotransaminase [AST], alanine aminotransferase [ALT], lactate dehydrogenase [LDH], alkaline phosphatase)

   4) Serum amylase, lipase

   5) Serum phosphate

   6) Serum lactate

   7) Sickle cell screen

   8) Fecal antigen assay, urea blood test or blood (less specific) for *Helicobacter pylori*

   9) Type and crossmatch

   10) Serial hematocrit

   11) Coagulation profile: prothrombin time (PT), partial thromboplastin time (PTT), international normalized ratio (INR)

   12) Urinalysis; urine culture, pregnancy test in female patients of childbearing age

   13) Stool for occult blood, parasites, white blood cell (WBC) count, mucus, protein, culture

   14) Enzyme-linked immunosorbent assay (ELISA) of stool

   b. Imaging studies

   1) Flat plate abdominal radiograph

   2) Upright abdominal radiograph

   3) Left lateral decubitus radiograph

   4) Cross-table lateral abdominal radiograph

   5) Posteroanterior (PA) chest upright radiograph (to detect thoracic involvement)

   6) Abdominal computed tomography (CT) scan

   7) Abdominal ultrasonography

      a) May consider focused assessment sonography for trauma (FAST) scan as indicated

   8) Magnetic resonance imaging (MRI)

   9) Barium enema

   10) Upper GI series

   11) Angiography

   12) Nuclear scanning

   13) Intravenous (IV) cholangiography

   14) IV urography or cystography

   15) Hepatobiliary iminodiacetic acid (HIDA) scan

   c. Other

   1) 12- to 15-lead electrocardiogram (ECG)

   2) Gastroscopy or endoscopy

   3) Sigmoidoscopy/proctoscopy/colonoscopy

   4) Abdominal paracentesis

   5) Esophageal manometry

B. ANALYSIS: DIFFERENTIAL NURSING DIAGNOSES/COLLABORATIVE PROBLEMS

1. Acute/chronic pain
2. Ineffective tissue perfusion
3. Impaired gas exchange
4. Deficient fluid volume
5. Anxiety/fear
6. Imbalanced nutrition
7. Constipation
8. Diarrhea
9. Risk for infection
10. Deficient knowledge

C. PLANNING AND IMPLEMENTATION/ INTERVENTIONS

1. Determine priorities of care

   a. Maintain airway, breathing, and circulation (see Chapter 1)

   b. Provide supplemental oxygen as indicated

   c. Establish intravenous (IV) access for administration of crystalloid fluid/blood products/medications as needed

   d. Obtain and set up necessary equipment and supplies

   e. Prepare for/assist with medical interventions

   f. Administer pharmacologic therapy as ordered

2. Relieve anxiety/apprehension

3. Allow significant others to remain with patient if supportive

4. Educate patient and significant others

D. EVALUATION AND ONGOING MONITORING

1. Continuously monitor and treat as indicated
2. Monitor patient responses/outcomes and modify nursing care plan as appropriate
3. If positive outcomes are not demonstrated, reevaluate assessment and/or plan of care

E. DOCUMENTATION OF INTERVENTIONS AND PATIENT RESPONSE

F. AGE-RELATED CONSIDERATIONS

1. Pediatrics
   a. Growth or development related
      1) Immature kidney function in infants limits their ability to concentrate and dilute urine and most often results in dehydration
      2) Higher percentage of water compared with body weight, higher metabolic rate, and increased insensible fluid loss make fluid, fluid/electrolyte, and acid-base balance more precarious
      3) Decreased glycogen stores along with the higher metabolic rate increase the risk of hypoglycemia
      4) Hypotension is a late sign of shock and does not appear until circulating blood volume is decreased by 25%
      5) Diarrhea is a major cause of metabolic acidosis; potassium, glucose, and calcium must be carefully monitored
   b. "Pearls"
      1) Avoid restraining the child as much as possible
      2) Use distraction such as television, movies, rhythmic breathing, and imagery for relaxation and pain control
      3) Pain medication may be administered in various ways: intravenously, suppositories, flavored syrup elixirs, pills, or capsules in ice cream
      4) When obtaining history, use face-to-face interviewing, ask specific questions to caregivers, and ask age-appropriate questions to child
      5) Oral replacement therapy (ORT) is the rehydration route of choice for children with mild to moderate dehydration who can tolerate oral fluids. Fluids of choice for ORT include glucose water, clear liquids, sports drinks, gelatin, oral electrolyte solution, broth, tea, or ice pops at 5 mL every 3–5 minutes
      6) IV fluid replacement to correct dehydration should be done with isotonic fluids and fluids containing chloride, glucose, water, sodium, and potassium
      7) IV fluid replacement with isotonic crystalloid solution for signs of shock at 20 mL/kg
      8) Obtain a history for trauma and consider if signs and symptoms could be associated with abuse
2. Geriatrics
   a. Aging related
      1) Obtaining a history from an elderly patient may be difficult secondary to impaired cognitive function, diminished vision, diminished hearing, and slower psychomotor responses
      2) Elderly patients usually do not present with classic signs and symptoms, because of aging changes or medications. They are inclined to underreport or be vague about symptoms
      3) An emergency department visit may be a crisis to elderly persons because they fear the loss of independence or that the visit may trigger a financial crisis
      4) Older patients have a reduced ability to adjust to extremes in environmental temperature. Care should be taken to minimize body exposure in the elderly
      5) Alterations in GI function associated with aging include increased gastric secretions and decreased gastric motility
      6) Slower metabolism of medications increases the risk of developing medication toxicities
      7) Decreases in stomach acid secretion and GI tract motility can lead to nutritional problems
      8) Obtain a history for trauma and consider if signs and symptoms could be associated with abuse

II. Specific Abdominal Emergencies

A. APPENDICITIS

Appendicitis is an inflammation or obstruction of the appendix, a blind pouch in the inferior part of the cecum. This can lead to compromised vascular supply of the vermiform appendix, causing ischemia, necrosis, or perforation. The resulting damage allows for bacterial invasion of the wall of the appendix and potential invasion of bacteria to the peritoneum triggering abscess formation or peritonitis. A high index of suspicion is important, because no specific assessment finding or diagnostic test can accurately identify appendicitis. Individuals of any age may be affected, with the highest incidence occurring in the late teen years and twenties; cases of perforation are more common in the young because of delays in diagnosis.

1. Assessment
   a. Subjective data collection
      1) History of present illness/chief complaint
         a) Pain
            (1) Pain with movement: position of comfort with hips and knees flexed
            (2) Initially dull, later may be colicky

(3) Early: poorly localized or periumbilical; later: localizes to right lower quadrant (RLQ). In the pregnant patient, the uterus displaces the appendix, and the pain may be in the right upper quadrant (RUQ)

b) Loss of appetite

c) Nausea/vomiting

d) Constipation

e) Last normal menstrual period: female patients of childbearing age

2) Past medical history

a) Current and preexisting diseases/illness

b) Allergies

c) Medications

b. Objective data collection

1) Physical examination

a) General appearance

(1) Elevated temperature: low-grade fever

(2) Moderate distress/discomfort (pain scale rating)

b) Inspection

(1) Vomiting (amount, color, odor)

c) Auscultation

(1) Bowel sounds: hypoactive

d) Palpation

(1) RLQ tenderness over McBurney's point

(2) Muscle rigidity and guarding

(3) Rovsing sign: left lower quadrant (LLQ) pressure will intensify RLQ pain

(4) Rebound tenderness, pain with movement, coughing if peritonitis present

2) Diagnostic procedures

a) CBC with differential: elevated WBC greater than 10,000 with neutrophilia in adults

b) Serum chemistries; C-reactive protein (CRP) >1 mg/dL common

c) Urinalysis; pregnancy test in female patients of childbearing age

d) Abdominal helical CT scan: most precise

(1) High degree of sensitivity and specificity

e) Abdominal ultrasonography

(1) Preferred diagnostic radiograph for pregnant female patients

(2) If negative, appendicitis may still be present

f) Kidney, ureter, bladder (KUB) radiograph

(1) Appendicolith (calcified deposits within the appendix) may be visualized (particularly in children with appendicitis): rare

(2) Overall poor sensitivity and specificity

2. Analysis: differential nursing diagnoses/collaborative problems

a. Acute pain

b. Risk for infection

c. Risk for fluid volume deficit

d. Anxiety/fear

3. Planning and implementation/interventions

a. Establish IV access for administration of crystalloid fluids/medications as needed

b. Allow patient position of comfort (often in fetal position)

c. Prepare for/assist with medical interventions

1) Initiate and maintain NPO status

2) Insert gastric tube and attach to suction as indicated

3) Assist with hospital admission and preparation for surgery

d. Administer pharmacologic therapy as ordered

1) Nonnarcotic analgesics

2) Narcotics

3) Antibiotics

4) Antipyretics

4. Evaluation and ongoing monitoring

a. Hemodynamic status

b. Pain relief

c. Bowel sounds

d. Intake and output

B. BOWEL OBSTRUCTION

An intestinal obstruction results in the inability of intestinal contents to flow normally along the intestinal tract. Obstruction may be partial, in which the bowel lumen is narrowed, or complete, in which the bowel lumen is closed. Causes include cancer, foreign bodies, strictures, hernias, postoperative peritoneal adhesions, volvulus, paralytic ileus, intussusception, Crohn's disease, congenital defects, stenosis, and neurogenic conditions. A bowel obstruction results in the accumulation of intestinal contents, fluids, and gas proximal to the obstruction. The absorption of fluids is decreased and gastric secretions are increased. Fluids and electrolytes are lost, and increasing pressure within the intestinal lumen causes a decrease in venous and arteriolar capillary pressure. This leads to edema, congestion, necrosis, and eventual rupture or perforation of the intestinal wall.

1. Assessment

a. Subjective data collection

1) History of present illness/chief complaint

a) Pain

(1) May have temporary relief after emesis

(2) Colicky, crampy, intermittent, wavelike

(3) Poorly localized

(4) Intermittent: rapid onset in small bowel, gradual onset in large bowel

2) Past medical history

a) Current or preexisting diseases/illness

b) History of abdominal surgery

c) Change in bowel habits

d) Medications

e) Allergies

b. Objective data collection
  1) Physical examination
    a) General appearance
      (1) Elevated temperature
      (2) Tachycardia and hypertension in early sepsis: may become hypotensive later
      (3) Moderate to severe distress/discomfort, critically ill
    b) Inspection
      (1) Abdominal distention: minimal (small intestine) to maximal (large intestine)
      (2) Vomiting: bilious, fecal material may be present if bacterial proliferation
    c) Auscultation
      (1) Bowel sounds
        (a) High-pitched peristaltic rush sounds proximal to the area of obstruction
        (b) Audible borborygmi (hyperactive bowel sounds)
        (c) Absent bowel sounds: late finding
    d) Palpation
      (1) Diffuse abdominal tenderness and rigidity
  2) Diagnostic procedures
    a) CBC with differential: possible leukocytosis with left shift
    b) Serum chemistries including BUN and creatinine
    c) Serum amylase and lipase: may be elevated with ischemia
    d) Urinalysis; pregnancy test in female patients of childbearing age
    e) Type and crossmatch
    f) Stool for occult blood
    g) Flat and upright abdominal radiograph
    h) Abdominal CT scan
    i) Barium studies
2. Analysis: differential nursing diagnoses/collaborative problems
  a. Pain
  b. Deficient fluid volume
  c. Imbalanced nutrition: less than body requirements
  d. Anxiety/fear
3. Planning and implementation/interventions
  a. Maintain airway, breathing, and circulation
  b. Provide supplemental oxygen as indicated
  c. Establish IV access for administration of crystalloid fluids/medications as needed
  d. Prepare for/assist with medical interventions
    1) Institute cardiac and pulse oximetry monitoring
    2) Initiate and maintain NPO status
    3) Insert gastric tube and attach to suction
    4) Insert indwelling urinary catheter as indicated by hemodynamic status or surgical urgency
    5) Assist with hospital admission and surgical intervention as indicated

  e. Administer pharmacologic therapy as ordered
    1) Antiemetics
    2) Antibiotics
    3) Nonnarcotic analgesics
    4) Narcotics
4. Evaluation and ongoing monitoring
  a. Hemodynamic status
  b. Breath sounds and pulse oximetry
  c. Cardiac rate and rhythm
  d. Pain relief
  e. Bowel sounds
  f. Intake and output

C. CHOLECYSTITIS

Cholecystitis is an inflammation of the gallbladder and is most frequently caused by gallstones that obstruct the cystic duct or common bile duct. Other causes include infectious agents or a tumor obstructing the biliary tract. Obstruction or acute inflammation of the bile ducts causes blockage of bile secretion and may possibly result in gangrene.

1. Assessment
  a. Subjective data collection
    1) History of present illness/chief complaint
      a) Pain
        (1) Aggravated by deep breathing
        (2) Sharp, constant: may be colicky
        (3) RUQ or epigastric; may be referred to right scapula and shoulder
        (4) Frequently occurs after ingestion of a large or fatty meal
      b) Indigestion, nausea, anorexia, vomiting
    2) Past medical history
      a) Current or preexisting diseases/illness
      b) Last normal menstrual period: female patients of childbearing age
      c) Fatty food diet
      d) Recent rapid weight loss
      e) Medications
      f) Allergies
  b. Objective data collection
    1) Physical examination
      a) General appearance
        (1) Elevated temperature: if infection present
        (2) Moderate distress/discomfort
      b) Inspection
        (1) Possible jaundice
      c) Auscultation
        (1) Bowel sounds: hypoactive or absent
      d) Palpation
        (1) RUQ tenderness, guarding, and rigidity
        (2) Murphy's sign: inability to take deep breaths during palpation beneath right costal arch below hepatic margin
    2) Diagnostic procedures
      a) CBC with differential: WBC count elevated
      b) Serum and urine bilirubin: elevated

c) ALT: elevated
d) Serum chemistries including glucose
e) Urinalysis; pregnancy test in female patients of childbearing age
f) Flat and upright abdominal radiographs
g) Abdominal ultrasonography
h) HIDA scan (cholescintigraphy)
i) Abdominal CT scan: if diagnosis not clear
j) Cholangiography

2. Analysis: differential nursing diagnoses/collaborative problems
   a. Pain
   b. Risk for infection
   c. Deficient fluid volume
   d. Deficient knowledge

3. Planning and implementation/interventions
   a. Establish IV access for administration of crystalloid fluids/medications as needed
   b. Prepare for/assist with medical interventions
      1) Initiate and maintain NPO status
      2) Insert gastric tube and attach to suction (questionable based on severity of the case)
      3) Assist with possible hospital admission
   c. Administer pharmacologic therapy as ordered
      1) Antiemetics
      2) Nonnarcotic analgesics
      3) Narcotics
      4) Antibiotics
   d. Educate patient/significant others
      1) Low-fat diet and medications
      2) Avoid causative factors

4. Evaluation and ongoing monitoring
   a. Hemodynamic status
   b. Pain relief
   c. Intake and output
   d. Bowel sounds

D. DIVERTICULITIS

Diverticulitis is an inflammation of colon diverticula, small mucosal pockets that may become obstructed with undigested food particles or fecal material. Bacteria and other irritating substances lead to inflammation and infection. Perforation of the thin walls of the diverticulum, leading to microscopic or frank bleeding, is also possible. Diverticulitis commonly involves the sigmoid colon and is seen predominantly in patients older than 50 years. A low-fiber diet causing low bulk stools is a contributing factor.

1. Assessment
   a. Subjective data collection
      1) History of present illness/chief complaint
         a) Pain
            (1) Aching, crampy
            (2) Vague, generalized abdominal pain; later localizes to LLQ
            (3) Usually abrupt onset but may be intermittent or present for days
         b) Change in bowel habits
         c) Anorexia
      2) Past medical history
         a) Current or preexisting diseases/illness
            (1) Diverticulosis or diverticulitis
         b) Medications
         c) Allergies
   b. Objective data collection
      1) Physical examination
         a) General appearance
            (1) Elevated temperature: low-grade fever
            (2) Moderate distress/discomfort
         b) Inspection
            (1) Occult blood in stool
         c) Auscultation
            (1) Bowel sounds: hyperactive/hypoactive
         d) Palpation
            (1) LLQ abdominal tenderness and guarding
            (2) Rectal tenderness
      2) Diagnostic procedures
         a) CBC with differential: WBC count elevated; erythrocyte sedimentation rate (ESR)
         b) Stool for occult blood: positive
         c) Urinalysis; pregnancy test in female patients of childbearing age
         d) Abdominal radiographs to rule out free air
         e) Abdominal CT scan
         f) Sigmoidoscopy GI consult—admitted or outpatient procedure
         g) Barium enema or colonoscopy: increased risk of perforation when done during initial episode, better for later evaluation of disease extent; GI consult—admitted or outpatient procedure

2. Analysis: differential nursing diagnoses/collaborative problems
   a. Acute pain
   b. Constipation
   c. Risk for infection
   d. Deficient knowledge

3. Planning and implementation/interventions
   a. Establish IV access for administration of crystalloid fluids/medications as needed
   b. Prepare for/assist with medical interventions
      1) Initiate and maintain NPO status: if unable to tolerate oral fluids
      2) Insert gastric tube and attach to suction as indicated if ileus
      3) Assist with hospital admission and prepare for surgery as indicated
   c. Administer pharmacologic therapy as ordered
      1) Analgesics
      2) Antibiotics
      3) Antispasmodics to relax smooth muscles
   d. Educate patient and significant others
      1) High-fiber diet and medications
      2) Avoid causative factors

4. Evaluation and ongoing monitoring
   a. Hemodynamic status
   b. Pain relief
   c. Intake and output
   d. Stools for appearance of blood or occult blood
   e. Bowel sounds

E. ESOPHAGEAL VARICES

Esophageal varices are dilated, submucosal veins of the lower esophagus that may extend into the upper esophagus and stomach. This condition occurs most often as a result of obstructed portal circulation associated with liver cirrhosis from alcoholism. Hemorrhage from ruptured esophageal varices is frequently the cause of death in patients with cirrhosis of the liver.

1. Assessment
   a. Subjective data collection
      1) History of present illness/chief complaint
         a) Pain
            (1) Dull
            (2) May have chest pain
            (3) Onset of discomfort may be gradual or sudden, constant or intermittent
         b) Ingestion of irritating fluids, salicylates, or drugs that erode the mucosa or interfere with cell replication
         c) Nausea and vomiting
      2) Past medical history
         a) Current or preexisting diseases/illness
            (1) Alcoholism, liver disease
            (2) Gastritis
            (3) Duodenal ulcer
            (4) Bleeding disorders
         b) Medications
         c) Allergies
   b. Objective data collection
      1) Physical examination
         a) General appearance
            (1) Level of consciousness, behavior, affect: restlessness, drowsiness
            (2) Tachycardia, hypotension,
            (3) Moderate to severe distress/discomfort, critically ill
         b) Inspection
            (1) Pallor
            (2) Hematemesis: bright red or brown; may be provoked by sneezing, coughing, straining at stool, lifting heavy objects, vomiting, or swallowing poorly chewed food
            (3) Melena
         c) Palpation
            (1) Hepatomegaly/splenomegaly
            (2) Ascites
            (3) Diaphoresis
      2) Diagnostic procedures

         a) CBC with differential: hemoglobin and hematocrit may be normal or decreased from blood loss
         b) Type and crossmatch
         c) Serum chemistries including glucose, BUN, and creatinine
         d) Liver function tests: frequently elevated
         e) Serial hematocrits
         f) Urinalysis; pregnancy test in female patients of childbearing age
         g) Stool for occult blood
         h) Serum ammonia level
         i) Coagulation profile: PT, PTT, INR, clotting time
         j) Emergent endoscopy—GI consult
         k) Chest radiograph
         l) Upper GI series—GI consult

2. Analysis: differential nursing diagnoses/collaborative problems
   a. Deficient fluid volume
   b. Pain
   c. Anxiety/fear
   d. Deficient knowledge

3. Planning and implementation/interventions
   a. Maintain airway, breathing, and circulation
   b. Provide supplemental oxygen as indicated
   c. Establish IV access for administration of crystalloid fluids/blood products/medications as needed
      1) Insert two large-bore IV catheters
      2) Infuse normal saline solution and blood products as indicated
   d. Prepare for/assist with medical interventions
      1) Institute cardiac and pulse oximetry monitoring
      2) Initiate and maintain NPO status
      3) Insert gastric tube and attach to suction
      4) Insert indwelling urinary catheter as indicated
      5) Endoscopy or mechanical tamponade with Sengstaken-Blakemore tube or other tubes. If balloon tamponade is to be done, prepare for endotracheal intubation prior to insertion Patient is taken to GI department for endoscopic therapy (sclerotherapy or variceal ligation)
      6) Assist with hospital admission and prepare for surgical admission if indicated
   e. Administer pharmacologic therapy as ordered
      1) Vasopressors (e.g., vasopressin [Pitressin])
      2) Vitamin K (AquaMEPHYTON)
      3) Analgesics

4. Evaluation and ongoing monitoring
   a. Hemodynamic status
   b. Breath sounds and pulse oximetry
   c. Cardiac rate and rhythm
   d. Pain relief
   e. Intake and output
   f. Gastric emesis for blood
   g. Stools for tarry appearance and/or occult blood

h. Hemoglobin and hematocrit
i. Serum electrolytes
j. Arterial blood gases

F. ESOPHAGITIS

Esophagitis is an inflammatory response of the mucosa of the esophagus related to a variety of stimuli, including achalasia, gastroesophageal reflux disease (GERD), infection, medications, or trauma. The response is of variable severity; the most severe is characterized by upper GI bleeding and stricture. Achalasia is impaired motility of the lower two thirds of the esophagus as a result of alteration in the neurologic functioning in the esophagus or lack of lower esophageal sphincter receptors. In GERD, the inflammation is caused by reflux of gastric secretions. Infections such as with *Candida*, herpes simplex, and cytomegalovirus can occur in the esophagus, most commonly in immunosuppressed people. Prolonged exposure to drugs such as NSAIDs, potassium chloride, quinidine, and antibiotics can irritate the esophagus, especially if not much fluid was used to swallow the pills or if the person was supine immediately after taking the medication.

1. Assessment
   a. Subjective data collection
      1) History of present illness/chief complaint
         a) Pain
            (1) May occur after taking pills, eating
            (2) Burning
            (3) Location: chest, epigastric, substernal
            (4) Intermittent or constant
         b) Reflux or heartburn
         c) Dysphagia
         d) Odynophagia
         e) Nausea or vomiting
      2) Past medical history
         a) Current or preexisting diseases/illness
            (1) Possible immunosuppression: human immunodeficiency virus (HIV), organ replacement, leukemia, lymphoma
            (2) Current radiation therapy
            (3) History of GERD
         b) Medications that may influence condition: NSAIDs, steroids, potassium chloride, antibiotics, or medications influencing achalasia such as anticholinergics or calcium channel blockers
         c) Allergies
   b. Objective data collection
      1) Physical examination
         a) General appearance
            (1) Mild to moderate distress/discomfort
         b) Inspection
            (1) Herpetic mouth or nose lesions if viral cause
            (2) Oral thrush
         c) Palpation
            (1) Slight epigastric tenderness

2) Diagnostic procedures
   a) Upper GI/barium swallow GI consult—admitted patient or outpatient procedure
   b) Endoscopy with biopsy GI consult—admitted patient or outpatient procedure
   c) Esophageal manometry GI consult—admitted patient or outpatient procedure
2. Analysis: differential nursing diagnoses/collaborative problems
   a. Acute/chronic pain
   b. Imbalanced nutrition: less than body requirements
   c. Deficient knowledge
3. Planning and implementation/interventions
   a. Establish IV access for administration of crystalloid fluid/blood products as needed
   b. Prepare for/assist with medical interventions
      1) Nutritional support as indicated: percutaneous endoscopic gastrostomy tube
      2) Assist with hospital admission for esophageal dilatation or surgery
   c. Administer pharmacologic therapy as ordered
      1) Analgesics
      2) Proton pump inhibitors
      3) Antibiotics
   d. Educate patient/significant others
      1) Diet of small, frequent meals and medications
      2) Avoid causative factors
4. Evaluation and ongoing monitoring
   a. Hemodynamic status
   b. Pain relief
   c. Intake and output

G. GASTRITIS

Gastritis is inflammation of the stomach that most often originates from ingestion of nonsteroidal antiinflammatory drugs (NSAIDs), alcohol, salicylates, steroids, caustic ingestion (acids, alkalis, or food with excessive seasoning), or ingestion of infected foods. Other causes include physical or emotional stress, tobacco, radiation, bacterial or viral infection, and diseases that affect the gastric mucosal cells. Chronic gastritis may be caused by *H. pylori*, which is present in 30% to 50% of the population. The gastric mucous membrane undergoes superficial erosion, causing excessive secretion of gastric juices containing acid and mucus. Acute episodes may cause epigastric pain, nausea, vomiting, diarrhea, anorexia, and eructations of gas. Chronic episodes of gastritis may lead to duodenal and gastric (peptic) ulcers, hemorrhage, pernicious anemia, pyloric obstruction, and perforation.

1. Assessment
   a. Subjective data collection
      1) History of present illness/chief complaint
         a) Pain
            (1) Relieved by intake of food
            (2) Squeezing, burning, dull, gnawing, colicky
            (3) Epigastric area

      (4) Sudden or gradual onset, may be chronic, intermittent, or constant
    b) Nausea and/or vomiting
      (1) Frequent nausea
      (2) Vomiting (blood, mucus, undigested food)
  2) Past medical history
    a) Current or preexisting diseases/illness
      (1) Ulcer disease, chronic indigestion, malignancy
      (2) Cardiovascular disease
      (3) Diabetes
    b) Consumption of alcohol or tobacco use
    c) Unusual or chronic tension or anxiety
    d) Ingestion of an irritant (spicy foods or alcohol)
    e) Medication use: NSAIDs, steroids, antacids, or OTC histamine-2 (H_2) blockers
    f) Allergies
 b. Objective data collection
  1) Physical examination
    a) General appearance
      (1) Possible positive orthostasis
      (2) Mild to moderate distress/discomfort
    b) Inspection
      (1) Hematemesis
    c) Auscultation
      (1) Bowel sounds: normal to hyperactive
    d) Palpation
      (1) Epigastric tenderness on palpation
      (2) Muscular guarding
  2) Diagnostic procedures
    a) Serum chemistries
    b) CBC with differential
    c) Coagulation profile (PT, PTT, INR)
    d) Urinalysis; pregnancy test in female patients of childbearing age
    e) Fecal antigen assay, urea breath test, or blood test (less specific) for *H. pylori*
    f) Radiograph flat and upright of abdomen (presence of free air)
    g) Stool examination for occult blood
    h) Upper GI series
    i) Upper endoscopy with biopsy
    j) Gastric analysis
2. Analysis: differential nursing diagnoses/collaborative problems
 a. Pain
 b. Risk for deficient fluid volume
 c. Deficient knowledge
3. Planning and implementation/interventions
 a. Establish IV access for administration of crystalloid fluid/medications as needed
 b. Prepare for/assist with medical interventions
  1) Initiate and maintain nothing by mouth (NPO) status
  2) Insert gastric tube and attach to suction as indicated

 c. Administer pharmacologic therapy as ordered
  1) Nonnarcotic analgesics
  2) Narcotics
  3) Antiemetics
  4) Antacids, histamine receptor antagonist, or proton pump inhibitors
  5) Anticholinergics
 d. Educate patient/significant others
  1) Regular diet on cessation of vomiting, medications
  2) Avoid causative factors
4. Evaluation and ongoing monitoring
 a. Hemodynamic status
 b. Pain relief
 c. Intake and output
 d. Gastric emesis for blood
 e. Bowel sounds
 f. Stools for tarry appearance and/or occult blood

H. GASTROENTERITIS/INFECTIOUS DIARRHEA

Gastroenteritis is an inflammation of the lining of the stomach and intestine. Eighty-five percent of cases are infectious, caused by viral, protozoan, bacterial, or parasitic agents. Gastroenteritis may also be caused by an imbalance in the normal flora of the gut, secondary to antibiotic therapy. Gastroenteritis usually runs an acute course with no sequelae. Infectious diarrhea may be caused by viral (rotavirus, Norwalk-type virus, parvovirus), protozoan (amoebic dysentery), bacterial (*Salmonella, Shigella dysenteriae, Escherichia coli, Staphylococcus aureus, Clostridium difficile*), or parasitic (*Trichinella*, tapeworm) agents. Traveler's diarrhea is infectious diarrhea that results from consumption of contaminated foods or water. Routes of infection include person-to-person contact, contact with feces such as with diaper changing, consumption of raw or inadequately prepared shrimp, shellfish, or meat. Noninflammatory diarrhea is caused by infectious agents (*C. difficile, Giardia lamblia, E. coli*) that produce enterotoxins that override the colon's capacity to absorb fluid, resulting in large amounts of watery diarrhea, abdominal cramping, and possibly nausea and vomiting. Inflammatory diarrhea is caused by agents such as rotavirus, Norwalk virus, *S. dysenteriae, Salmonella, E. coli,* and *Campylobacter jejuni.* They invade the intestinal mucosa and secrete toxins that destroy the intestinal mucosal epithelial cells and result in bloody diarrhea, lower abdominal cramping, and fever. Food poisoning is caused by bacterial toxins such as *S. aureus, Clostridium perfringens,* and *Bacillus cereus* and is characterized by a short (2- to 6-hour) incubation period and prominent vomiting. Numerous people may be affected in a single outbreak.

1. Assessment
 a. Subjective data collection
  1) History of present illness/chief complaint
    a) Pain
      (1) Secondary to increased peristalsis

      (2) Cramping, colicky

      (3) Diffuse

      (4) Usually resolves within 24 hours

    b) Nausea and/or vomiting and diarrhea

  2) Past medical history

    a) Current or preexisting diseases/illness

    b) Stool pattern: cramping diarrhea

    c) Travel to foreign country

    d) Recent dietary change

    e) Use of antibiotics

    f) Consumption of raw or inadequately cooked shrimp, shellfish, meat

    g) Employed in a day care center or custodial institution

    h) Medications

    i) Allergies

  b. Objective data collection

    1) Physical examination

      a) General appearance

        (1) Elevated temperature

        (2) Moderate distress/discomfort

      b) Inspection

        (1) Weak, malaise

        (2) Vomiting

        (3) Diarrhea

        (4) Blood or mucus in stools

      c) Auscultation

        (1) Bowel sounds: hyperactive

    2) Diagnostic procedures

      a) CBC with differential: leukocytosis

      b) Serum chemistries

      c) Urinalysis; pregnancy test in female patients of childbearing age

      d) Stool for WBC count; culture if positive for WBC count; occult blood; ova/parasites; rotavirus if prolonged diarrhea, travel history, or contact with day care

2. Analysis: differential nursing diagnoses/collaborative problems

  a. Deficient fluid volume

  b. Diarrhea

  c. Pain

  d. Deficient knowledge

3. Planning and implementation/interventions

  a. Maintain airway, breathing, and circulation

  b. Provide supplemental oxygen as indicated

  c. Establish IV access for administration of crystalloid fluid/medications as needed

    1) Normal saline solution boluses if unable to take oral rehydration

  d. Prepare for/assist with medical interventions

    1) Initiate and maintain NPO status until vomiting stops

    2) Oral rehydration: fluids with glucose, sodium, and potassium (i.e., sports drinks)

  e. Administer pharmacologic therapy as ordered

    1) Antiemetics

    2) Nonnarcotic analgesics

    3) Narcotics

    4) Antibiotics

    5) Anticholinergics

    6) Corticosteroids with parasitic gastroenteritis

  f. Educate patient/significant others

    1) Regular diet with cessation of vomiting

    2) Hand hygiene

    3) GI referral for further workup

4. Evaluation and ongoing monitoring

  a. Hemodynamic status

  b. Pain relief

  c. Intake and output

  d. Stools for tarry appearance and/or occult blood

  e. Bowel sounds

I. GASTROESOPHAGEAL REFLUX DISEASE

Gastroesophageal reflux disease (GERD) is the backflow of gastric contents into the esophagus. It is seen more predominantly with obesity and people who are more than 40 years old. It can be caused by decreased tone of the lower esophageal sphincter, slowed motility or peristalsis, or slowed gastric emptying. Approximately 50% of people with GERD will develop some degree of esophagitis. GERD can occur with or without a hiatal hernia, a condition in which muscle weakness causes the sphincter of the stomach to herniate above the diaphragm into the thoracic cavity.

1. Assessment

  a. Subjective data collection

    1) History of present illness/chief complaint

      a) Pain

        (1) Exacerbated by meals and activities that increase intraabdominal pressure, such as lifting, straining, or recumbent position

        (2) Burning sensation that moves up and down the esophagus

        (3) Epigastric; may radiate to back, neck, jaw, chest

        (4) Frequently occurs 30 to 60 minutes after meals

        (5) Sensation of "something stuck" in chest after eating

      b) Reflux

      c) Dysphagia: intermittent when lying or supine

    2) Past medical history

      a) Current or preexisting diseases/illness

        (1) Peptic ulcer disease

        (2) Cardiovascular disease

      b) Obesity or weight gain

      c) Use of tobacco products

      d) Consumption of caffeine, high-fat diet

      e) Medication history: NSAIDs, anticholinergic drugs, calcium channel blockers, salicylates, and long-term use of antacids or H_2 blockers

      f) Allergies

  b. Objective data collection

1) Physical examination
   a) General appearance
      (1) Hoarseness or laryngitis, belching
      (2) Mild to moderate distress/discomfort
   b) Palpation
      (1) Slight epigastric tenderness
2) Diagnostic procedures
   a) Serum chemistries
   b) Urinalysis; pregnancy test in female patients of childbearing age
   c) Endoscopy with biopsy: distinguish from peptic ulcer disease
   d) Esophageal manometry
   e) Ambulatory 24-hour pH monitoring
   f) Gastric secretions analysis
   g) Upper GI/barium swallow (limited value unless suspect stricture)
   h) ECG

2. Analysis: differential nursing diagnoses/collaborative problems
  a. Pain
  b. Deficient knowledge
  c. Risk for aspiration
  d. Anxiety/fear

3. Planning and implementation/intervention
  a. Administer pharmacologic therapy as ordered
    1) Antacids
    2) H_2-receptor antagonists or proton pump inhibitors
    3) Cholinergic medications
  b. Educate patient/significant others
    1) Diet: eat small meals; avoid caffeine, spicy foods, alcohol, chocolate, peppermint, high-fat foods
    2) Raise head of bed on 6- to 8-inch blocks
    3) Weight loss as indicated
    4) Avoid tobacco

4. Evaluation and ongoing monitoring
  a. Pain relief

J. INTUSSUSCEPTION

Intussusception occurs when a segment of the bowel telescopes within itself, causing a mechanical bowel obstruction, and is most commonly found in infants and small children. The incidence of intussusception is 1.5–4 cases per 1,000 live births, with a male-to-female ratio of 3:2. The highest incidence of idiopathic intussusception is in infants aged 9–24 months. A seasonal incidence has been described with peaks in the spring, summer, and middle of winter that correspond with occurrence of seasonal gastroenteritis and upper respiratory tract infections. Intussusception most commonly develops at or near the ileocecal valve or at the point of attachment of a colon tumor, polyp, or Meckel diverticulum. Without treatment, death can occur within 2–4 days because of the compromised vascular supply to the bowel and mesentery and the resulting gangrene and sepsis. Careful history taking and physical examination are essential because the classic presenting triad of vomiting, colicky abdominal pain, and red currant jelly stool occurs in less than 25% of all patients.

1. Assessment
  a. Subjective data collection
    1) History of present illness/chief complaint
      a) Pain
        (1) Occurs during peristalsis
        (2) Colicky, spasmodic
        (3) Diffuse
        (4) Out of proportion to physical examination
        (5) Explosive, sudden onset, episodic, with pain-free intervals
    2) Past medical history
      a) Current or preexisting diseases/illness
      b) Diarrhea
      c) Constipation
      d) Appetite changes
      e) Medications
      f) Allergies
  b. Objective data collection
    1) Physical examination
      a) General appearance
        (1) Level of consciousness, behavior, affect: lethargy, late finding
        (2) Elevated temperature: late finding
        (3) Mild to severe distress/discomfort, possibly critically ill
      b) Inspection
        (1) Paroxysms of acute abdominal pain followed by normal activity
        (2) Knees flexed up to abdomen, then relaxing as pain eases
        (3) Rectal blood or "currant jelly" stools (blood and mucus in stools): stools may appear normal but will usually test positive for occult blood
        (4) Vomiting food, mucus, and/or fecal matter
      c) Auscultation
        (1) Bowel sounds: hyperactive/hypoactive with "rushes" during pain episodes
      d) Palpation
        (1) Tender, palpable, "sausage-shaped" mass at site of intussusception in right lower and middle abdomen may be present
    2) Diagnostic procedures
      a) CBC with differential
      b) Serum chemistries
      c) Urinalysis
      d) Stool for occult blood: positive
      e) Type and cross (surgical intervention)
      f) Abdominal x-ray (three views: supine, prone, left decubitus)
      g) Abdominal ultrasonography

h) Barium enema with fluoroscopic examination (gold standard) or sonography-guided air enema may be both diagnostic and therapeutic; either test provides a high incidence of reduction of intussusception

2. Analysis: differential nursing diagnoses/collaborative problems
   a. Pain
   b. Ineffective tissue perfusion
   c. Risk for infection
   d. Risk for deficient fluid volume
   e. Anxiety/fear
3. Planning and implementation/interventions
   a. Establish IV access for administration of crystalloid fluid/medications as needed
   b. Prepare for/assist with medical procedures
      1) Initiate and maintain NPO status
      2) Insert gastric tube and attach to suction as indicated
      3) Insert indwelling urinary catheter
      4) Assist with hospital admission and surgical interventions as necessary
   c. Administer pharmacologic therapy as ordered
      1) Analgesics
      2) Antispasmodics
      3) Anticholinergics
   d. Educate patient/significant others
      1) Diet and medications
      2) Avoiding causative factors
4. Evaluation and ongoing monitoring
   a. Hemodynamic status
   b. Pain relief
   c. Bowel sounds
   d. Intake and output

K. IRRITABLE BOWEL SYNDROME

Irritable bowel syndrome (IBS), also called spastic colon, is the most common cause of chronic or recurrent abdominal pain not resulting from structural or biochemical factors. It is a disorder of intestinal motility influenced by a number of stimuli and increased sensitivity to abdominal stimuli. Signs and symptoms are first seen in early adulthood and in female patients more than in male patients. More than half of those with IBS have underlying depression or anxiety.

1. Assessment
   a. Subjective data collection
      1) History of present illness/chief complaint
         a) Pain
            (1) Precipitated by meals, fatigue, neuro-hormonal agents; may be relieved by defecation
            (2) Crampy, intermittent
            (3) Lower abdomen or LLQ
      2) Past medical history
         a) Current or preexisting diseases/illness
         b) Anorexia/weight loss

c) Anxiety or depression
d) Bowel pattern: diarrhea and/or constipation, mucous stools, frequent stools
e) Medications
f) Allergies

   b. Objective data collection
      1) Physical examination
         a) General appearance
            (1) Moderate distress/discomfort
         b) Inspection
            (1) Abdominal distention and bloating
         c) Auscultation
            (1) Bowel sounds: hyperactive/hypoactive
         d) Palpation
            (1) Tenderness in LLQ
      2) Diagnostic procedures (the following lab tests should be normal)
         a) CBC with differential
         b) Erythrocyte sedimentation count
         c) Serum albumin
         d) Stool for occult blood, ova and parasites
         e) Flexible sigmoidoscopy GI consult—admitted or outpatient procedure
         f) Barium enema GI consult—admitted or outpatient procedure
         g) Colonoscopy GI consult—admitted or outpatient procedure
         h) Test for lactose intolerance

2. Analysis: differential nursing diagnoses/collaborative problems
   a. Acute/chronic pain
   b. Deficient fluid volume
   c. Constipation and/or diarrhea
3. Planning and implementation/interventions
   a. Administer pharmacologic therapy as ordered
      1) Nonnarcotic analgesics
      2) Narcotics
      3) Anticholinergic or antispasmodic medications
      4) Antidiarrheal medications only for severe diarrhea
   b. Educate patient/significant others
      1) High-fiber diet and medications
      2) Avoid causative factors
4. Evaluation and ongoing monitoring
   a. Hemodynamic status
   b. Pain relief
   c. Intake and output
   d. Stools for appearance of blood or occult blood
   e. Bowel sounds

L. PANCREATITIS

Pancreatitis is an inflammation of the pancreas with accumulation or release of the digestive enzymes from the acinar cells into the surrounding tissue of the gland that leads to autolysis. Patients may present to the emergency department with either acute pancreatitis or exacerbations of chronic pancreatitis. Acute pancreatitis can arise from many causes, including mechanical obstruction (usually gallstones) of the biliary tract, injury, infection, alcoholism, and medications (glucocorticoids, thiazide diuretics, sulfonamides). Respiratory symptoms, such as atelectasis and pleural effusion, are often seen as complications of acute pancreatitis. Acute pancreatitis can occur at any age and affects more than 200,000 patients per year. Chronic pancreatitis is an inflammatory state that results in irreversible damage to pancreatic structure and function. Chronic pancreatitis commonly affects those older than age 45. In chronic pancreatitis, the organ's endocrine functions are preserved until late in the disease course; however, production of the pancreatic enzymes needed for the digestion of proteins, carbohydrates, and fats is diminished. Hypocalcemia may result as a complication of pancreatitis because the free fatty acids formed by the release of lipase into the soft tissue spaces bind the calcium and cause a decrease in ionized calcium.

1. Assessment
    a. Subjective data collection
        1) History of present illness/chief complaint
            a) Pain
                (1) Aggravated by eating, alcohol intake, walking or lying supine; unrelieved by antacids, better by leaning forward
                (2) Sharp, boring
                (3) Epigastric, abdominal, chest, radiation to back
                (4) Abrupt onset
            b) Loss of appetite
            c) Difficulty breathing
            d) Fever
        2) Past medical history
            a) Current and preexisting diseases/illness
            b) Previous episodes of pancreatitis
            c) Alcohol intake, especially recent binge drinking
            d) Recent gallbladder disease or endoscopic retrograde cholangiopancreatography (ERCP)
            e) Medications
            f) Allergies
    b. Objective data collection
        1) Physical examination
            a) General appearance
                (1) Hypotension and tachycardia resulting from acute hemorrhagic state and/or fluid loss into tissues and peritoneal cavity
                (2) Elevated temperature
                (3) Tachypnea
                (4) Severe distress/discomfort, critically ill
            b) Inspection
                (1) Abdominal distension
                (2) Bulky, fatty, foul-smelling stool
                (3) Jaundice
                (4) Vomiting, may be bile tinged
                (5) Signs of tetany as a result of hypocalcemia
            c) Auscultation
                (1) Bowel sounds: hypoactive or absent
                (2) Breath sounds: basilar crackles, rhonchi with cough from abdominal distention or pleural effusion
            d) Palpation
                (1) Tenderness over epigastria
        2) Diagnostic procedures
            a) CBC with differential: elevated WBC, decreased hemoglobin and hematocrit if hemorrhage
            b) Serum amylase and lipase: elevated (lipase remains elevated longer than amylase)
            c) Serum bilirubin, ALT, AST, alkaline phosphatase levels: may be elevated
            d) Serum chemistries including glucose, BUN, and creatinine
                (1) Elevated glucose
                (2) Decreased calcium: less than 8 mg/100 dL
            e) Urinalysis; pregnancy test in female patients of childbearing age
                (1) Elevated glucose
            f) Type and crossmatch
            g) KUB and upright abdominal flat plate radiograph
                (1) Indicates epigastric opacities
                (2) Upright position to exclude viscus perforation
            h) Chest radiograph
            i) Ultrasonography
                (1) Useful as screening test
                (2) May not be specific
            j) Abdominal CT scan: most reliable
            k) MRI
            l) 12- to 15-lead ECG
2. Analysis: differential nursing diagnoses/collaborative problems
    a. Deficient fluid volume
    b. Impaired gas exchange
    c. Pain
    d. Ineffective tissue perfusion
    e. Anxiety/fear
    f. Deficient knowledge
3. Planning and implementation/interventions
    a. Maintain airway, breathing, and circulation
    b. Provide supplemental oxygen as indicated
        1) Rapid-sequence intubation (RSI) and ventilatory support if impending respiratory failure
        2) High-flow oxygen
    c. Establish IV access for administration of crystalloid fluids/blood products/medication as needed

1) Infuse packed red blood cells if hemorrhagic pancreatitis
2) Normal saline solution boluses usually required

   d. Prepare for/assist with medical interventions
1) Advanced airway management and ventilatory support as indicated
   a) Nasal or oral intubation
   b) Supraglottic airway (e.g., King, Combitube, laryngeal mask airway)
   c) Surgical airway (e.g., cricothyrotomy)
2) Institute cardiac and pulse oximetry monitoring
3) Catheter placement and monitoring of pulmonary artery pressure (see Chapter 6)
4) Initiate and maintain NPO status
5) Insert gastric tube and attach to suction
6) Insert indwelling urinary catheter as indicated
7) Assist with hospital admission

   e. Administer pharmacologic therapy as ordered
1) RSI premedications: sedatives, analgesics, neuromuscular blocking agents
2) Nonnarcotic analgesics
3) Narcotics: avoid morphine if possible
4) Antibiotics
5) Antiemetics

4. Evaluation and ongoing monitoring
   a. Hemodynamic status
   b. Breath sounds and pulse oximetry
   c. Cardiac rate and rhythm
   d. Pain relief
   e. Intake and output
   f. Gastric emesis for blood
   g. Stools for tarry appearance and/or occult blood
   h. Bowel sounds

M. PYLORIC STENOSIS

Pyloric stenosis is the most common cause of intestinal obstruction in infancy. Also known as infantile hypertrophic pyloric stenosis (IHPS), it is diagnosed 95% of the time during the first 3–12 weeks of life. Marked hypertrophy and hyperplasia of the pylorus muscle and a narrowing of the gastric antrum occur, resulting in the obstruction. Causes of the condition are multifactorial involving both environmental and hereditary factors. These include genetics (e.g., abnormal myenteric plexus innervation and infantile hypergastrinemia), exposure to macrolide antibiotics, and nitric oxide synthase deficiency. The incidence of infantile hypertrophic pyloric stenosis is 2–4 per 1,000 live births. The condition is more common in the white population, and there is a 4:1 male-to-female predominance with 30% of the patients being first-born male children. Delays in diagnosis can lead to dehydration, shock, and mortality.

1. Assessment
   a. Subjective data collection
1) History of present illness/chief complaint
   a) Projectile vomiting: intermittent or occurring after each feeding

   b) Poor weight gain, weight loss from birth
   c) Continual hunger
   d) Constipation
2) Past medical history
   a) Current or preexisting diseases/illness
   b) Prenatal course
   c) Delivery complications

   b. Objective data collection
1) Physical examination
   a) General appearance
   (1) Level of consciousness, behavior, affect: lethargy
   (2) Hypotension, tachycardia
   (3) Malnourished
   (4) Moderate distress/discomfort, possibly critically ill
   b) Inspection
   (1) Jaundice
   (2) Gastric peristalsis prior to emesis
   c) Auscultation
   (1) Bowel sounds: hypoactive with possible increase prior to emesis
   d) Palpation
   (1) Mobile, hard pylorus: "olive"-shaped mass in RUQ
2) Diagnostic procedures
   a) Serum chemistries: hypochloremia, hypokalemia
   b) Urinalysis
   c) Arterial blood gases: metabolic alkalosis
   d) Bilirubin: elevated unconjugated level
   e) Abdominal ultrasonography
   f) Upper GI imaging (performed if ultrasonography is nondiagnostic)

2. Analysis: differential nursing diagnoses/collaborative problems
   a. Deficient fluid volume
   b. Acute pain
   c. Imbalanced nutrition

3. Planning and implementation/interventions
   a. Maintain airway, breathing, and circulation
   b. Provide supplemental oxygen as indicated
   c. Establish IV access for administration of crystalloid fluids
1) Initial normal saline solution bolus of 20 mL/kg infused immediately
2) Maintenance solutions: 5% dextrose, 0.25% sodium chloride, or 0.33% sodium chloride

   d. Prepare for/assist with medical interventions
1) Institute cardiac and pulse oximetry monitoring
2) Initiate and maintain NPO status
3) Insert gastric tube and attach to suction
4) Insert indwelling urinary catheter
5) Surgical correction is considered the standard of care for IHPS

   e. Administer pharmacologic therapy as ordered

1) Potassium chloride, 2–4 mEq/100 mL
2) Atropine sulfate IV, oral: may reduce need for surgery by relaxing the pyloric musculature
4. Evaluation and ongoing monitoring
   a. Level of consciousness
   b. Hemodynamic status
   c. Breath sounds and pulse oximetry
   d. Cardiac rate and rhythm
   e. Pain relief
   f. Bowel sounds
   g. Intake and output

N. ULCERS

An ulcer results from the sloughing of the mucous membrane of the esophagus, stomach, or duodenum. The origin is poorly understood, but ulcers commonly occur in areas of the GI tract that are exposed to hydrochloric acid and pepsin. Duodenal ulcers occur most frequently in persons age 30 and 55 years, whereas gastric ulcers are more common in those age 55 to 70 years. Of persons with ulcers, 75% to 95% also have gastritis associated with *H. pylori*. Ulcers are more common in men, smokers, and persons who take NSAIDs regularly.

1. Assessment
   a. Subjective data collection
      1) History of present illness/chief complaint
         a) Pain
            (1) Associated with eating or fasting
            (2) Squeezing, indigestion, gnawing, colicky, aching, feeling full
            (3) Epigastric, may radiate to midback
            (4) Duodenal ulcer pain typically is felt before meals and relieved by food or antacids; gastric ulcer pain usually occurs after eating
      2) Past medical history
         a) Current or preexisting diseases/illness
            (1) Ulcer disease, recurring or chronic gastritis
            (2) Bleeding tendencies
         b) Consumption of alcohol, caffeine, and tobacco use
         c) Chronic ingestion of irritants or drugs (NSAIDs, aspirin)
         d) Change in appetite
         e) Medications
         f) Allergies
   b. Objective data collection
      1) Physical examination
         a) General appearance
            (1) Moderate distress/discomfort
         b) Inspection
            (1) Vomiting
            (2) Hematemesis
         c) Auscultation
            (1) Bowel sounds: hypoactive or absent
         d) Palpation
            (1) Midepigastric tenderness
            (2) Muscular guarding
      2) Diagnostic procedures
         a) CBC with differential
         b) Serum chemistries
         c) Urinalysis; pregnancy test in female patients of childbearing age
         d) Type and crossmatch
         e) Liver enzymes, amylase
         f) Upper GI barium contrast study
         g) Upper endoscopy with biopsy
         h) Stool for occult blood
         i) Gastric analysis
2. Analysis: differential nursing diagnoses/collaborative problems
   a. Pain
   b. Risk for deficient fluid volume
   c. Anxiety/fear
   d. Deficient knowledge
3. Planning and implementation/interventions
   a. Maintain airway, breathing, and circulation
   b. Provide supplemental oxygen as indicated
   c. Establish IV access for administration of crystalloid fluid/blood products/medications as indicated
      1) Administer normal saline solution bolus(es)
      2) Replace electrolytes as needed
      3) Administer blood products
   d. Prepare for/assist with medical interventions
      1) Institute cardiac and pulse oximetry monitoring
      2) Initiate and maintain NPO status initially
      3) Insert gastric tube—may be inserted and removed, or attached to suction
      4) Assist with hospital admission and surgical intervention as indicated
   e. Administer pharmacologic therapy as ordered
      1) Nonnarcotic analgesics
      2) Narcotics
      3) Antiemetics
      4) Antacids
      5) Histamine receptor antagonists or proton pump inhibitors
      6) Antibiotics for *H. pylori*
   f. Educate patient/significant others
      1) Bland, low-fiber and/or low-fat diet and medications
      2) Avoid causative factors
      3) Avoid caffeine, alcohol, smoking
4. Evaluation and ongoing monitoring
   a. Hemodynamic status
   b. Pain relief
   c. Intake and output
   d. Gastric emesis for blood
   e. Stools for tarry appearance and/or occult blood
   f. Bowel sounds

Bibliography

Ackley B, Ladwig Gail, B: *Nursing diagnosis handbook: A guide to planning care*, 10th ed., St. Louis, MO, 2013, Mosby Elsevier.

Carpentino, JL: *Nursing diagnosis: Application to clinical practice*, 14th ed., Philadelphia, PA, 2012, Lippincott Williams, & Wilkins.

Cartwright DL, Knudson MP: Diagnostic imaging of acute abdominal pain in adults, *American Family Physician* 91(7):452–459, 2015.

Holten KB, Wetherington A, Bankston L: Diagnosing the patient with abdominal pain and altered bowel habits: Is it irritable bowel syndrome? *American Family Physician* 67(10):2157–2162, 2003.

Howell JM, Eddy OL, Lukens TW, Weingart SD, Decker WW: Clinical policy: Critical issues in evaluation and management of emergency department patients with suspected appendicitis, *Annals of Emergency Medicine* 55(1):71–116, 2010.

Jarvis C: In Abdomen, editor: *Physical examination & health assessment*, 7th ed., St. Louis, MO, 2015, Elsevier Saunders.

Kamin R, Nowicki T, Courtney D, Powers R: Pearls and pitfalls in the emergency department evaluation of abdominal pain, *Emergency Medicine Clinics of North America* 21(1):61–70, 2003.

Kuo D, Rider A, Estrada P, Kim D, Pillow M: Acute pancreatitis: What's the score? *Journal of Emergency Medicine* 48(6):762–770, 2015.

Marx J, Hockberger RS, Walls RM: In *Rosen's emergency medicine: Concepts and clinical practice*, 8th ed., St. Louis, MO, 2013, Mosby.

McCollough M, Sharieff G: Abdominal surgical emergencies in infants and young children, *Emergency Medicine Clinics of North America* 21(4):909–914, 2003. 921–924.

McNamara R, Dean A: Approach to acute abdominal pain, *Emergency Medicine Clinics* 29(2):159–173, 2011.

Mulligan C: Update on diverticular disease and implications for primary care, *The Journal for Nurse Practitioners* 11(9):883–888, 2015.

Nettina S, Shivan JC: Pediatric gastrointestinal and nutritional disorders. In *Lippincott manual of nursing practice*, 10th ed., Amber, PA, 2014, Lippincott Williams & Wilkins.

Old J, Dusing R, Yap W, Dirks J: Imaging for suspected appendicitis, *American Family Physician* 71(1):71–78, 2005.

Privette T, Carlisle M, Palma J: Emergencies of the liver, gallbladder, and pancreas, *Emergency Medicine Clinics of North America* 29(2):293–317, 2011.

Schroeder B: Evaluation of epigastric discomfort and management of dyspepsia and GERD, *American Family Physician* 68(6):1215–1216, 2003.

Tierney L, McPhee S, Papadikis M: *Current medical diagnosis and treatment*, 45th ed., New York, NY, 2006, McGraw-Hill.

Yusoff I, Barkun J, Barkun A: Diagnosis and management of cholecystitis and cholangitis, *Gastroenterology Clinic of North America* 32(4):1145–1151, 2003.

CHAPTER 12
Cardiovascular Emergencies

Joanne E. Navarroli, MSN, RN CEN

I. General Strategy

A. ASSESSMENT

1. Primary and secondary assessment/resuscitation (see Chapter 1)
2. Focused assessment
   a. Subjective data collection
      1) History of present illness/chief complaint
         a) Pain: PQRST (see Chapter 8)
            (1) Provocation
            (2) Quality
            (3) Region/radiation
            (4) Severity of symptoms
            (5) Temporal factors
               (a) Onset: when symptoms started
               (b) Duration: length of time symptoms lasted; constant versus intermittent
               (c) Changes over time (e.g., from dull to sharp)
               (d) Temporality: symptoms associated with a particular time of day, time of year
               (e) Frequency: first episode or frequent or chronic problem
         b) Dyspnea
            (1) Dyspnea on exertion (DOE)
            (2) Dyspnea when lying down (orthopnea)
            (3) Paroxysmal nocturnal dyspnea (PND)
         c) Cough
            (1) Dry, "cardiac" cough
            (2) Hemoptysis, or copious, pink, frothy sputum (pulmonary edema)
         d) Syncope, fatigue, weakness, lightheadedness
         e) Palpitations
         f) Nausea, vomiting
         g) Headache
         h) Altered mental status, behavioral changes
         i) Activity limitations, sleep disturbances
         j) Efforts to relieve symptoms
            (1) Home remedies
            (2) Alternative therapies
            (3) Medications
               (a) Prescription
               (b) OTC/herbal
      2) Past medical history
         a) Current or preexisting diseases/illness
            (1) Acute coronary syndromes (ACSs)
               (a) Angina: stable, unstable
               (b) Previous myocardial infarction (MI)
            (2) Hypertension (HTN)
            (3) Heart failure
            (4) Pulmonary disease
            (5) Diabetes mellitus
            (6) Renal disease

(7) Vascular disease: arterial or venous
  (a) Peripheral
  (b) Cerebral
b) Cardiac surgery or other cardiac interventions
c) Congenital anomalies
d) Substance and/or alcohol use/abuse
e) Smoking
f) Last normal menstrual period: female patients of childbearing age
g) Current medications
  (1) Prescription
    (a) Nitrates
    (b) Beta blockers
    (c) Calcium channel blockers
    (d) Antihypertensives
    (e) Digitalis glycosides
    (f) Diuretics
    (g) Angiotensin-converting enzyme (ACE) inhibitors
    (h) Antidysrhythmics
    (i) Anticoagulants
    (j) Antiplatelet agents (aspirin, clopidogrel [Plavix®])
    (k) Warfarin (Coumadin), heparin
    (l) Steroids
    (m) Pulmonary-specific drugs
    (n) Erectile dysfunction medications
  (2) OTC/herbal
h) Allergies
3) Psychological/social/environmental factors
a) Unmodifiable
  (1) Age: the incidence of cardiac disease increases with age
  (2) Gender: male sex predominates, particularly among younger patients
  (3) Genetics: family history is a strong predictor of cardiac disease
  (4) Race/ethnicity: blacks/African-Americans have a higher incidence than whites, American Indians, or Asians
b) Modifiable
  (1) Blood pressure
  (2) Obesity, diet
  (3) Dyslipidemia
  (4) Smoking
  (5) Sedentary lifestyle
  (6) Stress
  (7) Possible/actual assault, abuse, or intimate partner violence situations (see Chapters 3 and 40)
b. Objective data collection
  1) General appearance
  a) Level of consciousness, behavior, affect
  b) Vital signs
    (1) Respiratory rate, effort, pattern

(2) Blood pressure
  (a) Both arms: significant differences greater than 10 mm Hg
  (b) Orthostasis: supine, sitting, standing
(3) Peripheral pulses: bounding, normal, diminished, absent
c) Odors
d) Gait
e) Hygiene
f) Level of distress/discomfort
2) Inspection
a) Skin color: cyanosis
  (1) Central: present when cardiac output is severely decreased
  (2) Peripheral: indicates decreased blood flow to the periphery
b) Edema
  (1) Dependent: extremities, sacrum
  (2) Pitting: cardiac
c) Clubbing of the fingers: associated with congenital heart disease
d) Pupils
  (1) Size
  (2) Equality
  (3) Reaction to light
e) Neck veins: flat, normal, or distended (jugular venous distention [JVD])
  (1) Inspect for JVD with patient supine at a 45-degree angle. With patient head turned to one side inspect for pulsation or distention. Distention appears as waves while pulsations are carotid pulse. To verify pulsation, palpate radial pulse while watching neck to see if pulsation and pulse coincide
  (2) Flat at 45-degree angle indicative of hypovolemia
f) Thorax
  (1) Configuration: symmetry, deformities, anteroposterior diameter, kyphosis, chest wall movement with respiration
  (2) Scars or objects: surgical incision, pacemaker, automatic implanted cardioverter-defibrillator (AICD), implanted venous catheter, medication patch
g) Precordium: abnormal precordial movements (e.g., heaves, lifts)
h) Epigastric and abdominal pulsations, ascites, venous distention
i) Cardiac dysrhythmias on monitor
3) Auscultation
a) Breath sounds
  (1) Depth
  (2) Equality
  (3) Location of bronchial, vesicular, and bronchovesicular sounds

(4) Adventitious sounds: crackles (fine or coarse), wheezes, friction rub (harsh, grating sound that is often positional)

b) Heart sounds

(1) Apical heart rate

(a) Rate: regular, tachycardia, or bradycardia

(b) Rhythm: regular, regularly irregular, or irregularly irregular

(2) Auscultatory sites: aortic valve (second right intercostal space [ICS]), pulmonic valve (second left ICS), tricuspid valve (lower left sternal border), mitral valve (apex), Erb point (third left ICS), epigastric area (below xiphoid). When auscultating heart tones also palpate radial pulse to ensure perfusion

(3) S_1 and S_2: S_1, mitral and tricuspid valves close; S_2, aortic and pulmonic valves close

(4) S_3 and S_4: S_3, can be normal in children, young adults, pregnant women, and some elderly patients; the presence of S_4 is always abnormal

(5) Murmurs: systolic or diastolic, location, grade (I to VI)

(6) Variations related to dysrhythmias: premature extra systoles, atrial fibrillation, complete heart block

(7) Abnormal cardiac sounds: pericardial friction rub, venous hum, click, carotid bruits

4) Palpation

a) Skin temperature, moisture

b) Capillary refill time

c) Areas of tenderness

d) Precordial area

(1) Point of maximal impulse (PMI); usually located in fifth left ICS at midclavicular line (MCL); size is normally 2 cm

(2) Thrills: feels like a purring cat

e) Epigastrium

(1) Differentiate between abdominal aorta and right ventricular (RV) pulsations

3. Diagnostic procedures

a. Laboratory studies

1) Complete blood count (CBC) with differential

2) Comprehensive metabolic panel includes electrolytes, liver function, kidney function (blood urea nitrogen [BUN] and creatinine), glucose, calcium, and proteins; also magnesium level will need to be added

3) Cardiac biomarkers (troponin I, troponin T, myoglobin, BNP B-type [or brain] natriuretic peptide)

4) Coagulation profile: prothrombin time, international normalized ratio (PT-INR); activated partial thromboplastin time (aPTT)

5) D-dimer

6) Erythrocyte sedimentation rate (ESR)

7) Digoxin level if pertinent to patient medication regimen

8) Arterial blood gas (ABG)

9) Urinalysis; pregnancy test in female patients of childbearing age

10) Serum and urine toxicology screen

11) Type and crossmatch

b. Imaging studies

1) Chest radiograph

a) Heart size and location

b) Presence of interstitial edema, pulmonary infiltrates, or pleural effusion

c) Mediastinal width

d) Aortic calcifications

2) Echocardiography

a) Transthoracic (TTE)

b) Transesophageal (TEE)

3) Coronary computed tomography (CT) scan

4) Cardiac magnetic resonance imaging (MRI)/magnetic resonance angiography (MRA)

5) Venous duplex scan

6) Abdominal sonography

7) Echocardiogram—cardiac ultrasound/Doppler study to evaluate blood flow and valves and provide 3-D images of the cardiovascular system as well as measure ejection fraction (EF)

c. Other testing

1) 12-lead, 15-lead, 18-lead, or right-side electrocardiogram (ECG)

2) Coronary angiogram/cardiac catheterization: invasive procedure used to diagnose and treat cardiovascular conditions such as acute myocardial infarction. Details of procedure and emergency nurse role will be described in acute coronary syndrome section

3) Exercise stress testing

4) Nuclear scintigraphy (e.g., thallium)

5) Aortography/venography

6) Echocardiogram with bubble study: invasive echocardiogram that uses saline with bubbles for patent foramen ovale (PFO) or atrial septal defect (ASD)

7) Electrophysiologic mapping

B. ANALYSIS: DIFFERENTIAL NURSING DIAGNOSES/COLLABORATIVE PROBLEMS

1. Decreased cardiac output

2. Ineffective tissue perfusion: cardiac, cerebral, renal, or peripheral

3. Acute pain

4. Excess fluid volume

5. Impaired gas exchange

6. Deficient knowledge

7. Anxiety

C. PLANNING AND IMPLEMENTATION/ INTERVENTIONS

1. Determine priorities of care
   a. Maintain airway, breathing, and circulation (see Chapter 1)
   b. Provide supplemental oxygen as indicated
   c. Establish intravenous (IV) access for administration of crystalloid fluid/medications as needed
   d. Obtain and set up equipment and supplies
   e. Prepare for/assist with medical interventions
   f. Administer pharmacologic therapy as ordered
2. Relieve anxiety/apprehension
3. Allow significant others to remain with patient if supportive
4. Educate patient/significant others

D. EVALUATION AND ONGOING MONITORING

1. Continuously monitor and treat as indicated
2. Monitor patient response/outcomes, and modify nursing care plan as appropriate
3. If positive patient outcomes are not demonstrated, reevaluate assessment and/or plan of care

E. DOCUMENTATION OF INTERVENTIONS AND PATIENT RESPONSE

F. AGE-RELATED CONSIDERATIONS

1. Pediatric
   a. Growth or development related
      1) Congenital heart disease
      2) Acquired heart disease (Kawasaki disease or rheumatic fever)
      3) Endocrine or metabolic disorders (e.g., diabetes, pheochromocytoma)
      4) Drug ingestion—accidental or intentional (e.g., tricyclic antidepressants, beta blockers, calcium channel blockers, digoxin, stimulants)
   b. "Pearls"
      1) Cardiac arrest in the pediatric population is usually the result of progressive deterioration in respiratory system leading to abnormal circulatory function, rather than the result of a sudden cardiac event
      2) Syncope—an abrupt and transient loss of consciousness in children and adolescents is a red flag that might indicate long QT syndrome (LQTS). Questions that need to be asked include:[1]
         a) Was there any associated chest pain or palpitations prior to fainting?
         b) Was there seizure-like activity or an aura?
         c) Did it occur during exercise?
         d) Is there a family history of sudden death?
      3) Commotio cordis causes sudden cardiac death from blunt trauma to the left anterior chest wall usually from a thrown or batted ball; occurs predominately in young male patients[2]
      4) The presence of heart failure, cardiogenic shock, or multiple dysrhythmias in the pediatric patient is usually related to congenital cardiac anomalies
      5) Autonomic immaturity contributes to bradydysrhythmias in infants
2. Geriatric
   a. Aging related
      1) Aging is an independent major risk factor for cardiovascular disease as seen with age-related changes to the vascular function (arterial stiffening) and cardiac function (heart rate, contraction)[3]
      2) The presence of chronic diseases may obscure or confound the cardiac picture
      3) Drug-related problems stem from ineffectiveness of medication, over/underdosing, adverse drug reactions, and drug-drug interactions
      4) Drug metabolism is altered (generally slowed) in the elderly; drug interactions may further decrease drug metabolism
      5) Drug-disease interactions cause a drug to exacerbate another disease process leading to potentially dangerous prescribing cascade[4]
      6) Older individuals have multiple physiologic differences (e.g., diminished responses to stress, decreased hepatic and renal function, changes in laboratory values) that must be taken into account during assessment
      7) Psychological and social differences: older adults may have different goals for their treatment plan regarding prolonging life and the use of life support
      8) Some older adults adapt so well to cardiac disease that signs that would otherwise be remarkable go undetected
      9) Arteriosclerotic changes in the aorta and peripheral circulation may make it difficult to palpate pulses
      10) Rhythm abnormalities are so common among elderly patients that they are often the patient's norm
      11) In older adults, the venodilatory effect of nitroglycerin is greater; because of normal mouth dryness, the onset of action for sublingual nitroglycerin can be prolonged, and nitroglycerin spray may be a better choice
      12) Adverse beta-blocker effects are more common and more severe in the elderly
   b. "Pearls"
      1) "Start low, go slow" when treating the elderly with pharmacologic agents

2) Concurrent use of multiple medications (polypharmacy) poses a variety of problems for the older patient; frequent reevaluation of all medications (medication reconciliation) is essential for preventing complications

3) In older patients, typical angina-equivalent symptoms include weakness, dyspnea, syncope, acute confusion, and stroke

4) Unexplained sinus tachycardia, cardiac asthma, and new-onset lower extremity edema have also been reported as angina equivalents in the elderly

5) Among the very elderly, assess for neurologic presentations of cardiovascular problems (e.g., acute mental status changes, new-onset weakness, stroke)

6) The incidence of asymptomatic MI in persons aged 75–84 years is more than 40%

II. Specific Medical Cardiovascular Emergencies

A. ACUTE AORTIC ANEURYSM—NONTRAUMATIC

An acute aortic aneurysm (AAA) is an abnormal deterioration of the tunica media leading to dilation of all layers of the aorta. An increased diameter of at least 50% constitutes an aneurysm. Most AAAs begin below the renal arteries and end above the iliac arteries. Aortic aneurysms are classified based on where they develop along the vasculature as well as shape of the protuberance. Classification of shape is either a fusiform aneurysm (circumferential, uniform equal swelling along an extended section) or a saccular aneurysm (a small bubble on only one side of the aorta). An aneurysm that develops in the thoracic area is known as a thoracic aortic aneurysm (TAA). TAAs account for roughly 25% of all aneurysms with approximately 40% occurring in the ascending aorta and another 35% occurring in the descending thoracic aorta. When the TAA arises in the upper abdomen it is call thoracoabdominal acute aneurysm (TAAA), making up 15% of all TAAs with the remaining 10% being in the aortic arch.[5]

AAAs arise in the abdominal area normally below the renal arteries accounting for 75% of aortic aneurysms. While AAAs are moderately common, patients are largely diagnosed incidentally, remaining asymptomatic until complications develop. The most common complication is a rupture, which is a complete loss of aortic wall integrity and constitutes a significantly fatal surgical emergency with an overall mortality rate of approximately 90%. Patients presenting with a ruptured AAA classically have complaints of sudden severe back, flank, and/or groin pain with or without abdominal pain. Other symptoms include altered mental status, cyanosis, mottling, syncope,

tachycardia, and/or hypotension. A palpable sometimes visual pulsatile abdominal mass may be present, and while this finding clinically substantiates an AAA it is found in less than 50% of all cases.[6]

Typically, AAAs occur in men older than 65 years of age with a history of smoking, hypertension, and atherosclerosis at a rate of 3:1 over females. Other risk factors include family history, acquired connective tissue disorders, or congenital diseases.

Aortic aneurysms are most often caused by damage to the artery's wall due to atherosclerosis, hypertension, congenital defect, smoking, trauma (see Chapter 39), and dissection.

Some patients have small AAAs that do not need immediate surgical intervention. Treatment goals for this subset of patients is to reduce expansion rate and rupture risk through aggressive management of hypertension. These patients largely can be managed outpatient but will need to be educated on symptoms, smoking cessation, and medications. Aneurysms 3–4 cm in diameter require annual imaging to monitor for further expansion. Aneurysms 4–4.5 cm in diameter should be evaluated every 6 months. Any AAA greater than 4.5 cm in diameter or expansion of greater than 1 cm in diameter in 1 year should be referred to a vascular surgeon for possible elective repair.[7]

While this presentation may require the patient to be moved to an operating suite rapidly, collection of as much subjective and objective data as possible may provide key information.

1. Assessment
   a. Subjective data collection
      1) History of present illness/chief complaint
         a) Pain—PQRST (see Chapter 8); classically patients report sudden onset of excruciating pain (Q) described as sharp, tearing, and or knifelike in (R) either substernal, neck, or throat if ascending dissection or interscapular, back, abdomen, flank, and/or lower extremities if descending dissection. Patients may also report migratory pain (T) if the dissection is extending
            (1) 5–10% of patients have no pain
            (2) In patients who have pain, opioids fail to substantially relieve pain
      2) Past medical history
         a) Current or preexisting diseases/illness
            (1) HTN
            (2) Marfan syndrome or other connective tissue disorder (these patients tend to be younger with an equal male-to-female distribution)
            (3) Congenital heart disease
         b) Age >60 years
         c) Family history
         d) Pregnancy
         e) Smoking and/or recreational drug use

b. Objective data collection
   1) Physical examination
      a) General appearance—severity of distress/discomfort
         (1) Level of consciousness, behavior, affect
         (2) Blood pressure (manual) taken in both arms[7]
            (a) May be normal with ruptured AAA as in retroperitoneal containment
            (b) Hypertension common in nonruptured AAA
            (c) Hypotension: SBP 80 mm Hg in 40% with ruptured AAA
      b) Inspection
         (1) Skin pallor, peripheral cyanosis, or diaphoresis
         (2) Pulsatile mass may be visible
      c) Auscultation
         (1) Heart sounds: precordial systolic murmur or a diastolic aortic valve murmur, noted at the right sternal border; muffled tones if tamponade is present
         (2) Breath sounds: possible crackles
      d) Palpation
         (1) Paresthesia, hemiplegia, paraplegia (if the spinal arteries are obstructed)
         (2) Diminished weak, thready peripheral pulses
   2) Laboratory studies
      a) CBC with differential
      b) Type and crossmatch
      c) Comprehensive metabolic panel includes electrolytes, liver function, kidney function (BUN, creatinine), glucose, calcium, and proteins
      d) Coagulation profile
      e) Urinalysis
   3) Imaging studies
      a) Bedside ultrasound
      b) Computed tomography (CT)
      c) Angiography
      d) Magnetic resonance imaging, for stable patients with known aneurysm and worsening symptoms as a comparison
      e) Chest radiograph
         (1) Widening of the aortic silhouette
         (2) Mediastinal widening
         (3) Intimal calcification
         (4) Left-sided pleural effusion
2. Analysis: differential nursing diagnoses/collaborative problems
   a. Acute pain
   b. Ineffective tissue perfusion: cerebral, renal, peripheral
   c. Anxiety

3. Planning and implementation/interventions
   a. Maintain airway, breathing, and circulation (see Chapter 1)
   b. Provide supplemental oxygen
   c. Establish IV access for administration of crystalloid fluid/medications/blood products
      1) Insert two large-bore IV catheters
      2) Anticipate packed red blood cell administration
   d. Prepare for/assist with medical interventions
      1) Institute cardiac and pulse oximetry monitoring
      2) Prepare for immediate transfer to operating suite
      3) If patient has a stable aneurysm, assist with hospital admission or possible discharge home based on size of aneurysm, symptoms, and comorbidities
   e. Administer pharmacological therapy as ordered
      1) Beta blockers (Labetalol) decrease arterial pressure and the force of LV ejection
      2) Nitroprusside (Nipride)
      3) Beta blockers or calcium channel blockers if beta blockade is contraindicated
      4) Narcotics
4. Evaluation and ongoing monitoring
   a. Level of consciousness
   b. Hemodynamic status
   c. Breath sounds and pulse oximetry
   d. Cardiac rate and rhythm
   e. Intake and output
   f. Peripheral neurologic status: paresthesia, decreased movement or strength, pain or tingling
   g. Pain relief

B. ACUTE AORTIC DISSECTION

Acute aortic dissection arises when a tear of the intimal layer of the aorta allows blood to surge into and subsequently dissect the tunica media, creating two lumens: the true lumen and a false lumen. The dissection of the tunica media is significant in that the medial layer provides the aorta distensibility, elasticity, and tensile strength to allow for an increase in volume without a significant increase in pressure. As the false lumen expands retrograde or anterograde, it blocks or diverts blood away from the true lumen decreasing the overall strength and distensibility of the aorta. Pathophysiology coupled with age and other risk factors initiates this potentially life-threatening situation. The most common site of dissection associated with the highest mortality rate is the ascending aorta, 90% of which develop within 10 cm of the aortic valve.[8,9] The second most common site is the descending thoracic aorta at the ligamentum arteriosum distal to the left subclavian artery. Only 5% of all dissections arise in the abdominal aorta. Regardless of where the dissection occurs, the formation of two lumens further restricts blood flow to major organs leading to acute myocardial infarctions, strokes, or even paralysis. Acute aortic dissection is a rare but critical condition typically affecting men three times more than women aged 60 to 80. Hypertension (HTN) is the primary risk factor seen in 70% of all cases. Additional risk factors include a preexisting aortic aneurysm, inflammatory diseases that cause vasculitis, trauma (see Chapter 39), and family history (first-degree relative). However, dissection can occur in young people especially those with genetically acquired connective tissue disorders such as Marfan syndrome (increases risk in pregnant females), Ehlers-Danlos syndrome (vascular), and Loeys-Dietz syndrome (identified in 2005) or congenital diseases such as coarctation of the aorta, bicuspid aortic valve, tetralogy of Fallot, and Turner syndrome. Other contributing factors for young people include extreme high-intensity weightlifting and cocaine use. Patient presentations are variable often mimicking other conditions with no one sign or symptom indicating a dissection. For instance, complaints of mild chest pain, anterior wall pain, neck/jaw pain, intrascapular, back or flank pain may mislead assessment. Other confounding symptoms include stroke symptoms including dysphagia, numbness, tingling and weakness, altered mental status, syncope, dyspnea, hemoptysis, or fever. Anxiety or premonition of dying along with history and symptoms should raise level of suspicion during assessment.

Initial treatment involves stabilizing the patient while safely reducing blood pressure and heart rate thus limiting spread of the dissection. Definitive treatment consists of surgical repair.

1. Assessment
   a. Subjective data collection
      1) History of present illness/chief complaint
         a) Pain—PQRST; classically patients report sudden onset of excruciating pain (Q) described as sharp, ripping or tearing and/or knifelike in (R) either substernal, neck, or throat if ascending dissection or interscapular, back, abdomen, flank, and/or lower extremities if descending dissection. Patients may also report migratory pain (T) if dissection is extending
            (1) Anterior chest—anterior arch or aortic root dissection
            (2) Substernal chest, neck, or jaw pain—ascending aorta and/or aortic arch with extension into the great vessels
            (3) Intrascapular, back, or flank pain described as tearing or ripping indicative of descending aorta
            (4) Mild chest pain; 5–10% of patients have no pain
            (5) In patients who have pain opioids fail to substantially relieve pain
      2) Past medical history
         a) Current or preexisting diseases/illness
            (1) HTN
            (2) Marfan syndrome or other connective tissue disorder (these patients tend to be younger with an equal male-to-female distribution)
            (3) Congenital heart disease
         b) Age greater than 60 years
         c) Family history
         d) Pregnancy
         e) Smoking and/or recreational drug use
   b. Objective data collection
      1) Physical examination
         a) General appearance—severity of distress/discomfort
            (1) Level of consciousness, behavior, affect; possibly comatose
            (2) Blood pressure (manual) taken in both arms
            (3) Significant right and left arm BP variation of 20 mm Hg
            (4) Hypertension in 70% of patients with distal dissection
            (5) Hypotension: common with proximal dissection
            (6) Pulse deficits decreased or absent carotid or peripheral pulses secondary to compression of true lumen; seen in 50% of proximal dissections
         b) Inspection
            (1) Skin pallor or diaphoresis
            (2) Peripheral cyanosis
         c) Auscultation
            (1) Heart sounds: precordial systolic murmur or a diastolic aortic valve murmur, noted at the right sternal border; muffled tones if tamponade is present
            (2) Breath sounds: possible crackles
         d) Palpation
            (1) Paresthesia, hemiplegia, paraplegia (if the spinal arteries are obstructed)
            (2) Diminished peripheral pulses
      2) Diagnostic procedures
         a) CBC with differential
            (1) Decreased hematocrit if rupture occurs
            (2) White blood cell count 12,000–20,000 cells/mm^{10}
         b) Type and crossmatch
         c) Comprehensive metabolic panel includes electrolytes, liver function, kidney function (BUN, creatinine), glucose, calcium, and proteins
         d) Coagulation profile
         e) Urinalysis
         f) Chest radiograph
            (1) Widening of the aortic silhouette
            (2) Mediastinal widening

(3) Intimal calcification

(4) Left-sided pleural effusion

g) Spiral CT (the most sensitive study)

h) MRI

i) 12- to 15-lead ECG

    (1) Normal in one third of patients

    (2) LV hypertrophy (if patient was previously hypertensive)

    (3) MI or coronary insufficiency secondary to coronary artery obstruction

j) Aortography

k) Transthoracic echocardiogram (TTE)—noninvasive echocardiogram

l) Transesophageal echocardiogram (TEE)—invasive echocardiogram using flexible endoscopy and ultrasound to provide 2D and 3D images of the posterior visualization of cardiac vasculature

2. Analysis: differential nursing diagnoses/collaborative problems

  a. Acute pain

  b. Ineffective tissue perfusion: cerebral, renal, peripheral

  c. Anxiety

3. Planning and implementation/interventions

  a. Maintain airway, breathing, and circulation (see Chapter 1)

  b. Provide supplemental oxygen

  c. Establish IV access for administration of crystalloid fluid/medications/blood products

    1) Insert two large-bore IV catheters

    2) Anticipate packed red blood cell administration

  d. Prepare for/assist with medical interventions

    1) Institute cardiac and pulse oximetry monitoring

    2) Insert gastric tube and attach to suction

    3) Insert indwelling urinary catheter

    4) Anticipate possible emergency thoracotomy

    5) Catheter placement and monitoring of arterial, central venous, or pulmonary wedge pressures (see Chapter 6)

    6) Assist with hospital admission and possible immediate operative intervention

  e. Administer pharmacologic therapy as ordered

    1) Nitroprusside (Nipride)

    2) Labetalol (Normadyne, Trandate): decreases both arterial pressure and the force of LV ejection

    3) Calcium channel blockers (verapamil [Isoptin, Calan] or diltiazem [Cardizem]) if beta blockade is contraindicated

    4) Narcotics

4. Evaluation and ongoing monitoring

  a. Level of consciousness

  b. Hemodynamic status

  c. Breath sounds and pulse oximetry

  d. Cardiac rate and rhythm

  e. Intake and output

  f. Peripheral neurologic status: paresthesia, decreased movement or strength, pain or tingling

  g. Pain relief

C. ACUTE ARTERIAL OCCLUSION

Acute disruption of arterial blood flow results when an embolus, thrombus, or trauma occludes the vessel. This is in contrast to chronic occlusions, which are much more common and are a complication of long-standing vascular disease. However, patients with a history of chronic PVD are at risk for acute occlusion. Emboli are the leading cause of acute arterial occlusion, and approximately 80% of these emboli originate in the heart. The femoral artery is the primary site for emboli to lodge, followed by the iliac, aortic, popliteal, mesenteric, brachial, and renal arteries. Occlusion secondary to thrombosis generally occurs at areas of stenosis. This stenosis may result from atherosclerosis, or it can be iatrogenic (e.g., an intraarterial catheter insertion site). Less common causes of acute arterial occlusion include trauma, vasospasm, cocaine use, thrombosis of vascular grafts, and dissecting aneurysms.

Regardless of the cause, sudden interruption of blood flow, without collateral circulation, leads to ischemia of the tissues supplied by the affected artery. If untreated, cellular necrosis occurs. This can lead to the development of gangrene and loss of the involved extremity. Therefore, timely recognition and treatment are imperative.

1. Assessment

  a. Subjective data collection

    1) History of present illness/chief complaint

      a) Pain (see Chapter 8)

        (1) Provocation

          (a) Movement/exercise

          (b) Pain at rest

        (2) Quality

          (a) Discomfort

          (b) Burning

          (c) Throbbing

        (3) Region/radiation

          (a) Radiates to region distal to occlusion

        (4) Severity

          (a) Excruciating

        (5) Timing

          (a) Sudden onset

          (b) Relentless

      b) Coldness below level of occlusion

      c) Numbness

      d) Paralysis

    2) Past medical history

      a) Current or preexisting diseases/illness

        (1) History of MI

        (2) Rheumatic heart disease

        (3) Atrial fibrillation

        (4) Patent foramen ovale

(5) Previous cardiac surgery
 (a) Mitral commissurotomy
 (b) Prosthetic cardiac valve
(6) LV aneurysm
(7) Chronic heart failure
(8) Cancer
 (a) Predisposition to thrombosis
 (b) Tumor embolization
(9) Peripheral atherosclerotic disease
 b) Recent knee arthroplasty
 c) Recent extremity trauma
 d) Recent placement of intraarterial catheter for monitoring or arteriography
 e) Medications
 f) Allergies
 b. Objective data collection
 1) Physical examination
 a) General appearance
 (1) Moderate to severe distress/discomfort
 b) Inspection (below site of occlusion)
 (1) Pallor, cyanosis, or mottled appearance
 (2) Paralysis (below site of occlusion)
 (3) Muscle rigor (with prolonged ischemia)
 (4) Petechiae (associated with microemboli)
 c) Palpation (below site of occlusion)
 (1) Pulselessness
 (2) Paresthesia
 (3) Coldness
 (4) Muscle tenderness to palpation
 2) Diagnostic procedures
 a) CBC with differential
 b) Coagulation profile: PT-INR, aPTT
 c) Arteriography
 (1) Conventional (intraarterial)
 (a) Digital subtraction angiography
 (2) CT angiography (CTA)
 (3) MR angiography (MRA)
 d) Doppler flow studies
 e) Ankle-brachial index (ABI): a comparison of ankle BP with arm pressure; ABI <0.30 is not compatible with limb viability
 f) ECG
2. Analysis: differential nursing diagnoses/collaborative problems
 a. Ineffective tissue perfusion
 b. Pain
 c. Anxiety
3. Planning and implementation/interventions
 a. Provide supplemental oxygen as indicated
 b. Establish IV access for administration of crystalloid fluids/medications
 c. Prepare for/assist with medical interventions
 1) Elevate head of bed to facilitate blood flow to ischemic extremity
 2) Institute cardiac and pulse oximetry monitoring
 3) Assist patient to find a position of comfort

4) Provide a warm environment: do not apply heat to ischemic area
5) Do not elevate an ischemic extremity
6) Assist with hospital admission for
 a) Percutaneous procedures
 (1) Balloon angioplasty
 (2) Balloon catheter extraction
 (3) Stenting
 b) Embolectomy
 c) Bypass grafting
 d. Administer pharmacologic therapy as ordered
 1) Anticoagulants
 2) Fibrinolytics
4. Evaluation and ongoing monitoring
 a. Hemodynamic status
 b. Extremity movement and sensation
 c. Skin temperature changes
 d. Pain relief

D. ACUTE CORONARY SYNDROMES

Acute coronary syndrome (ACS) is an umbrella term used when referring to patients presenting with symptoms associated with myocardial ischemia. Chest pain or other symptoms such as neck, arm, or jaw pain; difficulty breathing; palpitations; or fatigue develop as a result of decreased blood supply to the myocardium primarily caused by coronary artery disease (CAD), more specifically coronary atherosclerosis. Any reduction in blood flow to the heart initiates the myocardial ischemic process. If appropriate interventions are not initiated quickly and inadequate blood supply continues, ischemia leads to cell death, otherwise known as necrosis or infarction. ACS disease processes include unstable angina (UA), non-ST-segment elevation myocardial infarction (NSTEMI), and ST-segment elevation myocardial infarction (STEMI). Prolonged myocardial ischemia produces necrosis, referred to as myocardial infarction (MI). Most MIs occur as a result of coronary artery atherosclerosis, followed by rupture of an unstable atheromatous plaque, platelet activation, and fibrin clot formation. The resultant thrombosis interrupts blood flow and leads to an imbalance between myocardial oxygen supply and demand. Nonatherosclerotic causes of MI include coronary artery spasm, congenital abnormalities, coronary artery embolus, and connective tissue disorders.

Regardless of the initial cause, if the myocardial oxygen supply–demand imbalance is severe or persistent, ischemia will produce irreversible cellular damage. The subsequent impact on myocardial contractility, stroke volume, and ventricular function will depend on the duration of ischemia, the extent of myocardial tissue involvement, and the patient's preexisting cardiac status. Myocardial ischemia also stimulates catecholamine release, which increases peripheral vascular resistance, promotes tachycardia, and raises both preload and afterload. Because many other conditions produce symptoms similar to those of ACS, careful

Table 12.1

Acute Coronary Syndromes

Findings	Unstable Angina	NSTEMI	STEMI
Symptoms	Angina at rest (usually greater than 20 minutes) or previously diagnosed stable angina that has become more severe, prolonged, frequent, or occurs at a lower threshold	Chest pain or discomfort, nausea, vomiting, dyspnea, unexplained weakness, fatigue, dizziness, lightheadedness, syncope	
ECG changes	Transient ST-segment or T-wave changes may occur	Evidence of ischemia ST-segment depression T-wave abnormalities	Evidence of infarction ST-segment elevation: at or >2 mm in leads V_1, V_2, or V_3, ST-segment elevation: at or >1 mm in other leads New left bundle branch block
Troponin level	Normal	Elevated	Elevated

ECG, electrocardiogram; *NSTEMI*, non-ST-segment elevation myocardial infarction; *STEMI*, ST-segment elevation myocardial infarction.

examination and history taking are essential. Differential diagnosis is extensive, ranging from non-life-threatening musculoskeletal pain to significantly critical conditions such as tension pneumothorax. Other conditions that imitate ACS include inflammatory diseases of the heart, aortic dissection, pulmonary embolus, esophageal spasm or rupture, pneumonia, pleurisy, gastroesophageal reflux disease, and cardiac dysrhythmias. Because each of the three ACSs is produced by the same underlying disease process, these syndromes are distinguished physiologically only by the extent of myocardial injury. Risk factors, assessment parameters, and many interventions are identical for all patients with ACS.

Having appropriate treatment strategies in place when treating patients with ACS is paramount to decreased mortality and improved outcomes. Becoming a designated chest pain center allows each hospital to determine which designation best suits the available resources. The three different designations are based on a facility's ability to provide immediate primary percutaneous coronary intervention (PCI). Chest pain centers with primary PCI and resuscitation have primary PCI available 24 hours a day 7 days a week with early recognition and treatment including PCI with simultaneous therapeutic hypothermia or targeted temperature management (TTM) including patients who have return of spontaneous circulation (ROSC) after cardiac arrest. Chest pain centers with primary PCI have intervention available around the clock, with appropriate staff available within 30 minutes of STEMI activation. Chest pain centers that do not have PCI coverage available at all times have protocols in place that ensure that reperfusion intervention time does not exceed 120 minutes by having either a transfer plan in place or the ability to provide fibrinolytic therapy.[10]

With ongoing research and frequent changes to treatment modalities it is imperative to follow institutional guidelines when treating patients with cardiovascular presentations.

1. Assessment (Table 12.1)
   a. Subjective data collection
      1) History of present illness/chief complaint
         a) Pain or "discomfort" (see Chapter 8)
            (1) Provocative factors: activity that increases myocardial oxygen requirements
                (a) Physical activity/exercise
                (b) Emotional stress
                (c) Cold weather
                (d) After meals
                (e) Sexual activity
                (f) May occur at rest
            (2) Palliative factors: unrelieved by change in position or nitrate use
            (3) Quality: pain may be "different" from patient's usual angina; quality may be described as squeezing, crushing, stabbing, knifelike, heaviness, pressure, or "something sitting on my chest"; may also be described as tightness, burning, or indigestion, especially by women or older adults
            (4) Region/radiation: chest, substernal area, epigastrium, neck, infrascapular region, jaw, or ulnar aspect of the left arm or elbow producing tingling in the wrist, hand, and fingers
            (5) Severity of symptoms: can range from vague to severe; generally more intense than patient's usual angina
            (6) Temporal factors: time of onset; continuous or lasting more than 30 minutes; circadian variability (peaks from 6 a.m. to noon, usually in the first 2–3 hours after arising)
         b) Nausea or vomiting
         c) Dyspnea or orthopnea
         d) Diaphoresis
         e) Fatigue, sleep disturbances, and dyspnea, especially in women
         f) Weakness or dizziness, especially in older adults

g) Palpitations

h) Syncope

i) Feeling of impending doom

2) Past medical history

  a) Current or preexisting diseases/illness

    (1) Angina

    (2) Previous MI

    (3) HTN (increases cardiac workload)

    (4) Cerebral vascular disease/stroke

    (5) Diabetes mellitus: increases incidence of MI; patients are more likely to experience vague symptoms or "silent" MI

    (6) Dyslipidemia

  b) Previous cardiac interventions (e.g., angioplasty, valve replacement, coronary artery bypass grafting, stent insertion, pacemaker, or AICD placement)

  c) Thromboembolic event

  d) Other cardiac risk factors

    (1) Age: >65 years

    (2) Smoking

    (3) Obesity

    (4) Sedentary lifestyle

    (5) Recreational drug or alcohol use

  e) Medications

    (1) Recent use of erectile dysfunction medications

  f) Allergies

b. Objective data collection

1) Physical examination

  a) General appearance

    (1) Level of consciousness, behavior, affect: anxious, restless

    (2) Clenched fist against the sternum (Levine sign)

    (3) Tachycardia, bradycardia

    (4) Possible hypotension/hypertension

    (5) Tachypnea

    (6) Possible elevated temperature: initially normal, then begins to rise 4–8 hours after MI onset as a nonspecific response to tissue necrosis

    (7) Moderate to severe distress/discomfort, critically ill

  b) Inspection

    (1) Pale, diaphoretic, possible cyanosis or mottled coloring

    (2) Cardiac dysrhythmias on monitor

  c) Auscultation

    (1) Heart sounds

      (a) S_4 is almost universally present

      (b) S_3 indicates left ventricular (LV) dysfunction

      (c) Murmurs: may be transient or permanent; indicate valve dysfunction

      (d) Muffled sounds indicate effusion

    (2) Breath sounds: possible crackles, wheezes

2) Diagnostic procedures

  a) Cardiac biomarkers: elevated

    (1) Troponin proteins (cTnI and cTnT) most sensitive and specific for myocardial damage; they have replaced enzyme studies for the diagnosis of MI1, MI2

      (a) Troponin levels elevate 3–12 hours after MI onset, peak in 24 hours (cTnI) or 12–48 hours (cTnT), and return to normal in 5–12 days

      (b) Troponin elevation is not specific to MI; elevated levels are associated with several other disease states

      (c) cTnT may be elevated in patients with renal failure; cTnI is more cardio specific

      (d) Absence of troponin level elevation distinguishes UA from MI

  b) CBC with differential

  c) Comprehensive metabolic panel includes electrolytes, liver function, kidney function (BUN, creatinine), glucose, calcium, and proteins; also a magnesium level will need to be added

  d) Coagulation profile

  e) 12- to 18-lead ECG

    (1) ECG changes may not be apparent initially; the ECG may be completely normal, which does not rule out MI, especially shortly after occlusion

    (2) ECG findings reflect changes in the myocardium (Table 12.2)

    (3) Infarct location is determined by the presence of ECG changes in specific leads (Table 12.3); an infarct may involve more than one area of the heart

    (4) Right-sided ECG in patients with changes suggestive of inferior MI to determine presence of posterior MI

    (5) Repeat ECGs are helpful for detecting ongoing changes, which may lag behind symptoms

  f) Chest radiograph

  g) Echocardiogram: evaluate wall motion and perfusion; particularly useful in patients with NSTEMI

2. Analysis: differential nursing diagnoses/collaborative problems

  a. Acute pain

  b. Ineffective tissue perfusion: cardiac, peripheral

  c. Anxiety

3. Planning and implementation/interventions

  a. Maintain airway, breathing, and circulation (see Chapter 1)

    1) Initiate or continue ACLS per AHA 2015 protocols

    2) Intubation using rapid sequence intubation (RSI) and ventilatory support per protocols

Table 12.2

Electrocardiographic Signs of Myocardial Infarction

ECG Signs	Onset/Appearance	Area of Injury	Indicates
Tall, peaked T waves	Very early (hyperacute) sign	Subendocardium	Ischemia; will disappear if ischemia resolves
T-wave inversion	T wave appears deep and symmetrical	Myocardium	Ischemia; will disappear if ischemia resolves
ST-segment elevation	Elevation above the isoelectric line indicates acuteness of injury	Epicardium	Injury: the ST segment returns to the isoelectric line within hours or days
Significant Q waves	Appear within 24 hours of infarct Q waves are (1) at or greater than 0.04 second in duration, (2) greater than 25% of the R wave in depth, (3) or both	Myocardium	Infarct; may remain permanently

ECG, electrocardiogram.

Table 12.3

Infarct Location

Location	Lead Changes
Anterior	Leads V_1, V_2, V_3, or V_4 Septal: V_1 and V_2
Lateral	Leads I, aVL, V_5, V_6 Apical infarct: V_5, V_6
Posterior	"Reciprocal" V_1 and V_2 No Q wave, but tall R wave ST-segment depression Upright T wave
Inferior	Leads II, III, aVF
Right ventricular	Leads V_{4R}–V_{6R}

3) Advanced airway management and ventilatory support as indicated
  a) Nasal or oral intubation
  b) Supraglottic airway (e.g., King, Combitube, laryngeal mask airway)
  c) Surgical airway (e.g., cricothyrotomy)
4) Provide supplemental oxygen, as indicated
b. Establish a minimum access of two IV catheters for administration of crystalloid fluid/medications
c. Prepare for/assist with medical interventions
  1) Institute cardiac and pulse oximetry monitoring
  2) Prepare patient for reperfusion therapy: most patients experiencing an acute ST elevation myocardial infarction (STEMI) will need immediate coronary artery reperfusion of the infarcted artery(ies) with either primary percutaneous coronary intervention (PCI) or fibrinolytic therapy. Current guidelines recommend door to PCI of 90 minutes and door to fibrinolytic therapy of 30 minutes as this improves myocardial recovery and reduces mortality compared to no reperfusion[11]
    a) Primary PCI is cardiac catheterization/angiography with angioplasty of blocked coronary artery(ies). Despite being available in less than half of all U.S. hospitals, PCI is the reperfusion method of choice for STEMI with outcome/advantages from the procedure best realized within the first few hours of symptom onset
    b) Fibrinolytic (thrombolytic) therapy: well established, more commonly available reperfusion therapy used in the absence of primary PCI. These agents convert plasminogen to plasmin which in turn attacks fibrinogen and fibrin dissolving the clot and are given concurrently with antithrombin and antiplatelet agents
      (1) Absolute contraindications: any prior intracranial hemorrhage or malignant neoplasm, suspected aortic dissection, bleeding disorders, trauma, or pregnancy
      (2) Drugs may include fibrin-specific agents tenecteplase (TNK), alteplase (tPA), or reteplase (recombinant plasminogen activator [r-PA])
  3) As needed interventions
    a) Catheter placement and monitoring of pulmonary wedge pressure (see Chapter 6)
    b) Cardiac pacing, defibrillation, ventricular assist devices for patients in cardiogenic shock
    c) Insert gastric tube and attach to suction
    d) Insert indwelling urinary catheter
    e) Assist with hospital admission or transfer to an institution providing a higher level of care
d. Administer pharmacologic therapy as ordered
  1) RSI medications: sedatives, analgesics, neuromuscular blocking agents
  2) Aspirin: antiplatelet chewable unless administered prior to arrival either by self or prehospital care providers
  3) Clopidogrel (Plavix): antiplatelet loading dose 75 mg orally to patients 75 years or older, 300 mg orally to patients 75 years or younger

4) Sublingual nitroglycerin up to three doses, 5 minutes apart until symptoms are relieved, systolic BP falls below 90 mm Hg, or maximum dose has been reached. May hold for suspected right ventricular MI or in cases where erectile dysfunction medications have been taken within 24–48 hours

5) Metoprolol (Toprol, Lopressor) beta-blocker therapy reduces infarct size—hold for patients with known heart failure

6) Morphine sulfate 4–8 mg IV, may be repeated every 5–15 minutes for severe angina; also decreases preload and afterload as well as anxiety

7) Glycoprotein IIb/IIIa inhibitor (e.g., eptifibatide [Integrilin], abciximab [ReoPro]) platelet inhibitors used primarily in unstable angina and NSTEMI in conjunction with aspirin or heparin bolus for patients having invasive heart procedures

8) Antithrombin agents use either heparin (unfractionated heparin [UFH]) bolus followed by infusion or low-molecular-weight heparin (enoxaparin [Lovenox])

9) ACLS medications per protocols

10) Antidysrhythmics, vasopressors, vasodilators, and inotropic agents for patients in cardiogenic shock from MI

4. Evaluation and ongoing monitoring
   a. Airway patency
   b. Level of consciousness
   c. Hemodynamic status
   d. Breath sounds and pulse oximetry: pulmonary congestion may occur in patients with significant LV failure
   e. Changes in patient as a result of change in cardiac rate and rhythm such as ectopy, blocks, reperfusion dysrhythmias
   f. Pain relief
   g. Intake and output
   h. Internal/external bleeding in patients receiving fibrinolytic therapy

E. ANGINA, STABLE AND UNSTABLE

Unstable angina or acute chest pain is considered an acute coronary syndrome due to the nature and severity of the chest pain that strikes either at rest or with exertion secondary to myocardial ischemia and oxygen supply–demand imbalance. The most common cause is an atherosclerotic thrombus that is partially or completely occluding a coronary artery. Classically unstable angina differs from chronic stable angina in that the pain is new, does not follow a pattern, and is generally not relieved by rest or pain medication. Unstable angina is considered a medical emergency as it may be an indication NSTEMI (partial occlusion) or a STEMI (complete occlusion).

Variant or Prinzmetal angina is considered to be an unstable form of angina but is not treated as a medical emergency. The pain associated with this type of angina is the result of coronary artery spasm and can occur in patients with or without atherosclerotic changes. Symptoms often repeat cyclically, frequently at the same time each day. Variant angina occurs almost exclusively at rest and is not usually precipitated by physical exertion or emotional stress. The episodes tend to cluster at night, between midnight and 8 a.m. and can be triggered by alcohol ingestion, drinking iced liquids, rapid eye movement sleep, atrial pacing, nicotine, acetylcholine, or hyperventilation. Vasospastic angina is also associated with the use of stimulants, most commonly cocaine. Variant angina has been associated with other vasospastic disorders such as migraine headaches and Raynaud phenomena. Patients with variant angina are usually younger than those with chronic stable angina or UA. Women experience variant angina more frequently than men. The ST-segment elevation seen during a variant anginal episode returns to baseline once the pain is gone.

Chronic stable angina while not technically an ACS is still considered to be part of the coronary artery disease (CAD) continuum. As is true of ACSs, stable angina pain is the result of an imbalance between myocardial oxygen supply and demand. Atherosclerotic coronary arteries are the typical cause of stable angina, but the condition may also be produced by vasospasm. Like the pain of unstable angina or MI, stable angina is a poorly localized symptom of myocardial ischemia described as pain or discomfort in the chest or adjacent areas. It is associated with physical exertion, emotional stress, or exposure to extreme temperatures. Unlike unstable angina, the pain of stable angina is relieved after a few minutes of rest or sublingual nitroglycerin administration. Keep in mind that stable angina can become unstable angina if there is a change in the pain intensity, onset, and/or associated symptoms.

Importantly, patients with a history of stable angina usually self-treat. Persons who present to the emergency department are generally those with new-onset angina, worsening symptoms, or symptoms that patients are unable to self-manage. These individuals may be experiencing UA or MI and must initially be treated as patients with ACS.

1. Assessment
   a. Subjective data collection (see Acute Coronary Syndromes; other data specific to stable angina are noted here)
      1) History of present illness/chief complaint
         a) Pain or "discomfort" (see Chapter 8)
            (1) Provocative factors: activities that increase myocardial oxygen requirements
               (a) Physical or emotional stress
               (b) Stimulant use
               (c) May occur during sleep or at rest (variant angina)

(2) Palliative factors
- (a) Rest and/or cessation of activity
- (b) Sublingual nitroglycerin
- (c) Resolves spontaneously (variant angina)

(3) Quality: typically the same sensation, location, and intensity with each episode

(4) Region/radiation: chest, substernal area, epigastrium, neck, infrascapular region, jaw, or left arm; variant angina generally manifests as chest pain

(5) Severity: can range from vague to severe
- (a) Stable: commonly described as discomfort rather than pain; unchanged from "normal" anginal episode
- (b) Variant: extremely severe, referred to as pain

(6) Temporal factors
- (a) Stable: usually lasts 3–5 minutes
- (b) Variant: may occur at same time each day; attacks tend to cluster at night, between midnight and 8 a.m.; may awaken patient

2) Past medical history
- a) Current or preexisting diseases/illness
  - (1) Stable angina
- b) Stimulant use (e.g., cocaine, methamphetamine)
- c) Heavy smoker: common with variant-type angina

b. Objective data collection (see Acute Coronary Syndromes; other data specific to stable angina are noted here)
1) Physical examination
- a) Auscultation
  - (1) Breath sounds: transient pulmonary crackles may be associated with anginal episodes

2) Diagnostic procedures
- a) Cardiac biomarkers: the absence of troponin elevation distinguishes angina from MI; serial tests are indicated if patient does not quickly obtain symptom relief
- b) CBC with differential: anemia-induced angina
- c) ECG
  - (1) Stable angina: ST-segment depression may accompany pain
  - (2) Variant angina: ST-segment elevation occurs with pain; ST segment returns to baseline when pain subsides
  - (3) In patients with a cardiac history, ECG patterns of LV hypertrophy, old MI (significant Q waves), and nonspecific ST-segment and T-wave abnormalities may also be present

2. Analysis: differential nursing diagnoses/collaborative problems
- a. Acute pain
- b. Anxiety
- c. Risk for ineffective tissue perfusion

3. Planning and implementation/interventions (see Acute Coronary Syndromes; other interventions specific to stable angina are noted here)
- a. Administer pharmacologic therapy as ordered
  1) Sublingual nitroglycerin if patient's systolic BP is at least 90 mm Hg; failure to respond to nitroglycerin may be indicative of unstable angina
  2) Morphine sulfate
  3) Beta blockers: can exacerbate vasospasm in patients with vasospastic angina; propranolol (Inderal) is known to prolong the duration of variant angina episodes. If the patient's condition deteriorates after beta-blocker administration, consider that coronary artery spasm may be the cause of the angina
  4) Calcium channel blockers/antagonists (nifedipine, diltiazem, or verapamil) work best with variant angina. They prevent vasoconstriction and promote vasodilation, and are used as second-line therapy in patients with continued ischemia despite nitroglycerin and beta blockers. Use with caution in elderly patients taking digitalis as concomitant use increases risk of digitalis toxicity
- b. Educate patient/significant others
  1) Identification of anginal pain
  2) Discontinue any aggravating activity and rest at the onset of anginal pain
  3) Nitroglycerin tablet or spray: sublingual only, should sting or taste bitter, use one tablet/spray every 3–5 minutes up to three doses
     - a) If chest pain is not alleviated after three nitroglycerin doses (over a 15-minute period), seek emergency care
     - b) Do not administer nitroglycerin if an erectile dysfunction medication was taken within the last 24–48 hours
  4) Changes in pain that may indicate worsening of disease

4. Evaluation and ongoing monitoring
- a. Level of consciousness
  1) Evaluate for developing headache, which may be caused by cerebral vasodilation; headache often resolves with acetaminophen administration
- b. Hemodynamic status
  1) Evaluate BP frequently; peripheral vasodilation from nitroglycerin can produce hypotension
- c. Breath sounds and pulse oximetry
  1) Evaluate for developing heart failure resulting from calcium antagonists' negative inotropic effect

d. Cardiac rate and rhythm: development of reflex tachycardia

e. Pain relief

F. CARDIAC DYSRHYTHMIAS

Cardiac dysrhythmias are an aberrancy to the normal cardiac conduction system yielding sometimes chaotic and symptomatic dysrhythmias. Aberrancies are divided into three categories: (1) disorders of impulse formation, affecting automaticity, (2) disorders of impulse conduction, affecting reentry, or (3) a combination of both. Impulse formation disorders are caused by abnormal automaticity, a triggering activity, or afterdepolarizations. Disorders of impulse conduction are the result of a conduction delay or block, which can lead to bradycardia or a reentry tachycardia. Reentry occurs when an impulse reactivates myocardial tissue for a second or multiple times. This happens when a unidirectional block allows the impulse to conduct in only one direction. An afterdepolarization is a depolarization that follows the action potential of a cardiac cell.

Various factors contribute to cardiac dysrhythmias, most importantly coronary artery disease, atherosclerosis, and family history. Other chronic illnesses, metabolic imbalances, and medications including congenital disorders, heart failure, hypertension, diabetes, electrolyte abnormalities, sleep apnea, and certain medications contribute to risk for cardiac dysrhythmias. Furthermore, lifestyle choices such as tobacco use, excessive alcohol intake, drug use/abuse, obesity/diet, stress, and use of certain OTC supplements and herbal remedies are factors.

The types of dysrhythmias will be discussed in the following sections. The major consequence of any dysrhythmia is a decrease in cardiac output initiating serious consequences up to and including death. Therefore, the need for emergent dysrhythmia treatment, determined by the patient's hemodynamic status, is implemented immediately.

The following information pertains to all dysrhythmias.

1. Assessment
   a. Subjective data collection
      1) History of present illness/chief complaint
         a) Lightheadedness, dizziness, or syncope
         b) Fatigue, weakness, sleep disturbances
         c) Dyspnea
         d) Nausea, vomiting
         e) Pain (see Chapter 8)
         f) Severe hemodynamic compromise
         g) Pulselessness, cardiac arrest
      2) Past medical history: highly variable
         a) Current or preexisting diseases/illness
            (1) Cardiovascular disease
            (2) Pulmonary disease
            (3) Endocrine disease
            (4) Renal failure
            (5) Congenital disorder
            (6) Autoimmune disease
            (7) Infectious disease
         b) Trauma: blunt or penetrating forces
         c) Smoking/substance abuse history
   b. Objective data collection
      1) Physical assessment
         a) General appearance
            (1) Apneic or pulselessness
            (2) Level of consciousness, behavior, affect: alert, anxious, lethargic, comatose
            (3) Vital signs: normal or abnormal
            (4) Moderate to severe distress/discomfort, possibly critically ill
         b) Inspection
            (1) Jugular vein distention
            (2) Possible pale, ashen skin
            (3) Cardiac dysrhythmias on monitor
         c) Auscultation: heart and lungs
         d) Palpation
      2) Diagnostic procedures
         a) Electrocardiogram
         b) CBC with differential
         c) Comprehensive metabolic panel with magnesium level added
         d) Cardiac biomarkers
         e) Serum and urine toxicology screen
         f) Coagulation profile
         g) Chest radiograph
2. Analysis: differential nursing diagnoses/collaborative problems
   a. Decreased cardiac output
   b. Ineffective tissue perfusion
   c. Anxiety
3. Planning and implementation/interventions
   a. Maintain airway, breathing, and circulation (see Chapter 1)
      1) Initiate or continue ACLS per most current American Heart Association protocols
      2) Intubation and ventilatory support per protocols
      3) Provide supplemental oxygen as needed
   b. Establish IV access for administration of crystalloid fluid/medications
   c. Prepare for/assist with medical interventions
      1) Advanced airway management
         a) Nasal or oral intubation
         b) Supraglottic airway (e.g., King, Combitube, laryngeal mask airway)
         c) Surgical airway (e.g., cricothyrotomy)
      2) Institute cardiac and pulse oximetry monitoring
      3) Assist with application of vagal maneuvers
         a) Valsalva maneuver
         b) Unilateral carotid massage
      4) Insert gastric tube and attach to suction as indicated

Box 12.1

Premature Atrial Complexes

Rhythm

Rate: 60–100 beats/minute
Rhythm: Irregular because of premature beats
P waves: Present; premature beats have differing shapes
QRS complexes: Present; normal duration

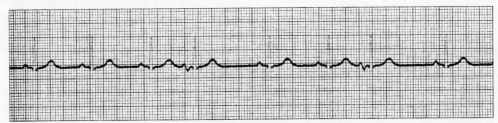

Premature atrial complexes. *From Kitt, S. (1990). Emergency nursing: A physiologic and clinical perspective. Philadelphia: Saunders.*

5) Insert indwelling urinary catheter as indicated
6) Utilize transcutaneous cardiac pacing as indicated
7) Assist with transvenous pacemaker insertion as indicated
8) Assist with synchronized cardioversion as indicated
   a) Begin at 50–100 joules (J) in adults; 0.5–1 J/kg in pediatrics
   b) Increase the energy dose as needed. In adults, give up to 360 J (monophasic) or the manufacturer's recommended biphasic equivalent
9) Assist with defibrillation as indicated
   a) Monophasic defibrillator: 360 J in adult patients; 2 J/kg first shock and 4 J/kg for subsequent shocks in pediatric patients
   b) Biphasic defibrillator: 120–200 J
10) Assist with therapeutic hypothermia or targeted temperature management (TTM); see details under Cardiac Arrest and Postresuscitation Care

ATRIAL DYSRHYTHMIAS

Premature Atrial Complexes. A premature atrial complex or contraction (PAC) occurs when an ectopic focus in the atria conducts a beat before the next beat was due (Box 12.1). Transient PACs are often related to the use of stimulants (e.g., caffeine, alcohol, nicotine, cocaine) or anxiety. However, they also occur in association with more serious conditions such as atrial enlargement, pericarditis heart failure, myocardial ischemia or infarction, hypoxemia, electrolyte abnormalities, chronic obstructive pulmonary disease (COPD), fever, and infections. Certain medications, such as digitalis, can stimulate PACs. Because PACs indicate atrial irritability, they may precede supraventricular tachycardia, atrial flutter, or atrial fibrillation. Rarely do PACs produce ventricular dysrhythmias.

Atrial Flutter. Atrial flutter, like all atrial tachycardias, occurs when an irritable focus within the atria takes over as the pacemaker or is more commonly the result of atrial impulse reentry. Atrial flutter is characterized by an atrial depolarization rate of 250–350 beats/minute (Box 12.2). Typically, many of the atrial impulses fail to conduct to the ventricles, thus producing a ventricular rate that is slower than the atrial rate.

The ratio of atrial impulses to ventricular contractions is usually 2:1 but can be 3:1 or 4:1. P waves on the ECG have a "saw tooth" appearance and are referred to as flutter waves. Atrial flutter is often associated with underlying heart disease, valvular disorders, rheumatic or ischemic heart disease, cardiomyopathy, and atrial dilation. Atrial flutter may also be caused by stimulation of sympathetic nervous system, pulmonary embolism, cardiac surgery, or thyrotoxicosis. Atrial flutter is usually a transient rhythm; the condition will either convert to a normal sinus rhythm or progress to atrial fibrillation.

Atrial Fibrillation. Atrial fibrillation is characterized by a chaotic atrial rhythm associated with an irregular ventricular response (Box 12.3). It may result from multiple irritable foci or from multiple areas of impulse reentry. In atrial fibrillation, the electrical activity of the atria is variable and rapid, with a rate of 400–700 beats/minute. This electrical activity produces small waves in the atria but no effective atrial contractions. Only a few of the stimuli are conducted through the AV node to the ventricles. The ventricular response rate is generally between 100 and 180 beats/minute.

Part 2

Box 12.2

Atrial Flutter

Rhythm

Rate: 240–360 beats/minute
Rhythm: Regular or irregular
P waves: Saw-toothed pattern (flutter waves)
QRS complexes: Present; normal duration
P/QRS relationship: Variable ventricular response; ventricular response may be regular or irregular depending on rate
PR interval: Unable to determine

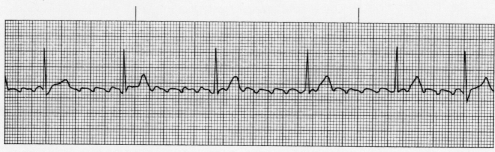

Atrial flutter. *From Kitt, S. (1990).* Emergency nursing: A physiologic and clinical perspective. *Philadelphia: Saunders.*

Box 12.3

Atrial Fibrillation

Rhythm

Atrial Rate: 400 beats/minute or greater
Rhythm: Irregular
P waves: Unidentifiable, erratic
QRS complexes: Present; normal or abnormal duration
P/QRS relationship: Unidentifiable
PR interval: Unable to determine

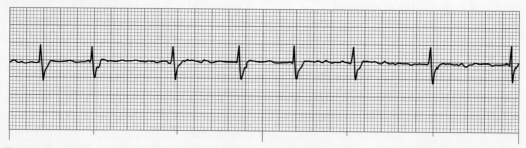

Atrial fibrillation. *From Kitt, S. (1990).* Emergency nursing: A physiologic and clinical perspective. *Philadelphia: Saunders;* Aehlert, B. (2013). ECGs made easy (5th ed.). St. Louis, MO: Elsevier.

Atrial fibrillation may be associated with heart failure, atrial enlargement, HTN, thyrotoxicosis, CAD, or rheumatic heart disease. Atrial fibrillation is clinically significant for the following reasons: (1) the loss of atrial contraction causes stroke volume to decrease by 20–30%; (2) when fibrillating, the atria are unable to empty completely, resulting in blood pooling, possible clot formation, and potential emboli release; and (3) if the ventricular response is rapid, the patient may quickly experience heart failure, syncope, or angina as a result of reduced cardiac output.

The ultimate goal of treatment is to restore normal rhythm by either treating underlying disorder or through synchronized cardioversion. However, synchronized cardioversion is

Box 12.4

Supraventricular Tachycardia

Rhythm

Rate: 100–280 beats/minute; may exceed 300 beats/minute in small children
Rhythm: Regular
P waves: Present: may be distorted in shape or buried in QRS complex
QRS complexes: Present; normal duration usually
P/QRS relationship: P wave for each QRS complex, but may be buried
PR interval: Short or unable to determine

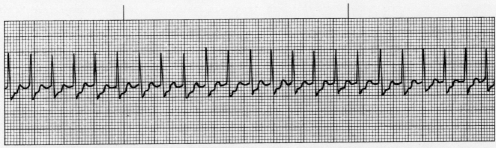

Paroxysmal supraventricular tachycardia/narrow complex tachycardia. *From Kitt, S. (1990). Emergency nursing: A physiologic and clinical perspective. Philadelphia: Saunders.*

not recommended in patients with known digitalis toxicity or those who have known AFib of greater than 48 hours. A transesophageal echocardiogram (TEE) to visualize atria for thrombus along with proper anticoagulation therapy should be done prior to cardioversion. After cardioversion, patients need to be anticoagulated for 4 weeks. Secondary treatment goals address rate control through medication management (beta blockers, calcium channel blockers, or digoxin), which allows the ventricles enough time to empty completely thus decreasing the risk of thrombi formation and stroke.[12]

Supraventricular Tachycardia/Narrow Complex Tachycardia. The term *supraventricular tachycardia* is used to describe any rapid rhythm (sinus tachycardia, atrial flutter, atrial fibrillation, multifocal atrial tachycardia) that originates above the level of the ventricles that has an abrupt onset and termination (paroxysmal) (Box 12.4). PSVT is a reentrant tachycardia usually generated by the AV node, but it may be either atrial or junctional in origin. SVT is a common arrhythmia requiring treatment in the pediatric population, and it is frequently seen in young persons without organic heart disease.[13] Some patients are born with accessory conduction system pathways that predispose them to reentrant rhythms. This includes pediatric patients with congenital conduction abnormalities that cause Wolff-Parkinson-White (WPW) or Long-Ganong-Levine (LGL) syndromes. Other causes of SVT include hypoxia, ischemia, electrolyte imbalances, heart failure, rheumatic heart disease, acute pericarditis,

MI, stimulant use, and mitral valve prolapse. As is true of any tachydysrhythmia, the primary consequence of SVT is a shortened diastolic filling time, which subsequently decreases cardiac output. This is generally well tolerated by young, healthy patients but poorly tolerated by those with significant disease.

a. Atrioventricular node conduction disturbances/heart block atrioventricular (AV) heart blocks are conduction defects that disrupt/block/delay the sinus impulse through the AV node causing atrial depolarization to the ventricles to fail. Myocardial and systemic disease processes that might lead to AV blocks include endocarditis, valve calcification/replacement, congenital defect repairs, sarcoidosis, myxedema, hemochromatosis, Lyme disease, and ankylosing spondylitis. Medications such as beta blockers, calcium channel blockers, or digitalis intended to block the AV node may also be a contributing factor. While a block may occur at any site along the conduction pathway, the most common site is between the atria and the ventricles. Treatment for AV blocks varies based on degree and symptomatology. Keep in mind if a patient's condition worsens after treatment with atropine or isoproterenol the block may be originating in the His-Purkinje system.[14] Heart blocks are classified by severity: first degree, second degree (type I and type II), and third degree.

First-Degree Atrioventricular Block

Rhythm

Rate: Usually 60–100 beats/minute
Rhythm: Regular
P waves: Present, usually normal shape
QRS complexes: Present; normal duration
P/QRS relationship: P waves precedes each QRS complex
PR interval: >0.20 second

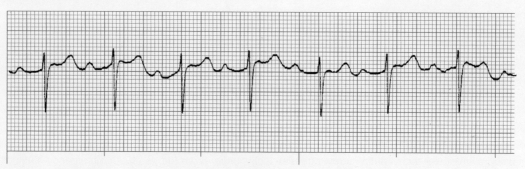

First-degree block. *From Kitt, S. (1990).* Emergency nursing: A physiologic and clinical perspective. *Philadelphia: Saunders; Aehlert, B. (2013).* ECGs made easy (5th ed.). *St. Louis, MO: Elsevier.*

First-Degree Atrioventricular Block. First-degree AV block is characterized by a prolonged PR interval in an otherwise normal-appearing cardiac rhythm (Box 12.5). A P wave precedes each QRS, but the PR interval is longer than 0.20 second. This delay usually takes place in the AV node, but can occur in the His-Purkinje system. First-degree AV block may occur in healthy persons. However, it is also associated with pathologic conditions such as hypokalemia, myocardial ischemia or infarction, rheumatic heart disease, and excess vagal stimulation. Additionally, cardiac medications (digitalis, quinidine, and procainamide) may produce this dysrhythmia. First-degree AV block is often an incidental finding, rarely producing symptoms, and has no specific treatment except treating the underlying cause. In the presence of myocardial ischemia, monitor patients for deterioration.

Second-Degree Atrioventricular Block. There are two types of second-degree AV heart blocks: Mobitz type I and Mobitz type II. Mobitz type I (Wenckebach) second-degree AV block is characterized by a progressive increase in the length of the PR interval. Eventually, usually after three to five beats, one of the impulses fails to conduct to the ventricles, and the QRS is "dropped" (Box 12.6). The process usually repeats, resulting in a "grouped-beats" pattern on the ECG. A Mobitz type I AV block almost always occurs as a result of impulse transmission delay through the AV node. This rhythm

is associated with increased parasympathetic tone, myocardial ischemia or infarction, and the effects of certain drugs (e.g., digitalis, propranolol). If Mobitz type I AV block occurs in the presence of an MI, it is generally transient and rarely requires temporary pacing.

Second-Degree Atrioventricular Block: Mobitz Type II. A Mobitz type II second-degree AV block is caused by a conduction delay below the level of the AV node, either at the bundle of His or, more commonly, in the bundle branches (Box 12.7). This rhythm occurs less frequently than a Mobitz type I and is associated with a higher mortality. The PR interval is constant with more nonconducting P waves than QRS complexes with symptomatology attributed to the ventricular rate. In the presence of an acute MI, patients with Mobitz type II AV block may require pacing (temporary or permanent).

Third-Degree (Complete) Atrioventricular Block. Third-degree AV block is characterized by a complete absence of conduction between the atria and the ventricles. While both the atrial and ventricular rhythms are regular, P waves are not conducting through the AV node, leaving the ventricles to be controlled by an independent pacemaker (Box 12.8). Third-degree blocks may be transient needing no treatment or life-threatening needing immediate intervention depending on the level of the block. Causes of third-degree AV block include MI, digitalis toxicity, congenital anomalies, and various cardiac disease states.

Box 12.6

Second-Degree Atrioventricular Block: Mobitz I (Wenckebach)

Rhythm

Rate: Atrial rate is greater than ventricular rate
Rhythm: Irregular
QRS complexes: When present, normal duration
P/QRS relationship: QRS complex follows P wave until dropped
PR interval: Lengthens with each QRS complex until complex dropped; pattern then repeats

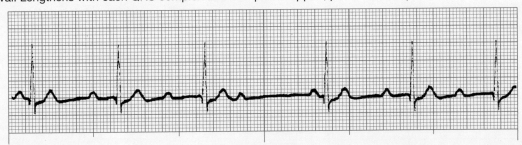

Second-degree block, Mobitz type I. *From Kitt, S. (1990). Emergency nursing: A physiologic and clinical perspective. Philadelphia: Saunders; Aehlert, B. (2013). ECGs made easy (5th ed.). St. Louis, MO: Elsevier.*

Box 12.7

Second-Degree Atrioventricular Block: Mobitz II

Rhythm

Rate: Atrial: 60–100 beats/minute; ventricular slower than atrial
Rhythm: Usually regular but may be irregular
P waves: Some P waves not followed by QRS complex
QRS complexes: Normal or prolonged duration when present
P/QRS relationship: One or more P waves for each QRS complex
PR interval: Normal or lengthened for each conducted QRS complex

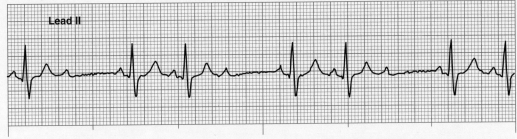

Second-degree block, Mobitz type II. *From Kitt, S. (1990). Emergency nursing: A physiologic and clinical perspective. Philadelphia: Saunders; Aehlert, B. (2013). ECGs made easy (5th ed.). St. Louis, MO: Elsevier.*

JUNCTIONAL DYSRHYTHMIAS

Premature Junctional Complex. A premature junctional complex or contraction (PJC) occurs when an ectopic focus in the AV junction conducts an electrical impulse before the next expected sinus impulse (Box 12.9). PJCs result in retrograde atrial depolarization. Consequently, the P wave may be seen before, during, or after the QRS complex. Because conduction through the ventricles is usually unimpaired, the QRS has a normal morphology. PJCs can occur in response to increased vagal tone, myocardial

---

Box 12.8

Third-Degree (Complete) Atrioventricular Block

....

Rhythm

Rate: Atrial rate 60–100 beats/minute; ventricular rate <60 beats/minute
Rhythm: Regular
P waves: Present, some not followed by QRS complex
QRS complexes: Present; may be normal duration or >0.12 second
P/QRS relationship: No relationship
PR interval: Inconsistent or nonexistent

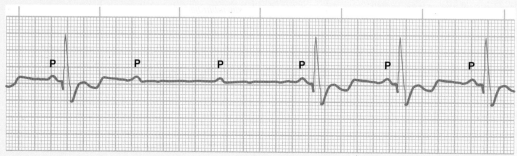

Third-degree block. *From Kitt, S. (1990). Emergency nursing: A physiologic and clinical perspective. Philadelphia: Saunders; Aehlert, B. (2013). ECGs made easy (5th ed.). St. Louis, MO: Elsevier.*

Box 12.9

Premature Junctional Complex

....

Rhythm

Rate: Bradycardic to normal depending on underlying rhythm
Rhythm: Irregular
P waves: May be absent, retrograde (behind QRS complex), or immediately prior to QRS complex; frequently inverted
QRS complexes: Present; normal duration
P/QRS relationship: Absent, retrograde, or immediately preceding QRS complex
PR interval: None, or <0.12 second if P-wave QRS complex

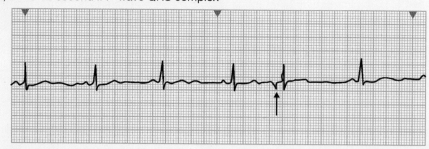

Junctional rhythm/junctional tachycardia. *From Kitt, S. (1990). Emergency nursing: A physiologic and clinical perspective. Philadelphia: Saunders.*

---

irritability (resulting from CAD or MI), stimulant ingestion (e.g., caffeine, nicotine, cocaine), and the use of certain medications, particularly digitalis. Treatment of PJCs is rarely necessary. Interventions are directed at removing the offending stimulus.

Junctional Rhythm and Junctional Tachycardia. Junctional rhythms occur when the AV node takes over from the sinoatrial (SA) node as the heart's pacemaker. If the SA node discharge rate falls to less than the AV node's intrinsic rate of 40–60 beats/minute, the AV node takes

Junctional Escape Rhythm

Rhythm

Rate: 40–60 beats/minute
Rhythm: Regular
P waves: May be absent, retrograde (behind QRS complex), or immediately prior to QRS complex; frequently inverted
QRS complexes: Present; normal duration
P/QRS relationship: Absent, retrograde, or immediately preceding QRS complex
PR interval: None, or <0.12 second if P-wave QRS complex

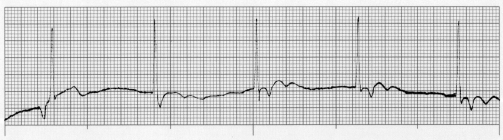

Junctional rhythm/junctional tachycardia. *From Kitt, S. (1990). Emergency nursing: A physiologic and clinical perspective. Philadelphia: Saunders; Aehlert, B. (2013). ECGs made easy (5th ed.). St. Louis, MO: Elsevier.*

over and becomes the heart's pacemaker. The resultant rhythm consists of junctional escape beats (Box 12.10). Junctional tachycardia occurs when the junction is acting as the pacemaker, but at a rate higher than its intrinsic rate (usually >70 beats/minute) and faster than the SA impulse rate. The most common cause of junctional rhythms is digitalis toxicity. Other causes include IWMI, heart disease, and hypokalemia. Symptoms vary depending on the rate, cause, and the patient's underlying cardiovascular status. Slow rates compromise cardiac output and may allow breakthrough ventricular dysrhythmias. Rapid rates can decrease cardiac output by reducing diastolic filling time. Patients with junctional rhythms may also experience symptoms related to loss of the atrial contribution to cardiac output. Treatment focuses on identifying the cause and providing supportive care as necessary.

SINUS DYSRHYTHMIAS

Sinus Bradycardia. Sinus bradycardia is characterized by a sinus node discharge rate of <60 beats/minute in an adult. Sinus bradycardia (Box 12.11) may be normal in athletes and during sleep, or it may be a response to vagal stimulation. Other causes include IWMI, eye surgery, increased intracranial pressure, myxedema, hypoxia, hypothermia, obstructive jaundice, anorexia nervosa, and medications (cardiac glycosides, beta blockers, calcium channel blockers). In most cases, sinus bradycardia is a benign dysrhythmia and requires treatment only if the patient is exhibiting signs of low cardiac output.

Sinus Tachycardia. Sinus tachycardia is characterized by a sinus node discharge rate of >100 beats/minute (Box 12.12). Sinus tachycardia is a normal physiologic response to any demand for an increase in cardiac output including exercise, anxiety, fever, hypovolemia, anemia, and tissue ischemia. Therefore, management of sinus tachycardia primarily involves identifying and treating the underlying disorder and not the heart rate itself. Sympathomimetic and parasympatholytic drugs can also produce sinus tachycardia. Examples of these agents include atropine, epinephrine, dopamine (Inotropin), cocaine, methamphetamine, and caffeine.

VENTRICULAR DYSRHYTHMIAS

Long QT Syndrome. Long QT syndrome (LQTS) is a condition affecting the myocardial electrical system, specifically the ventricular activity that controls depolarization and repolarization. LQTS arises when the ion channels are not functioning properly, interrupting ion flow into and out of the heart, thus delaying timely recharge of the electrical system before the next cycle. This defect precipitates prolongation of the QT interval which in turn increases the risk for life-threatening ventricular dysrhythmias, predominantly torsades de pointes (TdP) and/or sudden cardiac death (SDC).

Long QT syndrome is either congenital or acquired. Congenital LQTS is rare, affecting 1 in 5,000 persons in the United States, and is discovered during childhood or young adulthood but seldom after 40 years of age. Congenital LQTS stems from autosomal dominant or recessive gene mutations of the cardiac potassium, sodium, or calcium ion

Box 12.11

Sinus Bradycardia

Rhythm

Rate: <60 beats/minute
Rhythm: Regular
P waves: Present
QRS complexes: Present; normal duration
P/QRS relationship: P wave precedes each QRS complex
PR interval: Normal
Assessment
Assess for findings consistent with inferior wall myocardial infarction
Consider obtaining right-sided electrocardiogram

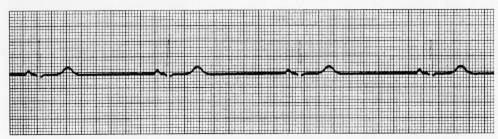

Sinus bradycardia. *From Kitt, S. (1990).* Emergency nursing: A physiologic and clinical perspective. *Philadelphia: Saunders.*

Box 12.12

Sinus Tachycardia

Rhythm

Rate: 100–180 beats/minute
Rhythm: Regular
P waves: Present; may be merged with preceding T wave
QRS complexes: Present; normal duration
P/QRS relationship: P wave precedes each QRS complex
PR interval: Normal

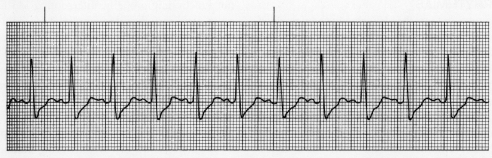

Sinus tachycardia. *From Kitt, S. (1990).* Emergency nursing: A physiologic and clinical perspective. *Philadelphia: Saunders.*

channels. There are currently 12 identified classifications of ion abnormalities with the most common being LQTS 1 to LQTS5; and LQTS3 creating the highest risk. Risk factors for congenital LQTS include congenital heart disease, infants who are deaf at birth, and first-degree family members who have known LQTS or have had unexplained syncope or SCD.[15]

Acquired LQTS develops as a consequence of drug therapy, electrolyte imbalances such as hypokalemia, hyponatremia, hypomagnesemia, or hypocalcemia, as well as bradyarrhythmias. In addition to antiarrhythmic medications (quinidine, amiodorone, procainamide) that are known to prolong the QT interval are other medications such as antipsychotics (lithium, phenothiazines), antihistamines (diphenhydramine), antibiotics (quinolones, azithromycin), antidepressants (fluoxetine), and antiemetics (ondansetron, phenothiazines). Acquired and congenital LQTS overlap in patients who are taking medications that delay myocardial repolarization who have an undiagnosed congenital LQTS. Additional risk factors for acquired LQTS include heart failure, myocardial infarction, myocarditis, electrolyte imbalances, and rheumatic fever.

The most common symptoms include unexplained syncope, palpitations, seizures, and SCD or unexplained bradycardia in newborns and infants. Symptoms can appear during physical or emotional stress, upon being startled or awakened suddenly, and even while sleeping, which manifests as unusually loud gasping sounds.

Diagnosis of LQTS is rendered by measuring the QT interval on an electrocardiogram (ECG) which is best evaluated in lead II or V_5 from the beginning of the QRS complex to the end of the T wave. Normally, the QT interval is 0.36–0.44 second across approximately 9–11 boxes. Because the QT interval varies with heart rate (higher heart rate equals shorter QT), a corrected QT (QTc) needs to be calculated using the R–R interval and Bazett square root formula. QTc is equal to QT interval in seconds divided by the square root of the preceding R–R interval in seconds or QTc = QT interval / √ R–R interval. QTc is normally <0.44 and is linked to higher risk of TdP if >0.50.[16]

Further testing is necessary and may include genetic testing, exercise stress test, echocardiogram, Holter monitor, or other drug-induced provocative studies. Treatment options include beta blockers, ICD or AED, or left cardiac sympathectomy denervation (LCSD).

Premature Ventricular Contractions. A premature ventricular complex or contraction (PVC) is a beat initiated by one of the ventricles prior to the next expected sinus beat (Box 12.13). PVCs are characterized by a QRS complex that is bizarre in shape and has a duration that exceeds 0.12 second. These beats are usually caused by conditions that enhance ventricular automaticity, such as anxiety, hypoxia, electrolyte imbalance (e.g., hypokalemia), infection, myocardial ischemia, cardiac disease, medications (e.g., digitalis, phenothiazines, tricyclic antidepressants), and irritation from a pacemaker malfunction.

The prevalence of ectopic ventricular activity increases with age and is more common in male patients. PVCs are considered benign if they are occasional, unifocal, and occur in an asymptomatic patient without cardiac disease. However, PVCs may initiate ventricular fibrillation (VF) when they are multifocal (arising from different ventricular sites), have a frequency of more than six per minute (which may be a conservative number), occur in couplets (pairs of PVCs), occur close to the preceding T wave, or occur in patients experiencing an acute MI. Three or more PVCs in a row constitute a run of ventricular tachycardia (VT).

Box 12.13

Premature Ventricular Contraction
....

Rhythm

Rate: Variable
Rhythm: Irregular because of premature beats
P waves: Present with each sinus conducted QRS complex; not present with premature QRS complex
QRS complexes: Normal duration of sinus conducted complexes; >0.12 second in premature complexes
PR interval: Normal with sinus beats; missing with premature complexes

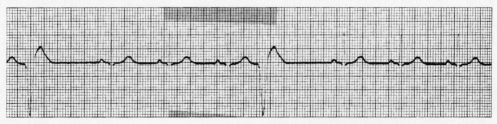

Premature ventricular contractions. *From Kitt, S. (1990).* Emergency nursing: A physiologic and clinical perspective. *Philadelphia: Saunders.*

Ventricular Tachycardia. Ventricular tachycardia (VT) is a dysrhythmia characterized by a series of three or more successive ventricular beats at a rate >100 beats/minute (Box 12.14). A patient's ability to tolerate this rhythm will depend on the rate and duration of the tachycardia as well as the extent of underlying cardiovascular disease. The primary cause of VT is acute MI; other causes include cardiomyopathy, primary conduction disturbances, valvular heart disease, congenital heart disease, LV hypertrophy, digitalis and quinidine toxicity, hypoxia, and hypokalemia. In the pediatric population, VT is an uncommon rhythm. When VT does occur in this age group, causes include underlying structural deficits, a prolonged QT interval, hypoxia, acidosis, electrolyte imbalances, and poisoning, particularly tricyclic antidepressants and cardiac medications. VT is considered sustained when it lasts longer than 30 seconds or requires termination because of hemodynamic collapse. VT is considered nonsustained if its duration is fewer than 30 seconds and it terminates spontaneously.

Torsades de Pointes. Torsades de pointes (TdP or torsades) is a distinctive form of polymorphic VT distinguished by QRS complexes that rapidly and irregularly spiral around the isoelectric baseline. Torsades is potentially life threatening with LQTS and is also the result of other etiologies including drug-drug interactions, drug toxicities, and antidysrhythmic agent medications that prolong ventricular repolarization. Additional triggers include electrolyte imbalances, specifically magnesium and potassium, frequently seen in malnourished and chronic alcoholics, congenital heart anomalies, and congenital catecholamine-induced polymorphic ventricular tachyarrhythmia (autosomal dominant gene mutations similar to LQTS). Clinical manifestations of TdP depend on rate and duration which may terminate spontaneously or deteriorate to ventricular tachycardia or fibrillation, or present as sudden cardiac death. TdP is more common in women than men. Treatment involves correcting prolonged QT by identifying the offending agent and preventing recurrence of TdP or deterioration. This is usually accomplished through the administration of 2 grams magnesium intravenously.

Ventricular Fibrillation. Ventricular fibrillation (VF) is a lethal dysrhythmia characterized by disorganized electrical activity of the ventricles, which produces only ineffective ventricular quivering (Box 12.15). There is no cardiac output or pulse with VF. The terms "coarse" and "fine" are sometimes used to describe the size or amplitude of the waveforms in VF. Generally, coarse VF is considered more recent in onset and may possibly be corrected more readily. Fine VF indicates VF of longer duration and is considered more difficult to reverse. VF is a life-threatening condition treated following advanced cardiac life support (ACLS) guidelines as outlined by the American Heart Association (AHA) which places emphasis on excellent effective uninterrupted chest compressions along with early defibrillation to ensure sufficient perfusion with the ultimate goal of a successful resuscitation known as return of spontaneous circulation (ROSC).[17] The most common cause of VF is acute MI. Other causes include hypoxia,

---

Box 12.14

Ventricular Tachycardia

Rhythm

Rate: 100–250 beats/minute
Rhythm: Regular
P waves: Usually not seen
QRS complexes: >0.12 second and bizarrely shaped
P/QRS relationship: None
PR interval: None

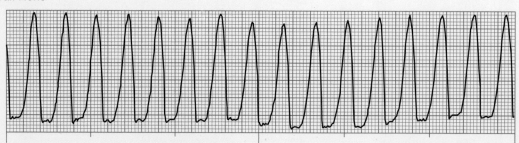

Ventricular tachycardia. *From Kitt, S. (1990).* Emergency nursing: A physiologic and clinical perspective. *Philadelphia: Saunders; Aehlert, B. (2013).* ECGs made easy *(5th ed.). St. Louis, MO: Elsevier.*

electrical shock, sudden cardiac death, and digitalis or quinidine toxicity. VF is an uncommon event in pediatric patients and is especially rare in infants.

Ventricular Asystole. Asystole is the complete absence of electrical and mechanical cardiac function (Box 12.16). It generally results from severe end-stage disease or follows prolonged cardiac arrest. Asystole has a grim prognosis, and its presence usually confirms death. Treatment is focused on identifying a possibly reversible cause and managing it aggressively following advanced cardiac life support (ACLS) guidelines as outlined by the American Heart Association (AHA). The 2015 guidelines place emphasis on excellent effective uninterrupted chest compressions to provide sufficient perfusion. Defibrillation is not recommended for asystole.

G. CARDIAC ARREST AND POSTRESUSCITATION CARE

Cardiac arrest or cardiopulmonary arrest occurs as an unexpected interruption of mechanical activity affecting normal blood flow substantiated by the absence of palpable central pulses. It is estimated that over 60% of all cardiac arrests are directly caused from an acute myocardial infarction. Cardiopulmonary resuscitation (CPR) is initiated either prehospital or inhospital followed with advanced cardiac life support (ACLS) guidelines as outlined by the American Heart Association (AHA). Principles of management of CPR as outlined in the 2010 and 2015 AHA guidelines place emphasis on excellent effective uninterrupted chest compressions along with early defibrillation to ensure sufficient perfusion

with the ultimate goal of a successful resuscitation known as return of spontaneous circulation (ROSC).[18]

When a cardiac arrest patient has ROSC there are essential standards of postcardiac arrest care. Management principles include interventions to optimize cardiopulmonary and neurologic function keeping in mind that not all critical postcardiac arrest care interventions are appropriate for all patient types.[19]

1. Identify and treat acute coronary syndrome by obtaining a 12-lead electrocardiogram (ECG)
   a. Prepare patient for emergent reperfusion therapy to prevent further complications
2. Preferred method for reperfusion: coronary angiography/angioplasty
3. Augment perfusion of vital organs by immediately correcting hypotension and maintaining hemodynamic stability
4. Implement therapeutic hypothermia or targeted temperature management (TTM) for those patients who remain comatose after ROSC[20]
   a. Goal-directed therapy intended to decrease cerebral metabolism and cerebral cell death thus preserving neurologic function
   b. Since the target temperature of 32–34°C should be reached within 3 hours of ROSC, the induction phase of TTM ideally should begin in the emergency department
   c. Important exclusion criteria
      1) Recent (within 14 days) major surgery: increased risk of bleeding

---

Box 12.15

Ventricular Fibrillation

Rhythm

Rate: Indeterminable
Rhythm: Irregular
P waves: None
QRS complexes: None
P/QRS relationship: None
PR interval: None

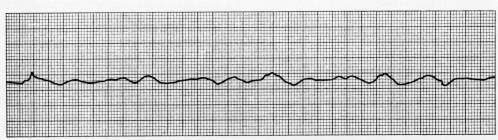

Ventricular fibrillation. *From Kitt, S. (1990).* Emergency nursing: A physiologic and clinical perspective. *Philadelphia: Saunders.*

Box 12.16

Ventricular Asystole

Rhythm

Rate: None

Rhythm: None

P waves: Usually none

P/QRS relationship: None

PR interval: None

Ventricular asystole. *From Kitt, S. (1990). Emergency nursing: A physiologic and clinical perspective. Philadelphia: Saunders; Aehlert, B. (2013). ECGs made easy (5ᵗʰ ed.). St. Louis, MO: Elsevier.*

2) Known bleeding disorders: hypothermia may impair the clotting system

3) Preexisting coma prior to cardiac arrest or from other causes such as drug overdose

5. Monitor for dysrhythmias and changes in neurological function

6. Prepare patient for admission to intensive care unit or transfer to appropriate facility

7. Educate: keep patient and family informed about medications and treatment plan throughout

H. CARDIAC IMPLANTABLE ELECTRONIC DEVICE MALFUNCTION

Pacemakers and implantable cardioverter-defibrillators (ICDs), collectively known as cardiac implantable electronic devices (CIEDs), are surgically placed medical devices intended to monitor and treat potentially life-threatening dysrhythmias or heart failure. The type of CIED inserted is based on the severity of symptoms and the desired outcomes. Devices include single, dual, and triple chamber, which indicates the number of leads that carry impulses. Each device is then programmed to indicate chamber paced, chamber sensed, sensing response, programmability, and antitachycardia functions. Patients who present with a malfunctioning device will complain of dizziness or syncope, palpitations, shortness of breath, confusion, fatigue, hiccups, or being shocked.

Triggers for malfunction include battery depletion, loose or fractured wire, and electrode-tissue interface issues. Problems with the pulse generator/circuit failure lead to failure to sense and failure to capture both electrically and mechanically. Electromagnetic interference, extracardiac stimulation, or underlying cardiac events such as electrolyte imbalances or acute myocardial infarction will produce device malfunction. In some cases, malfunction of a device is attributed to the patient subconsciously or deliberately manipulating the pocket device, known as twiddler's syndrome. This causes the leads to twist around the pulse generator leading to lead fracture or dislodgement.

For symptomatic dysrhythmias, including pacemaker-mediated tachycardia (PMT) or hypotension, initial assessment and management according to advanced cardiac life support (ACLS) guidelines should be instituted in addition to placing a magnet on the device. Asymptomatic patients should have an emergent electrocardiogram (EKG) and interrogation of the device as well as continuous monitoring with assessment following guidelines listed under Cardiac Dysrhythmias.

I. CARDIOGENIC SHOCK (SEE CHAPTER 29)

J. CARDIOMYOPATHY

Cardiomyopathy is a term used to describe many disorders, systemic diseases, and processes that affect the myocardium. Cardiomyopathies are classified based on how the condition affects the heart. Dilated cardiomyopathy is the most common in the aged population, affecting the left ventricle's ability to pump blood. Hypertrophic cardiomyopathy (HCM) is the result of thickened myocardium which affects 1 in 500 people of any age group equally between males and females. Unfortunately, HCM is a common cause in young athletes' sudden cardiac death.[21] Restrictive cardiomyopathy (RCM) is rare and affects the ventricles' ability to fill and relax properly between cycles. Patients with cardiomyopathy present with symptoms of heart failure, manifested by a reduction in LV contractility and cardiac output. The causes of cardiomyopathy are diverse and include acute, subacute, and chronic diseases, alcoholism, and toxin exposure. The toxic agents most frequently associated with cardiomyopathy are heavy metals, doxorubicin, cocaine, and methamphetamines. Infectious causes include human immunodeficiency virus (HIV), viral endocarditis/myocarditis, parasites, and protozoa. Certain high cardiac output states (e.g., anemia, thyrotoxicosis, pregnancy, collagen vascular diseases) can also cause cardiomyopathy.

1. Assessment
   a. Subjective data collection
      1) History of present illness/chief complaint
         a) Fatigue
         b) DOE, orthopnea, PND
         c) Edema
      2) Past medical history
         a) Current or preexisting diseases/illness
            (1) HTN
            (2) Angina
            (3) CAD
            (4) Anemia
            (5) Thyroid dysfunction
            (6) Breast cancer
         b) Exposure to high-risk medications
         c) Substance abuse (tobacco, alcohol, illicit drugs)
         d) Medications
         e) Allergies
   b. Objective data collection
      1) Physical examination
         a) General appearance
            (1) Tachypnea
            (2) Tachycardia
            (3) HTN
            (4) Moderate to severe distress/discomfort
         b) Inspection
            (1) Jugular venous distention
            (2) Peripheral edema
            (3) Possible cardiac dysrhythmias on monitor
         c) Auscultation
            (1) Breath sounds: crackles and/or wheezes
            (2) Heart sounds: S_3 gallop
         d) Palpation
            (1) Enlarged liver or hepatojugular reflex
      2) Diagnostic procedures
         a) Cardiac biomarkers: differentiates ischemic heart disease from dilated cardiomyopathy
         b) BNP: possible elevation
         c) Thyroid function tests
         d) CBC with differential
         e) Urinalysis; pregnancy test in female patients of childbearing age
         f) Serum and urine toxicology screen
         g) Chest radiograph
            (1) Cardiomegaly
            (2) Pulmonary infiltrates
         h) ECG
            (1) Differentiates dilated cardiomyopathy from ischemic heart disease
         i) Echocardiogram
            (1) Differentiates dilated cardiomyopathy from restrictive and hypertrophic cardiomyopathy
            (2) Identifies LV enlargement and chamber sizes
         j) Endomyocardial biopsy
2. Analysis: differential nursing diagnoses/collaborative problems
   a. Ineffective breathing pattern
   b. Excess fluid volume
   c. Ineffective tissue perfusion: renal, cerebral, cardiopulmonary, GI, peripheral
3. Planning and implementation/interventions
   a. See Heart Failure and Cardiogenic Pulmonary Edema
4. Evaluation and ongoing monitoring
   a. See Heart Failure and Cardiogenic Pulmonary Edema

K. HEART FAILURE AND CARDIOGENIC PULMONARY EDEMA

Heart failure (previously referred to as congestive heart failure [CHF]) is a broad diagnosis that can be a complication of any type of cardiac disease. Heart failure may be caused by inadequacy of the heart itself, but it can also occur in the presence of near-normal cardiac function under conditions of high demand such as hyperthyroidism, renal failure, or severe anemia. The most common causes of heart failure are CAD, chronic HTN, and diabetes. When severe, both cardiomyopathy and myocarditis can produce heart failure. In the pediatric population, heart failure is usually associated with a congenital defect.

The clinical syndrome of heart failure is the result of complex interactions among the body's renal, pulmonary, cardiovascular, and neurohormonal systems. When malfunction of any of these systems impairs the heart's ability to pump enough blood to meet the body's metabolic needs, heart failure ensues. Low cardiac output causes selective upregulation of the sympathetic nervous system and the renin-angiotensin axis that leads to release of vasopressin and atrial natriuretic peptide. This produces volume expansion, which induces vasoconstriction and further limits cardiac output.

The spectrum of heart failure ranges from acute and dramatic to chronic and insidious. Heart failure can also be categorized as right sided/left sided, systolic/diastolic, and low output/high output. Ultimately, heart failure leads to intravascular and interstitial volume overload causing decreased tissue perfusion. Left-sided heart failure produces pulmonary edema. When LV failure occurs (as the result of either mechanical overload or MI), the subsequent pulmonary HTN causes fluid to accumulate in the interstitium and alveoli. Severe or long-standing pulmonary HTN then compromises the right ventricle, leads to right-sided failure as well, and produces signs of venous congestion.

Emerging trends in management of patients with cardiomyopathies and significant heart failure is the use of biventricular pacemakers to provide cardiac resynchronization therapy (CRT). These three lead pacers treat the ventricular conduction defects that cause uncoordinated contraction of the ventricles, thereby increasing cardiac output.[22]

1. Assessment
   a. Subjective data collection
      1) History of present illness/chief complaint
         a) DOE
         b) Fatigue and weakness
         c) PND
         d) Orthopnea
         e) Weight gain
         f) Extremity swelling
         g) Palpitations
         h) Reduced exercise capacity
         i) Nocturia
         j) GI symptoms: nausea, anorexia, bloating, constipation
      2) Past medical history
         a) Current or preexisting diseases/illness
            (1) CAD/MI: produces an acute decrease in ventricular function
            (2) HTN: causes an increase in afterload
            (3) Diabetes mellitus: microvascular disease leads to poor cardiac function
            (4) Valve dysfunction (stenosis or regurgitation): may be either acute or a chronic, progressive disorder
            (5) Dysrhythmias: any dysrhythmia significant enough to reduce cardiac output; it may be acute (e.g., paroxysmal supraventricular tachycardia [PSVT]) or chronic (e.g., atrial fibrillation)
            (6) Endocrine disorders: any disorder that increases cardiac workload (e.g., thyroid disease)
            (7) Cardiomyopathy (ischemic, viral, dilated, hypertrophic, alcoholic, restrictive, peripartum, or idiopathic): weakens the heart muscle and changes muscular structure
            (8) Connective tissue disorders (e.g., Marfan syndrome): faulty connective tissue causes the heart muscle to weaken and stretch
            (9) Congenital heart defects
         b) Toxin ingestion: may have cardiac depressant effects
         c) Medications
         d) Allergies
   b. Objective data collection
      1) Physical examination
         a) General appearance
            (1) Level of consciousness, behavior, affect: anxious
            (2) Tachypnea, tachycardia
            (3) Malnourished, cachectic (with chronic heart failure)
            (4) Moderate to severe distress/discomfort, critically ill
         b) Inspection
            (1) Orthopnea
            (2) Edema: extremities, anasarca, ascites
            (3) Jugular venous distention
            (4) Dusky skin color
            (5) Cardiac dysrhythmias on monitor
         c) Auscultation
            (1) Breath sounds: crackles, wheezes
            (2) Heart sounds: S$_3$ gallop
         d) Palpation
            (1) Hepatomegaly
      2) Diagnostic procedures
         a) CBC with differential: anemia—decreased erythrocytes cause an increased cardiac workload, which can precipitate failure
         b) Serum chemistries including glucose, BUN, and creatinine
            (1) Hyponatremia: in severe heart failure
            (2) Hypokalemia: if the patient is taking diuretics
            (3) BUN and creatinine: elevated
         c) BNP: elevated; BNP is an endogenously generated peptide activated in response to ventricular volume expansion
         d) Liver function tests: abnormal as a result of hepatic congestion
         e) ABGs
         f) Urinalysis: proteinuria and high urine specific gravity
         g) Chest radiograph
            (1) Cardiomegaly
            (2) Pulmonary edema
            (3) Pleural effusion
         h) ECG
            (1) Acute failure: acute MI, ischemia, conduction defects
            (2) Chronic failure: ventricular hypertrophy, atrial enlargement, axis deviation
         i) Echocardiography can distinguish systolic dysfunction from diastolic dysfunction; findings include
            (1) Cardiac hypertrophy
            (2) Valve dysfunction
            (3) Wall motion abnormalities
            (4) Ejection fraction measurement
2. Analysis: differential nursing diagnoses/collaborative problems
   a. Ineffective breathing pattern
   b. Excess fluid volume
   c. Ineffective tissue perfusion: renal, cerebral, cardiopulmonary, GI, peripheral
3. Planning and implementation/interventions
   a. Maintain airway, breathing, and circulation (see Chapter 1)

b. Provide supplemental oxygen
  1) RSI and ventilatory support for patients with respiratory compromise
  2) Bilevel positive airway pressure (BiPAP) ventilation
  3) Continuous positive airway pressure (CPAP) ventilation
  4) High-flow oxygen
c. Establish IV access for administration of crystalloid fluid/medications
  1) Minimal fluid administration
d. Prepare for/assist with medical interventions
  1) Advanced airway management
    a) Nasal or oral intubation
    b) Supraglottic airway (e.g., King, Combitube, laryngeal mask airway)
    c) Surgical airway (e.g., cricothyrotomy)
  2) Place the patient in a high Fowler's position or other position of comfort
  3) Institute cardiac and pulse oximetry monitoring
  4) Catheter placement and monitoring of pulmonary wedge and arterial pressures (see Chapter 6)
  5) Insert gastric tube and attach to suction
  6) Insert indwelling urinary catheter
  7) Assist with hospital admission
e. Administer pharmacologic therapy as ordered
  1) RSI premedications: sedatives, analgesics, neuromuscular blocking agents
  2) Diuretics
    a) Furosemide (Lasix): decreases preload by increasing venous capacitance and reduces blood volume through diuresis
    b) Administer cautiously in older adults; they are prone to diuretic-induced hypokalemia and hyponatremia
  3) Morphine sulfate
    a) Reduces myocardial workload by increasing venous capacitance, decreasing afterload, limiting anxiety, and minimizing sympathetic stimulation
    b) Use with caution in acutely dyspneic patients
    c) Avoid in patients with decreased level of consciousness, hypercarbia, or hypotension
  4) Vasodilators
    a) Venodilators (e.g., nitroglycerin, isosorbide dinitrate [Isordil]) increase venous pooling; nitroglycerin is preferred for treatment of pulmonary edema in patients with CAD because it also improves coronary artery blood flow; in acute settings, sublingual or IV nitroglycerin is recommended over paste or oral forms because of inconsistent absorption
    b) Arteriolar dilators (e.g., hydralazine [Apresoline], minoxidil [Loniten]) act on the arteries to decrease systemic arterial resistance; these agents are usually administered concurrently with venodilators; because hydralazine increases renal blood flow, it may be a good choice for patients who cannot tolerate an ACE inhibitor
    c) Combined dilators (e.g., nitroprusside [Nipride], nesiritide [Natrecor]) dilate both veins and arteries, reducing preload and afterload; onset of action is rapid; nitroprusside can cause cardiac ischemia in the setting of CAD by reducing coronary vessel filling; nesiritide also promotes diuresis and increases cardiac output through reflex vasodilation
    d) ACE inhibitors (e.g., captopril [Capoten], enalapril [Vasotec], lisinopril [Zestril]) block the formation of angiotensin II, a vasoconstrictor; ACE inhibitors also limit aldosterone production, which decreases preload by increasing sodium and water excretion; ACE inhibitors have been shown to reduce mortality and directly improve cardiac function in patients with heart failure. Avoid overdiuresis before ACE inhibitor use to prevent hypotension or renal insufficiency. Hypotension can usually be easily treated with fluids. ACE inhibitors are cleared by the kidneys; dose adjustment may be necessary in patients with renal failure
  5) Positive inotropic agents include cardiac glycosides (digitalis [Lanoxin]), sympathomimetic agents (dopamine [Intropin], dobutamine [Dobutrex]), and phosphodiesterase inhibitors (amrinone [Inocor], milrinone [Primacor])
    a) Actions
      (1) Increase contractility and cardiac output
      (2) Decrease myocardial workload
      (3) Improve oxygen delivery to tissues
    b) Dobutamine is the drug of choice for normotensive patients in pulmonary edema
    c) Dopamine is useful for pulmonary edema patients with hypotension; at higher infusion rates, dopamine produces peripheral vasoconstriction
    d) Digoxin is not recommended for the acute management of heart failure; use cautiously in older adults; dosages are determined by body size and renal function
    e) Phosphodiesterase inhibitors are classified as inodilators because they possess both positive inotropic and vasodilator effects
  6) Bronchodilators
    a) In patients with wheezing, "cardiac asthma"
f. Educate patient and significant others
  1) Secondary/contributing causes of heart failure may be minimized by weight loss, dietary changes, smoking cessation, use of lipid-lowering agents, alcohol intake reduction, or use of antihypertensive medications

4. Evaluation and ongoing monitoring
    a. Level of consciousness
    b. Hemodynamic status
    c. Breath sounds and pulse oximetry
    d. Cardiac rate and rhythm
    e. Respiratory effort
    f. Intake and output

L. HYPERTENSIVE CRISES

Hypertension (HTN) is a chronic condition that develops over time as a result of increased force of blood against arterial walls. According to the American Heart Association, normal blood pressure is <120/80 with hypertension stage 1 at 140/90. While HTN may cause symptomatology in patients, it is not considered a medical emergency.[23] Hypertensive crises include hypertensive urgency, hypertensive emergency, and malignant hypertension. Regardless of which spectrum hypertensive crisis falls to it is defined as either systolic BP >180 mm Hg or diastolic BP >110 mm Hg in an adult patient.[23] Hypertensive crises can be emergent or urgent and are differentiated by organ damage. While both conditions require immediate medical attention to lower blood pressure, hypertensive emergency constitutes a medical emergency due to the rapid rise in pressure and the acute neurologic and cardiovascular organ deterioration that requires aggressive treatment to decrease morbidity and mortality. Hypertensive urgency symptoms may include severe headache, shortness of breath, nosebleeds, or severe anxiety. While these patients will need oral medication to lower blood pressure, they will not require hospitalization. Hypertensive emergency presents with symptoms indicating organ damage such as ischemic or hemorrhagic stroke, hypertensive encephalopathy, MI, pulmonary edema, aortic dissection, or eclampsia (pregnancy induced). Treatment for emergencies is dependent on what system is affected and the desired outcomes. Use of specific agents will lower blood pressure either rapidly or slowly, but will always require hospitalization and continuous monitoring.

Malignant hypertension is considered a hypertensive crisis that uses comparable therapies as urgency and emergency but may or may not have similar presenting symptoms. Malignant hypertension patients will have retinal papilledema, flame-shaped hemorrhages and exudates, as well as a hallmark sign of fibrinoid necrosis of the arterioles occurring systemically, but more specifically affecting the renal system. Other symptoms may include impaired renal function with hematuria, confusion, encephalopathy, intravascular coagulation issues, and weight loss.[24]

Treatment guidelines exist but are dependent on the patient's clinical condition, degree of end-organ impairment, fluid status, and comorbidities with no clear consensus on the acute or emergent management. What is known is that blood pressure must be lowered cautiously to avoid organ hypoperfusion and tissue ischemia. Not all patients with a hypertensive crisis require hospitalization but those that do will require continuous monitoring in an intensive care unit or intermediate (telemetry) setting.

1. Assessment
    a. Subjective data collection
        1) History of present illness/chief complaint
            a) Pain (see Chapter 8)
                (1) Headache
                (2) Chest pain
            b) Dizziness
            c) Visual complaints
            d) Symptoms of heart failure
            e) Patients may be asymptomatic
        2) Past medical history
            a) Current or preexisting diseases/illness
                (1) HTN
                    (a) Undiagnosed
                    (b) Poorly controlled
                    (c) Sudden discontinuation of antihypertensive agents
                (2) Renal disease
                (3) Adrenal disease (pheochromocytoma)
            b) Pregnancy (pregnancy-induced HTN/eclampsia)
            c) Sympathetic drug use
            d) Medications
            e) Allergies
    b. Objective data collection
        1) Physical examination
            a) General appearance
                (1) Level of consciousness, behavior, affect: drowsiness, seizures, confusion, lethargy, stupor, may progress to coma
                (2) Diastolic BP often >130 mm Hg
                (3) Hemiparesis
                (4) Moderate to severe distress/discomfort
            b) Inspection
                (1) Retinopathy
                    (a) Optic hemorrhages and exudates
                    (b) Papilledema: indicates accelerated-malignant HTN
            c) Auscultation
                (1) Heart sounds: prominent apical pulse; S_3, S_4
                (2) Breath sounds: crackles
                (3) Abdominal bruits
        2) Diagnostic procedures
            a) Comprehensive metabolic panel includes electrolytes, liver function, kidney function (BUN, creatinine), glucose, calcium, and proteins; a magnesium level may need to be added
            b) CBC with differential
            c) Urinalysis; pregnancy test in female patients of childbearing age
            d) Chest radiograph
            e) 12- to 15-lead ECG
                (1) Ischemic changes
                (2) Axis deviation

(3) LV hypertrophy

(4) ST-segment and T-wave abnormalities

    f) Head CT scan

2. Analysis: differential nursing diagnoses/collaborative problems

  a. Ineffective tissue perfusion: cerebral, renal

  b. Impaired gas exchange

3. Planning and implementation/interventions

  a. Maintain airway, breathing, and circulation (see Chapter 1)

  b. Provide supplemental oxygen

  c. Establish IV access for administration of crystalloid fluid/medications

  d. Prepare for/assist with medical interventions

    1) Institute cardiac and pulse oximetry monitoring

    2) Catheter placement and monitoring of arterial pressure (see Chapter 6)

    3) Insert gastric tube and attach to suction as indicated

    4) Insert indwelling urinary catheter as indicated

    5) Assist with hospital admission

  e. Administer pharmacological therapy as ordered

    1) Nitroprusside (Nipride)

      a) The mainstay of treatment for most patients with hypertensive emergencies

      b) Administered as a continuous IV infusion; titrate to effect

      c) Rapid onset of action and short duration of effects

      d) Produces arterial and venous dilation, decreasing both preload and afterload

      e) Close observation of patients for hypotension

    2) Nitroglycerin

      a) Preferred in patients with CAD or cardiac ischemia because of its ability to dilate coronary arteries

      b) Vasodilates venous vessels more than arterial vessels, reducing preload

      c) May cause tachycardia and, occasionally, bradycardia

    3) Labetalol (Normodyne, Trandate)

      a) Alpha and beta blocker (noncardioselective)

      b) Onset and cessation of action are slower than nitroprusside or nitroglycerin

      c) Indicated for patients with sympathomimetic overdose because it blocks both alpha and beta effects

      d) Contraindicated in patients with heart failure, second- or third-degree block, bradycardia, or reactive airway disease

    4) Hydralazine (Apresoline)

      a) Vasodilator, mostly arterial

      b) Medication of choice in eclampsia; not indicated for other hypertensive emergencies

    5) Phentolamine (Vasomax, Regitine)

      a) Alpha and beta blocker

      b) Used in patients with catecholamine crisis (pheochromocytoma)

    6) Propranolol (Inderal) or esmolol (Brevibloc)

      a) Short-acting beta blockers

      b) Not the primary agents for treatment of hypertensive emergencies; should not be used for stimulant-induced hypertensive emergencies because they do not block alpha effects

      c) Propranolol is preferred over esmolol for treatment of HTN associated with aortic dissection

    7) Diuretics

    8) Morphine sulfate

4. Evaluation and ongoing monitoring

  a. Level of consciousness

  b. Hemodynamic status: measure BP every 5 minutes until stable

  c. Breath sounds and pulse oximetry

  d. Cardiac rate and rhythm

  e. Intake and output

M. INFECTIVE ENDOCARDITIS

Infective endocarditis is a disease of the endocardium and heart valves. This disorder is classified by cause into four categories: (1) native valve infective endocarditis, (2) prosthetic valve infective endocarditis, (3) infective endocarditis in IV drug users, and (4) nosocomial infective endocarditis. Endocarditis in the pediatric patient is uncommon and is primarily associated with congenital heart abnormalities, particularly following surgical repair.

Endocardial infection may be either subacute or acute, depending on the progression and virulence of the offending pathogen. Subacute bacterial endocarditis (SBE) usually occurs in patients with congenital or acquired valvular heart disease. It evolves over several weeks or months and patients tend to be less toxic than those with acute disease. Acute bacterial endocarditis (ABE) is differentiated from SBE by its greatly accelerated onset (days to weeks). ABE generally affects normal heart valves, and patients can present as extremely toxic, with disseminated infection. *Staphylococcus aureus* is the most common ABE pathogen and *Streptococcus viridans* is the most frequent causative organism in those with SBE. Nevertheless, many bacteria, fungi, mycobacteria, and a host of other organisms may produce infective endocarditis.

Pathogens originate in the upper airway, genitourinary tract, GI system, or the skin. Risk factors include valvular disease (particularly mitral valve prolapse), congenital heart defects, rheumatic heart disease, prosthetic heart valves, body piercing, IV drug use, and long-term venous access devices. Pathologic changes include cardiac endothelial alterations that cause platelet and fibrin deposition. Circulating organisms then colonize the damaged tissue. Further organism growth, coupled with platelet-fibrin aggregation, results in the formation of valvular vegetations.

Local cardiac damage may be catastrophic. Infective endocarditis can destroy the valve, extend to adjacent structures, rupture the chordae tendineae, and form abscesses or fistulas throughout the cardiac vessels and chambers. The consequences of these changes include progressive heart failure, conduction disturbances, and dysrhythmias. In addition, valvular vegetations can embolize. This sheds microorganisms into circulation, which results in infecting or infarcting of tissue at any distal site including the brain, kidneys, lungs, spleen, bones, and joints.

1. Assessment
   a. Subjective data collection
      1) History of present illness/chief complaint
         a) Fever
            (1) Low grade and remittent with SBE
            (2) Acute and abrupt (<102°F [38.9°C]) and associated with chills in ABE
         b) Anorexia, weight loss
         c) Night sweats
         d) Arthralgia/myalgia
         e) Fatigue/malaise
         f) Dyspnea, cough
         g) Pain (see Chapter 8)
            (1) Pleuritic
            (2) Abdominal
            (3) Back
         h) Hemoptysis
         i) Headache/signs of stroke
         j) Confusion
      2) Past medical history
         a) Current or preexisting diseases/illness
            (1) Cardiac surgery, especially prosthetic heart valve insertion
            (2) Congenital or acquired valve disease
            (3) Rheumatic heart disease
            (4) Cardiac pacemaker insertion
            (5) Recent GI or genitourinary disorder
         b) IV drug abuse
         c) Poor dental hygiene
         d) Body piercings, tattooing
         e) Patients with valve disease (or a prosthetic valve) who underwent a recent dental procedure without taking prophylactic antibiotics
         f) Medications
         g) Allergies
   b. Objective data collection
      1) Physical examination
         a) General appearance
            (1) Level of consciousness, behavior, affect: changes associated with embolic stroke
            (2) Elevated temperature: may be absent in older adults, debilitated patients, and those with chronic renal failure
            (3) Tachycardia
            (4) Moderate to severe distress/discomfort
         b) Inspection
            (1) Janeway lesions: petechial lesions on palms or soles
            (2) Roth spots: hemorrhage in the retina with a white center; seen on ophthalmic examination
            (3) Osler nodes: painful fingertips lesions
            (4) Splinter hemorrhages of the nails (caused by emboli)
            (5) Petechiae of the conjunctiva, palate, neck, upper trunk, or extremities
            (6) Clubbing: thickening of the flesh under toe and finger nails; seen with long-standing SBE
            (7) Peripheral edema in advanced disease
         c) Auscultation
            (1) Heart sounds: murmur
            (2) Breath sounds: crackles in advanced disease
         d) Palpation
            (1) Splenomegaly from emboli in spleen: more common with SBE
      2) Diagnostic procedures
         a) CBC with differential: elevated WBC, anemia common with SBE
         b) Blood cultures
            (1) Most important test for determining diagnosis
            (2) May require four to six culture specimens (aerobic, anaerobic, fungal)
         c) Comprehensive metabolic panel includes electrolytes, liver function, kidney function (BUN, creatinine), glucose, calcium, and proteins; a magnesium level may need to be added
         d) ESR: elevated in both SBE and ABE
         e) Urinalysis: proteinuria and microscopic hematuria are common; pregnancy test
         f) Head CT or MRI: for patients with neurologic deficits
         g) ECG: conduction abnormalities may be present in patients with a septal abscess
         h) Echocardiogram: used to visualize valve dysfunction, regurgitation, the mobility and extent of vegetations, and myocardial abscesses
2. Analysis: differential nursing diagnoses/collaborative problems
   a. Infection
   b. Decreased cardiac output
   c. Anxiety
3. Planning and implementation/interventions
   a. Maintain airway, breathing, and circulation (see Chapter 1)
   b. Provide supplemental oxygen
   c. Establish IV access for administration of crystalloid fluid/medications

d. Prepare for/assist with medical interventions
  1) Institute cardiac and pulse oximetry monitoring
  2) Possible catheter placement and monitoring of pulmonary wedge pressure if patient is in heart failure (see Chapter 6)
  3) Insert indwelling urinary catheter as indicated
  4) Assist with hospital admission
e. Administer pharmacologic therapy as ordered
  1) Antipyretics
  2) Antibiotics after obtaining blood cultures
4. Evaluation and ongoing monitoring
  a. Level of consciousness
  b. Hemodynamic status
  c. Breath sounds and pulse oximetry
  d. Cardiac rate and rhythm
  e. Intake and output
  f. Fever control

N. MYOCARDITIS

Myocarditis is characterized by inflammation and destruction of cardiac muscle. Patients may present as nearly asymptomatic, in severe heart failure, or with sudden death from dysrhythmias. The causes of myocarditis are numerous and can be roughly divided into infectious, toxic, and immunologic. Viral infections are the predominant cause in North America. Causes of toxic myocarditis include both pharmacologic and environmental agents. Common drugs associated with myocarditis include penicillin, ampicillin, hydrochlorothiazide, methyldopa, sulfonamides, lithium, doxorubicin, cocaine, and acetaminophen. Environmental toxins include lead, arsenic, carbon monoxide, and insect venoms. Immunologic and inflammatory causes of myocarditis include connective tissue disorders such as systemic lupus erythematosus, rheumatoid arthritis, dermatomyositis, and Kawasaki disease.

1. Assessment
  a. Subjective data collection
    1) History of present illness/chief complaint
      a) Most cases of myocarditis are subclinical
      b) History of a viral infection in the past 2 weeks (present in more than one half of patients)
      c) Fatigue, mild dyspnea, orthopnea, myalgias, arthralgias, and malaise
      d) Chest pain or discomfort; palpitations
    2) Past medical history
      a) Current or preexisting diseases/illness
      b) Medications
      c) Allergies
  b. Objective data collection
    1) Physical examination
      a) General appearance
        (1) Tachycardia, tachypnea
        (2) Elevated temperature: present in 20% of patients
        (3) Hypotension
        (4) Moderate to severe distress/discomfort
      b) Inspection
        (1) Jugular venous distention (see Chapter 1)
        (2) Ascites
        (3) Peripheral edema
        (4) Possible cardiac dysrhythmias on monitor
      c) Auscultation
        (1) Breath sounds: bibasilar crackles
        (2) Heart sounds: S_3, summation gallop, murmur, or pleural friction rub
    2) Diagnostic procedures
      a) Cardiac biomarkers; rarely elevated but serve to rule out ACS
      b) ESR: elevated in 60% of acute cases
      c) CBC with differential: leukocytosis; present in 25% of patients
      d) Virology culture: viruses isolated from other body sites suggest myocarditis
      e) If a systemic disorder (e.g., systemic lupus erythematosus) is suspected, consider antinuclear antibodies (ANA) and other collagen vascular disorder tests
      f) Chest radiograph
        (1) Cardiomegaly
        (2) Pulmonary edema, pleural effusion
      g) ECG
        (1) Sinus tachycardia is the most frequent finding
        (2) ST-segment elevation without reciprocal depression
        (3) Decreased QRS amplitude and transitory Q-wave development
        (4) Conduction delays; second-degree block Mobitz I, Mobitz II, or complete heart block
        (5) Left or right bundle branch block (in 20% of patients)
      h) Echocardiography
        (1) LV impairment, reduced ejection fraction
        (2) Wall motion abnormalities
        (3) Pericardial effusion
        (4) Ventricular thrombus (in 15% of patients)
      i) MRI: very sensitive and specific for myocarditis
2. Analysis: differential nursing diagnoses/collaborative problems
  a. Acute pain
  b. Decreased cardiac output
  c. Anxiety
3. Planning and implementation/interventions
  a. Provide supplemental oxygen
  b. Establish IV access for administration of crystalloid fluid/medications
  c. Prepare for/assist with medical interventions
    1) Institute cardiac and pulse oximetry monitoring
    2) Pacemaker placement in patients with Mobitz II or complete heart block

3) Assist with possible hospital admission
d. Administer pharmacologic therapy as ordered
   1) Avoid sympathomimetic and beta-blocker drugs, as they increase extent of myocardial necrosis and mortality
   2) Antipyretics
e. Educate patient/significant others
   1) Limit activities for approximately 6 months
4. Evaluation and ongoing monitoring
   a. Hemodynamic status
   b. Breath sounds and pulse oximetry
   c. Cardiac rate and rhythm
   d. Fever control

O. PERICARDITIS

Pericarditis (inflammation of the pericardium) is a common disorder that is most frequently idiopathic. However, pericarditis can develop as a result of bacterial, viral, or fungal infections; autoimmune diseases; MI; connective tissue disorders (systemic lupus erythematosus, rheumatoid arthritis); renal failure; mediastinal injury; neoplastic disorders; and radiation therapy and following percutaneous procedures or the use of certain medications (e.g., hydralazine [Apresoline], procainamide [Pronestyl]). The acute changes seen with pericarditis include infiltration of polymorphonuclear leukocytes into the pericardium, increased pericardial vascularity, and fibrin deposition. The inflammation can extend to adjacent structures and may produce an exudate. Signs and symptoms of pericarditis depend on its cause, the type of effusion, and the effusion volume. Pericarditis is more common in men than women and is seen more often in adults than children.

Patients with uncomplicated pericarditis experience pleuritic chest pain that radiates to the left shoulder. The pain may be relieved by leaning forward. Pericarditis is generally a mild disorder that resolves spontaneously, although treatment with a nonsteroidal antiinflammatory drug or corticosteroids may be helpful. When a large pericardial effusion is produced, cardiac function may be compromised, and cardiac tamponade can occur. In cases of persistent inflammation, the pericardium becomes fibrous or calcified, resulting in cardiac constriction. Drainage or surgical intervention is necessary in patients with complicated pericarditis. Chest radiographs, Doppler studies, M-mode echocardiography, and laboratory tests confirm the diagnosis and provide information about the origin and extent of effusion.

Management depends on the underlying cause. Viral, idiopathic, post-MI, and postpericardiotomy pericarditis are usually self-limiting conditions. Recurrent pericarditis is the most common and most troublesome complication of this disorder. However, patients may suffer hemodynamic compromise secondary to cardiac compression as a result of effusion (pericardial tamponade), fibrosis formation (cardiac restriction), or a combination of both.

1. Assessment
   a. Subjective data collection
      1) History of present illness/chief complaint
         a) Chest pain (see Chapter 8)
            (1) Provocative factors
               (a) Deep inspiration
               (b) Recumbent position
               (c) Coughing
               (d) Movement
               (e) Swallowing
            (2) Palliative factors
               (a) Sitting up and leaning forward
            (3) Quality
               (a) Severe, sharp, pleuritic
               (b) May radiate to the neck, arms, or left shoulder
               (c) Oppressive
               (d) Dull ache
            (4) Region/radiation
               (a) Retrosternal
               (b) Left precordial regions
               (c) Radiates to the back, neck, or side
               (d) Epigastric
            (5) Timing
               (a) Sudden in onset
               (b) Persists for days
         b) General malaise, weight loss
         c) Fever/chills: maximal on the first day
         d) Dyspnea, cough
      2) Past medical history
         a) Current or preexisting diseases/illness
            (1) Tuberculosis: may infect the pericardium
            (2) Congenital anomalies: congenital pericardial cysts
            (3) Immune or collagen disorders: systemic lupus erythematosus, rheumatic fever
            (4) Recent MI (Dressler syndrome)
            (5) Neoplastic disease: radiation therapy, adenocarcinoma of the breast
            (6) Uremia: pericarditis is common in patients receiving hemodialysis
         b) Cardiac surgery: postpericardiotomy syndrome
         c) Cardiac trauma: blunt or penetrating forces
         d) Medications: hydralazine (Apresoline), procainamide (Pronestyl), and anticoagulants
         e) Allergies
   b. Objective data collection
      1) Physical examination
         a) General appearance
            (1) Tachycardia, tachypnea
            (2) Elevated temperature: in pediatric patients, temperature may be very high or low grade

(3) Moderate distress/discomfort
b) Auscultation
   (1) Heart sounds: pericardial friction rub
      (a) Hallmark of acute pericarditis, but it is frequently absent
      (b) Heard best at end expiration, left of the lower sternal border, with the patient leaning forward
      (c) Raspy or creaking sound; occasionally has a "leathery" quality and is not associated with the respiratory cycle
      (d) Triphasic and transient
         (i) Ventricular systole
         (ii) Ventricular diastole
         (iii) Atrial systole
2) Diagnostic procedures
   a) CBC with differential: elevated WBC
   b) Troponin I: used to distinguish pericarditis from ACS, but levels may be elevated in acute pericarditis if there is myocardial involvement
   c) Comprehensive metabolic panel includes electrolytes, liver function, kidney function (BUN, creatinine), glucose, calcium, and proteins; a magnesium level may need to be added
   d) Blood cultures
   e) Pericardial fluid analysis: Gram stain and aerobic/anaerobic cultures
   f) Urinalysis; pregnancy test in females of childbearing age
   g) Chest radiograph
   h) ECG: findings vary throughout the course of the disease
      (1) ECG changes occur in approximately 90% of patients with acute pericarditis
      (2) Changes are seen in the inferior leads (II, III, and aVF) and sometimes in the apical leads (V_5, V_6)
      (3) Four stages
         (a) ST-segment elevation (early) concave shape, upright T waves, usually present in all leads except aVR and V_1
         (b) T waves flatten; ST segment returns to baseline after several days
         (c) T-wave inversion
         (d) T waves return to normal; this may take weeks or months
   i) Echocardiograms (TTE or TEE) are the most sensitive and accurate diagnostic tests for pericarditis
2. Analysis: differential nursing diagnoses/collaborative problems
   a. Pain

   b. Risk for infection
   c. Anxiety
3. Planning and implementation/interventions
   a. Provide supplemental oxygen
   b. Establish IV access for administration of crystalloid fluids/medications
   c. Prepare for/assist with medical interventions
      1) Institute cardiac and pulse oximetry monitoring
      2) Assist the patient to assume a position of comfort
      3) Assist with possible pericardiocentesis
      4) Assist with possible hospital admission
   d. Administer pharmacologic therapy as ordered
      1) Antiinflammatory agents (e.g., aspirin, ibuprofen [Advil, Motrin], indomethacin [Indocin], corticosteroids)
      2) Antipyretics
      3) Antibiotics
      4) Colchicine
      5) Diuretics for constrictive pericarditis
4. Evaluation and ongoing monitoring
   a. Hemodynamic status
   b. Breath sounds and pulse oximetry
   c. Cardiac rate and rhythm
   d. Pain relief
   e. Intake and output

P. PERIPHERAL VASCULAR DISEASE

The peripheral circulation is defined as any circulation external to the heart and brain with disease processes affecting both peripheral veins and arteries. Peripheral venous disease will be discussed in the next section. Peripheral vascular disease (PVD) or peripheral artery disease (PAD) is a narrowing or occlusion of the arteries outside the heart as a result of thickening of the intimal wall of the small arteries and arterioles caused primarily by arteriosclerosis. Arteriosclerosis is a general term, whereas atherosclerosis is a specific type of hardening caused by the accumulation of fats, cholesterol, and other substances creating plaque in medium and large arteries. The insidious process begins early in life and is accelerated based on risk factors and lifestyle choices such as heredity, gender (male more prominent), age, smoking, hypertension, hyperlipidemia, diabetes, and obesity. Because atherosclerosis is a systemic disease process, patients with PVD are also at increased risk of coronary artery disease (CAD), aneurysms, and stroke. Symptoms of PVD are commonly not seen until later in life (40–60 years of age) when there is marked narrowing from disease progression that restricts blood flow. The decreased blood flow and tissue perfusion associated with PVD causes pain, skin discoloration, and decreased peripheral pulses.

Other associated PVD disorders include Raynaud and Buerger (thromboangiitis obliterans). Raynaud disease is a circulatory disorder of the arteries that severely reduces blood flow as the result of episodic intense vasospasm of the digits (fingers most common), tip of the nose, or ears generally in response to extreme cold, emotional stress, and/or smoking. Women are more prone to Raynaud disease than are men, as are persons who dwell in colder climates. Ischemia results from episodic vasospasms causing pallor, followed by cyanosis, coldness, numbness, tingling, and possible decreased motor function in the affected area. Episodes may last from a few minutes to a few hours. As vasospasm and ischemia resolve, hyperemia produces intense rubor and throbbing pain. Afterward, there is a return to normal color.

Raynaud disease is divided into two types. Primary Raynaud disease has no known cause and tends to be the less severe form of this condition. Secondary Raynaud disease, also called Raynaud phenomenon, is associated with previous vessel injury or connective tissue diseases such as scleroderma. Chronic and frequent exacerbations lead to ischemic changes, including thickening of the fingertips and nails, skin ulcers, and in rare cases can lead to gangrene. While there is no cure for Raynaud disease, treatment plans aim to decrease pain and vasospastic events. Calcium channel blockers and vasodilation creams are sometimes prescribed to relax and open small blood vessels in the hands and feet reducing frequency and severity of episodes thus reducing ischemic injury. Patients should be educated to avoid beta blockers and OTC cold medications such as pseudoephedrine as these types of medications increase the risk of spasms.

Thromboangiitis obliterans, Buerger disease, is an occlusive, chronic, inflammatory disorder of the small and medium-size arteries, veins, and surrounding nerves. Buerger disease triggers decreased blood flow first in the hands and feet that results in ischemia and pain. As the disease progresses to the arms and legs, intermittent claudication, decreased or absent peripheral pulses, and changes in skin color from cyanotic to reddish blue occur. Eventually episodes of decreased blood flow cause the skin to become thin and shiny where infection, skin ulcers, and gangrene may develop. While rare in the United States, this condition is common in the Middle and Far East regions where heavy use of tobacco, specifically hand-rolled cigarettes, among males under the age of 40 is customary. Treatment priorities include absolute cessation of any and all tobacco and nicotine products. Other regimens may be used to increase blood flow to the affected extremity and to prevent further injury.

1. Assessment
   a. Subjective data collection
      1) History of present illness/chief complaint
         a) Pain (see Chapter 8)
            (1) Palliative/provocative
               (a) Cold environment
               (b) Stress
               (c) Exercise
               (d) Relieved by removal or discontinuation of the offending stimulus
            (2) Quality: severe/throbbing
            (3) Radiation/region
               (a) Fingers, toes
               (b) Calf, foot
            (4) Timing
               (a) After exercise
               (b) During stressful situations
               (c) Exposure to cold
      2) Past medical history
         a) Current or preexisting diseases/illness
         b) Smoking
         c) Medications
         d) Allergies
   b. Objective data collection
      1) Physical assessment
         a) General appearance: moderate to severe discomfort
         b) Inspection
            (1) Extremity rubor (redness)
            (2) Thin, shiny skin
            (3) Thickened fingertips and nails
            (4) Extremity ulcerations or areas of necrosis
            (5) Pallor, cyanosis of area
         c) Palpation
            (1) Coldness to touch
            (2) Decreased/absent pulses
      2) Diagnostic procedures
         a) CBC with differential
         b) Antinuclear antibodies (ANA): positive result indicates autoimmune component
         c) Doppler flow studies
         d) Arteriogram
         e) Magnetic resonance angiogram (MRA)
         f) Ankle-brachial index (ABI): a comparison of ankle BP with arm pressure; an ABI <0.30 is not compatible with limb viability
2. Analysis: differential nursing diagnoses/collaborative problems
   a. Ineffective tissue perfusion
   b. Pain
   c. Anxiety
3. Planning and implementation/interventions
   a. Provide supplemental oxygen as indicated
   b. Establish IV access for administration of crystalloid fluid/medications
   c. Prepare for/assist with medical interventions
      1) Remove any precipitating stimuli (e.g., stress, cold)
      2) Provide a warm environment
      3) Do not elevate the ischemic extremity
      4) Assist with possible hospital admission

d. Administer pharmacologic therapy as ordered
  1) Calcium channel blockers
  2) Adrenergic blocking agents
  3) Nonnarcotic analgesics
  4) Narcotics
e. Educate: keep patient/family informed about medications and treatment plan throughout
4. Evaluation and ongoing monitoring
  a. Hemodynamic status
  b. Extremity movement and sensation
  c. Skin temperature changes
  d. Pain relief

Q. RIGHT VENTRICULAR INFARCTION

Like LV infarction, RV infarction (RVI; STEMI or NSTEMI) is an ACS; however, the diagnosis and treatment vary somewhat from those of a typical left-sided ACS event. RVI most commonly occurs as a result of occlusion of the proximal right coronary artery. In patients with atypical coronary perfusion, RVI can be caused by occlusion of either the left circumflex or the left anterior descending artery. Isolated RVI is a rare event; it is generally associated with inferior wall (IW) MI and occurs in 30–50% of the population with IWMI. RVI with IWMI has a higher mortality than IWMI alone.

Injury to the right ventricle causes RV dilation and decreased contractility. The inability to pump venous blood efficiently into the pulmonary vasculature reduces blood flow to the left ventricle, which leads to a drop in cardiac output. The symptoms of RVI range from mild to life threatening; if the reduction in preload is profound, cardiogenic shock will result. The right ventricle's inability to move blood forward also results in venous HTN. The clinical triad of arterial hypotension, clear lung sounds, and increased jugular venous pressure is highly suggestive of RVI. Unfortunately, these classic findings occur in only one fourth of patients with RVI. As with all MIs, management focuses on early reperfusion. However, in patients with RVI, RV preload must be maintained using IV fluids, ventricular contractility must be augmented using inotropes, and afterload must be reduced using vasodilators, especially if concomitant LV injury and failure are present. The administration of nitrates, diuretics, and morphine sulfate should be avoided because of their preload-reducing effects.

1. Assessment
  a. Subjective data collection (see Acute Coronary Syndromes)
  b. Objective data collection (see Acute Coronary Syndromes; other data specific to RVI are noted here)
    1) Physical examination
      a) General appearance/vital signs
        (1) Bradycardia secondary to inferior wall MI
        (2) Hypotension if concomitant LV damage

      b) Inspection
        (1) Peripheral edema: extent depends on the degree of right heart failure
        (2) Jugular venous distention (see Chapter 1)
      c) Auscultation
        (1) Breath sounds: clear
        (2) Heart sounds: S_3, tricuspid regurgitation
    2) Diagnostic procedures
      a) ECG including right-sided leads
        (1) ST elevation in leads II, III, and aVF indicate IW involvement: highly suggestive of RVI
        (2) ST elevation in V_4R: highly sensitive and specific for RVI
        (3) Right bundle branch block or third-degree heart block: common conduction defects associated with RVI
        (4) Atrial fibrillation: may be present in patients with concurrent atrial infarction or dilation
      b) Echocardiography: detect RV dilatation and RV wall motion defects
2. Analysis: differential nursing diagnoses/collaborative problems
  a. See Acute Coronary Syndromes
3. Planning and implementation/interventions (see Acute Coronary Syndromes; other interventions specific to RVI are noted here)
  a. Establish IV access for administration of crystalloid fluid/medications
    1) Administer normal saline solution boluses as necessary for the treatment of hypotension
  b. Administer pharmacologic therapy as ordered
    1) Inotropic support: dobutamine (Dobutrex) if 1–2 L of fluid fails to improve patient's cardiac output
4. Evaluation and ongoing monitoring
  a. Level of consciousness
  b. Hemodynamic status
  c. Breath sounds and pulse oximetry
  d. Cardiac rate and rhythm changes
    1) Bradycardia
    2) Right bundle branch block
    3) AV blocks
    4) Atrial fibrillation
  e. Pain relief
  f. Intake and output

R. VENOUS THROMBOEMBOLISM

Venous thromboembolism (VTE), also known as peripheral venous thrombosis, is an occlusion of a vein by a thrombus restricting blood outflow. While VTEs include both deep vein thrombosis (DVT) and pulmonary embolism (PE), the focus of this section will be on DVTs, with PEs being discussed at length in Chapter 28. The majority of DVTs occur in the lower extremities and are classified as proximal or distal. Distal vein thrombi arise in the calf, while proximal vein thrombi involve the popliteal, femoral, or iliac veins. DVTs occurring in the popliteal vein or above have a higher risk of developing a PE if not treated appropriately. Virchow triad delineates the triggers often associated with development of DVT/VTE to include (1) hypercoagulable states such as cancer, pregnancy, sepsis, surgery, and/or trauma; (2) vascular endothelial injury caused by atherosclerosis, immune response, surgery, trauma, and/or venipuncture; and (3) circulatory stasis subsequent to aging, inherited conditions such as factor V Leiden, atrial fibrillation, left ventricular dysfunction, immobility, use of hormone therapy or birth control pills, or venous insufficiency. Signs and symptoms of DVTs vary among presenting patients, including but not limited to swelling, pain, or tenderness in one or both legs; and warm, red, or discolored skin.

VTEs related to recent hospitalization occur in approximately half of all adult cases. These cases are then 40 times more likely to suffer another event than compared to those unaffected by VTEs. Since VTEs are the third most common cardiovascular illness behind acute coronary syndrome (ACS) and stroke affecting 1 in 1,000 in the United States annually,[25] it is important to note that there are potential long-term complications, including chronic thromboembolic pulmonary hypertension (CTEPH) and postthrombotic syndrome (PTS). Chronic thromboembolic pulmonary hypertension is a rare form of pulmonary hypertension that may develop in patients who have experienced a pulmonary embolism and generally appears within 6 months but up to 2 years after the initial PE.[26]

Postthrombotic syndrome (PTS) is considered the most common long-term complication of a DVT occurring in the limb that was previously affected within 6 months of initial insult but up to 2 years after the initial DVT. Signs and symptoms manifest as a result of chronic venous insufficiency varying from minor leg discomfort, swelling, and hyperpigmentation up to more severe complications such as venous claudication, chronic debilitating pain, intractable edema, and skin ulcerations. Assessment includes past history for DVTs, physical assessment of affected limb, and current treatment plan. Treatment of PTS is geared toward secondary prevention by maximizing anticoagulation effects while treating the initial DVT.

1. Assessment
   a. Subjective data collection
      1) History of present illness/chief complaint
         a) Pain (see Chapter 8)
            (1) Provocation: walking
            (2) Quality: aching, throbbing
            (3) Region: localized to the point of occlusion
            (4) Severity: moderate
            (5) Timing: constant
         b) Swelling at and below site of occlusion
         c) Deep muscle tenderness
         d) Mild temperature elevation
      2) Medical history
         a) Current or preexisting diseases/illness
            (1) Heart failure
            (2) Thrombotic hematologic disorders
            (3) Malignancies
            (4) Venous disorders
            (5) Recent MI
         b) Recent trauma, injury, or surgery
         c) Current pregnancy or postpartum
         d) Recent prolonged immobility (bedrest or travel)
         e) Obesity
         f) Hormone therapy including oral contraceptives
   b. Objective data collection
      1) Physical examination and general appearance
         a) Degree of distress/discomfort
         b) Inspection
            (1) Extremity erythema
            (2) Extremity swelling/induration
            (3) Asymmetrical extremity size
            (4) Pain in calf with dorsiflexion of the foot (Homan sign)
         c) Palpation
            (1) Warmth of area
            (2) Deep muscle tenderness on palpation
      2) Diagnostics
         a) Laboratory
            (1) CBC with differential
            (2) D-dimer
            (3) Coagulation profile: PT-INR, aPTT
         b) Imaging
            (1) Venous duplex scan: combines vascular and Doppler ultrasound techniques to provide both images and evaluation of blood flow through arteries and veins
            (2) Venography: used if ultrasound is unremarkable. Invasive exam where dye is injected into a leg vein and an x-ray is taken to show blood flow
            (3) Other imaging used if symptoms indicate possible PE
            (4) Computed tomography: chest CT or spiral CT
            (5) Ventilation-perfusion (VQ) scan: nuclear medicine study to measure air and blood flow of the lungs
            (6) Impedance plethysmography (IPG): manometric electrode impedance exam that estimates blood flow of affected extremity
2. Analysis: differential nursing diagnoses/collaborative problems
   a. Ineffective tissue perfusion
   b. Pain
3. Planning and implementation/interventions
   a. Institute cardiac and pulse oximetry monitoring
   b. Provide supplemental oxygen as indicated

c. Establish IV access for administration of crystalloid fluids/medications

d. Administer pharmacologic therapy as ordered

   1) Initiate appropriate anticoagulant therapy

      a) Unfractionated heparin (UFH): heparin

      b) Low-molecular-weight heparin (LMWH): enoxaparin (Lovenox)

      c) Direct factor Xa inhibitors: rivaroxaban (Xarelto), (Arixtra) (Fondaparinux Sodium)

      d) Direct thrombin inhibitors: dabigatran (Pradaxa)

   2) Nonnarcotic analgesics

   3) Fibrinolytics

e. Monitor for worsening symptoms that might indicated PE

   1) Sudden sharp chest pain

   2) Rapid breathing, shortness of breath, or cough

   3) Severe lightheadedness or sudden syncopal episode

f. Elevate the affected extremity

g. Apply stockings or compression device as directed

h. Prepare for admission or discharge home

i. Educate: keep patient and family informed about medications and treatment plan throughout

4. Evaluation and ongoing monitoring

References

1. Sovari AA: Long QT syndrome. Medscape Nurses. Retrieved from http://emedicine.medscape.com/article/157826-overview, 2014, April.

2. Link MS: Commotio cordis ventricular fibrillation triggered by chest impact–induced abnormalities in repolarization. *Circulation: Arrhythmia and Electrophysiology*, 425–432, 2012, April. Retrieved from http://circep.ahajournals.org/content/5/2/425.full.pdf.

3. Webb RC, Inscho EW: Age-related changes in the cardiovascular system. In Prisant LM, editor: *Clinical hypertension and vascular diseases: Hypertension in the elderly*, Totowa, NJ, 2005, Springer, pp 11–21.

4. Ruscin M, Linnebur SA: Drug-related problems in the elderly, *Merck Manuals Professional*, 2015. Retrieved from http://www.merckmanuals.com/professional/geriatrics/drug-therapy-in-the-elderly/drug-related-problems-in-the-elderly.

5. Danyi P, Elefteriades JA, Jovin IS: Medical therapy of thoracic aortic aneurysms. Are we there yet? *Circulation*, 1469–1474, 2011, September 27. Retrieved from http://circ.ahajournals.org/content/124/13/1469.full.pdf.

6. The Society of Thoracic Surgeons: Aortic aneurysms. Retrieved from http://www.sts.org/patient-information/aneurysm-surgery/aortic-aneurysms, 2015.

7. Rahimi SA: Abdominal aortic aneurysm. Retrieved from http://emedicine.medscape.com/article/1979501-overview, 2015, September 28.

8. Braverman AC: Acute aortic dissection clinician update. *Circulation*, 184–188, 2010, July 13. Retrieved from http://circ.ahajournals.org/content/122/2/184.full.pdf.

9. Criado FJ: Aortic dissection: a 250-year perspective, *Texas Heart Institute Journal* 38(6):694–700, 2011. Retrieved from http://www.ncbi.nlm.nih.gov/pmc/articles/PMC3233335/pdf/20111200s00023p694.pdf.

10. SCPC: Chest pain center accreditation. Society of Cardiovascular Patient Care. Retrieved from http://www.scpcp.org/services/cpc.aspx, 2015.

11. O'Gara PT, Kushner FG, Ascheim DD, Casey DE, Chung MK, deLemos JA, Tamis-Holland: 2013 ACCF/AHA guideline for the management of ST-elevation myocardial infarction: a report of the American College of Cardiology Foundation/American Heart Association Task Force on Practice Guidelines. *The Journal of the American College of Cardiology*, 61(4): e78–e140, 2013, January. Retrieved from http://content.onlinejacc.org/article.aspx?articleid=1486115.

12. Beinart SC, Rottman JN: Synchronized electrical cardioversion. Retrieved from http://emedicine.medscape.com/article/1834044-overview#a1, 2014, October.

13. Page RI, Joglar JA, Al-Khatib SM, Caldwell MA, Calkins H, Conti JB, Hammill SC: 2015 ACC/AHA/HRS guideline for the management of adult patients with supraventricular tachycardia: executive summary. *Circulation*. Retrieved from http://circ.ahajournals.org/content/early/2015/09/22/CIR.0000000000000310.full.pdf, 2015, September 23.

14. Sandesara CM, Rottman JN: Atrioventricular block. Retrieved from http://emedicine.medscape.com/article/151597-overview, 2014, December 18.

15. Abrams DJ, MacRae C: Long QT syndrome, *Circulation*, 1524–1529, 2014. Retrieved from http://circ.ahajournals.org/content/129/14/1524.full.pdf.

16. Cox, NK. (2011, March/April). The QT interval: How long is too long? *Nursing Made Incredibly Easy!*, 17–21. Retrieved from http://www.omnimedicalsupply.com/QRS/The%20QT%20interval.pdf.

17. American Heart Association: Adult cardiac arrest circular algorithm—2015 Update. Retrieved from http://eccguidelines.heart.org/wp-content/uploads/2015/10/2010-Integrated_Updated-Circulation-ACLS-Cardiac-Arrest-Circular-Algorithm.pdf, 2015b.

18. American Heart Association. Adult cardiac arrest algorithm—2015 Update. Retrieved from http://eccguidelines.heart.org/wp-content/uploads/2015/10/ACLS-Cardiac-Arrest-Algorithm.pdf, 2015ba.

19. Callaway CW, Donnino MW, Fink EL, Geocadin RG, Golan E, Kern KB, Zimmerman JL et al.: Part 8: Post–cardiac arrest care: 2015 American Heart Association Guidelines Update for Cardiopulmonary Resuscitation and Emergency Cardiovascular Care. *Circulation*, 132(2): S465–S482, 2015, November 3. Retrieved from http://circ.ahajournals.org/content/132/18_s.

20. Deckard ME, Ebright PR: Therapeutic hypothermia after cardiac arrest: what, why, who, and how cooling patients can improve their neurologic outcome. *American Nurse Today*, 6(7): 23–28, 2011, July. Retrieved from http://www.americannursetoday.com/assets/0/434/436/440/7986/7988/7990/8014/b12fb51c-3u12-456f-abae-56b7972846d1.pdf.

21. American Heart Association: Hypertrophic cardiomyopathy. Retrieved from http://www.heart.org/HEARTORG/Conditions/More/Cardiomyopathy/Hypertrophic-Cardiomyopathy_UCM_444317_Article.jsp#.VmUQvT90zIU, 2015, August.

22. Cooper KL: Biventricular pacemakers in patients with heart failure. *Critical Care Nurse*, 35(2): 20–27, 2015, April. Retrieved from http://www.aacn.org/wd/Cetests/media/C1523.pdf.

23. American Heart Association: Understanding blood pressure readings. Retrieved from http://www.heart.org/HEARTORG /Conditions/HighBloodPressure/AboutHighBloodPressure/ Understanding-Blood-Pressure-Readings_UCM_301764_A rticle.jsp#.VmTYZD90zIU, 2015, October 22.

24. Hopkins C, Brenner BE: Hypertensive emergencies. Retrieved from http://emedicine.medscape.com/article/1952052-over-view, 2015, August.

25. Mozaffarian D, Benjamin EJ, Go AS, Arnett DK, Blaha MJ, Cushman M, Lackland D et al.: Heart disease and stroke statistics—2015 update. A report from the American Heart Association. *Circulation*, e30–e535, 2015, January 27. Retrieved from http://circ.ahajournals.org/content/131/4/e29.full.pdf.

26. International Society on Thrombosis and Haemostasis (ISTH) Steering Committee: Thrombosis: a major contributor to the global disease burden, *Journal of Thrombosis and Haemostasis*, 1580–1590, 2014. Retrieved from http://www .worldthrombosisday.org/assets/_control/content/files/Thr ombosis%20Global%20Burden%20of%20Disease.pdf.

Bibliography

American Heart Association: Top ten things to know about the management of ST-elevation myocardial infarction. Retrieved from ht tp://my.americanheart.org/idc/groups/ahaecc-public/@wcm/@s op/@smd/documents/downloadable/ucm_447534.pdf, 2013.

CDC. (n.d.). Aortic aneurysm fact sheet. Retrieved from http:// www.cdc.gov/dhdsp/data_statistics/fact_sheets/docs/fs_aorti c_aneurysm.pdf.

Dupras D, Bluhm J, Felty C, Hansen C, Johnson T, Lim K, Skeik N: Venous thromboembolism diagnosis and treatment, *Institute for Clinical Systems Improvement*, 2013. Retrieved from https:/ /www.icsi.org/_asset/5ldx9k/VTE01.

Elefteriades JA, Farkas EA: Thoracic aortic aneurysm clinically pertinent controversies and uncertainties. *Journal of the American College of Cardiology*, 55(9), 841–857, 2010, March 2. Retrieved from http://content.onlinejacc.org/article.aspx?articleid=1140497.

Frazier A, Hunt EA, Holmes K: Pediatric cardiac emergencies: children are not small adults. *Journal of Emergencies, Trauma, and Shock*, 4(1), 2011, Jan-Mar. Retrieved from http://www. ncbi.nlm.nih.gov/pmc/articles/PMC3097588/#.

Friedman KG, Alexander ME: Chest pain and syncope in children: a practical approach to the diagnosis of cardiac disease. *Journal of Pediatrics*, 163(3), 896–901, 2013, September. Retrieved from http://www.ncbi.nlm.nih.gov/pmc/articles/.

Go JS (n.d.): Reperfusion therapy for acute myocardial infarction. Retrieved from https://www.heart.org/idc/groups/heart-public/ @wcm/@mwa/documents/downloadable/ucm_465029.pdf.

Goldenberg I, Moss AJ, Zareba W: QT interval: how to measure it and what is "normal.", *Journal of Cardiovascular Electrophysiology*, 333–336, 2006. Retrieved from http://www.medscape. com/viewarticle/525633.

Jneid H, Anderson JL, Wright RS, Adams CD, Bridges CR, Casey DE: 2012 ACCF/AHA focused update of the guideline for the management of patients with unstable angina/non–ST-elevation myocardial infarction. *Circulation*, 875–910, 2012, August 14. Retrieved from http://circ.ahajournals.org/content/126/7/875.full.pdf.

Kahn SR, Comerota AJ, Cushman M, Evans NS, Ginsberg JS, Goldenberg NA, Weitz J et al.: The post-thrombotic syndrome: evidence-based prevention, diagnosis, and treatment strategies. *Circulation*, 1636–1661, 2014, October 28. Retrieved from http:/ /circ.ahajournalorg/content/130/18/1636.full.pdf.

Nelson BP: Thoracic aneurysms. Retrieved from http://emedicine. medscape.com/article/761627-overview, 2015, October.

Overbaugh KJ: Acute coronary syndrome. *American Journal of Nursing*, 42–52, 2009, May. Retrieved from http://alliedhealth.ceconn ection.com/files/AcuteCoronarySyndrome-1404755986278.pdf.

Rab T, Kern KB, Tamis-Holland JE, Henry TD, McDaniel M, Dickert NW, Ramee S: Cardiac arrest a treatment algorithm for emergent invasive cardiac procedures in the resuscitated comatose patient. *Journal of the American College of Cardiology*, 66(1): 62–73, 2015, July.

Raghavan SS: Pediatric long QT syndrome. Retrieved from http://emedicine.medscape.com/article/891571-overview, 2014, June 26.

Rivera-Bou WL: Thrombolytic therapy. Retrieved from http://emed icine.medscape.com/article/811234-overview#a1, 2014, March.

Rosendorff C, Lackland DT, Allison M, Aronow WS, Black HR, Blumenthal RS, Long J: Treatment of hypertension in patients with coronary artery disease: a scientific statement from the American Heart Association, American College of Cardiology, and American Society of Hypertension, *Circulation*, e435–e470, 2015. Retrieved from http://circ.ahajournals.org/conten t/131/19/e435.full.pdf.

Saliba E, Sia Y, Dore A, Hamamsy IE: The ascending aortic aneurysm: When to intervene? *IJC Heart & Vasculature*, 6: 91–100, 2015, January. Retrieved from http://www.ijcha-journal.com/article/ S2352-9067(15)00010-X/pdf.

Schulman S, Kakkar AK, Goldhaber SZ, Schellong S, Eriksson H, Mismetti P, Kearon CC: Treatment of acute venous thromboembolism with dabigatran or warfarin and pooled analysis. *Circulation*, 2013, December 16. Retrieved from http://circ.a hajournals.org/content/early/2013/12/10/CIRCULATIONAH A.113.004450.full.pdf.

Society of Vascular Surgery: Thoracic aortic aneurysm. Retrieved from https://www.vascularweb.org/vascularhealth/Pages/thor acic-aortic-aneurysm.aspx, 2010.

University of Pennsylvania Hospital System: Clinical guideline: post cardiac arrest targeted temperature management. Retrieved from https://www.med.upenn.edu/resuscitation/hy pothermia/documents/PennsylvaniaHospitalTTMPolicyforC CandED41614FinalRevision.pdf, 2014, February.

Vincent GM (n.d.): Sudden loss of consciousness (syncope) and sudden death in children. Sudden Arrhythmia Death Syndromes Foundation (SADS). Retrieved from https://www.goo gle.com/search?q=abrupt+brief+loss+of+consciousness#.

Yarlagadda C: Pacemaker malfunction treatment & management. Retrieved from http://emedicine.medscape.com/artic le/156583-treatment, 2014, December.

Yates MC, Syamasundar RP: Pediatric cardiac emergencies. *Emergency Medicine*, 3(6), 2013, November. Retrieved from http://www.omicsgroup.org/journals/pediatric-cardiac-emergencies-2165-7548.1000164.pdf.

Zierler BK: Ultrasonography and diagnosis of venous thromboembolism, *Circulation*, 2004. Retrieved from http://circ.ahajo urnals.org/content/109/12_suppl_1/I-9.full.pdf.

CHAPTER 13

Dental, Ear, Nose, and Throat Emergencies

Jeff Solheim, MSN, RN, CEN, CFRN, FAEN

MAJOR TOPICS

General Strategy
Assessment
Analysis: Differential Nursing Diagnoses/Collaborative Problems
Planning and Implementation/Interventions
Evaluation and Ongoing Monitoring
Documentation of Interventions and Patient Response
Age-Related Considerations

Specific Dental Emergencies
Acute Necrotizing Ulcerative Gingivitis (Trench Mouth)
Dental Abscess
Ludwig Angina
Odontalgia
Pericoronitis
Postextraction Pain and Bleeding
Tooth Eruption

Specific Ear Emergencies
Acute Otitis Externa

Acute Otitis Media
Labyrinthitis
Meniere Disease
Otic Foreign Body
Ruptured Tympanic Membrane

Specific Nose Emergencies
Epistaxis
Nasal Foreign Body
Rhinitis

Specific Throat Emergencies
Epiglottitis
Exudative Pharyngitis
Laryngeal Foreign Body
Laryngitis
Peritonsillar Abscess
Pharyngitis
Retropharyngeal Abscess

I. General Strategy

A. ASSESSMENT

1. Primary and secondary assessment/resuscitation (see Chapter 1)
2. Focused assessment
   a. Subjective data collection
      1) Chief complaint
         a) In quotes
         b) Use patient's own words
      2) History of present illness
         a) Pain: PQRST (see Chapter 8)
         b) Bleeding or hemorrhage: estimated blood loss, syncope, or dizziness
         c) Shortness of breath or obstructed airway
         d) Swelling or edema: goiter, glands, lymphadenopathy
         e) Hoarseness
         f) Foreign body aspiration or insertion
         g) Facial asymmetry or bony dislocation

      h) Fever, chills
      i) Nausea, vomiting
      j) Paresthesia, facial numbness
      k) Dysphasia, dysphagia, muffled voice
      l) Foul odor or bad taste in mouth
      m) Loss of hearing
      n) Tinnitus or vertigo
      o) Trismus: spasm of masticatory muscles resulting in difficulty in opening mouth
      p) Injury: mechanism and time (see Chapter 31)
      q) Discharge or drainage: ears, nose, or mouth
      r) Pruritus
      s) Neck pain
      t) Drooling
      u) Bleeding gums
      v) Excessive or decreased salivation
      w) Headache
      x) Dyspnea
      y) Difficulty with sleeping in supine position

z) Efforts to relieve symptoms
   (1) Home remedies
   (2) Alternative therapies
   (3) Medications
     (a) Prescription
     (b) OTC/herbal/vitamins

3) Past medical history
  a) Current or preexisting diseases/illness
   (1) Hypertension
   (2) Cardiopulmonary disease
   (3) Atherosclerosis
   (4) Neurologic disease
   (5) Cancer of head and neck
   (6) Hematologic disease
   (7) Diabetes
   (8) Immunosuppressive conditions with or without chemotherapy or radiation
  b) Surgical history including dental, brain, or ear, nose, and throat (ENT)
  c) Previous injury or fractures
  d) Previous dental or ENT infections
  e) Exposure to noxious agents
  f) Denture use
  g) Substance and/or alcohol use/abuse
  h) Last normal menstrual period: female patients of childbearing age
  i) Current medications
   (1) Prescription
   (2) OTC/herbal/vitamins
  j) Allergies
   (1) Medication
   (2) Food
   (3) Environmental factors (e.g., cats, pollen)
  k) Immunization status

4) Psychological, social, and environmental factors
  a) Infrequent dental care or lack of maintenance (e.g., flossing and brushing)
  b) Poor nutrition
  c) Contact sports without correct mouth protectors
  d) Swimming in contaminated water
  e) Trauma resulting from attempts to clean or scratch an itching ear
  f) Blast injuries
  g) Air travel with upper respiratory tract infection without premedication
  h) Possible/actual abuse, assault, or intimate partner violence situations (see Chapters 3 and 40)
  i) Unsanitary living conditions
  j) Contact with sick individuals
  k) Tobacco use including smoking and chewing
  l) Occupational exposures (e.g., gases, fumes)

b. Objective data collection
1) General appearance
  a) Level of consciousness, behavior, affect
  b) Vital signs
  c) Odors, smells
  d) Gait
  e) Hygiene
  f) Level of distress/discomfort

2) Inspection
  a) External ear
   (1) Position, size, symmetry
   (2) Skin color
   (3) Lumps, deformities, skin lesions
   (4) Edema, erythema, drainage
  b) Ear canal and drum
   (1) Discharge, foreign bodies, redness of the skin, or swelling
   (2) Presence of cerumen
  c) Tympanic membrane (TM): necessitates use of otoscope
   (1) Pull the auricle upward and backward (adult) or downward and backward (children)
   (2) Color: pearly gray (normal), red, white, or yellow
   (3) Translucency: transparent (normal), opaque
   (4) Position: neutral (normal), retracted, bulging
   (5) Landmark identification: cone of light at 5 o'clock position
   (6) Mobility: use pneumatic otoscope and insufflator
  d) External nose
   (1) Position, shape, symmetry
   (2) Drainage/odor(s)
   (3) Ecchymosis
  e) Internal nose (use otoscope with large ear speculum)
   (1) Nasal septum: deviation, inflammation, or perforation
   (2) Inferior and middle turbinates and middle meatus: color and any swelling, bleeding, or exudate
  f) Mouth and pharynx
   (1) Teeth: number, color, form, and occlusion
   (2) Lips: color, symmetry, moisture, and surface characteristics
   (3) Oral buccal mucosa/oropharynx: color, landmarks, surface characteristics, and structures
   (4) Gingiva: color and surface characteristics
   (5) Tongue: symmetry, movement, color, surface characteristics, and ventral surface
   (6) Hard and soft palates: color, surface characteristics, and landmarks

g) Paranasal sinuses: soft tissue over sinus area for erythema or swelling
h) Neck: symmetry of structures and abnormalities
3) Palpation
   a) Skin temperature, moisture, and turgor
   b) Sinus tenderness
   c) Temporomandibular joint (TMJ): mobility and crepitus
   d) Lymph nodes: size, shape, mobility, consistency, tenderness
   e) Thyroid gland: size, shape, consistency, tenderness
3. Diagnostic procedures
   a. Laboratory studies
      1) Complete blood count (CBC) with differential
      2) Erythrocyte sedimentation rate (ESR)
      3) Coagulation profile
      4) Aerobic and anaerobic cultures if suspected infection
      5) *Streptococcus* screen/culture
      6) Arterial blood gases (ABGs)
   b. Imaging studies
      1) Dental
         a) Mandibular panoramic radiograph (Panorex)
         b) Chest radiograph: rule out aspiration of foreign body in lungs if teeth are missing
         c) Facial series radiograph: to detect fractures
      2) ENT
         a) Nasal bones radiograph: usually not indicated, diagnosis usually based on clinical presentation
         b) Facial bones radiograph with Waters, view
         c) Cervical spine (C-spine) radiograph and odontoid view with neck trauma
         d) Chest radiograph
         e) Computed tomography (CT) scan
         f) Magnetic resonance imaging (MRI)

B. ANALYSIS: DIFFERENTIAL NURSING DIAGNOSES/COLLABORATIVE PROBLEMS

1. Acute/chronic pain
2. Anxiety/fear
3. Risk for infection
4. Risk for deficient fluid volume
5. Ineffective tissue perfusion
6. Deficient knowledge
7. Risk for ineffective airway clearance
8. Risk for ineffective breathing pattern

C. PLANNING AND IMPLEMENTATION/INTERVENTIONS

1. Determine priorities of care
   a. Maintain airway, breathing, circulation (see Chapters 1 and 32)

   b. Provide supplemental oxygen as indicated
   c. Establish intravenous (IV) access for administration of crystalloid/blood products/medications as needed
   d. Obtain and set up equipment and supplies
   e. Prepare for/assist with medical interventions
   f. Administer pharmacologic therapy as ordered
2. Relieve anxiety/apprehension
3. Allow significant others to remain with patient if supportive
4. Educate patient and significant others

D. EVALUATION AND ONGOING MONITORING

1. Continuously monitor and treat as indicated
2. Monitor patient response/outcomes, and modify nursing care plan as appropriate
3. If positive outcomes are not demonstrated, reevaluate assessment and/or plan of care

E. DOCUMENTATION OF INTERVENTIONS AND PATIENT RESPONSE

F. AGE-RELATED CONSIDERATIONS

1. Pediatric
   a. Growth or development related
      1) The most common diagnoses for pediatric patients include acute upper airway respiratory infections, otitis media, and Eustachian tube disorders.[1] Pediatric patients have larger tongues than adults do, when compared to the size of the oral cavity, and the internal diameter of the airway is smaller, thus making them more vulnerable to airway obstructions. Infants are obligate nose breathers, making nasal congestion a potential source of respiratory distress. Children are also curious and tend to put things in their mouth, increasing the risk of airway obstruction. One study showed that 18% of all health care visits in children 14 years and younger involved foreign body ingestion.[2] Children between the ages of 6 months and 4 years constitute the highest age group for foreign body ingestion. It also remains the third most common cause of unintentional injury in children less than 1 year of age.[3,4]
      2) Irritability and lack of feeding in infants should not be overlooked as potential signs of dental and ENT emergencies
   b. "Pearls"
      1) Persistent cough or chronic wheezing may be indicative of an aspirated foreign body
      2) Difficulty with feeding may be indicative of a significant ENT emergency

3) Abrupt onset of upper respiratory and pulmonary symptoms suggests foreign body ingestion
4) Listen to the child's caregiver; he/she can provide valuable insight

2. Geriatric
   a. Aging related
      1) Difficulty in mastication, loss of sensation in mouth, and dry mouth may contribute to obstructions and infections
      2) Acuity of hearing diminishes with age and may be difficult to assess in the emergency department
   b. "Pearls"
      1) Malignant external otitis media and cholesteatoma should be considered in elderly patients and in diabetic patients with earache or recurrent ear infections
      2) Most dental and ENT trauma in the elderly is related to falls, visual changes occurring with age, motor vehicle crashes, and assaults

II. Specific Dental Emergencies

A. ACUTE NECROTIZING ULCERATIVE GINGIVITIS (TRENCH MOUTH)

Acute necrotizing ulcerative gingivitis (ANUG) is a noncontagious infection commonly referred to as trench mouth or Vincent angina. ANUG is associated with poor oral care, immunosuppression, existing gingivitis, emotional stressors, malnutrition, and smoking. It is commonly seen in adolescents and young adults but can occur in all age groups. ANUG is characterized by the acute onset of fetid breath, pain, and an ulcerative necrotic slough of the gingiva. The patient may be febrile with lymphadenopathy. Ulcerations may develop within the gingival tissue and may form a gray membrane that bleeds with pressure or when removed. Treatment measures include local debridement, good oral hygiene with half-strength hydrogen peroxide (H_2O_2) or oral chlorhexidine (e.g., Peridex) rinses, antibiotics, and adequate nutrition. Efforts to avoid irritation should be encouraged, and analgesics should be provided after initial debridement to minimize pain. Recovery usually occurs within 24 hours. Patients may require gingival curettage.

1. Assessment
   a. Subjective data collection
      1) Chief complaint
      2) History of present illness
         a) Pain (see Chapter 8)
         b) Fever, chills, malaise
         c) Bleeding gums
         d) Halitosis, foul metallic taste
         e) Referred earache

3) Past medical history
   a) Current or preexisting diseases/illness
      (1) Immunosuppression
      (2) Gum disease or pharyngeal infection
   b) Previous dental injury
   c) Poor nutrition
   d) Dental habits
   e) Medications
   f) Allergies
4) Past surgical history

b. Objective data collection
   1) Physical examination
      a) General appearance
         (1) Odors: fetid breath
         (2) Elevated temperature: >100.4°F (38°C)
         (3) Mild distress/discomfort
      b) Inspection
         (1) Spontaneous gingival bleeding
         (2) Dental papillae ulceration
         (3) Edematous gums
         (4) Poor oral hygiene
         (5) Gray pseudomembranous ulcers on pharyngeal structures
      c) Palpation
         (1) Cervical lymphadenopathy

2. Analysis: differential nursing diagnoses/collaborative problems
   a. Acute/chronic pain
   b. Infection
3. Planning and implementation/interventions
   a. Administer pharmacologic therapy as ordered
      1) Topical or local anesthetics
      2) Antibiotics
      3) Nonnarcotic analgesics
      4) Antipyretics
   b. Educate patient and significant others
      1) Refer to dentist for definitive management of illness
      2) Instruct the patient about how to care for gums and teeth
4. Evaluation and ongoing monitoring
   a. Pain relief

B. DENTAL ABSCESS

A dental abscess occurs from the localized accumulation of pus in a cavity of a tooth. Gingival swelling results as plaque and debris collect in the space between the tooth and gingiva. Periodontal disease results when infections extend into the surrounding tissues, gingival epithelium, periodontal ligament, or alveolar bone. Periapical (alveolar) abscess (infection spread beyond the bone) and periodontal abscess (bony destruction at the periodontal membrane) result when bacterial, viral, or mycotic pathogens are able to colonize. Treatment measures are aimed at managing infection with antibiotics. In some cases, incision and drainage of the soft tissue are necessary to prevent involvement to the extending fascial areas of the head and neck.

1. Assessment
   a. Subjective data collection
      1) Chief complaint
      2) History of present illness
         a) Pain (see Chapter 8)
            (1) Affected tooth and surrounding tissue radiating to jaw, ear, neck
            (2) Mild to severe depending on extent of abscess
            (3) May not be relieved by analgesics
         b) Swelling of face or neck on affected side
         c) Fever or chills
         d) Malaise
         e) Foul breath
         f) Unpleasant taste in mouth
         g) Sore gums
      3) Past medical history
         a) Current or preexisting diseases/illness
         b) Previous dental abscess, dental caries, or gum disease
         c) Infrequent dental care or lack of maintenance
         d) Medications
         e) Allergies
      4) Past surgical history
   b. Objective data collection
      1) Physical examination
         a) General appearance
            (1) Level of consciousness, behavior, affect: agitation or restlessness
            (2) Elevated temperature: >100.4°F (38°C)
            (3) Moderate to severe distress/discomfort
         b) Inspection
            (1) Edematous face (if minor and localized abscess)
            (2) Edematous face and neck (if major and extending abscess)
            (3) Possible edema of pharynx and surrounding structure on affected side
            (4) Purulent drainage
         c) Palpation/percussion
            (1) Tenderness of affected tooth
            (2) Tenderness of gum line
      2) Diagnostic procedures
         a) CBC with differential: elevated white blood cell (WBC) count
         b) Mandibular panoramic radiograph (Panorex)
         c) Culture and sensitivity testing of any drainage: aerobic and anaerobic
         d) Soft tissue neck CT, if symptoms suggest more systemic than localized
2. Analysis: differential nursing diagnoses/collaborative problems
   a. Acute pain
   b. Infection
   c. Anxiety/fear
3. Planning and implementation/interventions
   a. Prepare for/assist with medical interventions
      1) Incision and drainage of abscess if fluctuant area is present, leaving drain in place
      2) Obtain culture and sensitivity testing of exudate
   b. Administer pharmacologic therapy as ordered
      1) Nonnarcotic analgesics
      2) Narcotics
      3) Antibiotics
      4) Antipyretics
   c. Educate patient and significant others
      1) Use warm normal saline mouth rinses every 1–2 hours while patient is awake
      2) Antibiotics are only a temporary treatment
      3) Emphasize the need for definitive care as soon as possible from dentist or endodontist
      4) Brushing and flossing daily
      5) Regular dental checkups twice a year
4. Evaluation and ongoing monitoring
   a. Pain relief

C. LUDWIG ANGINA

Ludwig angina is characterized as a rapidly progressive gangrenous cellulitis of the soft tissues of the neck and floor of the mouth, which is usually the result of a secondary dental infection involving the lower second and third molars. The primary site for infection is the submandibular space; however, its fast progression to other spaces in the neck such as submaxillary and sublingual areas can lead to airway management problems. Most patients have bilateral submandibular swelling and protrusion or elevation of the tongue, which can cause difficulty in talking and swallowing. The most common organisms include *Staphylococcus*, *Streptococcus*, and *Bacteroides* species. Treatment of the infection should be initiated as soon as possible, which often includes a combination of penicillin, clindamycin (Cleocin), and metronidazole. Incision and drainage is required in about 65% of patients to provide relief from swelling and infection and to further protect the airway.

1. Assessment
   a. Subjective data collection
      1) Chief complaint
      2) History of present illness
         a) Severe pain (see Chapter 8)
         b) Swelling of jaw and neck
         c) Fever or chills
         d) Malaise
         e) Difficulty in swallowing (dysphagia)
         f) Difficulty in talking (dysphasia)
      3) Past medical history
         a) Current or preexisting diseases/illness
         b) Dental infection and treatment
         c) Medications
         d) Allergies
      4) Past surgical history
   b. Objective data collection
      1) Physical examination

a) General appearance
  (1) Level of consciousness, behavior, affect: agitation
  (2) Tachypnea
  (3) Elevated temperature: >100.4°F (38°C)
  (4) Possible stridor
  (5) Severe distress/discomfort, critically ill
b) Inspection
  (1) Marked bilateral swelling of jaw and neck
  (2) Marked elevation of tongue and floor of mouth toward palate
  (3) Pallor or cyanosis
  (4) Trismus
  (5) Possible poor dental hygiene/multiple caries
c) Palpation
  (1) Firm induration of swollen soft tissue of the anterior neck
  (2) Diaphoresis
2) Diagnostic procedures
  a) CBC with differential: elevated WBC count
  b) ESR
  c) ABGs if cyanosis or respiratory distress is present
  d) Culture and sensitivity testing of exudate
  e) Soft tissue neck CT scan
2. Analysis: differential nursing diagnoses/collaborative problems
  a. Impaired gas exchange
  b. Acute pain
  c. Infection
  d. Anxiety/fear
  e. Risk for ineffective airway clearance
  f. Risk for deficient fluid volume
3. Planning and implementation/interventions
  a. Maintain airway, breathing, circulation (see Chapters 1 and 32)
  b. Provide supplemental oxygen as indicated
    1) Rapid-sequence intubation (RSI) and ventilatory support if airway compromise is present
    2) High-flow oxygen
  c. Establish IV access for administration of crystalloid fluids/medications as needed
  d. Prepare for/assist with medical interventions
    1) Advanced airway management
      a) Nasal or oral intubation
      b) Supraglottic airway (e.g., King, Combitube, laryngeal mask airway)
      c) Surgical airway (e.g., cricothyrotomy)
    2) Assist patient to Fowler position
    3) Institute cardiac and pulse oximetry monitoring
    4) Assist with intraoral incision and drainage of infected area: procedural sedation may be required
    5) Assist with hospital admission

e. Administer pharmacologic therapy as ordered
  1) RSI premedications: sedatives, analgesics, neuromuscular blocking agents
  2) Nonnarcotic analgesics
  3) Narcotics
  4) Antipyretics
  5) Antibiotic: pharyngeal culture obtained prior to antibiotic administration
  6) Procedural sedation medications
4. Evaluation and ongoing monitoring
  a. Airway patency
  b. Level of consciousness
  c. Hemodynamic status
  d. Breath sounds and pulse oximetry
  e. Cardiac rate and rhythm
  f. Pain relief

D. ODONTALGIA

Odontalgia, or toothache, is frequently the result of a cavity involving a portion of pulp tissue within the tooth. Pulpal inflammation (pulpitis) invades the soft tissue and produces pain that is provoked by eating sweets or changes in temperature, especially cold. Pain may begin suddenly or gradually, creating sharp to throbbing sensations. Pain may be localized or radiate to the ear, jaw, temple, or neck. If left untreated, the pulpal inflammation extends into the dentin and root apex, producing necrosis. This necrosis increases the risk for periapical and alveolar abscess, facial cellulitis, and tooth extraction. Treatment measures are aimed at relieving pain and ultimately preventing tooth decay from dental caries. Good oral hygiene is essential to prevent oral microbes, generated by diet, from invading tooth enamel and causing decay. When disease is present, it is important to rule out secondary complications that may be associated with abscessed teeth; if required, tooth extraction, root canal treatment, or incision and drainage may be performed. Antibiotics and analgesics can be administered until definitive treatment by a dentist is provided.

1. Assessment
  a. Subjective data collection
    1) Chief complaint
    2) History of present illness
      a) Pain (see Chapter 8)
        (1) In diseased tooth: dental caries
        (2) Referred to gum line, jaw, temple, ear, and neck
        (3) Sharp, shooting pain in early phase progressing to intense, persistent, throbbing pain with tooth exquisitely sensitive to touch during later phase (pulp damage)
        (4) More intense nocturnal pain from affected tooth
        (5) Begins with heat or cold stimulus and occurs spontaneously with continued worsening

(6) No relief with analgesics; irreversible pain indicates necessity for root canal treatment or extraction
  3) Past medical history
    a) Current or preexisting diseases/illness
    b) Previous dental caries, injuries, or gum disease
    c) Poor oral hygiene
    d) Substance abuse including but not limited to methamphetamines
    e) Medications
    f) Allergies
  4) Past surgical history including dental procedures
b. Objective data collection
  1) Physical examination
    a) General appearance
      (1) Fetid breath
      (2) Moderate distress/discomfort
    b) Inspection
      (1) Presence of tooth discoloration or obvious decay
      (2) Facial swelling/redness
    c) Palpation/percussion
      (1) Tenderness of tooth/gums
  2) Diagnostic procedures: frequently none
2. Analysis: differential nursing diagnoses/collaborative problems
  a. Acute pain
  b. Anxiety/fear
  c. Risk for infection
3. Planning and implementation/interventions
  a. Establish IV access for administration of crystalloid fluid/medications as needed
  b. Prepare for/assist with medical interventions
    1) Dental nerve block
  c. Administer pharmacologic therapy as ordered
    1) Antibiotics
    2) Nonnarcotic analgesics
    3) Narcotics
  d. Educate patient/significant others
    1) Explain disease process
    2) Stress importance of follow-up dental care, brushing and flossing daily
4. Evaluation and ongoing monitoring
  a. Pain relief

E. PERICORONITIS

Pericoronitis is inflammation of the gingival tissue surrounding the crown of a tooth. It is usually associated with erupting or impacted wisdom teeth or third molar. The space between the crown, overlying tooth, and gingival flap has a tendency to accumulate food and bacteria and thus cause increased inflammation. This is commonly seen in adults entering their third decade of life but can be found in teenagers as well. Pain is the primary symptom and may radiate to the ears, throat, and floor of the mouth.

General treatment measures consist of saline irrigations, warm mouth rinses, and pain control with analgesic medications. Occasionally, systemic symptoms occur and may include lymphadenopathy, fever, and fatigue. Antibiotics, debridement, excision of the gingival flap, or extraction of the molar may be necessary. Cellulitis, peritonsillar abscess, and Ludwig angina are rare complications that should be considered when systemic symptoms are present.

1. Assessment
  a. Subjective data collection
    1) Chief complaint
    2) History of present illness
      a) Pain (see Chapter 8)
        (1) Nonspecific, diffuse, extraoral pain or pain on biting down
        (2) Earache on affected side
      b) Discharge of pus from the gum near the tooth
      c) Bad smell or taste in the mouth
    3) Past medical history
      a) Current or preexisting diseases/illness
      b) Unerupted third molar tooth in area of discomfort or pain
      c) Medications
      d) Allergies
    4) Past surgical history
  b. Objective data collection
    1) Physical examination
      a) General appearance
        (1) Elevated temperature: >100.4°F (38°C)
        (2) Mild to moderate distress/discomfort
      b) Inspection
        (1) Submandibular lymphadenopathy
        (2) Red, inflamed gums or draining fluid or pus around crown of partially erupted tooth
    2) Diagnostic procedures
      a) Mandibular panoramic radiograph (Panorex)
      b) CT scan, if more systemic symptoms are present
2. Analysis: differential nursing diagnoses/collaborative problems
  a. Acute pain
  b. Risk for infection
3. Planning and implementation/interventions
  a. Prepare for/assist with medical interventions
    1) Apply gentle massage to overlying gingival tissue with finger
    2) Irrigate under pericoronal flap with warm normal saline to remove debris
    3) Assist with draining of abscess, if present
  b. Administer pharmacologic therapy as ordered
    1) Antibiotic therapy if infection present
    2) Antipyretics
    3) Nonnarcotic analgesics
    4) Narcotics

c. Educate patient and significant others
   1) Dental referral for debridement of pericoronal flap or tooth extraction and follow-up therapy
   2) Brushing and flossing daily
   3) Regular dental checkups twice a year
4. Evaluation and ongoing monitoring
   a. Pain relief

F. POSTEXTRACTION PAIN AND BLEEDING

Pain and swelling are generally present up to 24 hours after a tooth extraction. This condition is known as periostitis and usually responds well to analgesics, particularly NSAIDs. However, pain lasting more than 2–3 days may be caused by alveolitis, commonly referred to as "dry socket" syndrome. Pain may radiate to the ear on the affected side and may last from days to weeks. It is most commonly found in patients who have had the mandibular posterior teeth removed and results from loss of the healing blood clot and localized infection. Alveolitis is best treated with irrigation of the socket and topical analgesic medication or gauze moistened with eugenol (oil of cloves) that is changed daily. Fever or swelling should be reported. Antibiotic therapy should be initiated, and the patient should be referred to a dentist within 24 hours for definitive management and monitored for complications such as osteomyelitis of the jaw.

Postextraction bleeding may occur from small vessels that continue to bleed after a tooth extraction. After the clot is removed, a pressure dressing using cotton wrapped in gauze may be applied directly to the extraction site for approximately 60 minutes.[5] This may be repeated until the bleeding resolves. If bleeding continues, the site may be anesthetized using lidocaine with epinephrine and sutured. In addition, oxidized cellulose, topical thrombin in a gelatin sponge, or microfibrillar collagen can be placed in the socket to act as a hemostatic agent and to tamponade bleeding. A patient with prolonged bleeding should be referred to the oral surgeon for definitive treatment.

1. Assessment
   a. Subjective data collection
      1) Chief complaint
      2) History of present illness
         a) Tooth extraction usually within previous 24 hours if bleeding present
         b) Severe pain several days after tooth extraction (dry socket)
      3) Past medical history
         a) Current or preexisting diseases/illness
         b) Previous difficult extractions
         c) Smoking history
         d) Medications
            (1) Drugs with antiplatelet activity (e.g., aspirin, clopidogrel, rivaroxaban)
         e) Allergies

   f) Drinking from a straw after extraction (creates negative pressure in the oral cavity)
   g) Excessive spitting after extraction
      4) Past surgical history
   b. Objective data collection
      1) Physical examination
         a) General appearance
            (1) Mild to moderate distress/discomfort
         b) Inspection
            (1) Bleeding from socket
            (2) Socket healing: may be delayed in dry socket syndrome
      2) Diagnostic procedures
         a) Clot removal from socket
2. Analysis: differential nursing diagnoses/collaborative problems
   a. Risk for deficient fluid volume
   b. Acute pain
   c. Anxiety/fear
   d. Risk for infection
3. Planning and implementation/interventions
   a. Prepare for/assist with medical procedures
      1) Control bleeding
         a) Have patient bite on gauze over extraction site for 60 minutes
   b. Administer pharmacologic therapy as ordered
      1) Nonnarcotic analgesics
      2) Narcotics
      3) Pack socket with local anesthetic
      4) Site may be infiltrated with 2% lidocaine with 1:100,000 epinephrine
   c. Educate patient and significant others
      1) Bite on gauze over extraction site if bleeding reoccurs
      2) Refer to dentist or oral surgeon for follow-up
      3) Avoid eating hard or hot foods
4. Evaluation and ongoing monitoring
   a. Bleeding control
   b. Pain relief

G. TOOTH ERUPTION

Tooth pain is commonly experienced when the primary teeth in infants and children are erupting from the gums. Tooth eruption generally begins at 6 months of age.[6] Eruption of the primary teeth during infancy tends to be more painful than eruption of secondary teeth later in childhood, although eruption of the large molars in adolescence and the second decade of life can be painful. Management is supportive and directed toward pain control and adequate hydration. Analgesia (both oral and topical) and NSAIDs are used to alleviate discomfort.

1. Assessment
   a. Subjective data collection
      1) Chief complaint
      2) History of present illness
         a) Pressure or tenderness of erupting tooth

b) Irritability, agitation, crying

c) Disrupted sleep

d) Decreased fluid intake

3) Past medical history

a) Current or preexisting diseases/illness

b) Similar occurrences

c) Medications

d) Allergies

4) Past surgical history

b. Objective data collection

1) Physical examination

a) General appearance

(1) Level of consciousness, behavior, affect: fussy/crying

(2) Mild to moderate distress/discomfort

b) Inspection

(1) Drooling

(2) Circumoral rash around mouth

(3) Reddened, edematous tissues over erupting tooth

c) Palpation

(1) Tenderness on palpation of affected gum area

2. Analysis: differential nursing diagnoses/collaborative problems

a. Acute pain

b. Anxiety/fear

3. Planning and implementation/interventions

a. Prepare for/assist with medical interventions

1) Apply gentle massage to overlying gingival tissue with finger or teething ring

2) Place ice chips wrapped in a cloth over gingival tissue

b. Administer pharmacologic therapy as ordered

1) Topical anesthetic: benzocaine (e.g., Orajel or Numzit)

2) Nonnarcotic analgesics

c. Educate patient and significant others/parents

1) Use warm saline mouth rinses

2) Soft diet

3) Dental referral if eruption site remains soft or swollen: probable eruption cyst, which may rupture and bleed

4) Brushing and flossing daily

5) Regular dental checkups twice a year

4. Evaluation and ongoing monitoring

a. Pain relief

III. Specific Ear Emergencies

A. ACUTE OTITIS EXTERNA

Acute otitis externa (AOE), commonly referred to as "swimmer's ear," is an inflammatory condition of the external auditory canal and auricle of the ear. This inflammatory reaction promotes swelling and maceration of the stratum corneum of the skin, causing pruritus, swollen lymph nodes, and pain in the involved area. Exudate may or may not be present initially. Movement of the external ear and auricle and pressure on the tragus, mastoid, parotid area, and upper neck further aggravate the pain response. The etiologic agents include infection (viral, fungal, or bacterial), perforation, foreign body, and dermatosis. Gram-negative bacteria (e.g., *Pseudomonas*) that produce a green exudate visualized in the external canal may cause infections. Yellow exudate or crusting may represent *Staphylococcus aureus*. Other infections associated with fungal pathogens, including *Aspergillus* or *Candida*, produce a fluffy white to black material similar to that of bread mold. Chronic dermatologic disorders, such as eczema, can lead to cellulitis in the affected ear canal. Malignant otitis should be considered in any diabetic patient. General principles for treatment of AOE consist of cleaning debris of the external auditory canal with a cotton-tipped applicator, suctioning, and applying or instilling an antibiotic-steroid solution or powder for bacterial and fungal infections for approximately 1 week. An ear wick (otowick) saturated with antibiotic solution may be placed in the external canal of some patients in which the swelling is too significant to allow for adequate instillation of the topical antibiotic. The ear wick generally falls out in 2–3 days as the swelling of the canal resolves. Most episodes of AOE resolve within 7 days after treatment is started. When persistent infections occur, cultures of the ear should be taken to identify the underlying pathogens. Additional treatment includes protecting the external ear canal from excessive moisture when bathing. Swimming and frequent cleansing of the ear canal using cotton-tipped applicators should be avoided until the infection has resolved. Patients with persistent infections should be referred to an otolaryngologist.

1. Assessment

a. Subjective data collection

1) Chief complaint

2) History of present illness

a) Pain (see Chapter 8)

(1) Localized to the outer ear and external canal

(2) Radiation to affected side of head, jaw, and neck

(3) Moderate to severe pain with movement of external ear (pinna and tragus)

(4) Poor response to OTC analgesics and NSAIDs

b) Impaired or diminished hearing: conductive hearing loss

c) Swelling, redness, discharge, or debris in external and outer ear

d) Tender, enlarged lymph nodes over cervical preauricular and postauricular areas

e) Pruritus: 1–3 days of progressive ear itching

f) Low-grade fever

g) Malaise
h) Pressure or sensation of fullness in ear
3) Past medical history
 a) Current or preexisting diseases/illness
  (1) Prior ear infection
  (2) Recent upper respiratory tract infection
 b) Recent swimming or water submersion
 c) Recent use of objects to clean or irrigate ears
 d) Medications
 e) Allergies
4) Past surgical history
b. Objective data collection
 1) Physical examination
  a) General appearance
   (1) Elevated temperature: ≥100.4°F (38°C)
   (2) Decreased hearing: distinguish between sensorineural and conductive loss
   (3) Moderate distress/discomfort
  b) Inspection
   (1) Purulent drainage from external ear canal
   (2) Edema, tenderness, and erythema of ear canal
   (3) Cellulitis
   (4) TM usually normal appearing
  c) Palpation
   (1) Pain with movement of auricle, tragus, and pinna
   (2) Periauricular, cervical lymphadenopathy
 2) Diagnostic procedures
  a) Whisper voice test to determine hearing loss
  b) Tuning fork tests (Rinne or Weber test): differentiates conductive from sensorineural hearing loss
  c) Gram stain and culture of any discharge from ear canal
2. Analysis: differential nursing diagnoses/collaborative problems
 a. Acute pain
 b. Infection
3. Planning and implementation/interventions
 a. Speak slowly and clearly toward healthy ear while directly facing patient
 b. Administer pharmacologic therapy as ordered: insert ear wick when ear canal is too acutely swollen to distribute medication evenly in canal
  1) Nonnarcotic analgesics
  2) Narcotics
  3) Topical antibiotics
  4) Topical steroid solution (suspension)
  5) Antipyretics
 c. Educate patient and significant others
  1) Apply warm, moist compress to affected ear
  2) Keep ear canal dry with use of ear plugs and avoid over cleaning

  3) Use topical acidifying solutions such as VoSol or vinegar drops
4. Evaluation and ongoing monitoring
 a. Pain relief

B. ACUTE OTITIS MEDIA

Acute otitis media (AOM) is a disease of the middle ear that results from a bacterial infection. Common pathogens include *Streptococcus pneumoniae*, *Haemophilus influenzae*, *Streptococcus pyogenes*, and *Moraxella catarrhalis*. Barotrauma, eustachian tube dysfunction, and serous otitis media can precipitate AOM. Most cases of AOM involve a concurrent upper respiratory tract infection. As the eustachian tube swells, fluid accumulates, thus preventing effective drainage and allowing bacteria to proliferate. Although AOM is commonly seen in infants and children, all age groups may be affected. Patients with AOM complain of severe earache, ear pressure, and decreased hearing, and they may present with fever. Infants and children with AOM are observed tugging at their ears. Physical examination reveals an erythematous and dull TM with poorly visualized landmarks or dull light reflex. The TM has decreased mobility and may appear as a bulge caused by increased pressure as fluid accumulates within the middle ear. In these cases, rupture of the TM may occur; this results in a significant decrease in pain as pressure is reduced and drainage is released. Healing of the TM is usually spontaneous, and scar tissue may later be found on visual examination. Although rare, complications related to AOM include mastoiditis and meningitis. Treatment of AOM consists of observational treatment, pain control, adequate hydration, and antibiotic therapy in selected cases. Antipyretics and NSAIDs should be given for pain and fever control. In patients who are immunocompetent or who have chronic recurrent AOM, tympanocentesis may be performed to identify the source of infection and to obtain fluid for culture. Surgical drainage of the middle ear (myringotomy) with the insertion of ear ventilating tubes may be considered when complications such as meningitis, mastoiditis, osteomyelitis, facial paralysis, or intracranial abscess result from AOM or chronic recurrent episodes of AOM.

1. Assessment
 a. Subjective data collection
  1) Chief complaint
  2) History of present illness
   a) Pain (see Chapter 8): otalgia (earache) that increases with prone position
    (1) Pulling at ear: infant or toddler
    (2) Verbal complaints: older child
   b) Sensation of fullness in ear
   c) Decreased hearing
   d) Irritability or malaise
   e) Fever or chills
   f) Anorexia or vomiting
   g) Diarrhea

            h) Vertigo or dizziness
            i) Recent air travel
        3) Past medical history
            a) Current or preexisting diseases/illness
                (1) Previous ear infections
                (2) Upper respiratory tract infection
            b) Medications
            c) Allergies
            d) Immunization status
        4) Past surgical history
    b. Objective data collection
        1) Physical examination
            a) General appearance
                (1) Level of consciousness, behavior, affect: restlessness, agitation
                (2) Elevated temperature
                (3) Diminished hearing: conductive loss
                (4) Moderate distress/discomfort
            b) Inspection
                (1) Purulent nasal discharge
                (2) Erythema of pharynx
                (3) Erythema of TM
                (4) Retracted or bulging TM
                (5) Blebs on eardrum surface (bullous myringitis)
                (6) White or yellow discoloration of TM
                (7) Excessive purulent drainage from ear if TM has ruptured
        2) Diagnostic procedures
            a) Pneumatic otoscopy
            b) Hearing tests
            c) Blood cultures: if septic appearing
2. Analysis: differential nursing diagnoses/collaborative problems
    a. Acute pain
    b. Infection
    c. Anxiety/fear
3. Planning and implementation/interventions
    a. Speak slowly and clearly toward healthy ear while directly facing patient
    b. Administer pharmacologic therapy as ordered
        1) Nonnarcotic analgesics
        2) Narcotics
        3) Antibiotics
        4) Antipyretics
    c. Educate patient and significant others/parents
        1) Follow-up within 2 weeks if improving
        2) Follow-up within 3 days if no improvement
4. Evaluation and ongoing monitoring
    a. Pain relief

C. LABYRINTHITIS

Labyrinthitis is an inflammatory response of the inner ear that is more common in adults than children and may involve the nerves connecting the inner ear to the brain. Both bacterial and viral infections can cause this inflammation, producing disturbances within the cochlea that result in tinnitus and dizziness. When the vestibular system is affected, symptoms include disturbances in balance and vision that may vary from mild to severe, depending on the severity of infection. Bacterial labyrinthitis may damage the labyrinth by infecting the middle ear or surrounding bone of the inner ear. Bacteria may invade the cochlea or vestibular system, thus resulting in inflammation. More serious symptoms are usually from chronic or untreated middle ear infections and/or inner ear trauma. Treatment measures are aimed at eliminating the bacteria with appropriate antibiotics. Surgery may be indicated to prevent further disease and complications when the middle or inner ear membranes are involved or have ruptured. Viruses may also invade the inner ear and cause inflammation to the labyrinth. Symptoms are sudden in onset, including symptoms of severe spontaneous vertigo. These viruses invade the inner ear through the blood stream and cause both local and systemic responses. Influenza, measles, mumps, rubella, polio, herpes, and Epstein-Barr viral infections have been associated with this disorder. Symptoms of this condition include hearing abnormalities, balance and gait instability, nausea, vomiting, and dizziness. Dizziness and the sensation of spinning (vertigo) are the most common symptoms described. The initial symptoms persist for several days but may continue in varying severity for 6 weeks or longer. Diagnosis is contingent on ruling out neurologic and cardiovascular disease, trauma, illicit drug or alcohol use, anxiety, allergies, and use of pharmacologic agents. Treatment of symptoms is supportive, with the use of antihistamines and antiemetics to manage dizziness and nausea.

1. Assessment
    a. Subjective data collection
        1) Chief complaint
        2) History of present illness
            a) Vertigo, especially with movement of head or body
            b) Nausea and vomiting
            c) Hearing abnormalities: tinnitus, sensitivity to loud noises, hearing loss
            d) Ear pressure
            e) Headache
            f) Malaise
        3) Past medical history
            a) Current or preexisting diseases/illness
                (1) Ear infection
                (2) Meningitis
                (3) Recent upper respiratory tract infection
                (4) Viral illness: measles, mumps, rubella; Epstein-Barr virus; polio; herpes; or influenza
                (5) Hypertension or arteriosclerosis
                (6) Systemic lupus erythematosus or vasculitis
                (7) Neurologic disorders

(8) Migraine headaches
(9) Meniere syndrome
(10) Secondary or tertiary syphilis
b) Smoking and excessive caffeine use
c) Head or ear trauma
d) Alcohol or substance abuse
e) Medications
f) Allergies
4) Past surgical history
b. Objective data collection
1) Physical examination
a) General appearance
(1) Altered gait: disequilibrium
(2) Decreased hearing but usually no loss
(3) Possible orthostasis
(4) Moderate distress/discomfort
b) Inspection
(1) Spontaneous horizontal nystagmus with peripheral features, away from side of disease; suppression of nystagmus with fixation
(2) Normal neurologic and neurovascular examination and infectious disease workup
2) Diagnostic procedures
a) Caloric testing: indicated if symptoms persist; should show absent or decreased response on affected side
b) MRI
c) Electronystagmography
d) Formal audiogram
e) Forced hyperventilation: done for 1–3 minutes to see whether symptoms can be reproduced
f) Dix-Hallpike (Nylen-Barany) test: positional maneuvers that are designed to reproduce vertigo
2. Analysis: differential nursing diagnoses/collaborative problems
a. Risk for injury
b. Risk for deficient fluid volume
c. Anxiety/fear
3. Planning and implementation/interventions
a. Establish IV access for administration of crystalloid fluid/medications as needed
b. Administer pharmacologic therapy as ordered
1) Antiemetics
2) Sedatives/anxiolytics
3) Antibiotics
c. Educate patient/significant others
1) Lie still with eyes closed during an acute exacerbation
2) Explain importance of safety in relation to this condition (e.g., driving, vertigo or falling)
4. Evaluation and ongoing monitoring
a. Hemodynamic status
b. Diminished disequilibrium

D. MENIERE DISEASE

Meniere disease is a condition thought to arise from abnormal fluid and ion homeostasis in the inner ear. Although the exact cause is unknown, it may result from a pathologic lesion termed endolymphatic hydrops. It usually presents between ages 20 and 40 but may begin at any age. The damage to the hearing and balance structures of the ear causes severe rotary vertigo, nausea, vomiting, and tinnitus. Meniere disease may be a sequela from a blow to the head, infection, allergies, or degeneration of the inner ear. An episode may last for several hours; recurrent symptoms last for weeks to months. The triad of characteristics of Meniere disease includes unilateral sensorineural loss, tinnitus, and episodic vertigo. Physical examination during an exacerbation may reveal spontaneous nystagmus unaffected by positional changes. When vertigo is present, dizziness, nausea, imbalance, and vomiting are common because of the affected vagal and vestibular impulses. Additional vagal system involvement may produce abdominal pain, diaphoresis, bradycardia, and pallor. Differential diagnoses that produce similar symptoms must be considered and include acoustic neuroma, viral labyrinthitis, multiple sclerosis, syphilitic vertigo, labyrinthine fistula, vestibular granuloma, and temporal bone fracture. Medical treatment involves symptom management using labyrinthine sedatives and antiemetics to control nausea and antihistamines to lower endolymphatic pressure by increasing blood flow to the inner ear and thereby minimizing vertigo. Diuretics may also be prescribed to stabilize body fluid levels and to avoid secondary fluctuations in the endolymph. Lifestyle interventions include maintaining an adequate diet that balances sugar and salt intake; avoiding caffeine, alcohol, and smoking can also reduce symptoms. Hydration is important to minimize symptoms; therefore, fluid lost during exercise or excessive heat should be replenished. Surgery may be considered when Meniere disease is severe and refractory to medical treatment. An endolymphatic shunt to decompress and relieve fluid pressure in the inner ear, labyrinthectomy to destroy the inner ear, ablation of vestibular hair cells, and vestibular neurectomy to section the vestibular nerve and disconnect it from the brain are options that may be considered.

1. Assessment
a. Subjective data collection
1) Chief complaint
2) History of present illness
a) Rotational vertigo; inability to ambulate without falling; feelings of spinning or of objects spinning around the patient
b) Nausea or vomiting
c) Diaphoresis
d) Tinnitus: roaring sensation or ringing in ears
e) Mild to severe hearing loss
f) Feeling of pressure or fullness in affected ear
g) Heightened sensitivity to loud sounds

h) Headache
i) Blurred vision
j) Symptoms are often episodic and recurring
3) Past medical history
  a) Current or preexisting diseases/illness
    (1) Otitis media
    (2) Arteriosclerosis
    (3) Leukemias, blood disorders
  b) Smoking or alcohol use
  c) Medications
  d) Allergies
4) Past surgical history
b. Objective data collection
  1) Physical examination
    a) General appearance
      (1) Altered gait: disequilibrium, falls toward affected ear
      (2) Decreased hearing in affected ear
      (3) Moderate distress/discomfort
    b) Inspection
      (1) Moist, pale skin
      (2) Nystagmus
    c) Symptoms are often episodic and recurring
  2) Diagnostic procedures
    a) Caloric tests to differentiate from intracranial lesion are considered but not usually performed
2. Analysis: differential nursing diagnoses/collaborative problems
a. Risk for injury
b. Risk for deficient fluid volume
3. Planning and implementation/interventions
a. Establish IV access for administration of crystalloid fluids/medications as needed
b. Administer pharmacologic therapy as ordered
  1) Vasodilators
  2) Antihistamine (meclizine [Antivert])
  3) Diuretics
  4) Oral sedative/antiemetic
  5) Steroids
  6) Anticholinergics
  7) Benzodiazepines
c. Educate patient/significant others
  1) Maintain bed rest or quiet environment
  2) Explain importance of safety in relation to this condition (e.g., driving, vertigo or falling)
  3) Avoid triggers (e.g., dietary [salt] and medication)
  4) Instruct patient to make position changes or other movements slowly and to limit activity
  5) Instruct patient to avoid alcohol and caffeine
  6) Provide ENT referral for possible surgical intervention: decompression of the sac, shunt
4. Evaluation and ongoing monitoring
a. Hemodynamic status
b. Diminished disequilibrium

E. OTIC FOREIGN BODY

Foreign bodies in the ear are commonly seen in children but can be found in adults as well. Foreign objects and material are inserted or introduced into the external canal, where they become lodged and produce local irritation and tissue inflammation. Foreign bodies can be removed with instruments, including forceps, hooks, and loops, or with syringe irrigation. In some cases, microscopic guidance to remove a foreign body is required when the object is directed medially toward the TM or is displaced deeper into the meatus. Irrigation of organic foreign bodies, such as peas and beans, should be avoided because they have a tendency to absorb moisture and swell, thus obliterating the canal and making removal difficult. Flying insects in the ear canal (such as mosquitoes or flies) may be removed by placing the patient in a darkened room and shining a light into the ear canal. If the insect is still able to fly, it is likely to fly towards the light. If the insect does not fly (such as a cockroach or spider), instill either mineral oil or 2% viscous lidocaine into the canal to first kill and immobilize the insect prior to irrigation or extraction.

1. Assessment
a. Subjective data collection
  1) Chief complaint
  2) History of present illness
    a) Discharge from ear: purulent or bloody
    b) Pain (see Chapter 8)
    c) Decreased hearing in ear
    d) Foul odor in ear
    e) Buzzing noise, sensation, feeling of fullness in ear
  3) Past medical history
    a) Current or preexisting diseases/illness
    b) Socioenvironmental conditions
    c) Medications
    d) Allergies
b. Objective data collection
  1) Physical examination
    a) General appearance
      (1) Level of consciousness, behavior, affect: agitation
      (2) Odors: foul odor from affected ear
      (3) Mild to moderate distress/discomfort
    b) Inspection
      (1) Visible foreign body in ear
      (2) Edema and erythema of ear canal
      (3) Purulent drainage or bleeding in affected ear canal
  2) Diagnostic procedures
    a) Otoscopic examination
2. Analysis: differential nursing diagnoses/collaborative problems
a. Pain
b. Anxiety/fear
c. Risk for infection

3. Planning and implementation/interventions
   a. Prepare for/assist with medical interventions
      1) Irrigation of canal
         a) Normal saline or water at body temperature
         b) Mixture of alcohol and water for organic material: less swelling
         c) Live insect: mineral oil or 2% viscous lidocaine
      2) Suction
      3) Direct instrumentation: syringe irrigation or microscopically guided removal
      4) Live insect: use flashlight to attract live insect out of canal
   b. Administer pharmacologic therapy as ordered
      1) Nonnarcotic analgesics
      2) Antibiotics
4. Evaluation and ongoing monitoring
   a. Foreign body removed
   b. Pain relief

F. RUPTURED TYMPANIC MEMBRANE

Although most TM perforations are caused primarily by infection, some cases may result from trauma, including impact injury and explosive acoustic trauma. Hearing may be reduced until healing occurs. Healing is usually spontaneous, and efforts to avoid getting the ear wet are advised to avoid secondary complications. When blunt trauma or barotrauma causes hemotympanum (blood behind an intact TM), resolution of symptoms may take up to several weeks. If hearing loss persists, surgical intervention may be indicated to improve symptoms.

1. Assessment
   a. Subjective data collection
      1) Chief complaint
      2) History of present illness
         a) Pain (see Chapter 8)
         b) Discharge from ear: bloody or purulent
         c) Transient vertigo at time of injury
         d) Tinnitus
         e) Hearing loss
         f) Fever or chills
         g) Nausea or vomiting
         h) Recent injury to ear, face, head
         i) Involvement in a motor vehicle collision with an airbag deployment
         j) Barotrauma: seen with air travel and a concurrent upper respiratory tract infection (rupture occurs most commonly on descent) and submersion injuries associated with quick water descent or scuba diving
      3) Past medical history
         a) Current or preexisting diseases/illness
            (1) Previous ear infections
         b) Medications
         c) Allergies
      4) Past surgical history

   b. Objective data collection
      1) Physical examination
         a) General appearance
            (1) Elevated temperature: 100°F (38.0°C) or greater possible
            (2) Altered gait: disequilibrium, ataxia
            (3) Decreased hearing in affected ear
            (4) Mild to moderate distress/discomfort
         b) Inspection
            (1) Tear or perforation of TM: slit-shaped or irregular defect
            (2) Discharge from ear: purulent or bloody
            (3) Nystagmus: may or may not be present
            (4) Other signs of trauma to head or ear
      2) Diagnostic procedures
         a) Otoscopic examination
         b) Hearing tests: tuning fork and voice tests
         c) Skull, temporal bone, and cervical spine radiographs, as indicated
2. Analysis: differential nursing diagnoses/collaborative problems
   a. Pain
   b. Risk for infection
3. Planning and implementation/interventions
   a. Speak slowly and clearly toward healthy ear while directly facing patient
   b. Prepare for/assist with medical interventions
      1) Removal of blood and debris from ear canal
   c. Administer pharmacologic therapy as ordered
      1) Nonnarcotic analgesics
      2) Narcotics
      3) Antibiotics
      4) Antipyretics
   d. Educate patient/significant others
      1) Keep ear canal dry
      2) Instruct not to place anything in the ear
      3) Provide follow-up with ENT specialist
4. Evaluation and ongoing monitoring
   a. Pain relief

IV. Specific Nose Emergencies

A. EPISTAXIS

Common causes of epistaxis include trauma, upper respiratory tract infections, dry environments, nasal foreign bodies, rhinitis, topical nasal medications such as antihistamines and corticosteroids, as well as intranasal drugs such as cocaine. Severe, frequent or recurring epistaxis may be an indication of a systemic bleeding disorder or untreated high blood pressure. Approximately 90% of epistaxis arises from in front of the nasal bones, in the area known as the anterior nasal septum. Most of the blood will exit the nari in these cases and be obvious. The remaining epistaxis occurs in the posterior nasal septum, especially in the elderly population.[7] The blood is more likely to drip down the throat and be less obvious externally in a posterior epistaxis; instead the patient may cough or vomit blood. Depending on the cause and severity of the bleeding, treatment ranges from simple direct pressure, topical vasoconstrictors and analgesics, nasal packing (with a hemostatic packing agent, gelatin foam, oxidized cellulose, or a posterior balloon device), or chemical cautery.

1. Assessment
   a. Subjective data collection
      1) Chief complaint
      2) History of present illness
         a) Duration, frequency, and amount of bleeding
         b) Bleeding site
            (1) Anterior: constant oozing
            (2) Posterior: more profuse and possible arterial hemorrhage, patient often spits out blood and has blood draining down throat
         c) Possibility of nasal foreign body
         d) Recent nasal trauma
         e) Nausea or vomiting (blood or blood clots)
      3) Past medical history
         a) Current or preexisting diseases/illness
            (1) Hypertension
            (2) Atherosclerosis or other vascular abnormalities (e.g., neoplasm, arteriovenous malformation)
            (3) Known bleeding disorders
            (4) Liver disease or alcohol abuse
            (5) Nasal trauma (including digital manipulation [nose picking])
            (6) Intranasal substance use (e.g., cocaine)
         b) Previous epistaxis
         c) Medications
            (1) Use of aspirin or anticoagulant medications
            (2) Intranasal medication use
         d) Allergies
      4) Past surgical history
   b. Objective data collection
      1) Physical examination
         a) General appearance
            (1) Level of consciousness, behavior, affect: anxiety
            (2) Elevated or normal blood pressure: possible orthostasis
            (3) Tachycardia
            (4) Fear of dying or sense of impending doom
            (5) Moderate to severe distress/discomfort, possibly critically ill
         b) Inspection
            (1) Bleeding from nostril(s)
            (2) Blood in oropharynx
            (3) Active bleeding points on nasal mucosa
            (4) Erythema and swelling of nasal mucosa and turbinates
            (5) Blood in auditory canal/eyes: blood migrates through Eustachian tube and perforated TM, or blood in corners of eyes as it passes through lacrimal ducts
      2) Diagnostic procedures
         a) CBC for recurrent epistaxis
         b) Coagulation profile: international normalized ratio (INR), prothrombin time (PT), partial thromboplastin time (PTT) if bleeding disorder suspected or patient taking warfarin (Coumadin)
         c) Type and crossmatch if significant bleeding
         d) CT scan if mass is suspected
         e) ECG in older population with posterior nasal bleeding
2. Analysis: differential nursing diagnoses/collaborative problems
   a. Risk for deficient fluid volume
   b. Anxiety/fear
   c. Risk for ineffective airway clearance
3. Planning and implementation/interventions
   a. Maintain airway, breathing, circulation (see Chapters 1 and 32)
   b. Provide supplemental oxygen as indicated
   c. Establish IV access for administration of crystalloid fluid/blood products/medications as needed
   d. Prepare for/assist with medical interventions
      1) Assist patient with positioning: high Fowler position, leaning forward
      2) Institute cardiac and pulse oximetry monitoring
      3) Assist in control of hemorrhage
         a) Apply direct pressure to nose—nasal clamp or manually; manual pressure applied with thumb and index finger pinching the nostrils firmly as close to the nasal bones as possible for at least 10 minutes
         b) Assist with anterior or posterior nasal packing
         c) Have suction equipment available
         d) Assist with cauterization
            (1) Chemical: Silver nitrate
            (2) Electrocautery or diathermy
         e) Hemostatic material: oxidized regenerated cellulose (Surgicel), absorbable gelatin sponge (Gelfoam), or petroleum gauze
      4) Assist with possible hospital admission
   e. Administer pharmacologic therapy as ordered
      1) Anesthetics
      2) Topical vasoconstrictors (e.g., lidocaine, epinephrine, cocaine solutions)
      3) Decongestants
      4) Vasoconstrictors
      5) Antihypertensive medications to control elevated blood pressure
   f. Educate patient and significant others
      1) Encourage follow-up with ENT if appropriate

2) Importance of avoiding nasal trauma
3) Importance of treating high blood pressure, if underlying cause
4. Evaluation and ongoing monitoring
   a. Airway patency
   b. Hemodynamic status
   c. Breath sounds and pulse oximetry
   d. Cardiac rate and rhythm
   e. Bleeding control

B. NASAL FOREIGN BODY

Nasal foreign bodies are most commonly seen in children and result from play with buttons, beans, pebbles, beads, and small toy parts. Of particular concern are button batteries inserted into the nose. An electrical current may form around the outside of the battery causing a local tissue burn. The burning process may continue until the battery is removed. Presenting features usually reveal unilateral nasal obstruction. Foul-smelling rhinorrhea may result from retention of the foreign body in the nose for an extended period of time. The nose may be swollen, tender, or bleeding from previous attempts at removal. Difficult breathing, stridor, lethargy, and failure to eat may be indicators of foreign body aspiration and should be managed immediately. Removal of a foreign body, once it is located, can be attempted by several methods. Having the parent gently blow into the child's mouth while occluding the unaffected nostril, simple nose blowing, or suctioning may cause enough pressure to release the foreign body. Forceps and hooked or looped instruments may also be used. In some cases, 1% phenylephrine is applied topically to minimize swelling of the nasal mucosa before retrieving a nasal foreign object. When retrieval is difficult, a 6- or 8-French (e.g., Fogarty) catheter may be passed beyond the obstruction. When the balloon is inflated and the catheter is withdrawn, the foreign body may be easily removed.

1. Assessment
   a. Subjective data collection
      1) Chief complaint
      2) History of present illness
         a) Verbal report of foreign body in nose
         b) Nose pain or swelling
         c) Purulent nasal discharge
         d) Foul smell from nose
      3) Past medical history
         a) Current or preexisting diseases/illness
         b) Previous foreign body insertion
         c) Medications
         d) Allergies
      4) Past surgical history
   b. Objective data collection
      1) Physical examination
         a) General appearance
            (1) Level of consciousness, behavior, affect: agitation
            (2) Odors: foul-smelling rhinorrhea
            (3) Mild distress/discomfort
            (4) Nasal wheezing during the respiratory cycle
         b) Inspection
            (1) Unilateral purulent nasal discharge
            (2) Visualization of foreign body: usually lodges between middle turbinate and septum
            (3) Edema of nasal mucosa
            (4) Unilateral bleeding from nose
      2) Diagnostic procedure
         a) Nasal examination with speculum
2. Analysis: differential nursing diagnoses/collaborative problems
   a. Pain
   b. Anxiety/fear
3. Planning and implementation/interventions
   a. Instruct patient to blow nose in attempt to dislodge and remove foreign object
   b. If patient is a child, instruct parent to occlude patent nostril, then forcefully blow air into child's open mouth; using a pediatric bag-mask-ventilation device is an alternative method
   c. Prepare for/assist with medical interventions
      1) Apply a topical vasoconstrictive agent (1% phenylephrine) and/or a topical anesthetic inside the involved nostril to minimize swelling before manual removal of the object
      2) Assist with removal of the foreign object using suction, forceps, or a balloon-tipped catheter
   d. Educate patient and significant others/parents
      1) Return to the emergency department if significant bleeding occurs
      2) Provide information regarding safety proofing of the environment
4. Evaluation and ongoing monitoring
   a. Pain relief
   b. Nasal bleeding after foreign body removal

C. RHINITIS

Rhinitis is an inflammatory condition of the nasal mucosa characterized by nasal membrane edema, vasodilation, discharge, and obstruction. It is frequently seen in patients with viral or bacterial upper respiratory tract infections. Other causes include allergies, vasomotor response, and atrophic changes. Rhinitis medicamentosa (rebound nasal congestion) is seen in patients who overuse over-the-counter topical decongestant nasal sprays (e.g., Afrin), have been taking antihypertensives, or snort cocaine. Rhinitis affects all age groups and is spread by direct droplet contact from viruses and bacteria that invade the respiratory system. Symptoms include nasal congestion, runny nose, sneezing, headache, malaise, and scratchy throat. Ocular irritations such as itching and swelling as well as a loss of smell and taste can also occur. Physical examination reveals a swollen, erythematous nasal mucosa and nasal discharge.

Symptom management is generally all that is needed to minimize discomfort. Oral decongestants, antihistamines, and topical corticosteroid nasal sprays are administered, and symptoms usually resolve within 7 days. If secondary bacterial infections result, as evidenced by a change in color of the nasal discharge, antibiotics may be prescribed. Bacterial invasion may occur from *S. pneumoniae, S. aureus, H. influenzae,* or *M. catarrhalis.* When conventional treatment methods fail, referral to the otolaryngologist or allergist should be considered.

1. Assessment
   a. Subjective data collection
      1) Chief complaint
      2) History of present illness
         a) Sneezing
         b) Postnasal drip
         c) Copious nasal discharge: thin, purulent, mucoid
         d) Nasal obstruction
         e) Muscle aches
         f) Malaise
         g) Headache
         h) Watery or itchy eyes
         i) Sore throat
         j) Mild fever or chills
      3) Past medical history
         a) Current or preexisting diseases/illness
            (1) Previous rhinitis
         b) Substance use (e.g., cocaine)
         c) Medications
         d) Allergies
      4) Past surgical history
   b. Objective data collection
      1) Physical examination
         a) General appearance
            (1) Mild distress/discomfort
         b) Inspection
            (1) Inflammation of throat and sinuses
            (2) Nasal mucosa erythematous, edematous, and congested
            (3) Injected sclera
            (4) Clear drainage from eyes: watery eyes
            (5) Thick nasal mucous membrane: chronic rhinitis
            (6) Pale turbinates: allergic rhinitis
            (7) Possible nasal polyps
      2) Diagnostic procedures
         a) Nasal speculum examination
         b) Imaging: possible sinus radiographs, coronal CT scan, MRI, lateral neck films to evaluate soft tissue abnormalities such as hypertrophy of adenoids, nasal cytology, and rhinoscopy
2. Analysis: differential nursing diagnoses/collaborative problems
   a. Risk for ineffective breathing pattern (infants)
   b. Infection

3. Planning and implementation/interventions
   a. Administer pharmacologic therapy as ordered
      1) Nonnarcotic analgesics
      2) Antipyretics
      3) Nasal decongestants
      4) Antihistamines: oral, nonsedating versus sedating
      5) Corticosteroids: intranasal or oral
      6) Leukotriene modifiers (e.g., montelukast sodium [Singulair])
   b. Educate patient/significant others
      1) Maintain adequate humidification in home environment
      2) Use nasal decongestants for 2–3 days only, to prevent rebound nasal congestion
      3) Increase fluid intake
      4) Avoid triggers and control allergens
4. Evaluation and ongoing monitoring
   a. Hemodynamic status
   b. Airway patency: infants

V. Specific Throat Emergencies

A. EPIGLOTTITIS

Epiglottitis, or supraglottitis, is an infection and inflammation involving the epiglottis, vallecula, arytenoids, and aryepiglottic folds. It is frequently caused by *H. influenzae* type B (HiB), but group A streptococci and *H. parainfluenzae* organisms have been implicated in the adult population. Less common causes include candidal organisms and thermal injury from smoking or sidestream exposure to crack cocaine, ingestion of hot liquids, and scald burns. The epidemiology of epiglottitis has changed. Originally it was considered an adult disease, but it has changed to become a predominately pediatric illness, occurring in children between the ages of 2 and 7 years. The median pediatric age for developing epiglottis, in the United States, has increased from 35 months to 80 months. Since the introduction of the HiB vaccine, the pediatric incidence has decreased dramatically in those countries that immunize children with HiB. The adult incidence has remained constant, with the average age of onset being 45 years. The illness has an abrupt onset of fever and severe sore throat. Male patients tend to be affected more frequently than female patients, with a 3:1 ratio. There is no season typically associated with epiglottitis. The mortality rate in the pediatric population has decreased to less than 1%, whereas it remains at approximately 7% in adults. Airway obstruction is the major life-threatening problem, develops more quickly in children, and must be addressed immediately.

1. Assessment
   a. Subjective data collection
      1) Chief complaint
      2) History of present illness
         a) Fever

Part 2

b) Pain (see Chapter 8)
  (1) Severe sore throat
  (2) Dysphagia
  (3) Odynophagia: pain with eating/swallowing
c) Muffled voice
d) Cough
e) Dyspnea
f) Sudden onset of symptoms: over previous 12–24 hours
3) Past medical history
  a) Current or preexisting diseases/illness
  b) Recent, or exposure to, upper respiratory infection: usually no prodromal history
  c) Medications
  d) Allergies
  e) Immunization status
4) Past surgical history
b. Objective data collection
  1) Physical examination
    a) General appearance
      (1) Level of consciousness, behavior, affect: anxiety, confusion
      (2) Elevated temperature
      (3) Tripod positioning: in children, sitting up with neck extended in sniffing position
      (4) Stridor: late finding
      (5) Drooling
      (6) Severe distress/discomfort, critically ill
    b) Inspection
      (1) Absent or mild posterior pharynx erythema: in adults; do not examine in children
    c) Palpation
      (1) Cervical lymphadenopathy
      (2) Tenderness over larynx: in adults
  2) Diagnostic procedures: delay obtaining laboratory studies until airway is secure in children
    a) CBC with differential: elevated WBC count
    b) Blood culture
    c) Lateral soft tissue neck radiograph
      (1) May need to be obtained at bedside
      (2) Thumbprint sign: edema of epiglottis
    d) Nasopharyngoscopy: direct fiberoptic visualization in adults
    e) Chest radiograph: after airway secure
2. Analysis: differential nursing diagnoses/collaborative problems
  a. Risk for ineffective airway clearance
  b. Acute pain
3. Planning and implementation/interventions
  a. Maintain airway, breathing, circulation (see Chapters 1 and 32)
  b. Provide supplemental oxygen
    1) RSI and ventilatory support if airway compromise is present: for children, best performed in operating suite by pediatric specialist

2) High-flow oxygen: adults
3) Blow-by oxygen: children
c. Establish IV access for administration of crystalloid fluid/medications
  1) Performed after airway secured in children
d. Allow parents to remain with and hold child; minimize environmental stimuli
e. Prepare for/assist with medical procedures
  1) Advanced airway management
    a) Nasal or oral intubation
    b) Supraglottic airway (e.g., King, Combitube, laryngeal mask airway)
    c) Surgical airway (e.g., cricothyrotomy)
  2) Institute cardiac and pulse oximetry monitoring
  3) Assist with obtaining ENT consultation
  4) Assist with hospital admission
f. Administer pharmacologic therapy as ordered
  1) RSI premedications: sedatives, analgesics, neuromuscular blocking agents
  2) Antibiotics
4. Evaluation and ongoing monitoring
  a. Airway patency
  b. Level of consciousness
  c. Hemodynamic status
  d. Breath sounds and pulse oximetry
  e. Cardiac rate and rhythm
  f. Pain relief

B. EXUDATIVE PHARYNGITIS

Organisms responsible for pharyngitis can also affect the tonsils and cause infection. As part of the lymphatic system, tonsils are considered filters for circulating bacteria, lymph, and other foreign material that aid in fighting infections. As bacteria invade the nose and mouth, inflammation and enlargement of the palatine, lingual, and pharyngeal tonsils can occur, causing acute tonsillitis. Infection can be trapped within these structures and may result in sore throat, difficulty in swallowing, fever, chills, cervical lymphadenopathy, and fetid breath. Treatment measures include the use of antibiotics, analgesics, and warm saltwater gargles. Chronic exudative pharyngitis may occur in some patients and may necessitate surgical removal of the tonsils to avoid recurrent or relapsing infection from sore throat.
1. Assessment
  a. Subjective data collection
    1) Chief compliant
    2) History of present illness
      a) Pain (see Chapter 8)
        (1) Mild to severe throat pain: rapid onset
        (2) Pain or difficulty in swallowing
        (3) Referred pain to ear and neck
      b) Recent, or exposure to, upper respiratory tract or other infections
      c) Fever or chills
      d) Fatigue, myalgia, arthralgia
      e) Headache
      f) Nausea or vomiting

3) Past medical history
   a) Current or preexisting diseases/illness
   b) Previous infections of pharynx or tonsils
   c) Medications
   d) Allergies
   e) Immunization status
4) Past surgical history
b. Objective data collection
  1) Physical examination
   a) General appearance
    (1) Tachycardia
    (2) Elevated temperature
    (3) Moderate distress/discomfort
   b) Inspection
    (1) Red and swollen tonsils: petechiae to tonsils, pharynx, or palate
    (2) Purulent exudate on tonsillar crypts
    (3) Erythematous oropharynx
    (4) Flushed face
    (5) Inflammation and enlargement of pharyngeal or lingual tonsils
   c) Palpation
    (1) Enlarged and tender anterior cervical and submandibular lymphadenopathy
  2) Diagnostic procedures
   a) Rapid *Streptococcus* screen as indicated
   b) Culture and sensitivity testing of exudate
2. Analysis: differential nursing diagnoses/collaborative problems
a. Pain
b. Infection
3. Planning and implementation/interventions
a. Maintain airway, breathing, circulation (see Chapters 1 and 32)
b. Administer pharmacologic therapy as ordered
  1) Antibiotics
  2) Antitussives
  3) Steroids
  4) Antipyretics
c. Educate patient/significant others/parents
  1) Use warm saline throat irrigations
  2) Instruct on importance of adequate diet and rest
4. Evaluation and ongoing monitoring
a. Hemodynamic status
b. Pain relief

C. LARYNGEAL FOREIGN BODY

Foreign body aspiration is a common cause of accidental death in the United States among children 6 years of age and younger. Foreign bodies or objects such as peanuts, hotdogs, marshmallows, grapes, vegetables, seeds, and metal or plastic objects can obstruct the main stem bronchi or distal trachea near the carina and esophagus. Button batteries that are caught in the airway may form an electrical current around the outside of the battery, causing a local tissue burn. The burning process may continue until the battery is removed. Patients who

have ingested or inhaled a foreign body may present with a variety of symptoms, including wheezing, stridor, coughing, failure to eat or drink, and apnea. With any suspected foreign body, airway management is the priority until location of the foreign body is confirmed. Treatment and removal of the foreign body are dependent on its location. Radiographs are used to locate the foreign body and to assist in determining the type of treatment necessary. Emergency department management may include direct laryngoscopy to visualize the foreign body and facilitate removal with the use of Magill forceps. When indicated, removal of a foreign body can be achieved with a variety of methods, including rigid esophagoscopy, balloon-tipped catheter, bougienage, flexible endoscopy, and pharmacologic agents. The use of a foreign body airway obstruction maneuver (e.g., Heimlich maneuver), or chest and abdominal thrusts, can prevent unnecessary deaths associated with foreign body ingestion and aspiration.

1. Assessment
a. Subjective data collection
  1) Chief complaint
  2) History of present illness
   a) Pain (see Chapter 8)
   b) Vocal changes
   c) Drooling
   d) Coughing
   e) Difficulty in swallowing or breathing
   f) Difficulty in talking or inability to talk
   g) Recent ingestion of foreign object or food
   h) Diminished ability or inability to take oral fluids/food
  3) Past medical history
   a) Current or preexisting diseases/illness
   b) Medications
   c) Allergies
  4) Past surgical history
b. Objective data collection
  1) Physical examination
   a) General appearance
    (1) Level of consciousness, behavior, affect: agitation to unconscious
    (2) Tachypnea and increased respiratory effort to apnea
    (3) Tachycardia
    (4) Stridor
    (5) Possible drooling
    (6) Mild to severe distress/discomfort
   b) Inspection
    (1) Foreign body visible in pharynx or larynx
    (2) Retractions
    (3) Cyanosis
    (4) Skin cool and moist
    (5) Hemoptysis or hematemesis
   c) Auscultation
    (1) Breath sounds: wheezes

2) Diagnostic procedures
    a) Indirect laryngoscopy
    b) Anteroposterior and lateral chest radiographs with end-inspiratory and end-expiratory views; decubitus views as indicated
    c) Soft tissue radiograph of neck
    d) Examination with radiopaque contrast material

2. Analysis: differential nursing diagnoses/collaborative problems
  a. Risk for ineffective airway clearance
  b. Anxiety/fear

3. Planning and implementation/interventions
  a. Maintain airway, breathing, circulation (see Chapters 1 and 32)
    1) Finger sweep of mouth (age dependent)
    2) Foreign body airway obstruction maneuver (e.g., Heimlich maneuver) or abdominal chest thrust for apnea
  b. Provide supplemental oxygen as indicted
  c. Establish IV access for administration of crystalloid fluid/medications as needed
  d. Prepare for/assist with medical interventions
    1) Possible cricothyrotomy/tracheotomy
    2) Elevate head of bed 60–90 degrees
    3) Minimize environmental stimuli
    4) Indirect laryngoscopy
    5) Assist with foreign body removal procedures
      a) Rigid esophagoscopy
      b) Balloon-tipped catheter
      c) Bougienage: pushes esophageal coin ingestions into the stomach
      d) Flexible endoscopy
    6) Institute cardiac and pulse oximetry monitoring
    7) Assist with hospital admission as needed
  e. Administer pharmacologic therapy as ordered

4. Evaluation and ongoing monitoring
  a. Airway patency
  b. Level of consciousness
  c. Hemodynamic status
  d. Breath sounds and pulse oximetry
  e. Cardiac rate and rhythm

D. LARYNGITIS

Viral infection is the most frequent cause of hoarseness, more commonly referred to as laryngitis. Excessive use of voice, irritating inhaled or ingested substances, bacterial infections, and allergies can produce similar symptoms affecting the larynx and vocal cords. The constant urge to clear the throat and tickling sensations in the pharynx are often described. As inflammation of the mucous membranes increases, symptoms worsen. The voice sounds harsh and raspy. When significant edema is present, there is stridor or airway impairment, and emergency measures should be taken to prevent further airway obstruction. Differential diagnoses such as polyps, lesions, or tumors must be considered, and further examination by direct laryngoscopy must be performed to rule out disease. Treatment involves voice rest and use of corticosteroids to suppress inflammation, expectorants to liquefy secretions, and antibiotics to treat suspected bacterial infections.

1. Assessment
  a. Subjective data collection
    1) Chief complaint
    2) History of present illness
      a) Dry, tickling sensation in throat
      b) Partial or complete loss of voice, hoarseness
      c) Fever or chills
      d) Pain (see Chapter 8): sore throat
      e) Dyspnea: increasing dyspnea may be a sign of edematous laryngitis or croup
      f) Difficulty in swallowing
      g) Dry cough
      h) Minor discomfort
      i) Anorexia
    3) Past medical history
      a) Current or preexisting diseases/illness
      b) Recent, or exposure to, upper respiratory tract or other infections
      c) Injury
      d) Medications
      e) Allergies
      f) Immunization status
    4) Past surgical history
  b. Objective data collection
    1) Physical examination
      a) General appearance
        (1) Level of consciousness, behavior, affect: restlessness
        (2) Dysphonia or aphonia
        (3) Elevated temperature: >100.4°F (38°C)
        (4) Possible stridor
        (5) Mild distress/discomfort
      b) Inspection
        (1) Reddened larynx and vocal cords
        (2) Swelling of larynx and epiglottis
        (3) Dyspnea
        (4) Granulation of mucous membrane lining larynx (chronic)
        (5) Postnasal drip and rhinorrhea
    2) Diagnostic procedures
      a) Throat culture and sensitivity testing as indicated
      b) CBC with differential

2. Analysis: differential nursing diagnoses/collaborative problems
  a. Pain
  b. Infection
  c. Potential airway obstruction

3. Planning and implementation/interventions
  a. Provide warm room that is adequately humidified
  b. Instruct patient to maintain voice rest

c. Administer pharmacologic therapy as ordered
  1) Antibiotic: often in combination with oral or inhaled steroids
  2) Antitussive agents
  3) Nonnarcotic analgesics
  4) Topical anesthetic agent: viscous lidocaine 2% or phenol (Chloraseptic) spray
  5) Antipyretics
  6) Throat lozenges
d. Educate patient/significant others
  1) Apply ice bag to anterior aspect of patient's neck
4. Evaluation and ongoing monitoring
  a. Hemodynamic status
  b. Pain relief

E. PERITONSILLAR ABSCESS

Peritonsillar abscess results from an infection that penetrates the tonsillar capsule and superior constrictor muscle and invades the surrounding areolar tissue. Severe sore throat, painful or difficult swallowing, trismus, and uvular deviation are common features found in peritonsillar abscess. Streptococci bacteria are generally the pathogens responsible for this infection. Physical examination reveals the tonsil enlarged and erythematous, with the uvula displaced. Patients frequently demonstrate a muffled, "hot potato" voice and may be unable to swallow their own saliva. Providing drainage may produce immediate relief by aspirating pus from the peritonsillar fold located superior and medial to the upper pole of the tonsil. Incision and drainage are sometimes performed in the emergency department, and care must be taken to avoid complications involving the retropharyngeal, deep neck, and posterior mediastinal spaces. Antibiotics and warm saline irrigations aid in reducing infection and promoting comfort. Tonsillectomy is performed when infections are relapsing and peritonsillar abscess is recurrent.

1. Assessment
  a. Subjective data collection
    1) Chief complaint
    2) History of present illness
      a) Pain (see Chapter 8)
        (1) Sore throat
        (2) Pain on swallowing
        (3) Ipsilateral ear fullness or otalgia
      b) Fever or chills
      c) Pus on tonsils
      d) Difficulty in opening mouth or eating
      e) Drooling or inability to swallow
      f) Muffled, "hot potato" voice
      g) Difficulty breathing
      h) Fetid breath
    3) Past medical history
      a) Current or preexisting diseases/illness
      b) Recent, or exposure to others with, upper respiratory tract infection or tonsillitis

      c) Medications
      d) Allergies
    4) Past surgical history
  b. Objective data collection
    1) Physical examination
      a) General appearance
        (1) Elevated temperature
        (2) Tachypnea
        (3) Possible drooling
        (4) Fetid breath
        (5) Moderate to severe distress/discomfort; critically ill
      b) Inspection
        (1) Enlarged affected tonsil
        (2) Displacement of uvula toward nonaffected side
        (3) Edema and erythema of soft palate
        (4) Trismus
        (5) Torticollis: contracted state of cervical muscles, resulting in twisting of neck in abnormal position
        (6) Tonsillar or posterior pharynx exudate
      c) Palpation
        (1) Enlarged and tender cervical lymphadenopathy
    2) Diagnostic procedures
      a) Needle aspiration of suspected abscess
      b) Culture and sensitivity testing of exudate from abscess
      c) Soft tissue neck CT
2. Analysis: differential nursing diagnoses/collaborative problems
  a. Risk for ineffective airway clearance
  b. Pain
3. Planning and implementation/interventions
  a. Maintain airway, breathing, circulation (see Chapters 1 and 32)
  b. Provide supplemental oxygen as indicated
  c. Establish IV access for administration of crystalloid fluids/medications as needed
  d. Prepare for/assist with medical interventions
    1) Elevate head of bed 60–90 degrees
    2) Provide warm saline throat irrigations
    3) Aspiration or incision and drainage of abscess
    4) Assist with possible hospital admission
  e. Administer pharmacologic therapy as ordered
    1) Antibiotics
    2) Topical anesthetic throat spray
    3) Local anesthetic injection
    4) Nonnarcotic analgesics
    5) Narcotics
    6) Antipyretics
  f. Educate patient and significant others
    1) Apply ice collar to neck
    2) Return to emergency department for worsening condition

4. Evaluation and ongoing monitoring
   a. Airway patency
   b. Hemodynamic status
   c. Pain relief

F. PHARYNGITIS

Pharyngitis is an inflammation of the pharynx, and patients with this condition will likely present to the emergency department complaining of a sore throat. Pharyngitis accounts for 1–2% of all outpatient visits. Approximately 30 million cases of pharyngitis are diagnosed annually in the United States, with over 50% in patients between 5 and 24 years of age. It is most likely to occur in the cold months, with rhinovirus being the most likely cause in the fall and spring, coronavirus in the winter, and influenza between December and April. Pharyngitis is viral 25–45% of the time, in which case it will likely be associated with symptoms such as coryza, conjunctivitis, cough, and hoarseness requiring nothing more than symptomatic treatment. Pharyngitis can also be bacterial, with 15–30% of cases being caused by *Streptococcus* group A. Bacterial pharyngitis may cause serious complications including peritonsillar and retropharyngeal abscesses, cervical lymphadenitis, sinusitis, otitis media, mastoiditis, rheumatic fever, and glomerulonephritis. Prompt treatment with appropriate antibiotics minimizes the risk of these complications in cases of bacterial pharyngitis. Although uncommon, some noninfectious causes of pharyngitis should be considered, including chemical irritation (from smoking or second-hand smoke), allergic rhinitis, gastroesophageal reflux disease, and postnasal drainage.[8]

1. Assessment
   a. Subjective data collection
      1) Chief complaint
      2) History of present illness
         a) Pain (see Chapter 8)
            (1) Mild to severe sore throat, exacerbated by swallowing
            (2) Referred to ears, neck, and jaw
         b) Difficulty in swallowing or talking
         c) Fever or chills
         d) Recent, or exposure to, upper respiratory tract or other infections
         e) Harsh cough
         f) Anorexia
         g) Fatigue
         h) Body aches: muscle and joint pain
         i) Feeling of fullness in head or headache
      3) Past medical history
         a) Current or preexisting diseases/illness
         b) Smoking or inhaled substance abuse
         c) Medications
         d) Allergies
         e) Immunization status
      4) Past surgical history
   b. Objective data collection
      1) Physical examination
         a) General appearance
            (1) Nasal speech
            (2) Possible elevated temperature
            (3) Foul breath odor
            (4) Mild to moderate distress/discomfort
         b) Inspection
            (1) Enlarged tonsils
            (2) Erythema or exudate of pharynx or tonsils, suggestive of a viral etiology
            (3) Pharyngeal exudate or petechiae, suggestive of a bacterial etiology
            (4) Flushed face or hot skin
         c) Palpation
            (1) Cervical lymphadenopathy
      2) Diagnostic procedures
         a) Rapid *Streptococcus* screen if available
         b) Throat culture and sensitivity testing
2. Analysis: differential nursing diagnoses/collaborative problems
   a. Pain
   b. Infection
3. Planning and implementation/interventions
   a. Administer pharmacologic therapy as ordered
      1) Antipyretics
      2) Nonnarcotic analgesics
      3) Topical anesthetic agents
      4) Steroids
      5) Antibiotics
   b. Educate patient/significant others
      1) Use warm saline throat irrigations/gargle
      2) Instruct patient on importance of adequate rest and fluid intake
      3) Soft cool foods may feel comforting
      4) Viral infections should resolve within 3–7 days
4. Evaluation and ongoing monitoring
   a. Hemodynamic status
   b. Pain relief

G. RETROPHARYNGEAL ABSCESS

The retropharyngeal space lies posterior to the pharynx, nasopharynx, oropharynx, hypopharynx, larynx, and prevertebral fascia and lateral to the carotid sheaths; the buccopharyngeal fascia binds it anteriorly. It extends superiorly to the base of the skull and inferiorly to the mediastinum. The aerobic, anaerobic, gram-positive, and gram-negative organisms of beta-hemolytic streptococci, *S. aureus, Bacteroides, Veillonella,* and *Haemophilus parainfluenzae* are the usual causes of abscesses within this deep space of the neck. The abscess develops secondarily from a contiguous spreading of upper respiratory infections, pharyngitis, sinusitis, or otitis, but it can also occur from instrumentation trauma (e.g., intubation or foreign body ingestion and retrieval) and penetrating injury forces (e.g., falling down with an object in the mouth such as a Popsicle stick). Persons who are immunocompromised or who have chronic medical conditions such as diabetes, cancer, or alcoholism are at a greater risk for developing a retropharyngeal abscess. Classically, this condition was primarily seen in children between the ages of 6 months and 6 years. However, the incidence of retropharyngeal abscess in children has decreased in recent years possibly because of the use of antibiotics in treating upper respiratory infections. The adult incidence is now on the rise. Boys and men are affected more often than girls and women. This space-occupying abscess has the potential to cause airway occlusion, erosion of the carotid artery, jugular venous thrombosis, epidural abscess, pneumonia, mediastinitis, and aspiration.

1. Assessment
   a. Subjective data collection
      1) Chief complaint
      2) History of present illness
         a) Adults
            (1) Fever
            (2) Pain (see Chapter 8)
               (a) Sore throat
               (b) Neck pain and stiffness
               (c) Dysphagia
               (d) Odynophagia: pain with eating
               (e) Trismus
            (3) Dyspnea
         b) Infants and children
            (1) Fever
            (2) Pain (see Chapter 8)
               (a) Sore throat
               (b) Odynophagia
            (3) Cough
            (4) Neck stiffness
            (5) Neck swelling
            (6) Poor fluid intake
            (7) Behavior changes: lethargy
      3) Past medical history
         a) Current or preexisting diseases/illness
            (1) Tonsillitis
            (2) Pharyngitis
            (3) Otitis media
         b) Recent, or exposure to, upper respiratory infection
         c) Medications
         d) Allergies
         e) Immunization status
      4) Past surgical history
   b. Objective data collection
      1) Physical examination
         a) General appearance
            (1) Level of consciousness, behavior, affect: agitation to lethargy
            (2) Stridor
            (3) Drooling
            (4) Elevated temperature
            (5) Severe distress/discomfort, critically ill
         b) Inspection
            (1) Torticollis: in infants and children
            (2) Posterior pharyngeal edema: adults
         c) Palpation
            (1) Cervical lymphadenopathy
            (2) Neck mass: may rupture with palpation
      2) Diagnostic procedures
         a) CBC with differential: elevated WBC count
         b) Blood cultures
         c) C-reactive protein: elevated
         d) Lateral soft tissue neck radiograph
            (1) Swelling >7 mm at C2 and >14 mm at C6: both adults and children
            (2) Gas in tissues, or possible foreign bodies: rare
         e) Neck CT scan with contrast
         f) Chest radiograph: aspiration pneumonia and mediastinitis
2. Analysis: differential nursing diagnoses/collaborative problems
   a. Risk for ineffective airway clearance
   b. Acute pain
3. Planning and implementation/interventions
   a. Maintain airway, breathing, circulation (see Chapters 1 and 32)
   b. Provide supplemental oxygen
      1) RSI and ventilatory support if airway compromise is present
      2) High-flow oxygen: adults
      3) Blow-by oxygen: children
   c. Establish IV access for administration of crystalloid fluid/medications
   d. Prepare for/assist with medical procedures
      1) Advanced airway management
         a) Nasal or oral intubation
         b) Supraglottic airway (e.g., King, Combitube, laryngeal mask airway)
         c) Surgical airway (e.g., cricothyrotomy)
      2) Institute cardiac and pulse oximetry monitoring
      3) Assist with obtaining ENT consultation
      4) Assist with hospital admission
   e. Administer pharmacologic therapy as ordered
      1) RSI premedications: sedatives, analgesics, neuromuscular blocking agents
      2) Antibiotics
4. Evaluation and ongoing monitoring
   a. Airway patency
   b. Level of consciousness
   c. Hemodynamic status
   d. Breath sounds and pulse oximetry
   e. Cardiac rate and rhythm
   f. Pain relief

References

1. Centers for Disease Control and Prevention: *National Hospital Ambulatory Medical Care Survey: 2010 emergency department summary tables*. Retrieved from http://www.cdc.gov/nchs/data/ahcd/nhamcs_emergency/2010_ed_web_tables.pdf, 2015.
2. Susy Safe Working Group: The Susy Safe project overview after the first four years of activity, *International Journal of Pediatric Otorhinolaryngology* 76:S3–S11, 2012, May 14.
3. Conners GP: Pediatric foreign body ingestion, 2015, August 3. Retrieved from http://emedicine.medscape.com/article/801821-overview#a6.
4. Concepcion E: Pediatric airway foreign body. Retrieved from http://emedicine.medscape.com/article/1001253-overview#a6, 2015, October 13.
5. Murchison DF: Postextraction problems. Retrieved from http://www.merckmanuals.com/professional/dental-disorders/dental-emergencies/postextraction-problems, 2014, July.
6. American Dental Association: (n.d.). Eruption charts. Retrieved from http://www.mouthhealthy.org/en/az-topics/e/eruption-charts.
7. Bontempo LJ: Maxillofacial disorders. In Adams JG, editor: *Emergency medicine*, Philadelphia, PA, 2013, Mosby-Elsevier, pp 259–267.
8. Talledo K, Alcaide M: *Pharyngitis*. First Consult. Retrieved from https://www.clinicalkey.com/#!/content/medical_topic/21-s2.0-1014283, 2013, November 15.

Bibliography

Amsterdam JT: Oral medicine. In Marx JA, Hockberger RS, Walls RM, editors: *Rosen's emergency medicine*, Philadelphia, PA, 2014, Mosby-Elsevier, pp 895–908.
Ball JW, Dains JE, Flynn JA, Solomon BS, Stewart RW: Ears, nose, and throat. In Ball JW, editor: *Seidel's guide to physical examination*, Philadelphia, PA, 2015, Mosby-Elsevier, pp 231–259.
Besdine R: Physical changes with aging. In Porter RS, Kaplan JL, editors: *The Merck manual*, Kenilworth, IL, 2015, Merck & Co.
Bontempo LJ: Maxillofacial disorders. In Adams JG, editor: *Emergency medicine*, Philadelphia, PA, 2013, Mosby-Elsevier, pp 259–267.
Corren J, Baroody FM, Pawankar R: Allergic and nonallergic rhinitis. In Adkinson NF, Bochner BS, Burks AW, Busse WW, Holgate ST, O'Hehir RE, editors: *Middleton's allergy: Principles and practice*, Philadelphia, PA, 2014, Mosby-Elsevier, pp 664–685.
Ferri FF: *Advisor, Ferri's clinical*, Philadelphia, PA, 2016, Mosby-Elsevier.
Herdman TH, Kamitsuru S: *Nursing diagnosis: Definitions and classification 2015–2017*, Sussex, UK, 2014, Wiley Blackwell.
Howard ML: *Middle ear, tympanic membrane, perforations*. Retrieved from http://emedicine.medscape.com/article/858684-overview, 2015, July 14.
Melio FR, Berge LR: Upper respiratory tract infections. In Marx JA, Hockberger RS, Walls RM, editors: *Rosen's emergency medicine*, Philadelphia, PA, 2014, Mosby-Elsevier, pp 965–977.
Pfaff JA, Moore GP: Otolaryngology. In Marx JA, Hockberger RS, Walls RM, editors: *Rosen's emergency medicine*, Philadelphia, PA, 2014, Mosby-Elsevier, pp 931–940.
Seemungal B, Kaski D, Lopez-Escamez JA: Early diagnosis and management of acute vertigo from vestibular migraine and Meniere's disease, *Neurologic Clinics* 33(3):619–628, 2015, August 1.
Talledo K, Alcaide M: *Pharyngitis. First Consutl*. Retrieved from https://www.clinicalkey.com/#!/content/medical_topic/21-s2.0-1014283, 2013, November 15.
Thabet MH, Basha WM, Askar S: Button battery foreign bodies in children: Hazards, management, and recommendations, *Biomed Research International*1–7, 2013.
Thomas SH, Goodloe JM: Foreign bodies. In Marx JA, Hockberger RS, Walls RM, editors: *Rosen's emergency medicine*, Philadelphia, PA, 2014, Mosby-Elsevier, pp 767–784.
Waitzman AA: *Otitis externa*. Retrieved from http://emedicine.medscape.com/article/994550-overview, 2015, August 13.

CHAPTER 14

Endocrine Emergencies

Walter A. Perez, MSN, CEN, CCRN

I. General Strategy

A. ASSESSMENT

1. Primary and secondary assessment/resuscitation (see Chapter 1)
2. Focused assessment
   a. Subjective data collection
      1) History of present illness/chief complaint
         a) Pain: PQRST (see Chapter 8)
         b) Fatigue, malaise
         c) Vomiting
         d) Altered mental status or decreased level of consciousness
         e) Fever
         f) Dyspnea
         g) Weakness
         h) Weight loss
         i) Associated symptoms: anorexia, pruritus, diarrhea
         j) Efforts to relieve symptoms
            (1) Home remedies
            (2) Alternative therapies
            (3) Medications
               (a) Prescription
               (b) OTC/herbal
      2) Past medical history
         a) Current or preexisting diseases/illness
            (1) Diabetes
            (2) Coronary heart disease
            (3) Renal disease
            (4) Thyroid disease or surgery
            (5) Alcoholism
         b) Recent major trauma
         c) Previous similar episodes
         d) Health maintenance practices
         e) Smoking history
         f) Substance and/or alcohol use/abuse
         g) Last normal menstrual period: female patients of childbearing age
         h) Current medications
            (1) Prescription
            (2) OTC/herbal
         i) Allergies
      3) Psychological, social, and environmental factors
         a) Age: illness more severe in very young and very old
         b) Family history
         c) Stressors: surgery, trauma, illness, psychosocial factors
         d) Possible/actual assault, abuse, or intimate partner violence situations (see Chapters 3 and 40)
   b. Objective data collection
      1) General appearance
         a) Level of consciousness, behavior, affect
         b) Vital signs, including orthostatic blood pressure and pulse
         c) Odors: breath and body
         d) Gait
         e) Hygiene

f) Level of distress/discomfort
g) Height and weight
2) Inspection
  a) Skin color
  b) Pupil size, reactivity
  c) Neck veins
  d) Mucous membranes
3) Auscultation
  a) Breath sounds: clear, wheezes, crackles, adventitious sounds
  b) Bowel sounds: normal, hyperactive, hypoactive, absent, bruits or vascular sounds
  c) Heart sounds: S_1 and S_2, rhythm/regularity, other sounds (e.g., murmurs)
4) Palpation
  a) Abdominal distention
  b) Areas of edema
  c) Areas of tenderness
  d) Areas of hyperthermia
  e) Arteries: equality of peripheral pulses
  f) Veins: venous filling and varicosities
  g) Lymph nodes
3. Diagnostic procedures
  a. Laboratory studies
    1) CBC with differential
    2) Serum chemistries including glucose, BUN, creatinine
    3) Arterial blood gas (ABG) values
    4) Urinalysis; pregnancy test in female patients of childbearing age
    5) Alcohol level
    6) Serum and urine toxicology screen: therapeutic level and toxic ingestions
    7) Coagulation profile: partial thromboplastin time (PTT) and prothrombin time (PT)
    8) Liver enzyme levels
    9) Serum ketone levels
    10) Serum osmolality
    11) Cultures: blood, sputum, wound, throat, nasopharyngeal, viral
    12) Thyroid function studies
    13) Cortisol level
  b. Imaging studies
    1) Chest radiograph
    2) Head CT scan, as indicated by history and presentation
    3) Abdominal CT scan
  c. Other
    1) 12- to 15-lead ECG
    2) Lumbar puncture, as indicated

B. ANALYSIS: DIFFERENTIAL NURSING DIAGNOSES/COLLABORATIVE PROBLEMS

1. Impaired gas exchange
2. Ineffective breathing pattern
3. Decreased cardiac output
4. Deficient fluid volume
5. Ineffective tissue perfusion
6. Decreased intracranial adaptive capacity
7. Risk for infection
8. Deficient knowledge

C. PLANNING AND IMPLEMENTATION/INTERVENTIONS

1. Determine priorities of care
  a. Maintain airway, breathing, circulation (see Chapter 1)
  b. Provide supplemental oxygen as indicated
  c. Establish IV access for administration of crystalloid fluid/medications as needed
  d. Obtain and set up equipment and supplies
  e. Prepare for/assist with medical interventions
  f. Administer pharmacologic therapy as ordered
2. Relieve anxiety/apprehension
3. Allow significant others to remain with patient if supportive
4. Educate patient and significant others

D. EVALUATION AND ONGOING MONITORING

1. Continuously monitor and treat as indicated
2. Monitor patient response/outcomes, and modify nursing care plan as appropriate
3. If positive patient outcomes are not demonstrated, reevaluate assessment and/or plan of care

E. DOCUMENTATION OF INTERVENTIONS AND PATIENT RESPONSE

F. AGE-RELATED CONSIDERATIONS

1. Pediatrics
  a. Growth or development related
    1) Neonates, infants, and toddlers are more susceptible to illness and injury but also have more recuperative capacity
    2) Infants have decreased glycogen stores in comparison with adults
    3) Brain development is not complete until about age 20, so more susceptibility to injury exists
    4) Fluid and electrolyte composition: 75–80% of body weight in infants is fluid, making them more susceptible to dehydration
  b. "Pearls"
    1) Pediatric patients are developmentally unable to care for themselves during illness (e.g., maintaining adequate fluid intake)
    2) Inborn errors of metabolism may manifest as severe metabolic acidosis between the second and fifth day of life; late-onset errors of metabolism may manifest as gastroenteritis or recurrent "culture-negative" sepsis in toddlers

3) Parents know their children better than anyone: it is essential to listen to them
4) Most therapeutic choice is often reassurance
2. Geriatrics
   a. Aging-related
      1) In healthy elderly people, physiologic decreases in function are usually apparent only under stress
      2) Reserve capacity for responding to stress decreases
      3) Immune system is compromised
      4) Reduced ability to metabolize and clear medications leads to frequent occurrence of toxicity and adverse reactions
      5) Neurologic system: loss of nonreplicating cells (neurons) may lead to permanent deficit
         a) Dopaminergic neurons are lost, impairing gait and balance and increasing susceptibility to side effects of medication
         b) Loss of other neurotransmitter systems leads to autonomic dysfunction and alterations in neuroendocrine control and mental function
      6) Cardiovascular system
         a) Decreases in heart rate are accompanied by increases in end diastolic and end systolic volumes; reserve mechanisms to increase cardiac output are used routinely and may be overwhelmed by illness
         b) Baroreceptor reflex sensitivity decreases, altering response of system to changes in intravascular volume
            (1) Greater risk exists during rapid volume expansion
            (2) Orthostatic hypotension is more prevalent
      7) Pulmonary system: elasticity of small airways is lost
         a) Increasing tendency for alveoli to collapse
         b) By age 65, not all alveoli are open during regular breathing, thus increasing susceptibility to atelectasis and pneumonia
      8) Endocrine system
         a) Glucose intolerance, insulin resistance, and abnormal regulation of insulin secretion occur
         b) Metabolic clearance of thyroid hormone decreases; in thyroid disease, must decrease dose of exogenous thyroxine obtained from thyroid medication
         c) Decreased estrogen level alters bone metabolism, leading to osteoporosis
      9) Fluid and electrolytes: adaptive mechanisms are impaired, although balance (volume and number of solutes) is unchanged
         a) Nephron loss and decrease in renin and aldosterone levels contribute to increased sodium loss before compensatory mechanisms can be fully activated

         b) Decreased glomerular filtration rate, baroreceptor reflex sensitivity, and insulin and beta-adrenergic responsiveness increase risk of hyperkalemia
         c) Water conservation and urine-concentrating ability, as well as thirst mechanism, are impaired, resulting in increased susceptibility to dehydration
         d) Increased osmoreceptor sensitivity with higher set point for vasopressin (antidiuretic hormone) increases risk of syndrome of inappropriate antidiuretic hormone (SIADH) in patients taking certain drugs and in pulmonary and neurologic diseases
      10) Renal system: renal blood flow, glomerular filtration rate, and creatinine clearance are decreased
      11) Vision and hearing
         a) Decreased visual acuity, changes in refractive power, loss of accommodation, cataracts, and decreased tear secretion influence ability to see adequately
         b) Hearing loss occurs as a result of changes in peripheral auditory system and cerebral cortex
   b. "Pearls"
      1) Decreased activity and less emotional involvement in activity or roles occur
      2) Elderly patients have increased concern with immediate environment, health, and factors affecting them directly

II. Specific Endocrine Emergencies

A. ADRENAL CRISIS

Adrenal insufficiency occurs when the adrenal cortex ceases to produce glucocorticoid and mineralocorticoid hormones. Acute adrenal insufficiency or adrenal crisis can occur in response to an acute stressor, such as infections, hemorrhage, trauma, surgery, burns, pregnancy, or abrupt cessation of long-term steroid use. Primary causes of adrenal insufficiency may include autoimmune adrenalitis (Addison disease), tuberculosis, acquired immunodeficiency syndrome (AIDS), metastatic lung or breast cancer, and adrenal hemorrhage. Secondary causes of adrenal insufficiency may include sarcoidosis, pituitary tumor, chronic steroid use, pituitary stroke, and rarely, postpartum pituitary necrosis. Adrenal crisis should be suspected in patients who have hypotension unresponsive to fluid resuscitation and vasopressor medications, hyponatremia, or hyperkalemia. Death occurs because of circulatory collapse and hyperkalemia-induced dysrhythmia.
1. Assessment
   a. Subjective data collection

1) History of present illness/chief complaint
   a) Fever
   b) Pain (see Chapter 8): nonspecific abdominal pain; may simulate acute abdomen
   c) Nausea, vomiting, diarrhea
2) Past medical history
   a) Current or preexisting diseases/illness
      (1) Primary adrenal insufficiency
      (2) Possible hypothyroidism
   b) Abnormal skin coloring
   c) Weakness, fatigue, lethargy
   d) Anorexia and weight loss
   e) Salt craving
   f) Recent stressful events
   g) Medications: recent discontinuation of cortisol medication
   h) Allergies
b. Objective data collection
   1) Physical examination
      a) General appearance
         (1) Level of consciousness, behavior, affect: confusion
         (2) Hypotension, but may have warm extremities
         (3) Tachycardia
         (4) Tachypnea
         (5) Orthostasis
         (6) Elevated temperature
         (7) Severe distress/discomfort, critically ill
      b) Inspection
         (1) Hyperpigmentation of skin
      c) Auscultation
         (1) Heart sounds: very soft
   2) Diagnostic procedures
      a) CBC with differential
      b) Serum chemistries including glucose, BUN, creatinine
         (1) Hyponatremia
         (2) Hyperkalemia
         (3) Hypercalcemia
         (4) Blood glucose level: hypoglycemia
         (5) BUN: elevated (azotemia secondary to dehydration): creatinine
      c) Urinalysis; pregnancy test in female patients of childbearing age
      d) Blood cultures
      e) Plasma cortisol level: diagnostic if low
      f) Adrenocorticotropic hormone (ACTH) level: stimulation test
         (1) Elevated: primary adrenal insufficiency
         (2) Decreased: secondary adrenal insufficiency
      g) ECG
         (1) Low voltage
         (2) Flat or inverted T wave
         (3) Prolonged QT interval, QRS complex, or PR interval

h) Chest radiograph
i) Abdominal CT scan: if diagnosis not clear
   (1) May indicate adrenal hemorrhage, calcification, or metastasis
j) Head CT scan

2. Analysis: differential nursing diagnoses/collaborative problems
   a. Deficient fluid volume
   b. Ineffective tissue perfusion: cardiopulmonary and cerebral
3. Planning and implementation/interventions
   a. Maintain airway, breathing, circulation (see Chapter 1)
   b. Provide supplemental oxygen as indicated
   c. Establish IV access for administration of crystalloid fluid/medications as needed
      1) Rapid infusion of normal saline solutions or lactated Ringer solution
      2) Maintenance volume replacement: dextrose 5% in normal saline solution
   d. Obtain initial weight if possible, especially if patient will be in emergency care area for prolonged period
   e. Prepare for/assist with medical interventions
      1) Institute cardiac and pulse oximetry monitoring
      2) Insert gastric tube and attach to suction as indicated
      3) Insert indwelling urinary catheter as indicated
      4) Assist with hospital admission and other procedures as indicated by underlying cause of crisis (acute stressor)
   f. Administer pharmacologic therapy as ordered
      1) Intravenous crystalloids
      2) Hydrocortisone (Solu-Cortef) 100 mg IV (2 mg/kg for children) immediately, then every 8 hours
      3) Dexamethasone (Decadron)
         a) May be administered instead of hydrocortisone if reason for crisis is unknown
         b) Does not interfere with subsequent ACTH stimulation testing
      4) Corticotropin
      5) Dextrose 50%
      6) Possible electrolyte replacement
      7) Vasopressors
      8) Fludrocortisone acetate (Florinef): if hypotension, hyponatremia, and hyperkalemia persist after initial treatment
      9) Levothyroxine (Synthroid): if concurrent hypothyroidism present
4. Evaluation and ongoing monitoring
   a. Level of consciousness: brain dehydration and injury can develop with rising sodium levels
   b. Hemodynamic status, including orthostatic blood pressure and pulse
   c. Breath sounds and pulse oximetry
   d. Cardiac rate and rhythm
   e. Intake and output
   f. Electrolytes and glucose levels

B. DIABETIC KETOACIDOSIS

Diabetic ketoacidosis (DKA) is a result of insulin deficiency and stress hormone excess. It typically occurs in diabetes mellitus type 1, formally insulin dependent, but it may also occur in type 2 formally non-insulin-dependent diabetes. Lack of insulin causes decreased cellular glucose uptake, release of free fatty acids, and increased gluconeogenesis by the liver. Hyperglycemia promotes osmotic diuresis with dehydration, hyperosmolality, and electrolyte depletion. Counterregulatory (stress) hormones (glucagon, catecholamines, cortisol, and growth hormone) have antiinsulin effects and stimulate the release of free fatty acids. Free fatty acids are converted to ketone bodies. Infection and stressful events are the usual precipitating factors, along with omission of insulin and new-onset diabetes. Complications of therapy such as cerebral edema, hypoglycemia, and electrolyte imbalance may contribute to death during treatment.

1. Assessment
   a. Subjective data collection
      1) History of present illness/chief complaint
         a) Gradual onset from 24 hours to 2 weeks
         b) Preceding bacterial or viral illness, current infectious process, or significant stress
         c) Nausea and vomiting
         d) Pain (see Chapter 8): abdominal pain, usually generalized
         e) Fever
         f) Polyuria, polydipsia, and polyphagia
         g) Lethargy, weakness, and fatigue
         h) Decreasing level of consciousness and altered mental status
         i) Weight loss
         j) Dehydration
      2) Past medical history
         a) Current or preexisting diseases/illness
            (1) Diabetes
            (2) Cardiovascular disease
         b) Discontinuance or decreased dose of insulin or oral hypoglycemic agents
         c) Ingestion of other medications or substances such as salicylate, methanol, ethylene glycol, or paraldehyde; other causes of increased anion gap acidosis
         d) Recent urinary tract infection
         e) Complicated pregnancy
         f) Recent trauma, injury, surgery
         g) Recent stressful events
         h) Obesity
         i) Previous similar episodes
         j) Medications: steroids, thiazides, antipsychotics, sympathomimetics
   b. Objective data collection
      1) Physical examination
         a) General appearance
            (1) Level of consciousness, behavior, affect: confusion, coma
            (2) Tachycardia
            (3) Orthostasis or frank hypotension
            (4) Kussmaul respirations
            (5) Fruit odor: acetone of breath
            (6) Severe distress/discomfort, critically ill
         b) Inspection
            (1) Dry, hyperthermic, flushed skin
            (2) Dry mucous membranes
         c) Palpation
            (1) Poor skin turgor
      2) Diagnostic procedures
         a) Serum chemistries including glucose, BUN, creatinine
            (1) Glucose level: usually >300 mg/dL (pregnancy and alcohol ingestion are associated with "euglycemic DKA")
            (2) Sodium, chloride, potassium: decreased
            (3) Bicarbonate level <15 mEq/L
            (4) BUN and creatinine levels: normal unless advanced renal disease or severe dehydration is present
            (5) Elevated anion gap ($Na^+ - [Cl^- + HCO_3]$): normal 10–14 mEq/L
         b) Serum osmolality: >320 mOsm/kg
         c) Serum ketones
         d) Serum lactate
         e) Serum acetone level: elevated
         f) Venous or arterial pH <7.3 (arterial pH is about 0.03 above venous)
         g) CBC with differential: white blood cell (WBC) count >25,000, or marked left shift, suggests underlying bacterial infection
         h) Serum phosphorus: if patient at risk for hypophosphatemia (e.g., poor nutritional status, chronic alcoholism)
         i) Serum amylase: may be elevated with associated pancreatitis
         j) Cultures as indicated
         k) Urinalysis: increased glucose and ketone levels; pregnancy test in female patients of childbearing age
         l) Chest radiograph
         m) Head CT scan: especially in children with altered mental status
         n) ECG
2. Analysis: differential nursing diagnoses/collaborative problems
   a. Ineffective tissue perfusion: cerebral
   b. Deficient fluid volume
   c. Anxiety/fear
   d. Deficient knowledge
3. Planning and implementation/interventions
   a. Maintain airway, breathing, circulation (see Chapter 1)
   b. Provide supplemental oxygen as indicated
   c. Establish IV access for administration of crystalloid fluids/medications as needed

1) Insert two large-bore intravenous catheters
2) Infuse normal saline solutions at rate of 1 L in 1–2 hours
3) Normosol-R, a balanced electrolyte solution, may be infused if patient severely dehydrated; decreases development of hyperchloremic acidosis
4) 0.45% sodium chloride solution infused at 200–1,000 mL/hour after initial stabilization
5) Infuse solutions with added dextrose when blood glucose level is <250 mg/dL to prevent hypoglycemia

d. Prepare for/assist with medical interventions
1) Institute cardiac and pulse oximetry monitoring
2) If patient has decreased level of consciousness, insert gastric tube and attach to suction to help control vomiting
3) Insert indwelling urinary catheter
4) May need to restrain confused patient per institutional protocols
5) Assist with hospital admission
   a) If noncompliance is suspected, alert hospital nursing staff to address issue when patient recovers

e. Administer pharmacologic therapy as ordered
1) Regular insulin, as prescribed, to maintain serum glucose between 150 and 200 mg/dL until resolution of the ketosis
   a) IV bolus of 0.1–0.15 unit/kg (approximately 10 units); if awake, may give patient half by IV route and half subcutaneously
   b) IV maintenance dose with infusion pump at 0.1 unit/kg/hour; to saturate the tubing, run the first 50 mL of the insulin drip through the tubing and discard that fluid
   c) Children: 0.1 unit/kg/hour IV drip
2) Sodium bicarbonate ($NaHCO_3$) as prescribed, if pH <7
3) Potassium: 20–40 mEq replacement when serum level is <5.5 mEq/L (hypokalemia develops rapidly with insulin treatment)
4) Phosphate replacement of 20–30 mEq/L in select patients with level <1 mg/dL
5) Antibiotics for documented or suspected treatable infections
6) Antiemetics

4. Evaluation and ongoing monitoring
a. Level of consciousness: continually assess neurologic status; monitor for signs of cerebral edema (occurs from too-rapid resolution of acidosis and hypoglycemia), lactic acidosis, and arterial thrombosis (e.g., stroke, MI)
b. Hemodynamic status every 15–60 minutes until patient is stable

c. Breath sounds and pulse oximetry: respiratory distress syndrome; occurs with overzealous fluid administration
d. Cardiac rate and rhythm
e. Glucose every hour and potassium every 2 hours
f. Intake and output
g. Fluid and electrolyte balance achieved: pH that gradually returns to normal range, serum glucose level of 100–200 mg/dL, potassium level of 4–5 mEq/L, and serum osmolality of 285–300 mOsm/kg

C. HYPERGLYCEMIC HYPEROSMOLAR SYNDROME

Hyperglycemic hyperosmolar syndrome (HHS) is characterized by progressive hyperglycemia and hyperosmolarity. It is more common in older patients with type 2 or undiagnosed diabetes. The patient is unable to maintain adequate hydration. Ketoacidosis generally does not develop because there is enough endogenous insulin present to inhibit ketogenesis. Often, HHS is precipitated by infection, stroke, or sepsis. It may also be the initial presentation in a patient with new-onset type 2 diabetes mellitus. Identification of the precipitating illness is critical, and treatment must be concurrent with management of the HHS. The mortality rate is high despite aggressive therapy.

1. Assessment
a. Subjective data collection
1) History of present illness/chief complaint
   a) Insidious onset: from days to weeks
   b) Recent illness or infection
   c) Thirst
   d) Reduced fluid intake
   e) Polyuria or oliguria
2) Past medical history
   a) Current or preexisting diseases/illness
      (1) Non-insulin-dependent diabetes
      (2) Elderly patient with undiagnosed diabetes
      (3) Immunosuppression illnesses
      (4) Stroke
      (5) Myocardial infarction
   b) Visual changes: visual loss, hallucinations
   c) Limited mobility conditions: diminished ability to provide adequate hydration
      (1) Neglect/abuse
   d) Recent stressful events
   e) Medications: oral hypoglycemic agents, diuretics, medicines producing insulin inhibition or hyperglycemic effects
      (1) Beta blockers
      (2) Histamine 2 (H_2) blockers
   f) Noncompliance with diabetic therapy
   g) Allergies
b. Objective data collection
1) Physical examination

a) General appearance
  (1) Level of consciousness, behavior, affect: confusion and altered mental status are most prominent physical findings; drowsiness, weakness, and/or lethargy to seizure, delirium, coma
  (2) Hypotension: late indicator of profound dehydration
  (3) Tachycardia: early indicator of dehydration
  (4) Possible subnormal or elevated temperature
  (5) Severe distress/discomfort, critically ill
b) Inspection
  (1) Dry skin and mucous membranes: profound dehydration
  (2) Muscle fasciculations
  (3) Nystagmus
c) Palpation
  (1) Hemiparesis/hemisensory deficits
  (2) Poor skin turgor
2) Diagnostic procedures
a) Serum chemistries including glucose, BUN, creatinine
  (1) Glucose level: >600 mg/dL
  (2) Hypernatremia or hyponatremia resulting from dehydration
  (3) Potassium level: normal to high initially; hypokalemia develops with insulin therapy
  (4) BUN and creatinine levels: elevated as a result of prerenal azotemia and dehydration
b) Serum osmolality: >320 mOsm/kg
c) CBC with differential
d) ABGs/venous blood gases
  (1) Normal partial pressure of arterial oxygen (PaO_2)
  (2) pH >7.3
e) Serum ketone level: normal to slightly elevated
f) Cultures if infection source not obvious
g) Creatine phosphokinase (CPK) with isoenzymes: indicators of acute myocardial infarction, rhabdomyolysis
h) Coagulation profile: PT, activated PTT (aPTT)
i) Urinalysis: elevated glucose level, small ketonuria, elevated specific gravity, possible leukocytes, pregnancy test in female patients of childbearing age
j) Chest radiograph
k) Head CT scan
2. Analysis: differential nursing diagnoses/collaborative problems

a. Risk for injury
b. Risk for ineffective airway clearance
c. Ineffective tissue perfusion: cerebral, peripheral
d. Deficient fluid volume
e. Risk for infection
3. Planning and implementation/interventions
a. Maintain airway, breathing, circulation (see Chapter 1)
b. Provide supplemental oxygen as indicated
c. Restoring hemodynamic stability
  1) Insert large-bore intravenous catheter for rehydration, 0.9% NaCl at a rate of 15–20 mL/kg/h during the 1 hour (unless contradicted such as cardiac disease)
  2) If serum sodium is normal or elevated, infuse 0.45% sodium chloride solution at 4–14 mL/kg/hour
  3) If serum sodium is low, infuse 0.9% normal saline solution at 4–14 mL/kg/hour
  4) Infuse solutions containing dextrose once serum glucose reaches 300 mg/dL
d. Prepare for/assist with medical interventions
  1) Advanced airway management
  2) Elevate head of bed to 30 degrees if possible
  3) Institute cardiac and pulse oximetry monitoring
  4) Catheter placement and monitoring of central venous, arterial, or pulmonary artery pressures (see Chapter 6)
  5) Insert gastric tube and attach to suction
e. Administer pharmacologic therapy as ordered
  1) RSI premedications: sedatives, analgesics, neuromuscular blocking agents
  2) Regular insulin as indicated
    a) Intravenous maintenance with infusion pump at 0.1 unit/kg/hour with or without an initial bolus of 0.15 unit/kg; to saturate the tubing, run the first 50 mL of the insulin drip through the tubing and discard that fluid
  3) Potassium replacement as indicated
    a) 20 mEq added to each 1 L of fluid to maintain serum potassium of 4–5 mEq/L
  4) Low-dose heparin as indicated
4. Evaluation and ongoing monitoring
a. Airway patency
b. Continually reassess neurologic status, and monitor for signs of cerebral edema and seizures
c. Hemodynamic status every 15–60 minutes until patient stable
d. Breath sounds and pulse oximetry
e. Cardiac rate and rhythm
f. Fluid and electrolyte balance achieved: serum glucose level of 100–200 mg/dL, potassium level of 4–5 mEq/L, serum osmolality of 285–300 mOsm/kg
g. Intake and output
h. Peripheral cyanosis

D. HYPOGLYCEMIA

Hypoglycemia, the most common endocrine emergency, is a decrease in the serum glucose level to <70 mg/dL in male patients and <40 mg/dL in infants and children. A rapid reduction in glucose levels does not allow time for activation of ketogenesis to provide an alternative energy substrate. Hypoglycemia can lead to symptoms of sympathetic-adrenal activation (anxiety, tremor, sweating, nausea, tachycardia, and palpitations). Extreme low glucose results in hypoxia and eventual coma. Very young and elderly persons are more susceptible to experiencing low blood glucose. Lack of glucose causes permanent brain dysfunction. Any person with an altered level of consciousness should be considered to have hypoglycemia until proven otherwise.

1. Assessment
   a. Subjective data collection
      1) History of present illness/chief complaint
         a) Rapid onset
         b) No recent food intake
         c) Alcohol ingestion in last 36 hours
         d) Hunger, nausea
         e) Weakness, dizziness
         f) Lethargy
         g) Shakiness
         h) Anxiety
         i) Headache
         j) Altered mental status
      2) Past medical history
         a) Current or preexisting diseases/illness
            (1) Diabetes
         b) Insulin: increased dosage (easily reversed)
         c) Oral hypoglycemic agents: long half-life (difficult to reverse)
         d) Increase in physical exercise
         e) Medications and toxin exposures (Box 14.1)
         f) Surgery, other illnesses (Box 14.2)
         g) Allergies
   b. Objective data collection
      1) Physical examination
         a) General appearance
            (1) Level of consciousness, behavior, affect: confusion, shakiness, slurred speech, combative, seizures, comatose
            (2) Shallow respirations but normal rate
            (3) Subnormal or elevated temperature
            (4) Moderate to severe distress/discomfort
         b) Inspection
            (1) Cool, diaphoretic skin
            (2) Pale color
            (3) Dilated pupils
            (4) Hemiplegia or other signs of stroke
      2) Diagnostic procedures
         a) Serum glucose level
         b) Serum chemistry levels: normal
         c) Urinalysis: normal pregnancy test in females of childbearing age

---

Box 14.1

Medications and Toxins that May Cause Hypoglycemia

Medications
Alcohol
Amphotericin B
Angiotensin-converting enzyme (ACE) inhibitors
Beta blockers
Bishydroxycoumarin
Diazoxide
Fluoxetine
Haloperidol
Insulin
Lithium
Methotrexate
Pentamidine
Phenytoin
Propoxyphene
Quinine
Salicylates
Sertraline
Sulfonamide
Sulfonylureas
Tricyclic antidepressants

Herbal Remedies
Ginseng, panax ginseng

Toxins
Carbamate
Insecticides
Methanol
Organophosphates

Box 14.2

Other Causes of Hypoglycemia

Alcoholism
Enzyme deficiency
Gastrointestinal surgery
Hepatic, renal, or cardiac failure
Insulinoma
Islet cell tumor
Leukemia
Lymphoma
Pregnancy
Sarcoma (e.g., fibrosarcoma, mesothelioma, liposarcoma)
Sepsis
Starvation

d) ABG: normal pH

e) Serum alcohol level

f) Possible C-peptide measurement: elevated in insulinoma, normal or low with exogenous insulin, elevated with oral sulfonylureas

g) Possible liver function tests and serum insulin, cortisol, and thyroid levels

h) Chest radiograph

i) Abdominal CT scan or sonography

2. Analysis: differential nursing diagnoses/collaborative problems

a. Imbalanced nutrition: less than body requirements

b. Ineffective tissue perfusion: cerebral

c. Deficient knowledge

d. Risk for ineffective airway clearance

3. Planning and implementation/interventions

a. Maintain airway, breathing, circulation (see Chapter 1)

b. Provide supplemental oxygen as indicated

c. Hemodynamic stability

1) Administer 5% dextrose in water solution if patient is unresponsive or unable to take oral solution

d. Prepare for/assist with medical interventions

1) Suction oropharynx as necessary

2) Advanced airway management

3) Institute cardiac and pulse oximetry monitoring

4) Assist with hospital admission if hypoglycemia results from oral agents because of prolonged drug half-life

e. Administer pharmacologic therapy as ordered

1) Intramuscular (IM) or IV thiamine if patient is malnourished

2) Oral glucose solution if gag reflex is present

3) IV 50% dextrose in water solution; if no response, repeat; 25% dextrose in water solution if patient is <2 years old; 10–12.5% dextrose in water for neonates

4) Glucagon IM or subcutaneous glucagon if unable to establish IV access; 1 mg and may repeat twice; not effective in alcohol-induced hypoglycemia (no glycogen stores left)

f. Educate patient and significant others

1) Review mechanism of disease process with patient and significant others

2) Reinforce need to eat regularly

3) Carry quick glucose foods: simple carbohydrates (hard candy, sugar, orange juice, soft drinks made with sugar), not complex carbohydrates (e.g., candy bars) because fat retards ability to use glucose

4) Decrease insulin dosage if exercising

5) Avoid alcohol consumption while fasting; patients with alcoholism need to eat when binge drinking

6) Refer to social service or appropriate community agency as necessary

7) Instruct patient in signs and symptoms that indicate inadequate nutrition and necessitate return to emergency care setting

a) Persistent symptoms of hypoglycemia in spite of adequate food intake

b) Seizure

c) Failure to return to normal mental status after hypoglycemic episode

4. Evaluation and ongoing monitoring

a. Airway patency

b. Level of consciousness

c. Hemodynamic status

d. Breath sounds and pulse oximetry

e. Serum glucose level of 90–140 mg/dL

E. MYXEDEMA CRISIS

Myxedema crisis, or coma, the most severe manifestation of hypothyroidism, causes marked impairment of central nervous system function and cardiovascular decompensation. Recognition of this illness is hampered by its insidious onset and rarity. It typically occurs in patients with undiagnosed and untreated hypothyroidism of long duration. Precipitating factors include serious infection (pneumonia and urinary tract infection are common), recent sedative or tranquilizer use, stroke, exposure to cold environment, and discontinuance of thyroid hormone replacement. Ninety percent of cases occur during winter months. This prevalence may be related to the diminished ability to sense temperature changes with advanced age.

1. Assessment

a. Subjective data collection

1) History of present illness/chief complaint

a) Recent illness

b) Progressive decline in intellectual status

c) Apathy, self-neglect

d) Emotional lability

e) Anorexia

f) Weight gain

2) Past medical history

a) Current or preexisting diseases/illness

(1) Hypothyroidism or thyroid surgery

b) Medications: thyroid replacement hormone, recent use of tranquilizers and sedatives

b. Objective data collection

1) Physical examination

a) General appearance

(1) Level of consciousness, behavior, affect: decreased mental status, depressed mental acuteness, confusion, psychosis

(2) Deep, coarse voice

(3) Hypothermia, usually <95.9°F (35.5°C)

(4) Bradycardia with distant heart sounds, and cardiac output

(5) Hypoventilation

(6) Hypotension

(7) Severe distress/discomfort, acutely ill

b) Inspection
   (1) Pale, edematous face with periorbital edema
   (2) Macroglossia
   (3) Dry, cold, pale skin
   (4) Nonpitting extremity edema
   (5) Thin eyebrows
   (6) Scar from prior thyroidectomy
2) Diagnostic procedures
   a) Serum chemistries including glucose, BUN, creatinine
      (1) Hyponatremia, hypochloremia
      (2) Glucose: variable hypoglycemia
      (3) BUN and creatinine: elevated
   b) ABG: hypoventilation, hypoxia, hypercarbia
   c) Thyroid studies: low thyroxine (T_4), elevated thyrotropin (thyroid-stimulating hormone [TSH])
   d) CBC with differential: anemia and decreased WBC count
   e) Pretreatment plasma cortisol level
   f) Urinalysis; pregnancy test in female patients of childbearing age
   g) ECG
      (1) Low voltage
      (2) Sinus bradycardia
      (3) Prolonged QT interval
      (4) Possible effusion findings: prolonged PR interval, T-wave abnormalities, and electrical alternans
   h) Chest radiograph
   i) Acute abdominal radiographs
   j) Head CT scan
2. Analysis: differential nursing diagnoses/collaborative problems
   a. Risk for ineffective airway clearance
   b. Ineffective breathing pattern
   c. Decreased cardiac output
   d. Ineffective tissue perfusion: peripheral, cerebral
   e. Ineffective thermoregulation
3. Planning and implementation/interventions
   a. Maintain airway, breathing, circulation (see Chapter 1)
   b. Provide supplemental oxygen as indicated
      1) RSI and ventilatory support in patient with respiratory compromise
      2) High-flow oxygen
   c. Establish IV access for administration of crystalloid fluid/medications as needed
      1) Hypertonic saline solution
      2) Crystalloid solutions
      3) Warmed whole blood
   d. Prepare for/assist with medical interventions
      1) Advanced airway management
         a) Nasal or oral intubation
         b) Supraglottic airway (e.g., King, Combitube, laryngeal mask airway)
         c) Surgical airway (e.g., cricothyrotomy)
      2) Institute cardiac and pulse oximetry monitoring
      3) Maintain normothermic body temperature
         a) Use passive rewarming with blankets and increased room temperature
         b) Avoid rapid rewarming
      4) Institute seizure precautions
      5) Insert gastric tube and attach to suction if indicted
      6) Insert indwelling urinary catheter if indicted
      7) Assist with hospital admission
   e. Administer pharmacologic therapy as ordered
      1) RSI premedications: sedatives, analgesics, neuromuscular blocking agents ready if needed
      2) Intravenous thyroid hormone (*either T_4 or T_3 can be used, but in severe myxedema coma*)
         a) IV T_4 (levothyroxine) at 4 micrograms/kg, followed in 24 hours by 100 micrograms IV, then 50 micrograms IV until oral medication is tolerated (switch to 50–200 micrograms/day PO when patient is ambulatory)
         b) IV T_3 (liothyronine or triiodothyronine) for myxedema coma at 20 micrograms followed by 10 micrograms IV every 8 hours until patient is conscious (given because of risk of decreased T_3 generation from T_4 in severely hypothyroid patients); start with no more than 10 micrograms IV for the elderly or those with coronary artery disease
      3) Glucocorticoids (to prevent adrenal crisis)
      4) Vasoconstrictors
4. Evaluation and ongoing monitoring
   a. Airway patency
   b. Level of consciousness
   c. Hemodynamic status
   d. Breath sounds and pulse oximetry
   e. Cardiac rate and rhythm
   f. Intake and output

F. THYROID STORM

Thyroid storm or thyrotoxic crisis is an extreme and rare form of thyrotoxicosis with a high mortality rate. The classic triad of thyroid storm is high fever, central nervous system dysfunction or cerebral encephalopathy, and exaggerated tachycardia out of proportion to fever. Precipitants can include thyroid surgery, infection, trauma, stress, or radioactive iodine administration. The most common underlying cause of hyperthyroidism in cases of thyroid storm is Grave disease. Elderly patients may have apathetic hyperthyroidism in which symptoms go unrecognized and therefore are at higher risk for thyroid storm. Factors known to precipitate thyroid storm include infection, surgery, trauma, radioactive iodine treatment, pregnancy, anticholinergic and adrenergic drugs, thyroid hormone ingestion, and diabetic ketoacidosis.

1. Assessment
   a. Subjective data collection
      1) History of present illness/chief complaint
         a) Fever
         b) Nausea, vomiting, diarrhea
         c) Pain (see Chapter 8): abdominal
         d) Worsening of thyrotoxicosis symptoms
         e) Anxiety, restlessness, nervousness, irritability, possible coma
         f) Generalized weakness
         g) Precipitating event or recurrent illness
      2) Past medical history
         a) Current or preexisting diseases/illness
            (1) Thyrotoxicosis
            (2) Thyroid disease
            (3) Diabetes
         b) Easy fatigability
         c) Weight loss
         d) Sweating
         e) Body heat loss and heat intolerance
         f) Recent surgery or injury
         g) Current pregnancy
         h) Medications
         i) Allergies
   b. Objective data collection
      1) Physical examination
         a) General appearance
            (1) Level of consciousness, behavior, affect: delirium, agitation, confusion, coma
            (2) Elevated temperature: temperature may exceed 104°F (40°C)
            (3) Tachycardia (120–200 beats/minute), systolic hypertension, and widened pulse pressure
            (4) Severe distress/discomfort, critically ill
         b) Inspection
            (1) Hyperdynamic precordium
            (2) Spider angiomas
            (3) Tremulousness
            (4) Thin, silky hair
            (5) Eye signs
               (a) Lid lag
               (b) Stare
               (c) Exophthalmos
               (d) Periorbital edema
            (6) Jaundice
         c) Auscultation
            (1) Breath sounds: crackles secondary to heart failure
         d) Palpation
            (1) Warm, moist, velvety skin; becomes dry as dehydration develops
            (2) Enlarged thyroid gland with thrill or bruit
            (3) Hepatic tenderness

      2) Diagnostic procedures
         a) Thyroid function studies
            (1) T_4: elevated level
            (2) Triiodothyronine (T_3): elevated resin uptake
            (3) TSH: decreased level
         b) Serum cholesterol level: decreased
         c) Serum chemistries including glucose, BUN, creatinine
            (1) Glucose: increased
         d) CBC with differential: increased WBC count with left shift indicating bacterial infection
         e) Hepatic studies: increased liver enzymes
         f) Urinalysis; pregnancy test in female patients of childbearing age
         g) Cultures as indicated
         h) Chest radiograph
         i) Head CT scan
         j) ECG: rapid atrial fibrillation
2. Analysis: differential nursing diagnoses/collaborative problems
   a. Decreased cardiac output
   b. Impaired gas exchange
   c. Ineffective tissue perfusion
   d. Risk for deficient fluid volume
   e. Hyperthermia
   f. Deficient knowledge
   g. Anxiety/fear
3. Planning and implementation/interventions
   a. Maintain airway, breathing, circulation (see Chapter 1)
   b. Provide supplemental oxygen as indicated
   c. Establish IV access for administration of crystalloid fluids/medications as needed
      1) 5% dextrose and isotonic solution: dextrose solutions preferred because of continuous high metabolic demand and to replenish glycogen stores
   d. Prepare for/assist with medical procedures
      1) Institute cardiac and pulse oximetry monitoring
      2) Catheter placement and monitoring of central venous or pulmonary artery pressures (see Chapter 6)
      3) Maintain normothermic body temperature: use cooling blanket and cold packs to control hyperthermia
      4) Assist with hospital admission
         a) If patient is noncompliant with medication regimen, alert hospital staff to address issue after patient recovers
   e. Administer pharmacologic therapy as ordered
      1) Symptom control
      2) Antipyretics: acetaminophen (Tylenol) only; avoid aspirin because it displaces thyroid hormone from binding sites
      3) Dextrose 50%

4) Thionamides used for the treatment of thyrotoxicosis are either propylthiouracil (PTU) or methimazole (MMI)

5) Glucocorticoids; hydrocortisone: block conversion of T_4 to T_3 to improve survival rates

6) Iodine, Lugol solution, potassium iodide: inhibit hormone release

7) Propranolol, atenolol, or esmolol: administer by IV route to keep heart rate <100 beats/minute; lessens adrenergic effects

8) Digitalis: if beta-blocker medications contraindicated by medical conditions (e.g., asthma, pregnancy, diabetes, heart failure)

9) Antibiotics

10) Vitamins and thiamine

11) Sedatives

4. Evaluation and ongoing monitoring
   a. Level of consciousness
   b. Hemodynamic status
   c. Breath sounds and pulse oximetry
   d. Cardiac rate and rhythm
   e. Signs of hydration
   f. Electrolyte levels
   g. Intake and output

Bibliography

American Diabetes Association: Standards of medical care in diabetes—2015: summary of revisions, *Diabetes Care* 38:S4, 2015.

Bickley LS: *Bates' guide to physical exam and history taking*, ed 11, Philadelphia, PA, 2012, Lippincott, Williams and Wilkins.

Devereaux D, Tewelde SZ: Hyperthyroidism and thyrotoxicosis, *Emerg Med Clin of North Am* 32(2):277–292, 2014.

Godara H: *The Washington manual of medical therapeutics*, Philadelphia, PA, 2014, Lippincott, Williams & Wilkins.

Kasper D: *Harrison's principles of internal medicine*, ed 19, New York, NY, 2015, McGraw Hill.

Tintinalli JE, Stapczynski J, Ma O, Cline DM, Cydulka RK, Meckler GD: *Tintinalli's emergency medicine: a comprehensive study guide*, ed 7, New York, NY, 2012, McGraw-Hill.

CHAPTER 15

Environmental Emergencies

Kathleen Flarity, DNP, PHD, CEN, CFRN, FAEN

I. General Strategy

A. ASSESSMENT

1. Primary and secondary assessment/resuscitation (see Chapter 1)
2. Focused assessment
   a. Subjective data collection
      1) History of present illness/injury/chief complaint
         a) Mechanism of environmental exposure
         b) Environmental factors
            (1) Ambient temperature
            (2) Enclosed space
            (3) Water exposure: type and temperature
            (4) Wet bulb globe temperature (WBGT) index
            (5) Type of insect, animal, or reptile that lives in environment in which patient was found
            (6) Type of clothing/prevention used by patient
         c) Exposure
            (1) Time of exposure or when injury occurred
            (2) Length of time in environment or since incident occurred (e.g., time of submersion)
            (3) Underlying factors predisposing patient to exposure/injury: mental status, use of alcohol or mind-altering substances, lack of available shelter or appropriate clothing, activity before exposure/injury
         d) Pain (see Chapter 8)
            (1) Location of injury and severity of pain
            (2) Radiation with injury or toxicity, especially with envenomation
         e) Rash
         f) Pruritus
         g) Efforts to relieve symptoms
            (1) Home remedies
            (2) Alternative therapies
            (3) Medications
               (a) Prescription
               (b) OTC/herbal
      2) Past medical history
         a) Current or preexisting diseases/illness
            (1) Anaphylaxis
            (2) Alcoholism
            (3) Spinal cord injury
            (4) Central nervous system disorders (e.g., stroke, seizures)
            (5) Asthma

(6) Diabetes mellitus

(7) Cardiovascular disease

(8) Hepatic disease

(9) Hypoadrenalism

(10) Parkinsonism

(11) Hyperthyroidism

(12) Raynaud disease

(13) Cystic fibrosis

(14) Scleroderma

(15) Ectodermal dysplasia

(16) Malaria

(17) Viral infection (e.g., pneumonia, mononucleosis)

(18) Inflammation (e.g., fever)

(19) Malignant hyperthermia

(20) Sickle cell trait

b) Prior environmental injury (hypothermia, hyperthermia)

c) Substance and/or alcohol use/abuse

d) Smoking history

e) Last normal menstrual period: female patients of childbearing age

f) Current medications

  (1) Prescriptions/drug use

    (a) Diuretics

    (b) Anticholinergics (e.g., atropine)

    (c) Beta blockers (e.g., propranolol)

    (d) Amphetamines (e.g., Ecstasy)

    (e) Ergogenic aids (e.g., ephedra)

    (f) Phenothiazines

    (g) Antihistamines

    (h) Tricyclic antidepressants

    (i) Monoamine oxidase (MAO) inhibitors

    (j) Sympatholytic antihypertensives

    (k) Steroids

    (l) Immunosuppressive drugs

    (m) Anticoagulants

  (2) OTC/herbal

g) Allergies

h) Immunization status

i) History of previous rabies immunization

j) History of previous antivenom therapy

3) Psychological/social/environmental factors

a) Alterations in ability to perceive environmental threats

  (1) Age (infants, small children, older adults)

    (a) Pediatric: decision making limited to developmental level

    (b) Older adult: disease process altering ability for decision making/self-care

  (2) Psychiatric illness

  (3) Use of any substance that alters patient's ability to react to environment

b) Physical factors

  (1) Obesity

  (2) Malnutrition

  (3) Lack of psychological and physical preparation

c) Social risk factors

d) Poor physical fitness level

e) Lack of acclimatization

f) Dehydration

  (1) Homelessness or lack of appropriate shelter

  (2) Lack of appropriate clothing

  (3) Possible/actual assault, abuse, intimate partner violence situations (see Chapters 3 and 40)

g) Occupational risk factors

  (1) Firefighters, emergency medical services (EMS), and rescue personnel

  (2) Outside laborers

  (3) Occupations that involve exposure to excessive heat or cold

  (4) Hazardous material workers

  (5) Military personnel

h) Recreational risk factors

  (1) Amateur athletics

  (2) Long-distance running

  (3) Vigorous exercise

  (4) Heavy exertion

  (5) Cold weather sports

  (6) Hiking/walking in unfamiliar areas

i) Environmental risk factors

  (1) Weather conditions

    (a) High ambient temperature: >100.4°F (38°C) or <32°F (0°C)

    (b) Prolonged heat wave

  (2) Wind and wind chill factor

  (3) High humidity

  (4) Contact with metal or water

  (5) Enclosed area

    (a) Temperature

    (b) Ventilation

  (6) Animals, insects, spiders, aquatic animals, or reptiles indigenous to the specific environment

  (7) Raising or working with exotic pets

b. Objective data collection

1) General appearance

a) Level of consciousness, behavior, affect

b) Vital signs

c) Odors

d) Gait

e) Hygiene

f) Level of distress/discomfort

2) Inspection

a) Airway: patent, maintainable, not maintainable; angioedema

b) Erythema of the face, palate

c) Respiratory effort

d) Pupillary function

e) External injuries

f) Skin appearance
(1) Edema
(2) Ulceration
(3) Rash
(4) Urticaria
(5) Ticks
(6) Fang/bite marks
(7) Stingers
g) Bites/wounds
(1) Size
(2) Shape
(3) Depth
(4) Visible skin structures: muscle, subcutaneous tissues
3) Auscultation
a) Breath sounds
b) Heart sounds
c) Bowel sounds
4) Palpation
a) Peripheral and central pulses
b) Skin temperature
c) Area tenderness
d) Motor/sensory
3. Diagnostic procedures
a. Laboratory studies
1) Complete blood count (CBC) with differential
2) Serum chemistries including glucose, BUN, creatinine
3) Liver profiles
4) Coagulation profiles
5) Type and crossmatch
6) Arterial blood gas (ABG)
7) Creatine kinase (CK)
8) Thyroid profile
9) Urinalysis; pregnancy test in female patients of childbearing age
10) Serum and urine toxicology screen
b. Imaging studies: as indicated by injury
1) Plain radiograph
2) Computed tomography (CT) scan
3) Magnetic resonance imaging (MRI)
c. Other
1) 12- to 15-lead electrocardiogram (ECG)

B. ANALYSIS: DIFFERENTIAL NURSING DIAGNOSES/COLLABORATIVE PROBLEMS

1. Ineffective airway clearance
2. Impaired gas exchange
3. Deficient fluid volume
4. Hyperthermia
5. Hypothermia
6. Impaired skin integrity
7. Acute pain
8. Risk for infection
9. Deficient knowledge

C. PLANNING AND IMPLEMENTATION/INTERVENTIONS

1. Determine priorities of care
a. Maintain airway, breathing, circulation (see Chapters 1 and 32)
b. Provide supplemental oxygen as indicated
c. Establish intravenous (IV/IO) access for administration of crystalloid fluid/blood products/medications as needed
d. Obtain and set up equipment and supplies
e. Prepare for/assist with medical interventions
f. Administer pharmacologic therapy as ordered
2. Relieve anxiety/apprehension
3. Allow significant others/caregivers to remain with patient if supportive
4. Educate patient and significant others/caregivers

D. EVALUATION AND ONGOING MONITORING

1. Continuously monitor and treat as indicated
2. Monitor patient response/outcomes, and modify nursing care plan as appropriate
3. If positive patient outcomes are not demonstrated, reevaluate assessment and/or plan of care

E. DOCUMENTATION OF INTERVENTIONS AND PATIENT RESPONSE

F. AGE-RELATED CONSIDERATIONS

1. Pediatrics
a. Growth or development related
1) Death from drowning is among the leading causes of death in children[1,2,3]
2) Infants and small children have small airways, which are more easily obstructed by edema[4]
3) Children have a large ratio of body surface area to body weight and lose body heat more easily[4,5]
4) Children have less adipose tissue to maintain body heat and to provide insulation[4]
5) Infants <3 months of age are unable to produce heat through shivering and must burn brown fat for thermogenesis[4]
6) Children are dependent on caregivers to educate and protect them about the environment in which they live[4]
7) The potential for maltreatment should be considered (e.g., drowning may occur as a result of lack of supervision)[4]
8) Children's healing responses are more rapid than those of adults
b. "Pearls"
1) Children are curious and want to explore their environment; they may be exposed to danger from the environment with little fear of the

consequences of their actions (e.g., young children may not be afraid of a dog they do not know and may approach the animal without fear)[4]

2) Adolescents may take more risks because of peer pressure (potential consequences of this behavior include drowning as a result of swimming while intoxicated)[4]

3) Children are at a greater risk for injury from heat and cold emergencies because of their immature nervous system and dependency on caregivers to maintain the environment around them[4,5]

4) Children are at greater risk for complications from envenomation because of their smaller size and lower body weight[4]

2. Older adult
   a. Aging related
      1) A decrease in elasticity of lung tissue and a decrease in amount of alveoli may contribute to a limited ability to respond to toxic inhalation exposures[6]
      2) Cardiovascular changes that occur with aging cause decreased distensibility of blood vessels, increased systemic resistance, decreased cardiac output, and decreased response to stress[6]
      3) Increased risk for hyperthermia or hypothermia because of an inability to vasodilate or vasoconstrict blood vessels; decreased cardiac output; and decreased subcutaneous tissue[6,7]
      4) Delayed and diminished sweat response[6]
      5) Thirst mechanism becomes less efficient with aging, as does the kidney's ability to concentrate urine, thus increasing the risk of heat-related dehydration[4,5]
      6) Inactivity and immobility increase susceptibility to hypothermia by suppressing shivering and reducing heat-generating muscle activity[6,7]
      7) Medications such as beta blockers can interfere with the body's ability to increase heart rate in response to environmental emergencies[8]
   b. "Pearls"
      1) Older adult patients have thinner skin and may sustain more serious injury from bites[6]
      2) Fluid overload during resuscitation can cause serious consequences
      3) Older adult patients with altered mental status are dependent on caregivers to protect them from danger in the surrounding environment[6]

II. Specific Environmental Emergencies

A. AQUATIC ORGANISM INJURIES

Aquatic organisms usually do not prey on people but will inflict injury when they are disturbed. When disturbed, these creatures may bite or sting, causing mechanical injury and/or envenomation. Some of the most toxic substances

to humans are found in marine organisms. These wounds may also become infected from contaminated water.[9,10]

There are three types of aquatic organisms: (1) creatures that bite and may cause envenomation such as sharks, barracudas, moray eels, octopi, sea snakes, sea lions, and killer whales; the bite wounds vary from punctures to large, avulsion-type wounds; (2) creatures that sting (coelenterates) by means of nematocysts or stinging capsules and produce a wound and envenomation, such as jellyfish, hydrozoans (Portuguese man-of-war), anemones, hydrozoan fire corals, sea wasps, and box jellyfish; and (3) creatures that have spines, which produce traumatic puncture wounds and release toxins from venom sacs such as stingrays, scorpion fish, lionfish, sea urchins, and catfish.[9,11,12,13]

Envenomation from aquatic organisms can result in a variety of symptoms ranging from localized tissue irritation to death. In addition to envenomation, some stings and bites may cause an anaphylactic reaction. Wounds from spiny animals have a high incidence of ulceration, necrosis, and secondary infection. The venom can produce paresthesia, muscle weakness, hypotension, tachycardia, seizures, and cardiopulmonary arrest. People at risk include snorkelers, unprotected divers, and people walking along the beach. It is important to remember that even dead organisms may be able to inflict an injury, and health care providers and rescuers are at risk of being bitten or stung if appropriate precautions are not taken. [9,11,13]

1. Assessment
   a. Subjective data collection
      1) History of present injury/chief complaint
         a) Description, circumstances, time of incident
         b) Unexplained collapse while in water
         c) Geographic area of incident
         d) Description of aquatic organism
         e) Location of injury
         f) Extent of bleeding
         g) Subjective complaints of discomfort
         h) Nausea, vomiting
         i) Muscle weakness, stiffness
         j) Pain (see Chapter 8)
      2) Past medical history
         a) Current and preexisting diseases/illness
            (1) Cardiovascular disease
            (2) Diabetes
         b) Medications
         c) Allergies
         d) Immunization status
   b. Objective data collection
      1) Physical examination
         a) General appearance
            (1) Possible anaphylaxis
            (2) Possible cardiac/respiratory arrest
            (3) Level of consciousness, behavior, affect: seizures
            (4) Possible stridor

(5) Hypotension

(6) Paralysis

(7) Moderate to severe distress/discomfort

   b) Inspection

     (1) Location of wound

     (2) Urticaria

     (3) Bites: size of wound, depth of tissues involved, visible structures, foreign bodies, function of involved part

     (4) Stings: extent of body affected, urticarial lesions, adhered tentacles, barbs, swelling, redness, pain

     (5) Spines: extent of wound, spines, welts, streaks, redness, swelling

 2) Diagnostic procedures

   a) CBC with differential if indicated

   b) ECG

   c) Radiograph examination of affected area if retained parts are suspected or deeper structures involved

   d) Press transparent tape against affected area to obtain nematocysts for species identification

   e) Wound culture and sensitivity if infection suspected

2. Analysis: differential nursing diagnoses/collaborative problems

  a. Risk for ineffective airway clearance

  b. Ineffective breathing

  c. Acute pain

  d. Impaired skin integrity

  e. Risk for infection

  f. Deficient knowledge

3. Planning and implementation/interventions

  a. Maintain airway, breathing, circulation (see Chapters 1 and 32)

   1) Initiate or continue BLS and ALS per protocols if respiratory/cardiac arrest is present

  b. Provide supplemental oxygen as indicated

  c. Establish IV/IO access for administration of crystalloid fluid/medications as needed

  d. Prepare for/assist with medical interventions

   1) Treat anaphylaxis (see discussion of insects in Bites and Stings and Chapters 21 and 28)

   2) Aquatic bite wound care

    a) Cleanse wound with mild antiseptic soap

    b) Irrigate with copious amounts of normal saline

    c) Assist with or administer local anesthetic

    d) Assist or perform wound debridement and closure as indicated by the location and type of wound

    e) Apply appropriate dressing

   3) Coelenterate (e.g., jellyfish) sting wound care

    a) Immediately rinse wound with sea/saltwater[9,11]

    b) Do not rub area or use fresh water because this will stimulate the nematocysts that have not already fired

    c) Remove tentacles with gloved hand and forceps or hemostats

    d) Apply acetic acid 5% (vinegar) to inactivate the toxin

    e) Isopropyl alcohol 40–70% may be used as an alternative, but not for box jellyfish stings

    f) After soaking wound in vinegar or alcohol, remove remaining nematocysts by applying shaving cream or a paste with baking soda, flour, or talc, and shave the area

    g) A papain paste of meat tenderizer may be used for the pruritic dermatitis caused by larval forms of certain coelenterates

   4) Stingray wound care

    a) Immediate immersion of affected part in hot water 110–115°F (43.7–46.5°C) for 60–90 minutes for pain relief and deactivation of the heat susceptible venom [9,11,12,14]

    b) Radiology or otherwise imaged for foreign body

    c) Wound is cleansed, explored, and thoroughly debrided; may be packed open for delayed primary closure or sutured loosely[8,9,11,15]

   5) Scorpion fish and lionfish wound care

    a) Immediate immersion of affected part in hot water 110–115°F (43.7–46.5°C) for 60–90 minutes for pain relief and deactivation of the heat-susceptible venom [8,9,11,13]

    b) Wound should be explored to remove any retained spine fragments

   6) If evidence of a deeply retained spine or suspected foreign body, the wound should be surgically explored in the operating room with magnification; vigorous warmed saline irrigation should be performed, and the wound should be allowed to heal open with provision for adequate drainage[8,11,12,16]

  e. Administer pharmacologic therapy as ordered

   1) ALS medications per protocols if cardiopulmonary arrest or anaphylaxis occurs

   2) Topical anesthetics, antihistamines, and corticosteroid ointments may be applied after nematocyst removal to decrease pain

   3) Antivenom (available from Australia's Commonwealth Serum Laboratories for serious stings from stonefish and box jellyfish envenomations) as indicated[8]

   4) Nonnarcotic analgesics

   5) Narcotics

   6) Prophylactic antibiotics are recommended for many aquatic injuries because of the high incidence of ulceration, necrosis, and secondary infection[8,11]

   7) Tetanus immunization

  f. Educate patient/significant others

1) Wound care
2) Signs and symptoms of infection
3) Medication administration
4) Follow-up care
5) Prevention
   a) Remain far away from aquatic organisms that can inflict injury
   b) Wear protective clothing such as "stinger suits" and gloves
   c) Do not attempt to move dead aquatic organisms
4. Evaluation and ongoing monitoring
  a. Airway patency
  b. Level of consciousness
  c. Hemodynamic status
  d. Breath sounds and pulse oximetry
  e. Cardiac rate and rhythm
  f. Pain relief

B. BITES AND STINGS

A bite or a sting may produce a puncture wound or laceration and may cause serious complications, including anaphylaxis, envenomation, tissue damage, wound infection, and transmission of illnesses such as rabies or Lyme disease. Each year, thousands of patients are treated for bites and stings in the ED.[17,18,19] There are multiple sources of bites and stings, including mammals, reptiles, marine animals, insects, and spiders. Common sources of bites and stings in the United States are summarized in Table 15.1.

Occasionally, patients present to the ED after having been bitten or stung by an exotic insect or animal. People at greatest risk of being bitten or stung include young children, people working outside, and people unfamiliar with the insect or animal they are handling.[17,18,19]

HUMAN BITES (SEE CHAPTER 30)

DOMESTIC/WILD ANIMALS. Domestic and wild animal bites can produce deep lacerations, tearing, cutting, and crushing injuries and have the potential for infection and the transmission of diseases such as rabies. Animal bites, of all lacerations, are frequently contaminated with a broad variety of pathogens.[17–21] Animals, particularly dogs, can also produce crush injuries as a result of the power of their jaws closing on to an extremity or other exposed body part. Bite injuries may result in damage to the scalp, face, hands, and feet and may cause long-term scarring and loss of function.[17–21]

Most animal bites are from domestic dogs and cats.[17,18] There are approximately 20 animal bite–related deaths annually, mostly from dogs.[22] The majority (80–90%) of bites are inflicted by dogs. It is estimated that dogs bite 1.8% of all Americans, resulting in 4.7 million wounds annually.[22] More than 750,000 of these victims seek medical attention.[17,22] Domestic cats account for 5–15% of treated bites, although some studies report a figure as high as 25%. The bite location and affected populations vary by animal.[17] Cat bites occur most frequently in adult women on the extremities.[18,19] Most dog bites occur on the extremities; however, head, face, and neck bites are more common among children. Children, especially boys between the ages of 5 and 9 years, are at greatest risk of being bitten by animals, particularly dogs.[18,19] Dogs are bred to protect their territory, and when someone unfamiliar approaches them, they feel threatened and may bite in defense. Dog bites are also responsible for the majority of deaths reported from nonvenomous animals. Cats are another source of animal bites, and complications of cat bites may result from deep penetration leading to infection and cellulitis from the organism *Pasteurella*, which is carried in the cat's mouth. Although studies have shown that infections from cat bites are usually polymicrobial, *Pasteurella* is the most common organism.[18,19,20]

Wild animals, especially bats, are the most common source of human rabies infection in the United States. Other animals that may transmit rabies include skunks and raccoons. Knowing the rabies risk in the local area is important. The local animal control agency or health authority can provide information. Animal bites must be reported to health authorities, based on local and state regulations.

1. Assessment
  a. Subjective data collection
    1) History of present injury/chief complaint
      a) Type of animal that inflicted injury
      b) If the animal is known to the victim
      c) Provocation of animal
      d) Rabies status, if a domestic animal
      e) Time of injury
      f) Location of injury
      g) Extent of bleeding
      h) Pain (see Chapter 8)
    2) Past medical history
      a) Current or preexisting diseases/illness
        (1) Cardiovascular disease
        (2) Diabetes
        (3) Immunocompromised
      b) Medications
      c) Allergies
      d) Immunization status
  b. Objective data collection
    1) Physical examination

Table 15.1

Common Sources of Bites and Stings in the United States

Bites	Stings
Dogs	Bees
Cats	Wasps
Humans	Ants
Rodents	Scorpions
Horses	Some Marine Animals
Reptiles	
Bats	
Raccoons	
Skunks	
Spiders	

a) General appearance
  (1) Level of consciousness, behavior, affect: anxiety
  (2) Mild to moderate distress/discomfort
b) Inspection
  (1) Location of wound
  (2) Size of wound
  (3) Depth of wound
  (4) Obvious deep structure injury to tendons, muscles, bone, presence of foreign body (teeth)
c) Palpation
  (1) Neurovascular status of injured area
  (2) Function of injured area
2) Diagnostic procedures
  a) CBC with differential if indicated
  b) Wound culture and sensitivity of infected wounds if indicated (do not culture fresh wounds)
  c) Radiograph of injured area
2. Analysis: differential nursing diagnoses/collaborative problems
  a. Impaired skin integrity
  b. Risk for infection
  c. Acute pain
  d. Deficient knowledge
3. Planning and implementation/interventions
  a. Maintain airway, breathing, circulation (see Chapters 1 and 32)
  b. Provide supplemental oxygen as indicated
  c. Establish IV/IO access for administration of crystalloid fluid/medications as needed
  d. Prepare for/assist with medical interventions
    1) Provide wound care
      a) Control active bleeding
      b) Cleanse with mild antiseptic soap
      c) Pressure irrigate with copious amounts of normal saline
      d) Anesthetize wound as needed for patient comfort/pain management
      e) Evaluate for potential blunt trauma and injury to deeper and vital structures caused by penetrating teeth or claws[17–20]
      f) Wound should be carefully explored for tendon or bone involvement and foreign bodies such as teeth fragments
      g) Assist with or perform tissue debridement of obviously crushed and devitalized tissue
      h) Do not give prophylactic antibiotics for routine low-risk bite wounds
    2) Assist with or perform wound closure if indicated; delayed closure may be indicated to decrease risk of infection, but is determined by location and age of wound. Traditionally, animal bite wounds were left open to prevent secondary infections; however, providers should review factors that increase the risk of infection from animal bites[17,18,19]

a) Procedural sedation as needed
b) Selective treatment (wounds by risk factors)
  (1) Suture, staple, or use adhesive strips to close all skin wounds in the usual fashion, unless wounds are high risk (e.g., hand wounds, high-risk species, immunosuppressed patient)[15,17,19,23]
  (2) Culture infected wounds only if they show signs of established infection or if there is evidence of sepsis
  (3) Consider surgical consultation and delayed primary closure for high-risk wounds[15,17,23]
  (4) Strongly consider administration of prophylactic antibiotics to victims with high-risk wounds (amoxicillin–clavulanate as first line). To most effectively prevent wound infection, antibiotics should be started within 1 hour of injury[15,17,19,23]
  (5) After cleansing, cover the wound with sterile dressings
3) Assist in hospital admission if more extensive treatment required
e. Administer pharmacologic therapy as ordered
  1) Nonnarcotic analgesics
  2) Narcotics
  3) Procedural sedation medications
  4) Antibiotics
  5) Immunizations
    a) Tetanus immunization if >5 years since last immunization
    b) Rabies prophylaxis; if animal is suspected to be rabid (e.g., atypical behavior, high-risk species) assess need for rabies immune globulin and vaccine[6,24]
      (1) Rabies immune globulin (RIG): administer only if not previously vaccinated; 20 units/kg preferably infused around wound site, and residual volume administered intramuscularly (IM) at distant site[6,24]
      (2) Human diploid cell vaccine (HDCV), or rabies vaccine adsorbed (RVA): administer if not previously vaccinated; 1 mL IM deltoid on days 0, 3, 7, and 14[6,24]
      (3) HDCV or RVA: administer if previously vaccinated; 1 mL IM deltoid on days 0 and 3[6,24]
f. Educate patient and significant others
  1) Wound care
  2) Signs and symptoms of infection
  3) Medication administration
  4) Rabies prophylaxis schedule
  5) Follow-up care
  6) Bite injury prevention measures
    a) Be familiar with local animal behaviors
    b) Remain motionless when approached by an unfamiliar dog

c) If knocked down by a dog, roll into a ball and lie still

d) Do not keep dangerous animals where children can easily be exposed to them

4. Evaluation and ongoing monitoring
   a. Pain relief

SNAKES. Venomous snakebites are estimated at 7,000–8,000 in the United States per year with an annual incidence of 10 to 15 deaths.[8] Snakebites usually cause either a laceration or a puncture wound. Snakebites may become infected, but the major complication is envenomation. There are five families of venomous snakes but, with few exceptions, most fall into the families Viperidae (vipers and pit vipers) and Elapidae. The medically important North American venomous snakes are in the families Viperidae (subfamily Crotalinae, the pit vipers) and Elapidae (subfamily Elapinae [the coral snakes] and subfamily Hydrophiinae [the sea snakes]). In the United States, pit vipers are responsible for the majority of bites. Rattlesnakes are the most widespread pit vipers, found throughout much of North America. At least one species is found in each of the 48 contiguous states except Maine.[8,25,26,27] Pit vipers include timber and related rattlesnakes (*Crotalus*), massasauga and related rattlesnakes (*Sistrurus*), and copperheads and cottonmouths or water moccasins (*Agkistrodon*). The other large family of venomous snakes is the Elapidae, which includes coral snakes. Occasionally, a snake not native to the country bites a patient, whether it occurs at a zoo or in one's home where the reptile is kept as a pet. Snakebites most often occur in the lower extremities, but they also may involve the hands or the face. Dry bites occur in 20% of the cases and result in no significant symptoms. Following true Crotalinae envenomation, patients quickly develop burning pain and edema at the site. Ecchymoses and bullae develop after the edema spreads from the bite site.[8,25,26,27] Venom contains enzymes and proteins, which may cause local tissue damage, massive tissue edema, hypotension, coagulopathy, shock, and death. With *Elapidae* envenomation, little or no local reaction may be noted even with significant envenomation, although mild swelling or paresthesias may be present at the bite site. Symptom onset may be delayed 13 hours or longer. Patients with paresthesias and dysesthesias (unpleasant, abnormal sensations such as burning) are at greater risk for developing neuromuscular blockade and subsequent respiratory distress. People at risk for snakebites include snake handlers, hikers, campers, and intoxicated individuals. Adverse reactions that occur with new-generation antivenoms are less frequent and less severe than those reported with previous preparations.[8,25,26]

1. Assessment
   a. Subjective data collection
      1) History of present injury/chief complaint
         a) Description of incident
         b) Description and identification of the snake
            (1) Pit vipers have a triangular head with a pit between eyes and nostril (heat-sensing device), catlike elliptical pupils, two fangs that fold back when the mouth is closed, a single row of subcaudal scales on the underbelly, and interconnecting horny segments on the tail that function as a rattle on the rattlesnake
            (2) Coral snakes have red, yellow, and black bands; a black head; slender body; small, fixed fangs; and round, black eyes
               (a) The saying "red on yellow, kill a fellow; red on black, venom lack" differentiates coral snakes from harmless snakes, but applies only to *Micrurus fulvius* and *Micrurus fulvius tenere* found in the southern and eastern United States
         c) Location of bite
         d) Size and weight of victim
         e) Prehospital care provided
         f) Signs and symptoms before arrival
         g) Shortness of breath
         h) Weakness, paresthesia, diplopia, muscle pain
         i) Nausea and vomiting, diarrhea
         j) Time of incident
      2) Past medical history
         a) Current or preexisting diseases/illness
            (1) Cardiovascular disease
            (2) Diabetes
            (3) Immunocompromised
         b) Previous bite injury
         c) Previous administration of antivenom
         d) Medications
         e) Allergies
         f) Immunization status
   b. Objective data collection
      1) Physical examination
         a) General appearance
            (1) Level of consciousness, behavior, affect: anxiety, euphoria, confusion, seizures
            (2) Flaccid paralysis
            (3) Moderate to severe distress/discomfort
         b) Inspection
            (1) Appearance of wound
               (a) Pit viper: fang marks, semicircular teeth marks
               (b) Coral snake: scratch marks or tiny puncture marks
               (c) Nonvenomous: scratch marks, teeth marks
            (2) Ecchymosis, edema of area
            (3) Vesicles, bullae at or around bite site
            (4) Diaphoresis
            (5) Bleeding
      2) Diagnostic procedures
         a) CBC with differential
         b) Serum chemistries, CK

c) Type and crossmatch

d) Coagulation profile including platelets, fibrin split products

e) ABGs: if systemic symptoms present

f) Urinalysis: myoglobin

g) Wound culture and sensitivity

h) Radiograph of injured area as indicated: retained fangs

i) Chest radiograph: if history of pulmonary edema

j) EKG: if patient complains of chest pain, dyspnea, or has cardiac comorbidities

2. Analysis: differential nursing diagnoses/collaborative problems

a. Risk for ineffective airway clearance

b. Deficient fluid volume

c. Impaired skin integrity

d. Risk for infection

e. Acute pain

f. Anxiety/fear

g. Deficient knowledge

3. Planning and implementation/interventions

a. Maintain airway, breathing, circulation (see Chapters 1 and 32)

b. Provide supplemental oxygen

1) Patients with bites to the face or neck may require early endotracheal intubation to prevent loss of the airway caused by severe swelling

c. Establish IV/IO access for administration of crystalloid fluids/blood products/medications

1) With potential coagulopathy, venipuncture attempts should be minimized and noncompressible entry sites (e.g., subclavian vein) should be avoided[8]

2) As IV lines are placed, obtain blood draw for initial laboratory analysis (CBC, coagulation studies, electrolytes, renal and hepatic function studies, CK and blood typing and screening)[8]

d. Prepare for/assist with medical interventions

1) Immobilize affected part: do not apply tourniquets

2) Institute cardiac and pulse oximetry monitoring

3) Perform wound care, mark site of bite and perform serial measurements of increasing edema and redness; may need compartment measures

4) Determine the severity of envenomation and need for antivenom

5) Assist with hospital admission and possible fasciotomy for severe tissue injury

e. Administer pharmacologic therapy as ordered indications for antivenom and how administered

1) Antivenom: crotaline polyvalent immune fab (CroFab) most therapeutic when given within 4 hours of the bite; limited value after 12 hours.

Adverse reactions that occur with new-generation antivenom are less frequent and less severe than those reported with previous preparations[8,25,27]

2) Nonnarcotic analgesics

3) Narcotics

4) Antibiotics

5) Tetanus immunization

f. Educate patient and significant others

1) Wound care

2) Signs and symptoms of infection

3) Medication administration

4) Follow-up care

5) Prevention

a) Wear boots or high-top shoes when hiking

b) Do not attempt to pick up or provoke a snake

c) Be familiar with venomous species in areas where camping or hiking

4. Evaluation and ongoing monitoring

a. Airway patency

b. Level of consciousness

c. Hemodynamic status

d. Breath sounds and pulse oximetry

e. Cardiac rate and rhythm

f. Extremity edema progression

g. Neurovascular status distal to bite

h. Pain relief

INSECTS. The most common sources of venomous insects are members of the order Hymenoptera, including bees, wasps, and ants.[8] An insect sting causes a break in the skin and the deposit of a stinger, which contains an apparatus that injects venom into its victim. Venom is used for defense and to subdue the insect's prey. A serious complication of stings is anaphylaxis. Each year approximately 40 to 50 deaths occur per year in North America from Hymenoptera stings as the result of anaphylaxis occurring in victims with prior stings who developed specific immunoglobulin E (IgE) antibodies.[8] Anaphylaxis (see Chapters 21 and 28) is an acute allergic reaction that results from an exposure to a foreign protein to which the patient has already been sensitized. Signs and symptoms of anaphylaxis include facial or oral edema (angioedema), respiratory distress (stridor, wheezing, sternal retractions), and urticaria.[28] People at risk for insect stings include anyone who works outside, hikers, and campers.

1. Assessment

a. Subjective data collection

1) History of present injury/chief complaint

a) Type of insect

b) Description and location of sting(s)

c) Time incident occurred

d) Symptoms experienced after sting(s)

(1) Pain (see Chapter 8)

(2) Swelling, pruritus

(3) Shortness of breath

2) Past medical history
   a) Current or preexisting diseases/illness
      (1) Asthma
   b) Allergy to stings
   c) Medications
   d) Allergies
   e) Immunization status
b. Objective data collection
   1) Physical examination
      a) General appearance
         (1) Level of consciousness, behavior, affect: awake to comatose
         (2) Stridor
         (3) Hypotension, tachycardia
         (4) Mild to severe distress/discomfort
      b) Inspection
         (1) Appearance of skin site: redness, warmth, wheal formation, blisters
         (2) Presence of stinger
         (3) Cardiac dysrhythmias on monitor
      c) Auscultation
         (1) Breath sounds: wheezing if respiratory involvement
   2) Diagnostic procedures
      a) CBC with differential if indicated
      b) Wound culture and sensitivity if indicated
      c) Chest radiograph
      d) EKG
2. Analysis: differential nursing diagnoses/collaborative problems
   a. Risk for ineffective airway clearance
   b. Ineffective tissue perfusion
   c. Acute pain
   d. Deficient knowledge
3. Planning and implementation/interventions
   a. Maintain airway, breathing, circulation (see Chapter 1)
      1) Initiate or continue BLS and ALS per protocols if anaphylaxis/arrest is present
   b. Provide supplemental oxygen as indicated
      1) Intubation and ventilatory support in patients in respiratory/cardiac arrest
      2) High-flow oxygen
   c. Establish IV/IO access for administration of crystalloid fluids/medications as needed[29]
   d. Prepare for/assist with medical interventions
      1) Advanced airway management
         a) Nasal or oral intubation: supraglottic airway (e.g., King, Combitube, laryngeal mask airway)
         b) Surgical airway (e.g., cricothyrotomy)
      2) Remove stinger using a gentle, scraping motion with a credit card or similar tool. Do not squeeze or use tweezers; such techniques may cause contraction of the venom sac and release more contents into the puncture site[8]
      3) Clean area with mild antiseptic soap

4) Apply ice packs, baking soda paste, or aloe vera for comfort
5) Institute cardiac and pulse oximetry monitoring
6) Assist with hospital admission if respiratory difficulty or anaphylaxis. Persons with insect sting anaphylaxis require close observation, preferably in the hospital, over a period of 24 hours[8,28,29]
e. Administer medications as prescribed
   1) Epinephrine
      a) Epinephrine 1:1000 subcutaneously or IM at first indication of serious hypersensitivity. Adult dose is 0.3–0.5 mL, and for children <12 years 0.01 mL/kg, not to exceed 0.3 mL,[8,28] may repeat every 10–15 minutes
      b) In the presence of profound hypotension/shock, give 2–5 mL of a 1:10,000 epinephrine by slow IV push, or an infusion may be initiated by mixing 1 mg in 250 mL and infusing at a rate of 0.25–1 mL/minute[8,28]
      c) IV crystalloid solutions for hypotension/shock; pressor agents such as dopamine or norepinephrine may be required
      d) Fire ant bites: oral antihistamines and corticosteroids may provide some relief in severe cases. Because infection is common, topical antimicrobials (e.g., mupirocin) and prophylactic oral antibiotics are recommended. Breaking fire ant blisters should be avoided[8]
      e) Envenomation from multiple hymenopteran stings may require more aggressive therapy
   2) ALS medications per protocols
   3) Diphenhydramine (Benadryl)
   4) Histamine blockers
   5) β_2-selective inhaled agents
   6) Corticosteroids
   7) IV calcium gluconate (5–10 mL of 10% solution)
   8) Nonnarcotic analgesics
   9) Antibiotics
   10) Tetanus immunization
f. Educate patient and significant others
   1) Wound care
   2) Signs and symptoms of infection
   3) Signs and symptoms of anaphylaxis
   4) Follow-up care
   5) Prevention (e.g., wear light-colored clothing, use appropriate insect repellent)
   6) Patients with history of allergic reaction should carry an emergency kit, which includes injectable epinephrine and an oral antihistamine. Two commonly available epinephrine kits include Ana-Kit (Holister-Stier) and EpiPen/EpiPen JR (Center Laboratories)[8,28]

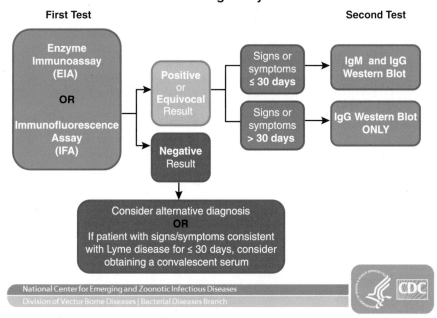

Two-Tiered Testing for Lyme Disease

First Test — **Second Test**

Enzyme Immunoassay (EIA) OR Immunofluorescence Assay (IFA) → Positive or Equivocal Result → Signs or symptoms ≤ 30 days → IgM and IgG Western Blot

Signs or symptoms > 30 days → IgG Western Blot ONLY

Negative Result → Consider alternative diagnosis OR If patient with signs/symptoms consistent with Lyme disease for ≤ 30 days, consider obtaining a convalescent serum

National Center for Emerging and Zoonotic Infectious Diseases
Division of Vector Borne Diseases | Bacterial Diseases Branch

CDC

FIG. 15.1 Two-tiered testing for Lyme disease. *(From Centers for Disease Control and Prevention. (2015). Two-step laboratory testing process. Available at* http://www.cdc.gov/LYME/DIAGNOSISTESTING/LABTEST/TWOSTEP/INDEX.HTML)

7) Teach patient strategies to help avoid future stings, including
   a) Do not wear perfumes or scented products when outside; stay away from flowers
   b) Avoid eating outside; keep drinks covered
   c) Keep garbage containers covered; stay away from rotting fruit or food
   d) Do not walk barefoot outside
   e) Keep windows closed or screened
4. Evaluation and ongoing monitoring
   a. Airway patency
   b. Hemodynamic status
   c. Breath sounds and pulse oximetry
   d. Cardiac rate and rhythm
   e. Extremity edema progression
   f. Pain relief

TICKS. Ticks are arthropods that attach and feed on the blood of mammals. Tick bites are often asymptomatic. Victims are frequently unaware of the presence of the insects because they are small and flat when not engorged with blood and may be in places difficult to view, such as one's head covered by hair. Various ticks transmit diseases such as Lyme disease, Rocky Mountain spotted fever, ehrlichiosis, tularemia, and Colorado tick fever.[8,30,31,32] Lyme disease is the most frequently reported vector-borne disease in the United States with 30,000 cases reported each year (Fig. 15.1).[30] Some ticks can inject neurotoxins, which may cause paralysis. As the length of time of attachment increases, the potential for infection also increases. People at risk for tick bites are children, outside workers (particularly in high-grass or wooded areas), hikers, and campers. There are three stages of Lyme disease with

TABLE 15.2

Stages and Symptoms of Lyme Disease

Stage	Symptoms
First Stage 1–4 weeks after tick bite	Bull's-eye rash on thigh, groin, or axilla Rash expansion (erythema chronicum migrans) Nonspecific flulike symptoms: headache, stiff neck, fatigue, joint and muscle aches
Second Stage 4–10 weeks after tick bite	Symptoms disappear in 2 weeks if not treated Systemic dissemination
Third Stage Weeks to years after tick bite	Monoarticular arthritis Multiple skin lesions Neurologic complications: memory loss, meningitis, poor motor coordination Cardiac involvement: atrioventricular block Meningoencephalitis Myocarditis Recurrent exacerbations of arthritis

(Data from Centers for Disease Control and Prevention. (2015). Educational materials. Lyme disease: What you need to know. http://www.cdc.gov/lyme/resources/brochure/lymediseasebrochure.pdf; Auerbach, P. S. (2012). Tick-borne diseases. In S. J. Traub and G. A. Cummins (Eds.), *Wilderness medicine* (954–975). St. Louis, MO: Elsevier.)

differing symptoms (Table 15.2).[30,32] Early, accurate diagnosis and treatment is the most effective way to avoid more serious illness and the potential for long-term complications related to Lyme. However, diagnostics are less than optimal for early Lyme disease, as it may take weeks for a detectable immune response to be sufficiently measured. Patients treated with appropriate antibiotics in the early stages of Lyme disease usually recover rapidly and completely.[30,31,32]

1. Assessment
    a. Subjective data collection
        1) History of present injury/chief complaint
            a) Walking in an area where ticks may be present
            b) Location of bite or where the tick was found
            c) Weakness, muscle and joint pain, progressive ascending paralysis
            d) Headache
            e) Photophobia
            f) Fever/chills
        2) Past medical history
            a) Current or preexisting diseases/illness
            b) Allergies
            c) Medications
            d) Immunization status
    b. Objective data collection
        1) Physical examination
            a) General appearance
                (1) Possible symmetrical ascending paralysis
                (2) Possible bulbar paralysis and respiratory failure
                (3) Mild to severe distress/discomfort
            b) Inspection
                (1) Tick attached to body
                (2) Skin rash initially on ankles and wrists; spreading to palms of hands and soles of feet, and later to axillae, trunk, and face
                (3) Cardiac dysrhythmia on monitor: atrioventricular blocks associated with Lyme disease
            c) Palpation
                (1) Paresthesia in the legs
        2) Diagnostic procedures
            a) CBC with differential
            b) Serum chemistries including glucose, BUN, creatinine
            c) Coagulation profile including PT, PTT, fibrin-split products
            d) Urinalysis; pregnancy test in female patients of childbearing age
            e) Lyme antibody titers; enzyme immunoassay (ELA) or immunofluorescence assay (IFA); if negative, consider alternative diagnosis or in cases where patient has had symptoms for <30 days, may treat and follow up with a convalescent serum. If first test yields positive or equivocal results, two options are available
                (1) If patient has had symptoms for ≤30 days, an IgM Western blot is performed
                (2) If patient has had symptoms for >30 days, the IgG Western blot is performed. The IgM should not be used if patient has been ill for >30 days[30,32]
            f) ECG

2. Analysis: differential nursing diagnoses/collaborative problems
    a. Ineffective airway clearance
    b. Acute pain
    c. Deficient knowledge
3. Planning and implementation/interventions
    a. Maintain airway, breathing, circulation (see Chapter 1)
    b. Provide supplemental oxygen as indicated
    c. Establish IV/IO access for administration of crystalloid fluids/medications as needed
    d. Prepare for/assist with medical interventions
        1) Patients with stage 3 Lyme disease may require pacemaker insertion for cardiac rhythm control
        2) Institute cardiac and pulse oximetry monitoring
        3) Remove tick
            a) Do not crush or squeeze tick
            b) Grasp tick with forceps as close to skin and mouthparts of tick as possible; gently pull or twist with steady, upward and outward pressure, and remove tick from skin[8,32]
            c) Examine the skin closely for any remaining parts; if head becomes disengaged or mouthparts remain, remove just as though these pieces were a splinter
            d) Applying heat or irritants to tick before removal is not recommended
            e) Save tick for species identification
        4) Clean site with mild antiseptic soap
    e. Administer pharmacologic therapy as ordered
        1) Nonnarcotic analgesics
        2) Antibiotics commonly used for oral treatment include doxycycline, amoxicillin, or cefuroxime axetil[30,32]
        3) Tetanus immunization
    f. Educate patient and significant others
        1) Wound care
        2) Medication administration
        3) Signs and symptoms of infection
        4) Follow-up care
        5) Prevention
            a) Wear protective clothing, long sleeves, and light colors
            b) Tuck pant legs into socks or boots
            c) Use tick repellents when outdoors in a known tick area
            d) Inspect all body parts carefully and regularly (at least twice daily)
4. Evaluation and ongoing monitoring
    a. Hemodynamic status
    b. Breath sounds and pulse oximetry
    c. Cardiac rate and rhythm
    d. Pain relief
    e. Pruritus intensity

SPIDERS. Awareness of the differential diagnosis is important for the management of suspected spider bites because the spider is rarely observed and identified. In general, spiders only bite humans in defense.[31,33,34] The two particular species of spiders in the United States that can cause significant problems with envenomation are the black widow (*Latrodectus mactans*) and the brown recluse (*Loxosceles reclusa*) spiders. Necrotic arachnidism occurs in wounds caused by the envenomation of various spiders, including the brown recluse spider, the hobo spider in the northwestern United States, and the jumping spider in the southern states. These spiders release a substance that results in tissue injury, necrosis, and thrombosis. Black widow spiders are found in all states except Alaska. They live in the ground in secluded, dark areas such as garages, barns, sheds, and outhouses. The venom of the black widow is a neurotoxin. When bitten by a black widow spider, patients feel a pinprick-like sensation, rapidly followed by a dull ache. Systemic symptoms generally occur 30 minutes after envenomation. These include abdominal symptoms mimicking those of an acute abdomen, hypertension, nausea, vomiting, and tachycardia.[31,33,34] The brown recluse spider is predominantly found in the southeastern United States, in such places as woodpiles or storage areas. The bite is often painless, with development of vesicles, bullae, and erythema after 1 to 3 hours. Pruritus and pain begin as the wound becomes hemorrhagic and erythematous. A painful, purple purpura develops and progresses to a necrotic ulcerating wound. This wound can extend deep into the tissue and can take a long time to heal.[31,33,34] Within 24 to 72 hours, systemic symptoms may begin, including fever, chills, nausea, vomiting, malaise, and myalgias. Most brown recluse spider bites heal within 2 to 3 months without medical intervention. Necrotic arachnidism or loxoscelism occurs in 10% of patients with envenomation. These cases may result in serious cutaneous injuries, with subsequent necrosis and tissue loss. Less often, severe systemic reactions may occur with hemolysis, coagulopathy, renal failure, and even death.[31,33,34] The excision of necrotic skin site may be advisable (especially for the rare large lesion) but only after 6 to 8 weeks of wound care, by which time an eschar has formed, adjacent tissues have recovered, and normal healing is possible. Early surgery usually is inadvisable. Several other spiders can cause a similar progression of symptoms. People at risk for spider bites include outside workers, anyone working in such areas as woodpiles, and children.[31,33,34]

1. Assessment
   a. Subjective data collection
      1) History of present injury/chief complaint
         a) History of spider bite or working in area where a spider may be found
         b) Black widow: complaint of sharp pinprick followed by dull ache
         c) Brown recluse: based on location
         d) Spider identification
            (1) Local findings of importance include anatomic location (spiders are more likely to bite defensively at sites where clothing binds tightly; thin skin is more readily envenomed than callous skin) and number of separate lesions (multiple bites suggest parasitic insect bite rather than spider bite)[33]
            (2) Black widow: shiny, black body with red hourglass or irregular markings on abdomen
            (3) Brown recluse: small, brown or tan, with dark band shaped like violin on cephalothorax
         e) Location of bite
         f) Time of bite
         g) Pain (see Chapter 8)
            (1) Black widow: severe pain 15–60 minutes after bite, increasing for 12–48 hours; pain in abdomen and back, paresthesias
         h) Nausea, vomiting
         i) Shortness of breath
      2) Past medical history
         a) Current or preexisting diseases/illness
            (1) Cardiovascular disease
            (2) Diabetes
         b) Medications
         c) Allergies
         d) Immunization status
   b. Objective data collection
      1) Physical examination
         a) General appearance
            (1) Systemic findings, depending on the species involved, may include changes in vital signs, diaphoresis, generalized rash, facial edema, gastrointestinal distress, muscle fasciculations, spasm or tenderness, or altered mental status. Possible seizure with black widow spider[8,31,33,34]
            (2) Mild to severe distress/discomfort
         b) Inspection
            (1) Black widow bite: swelling; presence of tiny fang marks; hypertension; paresthesias
            (2) Brown recluse bite: local reaction beginning in 2–8 hours; redness, blister formation, and ischemia; dark, firm center in 2–4 days; ulcer formation in 7–14 days
         c) Palpation
            (1) Paresthesias: black widow spider
            (2) Abdominal rigidity/guarding: black widow spider
      2) Diagnostic procedures
         a) For patients with significant local or systemic signs or symptoms
         b) CBC with differential
         c) Basic coagulation screening

d) Liver and renal function tests

e) Serum chemistries

f) Coagulation studies

g) Glucose-6-phosphate dehydrogenase (G6PD) level: if Dapsone is being considered for brown recluse envenomation

h) Urinalysis; pregnancy test in female patients of childbearing age

i) Wound discharge culture and sensitivity

j) Acute abdominal radiograph: diagnosis unclear in patient with abdominal pain

k) ECG

2. Analysis: differential nursing diagnoses/collaborative problems

   a. Pain

   b. Impaired skin integrity

   c. Risk for infection

   d. Deficient knowledge

3. Planning and implementation/interventions

   a. Maintain airway, breathing, circulation (see Chapter 1)

   b. Provide supplemental oxygen as indicated

   c. Establish IV/IO access for administration of crystalloid fluid/medications as needed

   d. Prepare for/assist with medical interventions (general supportive measures are the mainstays of therapy for most spider bites)

     1) Provide care for black widow envenomation

       a) Apply local cold compresses to decrease venom absorption

       b) Institute cardiac and pulse oximetry monitoring

     2) Provide care for brown recluse envenomation

       a) Clean area of bite with mild antiseptic soap

       b) Elevate affected extremity

       c) Perform wound care: necrotic lesions may need debridement after erythema has subsided; however, no sooner than 1 or 2 weeks after the bite, with close follow-up for several weeks. In severe cases skin grafting or plastic surgery may be needed when the wound is stable[31,33,34]

       d) Assist with possible hospital admission for hyperbaric therapy

   e. Administer pharmacologic therapy as ordered

     1) Analgesics/narcotics

     2) Muscle relaxants

     3) Antihistamines may help control itching but do not change the lesion[33]

     4) Hydration

     5) Antivenom

       a) Black widow antivenom after appropriate skin testing

       b) Brown recluse antivenom

     6) Corticosteroids are of unproved benefit and are generally not indicated although Dapsone has been used (brown recluse spider)

7) Surgical follow-up is indicated for debridement and management of extensive necrotic lesions

8) Antibiotics are not of value for simple venom injury, but are prescribed when bacterial cellulitis cannot be eliminated from the differential diagnosis

9) Tetanus immunization

   f. Educate patient/significant others

     1) Wound care

     2) Medication administration

     3) Signs and symptoms of infection

     4) Follow-up care

     5) Prevention (wear gloves when working in woodpiles, storage areas; shake out shoes or clothing when outside)

4. Evaluation and ongoing monitoring

   a. Hemodynamic status

   b. Breath sounds and pulse oximetry

   c. Cardiac rate and rhythm

   d. Pain relief

C. COLD-RELATED EMERGENCIES

In a cool environment, the body will attempt to maintain normothermia by conserving heat through vasoconstriction and producing heat through shivering. Risk factors for developing a cold-related emergency include extremes of age, ambient temperature, inappropriate clothing, wet clothing, water/metal contact, wind, and length of exposure. Alcohol, drugs such as phenothiazines, trauma, and illnesses such as diabetes pose additional risks for the development of cold-related emergencies. Cold-related emergencies include frostbite and hypothermia.[25,35]

FROSTBITE. Frostbite is tissue freezing, which is the formation of ice crystals in deep and/or superficial tissue. Ninety percent of frostbite cases involve the hands and feet; the cheeks, nose, ears, and penis are also commonly affected. Contributing factors include environmental (e.g., temperature, wind chill, length of exposure, altitude) and individual (e.g., genetics, comorbidities, alcohol, medications and drugs, clothing, previous frostbite injury).[25,36,37] The initial response to cold stress is peripheral vasoconstriction. Cooling increases blood viscosity and decreases capillary perfusion. It results in sludging and thrombosis of the vessels, decreased blood flow, and vascular stasis, which contribute to the development of tissue damage. Subsequently, alterations in vascular permeability lead to edema, progressive dermal ischemia, inflammatory mediator release, neutrophil adhesion, and endothelial damage.[25,36,37]

The degree of injury is a complex interaction of many variables. Frostbite may be divided into four degrees, based on the appearance after rewarming: first-degree injury with a central, pale area and surrounding erythema; second-degree injury with blisters surrounded by erythema and edema; third-degree with hemorrhagic blisters and eschar formation; and fourth-degree frostbite with necrosis and tissue loss. Any patient with frostbite must always be evaluated for hypothermia. Treatment includes rewarming of the affected part, pain management, and wound care.[25,36,37]

1. Assessment
   a. Subjective data collection
      1) History of present injury/chief complaint
         a) Patient age
         b) Cold ambient temperature
         c) Improper clothing; constricting clothing or clothing that does not cover high-risk areas (e.g., ears, nose, hands, fingers)
         d) Alcohol or drug intoxication
         e) Smoker
         f) Pain (see Chapter 8): in affected extremity
      2) Past medical history
         a) Current or preexisting diseases/illness
            (1) Cardiovascular disease
            (2) Diabetes
            (3) Raynaud disease
         b) History of cold injury
         c) Medications
         d) Allergies
         e) Immunization status
   b. Objective data collection
      1) Physical examination
         a) General appearance
            (1) Possible shivering
            (2) Possible subnormal temperature
            (3) Moderate to severe distress/discomfort
         b) Inspection
            (1) First-degree frostbite
               (a) Central pale area with surrounding erythema
               (b) Skin may be cyanotic
               (c) Edema
            (2) Second-degree frostbite
               (a) Blisters surrounded by erythema
               (b) Edema
               (c) Decreased sensation at the injured site
            (3) Third-degree frostbite
               (a) Hemorrhagic blisters
               (b) Eschar formation
               (c) Edema
            (4) Fourth-degree frostbite
               (a) Skin: cyanosis, necrosis, gangrene
               (b) Edema
         c) Palpation
            (1) Decreased sensation to the injured area
            (2) Nonpliable skin with third-degree frostbite
            (3) Decreased peripheral pulses
            (4) Motor function of the affected area

      2) Diagnostic procedures
         a) CBC with differential
         b) Coagulation profile: PT, PTT
         c) Serum chemistries including glucose, BUN, creatinine
         d) Liver profiles
         e) Serum and urine toxicology screen
         f) Urinalysis; pregnancy test in female patients of childbearing age
         g) Chest radiograph
         h) Affected extremity radiograph
         i) Compartment pressure monitoring of affected site if indicated
2. Analysis: differential nursing diagnoses/collaborative problems
   a. Impaired tissue integrity
   b. Ineffective tissue perfusion
   c. Risk for infection
   d. Hypothermia
   e. Acute pain
   f. Anxiety/fear
3. Planning and implementation/interventions
   a. Maintain airway, breathing, circulation (see Chapters 1 and 32)
   b. Provide supplemental oxygen
   c. Establish IV/IO access for administration of crystalloid fluids/medications
   d. Anticipate, assess, and treat patient for hypothermia, if present
   e. Obtain a complete set of vital signs, including temperature
   f. Prepare for/assist with medical interventions
      1) Because most tissue damage occurs during the thaw-and-refreeze cycle, rewarming is begun when the body part can be warmed and not reexposed to cold. Assess the frostbitten area carefully because the loss of sensation may cause the patient to be unaware of soft tissue injuries in that area[25,37]
         a) Remove wet clothing
         b) Remove jewelry, if present, from the affected area
         c) Obtain a patient history, including date of patient's last tetanus immunization
         d) Rewarm affected extremity in a warm 99–102°F (37–39°C) water bath in a container large enough to accommodate the frostbitten tissues without them touching the sides or bottom of the container[25,37]
         e) Water should be maintained at approximately 99–102°F (37–39°C) and gently circulated around the frostbitten tissue until the distal tip of the frostbitten part becomes pink or reddened.[25,37] Make no attempt to massage frostbitten parts

2) After thawing, tissues that were deeply frostbitten may develop blisters or appear cyanotic; blisters should not be broken and must be protected from injury[37]

3) Pain after rewarming usually indicates that viable tissue has been successfully rewarmed[37]

4) Rinse with sterile water 90–95°F (32.2–35°C)[37]

5) After rewarming, allow frostbitten tissues to dry in the warm air; avoid rubbing or towel drying[37]

6) Pad between affected digits, and bandage affected tissues loosely with a soft, sterile dressing; avoid putting undue pressure on the affected parts[37]

7) If possible rewarmed extremities should be kept at a level above the heart

8) Protect the rewarmed area from refreezing and other trauma; prevent blankets from pressing directly on the injured area[16,37]

9) Do not allow an individual who has frostbitten feet to walk; once frostbitten feet are rewarmed, the patient should be nonambulatory

10) Assist with hospital admission

g. Administer pharmacologic therapy as prescribed
1) Nonnarcotic analgesics
2) Narcotics
3) Consider vasodilator for severe frostbite (e.g., 400 mg IV chlorohydrate vasodilator [buflomedil])[37]
4) Ibuprofen (Motrin, Advil)
5) Aspirin or ibuprofen may help improve outcomes by blocking the arachidonic acid pathway
6) Antibiotics
7) Tetanus immunization

h. Educate patient/significant others
1) Hazards and effects of cold exposure
2) Need for protective clothing
3) Early signs and symptoms of frostbite
4) Avoidance of tobacco, caffeine, alcohol
5) Wound care

4. Evaluation and ongoing monitoring
a. Circulation, sensation, motor movement of involved digits
b. Pain relief

HYPOTHERMIA. Hypothermia has been defined as a core body temperature of less than 95°F (35°C). It is both a symptom and a clinical disease entity.[7,25,35] Hypothermia results when the body cannot maintain an adequate homeostasis temperature. It includes healthy patients with simple environmental exposure (primary), those with specific diseases that produce hypothermia (secondary), and those with predisposing conditions.[7,25,35] The body produces heat through cellular metabolism,

muscle activity, and shivering. Heat is lost through conduction, convection, evaporation, and radiation. The ambient temperature does not have to be very low to cause hypothermia. Hypothermia needs to be rapidly recognized and treated in an effort to avoid life-threatening complications such as apnea, ventricular fibrillation, and acidosis. There are multiple risk factors for hypothermia, including the following: age (pediatric patients because of their inability to shiver and decreased body fat and older adults because of the high incidence of cardiovascular disease and decreased body fat); medications, such as phenothiazines and neuromuscular blocking agents, which interfere with the patient's ability to shiver; alcohol; traumatic injury; shock; and diseases such as diabetes. The treatment of hypothermia focuses on returning the core body temperature to normal and providing supportive care. The method of rewarming is dependent on the severity of hypothermia.[7,25,35]

1. Assessment
a. Subjective data collection
1) History of present injury/chief complaint
a) Ambient temperature
b) Length of exposure
c) Patient's clothing
d) Exposure to water/metal
e) Trauma: blunt or penetrating forces
f) Administration of neuromuscular blocking agents
g) Patient age
2) Past medical history
a) Current or preexisting diseases/illness
(1) Alcoholism
(2) Hypothyroidism
(3) Malnutrition
(4) Diabetes
b) Medications
(1) Phenothiazines
(2) Barbiturates
c) Allergies
d) Immunization status
b. Objective data collection
1) Physical examination
a) General appearance
(1) Level of consciousness, behavior, affect: confusion to coma
(2) Subnormal temperature: best method/how to measure core temp
(a) Mild hypothermia: 93–95°F (35–36°C)
(b) Moderate hypothermia: 86–93°F (30–34°C)
(c) Severe hypothermia: <86°F (30°C)
(3) Hypoventilation
(4) Hypotension: difficult to detect blood pressure
(5) Moderate to severe distress/discomfort, possibly critically ill

b) Inspection
   (1) Fixed, dilated pupils
   (2) Pale, cyanotic skin
   (3) Paradoxical undressing: patient removes all clothing even though cold
   (4) Shivering diminished or absent at core body temperature of 86°F (30°C)
   (5) Cardiac dysrhythmias on monitor: bradycardia, atrial fibrillation, presence of an Osborn ("hump" between QRS complex and ST segment) or J wave, ventricular fibrillation

c) Palpation
   (1) Absence of reflexes

d) Auscultation
   (1) Breath sounds: crackles

2) Diagnostic procedures
   a) CBC with differential: increased hematocrit resulting from cold diuresis
   b) Coagulation profile including platelets, fibrin split products
   c) Serum chemistries including glucose, BUN, creatinine: hyperglycemia
   d) Liver profiles
   e) Serum and urine toxicology screen
   f) ABGs
   g) Urinalysis; pregnancy test in female patients of childbearing age
   h) Chest radiograph
   i) Head CT scan
   j) ECG

2. Analysis: differential nursing diagnoses/collaborative problems
   a. Ineffective airway clearance
   b. Impaired gas exchange
   c. Ineffective thermoregulation
   d. Deficient knowledge

3. Planning and implementation/interventions
   a. Maintain airway, breathing, circulation (see Chapters 1 and 32)
      1) Initiate or continue BLS and ALS per protocols if respiratory/cardiac arrest is present: medications and defibrillation may not be successful with body temperatures <86°F (30°C)[38]
   b. Provide supplemental oxygen
      1) RSI and ventilatory support in patient with compromised airway
      2) High-flow oxygen
   c. Establish IV/IO access for administration of crystalloid fluid/medications
      1) Infuse warmed normal saline solutions
   d. Prepare for/assist with medical interventions
      1) Advanced airway management
         a) Nasal or oral intubation
         b) Supraglottic airway (e.g., King, Combitube, laryngeal mask airway)

c) Surgical airway (e.g., cricothyrotomy)
2) Remove wet clothing and jewelry
3) Maintain normothermic body temperature
   a) Treat mild hypothermia 90–95°F (32.2–35°C) with passive rewarming
      (1) Warm blankets
      (2) Forced warm-air blankets and warmed environment (used with caution because peripheral vasoconstriction may place patient at risk for integument injury) and rewarming of extremities may place patient at risk for rewarming shock (afterdrop)[7,25,35]
      (3) Active external: prehospital body-to-body contact; application of heating devices such as fluid- or air-filled warming blankets; radiant lights
   b) Moderate hypothermia (82.5–90°F [28–32.2°C]) requires active core rewarming with warmed IV solutions, warmed oxygen, and warmed peritoneal lavage[7,25,35]
   c) Severe hypothermia (<82.5°F [28°C]) requires active core rewarming such as warmed IV solutions, warmed peritoneal lavage, warmed thoracotomy/mediastinal lavage
      (1) Consider cardiopulmonary bypass or continuous arteriovenous rewarming (CAVR) with a rapid fluid warmer if available[25,35]
4) Institute cardiac and pulse oximetry monitoring
5) Insert gastric tube and attach to suction
6) Insert indwelling urinary catheter
7) Continue resuscitation of a hypothermia victim until patient has been warmed to a minimum 86°F (30°C)
8) Assist with hospital admission
e. Administer pharmacologic therapy as ordered
   1) RSI premedications: sedatives, analgesics, neuromuscular blocking agents
   2) ALS medications per protocols
f. Educate patient and significant others
   1) Medical illness, medications, age
   2) Early signs and symptoms of hypothermia
   3) Prevention of hypothermia (e.g., proper clothing, recognizing when to seek shelter)

4. Evaluation and ongoing monitoring
   a. Airway patency
   b. Level of consciousness
   c. Hemodynamic status
      1) Monitor patient for rewarming shock (afterdrop), which occurs when cold blood from the periphery reaches the core after warming; can cause hypotension and dysrhythmias; may be avoided by warming the trunk and vascular areas first and then proceeding to extremities
   d. Breath sounds and pulse oximetry

e. Cardiac rate and rhythm
   1) Atrial fibrillation is a common dysrhythmia after exposure to cold weather, and premature ventricular contractions and ventricular fibrillation are frequent rewarming dysrhythmias. Careful handling of hypothermic patient is essential to prevent VF
f. Core temperature measurements continuously during rewarming efforts
g. Intake and output

D. DIVING EMERGENCIES (DYSBARISM)

Dysbarism refers to a group of disorders that occur as a result of pressure changes and breathing compressed gases while scuba diving.

BAROTRAUMA. Barotrauma is related to pressure changes in gas-filled structures of the body such as ear, tooth, sinus, gut, or chest. Symptoms of barotrauma depend on the affected area. Ear involvement may include intense pain, vertigo, nausea, vomiting, hearing deficit, and facial nerve palsy. The most serious type of barotrauma is pulmonary barotrauma of assent, which results from expansion of gas trapped in the lungs. If a diver does not allow the expanding gas to escape, a pressure differential develops between the intrapulmonary air space and the ambient pressure. The combination of overdistention of the alveoli and overpressurization causes the alveoli to rupture, producing a spectrum of injuries collectively referred to as pulmonary barotrauma, which manifests as chest pain, dyspnea, and subcutaneous emphysema.[8,25] The decreased ambient pressure causes expansion of lung gases and results in gas bubble entry into capillaries, with consequent gas embolism. Other barotrauma may involve pneumomediastinum, pneumothorax, and tension pneumothorax.[8,25]

DECOMPRESSION SICKNESS (TABLE 15.3). Decompression sickness (DCS), commonly known as "the bends," is a result of the expansion and release of dissolved nitrogen in the tissues. It occurs when ascent is too rapid after a dive that has been long enough to cause nitrogen tissue saturation. The gas bubbles form in supersaturated tissues and cause pain resulting from vascular occlusion, pressure, and nerve dysfunction. Nitrogen bubbles can form in joints, skin, peripheral nerves, or the spinal cord.[8,39]

ARTERIAL GAS EMBOLISM (SEE TABLE 15.3). Arterial gas embolism (AGE) results from air bubbles entering the pulmonary venous circulation from ruptured alveoli. When air is introduced into the pulmonary capillary blood, gas bubbles are showered into the left atrium, to the left ventricle, and subsequently into the systemic circulation.[8,25,39] Patients

Table 15.3

Decompression Sickness Types and Symptoms

Type	Symptoms
Decompression sickness (DCS) type I	Mild pains; beginning resolution within 10 min (niggles)
	Pruritus (skin bends)
	Skin rash with mottling or marbling appearance or papular/plaque-like violaceous (purple discoloration) rash
	Painless pitting edema; lymphatic involvement
	Anorexia, excessive fatigue
	Pain in joints (bends), tendons: dull, deep, throbbing, toothache-type; begins as mild but slowly intensifies; shoulder most commonly affected
Decompression sickness (DCS) type II	Pulmonary symptoms
	Hypovolemic shock
	Nervous system involvement
	Pain present in only 30% of cases
	Symptom onset may be delayed up to 36 hours
Arterial gas emboli (AGE)	Depends on travel of gas emboli
	Stroke, seizure, acute myocardial infarction
	Symptom onset: 10–20 min after surfacing

with AGE may exhibit significant neurologic deficits, such as confusion and seizures immediately after surfacing, and this condition can occur with any dive. The classic presentation is sudden onset of unconsciousness within minutes of reaching the surface after a dive. Symptoms occur immediately, and the effects are devastating. Approximately 4% of victims of AGE suffer immediate cardiac respiratory arrest and die; another 5% die in the hospital due to consequences of AGE or severe near drowning that can accompany AGE.[8] Consequences may include dysrhythmias, focal or general seizures, altered mental status or unconsciousness, and a variety of neurologic signs and symptoms, depending on the location of emboli.[8,25,39]

1. Assessment
   a. Subjective data collection
      1) History of present illness/chief complaint
         a) Description of incident
         b) Influences on presenting symptoms
            (1) Depth and length of the dive
            (2) Inert gas breathed
            (3) Delay to presentation
            (4) Adequacy of decompression
         c) Time elapsed since injury
         d) Prehospital care provided
         e) Pain (see Chapter 8)
         f) Vomiting
      2) Past medical history
         a) Current or preexisting diseases/illness
            (1) Cardiovascular disease

(2) Diabetes
   b) Medications
   c) Allergies
  b. Objective data collection
   1) Physical examination
    a) General appearance
     (1) Level of consciousness, behavior, affect: disorientation
     (2) Tachycardia
     (3) Tachypnea
     (4) Severe distress/discomfort, critically ill
    b) Inspection
     (1) Rashes or lesions
     (2) Ruptured tympanic membrane (hemotympanum)
     (3) Visual field deficit, nystagmus
     (4) Sharply defined area of pallor in tongue (Liebermeister sign)
    c) Palpation
     (1) Presence of subcutaneous emphysema
     (2) Bladder distention
     (3) Tracheal deviation: tension pneumothorax
    d) Auscultation
     (1) Breath sounds: diminished or absent if pneumothorax present
     (2) Heart sounds: Hamman sign (crackling/crunching noise synchronous with heartbeat)
   2) Diagnostic procedures
    a) ABGs
    b) If mental status changes
     (1) CBC with differential
     (2) Serum chemistries
     (3) Serum and urine toxicology screen
     (4) Carboxyhemoglobin
    c) If shock present, add
     (1) Type and screen/crossmatch
     (2) Coagulation profile: PT, PTT
    d) Chest radiograph
    e) Head CT or MRI scan
    f) ECG
    g) Diagnostic maneuvers for DCS (see Table 15.4)
2. Analysis: differential nursing diagnoses/collaborative problems
  a. Risk for ineffective airway
  b. Ineffective breathing pattern
  c. Impaired gas exchange
  d. Acute pain
  e. Deficient knowledge
3. Planning and implementation/interventions
  a. Maintain airway, breathing, circulation (see Chapters 1 and 32)
  b. Provide supplemental oxygen
   1) RSI and ventilatory support in patient with compromised airway

Table 15.4

Diagnostic Maneuvers for Identifying Decompression Sickness

Steps	Symptoms
Inflate blood pressure cuff to between 150 and 250 mm Hg over painful area	Temporary relief of pain: pressure increase forces nitrogen bubbles into fluid and away from joint
Milk muscle toward affected joint	Pain increases: milking pushes more nitrogen bubbles toward joint

   2) High-flow oxygen (10 L/min by nonrebreather face mask); supplemental oxygen enhances rate of resolution of inert gas bubbles and treats arterial hypoxemia[8,39]
  c. Establish IV/IO access for administration of crystalloid fluid/medications
  d. Prepare for/assist with medical interventions
   1) Place patient in left lateral, supine position
   2) Advanced airway management
    a) Nasal or oral intubation
    b) Supraglottic airway (e.g., King, Combitube, laryngeal mask airway)
    c) Surgical airway (e.g., cricothyrotomy)
   3) Needle decompression, chest tube, and/or thoracostomy
   4) Institute cardiac and pulse oximetry monitoring
   5) Insert gastric tube and attach to suction
   6) Insert indwelling urinary catheter
   7) Assist with admission to recompression chamber with hyperbaric oxygen therapy; all cases of suspected AGE must be referred for recompression treatment as rapidly as possible[8,25,39]
    a) Recompression to an environment of higher pressure promotes gas elimination and decreases the size of gas bubbles in the body
    b) Administer hyperbaric oxygen therapy according to standardized protocols published by the U.S. Navy. The Navy dive treatment tables are very effective, especially when recompression is initiated early. The treatment selected is based on severity of the patient's condition. The number of treatments is determined by physical examination and identifiable improvements from the baseline condition[8,39]
  e. Administer pharmacologic therapy as ordered
   1) RSI premedications: sedatives, analgesics, neuromuscular blocking agents
   2) Nonnarcotic analgesics
   3) Narcotics
4. Evaluation and ongoing monitoring
  a. Airway patency
  b. Level of consciousness

c. Hemodynamic status
d. Breath sounds and pulse oximetry
e. Cardiac rate and rhythm
f. Pain relief
g. Intake and output

E. HEAT-RELATED EMERGENCIES

Heat illnesses are best regarded as a continuum that transitions from the mild conditions of heat cramps and heat exhaustion to more serious conditions of heat injury and heatstroke.[25,40,41] Heat-related emergencies occur when the body is no longer able to regulate its body temperature through normal physiologic mechanisms. Thermoregulation occurs through the preoptic anterior hypothalamus. Information about body temperature is sent to the brain by peripheral and central thermoreceptors located in the skin, limb muscles, and spinal cord. The hypothalamus then initiates methods that help the body maintain a normal or tolerable body temperature. The body attempts to maintain a temperature of 98.6°F (37.1°C).[25,40,41] When the body is exposed to excessive heat, it will attempt to dissipate the heat by convection, radiation, or evaporation. Drugs, strenuous activity, and high ambient temperatures can increase internal heat production. Factors such as lack of acclimation, restrictive clothing, and high humidity affect the body's ability to manage excessive heat. As the body's temperature increases, there is stimulation of the sweat response to initiate evaporative heat loss. This is the body's primary mechanism of cooling. Sweating not only assists in cooling the body but also may cause loss of body weight, sodium, and potassium. If fluids and electrolytes are not replaced, dehydration can occur. The body also attempts to dissipate heat by shunting blood to the skin. There is an increase in heart rate, stroke volume, and cardiac output.[25,40,41] Additionally, the kidneys conserve fluid for evaporation by retaining salt and water. Under normal circumstances, with time to acclimate, these compensatory mechanisms assist the body in sustaining a normal temperature. However, if additional factors contribute to the heat stress, these mechanisms will fail, resulting in a heat-related emergency. People at risk for heat-related emergencies include the young, the older adult, and individuals not acclimated to hot weather.[25,41] Heat exhaustion and heat stroke represent progressive degrees of heat illness (Table 15.5).

HEAT CRAMPS. Heat cramps are usually brief but can cause agonizing pain in the skeletal muscles of the extremities and trunk. Cramps may be recurrent but are typically confined to the skeletal muscles that are involved in vigorous exercise in the heat.[25,41] Skeletal muscle spasms in the extremities may be sporadic, but they are painful and develop most frequently in persons who are usually in good health but not acclimatized to physical exertion in the environment and have not adequately replaced the fluids and electrolytes lost while sweating (see Table 15.5).[25,40,41]

However, heat cramps may also occur in fit athletes who are salt depleted. Heat cramps do not predispose to more serious heat illness and are not associated with complications beyond muscle soreness. The cause of heat cramps is not fully understood, but cramps are thought to occur in response to increased intracellular calcium release that stimulates actin-myosin filaments and muscle contraction.[41] Treatment includes cessation of the exertional activity, resting in a cool place, massage of the painful areas, and replacement of fluids with a balanced solution such as a commercially prepared sports drink (e.g., Gatorade). Salt tablets should be avoided because they may stimulate excess potassium loss and can cause gastrointestinal irritation.[25,41]

Table 15.5

Heat-Related Emergencies and Interventions

Emergency	Clinical Presentation	Interventions
Heat cramps	Brief, intermittent severe muscular cramps in muscles fatigued by heavy work, excessive fatigue, decreased coordination, nausea, vomiting, headache, dizziness	Place patient in cool environment and massage affected muscles; patient should rest until symptoms subside; administer intravenous salt solution: 0.9% normal saline 1,000 mL, over 1–3 hr or oral fluids of a balanced solution such as a commercially prepared sports drink (e.g., Gatorade). Increments of 0.1% saline solution 1–3 hr or 23.5% saline in 10–20 mL increments; or 0.1% saline solution orally; monitor electrolytes and magnesium levels, with replacement as needed
Heat exhaustion	Dehydration, malaise, weakness, flulike symptoms, thirst, tachycardia frontal headache, and muscle cramps	Fluid and electrolyte replacement based on serum electrolytes and calculation of water deficit; spontaneous cooling to 102°F (39°C); acetaminophen (Tylenol) or ibuprofen (Motrin, Advil) may be administered
Heat stroke	Hot, dry skin, altered level of consciousness, temperature ranges from 106°F (41.4°C) to 116°F (47°C); this is a neurologic emergency	Aggressive cooling to 102°F (39°C) within 1 hr; respiratory and cardiovascular support early

(Data from Leon, L. R., & Kenefick, R. W. (2012). Pathophysiology of heat-related illnesses. In *Wilderness medicine* (6th ed., chap 10); Auerbach, P. S. (2012). Pathophysiology of heat-related illnesses. In Leon, L. R., & Kenefick, R. W. (Eds.). *Wilderness medicine* (pp. 113–129). St. Louis, MO: Elsevier.)

HEAT EXHAUSTION (SEE TABLE 15.5). Heat exhaustion is a mild to moderate form of heat illness often precipitated by major exertion in hot weather. Peripheral vasodilatation occurs to dissipate heat, and fluids and electrolytes are lost through profuse sweating. Heat exhaustion is associated with moderate (>101.3°F [38.5°C]) to high (>104°F [40°C]) elevations in core temperature and an inability to sustain cardiac output.[25,41] Heat exhaustion may occur with or without exercise in hot environments and may progress to a moderately severe condition without associated organ damage. Heat exhaustion is often observed in older adults as a result of preexisting cardiovascular insufficiency, medications (e.g., diuretics), or inadequate water intake that leads to dehydration. On physical examination, the patient is pale, ashen, and sweating profusely. The patient may complain of fatigue, dizziness, headache, nausea, vomiting, malaise, hypotension, tachycardia, and severe thirst. Treatment includes placing the patient in a recumbent position in a cool environment and oral fluid hydration with electrolytes. Intravenous (IV) fluid administration may be warranted in severely dehydrated individuals.[25,41]

HEAT INJURY AND HEAT STROKE (SEE TABLE 15.5). Heat injury is a moderate to severe condition characterized by tissue (e.g., skeletal muscle) or organ (e.g., gut, kidney, spleen, liver) damage and hyperthermia (core temperature typically, but not always >104°F [40°C]).[25,41] Heat injury may progress to heatstroke if the patient is not rapidly cooled. Heat stroke is a medical emergency, with the patient presenting with profound CNS abnormalities, such as delirium, agitation, stupor, seizures, or coma, and severe hyperthermia (core temperature typically, but not always >104°F [40°C]). The patient is no longer able to dissipate heat because of failure of the central thermoregulation mechanisms. Morbidity is directly related to the amount of time the patient's body temperature remains elevated. Exertional heat stroke occurs primarily in young athletes. There is a history of extreme exertion in a hot environment with symptoms occurring over hours. Classic, or nonexertional, heat stroke more commonly occurs during periods of exposure to environmental temperatures exceeding 102.5°F (39.2°C) for a prolonged period of time.[25,40,41] Risk factors include age extremes, concurrent use of phenothiazines, and debilitation. There is a lack of acclimation, and the core body temperature rises to >106°F (41°C).[25,41] The patient's mental status ranges from confusion to coma, and the skin is hot and dry. Because of fluid loss, the patient is hypotensive and tachycardic. Patients with preexisting cardiovascular disease are prone to developing a hypodynamic state with a low cardiac index (output) and high systemic vascular resistance. Cardiovascular collapse may follow. Treatment includes stabilization of the patient's airway, breathing, and circulation, along with rapid cooling. There continues to be controversy about which cooling method is best. Immediately cool to <102.2°F (39°C) using cooling methods; removal of clothing,

covering the patient with wet sheets, and using a fan to enhance evaporative cooling; providing an ice water bath (conductive cooling); administering cool IV fluids; reestablishing normal CNS function; and avoiding antipyretics or drugs with liver toxicity.[25,41] Whatever cooling method(s) used, the patient's temperature must be closely monitored, and shivering must be controlled. Fluid and electrolyte imbalances must be corrected, and the patient must be monitored for cardia dysrhythmias, including ventricular aberrance and peaked T waves secondary to electrolyte imbalances. Muscle damage may occur at high temperatures; therefore, the patient must be monitored for symptoms of rhabdomyolysis (e.g., dark urine, muscle cramps). Clotting studies should be obtained to monitor the patient for development of disseminated intravascular coagulation (DIC), a potential complication of heat stroke.[25,41]

1. Assessment (heat exhaustion/heat stroke)
   a. Subjective data collection
      1) History of present injury/chief complaint
         a) Temperature of patient when found
         b) Relative humidity
         c) Wet bulb globe temperature (WBGT) index
         d) Type of activity in which patient was engaged
         e) Length of time in environment
         f) Risk factors for heat-related emergency
            (1) Age (infants, young children, older adults)
            (2) Exertion during hot weather
            (3) Lack of acclimation
            (4) Obesity
            (5) Physical conditioning
         g) Thirst
      2) Past medical history
         a) Current or preexisting diseases/illness
            (1) Alcoholism
            (2) Diabetes
            (3) Spinal cord injuries
            (4) Central nervous system disorders
            (5) Cardiovascular disease
         b) Substance and/or alcohol use/abuse
         c) Last normal menstrual period: female patients of childbearing age
         d) Medications
            (1) Phenothiazines
            (2) Tricyclic antidepressants
            (3) Antihistamines
            (4) Ethanol
            (5) Diuretics
         e) Allergies
   b. Objective data collection
      1) Physical examination
         a) General appearance
            (1) Level of consciousness, behavior, affect: confusion to coma
            (2) Abnormal posturing: limp; abnormal flexion/extension
            (3) Hypotension

(4) Tachycardia: rates commonly >130 beats/minute

(5) Tachypnea, hyperventilation

(6) Elevated core body temperature: >102.2°F (39°C)

(7) Moderate to severe distress/discomfort, possibly critically ill

b) Inspection

(1) Pale, ashen skin

(2) Diaphoresis/profuse sweating

(3) Pupils: nystagmus; fixed and dilated

c) Palpation

(1) Hot/dry skin (heat stroke)

(2) Moist skin (heat exhaustion)

(3) Tenderness in exerted muscles

(4) Weakness

d) Auscultation

(1) Breath sounds: crackles

2) Diagnostic procedures

a) CBC with differential: elevated WBC count

b) PT, PTT

c) Platelets, fibrin split products: decreased platelets with heat stroke

d) Serum chemistries including glucose, BUN, creatinine

(1) Hyponatremia

(2) Hypokalemia or hyperkalemia

(3) Hypoglycemia

e) Liver profiles: elevated aspartate aminotransferase (AST) and alanine aminotransferase (ALT) with heat stroke

f) CK

g) ABGs: lactic acidosis and respiratory alkalosis

h) Serum and urine toxicology screen

i) Urinalysis: myoglobin; pregnancy test in female patients of childbearing age

j) Chest radiograph

k) Head CT scan

l) ECG: bundle branch block, ischemic ST-segment and T-wave abnormalities

2. Analysis: differential nursing diagnoses/collaborative problems

a. Risk for ineffective airway clearance

b. Impaired gas exchange

c. Deficient fluid volume

d. Ineffective tissue perfusion

e. Ineffective thermoregulation

f. Deficient knowledge

3. Planning and implementation/interventions

a. Maintain airway, breathing, circulation (see Chapters 1 and 32)

b. Provide supplemental oxygen as indicated

1) Rapid-sequence intubation (RSI) and ventilatory support in patient with compromised airway

2) High-flow oxygen

c. Establish IV/IO access for administration of crystalloid fluid/medications

d. Prepare for/assist with medical interventions

1) Advanced airway management

a) Nasal or oral intubation

b) Supraglottic airway (e.g., King, Combitube, laryngeal mask airway)

c) Surgical airway (e.g., cricothyrotomy)

2) Maintain normothermic body temperature, using core temperature measurement

a) Aggressive cooling with heat stroke

(1) Goal is to cool to 102.2°F (39°C) within 1 hour

(2) Discontinue cooling when core temperature reaches 102.2°F (39°C) to avoid iatrogenic hypothermia

b) Place patient in cool environment

c) Remove patient's clothing, and spray or sponge patient with lukewarm water in an environment of air movement (large circulating fans)

d) Place padded ice packs along lateral aspects of patient's trunk and groin (monitor closely because it may increase shivering, heat production, and local tissue injury)

e) Methods to be used with caution include ice water immersion, gastric lavage, peritoneal lavage, rectal lavage, cardiopulmonary bypass, or hemodialysis

3) Institute cardiac and pulse oximetry monitoring

4) Insert gastric tube and attach to suction

5) Insert indwelling urinary catheter

6) Assist with hospital admission

e. Administer pharmacologic therapy as ordered

1) RSI premedications: sedatives, analgesics, neuromuscular blocking agents

2) Mannitol (Osmitrol) may be considered to reduce intracerebral swelling

3) Chlorpromazine (Thorazine) or benzodiazepines to reduce shivering

4. Evaluation and ongoing monitoring

a. Airway patency

b. Level of consciousness

c. Hemodynamic status

d. Body core temperature

e. Breath sounds and pulse oximetry

f. Cardiac rate and rhythm

g. Intake and output

EXERTIONAL HEATSTROKE. Exertional heatstroke (EHS) has a different etiology than classic heatstroke and typically affects young healthy populations that perform strenuous physical activity in hot weather. Examples are military and athletic populations who are highly motivated to perform strenuous physical activity in hot weather, which increases the risk for EHS.[25,41]

F. HIGH-ALTITUDE ILLNESS

The high-altitude environment exposes individuals to cold, low humidity; increased ultraviolet radiation; and decreased air pressure, all of which can cause problems.[42,43,44] High-altitude illness refers to a spectrum of conditions resulting from tissue hypoxia that may occur at altitudes anywhere from 4,900 feet (1,500 m) to extremes of >18,000 feet (5,500 m). As the partial pressure of oxygen decreases at high altitudes, there is less oxygen available to tissues as a result of incomplete hemoglobin loading; for example, at 10,000 feet (3,000 m) the inspired PO_2 is only 69% of sea-level value. The magnitude of hypoxic stress depends on altitude, rate of ascent, and duration of exposure. Altitude illness is divided into three syndromes: acute mountain sickness (AMS), high-altitude cerebral edema (HACE), and high-altitude pulmonary edema (HAPE).[42,43,44]

ACUTE MOUNTAIN SICKNESS. Acute mountain sickness (AMS) is the most common form of altitude illness, reported to affect 25% of visitors sleeping above 8,000 feet (2,500 m) in Colorado. AMS generally resolves with 24–72 hours.[4] For the partially acclimatized, AMS may result from an abrupt ascent to a higher altitude, overexertion, and/or use of respiratory depressants. Symptoms are described as being similar to an alcoholic hangover or viral syndrome.[42,43,44] Headache is the cardinal symptom, sometimes accompanied by fatigue, loss of appetite, nausea, weakness, and nausea/vomiting. Headache onset is usually 2–12 hours after arrival at a higher altitude and often during or after the first night. Preverbal children may develop loss of appetite, irritability, and pallor. AMS is usually self-limiting, with complete resolution within 24–72 hours of acclimatization. However, if continued assent to higher elevations occurs, the illness may worsen and progress to HACE.[42,43,44]

HIGH-ALTITUDE CEREBRAL EDEMA. High-altitude cerebral edema (HACE) is the clinical progression of the neurologic and cerebral signs of AMS. Symptoms of HACE include ataxia, severe lassitude, altered mental status, drowsiness, obtundation, stupor, and coma. Also evident are hallucinations, cranial nerve palsy, hemiparesis, seizures, hemiplegia, and various focal neurologic signs, including cortical blindness, aphasia, and an island-like blind spot in the visual field. The progression from AMS to HACE occurs over 12 hours to 4 days. Stroke may result from polycythemia, dehydration, increased ICP, cerebrovascular spasm, or other problems.[42,43,44]

HACE is a severe progression of AMS and is rare; it is most often associated with HAPE. In addition to AMS symptoms, lethargy becomes profound, with drowsiness, confusion, and ataxia on tandem gait test.[42] A person with HACE requires immediate descent; death from HACE can ensue within 24 hours of developing ataxia, if the person fails to descend.[42,43,44]

HIGH-ALTITUDE PULMONARY EDEMA. High-altitude pulmonary edema (HAPE) is a life-threatening condition that occurs at altitudes >8,000 feet (2,700 m). It usually develops within the first 4 days of ascent. Early symptoms include dry cough, dyspnea at rest, substernal pain, headache, anorexia, and lassitude. Later symptoms include tachypnea, wheezing, orthopnea, hemoptysis, tachycardia, pulmonary crackles and rhonchi, pink frothy sputum, mental changes, and ataxia. HAPE is believed to be a form of neurogenic pulmonary edema, which is a high-protein permeability edema.[42,43,44] HAPE can occur by itself or in conjunction with AMS and HACE; incidence is 1 per 10,000 skiers in Colorado and up to 1 per 100 climbers at >14,000 feet (4,270 m).[44] Initial symptoms are increased breathlessness with exertion, and eventually increased breathlessness at rest, associated with weakness and cough. Oxygen or descent is lifesaving.[42,43,44]

1. Assessment
   a. Subjective data collection
      1) History of present illness/chief complaint
         a) Description of incident
         b) Time elapsed since injury
         c) Altered gait
            (1) Ataxia is the clinical indicator used to denote progression from mild to severe AMS. Altered level of consciousness follows, with progression of confusion, disorientation, and impaired judgment
            (2) Coma may evolve within 24 hours after the development of ataxia
         d) Prehospital care provided
         e) Pain (see Chapter 8) and symptoms: in most cases, AMS symptoms begin approximately 12–24 hours after reaching altitude
         f) AMS is defined as a syndrome occurring in a setting of altitude gain accompanied by headache, and at least one of the following
            (1) Gastrointestinal symptoms (anorexia, nausea, vomiting)
            (2) Fatigue or weakness
            (3) Dizziness or lightheadedness
            (4) Difficulty sleeping (fragmented sleep)
            (5) Other symptoms
                (a) Irritability
                (b) Chills
                (c) Malaise, lassitude
                (d) Dyspnea on exertion
                (e) Tachycardia
                (f) Dry cough
                (g) Postural hypotension
                (h) Fluid retention and absence of normal urination
      2) Past medical history
         a) Current or preexisting diseases/illness
            (1) Cardiovascular disease (heart failure, myocardial ischemia, angina)

      (2) Diabetes
      (3) Sickle cell disease
      (4) Any form of pulmonary insufficiency
    b) Medications
    c) Allergies
  b. Objective data collection
    1) Physical examination
      a) General appearance
        (1) Level of consciousness, behavior, affect: confusion, irritability
        (2) Tachycardia
        (3) Tachypnea
        (4) Ataxia
        (5) Moderate to severe distress/discomfort
      b) Auscultation
        (1) Breath sounds: crackles
    2) Diagnostic procedures
      a) ABGs: possible respiratory alkalosis
      b) CBC with differential as indicated: possible mild leukocytosis
      c) Chest radiograph
      d) ECG: possible right-sided heart strain pattern
2. Analysis: differential nursing diagnoses/collaborative problems
  a. Risk for ineffective airway clearance
  b. Ineffective breathing pattern
  c. Ineffective tissue perfusion
  d. Acute pain
  e. Deficient knowledge
3. Planning and implementation/interventions
  a. Maintain airway, breathing, circulation (see Chapters 1 and 32)
  b. Provide supplemental oxygen
    1) High-flow oxygen
  c. Establish IV/IO access for administration of crystalloid fluid/medications as needed
  d. Prepare for/assist with medical interventions
    1) Institute cardiac and pulse oximetry monitoring
    2) Descent is the most effective treatment for all high-altitude illnesses, and a descent of only 1,600–3,200 feet (500–1,000 m) may alleviate the condition[42,43,44]
    3) Patients experiencing HAPE also require bed rest and supplemental oxygen. If the condition progresses to acute respiratory distress syndrome, intubation and mechanical ventilation are indicated. Portable hyperbaric chambers (Gamow bags) may be useful for patients who are unable to descend[42,44]
  e. Administer pharmacologic therapy as ordered
    1) Acetazolamide (Diamox) (also beneficial for prophylaxis in patients at moderate to high risk for AMS)
    2) Dexamethasone (Decadron)
    3) Aspirin

    4) Nifedipine
    5) Ibuprofen
    6) Phosphodiesterase-5 inhibitors can also selectively lower pulmonary artery pressure
4. Evaluation and ongoing monitoring
  a. Airway patency
  b. Level of consciousness
  c. Hemodynamic status
  d. Breath sounds and pulse oximetry
  e. Cardiac rate and rhythm

G. WATER-RELATED EMERGENCIES

DROWNING. Each year in the United States, more than 3,000 people die from drowning. Drowning is the leading cause of death for infants and young children between the ages of 1 and 4 years, and the second leading cause of unintentional injury deaths in children ages 1 to 14 years.[3,45,46] Drowning occurs whenever there is respiratory impairment from either submersion or immersion in liquid. The end result may be fatal or nonfatal.

SUBMERSION INJURIES. The true incidence of submersion injuries is unknown because many cases are not reported; however, it is estimated at 20 to 500 times the rate of drowning. A submersion emergency results when a person becomes hypoxic from submersion in a substance. The most common substance is water, but people have been submerged in dry chemicals and in grain. The populations at greatest risk for a submersion injury are children younger than 5 years and boys between the ages of 15 and 19 years. The primary risk factors related to submersion injuries include inability to swim, intoxication, seizures, trauma, hyperventilation before deep-water swimming, hypothermia, stroke, myocardial infarction, and child maltreatment and neglect.[2,25,45,46]

When a human is submerged, there is initial panic, followed by breath holding and hyperventilation, which result in aspiration and swallowing of fluid. It takes a very small amount of substance (e.g., water) to trigger this response. Hypoxia develops, and aspiration may lead to pulmonary injury. The injured lungs may begin shunting blood, thus causing further hypoxia. Subsequently, hypoxia contributes to cerebral injury, edema, and eventual brain death.[2,45,46]

1. Assessment
  a. Subjective data collection
    1) History of present injury/chief complaint
      a) Presence of risk factors
      b) Mechanism of injury (see Chapter 31): substance in which patient was found, entrapment, diving injuries, boating accidents, undertow or rip currents, cave diving
      c) Length of time submerged in substance
      d) Temperature of substance
      e) Fresh water versus saltwater
      f) Contributing factors: ability of the swimmer; water temperature; age and

health of the victim, including presence of mind-altering substances, panic, fatigue, exhaustion, showing off and risk-taking behaviors, suicidal behavior; child maltreatment

   2) Past medical history
     a) Current or preexisting diseases/illness
      (1) Cardiovascular disease
      (2) Central nervous system disease (e.g., seizures, stroke)
      (3) Diabetes
      (4) Intellectual disability
     b) Physical conditioning
     c) Medications
     d) Allergies
  b. Objective data collection
   1) Physical examination
     a) General appearance
      (1) Level of consciousness, behavior, affect: awake to comatose
      (2) Vital signs: normal to cardiac arrest
      (3) Possible subnormal temperature
      (4) Moderate to severe distress/discomfort, possibly critically ill
     b) Inspection
      (1) Pale, cyanotic skin
      (2) Gastric distention
      (3) Presence of other injuries (e.g., spinal cord injury)
      (4) Signs of maltreatment (e.g., bruising, rope burns)
     c) Palpation
      (1) Cool, clammy skin
     d) Auscultation
      (1) Breath sounds: crackles
   2) Diagnostic procedures
     a) ABGs: metabolic acidosis
     b) CBC with differential
     c) Coagulation profile including platelets, fibrin split products
     d) Serum chemistries including glucose, BUN, creatinine
     e) Liver profiles
     f) Serum and urine toxicology screen
     g) Urinalysis; pregnancy test in female patients of childbearing age
     h) Chest radiograph
     i) Head CT scan/MRI
     j) ECG
     k) Bronchoscopy: removal of significant sediment inhalation
2. Analysis: differential nursing diagnoses/collaborative problems
  a. Ineffective airway clearance
  b. Impaired gas exchange
  c. Ineffective breathing pattern
  d. Ineffective tissue perfusion: cerebral, peripheral
  e. Ineffective thermoregulation
  f. Deficient knowledge
3. Planning and implementation/interventions
  a. Maintain airway, breathing, circulation (see Chapters 1 and 32) with C-spine precautions if spinal injury suspected
   1) Initiate or continue BLS and ALS per protocols if respiratory/cardiac arrest is present
  b. Provide supplemental oxygen
   1) RSI and ventilatory support in patient with compromised airway
   2) High-flow oxygen
  c. Establish IV/IO access for administration of crystalloid fluid/medications
   1) Infused warmed normal saline solutions
  d. Prepare for/assist with medical interventions
   1) Advanced airway management
     a) Nasal or oral intubation
     b) Supraglottic airway (e.g., King, Combitube, laryngeal mask airway)
     c) Surgical airway (e.g., cricothyrotomy)
   2) Maintain normothermic body temperature with appropriate rewarming as indicated by patient's core body temperature (see the discussion of hypothermia in Cold-Related Emergencies)
   3) Institute cardiac and pulse oximetry monitoring
   4) Catheter placement and monitoring of central venous pressure (see Chapter 6)
   5) Insert gastric tube and attach to suction
   6) Insert indwelling urinary catheter
   7) Treat complications: respiratory distress syndrome and aspiration (see Chapter 28); increased intracranial pressure (ICP; see Chapter 35); seizures (see Chapter 22)
   8) Continue resuscitation of a submersion victim until patient has been warmed to a minimum of 86°F (30°C)
   9) Assist with hospital admission
   10) Notify appropriate authorities if child maltreatment suspected
  e. Administer pharmacologic therapy as ordered
   1) RSI premedication: sedatives, analgesics, neuromuscular blocking agents
   2) ALS medications per protocols
4. Evaluation and ongoing monitoring
  a. Airway patency
  b. Level of consciousness
  c. Hemodynamic status
  d. Breath sounds and pulse oximetry
  e. Cardiac rate and rhythm
  f. Intake and output

References

1. American Heart Association: Guidelines for cardiopulmonary resuscitation and emergency cardiovascular care, *Circulation*, 2010. http://circ.ahajournals.org/content/122/18_suppl_3/S640.full.

2. Auerbach PS: *Wilderness medicine*, ed 6, St. Louis, MO, 2012, Mosby.

3. Auerbach PS: Envenomation by aquatic invertebrates in wilderness medicine. In *Wilderness medicine*, ed 6, chap 80, pp 1596–1628. St. Louis, MO, 2012, Mosby.

4. Bartsch P, Swenson ER: Acute high-altitude illnesses, *New England Journal of Medicine* 369(17):1666–1667, 2013.

5. Boyer LV, Binford GJ, Degan JA: Spider bites. In *Wilderness medicine*, ed 6, chap 52, pp 975–996. St. Louis, MO, 2012, Mosby.

6. Bradford JE, Freer L: Bites and injuries inflicted by wild and domestic animals. In *Wilderness medicine*, ed 6, chap 56, pp 1102–1127, St. Louis, MO, 2012, Mosby.

7. Cantwell P: Drowning. Retrieved from http://emedicine.medscape.com/article/772753, 2015.

8. Cauchy E, Chetaille E, Marchand V, Marsigny B: Retrospective study of 70 cases of severe frostbite lesions: A proposed new classification scheme, *Wilderness and Environmental Medicine* 12:48–255, 2001.

9. Centers for Disease Control and Prevention: Rabies. Retrieved from http://www.cdc.gov/rabies/exposure/index.html, 2015.

10. Centers for Disease Control and Prevention: Unintentional drowning. Retrieved from http://www.cdc.gov/HomeandRecreationalSafety/Water-Safety/waterinjuries-factsheet.html, 2015.

11. Centers for Disease Control and Prevention: National Center for Injury Prevention and Control. (n.d.). Web-based Injury Statistics Query and Reporting System (WISQARS). Retrieved from http://www.cdc.gov/injury/wisqars.

12. Centers for Disease Control and Prevention: Hypothermia-related deaths—United States, 1999–2002 and 2005, *Morbidity and Mortality Weekly Report* 17/55(10):282–284, 2006.

13. Centers for Disease Control and Prevention: Heat stress illness hospitalizations–Environmental Public Health Tracking Program, 20 states, 2001–2010. Surveillance Summaries, *Morbidity and Mortality Weekly Report* 63:13, 2014, December 12.

14. Centers for Disease Control and Prevention: Nonfatal dog bite–related injuries treated in hospital emergency departments—United States, *Morbidity and Mortality Weekly Report* 52:605, 2003.

15. Centers for Disease Control and Prevention: Lyme disease. Retrieved from http://www.cdc.gov/lyme/resources/brochure/lymediseasebrochure.pdf, 2015.

16. Danzl D: Accidental hypothermia. In *Wilderness medicine*, ed 6, chap 6, pp 116–142. St. Louis, MO, 2012, Mosby.

17. Diaz J: The epidemiology, evaluation, and management of stingray injuries, *Journal of the Louisiana State Medical Society* 159:198, 2007.

18. Diving Alert Network (DAN): (n.d.). Education and resource materials. Available 24 hours/day from Duke University at 919-684-9111 or from DAN at 919-684-2948, and http://www.diversalertnetwork.org/about/ or http://anesthesia.duhs.duke.edu/divisions/dan.html.

19. Ellis E, Ellis C: Dog and cat bites, *American Family Physician* 90(4):239–243, 2014.

20. Emergency Nurses Association: *Emergency nursing core curriculum*, ed 6, Philadelphia, PA, 2007, Saunders.

21. Emergency Nurses Association: *Emergency nursing pediatric course provider manual*, ed 4, Philadelphia, PA, 2013, Saunders.

22. Emergency Nurses Association: *Trauma nursing core course provider manual*, ed 7, Philadelphia, PA, 2013, Saunders.

23. Endom EE: *Initial management of animal and human bites*. In Danzi DS, editor: Waltham, MA, 2011, UpToDate.

24. Estelle F, Simons S: Anaphylaxis: The acute episode and beyond, *The BMJ* 346, 2013. Retrieved from http://www.bmj.com/content/346/bmj.f602.

25. Flarity K, Hoyt S: Wound care and laceration repair for NPs in emergency care; Part I, *Advanced Emergency Nursing Journal* 32(4):1–14, 2010.

26. Freer L, Imray C: Frostbite. In Auerbach PS, editor: *Wilderness medicine*, ed 6, pp 181–201. Philadelphia, 2012, Mosby Elsevier.

27. Greenberg MI, Hendrickson RG, Silverberg M, Campbell C: *Greenberg's text-atlas of emergency medicine*, Philadelphia, PA, 2005, Lippincott Williams & Wilkins.

28. Hackett PH, Shlim DR: *Altitude illness*, Centers for Disease Control and Prevention, 2016. Retrieved from http://wwwnc.cdc.gov/travel/yellowbook/2016/the-pre-travel-consultation/altitude-illness.

29. Hackett PH, Roach RC: High-altitude medicine and physiology. In Auerbach PS, editor: *Wilderness medicine*, ed 6, pp 2–32. Philadelphia, PA, 2012, Mosby, Elsevier.

30. Haddad EV: Environmental dermatology: Skin manifestations of injuries caused by invertebrate aquatic animals, *Anais Brasileiros De Dermatologia* 88(4):496–506, 2013.

31. Hoyt S, Flarity K, Shanning SS: Wound care and laceration repair for NPs in emergency care, Part II, *Advanced Emergency Nursing Journal* 33(1):84–99, 2010.

32. Juckett G: Arthropod bites, *American Family Physician* 88(12):841–847, 2013.

33. Laosee OC, Gilchrist J, Rudd R: Drowning 2005–2009, *Morbidity and Mortality Weekly Report* 61(19):344–347, 2012.

34. Langley R, Mack K, Haileyesus T, Proescholdbell S, Annest J: National estimates of noncanine bite and sting injuries treated in US hospital emergency departments, 2001–2010, *Wilderness Environmental Medicine* 25:14–23, 2014.

35. Leon LR, Kenfick RW: Pathophysiology of heat related illness. In Auerbach PS, editor: *Wilderness medicine*, ed 6, St. Louis, MO, 2012, Mosby.

36. Markovchick V, Pons PT: In *Emergency medicine secrets*, ed 5, St. Louis, MO, 2011, Elsevier.

37. Morgan M, Palmer J: Dog bites, *The BMJ* 34(7590):413–417, 2007.

38. Norris R: Snake envenomations, coral. eMedicine. Retrieved from http://www.emedicine.com/emerg/topic542.htm, 2005.

39. Patterson JW: Marine injuries. In *Weedon's skin pathology*, ed 4, chap 28, pp 757–759. St. Louis, MO, 2016, Elsevier.

40. Payne KS, Schilli K, Meier K, Rader RK, Dyer JA, Mold JW, Stoecker MW: Extreme pain from brown recluse spider bites model for cytokine-driven pain, *JAMA Dermatology* 150(11):1205–1208, 2013.

41. Smith S, Sanders SF, Carr J, King TR, Zimmet L, Repasky TM, Ambrose HS: Bedside management considerations in the treatment of pit viper envenomation, *Journal of Emergency Nursing* 40(6):537–545, 2014.

42. Trickett R, Whitaker IS, Boyce DE: Sting-ray injuries to the hand: Case report, literature review and a suggested algorithm for management, *Journal of Plastic, Reconstructive and Aesthetic Surgery* 62:e3270, 2008.
43. Traub SJ, Cummins GA: Tick-borne diseases. In *Wilderness medicine,* ed 6, chap 51, pp 954–975. St. Louis, MO, 2012, Mosby.
44. Undersea and Hyperbaric Medical Society: (n.d.). Directory of approved chambers in the United States. Available at 301-942-2980 or https://www.uhms.org/resources/chamber-directory.html.
45. Vetrano SJ, Lebowitz JB, Marcus S: Lionfish envenomation, *Journal of Emergency Medicine* 23:379–382, 2002.
46. Swim Infant: National drowning statics. Retrieved from https://www.infantswim.com/assets/docs/NationalDrowningStatistics2011.pdf, 2011.

Bibliography

Rabies Prophylaxis in the Emergency Department: *Advanced Emergency Nursing Journal* 35(2):110–119, 2013. Retrieved from http://journals.lww.com/aenjournal/Fulltext/2013/04000/Rabies_Prophylaxis_in_the_Emergency_Department.5.aspx.

Part 2

CHAPTER 16
Facial and Ocular Emergencies

LaToria S. Woods, MSN, RN, APN, CCNS

I. General Strategy

A. ASSESSMENT

1. Primary and secondary assessment/resuscitation (see Chapter 1)
2. Focused assessment
   a. Subjective data collection
      1) History of present illness/chief complaint
         a) Pain: PQRST (see Chapter 8)
         b) Respiratory distress/shortness of breath
         c) Abnormal appearance of the eye
            (1) Eyelid swelling
            (2) Redness: lid, sclera, conjunctiva
            (3) Change in luster
            (4) Asymmetry
         d) Changes in visual acuity: normal to blindness
            (1) Decreased visual acuity from patient's "normal"
            (2) Decreased visual field from patient's "normal"
            (3) Blurring of vision
            (4) Diplopia
            (5) Cloudy or smoky vision
            (6) Photophobia
            (7) Foreign body sensation
         e) Tearing
         f) Itching
         g) Discharge color and consistency
         h) Efforts to relieve symptoms
            (1) Home remedies
            (2) Alternative therapies
            (3) Medications
               (a) Prescription
               (b) OTC/herbal
      2) Past medical history
         a) Current or preexisting disease/illness
            (1) Diabetes
            (2) Cardiovascular: recent cardiac catheterization
            (3) Hypertension
            (4) Sickle cell
            (5) Immunologic diseases, connective tissue disorders
         b) Ocular
            (1) Corrective lenses
               (a) Contact lenses or glasses
               (b) Worn at time of injury
               (c) Last eye examination/ocular evaluation
            (2) Past eye disease, injury, or surgery (cataract or LASIK)
            (3) Glaucoma
            (4) Chronic eye disease
            (5) Family history of eye disease
         c) Substance and/or alcohol use/abuse

    d) Current medications may cause ocular side effects
      (1) Prescription
        (a) Eye medication
        (b) Steroids
        (c) Parasympatholytic drugs
        (d) Narcotics
        (e) Anticoagulants
      (2) OTC/herbal
    e) Allergies
    f) Immunization status

3) Psychological, social, environmental factors and risk factors
    a) Behavior appropriate for age and developmental stage
      (1) School-age children susceptible to conjunctivitis because of close contact and contagious nature of disease
      (2) Contact lens wearers at greater risk for corneal abrasions, ulcers, and infections
    b) Occupation or profession
    c) Hobbies, avocation, recreational activities
      (1) Injuries occurring in the garden have increased potential for infection
      (2) Swimming may increase potential for ocular infections
    d) Possible/actual assault, abuse, or intimate partner violence situations (see Chapters 3 and 40)
    e) Sensory deficits/changes
      (1) Auditory
        (a) Ear pain
        (b) Hearing loss
        (c) Tinnitus (ringing in ears) or hyperacusis (abnormally acute hearing)
      (2) Visual
        (a) Decreased tearing
        (b) Partial or complete blindness
        (c) Visual field defects and decreased light perception
      (3) Tactile/kinesthetic
        (a) Decreased sensation
        (b) Facial pain and/or sensation of heaviness, numbness, tingling, and paresthesias
      (4) Gustatory
        (a) Impairment of taste
        (b) Loss of taste or metallic taste
      (5) Olfactory: unilateral or bilateral loss of smell
    f) Malocclusion or trismus (inability to open mouth)
    g) Facial asymmetry, swelling
    h) Recent viral illness
    i) Rash
    j) Fever/chills
    k) Nausea/vomiting
    l) Dizziness/vertigo
    m) Speech difficulties
    n) Excessive salivation
    o) Foreign body sensation
    p) Exposure to and/or ingestion of noxious agents
      (1) Contact substances
      (2) Inhalants
    q) Efforts to relieve symptoms
      (1) Home remedies
      (2) Alternative therapies
      (3) Medications
        (a) Prescription
        (b) OTC/herbal

4) Past medical history
    a) Current or preexisting diseases/illness
      (1) Neurologic disorders or diseases
      (2) Hypertension: may be secondary cause of epistaxis
      (3) Blood dyscrasias
    b) Previous dental or ear, nose, and throat surgery
    c) Smoking history
    d) Substance and/or alcohol use/abuse
    e) Last normal menstrual period: female patients of childbearing age
    f) Current medications
      (1) Prescription
        (a) Analgesics may affect neurologic assessment (e.g., slurred speech, altered level of consciousness)
        (b) Antibiotics
        (c) Anticoagulants
        (d) Psychotropic/phenothiazine drug reactions may cause inability to close mouth
      (2) OTC/herbal
    g) Allergies

5) Psychological, social, and environmental factors
    a) Age: some presentations more prone in specific age groups
    b) Infection: viral, bacterial, or fungal
    c) Stressors: surgery, trauma, illness, and psychosocial factors
    d) Possible/actual assault, abuse, or intimate partner violence situations (see Chapters 3 and 40)

b. Objective data collection
  1) General appearance
    a) Level of consciousness, behavior, affect
    b) Vital signs
    c) Odors
    d) Hygiene
    e) Level of distress/discomfort

2) Inspection—facial
    a) Possible drooling
    b) Symmetry of structures: size, position, and movement including palpebral fissures and nasolabial folds
    c) Herpetiform vesicular eruption
    d) Pupil reaction
3) Inspection—ocular: always use contralateral eye for comparison
    a) Visual acuity is the vital sign in ophthalmology. It is an essential part of the physical examination process to establish a baseline before treatment as well as for medicolegal reasons; exception to this rule involves patient with chemical injury, in which case irrigation first is mandatory; when possible, patients with glasses or contact lenses should have visual acuity tested with correction. Test each eye separately, then together. If vision is suboptimal, a pinhole testing device can determine whether a problem with acuity is caused by refractory error or another process
        (1) Exact assessment by a Snellen chart, picture chart, or "E" chart may be necessary for small children, nonverbal patients, or those who cannot read
            (a) Ambulatory: tested at distance of 20 feet
            (b) Nonambulatory: tested with hand-held Rosenbaum card at approximately 14 inches
        (2) Gross assessment by finger count at 4 feet, if vision is greater than 20/400
        (3) Ability to distinguish light or shadows
        (4) Visual fields, objects can be seen in the peripheral vision, confrontation
    b) Eyelid and adnexa, function, deformity, spasm, erythema, edema
    c) Eye/facial surface, to include upper and lower lids for lesions, erythema
    d) Tearing
    e) Discharge: clear, mucoid, purulent
    f) Pupils: should be equal, round, reactive to light and accommodation (PERRLA), measurement of pupil size
    g) Extraocular movements (EOMs): intact, limited, or painful
    h) Position and alignment of eyes
    i) Conjunctiva and sclera for color, inflammation, or edema
    j) Blood or white cells in anterior chamber
    k) Opaque, gray-white area of cornea
    l) Hazy cornea

4) Palpation
    a) Sensory deficits or changes
    b) Areas of tenderness
    c) Frontal/maxillary sinuses
    d) Intraocular pressure: palpation should not be performed if there is concern regarding integrity of globe; it may result in extrusion of ocular contents and may cause permanent visual loss; the procedure should be reserved for the emergency physician or ophthalmologist in suspected cases of acute glaucoma or central retinal artery occlusion
    e) Increased warmth of surrounding tissues/areas
5) Percussion
    a) Soft tissues over frontal sinuses
    b) Soft tissues over maxillary sinuses
3. Diagnostic procedures
  a. Laboratory studies
    1) Anaerobic or aerobic cultures of wounds
    2) Complete blood count (CBC) with differential
    3) Coagulation profile
    4) Arterial blood gas (ABG)
    5) Eye discharge culture
    6) Erythrocyte sedimentation rate (ESR)
    7) C-reactive protein (CRP)
    8) Serum glucose
    9) Coagulation profile
    10) Urinalysis; pregnancy test in female patients of childbearing age if surgery is imminent
  b. Imaging studies
    1) Facial bones radiograph: maxilla, mandible, zygoma, orbits, nasal bone
    2) Waters' view of facial bones and sinuses
    3) Panoramic oral radiograph (Panorex)
    4) Chest radiograph
    5) Computed tomography (CT) scan: head, sinuses, larynx
    6) Sonography
    7) Magnetic resonance imaging (MRI)
    8) Soft tissue (orbit films) for foreign body
    9) Skull radiographs with Waters' view, sinus involvement
    10) Ocular sonography
  c. Other
    1) 12- to 15-lead electrocardiogram (ECG)
    2) Direct ophthalmoscopic examination
    3) Tonometry: intraocular pressure measurement
    4) Slit-lamp examination
    5) Fluorescein staining: positive Seidel test if vitreous humor leakage present

B. ANALYSIS: DIFFERENTIAL NURSING DIAGNOSES/COLLABORATIVE PROBLEMS

1. Ineffective airway clearance
2. Risk for aspiration
3. Acute/chronic pain
4. Impaired skin integrity
5. Risk for infection
6. Anxiety/fear
7. Deficient knowledge
8. Ineffective coping
9. Inefficient tissue perfusion: ocular
10. Disturbed sensory perception: visual
11. Noncompliance
12. Self-care deficit

C. PLANNING AND IMPLEMENTATION/ INTERVENTIONS

1. Determine priorities of care
   a. Maintain airway, breathing, circulation (see Chapter 1)
   b. Provide supplemental oxygen as indicated
   c. Establish intravenous (IV) access for administration of crystalloid fluid/medications as needed
   d. Obtain and set up equipment and supplies
   e. Prepare for/assist with medical interventions
   f. Facilitate ophthalmology consultation as appropriate (Box 16.1)
   g. Administer pharmacologic therapy as ordered
2. Relieve anxiety/apprehension
3. Allow significant others to remain with patient if supportive
4. Educate patient and significant others

D. EVALUATION AND ONGOING MONITORING

1. Continuously monitor and treat as indicated
2. Monitor patient's responses and outcome, and modify nursing care plan as indicated

---

Box 16.1

Consultation Criteria

Patients with the following problems should be referred for ophthalmologic consultation:

Penetrating ocular trauma, including impaled objects, embedded foreign bodies, and ruptured globe

Chemical burns of the eye

Severe lid lacerations

Glaucoma

Central retinal artery occlusion

Retinal detachment

Orbital fracture

Hyphema or hypopyon

Preseptal/orbital cellulitis

---

3. If positive patient outcomes are not demonstrated, reevaluate assessment and/or plan of care

E. DOCUMENTATION OF INTERVENTIONS AND PATIENT RESPONSE

F. AGE-RELATED CONSIDERATIONS

1. Pediatric
   a. Growth or development related
      1) During the sixth and seventh years, maximal enlargement of the face occurs; primarily eruption of teeth and development of the midface influence facial proportions at that time
      2) May need to use picture chart or "E" chart (patient indicates direction to which "E" points)
      3) Delayed presentation may be problematic because children may not notice gradual visual loss
      4) Neonatal patients delivered vaginally may develop sexually transmitted diseases with *Neisseria gonorrhoeae*, *Chlamydia trachomatis*, and herpes simplex virus; usually develops within first month of life
   b. "Pearls"
      1) Explain honestly to children what is going to be done to them
      2) Limitation in verbal expressions presents a disadvantage in evaluation of children and complicates assessment
      3) Have great patience
      4) Infants and small children may need to be restrained in a blanket to reduce number of moving parts and facilitate examination
      5) A red eye is not always infectious
      6) Consider corneal abrasion as cause of crying in infants
2. Geriatric
   a. Aging related
      1) Changes associated with aging
         a) Perception
            (1) Visual acuity loss
            (2) Vision diminishes gradually until approximately 70 years and then more rapidly thereafter
            (3) Decreased ability to use standard charts for visual acuity as a result of physical impairment
            (4) Decreased accuracy of results from visual acuity testing
            (5) Decreased near vision is problematic for many older patients
            (6) Ability of eye to accommodate or adjust to distances decreases with age
            (7) Older adults frequently complain of eye dryness resulting from decrease in lacrimal secretions

(8) Cataracts become more common with advancing age, to the point at which approximately one in three people in their 80s are affected

(9) Geriatric population more likely to experience glaucoma, detached retina, and retinal bleeding

(10) Diminished hearing

(11) Decreased sense of taste

(12) Decreased sensitivity to touch

b) Consciousness

(1) Loss of short-term memory

(2) Slower thought processing

(3) Increased pain threshold

c) Musculoskeletal

(1) Muscle atrophy

(2) Decreased flexibility

2) Elderly patients tend to have deterioration in special senses

3) Chronic diseases add further limitations to aged patients

b. "Pearls"

1) Older adults may need home health referrals to help with administration of medications and environmental safety issues

II. Specific Facial Emergencies

A. BELL PALSY (IDIOPATHIC FACIAL PARALYSIS)

Bell palsy is defined as having an acute, peripheral facial paralysis on one side. The etiology is unknown, but accounts for 50% of cases in which people present with lower facial motor neuron paralysis. The frequency of occurrence is between 13 and 24 cases per 100,000. Autoimmune, infectious, vascular, genetic, entrapment, and metabolic causes have been suggested to contribute to the development of Bell palsy. The most popular theory stems from viral causation.[1] Herpes simplex virus (HSV) is thought to be the most common cause, followed by herpes zoster. Even though other viruses have been associated with Bell palsy, these are two of the most common.[1]

Many patients have indicated having a respiratory tract infection prior to being diagnosed with Bell palsy.[1] Symptoms associated with facial paresis frequently include postauricular ear pain or headache, abnormally acute hearing (hyperacusis), decreased tearing, and impairment of taste. A differential diagnosis for facial paralysis is Lyme disease. It is typically associated with bilateral facial nerve paralysis, not unilateral as seen with Bell palsy.[2] Immediate initiation of appropriate antibiotic therapy is required for those patients thought to have Lyme disease.[3]

The symptoms are presumed to be caused by swelling of the facial nerve. In the narrow course through the temporal bone, the nerve becomes compressed and ischemic.

Bell palsy in rare instances may be bilateral.[3] It is more common in young and middle-aged adults, those with diabetes mellitus, with a higher incidence presenting during pregnancy, particularly the last trimester or first week postpartum. Men and women are equally affected.[3] The symptoms of Bell palsy are usually self-limiting. Complete resolution occurs within several weeks in 80–90% of cases. Treatment commonly includes protecting the affected eye. Medications often include antiviral agents and a short course of oral steroids. Assessment and treatment for Bell palsy are listed in the section Herpes Zoster Oticus.

B. HERPES ZOSTER OTICUS (RAMSAY HUNT SYNDROME)

Herpes zoster oticus is a viral infection of the inner, middle, and external ear. It is characterized by unilateral facial paralysis, a herpetiform vesicular eruption, and vestibulocochlear dysfunction. The disease process involves a reactivation, along the dermatome, of the varicella-zoster virus (VZV) and may occur in immunocompromised individuals. It can be confused initially with Bell palsy until herpetiform vesicular eruptions occur. The vesicular eruptions may occur on the pinna, external auditory canal, tympanic membrane, soft palate, oral cavity, face, and neck as far down as the shoulder. The pain is considerably more severe than that associated with Bell palsy, and is often disproportionate to physical findings. Outcomes are worse than in Bell palsy, with a lower incidence of complete facial recovery and the possibility of permanent hearing loss. Treatment is similar to that of Bell palsy.[3]

1. Assessment (both Bell palsy and herpes zoster oticus)

a. Subjective data collection

1) History of present illness/chief complaint

a) Rapid, acute onset of symptoms

b) Viral prodrome

c) Sudden, unilateral facial weakness/paralysis (bilateral facial paralysis may occur but is rare; consider Lyme disease as a differential diagnosis)

d) Retroauricular and/or facial discomfort

e) Pain (see Chapter 8): facial and/or ear pain

f) Drooling and/or difficulty swallowing

g) Increased sensitivity to noise on involved side

h) Loss of taste; difficult to tell whether it is unilateral

i) Nausea/vomiting

2) Past medical history

a) Current or preexisting diseases/illness

(1) Diabetes and other diseases associated with immunosuppression

(2) Sarcoidosis

(3) Lyme disease (see Chapter 15)

b) Previous history of VZV infection

c) Medications

d) Allergies

b. Objective data collection
  1) Physical examination
    a) General appearance
      (1) Level of consciousness, behavior, affect: speech difficulties from facial paralysis
      (2) Possible drooling
      (3) Moderate distress/discomfort
    b) Inspection
      (1) Upward movement of eyeball on affected side when attempting to close eye (Bell phenomenon)
      (2) Facial paralysis can be complete or partial
      (3) Lid lag and inability to close eye on affected side
      (4) Decreased lacrimation on affected side
      (5) Drooping of mouth on affected side
      (6) Flattening of nasolabial fold on affected side
      (7) Positive corneal sensation but no blink on affected side
      (8) Inability to wrinkle forehead on affected side
      (9) Herpetiform vesicular lesions (Ramsay Hunt syndrome)
  2) Diagnostic procedures: performed to aid in the exclusion of other diagnoses that may be confused with Bell palsy (e.g., middle ear disease, middle ear tumor, eighth cranial nerve tumor, central nervous system disturbances, or Lyme disease) and to determine the site of the lesion causing facial paralysis; other diagnostic tests are conducted in the outpatient setting
    a) Lyme titer
    b) Mastoid radiograph: rule out temporal bone fractures
    c) CT scan if other facial abnormalities are suspected
2. Analysis: differential nursing diagnoses/collaborative problems
  a. Risk for ineffective airway clearance
  b. Acute pain
  c. Risk for injury to affected eye
  d. Anxiety
  e. Deficient knowledge
3. Planning and implementation/interventions
  a. Prepare for/assist with medical interventions
    1) Apply eye patch after instilling artificial tears and lubricant ointment, then gently close affected eyelid
  b. Administer pharmacologic therapy as ordered
    1) Lubricant ointment at night and artificial tears during the day to affected eye
    2) Nonnarcotic analgesics
    3) Narcotics
    4) Corticosteroid therapy

    5) Antiviral agents ONLY in combination with corticosteroid therapy
    6) Antiemetics
    7) Antibiotics if secondary bacterial infection of vesicles
  c. Educate patient and significant others
    1) Reassure patient/significant others that a stroke has not occurred and spontaneous recovery happens in a majority of cases within 3 weeks
    2) Use sunglasses and other protective eyewear
    3) Keep face warm and avoid drafts
    4) Use moist heat and facial massage
    5) Encourage passive and facial muscle exercise
    6) Possible use of facial sling to support sagging facial muscles
    7) Corneal protection: reinforce eye care
4. Evaluation and ongoing monitoring
  a. Airway patency
  b. Hemodynamic status
  c. Pain relief

C. PAROTITIS

Acute parotitis, or inflammation of the parotid gland, most often has a bacterial or viral origin, although it may be caused by calculi formation, human immunodeficiency virus (HIV), tuberculosis, or other infections and disease processes. Viral parotitis (mumps) occurs most commonly in children and is usually bilateral (see Chapter 20). The parotid glands, located in the buccal mucosa near the upper teeth, are stimulated by the action of chewing to release saliva into the mouth to moisten food.[4]
1. Assessment
  a. Subjective data collection
    1) History of present illness/chief complaint
      a) Pain (see Chapter 8)
        (1) Bacterial: progressively painful swelling of the gland; painful chewing
        (2) Viral: bilateral painful swelling over several days
      b) Fever
      c) Malaise
      d) Anorexia
    2) Past medical history
      a) Current or preexisting diseases/illness
      b) Medications
      c) Allergies
      d) Immunization status
  b. Objective data collection
    1) Physical examination
      a) General appearance
        (1) Elevated temperature
        (2) Moderate distress/discomfort
      b) Inspection
        (1) Localized swelling over parotid gland
        (2) Erythema
      c) Palpation

(1) Tenderness of parotid gland
(2) Purulent saliva released from Stensen duct when massaged
2) Diagnostic procedures
a) CBC with differential if patient appears toxic
b) Culture and sensitivity of purulent saliva
c) CT scan
d) Sonography
2. Analysis: differential nursing diagnoses/collaborative problems
a. Acute pain
b. Fatigue
c. Deficient knowledge
3. Planning and implementation/interventions
a. Prepare for/assist with medical interventions
1) Referral for definitive surgical intervention if indicated
b. Administer pharmacologic therapy as ordered
1) Nonnarcotic analgesics
2) Narcotics
3) Antibiotics
c. Educate patient and significant others
1) Apply moist heat to area
2) Gently massage gland to promote drainage
3) Use lemon drops or other agents to increase saliva production
4) Increase fluid intake
4. Evaluation and ongoing monitoring
a. Pain relief

D. SINUSITIS

Acute sinusitis is an inflammatory condition of the mucous membranes that line the nasal passage and paranasal sinuses lasting less than 4 weeks. Allergens, environmental irritants, and infection are a few predisposing factors. The most common cause is an upper respiratory infection (URI). The second most common cause in the occurrence of childhood acute sinusitis is allergic inflammation which includes allergic asthma, atopic dermatitis, allergic rhinitis, and ocular allergic diseases. Other conditions that may contribute to sinusitis include cystic fibrosis, immune disorders, abnormal ciliary function, nasal polyps, nasal foreign bodies (including indwelling nasal tubes), cleft palate, adenoidal hypertrophy, septal deviation, and gastroesophageal reflux disease.[5]

Symptoms can range from mild congestion to a severe, progressive infection with lethal complications. The maxillary sinus is most frequently affected. Acute sinusitis usually progresses over a period of 7–10 days. *Haemophilus influenzae* and *Streptococcus pneumoniae* are the common organisms involved in the adult population. *Moraxella catarrhalis*, in addition to *Haemophilus* and *Streptococcus*, are the responsible organisms in children. The immunocompromised person may develop sinusitis from the *Candida, Aspergillus,* or *Phycomyces* organisms.[4,6]

Bacterial disease is suggested by worsening symptoms after 5 days, persistent symptoms after 10 days, or initial improvement followed by more focal symptoms of sinus congestion and discomfort. Symptoms include nasal congestion, mucopurulent nasal drainage, pressure over the involved sinus, malaise, fever, and facial swelling. Complications of acute sinusitis include chronic sinusitis, orbital cellulitis, orbital abscess, epidural abscess, subdural empyema, meningitis, brain abscess, cavernous sinus thrombosis, and osteomyelitis of the frontal or maxillary bone. Because of these complications, aggressive medical management is often indicated.[3]

1. Assessment
a. Subjective data collection
1) History of present illness/chief complaint
a) Pain (see Chapter 8): over area of involved sinus
(1) Frontal: pain over forehead or around orbit, exacerbated when bending forward
(2) Maxillary: pain below eyes; pain over cheekbones, upper teeth, or upper jaw; ear pain; pain on chewing; and numbness over middle third of face; major site of infection in children
(3) Ethmoidal: pain at bridge of nose and behind eyes (retroocular) and mastoid pain; seen more frequently in children and associated with puffy eyes; may occur with maxillary sinusitis
(4) Sphenoidal: pain referred to the top of head and occipital area
(5) Headache: usually frontal and worsens with bending over or coughing
(6) Facial pain described as achy and dull
(7) Pressure sensation over involved sinuses
b) Fever: may or may not be present
c) Nasal quality to voice
d) Decreased appetite
e) Nausea
f) Nasal congestion/obstruction
g) Cough
h) Sore throat: may occur secondary to mouth breathing or postnasal drainage
2) Past medical history
a) Current or preexisting diseases/illness
(1) Diabetes
(2) Immunosuppression illnesses
(3) Hepatic, renal disease
(4) Deviated septum, nasal polyps, or enlarged turbinates
(5) Chronic or acute upper respiratory tract symptoms
(6) Recent cold that is not improving
(7) Recurrent otitis media in children
b) Recent molar extraction
c) Burns

d) Mouth odor in young children
e) Medications
f) Allergies
b. Objective data collection
1) Physical examination
a) General appearance
(1) Possible elevated temperature
(2) Fetid breath
(3) Moderate distress/discomfort
b) Inspection
(1) Red, swollen nasal mucosa
(2) Purulent nasal drainage, possibly blood tinged
(3) Conjunctivitis
(4) Opacification of sinuses to transillumination
(5) Puffy eyes in children
c) Palpation/percussion
(1) Tenderness over involved sinus areas
2) Diagnostic procedures
a) Sinus cultures: aerobic and anaerobic (e.g., via needle aspiration and/or cannulation of ostia); rarely performed in the emergency setting
b) Radiographs: reserved for complicated cases or patients unresponsive to previous therapy; includes Waters', Caldwell, submentovertical, and lateral views: evidence of active infection
(1) Presence of radiologic opacity
(2) Air-fluid level
(3) Mucosal thickening
c) Sinus CT scan: for patients with suspected complication or chronic sinusitis; tends to overdiagnose
2. Analysis: differential nursing diagnoses/collaborative problems
a. Acute pain
b. Risk for infection
c. Deficient knowledge
3. Planning and implementation/interventions
a. Acute uncomplicated sinusitis
1) Educate patient and significant others
a) Relieve obstruction using nasal/systemic decongestants, nasal steroids
(1) Local decongestants should be sprayed into each nostril as directed
(2) Local decongestants should not be used for more than 3–4 days, to avoid mucosal rebound effect
(3) If applicable, instruct parents on use of saline nose drops in children
b) Promote sinus drainage by keeping head of bed elevated
c) Apply heat to face to relieve pressure
d) Use room vaporizer

b. Acute complicated sinusitis
1) Establish IV access for administration of crystalloid fluid/medications
2) Prepare for/assist with medical interventions
a) Assist with hospital admission and possible surgical interventions
3) Administer pharmacologic therapy as ordered
a) Antibiotics
4. Evaluation and ongoing monitoring
a. Hemodynamic status
b. Pain relief

E. TRIGEMINAL NEURALGIA (TIC DOULOUREUX)

Trigeminal neuralgia is a neurologic disorder of the fifth cranial nerve of unknown origin. Any of the three nerve divisions can be affected. The second and third divisions, which innervate the maxillary and mandibular areas of the face, are more commonly affected. It is a syndrome characterized by excruciatingly painful paroxysms in one or more distributions of the trigeminal nerve. It is relatively uncommon; however, it is more common in women than in men. Individuals affected are most commonly between 50 and 69 years of age, and symptoms occur more frequently on the right side of the face. Structural lesions are believed to be the cause, allowing for repetitive firing in the nerve and its divisions. Exacerbations may be precipitated by exposure to cold and facial stimulus such as eating, drinking, washing the face, shaving, and applying makeup.[3,7]

1. Assessment
a. Subjective data collection
1) History of present illness/chief complaint
a) Pain (see Chapter 8)
(1) Similar to that from electrical shock occurring in distribution of one or more branches of trigeminal nerve (lower cheek, jaw, and, less commonly, forehead)
(2) Pain-free interval of minutes, hours, days, or longer; however, recurrences become more frequent and severe
(3) Unilateral during any single episode
(4) Triggered by light touch, vibration, chewing, shaving, face washing, or light breeze
b) Minimal to no sensory loss in distribution of trigeminal nerve
c) Right side affected more than left side
2) Past medical history
a) Current or preexisting diseases/illness
(1) Aneurysm
(2) Tumor
(3) Chronic meningeal inflammation
(4) Lesions of trigeminal nerve root
b) Previous, similar episodes
c) Frequently noncontributory
d) Medications
e) Allergies

b. Objective data collection
   1) Physical examination
      a) General appearance
         (1) Level of consciousness, behavior, affect: facial grimacing with episodes of pain
         (2) Moderate to severe distress/discomfort
      b) Palpation
         (1) Minimal or absent sensory loss along distribution of trigeminal nerve
         (2) Painful paroxysmal tic precipitated by touching of trigger zone on ipsilateral anterior aspect of face
   2) Diagnostic procedures
      a) Diagnosis may be made on basis of history and physical examination alone
      b) No further diagnostic tests are required unless intracranial lesion or other neurologic disorders are suspected
      c) MRI if atypical features are present
2. Analysis: differential nursing diagnoses/collaborative problems
   a. Acute pain
   b. Fatigue
   c. Deficient knowledge
3. Planning and implementation/interventions
   a. Prepare for/assist with medical interventions
      1) Referral for definitive surgical intervention if adequate pain relief not achieved pharmacologically
   b. Administer pharmacologic therapy as ordered
      1) Carbamazepine (Tegretol)
      2) IV phenytoin (Dilantin): sometimes successful in interrupting episodes
      3) Narcotics/analgesics: minimally effective
      4) Regional block: trigeminal nerve
   c. Educate patient/significant others
      1) Majority of patients with trigeminal neuralgia will respond to medical therapy within 48 hours
      2) Of these patients, 25–50% eventually fail to respond to drug therapy and require surgical intervention
      3) If exposing the affected cheek to sudden cold triggers neuralgia, avoid iced drinks, cold wind, swimming in cold water, and similar stimuli
4. Evaluation and ongoing monitoring
   a. Pain relief

III. Specific Medical Ocular Emergencies

A. ACUTE ANGLE-CLOSURE GLAUCOMA

Acute angle-closure glaucoma occurs when the distance or angle in the junction between the iris and the cornea becomes narrowed or is blocked completely. The aqueous fluid produced by the ciliary body is unable to exit through the canal of Schlemm. The precipitating factors of outflow obstruction are a gradual increase in pressure and sudden dilation of the pupil. Occurrences usually transpire in a darkened environment such as a movie theater.

If acute angle-closure glaucoma is not recognized and treated within hours of the onset of symptoms, blindness results from an increase in pressure causing damage to the optic nerve and decreased circulation to the retina. Patients with this emergent condition require immediate attention before permanent damage is incurred. This condition occurs in 100 per 100,000 cases, with a peak age group of 55–70 years. It may occur in younger people, especially those with a history of eye trauma or surgery.[8]

1. Assessment
   a. Subjective data collection
      1) History of present illness/chief complaint
         a) Red eye: entire conjunctiva is affected
         b) Pain (see Chapter 8): usually severe, sudden-onset, deep, unilateral
         c) Intense headache
         d) Blurred vision
         e) Halos around lights
         f) Photophobia
         g) Nausea and vomiting
         h) Abdominal pain, nonspecific
      2) Past medical history
         a) Current or preexisting diseases/illness
         b) Previous anterior uveitis/iritis
         c) Trauma: blunt or penetrating forces
         d) Medications
         e) Allergies
   b. Objective data collection
      1) Physical examination
         a) General appearance
            (1) Moderate to severe distress/discomfort
         b) Inspection
            (1) Visual acuity: decreased
            (2) Cornea: hazy, steamy, lusterless
            (3) Pupil on affected side: midposition, poorly reactive or fixed
            (4) Increased intraocular pressure: between 40 and 80 mm Hg (>20 mm Hg)
            (5) Unnatural globe appearance
            (6) Vomiting
         c) Palpation
            (1) Rocklike hardness of globe
      2) Diagnostic procedures
         a) Tonometry: intraocular pressure measurement
         b) Slit-lamp examination
         c) Gonioscopy per ophthalmology: examines the filtration angle of the anterior chamber of the eye

2. Analysis: differential nursing diagnoses/collaborative problems
   a. Acute pain
   b. Disturbed sensory perception: visual
   c. Ineffective tissue perfusion: ocular
   d. Anxiety/fear
   e. Deficient knowledge
3. Planning and implementations/interventions
   a. Establish IV access for administration of crystalloid fluid/medications as needed
   b. Prepare for/assist with medical interventions
      1) Referral to ophthalmologic consultant
      2) Definitive treatment: iridotomy
      3) Assist with possible hospital admission
   c. Administer pharmacologic therapy as ordered
      1) Nonnarcotic analgesics
      2) Narcotics
      3) Antiemetics
      4) Beta-adrenergic antagonists: eye drops and IV carbonic anhydrase inhibitor (e.g., acetazolamide [Diamox])
      5) Pilocarpine eye drops (e.g., Pilocar, Pilogel): 2% for light-colored eyes, 4% for dark-colored eyes
      6) IV osmotic diuretic agents: mannitol (Osmitrol)
4. Evaluation and ongoing monitoring
   a. Recheck intraocular pressure hourly
   b. Pain relief
   c. Visual acuity

B. ANTERIOR UVEITIS/IRITIS

Uveitis is defined as inflammation of one or all parts of the uveal tract, which includes the iris, ciliary body, and choroid. This inflammatory process usually includes the iris or uveal layer of the anterior segment of the eye and sometimes the ciliary body. This is commonly referred to as iritis or iridocyclitis. The symptoms include intense unilateral pain, conjunctival injection, edema, lacrimation, and photophobia. Posterior uveitis, also known as choroiditis, is rare with the exception of cytomegalovirus (CMV) in patients with acquired immunodeficiency syndrome (AIDS). Among the common predisposing conditions are a variety of systemic immune-mediated illnesses, including rheumatic diseases, systemic lupus erythematosus, ankylosing spondylitis, Reiter syndrome, and syphilis.[9,10]

More than 50% of patients have the human lymphocyte antigen HLA-B27 or HLA-B8. Although iritis may be seen as a sequela of injury, malignant disease, or medications, the condition is usually idiopathic. Pain in the affected eye is experienced when light is directed into the opposite eye because of consensual constriction of the irritated iris. The hallmark finding is the presence of inflammatory cells in the anterior chamber, visualized on slit-lamp examination. Without treatment, anterior uveitis can cause glaucoma, pupillary abnormalities, cataract formation, and macular dysfunction. Immediate referral to an ophthalmologist is recommended.[9,10]

1. Assessment
   a. Subjective data collection
      1) History of present illness/chief complaint
         a) Decreased visual acuity from patient's "normal," mildly blurred vision
         b) Unilateral pain (see Chapter 8): moderate to severe
         c) Edema of upper lid
         d) Red eye
         e) Intense photophobia
         f) Tearing
         g) Floating spots in the vision
      2) Past medical history
         a) Current or preexisting disease/illness
            (1) Rheumatoid arthritis
            (2) Ankylosing spondylitis
            (3) Syphilis
         b) Familial history of rheumatic disease
         c) Medications such as steroids and atropine drugs because these types of medications are used in treatment plan
         d) Allergies
   b. Objective data collection
      1) Physical examination
         a) General appearance
            (1) Moderate distress/discomfort
         b) Inspection
            (1) Visual acuity: decreased slightly
            (2) Intraocular pressure: low to minimally elevated
            (3) Pupils: miosis, small, irregular, sluggish reaction
            (4) Lacrimation
            (5) Ciliary flush: radiation of injected vessels outward from iris
            (6) Cornea: clear to hazy
            (7) Hypopyon: white cells/pus layering in the anterior chamber
         c) Palpation
            (1) Pain with application of eye pressure
      2) Diagnostic procedures
         a) Slit-lamp examination
         b) Fluorescein stain
         c) Tonometry: intraocular pressure measurement
2. Analysis: differential nursing diagnoses/collaborative problems
   a. Acute pain
   b. Disturbed sensory-perception: visual
   c. Anxiety/fear
   d. Deficient knowledge
3. Planning and implementation/interventions
   a. Prepare for/assist with medical interventions
      1) Provide darkened environment
      2) Apply warm compresses to eye

b. Administer pharmacologic therapy as ordered
   1) Topical steroid agents per ophthalmology
   2) Cycloplegic agents as prescribed for paralyzing ciliary muscle, thereby paralyzing accommodation and reducing ciliary spasms
c. Educate patient and significant others
   1) Shielding methods or use of dark glasses
   2) Instillation of medication
   3) Explain need to rest eyes
   4) Explain disease process in appropriate terms
   5) Follow-up plan of care with ophthalmologist
4. Evaluation and ongoing monitoring
   a. Visual acuity
   b. Pain relief

C. CENTRAL RETINAL ARTERY OCCLUSION

Central retinal artery occlusion is a sudden, painless, unilateral loss of vision caused by a blockage of the ophthalmic artery by an embolus. The embolus originates from atherosclerotic plaques in the carotid artery or from the cardiac valves. Events preceding the loss of vision include amaurosis fugax or a sudden temporary loss of vision lasting a few seconds to minutes. Prompt recognition of this ophthalmologic emergency and intervention within 1–2 hours of onset of symptoms are essential for preservation of vision. Although this condition generally occurs in the older population, ages 50–70 years, a history of thrombus or embolus may predispose young patients to this condition.[6,11]

1. Assessment
   a. Subjective data collection
      1) History of present illness/chief complaint
         a) Sudden, profound, unilateral loss of vision
         b) Painless
      2) Past medical history
         a) Current or preexisting diseases/illness
            (1) Cardiovascular disease
               (a) Hypertension
               (b) History of thrombus or embolus, stroke or transient ischemic attack (TIA)
               (c) Cardiac valve disease
               (d) Arteriosclerotic disease: most common underlying cause
               (e) Atrial fibrillation
            (2) Diabetes
            (3) Arteritis, giant cell
            (4) Sickle cell disease
         b) Trauma: blunt or penetrating forces
         c) IV substance use/abuse
         d) Medications
         e) Allergies
   b. Objective data collection
      1) Physical examination
         a) General appearance
            (1) Level of consciousness, behavior: anxious
            (2) Mild distress/discomfort, critically ill
         b) Inspection
            (1) Visual acuity limited to light perception or finger counting in affected eye
            (2) Afferent pupil defect
            (3) Retina: pale and edematous
      2) Diagnostic procedures
         a) Funduscopic examination
         b) Tonometry: intraocular pressure measurement
         c) CBC with differential
         d) Coagulation profile
         e) Serum glucose
2. Analysis: differential nursing diagnoses/collaborative problems
   a. Ineffective tissue perfusion: ocular
   b. Anxiety/fear
   c. Deficient knowledge
   d. Risk for injury
3. Planning and implementation/interventions
   a. Establish IV access for administration of crystalloid fluid/medications as needed
   b. Prepare for/assist with medical interventions
      1) Referral to ophthalmologic consultant
      2) Digital massage of globe: this therapy should be reserved for a physician
      3) Assist with hospital admission and possible surgery or transfer to an institution providing a higher level of care
   c. Administer pharmacologic therapy as ordered
      1) Ocular hypotensive drops, beta blockers
      2) Systemic acetazolamide (Diamox)
      3) Provide carbogen gas (95% oxygen plus 5% carbon dioxide), if available, for vasodilation in 3- to 10-minute treatments at 2-hour intervals for 24–48 hours (potentially harmful to patient with chronic obstructive pulmonary disease)
      4) Controversial intervention may include administration of anticoagulants, tissue plasminogen activator (tPA [Activase])
4. Evaluation and ongoing monitoring
   a. Hemodynamic status
   b. Visual acuity

D. CONJUNCTIVITIS

Conjunctivitis refers to any inflammatory condition of the membrane that lines the eyelids and covers the exposed surface of the sclera. Common causes include bacterial or viral inflammation, *Chlamydia*, *N. gonorrhoeae*, allergens, chemical burns, foreign bodies, ultraviolet or flash burns, exposure to irritants, and some systemic diseases. If the conjunctiva is injured or disrupted, the inflammatory process becomes evident with the infection of the cells. Common bacterial gram-positive and gram-negative organisms that cause conjunctivitis include streptococci, *Haemophilus influenzae*, staphylococci, pneumococci, and gonococci. Contact lens wearers require antibiotic coverage for *Pseudomonas* organisms.[10]

The common viral agents are adenovirsus types 3, 4, and 7, and herpes simplex. The inflammation causes marked hyperemia and discharge consistency from purulent to watery/clear. Neonates are at risk for chlamydia and *N. gonorrhoeae* from birth. Young children are at risk because of close proximity with other children and because of frequent hand-to-face contact with infrequent and ineffective handwashing.[10]

1. Assessment
   a. Subjective data collection
      1) History of present illness/chief complaint
         a) Redness of affected eye(s), abrupt onset
         b) Unilateral or bilateral involvement
         c) Pain (see Chapter 8): mainly irritation
         d) Foreign body sensation, "gritty" sensation
         e) Discharge
            (1) Purulent, mucopurulent, or thin/watery
            (2) Matting of eyelids and lashes after sleeping
         f) Itching/burning
         g) Eyelid edema
         h) Fever, pharyngitis (associated with viral illness), otitis media
      2) Past medical history
         a) Current or preexisting diseases/illness
         b) Recent upper respiratory tract infection
         c) Close contact with persons recently treated for like symptoms
         d) Medications
            (1) Steroids: may exacerbate local ocular infections; especially dangerous with herpes infections; therefore, not recommended
            (2) Previous antibiotic use may influence treatment choice
         e) Allergies: medication, environmental
   b. Objective data collection
      1) Physical examination
         a) General appearance
            (1) Mild distress/discomfort
         b) Inspection
            (1) Visual acuity: normal for patient
            (2) Cornea: clear
            (3) Pupil: normal
            (4) Conjunctiva: red or pink eye from congestion of conjunctival vessels
            (5) Chemosis: scleral swelling
            (6) Discharge: purulent or mucopurulent
            (7) Eyelid edema, mild
         c) Palpation
            (1) Enlarged preauricular lymph node(s), bacterial or viral infection
      2) Diagnostic procedures
         a) Culture of discharge if indicated
            b) Fluorescein stain: normal for bacterial, abnormal for viral herpes simplex as noted by a corneal dendrite
            c) Gram stain of discharge for identification of bacterial organisms if indicated
2. Analysis: differential nursing diagnoses/collaborative problems
   a. Acute pain
   b. Anxiety/fear
   c. Deficient knowledge
3. Planning and implementation/interventions
   a. Prepare for/assist with medical interventions
      1) Obtain culture of discharge if indicated
      2) Cleanse eyelids gently to remove debris
         a) Wipe from nose to outer corner of eye
         b) Warm compresses for bacterial infection; cool compresses for viral infection
      3) If herpes simplex virus present, assist with ophthalmology referral
   b. Administer pharmacologic therapy as ordered
      1) Bacterial infection: broad-spectrum antibiotics
      2) Fluoroquinolones for contact lens wearers
      3) Viral infection: nonsteroidal antiinflammatory drugs
      4) Allergic: antihistamines, topical vasoconstrictor
      5) Suspected gonococcal infection: aggressive systemic antibiotics must be instituted immediately to prevent severe ocular injury
   c. Educate patient/significant others
      1) Instillation of medication
      2) Frequent handwashing, aseptic technique
      3) Eye-cleansing procedure (cleanse lid line with baby shampoo)
      4) Avoid eye makeup, throw away previous products
      5) Follow-up care plans
      6) Prevention information: contagious nature of disease
4. Evaluation and ongoing monitoring
   a. Pain relief

E. PERIORBITAL/ORBITAL CELLULITIS

Acute redness and swelling of the eye and surrounding area must be evaluated to determine whether involvement is limited to the superficial soft tissue structures alone or whether there is extension into the globe and deeper structures. Periorbital, or preseptal, cellulitis is an infection of the superficial tissues of the eyelids and periorbital area. The symptoms include a swollen, erythematous eyelid with mild, diffuse, conjunctival injection. It may occur after injury such as a laceration or insect bite or as a complication of medical conditions such as sinusitis. It is usually caused by pneumococcal, staphylococcal, or streptococcal bacteria. In young children, the infection may be secondary to paranasal sinusitis caused by *H. influenzae*.[9,10]

Orbital cellulitis is more serious and involves the eye itself. It causes decreased visual acuity, proptosis (bulging eyeball), painful ocular movement, and additional edema. Diabetic and immunocompromised patients are at high risk for fungal infections, which can quickly become fatal. Orbital cellulitis represents a major ophthalmologic emergency and is potentially life threatening because the infection may extend into the cavernous sinus or the brain.[9,10]

1. Assessment
   a. Subjective data collection
      1) History of present illness/chief complaint
         a) Marked periorbital erythema
         b) Marked periorbital edema
         c) Pain (see Chapter 8): aching, severe, deep, aggravated by movement of eye
         d) Conjunctival injection
         e) Fever
      2) Past medical history
         a) Current or preexisting diseases/illness
         b) Recent upper respiratory tract infection, dental abscess, orbital fracture/trauma, hordeolum, dacryocystitis, or impetigo
         c) Medications
         d) Allergies
         e) Immunization status, especially *H. influenzae* type B (Hib)
   b. Objective data collection
      1) Physical examination
         a) General appearance
            (1) Elevated temperature: >98.6°F (37°C)
            (2) Moderate distress/discomfort
         b) Inspection
            (1) Visual acuity: decreased from patient's "normal"
            (2) Decreased pupillary reflexes
            (3) Afferent pupil defect
            (4) Erythema and swelling of the eyelids and surrounding structures
            (5) Paralysis or severe pain with EOM
      2) Diagnostic procedures
         a) Orbital CT scan: determine extent of infection
         b) Culture of discharge
         c) Gram stain of discharge: identification of bacterial organisms
         d) Blood cultures
         e) CBC with differential
         f) Lumbar puncture to rule out central nervous system infection/involvement in toxic-appearing patients
2. Analysis: differential nursing diagnoses/collaborative problems
   a. Acute pain
   b. Anxiety/fear
   c. Deficient knowledge
3. Planning and implementation/interventions
   a. Establish IV access for administration of crystalloid fluid/medications as needed
   b. Prepare for/assist with medical interventions
      1) Application of warm compresses
      2) Eyelid abscesses require surgical intervention
      3) Referral to ophthalmology consultant
      4) Assist with possible hospital admission for IV antibiotic therapy
   c. Administer pharmacologic therapy as ordered
      1) Parenteral antibiotics for moderate periorbital cellulitis and orbital cellulitis
      2) Antibiotic ointments
   d. Educate patient and significant others
      1) For mild periorbital cellulitis, oral antibiotics
      2) Importance of follow-up care within 24 hours
4. Evaluation and ongoing monitoring
   a. Hemodynamic status
   b. Pain relief

References

1. Buttaro TM, Trybulski J, Polgar Bailey P, Sandberg-Cook J: *Primary care*, ed 4, St. Louis, MO, 2013, Elsevier.
2. Glass GE, Tzafetta K: Bell's palsy: a summary of current evidence and referral algorithm, *Family Practice* 31(6):631–642, 2014.
3. Marx JA, Hockenberger RS, Walls RM, Biros MH, Danzl DF, Zink BJ: *Rosen's emergency medicine concepts and clinical practice*, ed 8, Philadelphia, PA, 2014, Saunders.
4. Shaw KN, Bachur RG, Chamberlain JM, Lavelle J, Nagler J, Shook JE: *Fleisher & Ludwig's textbook of pediatric emergency medicine*, ed 7, Philadelphia, PA, 2016, Wolter Kluwer.
5. Wolfson AB, Cloutier RL, Hendey GW, Ling LJ, Rosen CL: *Harwood-Nuss' clinical practice of emergency medicine*, ed 6, Philadelphia, PA, 2015, Wolters Kluwer.
6. Schaider JJ, Barkin RM, Hayden SR, Wolfe RE, Barkin AZ, Rosen P: *Rosen and Barkin's 5 minute emergency medicine consult*, ed 5, Philadelphia, PA, 2015, Wolters Kluwer Health.
7. Ferri FF: *Ferri's clinical advisor 2016: 5 books in 1*, Philadelphia, PA, 2016, Elsevier.
8. Adams JG, Barton ED, Collings JL, DeBlieux PMC, Gisondi MA, Sharma R: *Emergency medicine clinical essentials*, ed 2, Philadelphia, PA, 2013, Saunders.
9. Bickley LS: *Bates' guide to physical assessment and history taking*, ed 11, Philadelphia, PA, 2013, Wolters Kluwer Health, Lippincott Williams & Wilkins.
10. Kaiser PK, Friedman NJ, Pineda R: *The Massachusetts eye and ear infirmary illustrated manual of ophthalmology*, ed 4, China, 2014, Elsevier.
11. Tintinalli JE, Stapczynski JC, John Ma O, Cline DM, Cydulka RK, Meckler GD: *Tintinalli's emergency medicine: a comprehensive study guide*, ed 7, New York, NY, 2011, McGraw-Hill Companies, Inc.

CHAPTER 17

Fluid and Electrolyte Abnormalities

Betty L. Kuiper, PhDc, MSN, APRN, ACNS-BC, CEN

I. General Strategy

A. ASSESSMENT

1. Primary and secondary assessment/resuscitation (see Chapter 1)
   a. Subjective data collection
      1) History of present illness/chief complaint
         a) Pain: PQRST (see Chapter 8)
         b) Injury: mechanism (see Chapter 31) and time
         c) Fatigue, malaise
         d) Nausea, vomiting
         e) Altered mental status or decreased level of consciousness
         f) Fever
         g) Dyspnea
         h) Urticaria
         i) Edema: location and type
         j) Weakness
         k) Rash
         l) Cough
         m) Sore throat
         n) Other symptoms: anorexia, pruritus, diarrhea
         o) Efforts to relieve symptoms
            (1) Home remedies
            (2) Complementary alternative therapies
            (3) Medications
               (a) Prescription
                  (i) Anticoagulants
                  (ii) Insulin or oral hypoglycemic
                  (iii) Phenothiazines
                  (iv) Angiotensin-converting enzyme (ACE) inhibitors
                  (v) Beta blockers
                  (vi) Potassium-sparing diuretics
                  (vii) Angiotensin II receptor antagonists (or blockers) (ARBs)
                  (viii) Calcium channel blockers
                  (ix) Digitalis
                  (x) Bronchodilators
                  (xi) Tocolytic agents
                  (xii) Synthetic thyroid hormones
                  (xiii) Antibiotics (trimethoprim, penicillin G potassium)
               (b) OTC/herbal
                  (i) Decongestants
                  (ii) Acetaminophen or aspirin
            (4) Allergies
            (5) Immunization status
      2) Past medical history
         a) Current or preexisting diseases/illness
            (1) Vascular disease
            (2) Diabetes
            (3) Alcoholism
            (4) Sickle cell anemia
            (5) Hemophilia
            (6) Renal disease
               (a) Acute renal failure
               (b) Dialysis
               (c) Adrenal disease
            (7) Exposure to illness

(8) Splenectomy: alters immune system
(9) Infection: viral, bacterial, fungal, rickettsial, or parasitic
(10) Vitamin deficiency
(11) Malabsorption syndromes
b) Recent major injury
c) Previous similar episodes
d) Inadequately treated disease process
e) Last normal menstrual period: female patients of childbearing age
f) Smoking history
g) Substance and/or alcohol use/abuse
h) Current medications
3) Psychological/social/environmental factors
a) Age: illness more severe in very young and elderly
b) Family history
c) Gender: some disorders are gender linked
d) Race: may determine increased incidence
e) Possible/actual assault, abuse, or intimate partner violence situations (see Chapters 40 and 48)
f) Lifestyle
(1) Sedentary lifestyle
(2) Nutritional status: obesity and dietary excess or deficit
g) Stressors: surgery, trauma, illness, psychosocial factors
h) Climate or environment
i) Immobilization
b. Objective data collection
1) General appearance
a) Level of consciousness, behavior, affect
b) Vital signs, including orthostasis
c) Odors
d) Gait
e) Hygiene
f) Weight
g) Level of distress/discomfort
2) Inspection
a) Neck veins
b) Skin color, rash or urticaria
c) Mucous membranes
d) Evidence of trauma
e) Areas of erythema
3) Auscultation
a) Breath sounds: clear, wheezes, crackles
b) Bowel sounds: normal, hyperactive, hypoactive, absent
c) Heart sounds: S_1 and S_2, other sounds (e.g., murmurs), dysrhythmias
4) Palpation/percussion
a) Skin moisture, turgor
b) Areas of tenderness
c) Areas of edema

d) Areas of hyperthermia
e) Arteries: equality of peripheral pulses
f) Veins: venous filling and varicosities
g) Capillary refill
h) Lymph nodes
i) Muscle tone, strength
j) Deep tendon reflexes
2. Diagnostic procedures
a. Laboratory studies
1) Complete blood count (CBC) with differential
2) Serum chemistries including glucose, blood urea nitrogen (BUN), and creatinine
3) Arterial blood gases (ABGs)
4) Serum and urine toxicology: therapeutic level and toxic ingestion
5) Clotting profile: partial thromboplastin time (PTT), prothrombin time (PT)
6) Type and crossmatch
7) Serum ammonia level
8) Carboxyhemoglobin level
9) Serum uric acid
10) Liver enzymes
11) Sickle cell screen
12) Hepatitis screen
13) Serum ketone levels
14) Cerebrospinal fluid (CSF): cell count, glucose, and protein count, culture
15) Brain natriuretic peptide (BNP)
16) Urinalysis; pregnancy test in female patients of childbearing age
b. Imaging studies
1) Chest radiograph
2) CT scan
3) MRI scan
c. Other
1) 12- to 15-lead electrocardiogram (ECG)
2) Electroencephalogram (EEG)
3) Lumbar puncture

B. ANALYSIS: DIFFERENTIAL NURSING DIAGNOSES/COLLABORATIVE PROBLEMS

1. Ineffective airway clearance
2. Impaired gas exchange
3. Decreased cardiac output
4. Deficient/excess fluid volume
5. Ineffective tissue perfusion
6. Anxiety/fear
7. Fatigue
8. Impaired skin integrity
9. Deficient knowledge
10. Pain
11. Risk for infection
12. Risk for injury

C. PLANNING AND IMPLEMENTATION/ INTERVENTIONS

1. Determine priorities of care
   a. Maintain airway, breathing, circulation (see Chapter 1)
   b. Provide supplemental oxygen as indicated
   c. Establish intravenous (IV) access for administration of crystalloid fluid/blood products/medications; may consider intraosseus (IO) access as needed for clinical situation
   d. Obtain and set up equipment and supplies
   e. Prepare for/assist with medical interventions
   f. Administer pharmacologic therapy as ordered
2. Relieve anxiety/apprehension
3. Allow significant others to remain with patient if supportive
4. Educate patient/significant others

D. EVALUATION AND ONGOING MONITORING

1. Continuously monitor and treat as indicated
2. Monitor patient response/outcomes, and modify nursing care plan as appropriate
3. If positive patient outcomes are not demonstrated, reevaluate assessment and/or plan of care

E. DOCUMENTATION OF INTERVENTIONS AND PATIENT RESPONSE

F. AGE-RELATED CONSIDERATIONS

1. Pediatrics
   a. Growth or development related
      1) Children have a faster metabolic rate and greater oxygen demand per kilogram of body weight
      2) Neonates have higher sodium and chloride levels but lower potassium, magnesium, and phosphate levels than older children
      3) Fluid exchange rate is greater in neonates than in older children
      4) Dehydration can occur rapidly because of a larger body surface area, faster metabolic rate, and smaller extracellular fluid volume
   b. "Pearls"
      1) Dehydration in a previously healthy child is frequently the result of gastrointestinal (GI) losses from vomiting and diarrhea
      2) Most common type of dehydration is isotonic
      3) Normal urinary output in well-hydrated children is 1 mL/kg/hour and in newborns is 2 mL/kg/hour
      4) Neonates are prone to developing acidosis when under stress
      5) Neonates have limited fluid volume reserve
2. Geriatrics

   a. Aging related
      1) Decreased nutritional intake can occur because of mouth dryness, decreased appetite, poor fitting dentures, or lack of interest in eating; issues related to disability or difficulty with activities of daily living should be considered
      2) Total body water (TBW) decreases with age
      3) A decreased sense of "thirst" can lead to dehydration
   b. "Pearls"
      1) Chronic dehydration is more common in older adults
      2) Anorexia can be caused by hypercalcemia
      3) Hyponatremia is a common cause of delirium in the older adult
      4) Use of nutritional supplements (e.g., Ensure) can lead to hyponatremia

II. Specific Fluid Emergencies

A. DEHYDRATION

Fluid volume deficit is a TBW deficit that is associated with a loss of sodium accompanied by water. Isoosmolar fluid volume deficit occurs when sodium and water are lost in equal amounts. Hyperosmolar fluid volume deficit occurs when more fluid is lost than sodium, a condition resulting in higher serum osmolality than normal. Hypoosmolar fluid deficits occur from sodium deficiencies or free water excess, resulting in a lower than normal serum osmolality. Fluid deficit leads to conditions known as dehydration and hypovolemia. Dehydration is a disorder of water loss with or without loss of sodium and is frequently observed in critically ill patients. There are three types of dehydration: (1) isotonic, (2) hypotonic, and (3) hypertonic.

Isotonic dehydration, also termed isotonic fluid volume depletion, is a balanced depletion of water and sodium causing extracellular fluid loss. Causes include vomiting, diarrhea, and osmotic diuresis from elevated glucose levels. Total circulating volume is affected in isotonic dehydration as a result of overall fluid volume depletion.

Hypotonic dehydration, also termed extracellular fluid volume depletion, is a reduction in both sodium and water, with greater losses of sodium than water, which results in extracellular fluid loss. Causes include overuse of diuretics, chronic salt wasting, renal disease, and decreased intake of both salt and water. Circulation is affected in hypotonic dehydration because fluid moves intracellularly and decreases plasma volume.

Hypertonic dehydration, also known as intracellular or hypernatremic dehydration, is depletion in TBW content consequent to pathologic fluid losses, diminished water intake, or a combination of both. It results in hypernatremia (>145 mEq/L) in the extracellular fluid compartment, thereby drawing water from the intracellular fluids. The water loss is shared by all body fluid compartments, and relatively little reduction in extracellular fluids occurs. Thus, overall circulation is not compromised unless the loss is very large.

1. Assessment
   a. Subjective data collection
      1) History of present illness/chief complaint
         a) Nausea, vomiting, diarrhea
         b) Decreased intake
         c) Bleeding from any source
         d) Weight loss
         e) Polyuria, polydipsia
         f) Lassitude, fatigability, muscle cramps
         g) Postural dizziness and syncope
         h) Seizures, coma, confusion, syncope
         i) Unusual salt craving
         j) Trauma: blunt or penetrating forces
         k) Abdominal or chest pain (i.e., attributable to pancreatitis and decreased organ perfusion)
         l) Alcohol ingestion
         m) Fever
      2) Past medical history
         a) Current or preexisting diseases/illness
            (1) Diabetes
         b) Previous similar episodes
         c) Substance abuse
         d) Medications
         e) Allergies
   b. Objective data collection
      1) Physical examination
         a) General appearance
            (1) Level of consciousness, behavior, affect: confusion, lethargy, coma
            (2) Tachycardia, hypotension, orthostasis
            (3) Possible elevated temperature
            (4) Moderate to severe distress/discomfort
         b) Inspection
            (1) Lacerations, abrasions, ecchymosis, rashes, asymmetry, or edema
            (2) Petechiae
            (3) Bony deformities or angulation
            (4) Flattened external jugular veins
            (5) Sunken eyes
            (6) Pupils, including size, shape, equality, reactivity to light
            (7) Dry mucous membranes
            (8) Drainage or external bleeding
            (9) Respiratory rate, depth, work of breathing, use of accessory muscles, abdominal muscles, paradoxical chest wall movement
            (10) Abdominal distention
            (11) Venous access devices, feeding tubes or buttons
            (12) Weight loss
         c) Palpation/percussion
            (1) Skin temperature, moisture and turgor
               (a) Poor skin turgor: sternum or inner thigh in the elderly
            (2) Diminished peripheral pulses
            (3) Sunken fontanel
            (4) Skeletal muscle weakness
      2) Diagnostic procedures
         a) Serum osmolality: increased or decreased
         b) CBC with differential: hematocrit elevated or decreased
         c) Serum chemistries including glucose, BUN, creatinine
            (1) Sodium increased or decreased
         d) ABG analysis: metabolic alkalosis or metabolic acidosis
         e) Blood, urine, or CSF fluid cultures as appropriate
         f) Urinalysis; pregnancy test in female patients of childbearing age
         g) Radiograph studies as determined by history to rule out infection or trauma
         h) ECG
2. Analysis: differential nursing diagnoses/collaborative problems
   a. Deficient fluid volume
   b. Decreased cardiac output
   c. Ineffective tissue perfusion
   d. Deficient knowledge
3. Planning and implementation/interventions
   a. Maintain airway, breathing, circulation (see Chapter 1)
   b. Provide supplemental oxygen
   c. Establish IV/IO access for administration of crystalloid fluids/medications
      1) Rapidly infuse 1–2 L of normal saline solution in adults who have no cardiovascular disease
      2) Administer normal saline solution fluid challenge in older adults and monitor closely for fluid overload
      3) Infuse 20 mL/kg normal saline solution bolus in children; may repeat once
   d. Prepare for/assist with medical interventions
      1) Institute cardiac and pulse oximetry monitoring
      2) Provide oral fluid challenges
      3) Catheter placement and monitoring of central venous pressure (CVP) (see Chapter 6)
      4) Insert gastric tube and attach to suction as indicated
      5) Insert indwelling urinary catheter as indicated
      6) Assist with possible hospital admission
   e. Administer pharmacologic therapy as ordered
      1) Oral or IV sodium replacement
      2) IV sodium bicarbonate if pH <7.1
      3) Antiemetics
      4) Antidiarrheals

f. Educate patient/significant others
 1) Administer small, frequent amounts of oral fluids for 12–24 hours after vomiting stops, then advance diet as tolerated
 2) Continue feeding normally even when diarrhea is present
 3) Signs and symptoms that indicate need to return to emergency care setting
  a) Continued vomiting
  b) Continued diarrhea
  c) Elevated temperature
  d) Dry mucous membranes and skin
  e) Decreased urine output
  f) Sunken fontanel and sunken eyes
  g) Crying without tears (i.e., after 2–3 months old)
  h) Lethargy
  i) Postural dizziness
4. Evaluation and ongoing monitoring
 a. Level of consciousness
 b. Hemodynamic status including orthostasis
 c. Breath sounds and pulse oximetry
 d. Cardiac rate and rhythm
 e. Intake and output

III. Specific Electrolyte Emergencies

Electrolytes are divided into positively and negatively charged groups of cations (+) and anions (−). Electrolytes are found in intracellular and extracellular fluid and are critical for normal cellular metabolism and function. Sodium, the major extracellular cation, is responsible for maintaining plasma osmolarity, propagation and transmission of action potentials, maintaining acid-base balance, and maintaining electroneutrality. Potassium, the major intracellular cation, is responsible for electrical membrane excitability, maintaining acid-base balance, and regulating intracellular osmolarity. Calcium has several major roles; it is an essential component in the contractile processes (i.e., cardiac, skeletal, and smooth muscle), provides strength and density of teeth and bones, stabilizes excitable membranes, and is a cofactor in the clotting cascade. Magnesium is an important mineral component of the bony skeleton, a cofactor for many metabolic enzymes, and a regulator of ion channels and transporters in excitable tissues. Phosphorus has many critical roles and is a major component of bone mineral, phospholipids in cell membranes, and nucleic acids.

Direct measurement of intracellular electrolytes is not possible in the clinical setting, so the values are determined indirectly. Dietary excesses or deficits, prescribed medications, excess or lack of water ingestion, vomiting, and/or diarrhea may cause electrolyte abnormalities.

A. CALCIUM

Calcium is required for the proper functioning of muscle contraction, nerve conduction, hormone release, and blood coagulation. Serum calcium is present in three different forms: ionized, bound, and complexed. Approximately half of the plasma calcium is free ionized calcium. Slightly less than half the plasma calcium is bound to protein, primarily to albumin. The remaining small percentage is combined with nonprotein anions such as phosphate, citrate, and carbonate. The normal total calcium level is 9–10.5 mg/dL (4.5–5.3 mEq/L) in adults and 8.8–10.8 mg/dL in children. The normal ionized calcium level is 4.5–5.6 mg/dL (2.1–2.6 mEq/L) in adults and 4.8–5.52 mg/dL in children.

HYPOCALCEMIA. Hypocalcemia can occur primarily as a result of deficits of calcium intake, inhibition of calcium absorption from the GI tract, increased calcium excretion, decreased dietary intake of calcium, decreased vitamin D synthesis from sun exposure, lactose intolerance, malabsorption syndromes, renal failure, diarrhea/steatorrhea, or wound drainage.

Indirect causes of calcium deficits can include conditions that decrease the ionized fraction of calcium such as alkalosis, massive transfusion of citrated blood, hyperphosphatemia, immobility, acute pancreatitis, and the use of calcium chelators/binders. Indirect deficits of calcium can also be related to endocrine disorders that reduce parathyroid hormone (PTH) levels or to the removal or destruction of the parathyroid glands. The most common cause of a low total calcium level is hypoalbuminemia. Hypocalcemia occurs when the calcium level falls to <9 mg/dL (4.5 mEq/L).

1. Assessment
 a. Subjective data collection
  1) History of present illness/chief complaint
   a) Paresthesias followed by numbness
   b) Muscle cramps
   c) Hyperactive reflexes
   d) Altered dietary intake
   e) Acute anxiety and stress
   f) Infants: seizures, irritability, vomiting
  2) Past medical history
   a) Current or preexisting diseases/illness
    (1) Recent thyroidectomy or parathyroidectomy
    (2) Pancreatitis
    (3) Renal failure
    (4) Tumors
    (5) Chronic alcoholism
   b) Recent blood transfusions
   c) Previous toxic shock syndrome
   d) Infant prematurity or low birth weight
   e) Infant feeding of cow's milk, which elevates phosphate levels and decreases calcium levels
   f) Medications
   g) Allergies

b. Objective data collection
  1) Physical examination
    a) General appearance
      (1) Level of consciousness, behavior, affect: possible seizures
      (2) Hypotension, tachycardia
      (3) Decreased respiratory effort; hyperventilation
      (4) Stridor
      (5) Moderate distress/discomfort
    b) Inspection
      (1) Carpopedal spasm
        (a) Trousseau sign: carpal spasm after blood pressure cuff compression of arm
      (2) Muscle tetany
      (3) Muscle twitching, abdominal distention in infants
      (4) Cardiac changes on monitor
        (a) Prolonged QT and ST segments
        (b) T-wave inversion
    c) Auscultation
      (1) Breath sounds: wheezes
      (2) Bowel sounds: decreased to absent
    d) Palpation/percussion
      (1) Diminished peripheral pulses
      (2) Muscle weakness
      (3) Hyperreflexia
      (4) Chvostek sign: contraction of facial muscles when face tapped at angle of jaw
  2) Diagnostic procedures
    a) Serum chemistries including glucose, BUN, creatinine
      (1) Decreased calcium
      (2) Decreased magnesium
      (3) Decreased phosphate
    b) Urinalysis; pregnancy test in female patients of childbearing age
    c) ABGs: possible alkalosis
    d) Serum albumin level
    e) PTH level: decreased levels occur in hypoparathyroidism; increased levels may occur with other causes of hypocalcemia
    f) ECG
2. Analysis: differential nursing diagnoses/collaborative problems
  a. Pain
  b. Risk for ineffective airway clearance
3. Planning and implementation/interventions
  a. Maintain airway, breathing, circulation (see Chapter 1)
  b. Provide supplemental oxygen
  c. Establish IV access for administration of crystalloid fluids/medications
  d. Prepare for/assist with medical interventions
    1) Institute cardiac and pulse oximetry monitoring

    2) Insert gastric tube and attach to suction as indicated
    3) Insert indwelling urinary catheter as indicated
    4) Assist with possible hospital admission
  e. Administer pharmacologic therapy as ordered
    1) IV calcium gluconate or calcium chloride, as ordered
      a) Calcium gluconate: concentration 4.5 mEq of calcium
      b) Calcium chloride: concentration 13.5 mEq of calcium
      c) If dilution required for IV infusion, use 5% dextrose in water; saline solution increases calcium loss
    2) Nonnarcotic analgesics
    3) Narcotics
  f. Educate patient and significant others
    1) Eat well-balanced diet: foods rich in calcium
      a) Milk products
      b) Leafy green vegetables
    2) If condition is caused by hypoparathyroidism, omit milk products and other foods high in phosphorus
4. Evaluation and ongoing monitoring
  a. Level of consciousness
  b. Hemodynamic status
  c. Breath sounds and pulse oximetry
  d. Cardiac rate and rhythm
  e. Intake and output
  f. Serum electrolyte levels
  g. Pain relief

HYPERCALCEMIA. Serum calcium levels are maintained in a narrow range by the kidneys and the parathyroid gland. Any decrease in renal function or use of thiazide diuretics can reduce excretion of calcium; this reduction, in combination with an influx of calcium, results in hypercalcemia. Deterioration of renal function leads to increased calcium levels, which, in turn, can cause coma and eventual death. Hypercalcemia is known to occur as an end-stage event in patients with cancer.
1. Assessment
  a. Subjective data collection
    1) History of present illness/chief complaint
      a) Symptoms are usually absent unless calcium level is >11 mg/dL
      b) Anorexia, nausea, vomiting, constipation
      c) Pain (see Chapter 8): abdominal
      d) Weakness
      e) Depression, lethargy, confusion, psychosis, coma
      f) Weight loss
      g) Polyuria (from nephrogenic diabetes insipidus) and polydipsia
      h) Pruritus
      i) Bone pain

j) Fractures

k) Flank pain caused by renal calculi

  2) Past medical history

    a) Current or preexisting diseases/illness

      (1) Malignancy

      (2) Hyperparathyroid disease

      (3) Paget disease

      (4) Renal failure

    b) Prolonged immobilization

    c) Vitamin D or A overdose

    d) Medications

    e) Allergies

b. Objective data collection

  1) Physical examination

    a) General appearance

      (1) Level of consciousness, behavior, affect: lethargy, confusion, hallucinations, comatose

      (2) Hypertension, tachycardia

      (3) Moderate to severe distress/discomfort

    b) Inspection

      (1) Abdominal distention

      (2) Cardiac changes on monitor

        (a) Widened T wave

        (b) Shortened QT interval

        (c) Atrioventricular and bundle branch blocks

    c) Palpation/percussion

      (1) Profound muscle weakness

      (2) Hyporeflexia

  2) Diagnostic procedures

    a) Serum chemistries including glucose, BUN, creatinine

      (1) Increased calcium

      (2) Decreased sodium

      (3) Decreased phosphate

      (4) Decreased potassium

    b) Urinalysis; pregnancy test in female patients of childbearing age

    c) Serum albumin

    d) ABGs

    e) PTH: elevated

    f) ECG

2. Analysis: differential nursing diagnoses/collaborative problems

  a. Risk for deficient/excess fluid volume

  b. Risk for injury

  c. Pain

  d. Deficient knowledge

3. Planning and implementation/interventions

  a. Maintain airway, breathing, circulation (see Chapter 1)

  b. Provide supplemental oxygen

  c. Establish IV access for administration of crystalloid fluids/medications

    1) Insert large-bore IV catheter for rapid infusion of normal saline solutions

  d. Prepare for/assist with medical interventions

    1) Institute cardiac and pulse oximetry monitoring

    2) Catheter placement and monitoring of CVP or pulmonary artery pressure (see Chapter 6)

    3) Insert gastric tube and attach to suction as indicated

    4) Insert indwelling urinary catheter as indicated

    5) Assist with possible hospital admission, hemodialysis

  e. Administer pharmacologic therapy as ordered

    1) Furosemide (Lasix)

    2) Calcium-lowering medications

      a) Calcitonin (Calcimar)

      b) Pamidronate (Aredia)

    3) Malignancy-induced hypercalcemia

      a) Plicamycin (Mithracin)

      b) Gallium nitrate or zoledronic acid (Zometa)

    4) Corticosteroids

    5) Narcotics

4. Evaluation and ongoing monitoring

  a. Level of consciousness

  b. Hemodynamic status

  c. Cardiac rate and rhythm

  d. Breath sounds and pulse oximetry

  e. Intake and output

  f. Serum electrolyte levels

  g. Pain relief

B. MAGNESIUM

Magnesium is a coenzyme in carbohydrate and protein metabolism and is also involved in the metabolism of cellular proteins. Neuromuscular excitability is profoundly affected by fluctuations in serum magnesium levels. Approximately one half of the body's magnesium is located in bones, with the majority of the remaining magnesium contained within the cells. Most of the magnesium is bound to an ATPase molecule, which is important in phosphorylation of ATP (main source of energy for the body). Many factors that affect calcium levels also affect magnesium levels. Magnesium excretion is regulated through the kidneys. The normal range for magnesium is 1.3–2.1 mEq/L in adults, 1.4–1.7 mEq/L in children, and 1.4–2 mEq/L in newborns.

HYPOMAGNESEMIA. The primary causes of hypomagnesemia are related to decreased or insufficient intake of magnesium; chronic alcoholism is the most common. .Other causes of insufficient intake include prolonged IV feeding without magnesium supplements and excessive loss of magnesium through the GI tract (Crohn disease, celiac disease, diarrhea, steatorrhea), starvation, and malnutrition. Magnesium deficiencies can also result from increased renal excretion, pharmacologic therapy (cisplatin, aminoglycoside therapy, cyclosporin, diuretics), and use of citrate (found in blood products). Indirectly, magnesium deficits can be caused by intracellular shifts resulting from hyperglycemia, insulin administration, alkalosis, and sepsis.

Magnesium deficiency develops slowly and places the patient at risk for dysrhythmias, and it may be associated with hypokalemia. Clinical findings of hypomagnesemia resemble those seen in hypocalcemia.

1. Assessment
   a. Subjective data collection
      1) History of present illness/chief complaint
         a) Paresthesias
         b) Muscle cramps, twitches, fasciculations
         c) Inadequate nutritional intake
         d) Seizure, irritability
         e) Lethargy, weakness, fatigue
         f) Insomnia, mood changes, hallucinations, confusion
         g) Anorexia, nausea, vomiting
         h) Dysphasia
      2) Past medical history
         a) Current or preexisting diseases/illness
            (1) Chronic alcoholism
            (2) Crohn disease
            (3) Cancer
            (4) Colitis
            (5) Diabetes
            (6) Renal insufficiency
            (7) Cardiovascular disease
         b) Malnutrition
         c) Prolonged diarrhea
         d) Medications
            (1) Diuretics
            (2) Amphotericin B
            (3) Cisplatin
            (4) Digitalis
         e) Allergies
   b. Objective data collection
      1) Physical examination
         a) General appearance
            (1) Level of consciousness, behavior, affect: confusion, psychosis, seizures, comatose
            (2) Hypertension/hypotension
            (3) Tachycardia or bradycardia
            (4) Moderate to severe distress/discomfort
         b) Inspection
            (1) Muscle tetany
               (a) Trousseau sign: carpal spasm after blood pressure cuff compression of arm
            (2) Cardiac changes on monitor
               (a) T waves elevated
               (b) ST segment depressed
               (c) Ventricular dysrhythmias: premature ventricular contractions, tachycardia, torsades de pointes, fibrillation
         c) Palpation/percussion
            (1) Muscle weakness
            (2) Hyperreflexia
            (3) Chvostek sign: contraction of facial muscles when face tapped at angle of jaw
      2) Diagnostic procedures
         a) Serum chemistries including glucose, BUN, creatinine
            (1) Decreased magnesium
            (2) Decreased calcium
            (3) Decreased potassium
         b) Urinalysis; pregnancy test in female patients of childbearing age
         c) Serum albumin level: decreased
         d) Digitalis level if indicated: hypomagnesemia enhances toxicity
2. Analysis: differential nursing diagnoses/collaborative problems
   a. Decreased cardiac output
   b. Imbalanced nutrition: less than body requirements
   c. Risk for ineffective airway clearance
3. Planning and implementation/interventions
   a. Maintain airway, breathing, circulation (see Chapter 1)
   b. Provide supplemental oxygen
   c. Establish IV access for administration of crystalloid fluids/medications
   d. Prepare for/assist with medical interventions
      1) Institute cardiac and pulse oximetry monitoring
      2) Insert gastric tube and attach to suction as indicated
      3) Insert indwelling urinary catheter as indicated
      4) Assist with possible hospital admission
   e. Administer pharmacologic therapy as ordered
      1) Magnesium: oral, intramuscular, or IV
         a) IV: avoid dilution with normal saline
         b) IV: administer slowly to prevent potential cardiac or respiratory arrest
      2) Other electrolyte replacements
         a) Calcium gluconate
         b) Potassium chloride
   f. Educate patient and significant others
      1) Eat well-balanced diet: foods rich in magnesium
         a) Nuts and seeds
         b) Seafood and meat
         c) Leafy, green vegetables
         d) Wheat germ
         e) Bananas, oranges, grapefruit
         f) Peanut butter
         g) Chocolate
      2) If condition results from chronic alcoholism, refer to alcohol rehabilitation programs
4. Evaluation and ongoing monitoring
   a. Level of consciousness
   b. Hemodynamic status
   c. Cardiac rate and rhythm
   d. Breath sounds and pulse oximetry

e. Intake and output
f. Serum electrolyte levels

HYPERMAGNESEMIA. Conditions such as adrenal insufficiency and renal failure reduce excretion of magnesium through the kidneys. Patients with renal failure who ingest products containing magnesium (Maalox, Milk of Magnesia) can develop hypermagnesemia. Treatment of eclampsia in pregnant women can also lead to hypermagnesemia. The primary symptoms of hypermagnesemia are the result of depressed peripheral and central neuromuscular transmissions. The normal range for magnesium is 1.3–2.1 mEq/L in adults, 1.4–1.7 mEq/L in children, and 1.4–2 mEq/L in newborns.

1. Assessment
   a. Subjective data collection
      1) History of present illness/chief complaint
         a) Nausea and vomiting
         b) Altered mental functioning; drowsiness, lethargy, coma
         c) Sensation of heat
         d) Flushing, diaphoresis
         e) Muscle weakness or paralysis
         f) Paralysis of the respiratory muscles may occur when the magnesium level >10 mEq/L
      2) Past medical history
         a) Current or preexisting diseases/illness
            (1) Renal insufficiency or failure
            (2) Adrenocortical insufficiency
         b) Overdose of therapeutic magnesium
         c) Eclampsia
         d) Medications
         e) Allergies
   b. Objective data collection
      1) Physical examination
         a) General appearance
            (1) Possible respiratory and/or cardiac arrest
            (2) Level of consciousness, behavior, affect: lethargy to comatose
            (3) Hypotension, bradycardia
            (4) Moderate to severe distress/discomfort
         b) Inspection
            (1) Cardiac changes on monitor
               (a) Prolonged QT interval
               (b) Atrioventricular block
         c) Palpation/percussion
            (1) Muscle weakness
            (2) Loss of deep tendon reflexes
      2) Diagnostic procedures
         a) Serum electrolyte levels including glucose, BUN, creatinine
         b) Urinalysis; pregnancy test in female patients of childbearing age
         c) ECG

2. Analysis: differential nursing diagnoses/collaborative problems
   a. Ineffective airway clearance
   b. Decreased cardiac output
3. Planning and implementation/interventions
   a. Maintain airway, breathing, circulation (see Chapter 1)
      1) Initiate or continue basic life support (BLS) and advanced life support (ALS) if cardiac arrest present
   b. Provide supplemental oxygen
      1) Intubation and ventilatory support in respiratory/cardiac arrest patients
      2) High-flow oxygen
   c. Establish IV access for administration of crystalloid fluids/medications
      1) Infuse 0.45% sodium chloride solution
   d. Prepare for/assist with medical interventions
      1) Advanced airway management
         a) Nasal or oral intubation
         b) Supraglottic airway (e.g., King, Combitube, laryngeal mask airway)
         c) Surgical airway (e.g., cricothyrotomy)
      2) Institute cardiac and pulse oximetry monitoring
      3) Insert gastric tube and attach to suction as indicated
      4) Insert indwelling urinary catheter as indicated
      5) Assist with hospital admission, hemodialysis
   e. Administer pharmacologic therapy as ordered
      1) Diuretics and 0.45% sodium chloride solutions
         a) Enhances magnesium excretion in patients with adequate renal function
      2) IV calcium gluconate: 10 mL of 10% solution
         a) Antagonizes neuromuscular effects of magnesium
   f. Educate patient/significant others
      1) Minimize use of magnesium-containing medications
         a) Maalox
         b) Mylanta
         c) Gaviscon
4. Evaluation and ongoing monitoring
   a. Level of consciousness
   b. Hemodynamic status
   c. Breath sounds and pulse oximetry
   d. Cardiac rate and rhythm
   e. Intake and output
   f. Serum electrolyte levels

C. PHOSPHORUS

Phosphorus forms high-energy phosphate bonds in compounds such as adenosine triphosphate (ATP), is posttranslationally bound to proteins as an intracellular signal, and acts as a major pH buffer in urine and serum. Of the total body phosphorus content, 85% is in bone, 14% is in intracellular compartments, and only 1% is in extracellular fluid.

The normal concentration of phosphorus is 3–4.5 mg/dL (1–1.5 mM). Phosphorus is present in many foods, including meats, grains, and dairy products; and is absorbed in the small intestine. The kidneys excrete excess phosphorus, which is the principal mechanism by which the body regulates extracellular phosphate balance. Parathyroid hormone increases renal phosphate excretion by inhibiting the sodium-phosphate cotransporter in the proximal tubule, whereas vitamin D enhances intestinal phosphate absorption.

HYPOPHOSPHATEMIA. The primary causes of hypophosphatemia are alcoholism, burns, starvation, and diuretic use. Other causes of hypophosphatemia are TPN administration, refeeding after prolonged undernutrition, and severe respiratory alkalosis. Chronic hypophosphatemia is usually caused by hyperparathyroidism, hormonal disturbances (Cushing syndrome and hypothyroidism), electrolyte disorders (hypomagnesemia and hypokalemia), and long-term diuretic use. Phosphate deficiencies can also result from long-term ingestion of large amounts of phosphate-binding aluminium, usually in the form of antacids. Ingestion of aluminium is particularly prone to cause phosphate depletion when combined with decreased dietary intake and dialysis losses in phosphate in patients with end-stage renal disease. Hypophosphatemia is usually asymptomatic; however, patients may experience anorexia, muscle weakness, and osteomalacia. The muscle weakness of profound hypophosphatemia may be accompanied with rhabdomyolysis, especially in acute alcoholism.

HYPERPHOSPHATEMIA. Hyperphosphatemia is serum phosphate (PO_4) concentration >4.5 mg/dL (>1.46 mmol/L). Causes include chronic renal failure, hypoparathyroidism, and metabolic or respiratory acidosis. Clinical features may be due to accompanying hypocalcemia and include tetany. Diagnosis is by serum PO_4. Treatment includes restriction of PO_4 intake and administration of PO_4-binding antacids, such as Ca carbonate. The usual cause of hyperphosphatemia is a decrease in renal excretion of PO_4. Advanced renal insufficiency (GFR <30 mL/min) reduces excretion sufficiently to increase serum PO_4. Defects in renal excretion of PO_4 in the absence of renal failure also occur in pseudohypoparathyroidism and hypoparathyroidism. Hyperphosphatemia can also occur with excessive oral PO_4 administration and occasionally with overzealous use of enemas containing PO_4.

Hyperphosphatemia occasionally results from a transcellular shift of PO_4 into the extracellular space that is so large that the renal excretory capacity is overwhelmed. This transcellular shift occurs most frequently in diabetic ketoacidosis (despite total body PO_4 depletion), crush injuries, and nontraumatic rhabdomyolysis as well as in overwhelming systemic infections and tumor lysis syndrome.

1. Assessment
    a. Subjective data collection

1) History of present illness/chief complaint
    a) Anorexia
    b) Muscle weakness
    c) Inadequate nutritional intake
    d) Neuromuscular disturbances (progressive encephalopathy, seizures, coma)
    e) Rhabdomyolysis
2) Past medical history
    a) Current or preexisting diseases/illness
        (1) Alcoholism
        (2) Diabetes
        (3) Renal insufficiency
        (4) Dialysis
        (5) Diuretics use
        (6) Hematologic disturbances (hemolytic anemia and impaired leukocyte and platelet function
        (7) Allergies
b. Objective data collection
    1) Physical examination
        a) General appearance
            (1) Level of consciousness, behavior, affect: confusion, psychosis, seizures, comatose
            (2) Hypertension/hypotension
            (3) Tachycardia or bradycardia
            (4) Moderate to severe distress/discomfort
        b) Inspection
            (1) Muscle tetany
                (a) Trousseau sign: carpal spasm after blood pressure cuff compression of arm
            (2) Cardiac changes on monitor
                (a) T waves elevated
                (b) ST segment depression
                (c) Ventricular dysrhythmias: premature ventricular contractions, tachycardia, torsades de pointes, fibrillation
        c) Palpation/percussion
            (1) Muscle weakness
            (2) Hyperreflexia
            (3) Chvostek sign: contraction of facial muscles when face tapped at angle of jaw
    2) Diagnostic procedures
        a) Serum chemistries including glucose, BUN, creatinine
            (1) Decreased magnesium
            (2) Decreased calcium
            (3) Decreased potassium
        b) Urinalysis; pregnancy test in female patients of childbearing age
        c) Serum albumin level: decreased
        d) Digitalis level if indicated: hypomagnesemia enhances toxicity
2. Analysis: differential nursing diagnoses/collaborative problems
    a. Decreased cardiac output

b. Imbalanced nutrition: less than body requirements
c. Risk for ineffective airway clearance
3. Planning and implementation/interventions
a. Maintain airway, breathing, circulation (see Chapter 1)
b. Provide supplemental oxygen
c. Establish IV access for administration of crystalloid fluids/medications
d. Prepare for/assist with medical interventions
1) Institute cardiac and pulse oximetry monitoring
2) Insert gastric tube and attach to suction as indicated
3) Insert indwelling urinary catheter as indicated
4) Assist with possible hospital admission
e. Administer pharmacologic therapy as ordered
1) Phosphorus replacement: oral, intramuscular, or IV
a) IV: avoid dilution with normal saline
b) IV: administer slowly to prevent potential cardiac or respiratory arrest
2) Other electrolyte replacements
a) Calcium gluconate
b) Potassium chloride
f. Educate patient and significant others
1) Eat well-balanced diet: foods rich in phosphorus
a) Nuts and seeds
b) Seafood and meat
c) Leafy, green vegetables
d) Wheat germ
e) Bananas, oranges, grapefruit
f) Peanut butter
g) Chocolate
2) If the condition results from chronic alcoholism, refer to alcohol rehabilitation programs
4. Evaluation and ongoing monitoring
a. Level of consciousness
b. Hemodynamic status
c. Cardiac rate and rhythm
d. Breath sounds and pulse oximetry
e. Intake and output
f. Serum electrolyte levels

HYPOPHOSPHATEMIA TREATMENT.

1. Oral PO_4 replacement
2. IV PO_4 when serum PO_4 is <0.5 mEq/L or symptoms are severe
3. Oral treatment
a. Treatment of underlying disorder and oral PO_4 replacement are usually adequate in asymptomatic patients, even when serum concentration is very low
b. PO_4 can be given in doses up to about 1 g po tid in tablets containing Na+ or K+ PO_4
c. Oral Na+ or K+ PO_4 may be poorly tolerated because of diarrhea
d. Ingestion of 1 L low-fat or skim milk provides 1 g of PO_4 and may be more acceptable

e. Removal of the cause of hypophosphatemia may include stopping PO_4-binding antacids or diuretics or correcting hypomagnesemia.
4. Parenteral treatment
a. Parenteral PO_4 is usually given IV, administered in any of the following circumstances
1) When serum PO_4 is <0.5 mEq/L (<0.16 mmol/L)
2) Rhabdomyolysis, hemolysis, or CNS symptoms are present
3) Oral replacement is not feasible due to underlying disorder
NOTE: IV administration of KPO_4 (as buffered mix of K_2HPO_4 and KH_2PO_4) is relatively safe when renal function is well preserved. $NaPO_4$ (rather than KPO_4) preparations generally should be used in patients with impaired renal function. The usual parenteral dose of KPO_4 is 2.5 mg (0.08 mmol)/kg IV over 6 hours. Patients with alcoholism may require ≥1 g/day during TPN; supplemental PO_4 is stopped when oral intake is resumed. Serum Ca and PO_4 concentrations should be monitored during therapy, particularly when PO_4 is given IV or to patients with impaired renal function. In most cases, no more than 7 mg/kg (about 500 mg for a 70-kg adult) of PO_4 should be given over 6 hours. Close monitoring is done and more rapid rates of PO_4 administration should be avoided to prevent hypocalcemia, hyperphosphatemia, and metastatic calcification due to excessive Ca × PO_4 product.

HYPERPHOSPHATEMIA TREATMENT

1. PO_4 restriction
2. PO_4 binders
a. The mainstay of treatment in patients with renal failure is reduction of PO_4 intake, which is usually accomplished with avoidance of foods containing high amounts of PO_4 and with use of PO_4-binding drugs taken with meals
b. Because of the possibility of aluminum-related osteomalacia, Ca carbonate and Ca acetate replace aluminum-containing antacids in patients with end-stage renal disease
c. Because of the possibility of excessive Ca × PO_4 product causing vascular calcification in dialysis patients taking Ca-containing binders, a PO_4-binding resin without Ca, sevelamer, is widely used in dialysis patients in doses of 800–2,400 mg tid with meals
d. Lanthanum carbonate, another PO_4 binder that lacks Ca, can also be used in dialysis patients. It is given in doses of 500–1,000 mg tid with meals

D. POTASSIUM

Potassium is the most abundant intracellular cation, with only 2% of total body potassium located extracellularly. Potassium regulates cell membrane potential, cellular osmolality, and volume. Renal tubules are the primary control for potassium excretion; however, potassium can also be found in sweat, gastric juices, pancreatic juice, and bile. In an acute acidotic condition, potassium cations move from the intracellular spaces to the extracellular spaces in exchange for hydrogen cations. The opposite effect occurs in an alkalotic state, in which potassium moves intracellularly in exchange for hydrogen. Potassium abnormalities may be the result of vomiting and diarrhea, associated with diabetic ketoacidosis, or may be caused by massive crush injuries in which intracellular potassium is released from the damaged cells. The normal range for potassium levels is 3.5–5 mEq/L.

HYPOKALEMIA. Hypokalemia refers to serum potassium levels <3.5 mEq/L. Potassium decreases can result from inadequate potassium intake (e.g., NPO status) or excessive losses of potassium. Potassium loss can occur through the GI system (vomiting, diarrhea, fistulas, suction), the renal system (use of diuretics, increased mineralocorticoid levels) including nephritis, wound drainage, diaphoresis, heart failure, liver diseases, Cushing syndrome, and the use of various medications (e.g., digitalis, diuretics, corticosteroids corticosteroids, and laxatives).

1. Assessment
   a. Subjective data collection
      1) History of present illness/chief complaint
         a) Anorexia, nausea, vomiting
         b) Weakness and fatigue
         c) Leg cramps
         d) Shortness of breath
         e) Palpitations
         f) Urinary frequency
         g) Decreased oral intake and/or dietary intake of potassium
         h) Constipation
      2) Past medical history
         a) Current or preexisting diseases/illness
            (1) Cardiovascular disease
            (2) Renal disease
            (3) Ulcerative colitis
            (4) Diabetes
         b) Medications
            (1) Diuretics
            (2) Steroids
         c) Allergies
   b. Objective data collection
      1) Physical examination
         a) General appearance
            (1) Level of consciousness, behavior, affect: lethargy, confusion, comatose
            (2) Hypotension, orthostasis
            (3) Slowed, shallow respirations
            (4) Moderate to severe distress/discomfort
         b) Inspection
            (1) Abdominal distention
            (2) Cardiac changes on monitor
               (a) Sagging of the ST segment
               (b) T-wave depression
               (c) U-wave elevation
               (d) Premature ventricular and atrial contractions
               (e) Second- or third-degree atrioventricular block
               (f) Severe hypokalemia: ventricular fibrillation
         c) Auscultation
            (1) Bowel sounds: hypoactive, paralytic ileus
         d) Palpation/percussion
            (1) Muscle tenderness
            (2) Hyporeflexia, eventual flaccid paralysis
      2) Diagnostic procedures
         a) CBC with differential
         b) Serum chemistries including electrolytes, glucose, BUN, creatinine
         c) ABGs
         d) Serum osmolality
         e) Urinalysis; pregnancy test in female patients of childbearing age
         f) ECG
         g) Definitive neurologic studies: head CT scan, EEG, and lumbar puncture as indicated
2. Analysis: differential nursing diagnoses/collaborative problems
   a. Decreased cardiac output
   b. Deficient knowledge
3. Planning and implementation/interventions
   a. Maintain airway, breathing, circulation (see Chapter 1)
   b. Provide supplemental oxygen
   c. Establish IV access for administration of crystalloid fluids/medications
   d. Prepare for/assist with medical interventions
      1) Institute cardiac and pulse oximetry monitoring
      2) Insert gastric tube and attach to suction as indicated
      3) Insert indwelling urinary catheter as indicated
      4) Assist with possible hospital admission
   e. Administer pharmacologic therapy as ordered
      1) Potassium chloride replacement: oral or IV
         a) Administer slowly through peripheral veins to decrease local irritation
         b) Infusions >15 mEq/hour require cardiac monitoring
         c) Maximum dose 40 mEq/hour
   f. Educate patient/significant others
      1) Eat well-balanced diet: foods high in potassium
         a) Raw or steamed vegetables: spinach, Swiss chard, cauliflower, carrots
         b) Tomatoes
         c) Bananas
         d) Dried beans

2) Use caution with OTC medications/herbals
4. Evaluation and ongoing monitoring
   a. Level of consciousness
   b. Hemodynamic status
   c. Breath sounds and pulse oximetry
   d. Cardiac rate and rhythm
   e. Intake and output
   f. Serum electrolyte levels

HYPERKALEMIA. Hyperkalemia is characterized by excess serum potassium, exceeding 5.5 mEq/L. Effects of elevated serum potassium on the cardiovascular system are the most important manifestations of the condition, resulting in cardiac dysrhythmias. Hyperpolarization from excess extracellular potassium causes an inability of the action potential to perpetuate that leads to a cellular inability to repolarize. Ventricular asystole occurs as the terminal event.

1. Assessment
   a. Subjective data collection
      1) History of present illness/chief complaint
         a) Irritability, anxiety, confusion
         b) Palpitations
         c) Hyperexcitability
         d) Abdominal cramping, distention, diarrhea
         e) Weakness, especially of the lower extremities
         f) Numbness
         g) Crush/burn injury
      2) Past medical history
         a) Current or preexisting diseases/illness
            (1) Renal disease
            (2) Addison disease
            (3) Syndrome of hyporeninemic hypoaldosteronism
            (4) Tissue catabolism (fever, sepsis, trauma, fast-growing cancer, or recent surgery)
         b) Insulin deficiency, especially in patients with chronic renal failure
         c) Medications
            (1) Potassium-sparing diuretic use
            (2) ACE inhibitor use
            (3) Nonsteroidal antiinflammatory drugs (NSAIDs)
         d) Allergies
   b. Objective data collection
      1) Physical examination
         a) General appearance
            (1) Level of consciousness, behavior, affect: confusion
            (2) Tachycardia/bradycardia
            (3) Hypotension
            (4) Moderate to severe distress/discomfort
         b) Inspection
            (1) Abdominal distention
            (2) Cardiac changes on monitor
               (a) T-wave changes: elevated, peaked
               (b) Widened QRS complex
               (c) Prolonged PR interval
               (d) Ventricular dysrhythmias
         c) Auscultation
            (1) Bowel sounds: hyperactive/hypoactive
         d) Palpation/percussion
            (1) Muscle irritability
            (2) Flaccid paralysis
      2) Diagnostic procedures
         a) Serum chemistries including glucose, BUN, creatinine
         b) ABGs
         c) Urinalysis; pregnancy test in female patients of childbearing age
         d) Serum cortisol or cortisone stimulation test: used for the diagnosis of Addison disease
         e) ECG
2. Analysis: differential nursing diagnoses/collaborative problems
   a. Decreased cardiac output
   b. Anxiety/fear
   c. Deficient knowledge
3. Planning and implementation/interventions
   a. Maintain airway, breathing, circulation (see Chapter 1)
   b. Provide supplemental oxygen
   c. Establish IV access for administration of crystalloid fluids/medications
   d. Prepare for/assist with medical interventions
      1) Institute cardiac and pulse oximetry monitoring
      2) Insert gastric tube and attach to suction as indicated
      3) Insert indwelling urinary catheter as indicated
      4) Assist with possible hospital admission, peritoneal dialysis, or hemodialysis
   e. Administer pharmacologic therapy as ordered
      1) Monitor blood glucose and electrolyte levels
      2) Dextrose 50%, regular insulin
         a) Facilitates cellular entry of potassium
      3) Calcium gluconate: counteracts neuromuscular and cardiac effects of hyperkalemia
      4) Cation exchange resin sodium polystyrene sulfonate (Kayexalate) plus sorbitol solution
      5) Fludrocortisone (Florinef): increases urinary excretion of potassium
      6) Sodium bicarbonate if metabolic acidosis present
4. Evaluation and ongoing monitoring
   a. Level of consciousness
   b. Hemodynamic status
   c. Breath sounds and pulse oximetry
   d. Cardiac rate and rhythm
   e. Intake and output
   f. Serum electrolyte levels

E. SODIUM

Sodium is responsible for normal water balance and impulse conduction. Active transport by adenosine triphosphate

(ATP) is necessary to keep sodium in the extracellular space. Sodium is regulated by the renin-angiotension-aldosterone system, sympathetic nervous system (SNS), and in a less well-defined system, mediated by atrial natriuretic factor (ANF). Baroreceptor stimulation of the SNS leads to vasoconstriction, decreased glomerular filtration rate, and retention of sodium and water. Release of ANF by the atria leads to excessive sodium excretion and diuresis. The normal sodium level is 135–145 mEq/L.

HYPONATREMIA. Hyponatremia may result from either actual sodium deficits or dilutional causes. Sodium deficits resulting from dilutional effects can be caused by excess water intake, freshwater drowning, inappropriate antidiuretic hormone secretion, and psychogenic polydipsia or true sodium loss from hyperglycemia, heart failure, or burns. Causes of actual sodium deficits resulting from increased sodium excretion include diaphoresis, diuretic use, wound drainage, decreased secretion of aldosterone, hyperlipidemia, and renal disease. Causes of actual sodium deficits resulting from inadequate sodium intake include nothing by mouth (NPO) restrictions and a low-sodium diet. Symptoms related to hyponatremia usually do not occur unless the sodium level is <120–125 mEq/L.

1. Assessment
   a. Subjective data collection
      1) History of present illness/chief complaint
         a) Anorexia, nausea, vomiting, diarrhea
         b) Altered oral intake: immobility or inability to obtain oral fluids
         c) Altered dietary intake of sodium
         d) Excessive water consumption
         e) Trauma, burns, or neurologic injury or surgery
         f) Lethargy and apathy
         g) Thirst
         h) Confusion, personality changes
         i) Seizures and coma
         j) Weight change
         k) Fatigue and muscle cramps
         l) Dizziness
         m) Headache
         n) Poor peripheral pulses
         o) Skeletal muscle weakness
      2) Past medical history
         a) Current or preexisting diseases/illness
            (1) Cardiovascular disease
            (2) Pulmonary disease
         b) Previous or similar episodes
         c) Medications
            (1) Diuretics
         d) Allergies
   b. Objective data collection
      1) Physical examination
         a) General appearance

            (1) Level of consciousness, behavior, affect: seizure, confusion to comatose
            (2) Hypotension, tachycardia, orthostasis
            (3) Possible elevated temperature
            (4) Severe distress/discomfort, critically ill
         b) Inspection
            (1) Sunken eyes
            (2) Dry mucous membranes
            (3) Flattened jugular veins
         c) Auscultation/inspection
            (1) Breath sounds: crackles
         d) Palpation/percussion
            (1) Sunken fontanel
            (2) Poor skin turgor
            (3) Diminished deep tendon reflexes
      2) Diagnostic procedures
         a) CBC with differential
         b) Serum chemistries including glucose, BUN, creatinine
            (1) Sodium: <135 mEq/L
            (2) Chloride usually decreased
            (3) Bicarbonate: elevated or decreased to replace chloride
         c) Urinalysis; pregnancy test in female patients of childbearing age
         d) Chest radiograph
         e) Head CT scan
         f) ECG
2. Analysis: differential nursing diagnoses/collaborative problems
   a. Deficient/excess fluid volume
   b. Ineffective tissue perfusion: cerebral
   c. Risk for injury related to restlessness, seizure, or confusion
   d. Risk for ineffective airway clearance
   e. Deficient knowledge
3. Planning and implementation/interventions
   a. Maintain airway, breathing, circulation (see Chapter 1)
   b. Provide supplemental oxygen
      1) Rapid-sequence intubation (RSI) and ventilatory support for patient with compromised airway
      2) High-flow oxygen
   c. Establish IV/IO access for administration of crystalloid fluids/medications
   d. Prepare for/assist with medical interventions
      1) Advanced airway management
         a) Nasal or oral intubation
         b) Supraglottic airway (e.g., King, Combitube, laryngeal mask airway)
         c) Surgical airway (e.g., cricothyrotomy)
      2) Institute cardiac and pulse oximetry monitoring
      3) Insert gastric tube and attach to suction as indicated
      4) Insert indwelling urinary catheter as indicated

5) Initiate seizure precautions to protect patient as indicated
6) Apply restraints on combative patients per institutional protocols
7) Assist with hospital admission
   e. Administer pharmacologic therapy as ordered
1) RSI premedications: sedatives, analgesics, neuromuscular blocking agents
2) Electrolyte replacements
4. Evaluation and ongoing monitoring
   a. Airway patency
   b. Level of consciousness
   c. Hemodynamic status
   d. Breath sounds and pulse oximetry
   e. Cardiac rate and rhythm
   f. Intake and output
   g. Serum electrolyte levels

HYPERNATREMIA. Hypernatremia is less common than hyponatremia and can be caused by actual sodium excess or, indirectly, by decreased water intake or increased water loss. Indirect causes of decreased water intake are often related to NPO status. Increased water loss in excess of sodium can occur as a result of sweating, hyperventilation, infection, diaphoresis, diarrhea, diabetes insipidus, and/or fever. A true increase in sodium volume can be related to administration of sodium bicarbonate, normal saline, near drowning in saltwater, renal failure, use of corticosteroids, increased sodium ingestion, or hyperaldosteronism (Cushing syndrome).

Symptoms of hypernatremia are caused by hyperosmolarity. As the sodium level rises, cellular dehydration occurs. Brain cells shrink, resulting in central nervous system symptoms. As the brain shrinks, intracranial hemorrhage may occur from mechanical stress that tears vessels. The similarity of signs and symptoms among sodium disorders makes it very difficult to differentiate conditions without laboratory data. A serum sodium level of >145 mEq/L is considered hypernatremia. Hypernatremia in adults has a mortality of 40–60%.

1. Assessment
   a. Subjective data collection
1) History or present illness/chief complaint
   a) Anorexia, nausea, vomiting, diarrhea
   b) Altered oral intake
   c) Altered dietary intake of sodium
   d) Lethargy and apathy
   e) Thirst
   f) Confusion, seizures, coma (agitation may be present if hypovolemia also present)
   g) Neuromuscular excitability
   h) Weight change
   i) Fatigue and muscle cramps
   j) Dizziness
   k) Headache
   l) Thirst (major symptoms)
   m) Immobility or inability to obtain oral fluids

2) Past medical history
   a) Current or preexisting diseases/illness
      (1) Diabetes insipidus
   b) Previous similar episodes
   c) Medications
   d) Allergies
   b. Objective data collection
1) Physical examination
   a) General appearance
      (1) Level of consciousness, behavior, affect: confusion, seizures to coma
      (2) Hypotension and tachycardia, orthostasis
      (3) Severe distress/discomfort
   b) Inspection
      (1) Spontaneous muscle twitches
      (2) Tremors
      (3) Dry mucous membranes
      (4) Distended or flattened jugular veins
   c) Auscultation
      (1) Breath sounds: crackles
      (2) Heart sounds: S_3 gallop
   d) Palpation/percussion
      (1) Dry skin
      (2) Poor skin turgor
      (3) Muscle weakness, diminished deep tendon reflexes or hyperreflexia
2) Diagnostic procedures
   a) CBC with differential
   b) Serum chemistries with glucose, BUN, creatinine
      (1) Sodium: >145 mEq/L
      (2) Chloride: decreased or increased with sodium
      (3) Bicarbonate: elevated or decreased to replace chloride
      (4) Potassium: normal range 3.5–5 mEq/L; may be normal, decreased, or elevated
      (5) Magnesium: normal range 1.5–2 mEq/L; may be normal, decreased, or elevated
      (6) BUN: elevated if dehydration present
      (7) Creatinine level: normal
   c) Serum osmolality: increased
      (1) Infants: normal value 275–285 mOsm/kg
      (2) Adults: normal value 285–295 mOsm/kg
      (3) Symptoms develop at 320 mOsm/kg
      (4) Coma occurs at 360 mOsm/kg
   d) Urinalysis; pregnancy test in female patients of childbearing age
   e) Chest radiograph
   f) ECG
   g) Definitive neurologic studies: head CT scan, EEG, and lumbar puncture
2. Analysis: differential nursing diagnoses/collaborative problems
   a. Deficient/excess fluid volume
   b. Ineffective tissue perfusion: cerebral

c. Risk for injury related to restlessness, seizure, or confusion

d. Risk for ineffective airway clearance

e. Deficient knowledge

3. Planning and implementation/interventions

   a. Maintain airway, breathing, circulation (see Chapter 1)

   b. Provide supplemental oxygen

      1) RSI and ventilatory support for patient with compromised airway

      2) High-flow oxygen

   c. Establish IV/IO access for administration of crystalloid fluids/medications

      1) Hypoosmolar solution (0.2% or 0.45% sodium chloride; 5% dextrose in water) to decrease total body sodium

      2) Administer slowly to decrease serum sodium level 2 mEq/L/hour

   d. Prepare for/assist with medical interventions

      1) Advanced airway management

         a) Nasal or oral intubation

         b) Supraglottic Airway (e.g., King, Combitube, laryngeal mask airway)

         c) Surgical airway (e.g., cricothyrotomy)

      2) Institute cardiac, pulse oximetry, and frequent vital signs monitoring

      3) Insert gastric tube and attach to suction as indicated

      4) Insert indwelling urinary catheter as indicated

      5) Initiate seizure precautions to protect patient as indicated

      6) Apply restraints on combative patients per institutional protocols

      7) Assist with hospital admission

   e. Administer pharmacologic therapy as ordered

      1) RSI premedications: sedatives, analgesics, neuromuscular blocking agents

      2) Desmopressin acetate (DDAVP) nasal spray if caused by diabetes insipidus

      3) Furosemide (Lasix)

4. Evaluation and ongoing monitoring

   a. Airway patency

   b. Level of consciousness

   c. Hemodynamic status including orthostasis

   d. Breath sounds and pulse oximetry

   e. Cardiac rate and rhythm

   f. Intake and output

   g. Serum electrolyte levels

IV. Parenteral Administration

To help improve patient outcomes and safety, knowledge of parenteral fluids is essential when providing infusion therapy. This knowledge is vital since rapid and critical changes in fluid and electrolytes balance may be caused by infusates (see Table 17.1). A change in water content causes cells to swell or shrink. Tonicity refers to the tension or effect that the osmotic pressure of a solution, with impermeable solutes, exerts on cell size due to water movement across the cell membrane. Parenteral fluids are classified according to the tonicity of the fluid in relation to normal blood plasma (see Box 17.1). The osmolality of blood plasma is 290 mOsm/L and fluids that approximate 290 mOsm/L are considered isotonic. IV fluids with an osmolality >290 mOsm (+50 mOsm) are considered hypertonic; IV fluids with an osmolality <290 mOsm (−50 mOsm) are considered hypotonic. To provide safe parenteral fluid therapy, the nurse should be aware of the patient's clinical picture, physical status, and laboratory values. Box 17.2 contains laboratory values that are assessed during parenteral fluid therapy.

Table 17.1

Fluid Composition of Common Intravenous Fluids

	Human plasma	0.9% Sodium chloride	Hartmann's	Ringer's lactate	Ringer's acetate	Plasma-Lyte 148	Plasma-Lyte A pH 7.4	Sterofundin/ Ringerfundin
Osmolarity (mOsm/l)	275-295	308	278	273	276	295	295	309
pH	7.35-7.45	4.5-7.0	5.0-7.0	6.0-7.5	6.0-8.0	4.0-8.0	7.4	5.1-5.9
Sodium (mmol/l)	135-145	154	131	130	130	140	140	145
Chloride (mmol/l)	94-111	154	111	109	112	98	98	127
Potassium (mmol/l)	3.5-5.3	0	5	4	5	5	5	4
Calcium (mmol/l)	2.2-2.6	0	2	1.4	1	0	0	2.5
Magnesium (mmol/l)	0.8-1.0	0	0	0	1	1.5	1.5	1
Bicarbonate (mmol/l)	24-32							

Table 17.1

Fluid Composition of Common Intravenous Fluids—cont'd

	Human plasma	0.9% Sodium chloride	Hartmann's	Ringer's lactate	Ringer's acetate	Plasma-Lyte 148	Plasma-Lyte A pH 7.4	Sterofundin/ Ringerfundin
Acetate (mmol/l)	1	0	0	0	27	27	27	24
Lactate (mmol/l)	1-2	0	29	28	0	0	0	0
Gluconate (mmol/l)	0	0	0	0	0	23	23	0
Maleate (mmol/l)	0	0		0		0	0	5
Na:Cl ratio	1:21:1 to 1:54:1	1:1	1:18:1	1:19:1	1:16:1	1:43:1	1:43:1	1:14:1

(From Lobo, D. N., & Awad, S. (2014). Should chloride-rich crystalloids remain the mainstay of fluid resuscitation to prevent "pre-renal" acute kidney injury? *Kidney International, 86*, 1096–1105.)

BOX 17.1

Infusion of Fluids with Different Tonicities

Tonicity	Effect	Consequences
Isotonic fluid	Increases extracellular volume	Circulatory overload can result from isotonic fluid administration
Hypotonic fluid	Lowers the osmotic pressure of plasma	Water intoxication results when hypotonic fluid is infused beyond the patient's tolerance. Causes fluid to enter the cell
Hypertonic fluid	Increases osmotic pressure of plasma	Cellular dehydration may result from excessive infusions of hypertonic fluids. Pulls fluids from the cells

(Data from Weinstein, S., & Hagle, M. (2014). *Plumer's principles & practice of infusion therapy*. Philadelphia: Lippincott Williams & Wilkins.)

Box 17.2

Laboratory Values Assessed During Parenteral Fluid Therapy

Renal function and fluid volume changes	• Blood urea nitrogen (BUN) • Creatinine • Specific gravity • Urine osmolarity
Deviations from normal serum values	Serum electrolytes
Prior to replacement of RBC, WBC, and platelets	Complete blood count
Acid-base balance	Arterial blood gases
Evaluation prior to plasma volume expanders	Coagulation studies
Osmotic diuresis	Serum glucose

The nurse's responsibility requires monitoring the fluid and electrolyte status of the patient as well as the progress of the infusion. Greater emphasis must be placed on the causes and effects of fluid and electrolyte abnormalities so that these imbalances may be anticipated and recognized before they become alarming.

(Data from Alexander, M., Corrigan, A., Gorski, L., Hankins, J., & Perucca, R. (Eds.). (2010). Infusion nursing: An evidence-based approach (3rd ed.). St. Louis, MO: Elsevier.)

Bibliography

Evidence-based management of potassium disorders in the emergency department: *Emergency Medicine Practice* 14(2), 2015. Retrieved from http://www.ebmedicine.net/index.php.

Lobo DN, Awad S: Should chloride-rich crystalloids remain the mainstay of fluid resuscitation to prevent "pre-renal" acute kidney injury? *Kidney International* 86:1096–1105, 2014. http://dx.doi.org/10.1038/ki.2014.105.

Loscalzo L, editors: *Harrison's principles of internal medicine,* ed 19. Retrieved from http://accessmedicine.mhmedical.com.ezproxy.uky.edu/content.aspx?bookid=1130&Sectionid=79726591.

McCurdy M, Shanholtz C: Oncologic emergencies, *Critical Care Medicine* 40(7):2212–2222, 2012. http://dx.doi.org/10.1097/CCM.0b013e31824e1865.

Mount D: Fluid and electrolyte disturbances. In Kasper D, et al.: *Advances in diagnosis and management of hypokalemic and hyperkalemic emergencies.* Retrieved from http://accessmedicine.mhmedical.com/content.aspx?sectionid=79726591&bookid=1130&jumpsectionID=98706155&Resultclick=2.

Neumar RW, Shuster M, Callaway CW, Gent LM, Atkins DL, Hazinski MF: Part 1: Executive summary: 2015 American Heart Association guidelines update for cardiopulmonary resuscitation and emergency cardiovascular care, *Circulation* 132(2):S315–S367, 2015. http://dx.doi.org/10.1161/CIR.0000000000000252.

Porter R, Kaplan J, editors: *The Merck manual of diagnosis and therapy,* ed 19, Whitehouse Station, NJ, 2016, Merck Sharp & Dohme.

Seifter J: Potassium disorders. In *Goldman-Cecil medicine,* ed 25, Philadelphia, PA, 2016, Elsevier, pp 755–763.

Slotki I, Skorecki K: Disorders of sodium and water homeostatis. In *Goldman-Cecil medicine,* ed 25, Philadelphia, PA, 2016, Elsevier, pp 741–755.

Thakker R: The parathyroid glands, hypercalcemia and hypocalcemia. In *Goldman-Cecil medicine,* ed 25, Philadelphia, PA, 2016, Elsevier, pp 1649–1661.

Weinstein S, Hagle M: *Plumer's principles & practice of infusion therapy,* Philadelphia, PA, 2014, Lippincott Williams & Wilkins.

Yu A: Disorders of magnesium and phosphorus. In *Goldman-Cecil medicine,* ed 25, Philadelphia, PA, 2016, Elsevier, pp 774–778.

CHAPTER 18

Genitourinary Emergencies

Kathleen Sanders Jordan, DNP, MS, RN, FNP-BC, ENP-BC, SANE-P

I. General Strategy

A. ASSESSMENT

1. Primary and secondary assessment/resuscitation (see Chapter 1)
2. Focused assessment
   a. Subjective data collection
      1) History of present illness/chief complaint
         a) Pain: PQRST (see Chapter 8)
            (1) Suprapubic
            (2) Abdominal, flank, back
            (3) Testicular, scrotal, groin
         b) Change in urine/urinary elimination patterns
            (1) Frequency, dysuria, urgency
            (2) Hematuria
            (3) Odor
            (4) Oliguria/anuria
            (5) Dribbling/incontinence, difficulty initiating stream, enuresis, nocturia
         c) Discharge: vaginal, urethral, rectal (onset, color, character, odor, amount)
         d) Injury: mechanism (see Chapter 31), prehospital treatment, previous injuries, use of foreign objects
         e) Fever and chills
         f) Change in eating/feeding patterns (nausea, vomiting, anorexia)
         g) Tissue/skin changes (swelling, rash, turgor, deformity, pallor/cyanosis, open wounds)
         h) Lethargy or irritability
         i) Sexual history (active, orientation, safe sex practices)
         j) Efforts to relieve symptoms
            (1) Home remedies
            (2) Alternative therapies
            (3) Medications
               (a) Prescription
               (b) OTC
      2) Past medical history
         a) Current or preexisting diseases/illness
            (1) Renal disease
            (2) Urinary or pelvic infections
            (3) Sexually transmitted infections (STIs)
         b) Trauma: blunt or penetrating forces
         c) Surgery/urethral instrumentation
         d) Smoking history
         e) Substance and/or alcohol use/abuse
         f) Last normal menstrual period: female patients of childbearing age
         g) Current medications
            (1) Prescriptions
            (2) OTC/herbal
         h) Allergies
         i) Immunization status
      3) Psychological, social, and environmental risk factors
         a) Personal habits
            (1) Decreased fluid intake

(2) Immobility

(3) Poor perineal hygiene

(4) Unprotected sexual activity

(5) Multiple sexual partners

(6) New sexual partner in last 3 months

(7) Diet high in oxalates

  b) Other risk factors

(1) Pregnancy

(2) Spinal cord injury

(3) Use of lap restraint over distended abdomen

(4) Extremes of age

(5) Possible/actual assault, abuse, or intimate partner violence situations (see Chapters 3 and 40)

  b. Objective data collection

    1) General appearance

      a) Level of consciousness, behavior, affect, mood

      b) Vital signs

      c) Odors

      d) Gait

      e) Hygiene

      f) Level of distress/discomfort

    2) Inspection

      a) Guarding with movement

      b) Wound: open or closed

      c) Presence of visible foreign objects

      d) Presence of discharge, bleeding, inflammation, rash, lesions

    3) Auscultation

      a) Bowel sounds

      b) Breath sounds

      c) Fetal heart tones if pregnant

    4) Palpation/percussion

      a) Bladder distention

      b) Costovertebral angle (CVA) tenderness

      c) Abdomen: soft, nontender; tender, rigid, rebound, mass, guarding

      d) Testes and scrotum: equally descended; firm and mobile; presence of swelling or tenderness nodules, induration, mass

      e) Uterine distention

3. Diagnostic procedures

  a. Laboratory studies

    1) Urine dipstick: blood, leukocytes, nitrite, ketones, protein

    2) Urinalysis; pregnancy test in female patients of childbearing age; specific gravity

    3) Urine culture and sensitivity

    4) Renal stone analysis

    5) CBC with differential

    6) Serum chemistries including glucose, BUN, creatinine

    7) Liver function tests

    8) C-reactive protein, sedimentation rate (ESR)

    9) Antistreptolysin O (ASO) or anti-DNAase B titers

    10) ABG determination

    11) Coagulation profile: PT, PTT

    12) Serology: syphilis and HIV infection

    13) Gram stain of discharge

    14) Gonococcus (GC) culture; urine nucleic acid amplification test (NAAT)

    15) *Chlamydia* culture; urine nucleic acid amplification test (NAAT)

    16) Wet mount of discharge: saline and potassium hydroxide (KOH)

  b. Imaging studies

    1) Abdominal: kidney, urethra, bladder (KUB) radiograph

    2) CT scan

    3) Sonography

    4) Retrograde urethrogram

    5) Cystogram

    6) Intravenous pyelogram (IVP)

    7) MRI

    8) Renal arteriogram

    9) Doppler studies

  c. Other

    1) 12- to 15-lead ECG

B. ANALYSIS: DIFFERENTIAL NURSING DIAGNOSES/COLLABORATION PROBLEMS

1. Ineffective breathing pattern
2. Impaired tissue perfusion
3. Acute pain
4. Excess fluid volume
5. Deficient fluid volume
6. Deficient knowledge
7. Anxiety
8. Impaired urinary elimination
9. Risk for infection

C. PLANNING AND IMPLEMENTATION/ INTERVENTIONS

1. Determine priorities of care
  a. Maintain airway, breathing, circulation (see Chapter 1)
  b. Provide supplemental oxygen as indicated
  c. Establish IV access for administration of crystalloid fluid/medications as needed
  d. Obtain and set up equipment and supplies
  e. Prepare for/assist with medical interventions
  f. Administer pharmacologic therapy as ordered
2. Relieve pain and anxiety
3. Allow significant others to remain with patient if supportive
4. Educate patient and significant others

D. EVALUATION AND ONGOING MONITORING

1. Continuously monitor and treat as indicated
2. Monitor patient response/outcomes, and modify nursing care plan as appropriate
3. If positive outcomes are not demonstrated, reevaluate assessment and/or plan of care

E. DOCUMENTATION OF INTERVENTIONS AND PATIENT RESPONSE

F. AGE-RELATED CONSIDERATIONS

1. Pediatric
   a. Growth or development related
      1) Symptoms of urinary tract infection (UTI) in younger children are often nonspecific or generalized. They may include fever, lethargy, vomiting, diarrhea, or constipation. In infants <3 months of age, males are at greater risk than females. UTI must be a consideration in febrile illness without a source on any child who does not have urinary control
      2) Catheterization or suprapubic bladder aspiration should be used to obtain urine in boys <6 months of age and girls <2 years of age. A normal urinalysis does not exclude UTI or pyelonephritis. A bagged specimen cannot be correctly interpreted as either true infection or contamination. A urine culture is the standard of care for making the diagnosis
      3) Testicular torsion has two peak incidences: a small one in the neonatal period and a large one during puberty, although it can occur at any age
      4) Enuresis may be the presenting symptom of UTI
      5) The kidneys are injured more frequently in children than adults because of the proportionately larger size of children's kidneys and the incomplete ossification of ribs 10 and 11 until the third decade of life
   b. "Pearls"
      1) Symptoms of UTI may be subtle in infants, yet may be a cause of sepsis
      2) Child may fear punishment for insertion of foreign bodies
      3) STIs in children may indicate sexual abuse
2. Geriatric
   a. Aging related
      1) At risk for UTIs/calculi if immobile
      2) Epididymitis associated with bacterial causes
   b. "Pearls"
      1) May have decreased fluid intake, increasing risk for UTIs and calculi
      2) Prostatic hypertrophy may be cause of bladder distention
      3) As women age, occurrence of UTIs increases

II. Specific Genitourinary Emergencies

A. ACUTE KIDNEY INJURY (ACUTE RENAL FAILURE)

The term acute kidney injury (AKI) has replaced the term acute renal failure (ARF), because it has been recognized that any decline in kidney function, although not resulting in overt organ failure, is associated with increased morbidity and mortality. The term ARF is now reserved for severe AKI indicating the need for renal replacement therapy.

Acute kidney injury is defined as the deterioration in renal function that develops over a period of hours to days and results in the accumulation of nitrogenous wastes in the body. It leads to the disruption of extracellular fluid volume, electrolyte balance, and acid-base status. AKI is not a disease by itself, but a potential complication of many other disorders. It can also be superimposed on a patient with chronic kidney disease (CKD) and is classified into one of three categories, based on precipitating factors (Table 18.1). Prerenal disease, the most common cause of AKI, accounts for 40–80% of all cases. Up to 90% of the population who present to the ED have a reversible cause. It is the result of any condition that decreases renal perfusion and leads to the kidneys' inability to filter blood or regulate fluid and electrolytes. This may be caused by true volume depletion or decreased effective circulating volume. The goal of treatment is to correct the underlying cause and increase kidney perfusion. Postrenal disease (obstructive neuropathy) develops when an obstructive process impedes the outflow of urine. Subsequently, the retrograde flow of urine occurs through the urinary system, thus causing hydronephrosis and pressure on the renal parenchyma and leading to ischemia. Treatment is aimed at relieving the obstruction. Intrarenal disease results from damage to the renal blood vessels, glomeruli, or renal tubules, and it can result from untreated prerenal and postrenal causes as well as toxic exposures, trauma, and inflammation. Therapy consists of treating the underlying cause and preventing repeated toxic exposures. The most common fluid and electrolyte imbalances seen in AKI include hyperkalemia, hyponatremia, hypocalcemia, hyperphosphatemia, volume overload, and metabolic acidosis. Emergency dialysis is mandatory for those patients with severe fluid overload, intractable hypertension with pulmonary edema, and life-threatening metabolic derangements that do not respond to conservative medical management. Depending on the underlying cause and treatment course, AKI may be reversed or may result in chronic kidney disease, insufficiency, or failure.

1. Assessment
   a. Subjective data collection
      1) History of present illness/chief complaint

Table 18.1

Categories and Causes of the Three Types of Acute Kidney Injury

Pathologic Change	Causes
Prerenal	
Decreased blood flow to the kidneys leading to ischemia in the nephrons; prolonged hypoperfusion can lead to tubular necrosis and acute renal failure (ARF)	Conditions that cause decreased cardiac output: Shock Heart failure Pulmonary embolism Anaphylaxis Pericardial tamponade Sepsis
Intrarenal (Intrinsic)	
Actual tissue damage to the kidney caused by inflammatory or immunologic processes or from prolonged hypoperfusion	Acute interstitial nephritis Exposure to nephrotoxins Acute glomerulonephritis Vasculitis Hepatorenal syndrome Acute tubular necrosis (ATN) Renal artery or vein stenosis/thrombosis
Postrenal	
Obstruction of the urinary collecting system anywhere from the calices to the urethral meatus	Urethral or bladder cancer Renal calculi
Obstruction of the bladder must be bilateral to cause postrenal failure unless only one kidney is functional	Atony of bladder Prostatic hyperplasia or cancer Cervical cancer Urethral stricture

(From Ignatavicius, D. D., & Workman, M. L. (2002). *Medical-surgical nursing: Critical thinking for collaborative care* (4th ed., p. 1666). Philadelphia: Saunders.)

a) Recent volume loss: excessive vomiting, diarrhea, urination, hemorrhage, diaphoresis, and use of diuretics
b) Recent volume overload: decrease in urinary output, changes in body weight, edema, shortness of breath, hypertension, dyspnea on exertion, orthopnea, paroxysmal nocturnal dyspnea
c) Urinary frequency, urgency, or hesitancy; hematuria; flank pain
d) Recent increase in strenuous exercise
e) Mental status changes; seizures
f) Fever or other symptoms of constitutional illness
2) Past medical history
a) Current or preexisting diseases/illness
b) History specific to underlying causes
c) Recent use of radiocontrast agents
d) Recent blood transfusion

e) Medications
f) Allergies
b. Objective data collection
1) Physical examination
a) General appearance
(1) Level of consciousness, behavior, affect: confusion
(2) Tachycardia, hypertension, hypotension, orthostasis
(3) Severe distress/discomfort, critically ill
b) Inspection
(1) Jugular venous distention, peripheral edema
(2) Abdominal ascites
(3) Dialysis fistula, graft, or catheter
(4) Cardiac dysrhythmia on monitor
c) Auscultation
(1) Breath sounds: crackles, rhonchi
(2) Heart sounds: murmurs
d) Palpation/percussion
(1) Mucous membrane moisture, tissue turgor
(2) Abdominal/bladder distention, CVA tenderness
2) Diagnostic procedures
a) Urinalysis; pregnancy test in female patients of childbearing age
(1) Most important test in initial evaluation of AKI
(2) Reddish brown color: suggests acute glomerular nephritis, rhabdomyolysis or presence of myogloblin or hemoglobin
(3) Red blood cell (RBC) casts: pathognomonic for glomerular disease
(4) Uric acid crystals: may be present with acute tubular necrosis
(5) Calcium oxalate crystals: may be present in AKI
b) Serum chemistries: especially serum potassium, BUN, creatinine, calcium, phosphate, magnesium
(1) BUN: creatinine ratio >20:1 in prerenal disease
c) CBC with differential
d) Creatinine phosphokinase (CPK): rhabdomyolysis
e) Liver function tests
f) ABGs
g) ECG
h) Chest radiograph
i) Renal and/or abdominal sonography
j) Abdominal, kidney CT scan without contrast
k) IVP, retrograde pyelogram
l) Doppler scan: useful in detecting renal blood flow

m) Renal arteriogram
   (1) May not be performed because of dye load and risk of further renal damage
   (2) Aortorenal angiography: helpful in diagnosis of renal vascular disease

2. Analysis: differential nursing diagnoses/collaborative problems
  a. Ineffective breathing pattern
  b. Impaired gas exchange
  c. Ineffective tissue perfusion: renal
  d. Excess fluid volume
  e. Impaired urinary elimination
  f. Anxiety/fear
  g. Acute pain
  h. Deficient knowledge

3. Planning and implementation/interventions
  a. Maintain airway, breathing, circulation (see Chapter 1)
  b. Provide supplemental oxygen as indicated
    1) High-flow oxygen
  c. Establish IV access for administration of crystalloid fluids/medications as needed
    1) Administer fluids cautiously to avoid overload
  d. Prepare for/assist with medical interventions
    1) Institute cardiac and pulse oximetry monitoring
    2) Insert indwelling urinary catheter as needed
    3) Catheter placement and monitoring of pulmonary artery pressure (see Chapter 6)
    4) Assist with subclavian or femoral dual-lumen venous access placement for dialysis
    5) Assist with hospital admission for dialysis and possible surgery
  e. Administer pharmacologic therapy as ordered
    1) Antihypertensives
    2) Vasopressors
    3) Inotropic agents
    4) Potassium binding agents
      a) Temporary measures with a duration of action of approximately 4–6 hours
      b) Sodium polystyrene sulfonate (Kayexalate) for asymptomatic patients with a serum potassium >5.5 mEq/L
      c) Calcium gluconate intravenously (for cardiac and neuromuscular protection), insulin and glucose, and sodium bicarbonate for patients with a serum potassium >6.5 mEq/L or ECG abnormalities consistent with hyperkalemia
    5) Diuretics
    6) Nitrates
    7) Calcium channel blockers
    8) Nonnarcotic analgesics
    9) Narcotics

4. Evaluation and ongoing monitoring
  a. Level of consciousness
  b. Hemodynamic status
  c. Breath sounds and pulse oximetry
  d. Cardiac rate and rhythm
  e. Intake and output

B. EPIDIDYMITIS

Epididymitis is an inflammatory or infectious process of the epididymis, which lies on the posterior surface of the testicle. This condition most commonly affects men between the ages of 19 and 40, although it may occur in prepubertal boys and adolescents who are not sexually active. Epididymitis is most often caused by retrograde extension of organisms from the vas deferens. In men <35 years of age, epididymitis is most likely caused by a sexually transmitted pathogen, with *Chlamydia trachomatis* the most common. For men >35 years, epididymitis is often caused by coliform bacteria (*E. coli*) from an underlying obstructive urinary disease. Epididymitis can be present in the pediatric population and results from infection or from structural, neurologic, or functional abnormalities of the lower urinary tract. Complications include the formation of an epididymal abscess, which may progress to involve the testicle. Epididymitis may be difficult to differentiate from torsion or carcinoma.

1. Assessment
  a. Subjective data collection
    1) History of present illness/chief complaint
      a) Pain (see Chapter 8)
        (1) Gradual onset
        (2) Dull ache in the scrotum or lower abdomen
        (3) Increases with sexual activity
        (4) May decrease with scrotal elevation or support and application of ice
      b) Urinary frequency, urgency, or dysuria
      c) Nausea
      d) Fever and chills
      e) Urethral discharge: more commonly associated with STIs
    2) Past medical history
      a) Current or preexisting diseases/illness
      b) Recent urethritis and/or STI
      c) Recent urethral instrumentation
      d) Recent prostatectomy
      e) Unprotected sexual intercourse/multiple partners
      f) Medications
      g) Allergies
  b. Objective data collection
    1) Physical examination
      a) General appearance
        (1) Possible tachycardia, hypertension
        (2) Possible temperature elevation

(3) "Duck waddle" gait (to avoid touching
area while walking and causing pain)
(4) Mild to moderate distress/discomfort
b) Inspection
(1) Edematous epididymis and scrotum
(2) Scrotal erythema
(3) Urethral discharge
c) Palpation
(1) Scrotal warmth
(2) Scrotal tenderness
2) Diagnostic procedures
a) Urinalysis: may have pyuria (more common
with bacterial infection)
b) Urine culture and sensitivity: especially in
prepubertal and elderly patients
c) Gram stain and culture of urethral discharge
(STI or NAAT tests for *C. trachmatis* and *N.
gonorrhea*)
d) CBC with differential: elevated white blood
cell (WBC) count
e) Syphilis and HIV testing if associated STI
f) Doppler sonography or nuclear scan
2. Analysis: differential nursing diagnoses/collaborative
problems
a. Acute pain
b. Anxiety/fear
c. Deficient knowledge
3. Planning and implementation/interventions
a. Establish IV access for administration of crystalloid
fluids/medications as needed
b. Prepare for/assist with medical interventions
1) Obtain urethral discharge specimen prior to
urination
c. Administer pharmacologic therapy as ordered
1) Antibiotics
2) Analgesics
3) Antiinflammatory agents
d. Educate patient/significant others
1) Complete entire course of antibiotics
2) Follow up with urologist or primary care
provider in 5–10 days for repeat culture
3) Bed rest until pain free; begin ambulation with
scrotal support
4) Avoid lifting heavy objects or straining
during bowel movements (will increase
intraabdominal pressure and exacerbate
inflammatory process)
5) Return to work will be decided at follow-up
visit
6) Recognize and return for new or increasing
symptoms
a) Fever
b) Increasing abdominal pain
c) Continued dysuria, urethral discharge
7) Safe sexual practices (use condom with
intercourse, limit sexual partners)

4. Evaluation and ongoing monitoring
a. Hemodynamic status
b. Pain relief

C. FOREIGN BODIES

Foreign bodies may be placed in the urethra by patients of
all ages, but more commonly by young children. Placement
of foreign bodies in or around the urethra may result from
innocent exploration, from attempts to heighten sexual
experience, or in a patient unable to predetermine the outcome of such an act such as one with psychiatric or learning impairments. Embarrassment or fear of punishment
frequently delays the patient's request for help until pain or
infection is present.
1. Assessment
a. Subjective data collection
1) History of present injury/chief complaint
a) Pain (see Chapter 8)
(1) Urethral pain that may be sharp or dull
or sensation of pressure without relieving
factors
(2) May be constant or occur only on voiding
b) Patient admits to inserting foreign body into
urethra
c) Change in urinary patterns: inability to void,
dysuria, oliguria
2) Past medical history
a) Current or preexisting diseases/illness
(1) Psychiatric or learning impairments
b) Previous foreign body placement
c) Medications
d) Allergies
e) Immunization status
b. Objective data collection
1) Physical examination
a) General appearance
(1) Possible hypertension, tachycardia,
tachypnea
(2) Mild to moderate distress/discomfort
b) Inspection
(1) Urethral discharge (color, odor, consistency), blood at meatus
(2) Foreign object may be visible at urethral
meatus
2) Diagnostic procedures
a) Urinalysis: gross or occult hematuria
b) Urethral culture if object has been present for
prolonged time or signs of infection
c) Abdominal KUB radiograph
d) Cystoscope/retrograde urethrography
2. Analysis: differential nursing diagnoses/collaborative
problems
a. Acute pain
b. Impaired urinary elimination
c. Risk for infection
d. Anxiety/fear

3. Planning and implementation/interventions
   a. Establish IV for administration of crystalloid fluids/medications as needed
   b. Prepare for/assist with medical interventions
      1) Possible cystoscope/retrograde urethrography
      2) Procedural sedation
      3) Possible manual removal of object
      4) Assist with possible hospital admission and surgical removal of object
   c. Administer pharmacologic therapy as ordered
      1) Procedural sedation medications
      2) Nonnarcotic analgesics
      3) Narcotics
      4) Antibiotics
      5) Tetanus immunization
   d. Educate patient and significant others
      1) Medications: antibiotics, analgesics
      2) Maintain adequate urine output
      3) Hydration, force fluids
      4) Return if stream force declines, bloody urine does not resolve/improve, or urine output declines
4. Evaluation and ongoing monitoring
   a. Hemodynamic status
   b. Intake and output
   c. Pain relief

D. PRIAPISM

Priapism is a persistent, painful erection of the penis in the absence of sexual arousal lasting at least 4 hours. Priapism can occur in any age group. There is a bimodal peak occurring between 5 and 10 years in children and between 20 and 50 years in adults. This affects only the corpus cavernosa, whereas the corpus spongiosum of the glans penis remains flaccid. Priapism is classified as ischemic or nonischemic. Ischemic priapism is a urologic emergency. Urinary retention occurs in 50% of cases and requires the insertion of an indwelling urinary catheter. Treatment is aimed at immediate detumescence (relieving congestion and swelling to prevent endothelial inflammation and injury as well as to avoid long-term sequelae). Development of fibrosis and scarring in the cavernous spaces is related to the duration of priapism and can cause impotence. Priapism has been associated with several underlying disease states including leukemia, sickle cell crisis, multiple myeloma, tumor infiltration, spinal cord injuries, spinal anesthesia, carbon monoxide poisoning, malaria, and black widow spider bites. Several medications have also caused priapism, including those used for impotence (sildenafil citrate [Viagra], vardenafil hydrochloride [Levitra], tadalafil [Cialis], prostaglandin E [PGE], papaverine, phentolamine [Vasomax, Regitine], hydralazine [Apresoline]), calcium channel blockers, anticoagulants, phenothiazines, trazodone (Desyrel), cocaine, marijuana, and ethanol abuse. Treatment includes management of the underlying medical problem as indicated, including intracavernosal injection of a sympathomimetic drug. Phenylephrine is the sympathomimetic of choice. Intracavernosal aspiration may also be performed to relieve ischemic priapism. If the foregoing measures fail, placement of a surgical shunt may be necessary.

1. Assessment
   a. Subjective data collection
      1) History of present illness/chief complaint
         a) Pain (see Chapter 8): persistent, severe, penile pain related to number of hours of erection; intensity may increase with urinary retention and sexual intercourse
      2) Past medical history
         a) Current or preexisting diseases/illness
         b) Previous episode with spontaneous resolution
         c) Prolonged sexual stimulation
         d) Medications
         e) Allergies
   b. Objective data collection
      1) Physical examination
         a) General appearance
            (1) Level of consciousness, behavior: anxiety
            (2) Altered gait
            (3) Moderate to severe distress/discomfort
         b) Inspection
            (1) Penile erection
         c) Palpation
            (1) Bladder distention
      2) Diagnostic procedures
         a) CBC with differential and reticulocyte count
         b) Urinalysis, including toxicology screen
         c) Coagulation profile: PT/PTT
         d) Penile Doppler sonography
         e) Angiography
2. Analysis: differential nursing diagnoses/collaborative problems
   a. Acute pain
   b. Impaired urinary elimination
   c. Anxiety/fear
   d. Deficient knowledge
3. Planning and implementation/interventions
   a. Establish IV access for administration of crystalloid fluids/medications as needed
   b. Prepare for/assist with medical interventions
      1) Insertion of urinary catheter
      2) Aspiration/irrigation of corpus cavernosa
      3) Assist with obtaining urologic consult
      4) Assist with possible hospital admission and surgical intervention
   c. Administer pharmacologic therapy as ordered
      1) Nonnarcotic analgesics
      2) Narcotics
      3) Phenylephrine
   d. Educate patient/significant others
      1) Return if recurrence
      2) Return for signs and symptoms of infection: fever, redness, drainage

3) Follow-up appointment with urologist
4) Physical and sexual activity restrictions per physician
5) Medications as prescribed (antibiotics, anti-inflammatory agents, analgesics)

4. Evaluation and ongoing monitoring
   a. Pain relief
   b. Reduction of penile congestion and swelling

E. PROSTATITIS

Prostatitis is an infection or inflammation of the prostate gland. It is classified as acute bacterial, chronic bacterial, nonbacterial prostatitis, or prostatodynia. Most cases of prostatitis are nonbacterial in origin, meaning that the patient has signs and symptoms of inflammation, but no bacterial infection. Patients with prostatodynia have the complaints associated with prostatitis without the corresponding signs of infection. Acute bacterial prostatitis is the most common type of prostatitis encountered in the emergency department setting.

Acute bacterial prostatitis occurs most frequently in men aged 30–50 years. Those with diabetes mellitus or immunosuppressive conditions, or patients undergoing renal dialysis, are at risk. Frequently, the condition is the result of an ascending UTI, recent urinary instrumentation, or benign prostatic hypertrophy, but a hematogenous, lymphatic, or contiguous spread from the surrounding anatomy must also be considered. Acute bacterial prostatitis is characterized by the presence of acute inflammatory cells in both the prostate and the periglandular tissues and, if untreated, can lead to sepsis.

Eighty percent of the offending organisms involved in acute bacterial prostatitis are aerobic gram-negative bacteria. These include *E. coli, Enterobacter, Proteus, Serratia, Enterococcus,* and *Enterobacter*; however, in male patients <35 years old, *Neisseria gonorrhoeae* and *Chlamydia trachomatis* must be considered. In HIV-positive patients, the common pathogens include cytomegalovirus (CMV), *Mycobacterium tuberculosis,* and *Candida albicans.*

1. Assessment
   a. Subjective data collection
      1) History of present illness/chief complaint
         a) Fever/chills
         b) Urinary frequency, dysuria, hesitancy, incomplete voiding
         c) Pain (see Chapter 8)
            (1) Low back, suprapubic, abdominal
            (2) Scrotal, penile
            (3) Perineal, rectal
         d) Arthralgias, myalgias
         e) Malaise
         f) Genital discharge
      2) Past medical history
         a) Current or preexisting diseases/illness
            (1) Previous prostate infection
            (2) Diabetes

         b) Recent surgery or urinary instrumentation
         c) Medications
         d) Allergies
   b. Objective data collection
      1) Physical examination
         a) General appearance
            (1) Elevated temperature
            (2) Tachycardia, hypotension
            (3) Mild to moderate distress/discomfort
         b) Palpation
            (1) Nodular, boggy prostate gland
            (2) Edematous, tender prostate
      2) Diagnostic procedures
         a) CBC with differential: elevated WBC count in sepsis
         b) Serum chemistries: BUN, creatinine normal if renal function intact
         c) Urinalysis with culture and sensitivity
         d) Color Doppler sonography
         e) Transrectal sonography
         f) IV urography or voiding cystourethrogram if normal renal function
         g) Pelvic CT scan
2. Analysis: differential nursing diagnoses/collaborative problems
   a. Risk for infection
   b. Pain
   c. Impaired urinary elimination
3. Planning and implementation/interventions
   a. Establish IV access for administration of crystalloid fluid/medications as needed
   b. Prepare for/assist with medical interventions
      1) Insert urinary catheter for specimen collection
      2) Suprapubic bladder tube if obstruction present
      3) Assist with hospital admission as indicated
   c. Administer pharmacologic therapy as ordered
      1) Antibiotics
      2) Analgesics
   d. Educate patient/significant others
      1) Encourage sitz baths
      2) Use stool softeners
      3) Maintain hydration
4. Evaluation and ongoing monitoring
   a. Hemodynamic status
   b. Intake and output
   c. Pain relief

F. PYELONEPHRITIS

Pyelonephritis is an infection in the upper urinary tract involving the renal parenchyma. It occurs as the result of an ascending infection from the lower urinary tract. Approximately 80–95% of infections are caused by *E. coli.* Predisposing factors include recent instrumentation, urinary obstruction, anatomic abnormalities, previous UTIs (more than three in the past year), history of recent pyelonephritis, diabetes, immunosuppression, neurologic conditions, and pregnancy. It is more prevalent in infants, young women who are sexually active, and older men with obstructive uropathy. Pyelonephritis in pregnancy is associated with maternal and fetal complications, including preterm labor, premature delivery, hypertension and/or preeclampsia, maternal anemia, and amnionitis. Complications associated with untreated pyelonephritis include scarring of renal tissue, which may result in renal insufficiency and failure, perinephric abscess, and bacteremia.

1. Assessment
   a. Subjective data collection
      1) History of present illness/chief complaint
         a) Symptoms of UTI, including dysuria, urgency, frequency
         b) Pain (see Chapter 8): back, flank, and/or abdominal
         c) Fever, chills, myalgias, malaise, suprapubic pressure or tenderness
         d) Anorexia, feeding difficulties, nausea, and vomiting, especially in young children or infants: consider sepsis
         e) Lethargy or irritability, especially in children
         f) Enuresis in the previously toilet-trained child
      2) Past medical history
         a) Current or preexisting diseases/illnesses
            (1) Pregnancy or postpartum
            (2) Recurrent UTIs/pyelonephritis
            (3) Solitary kidney
         b) History of renal surgery or instrumentation of the genitourinary tract
         c) Last normal menstrual period in female patients of childbearing age
         d) Medications
         e) Allergies
   b. Objective data collection
      1) Physical examination
         a) General appearance
            (1) Level of consciousness, behavior, affect: lethargy or restlessness in infants and young children
            (2) Elevated temperature
            (3) Tachycardia, hypotension
            (4) Moderate distress/discomfort
         b) Inspection
            (1) Dry mucous membranes
         c) Palpation/percussion
            (1) CVA or suprapubic tenderness
      2) Diagnostic procedures
         a) Urinalysis: may require catheterization or suprapubic bladder aspiration when unable to obtain adequate clean catch such as in menstruation, infants, or the elderly
         b) Urine culture and sensitivity
         c) Urine pregnancy test in female patients of childbearing age
         d) CBC with differential
         e) Serum chemistries including glucose, BUN, creatinine
         f) C-reactive protein (CRP)
         g) Blood cultures
         h) Abdominal radiograph (KUB) if obstruction suspected
         i) Renal CT scan
         j) Renal sonography
         k) IVP if obstruction or renal disease suspected
2. Analysis: differential nursing diagnoses/collaborative problems
   a. Deficient fluid volume
   b. Acute pain
   c. Anxiety/fear
   d. Deficient knowledge
3. Planning and implementation/interventions
   a. Establish IV access for administration of crystalloid fluid/medications as needed
   b. Prepare for/assist with medical interventions
      1) Insert urinary catheter or perform suprapubic aspiration for specimen collection
      2) Insert gastric tube and attach to suction for continual vomiting
      3) Assist with hospital admission if unable to take oral fluids or if septic appearing
   c. Administer pharmacologic therapy as ordered
      1) Antibiotics
      2) Analgesics
      3) Antipyretics
   d. Educate patient/significant others
      1) Provide information regarding prevention of recurrence (see UTIs)
4. Evaluation and ongoing monitoring
   a. Hemodynamic status
   b. Intake and output

G. TESTICULAR TORSION

Testicular torsion is a true urologic emergency that results in strangulation of the testicle because of twisting of the spermatic cord structures. This leads to obstruction of the arterial blood supply with subsequent necrosis and atrophy of the testicle. It most commonly results from a congenital abnormality of the testicle involving an abnormality of the normal posterior anchoring in the scrotal sac (bell clapper deformity). There is an abnormally high attachment of the tunica vaginalis (outer covering of the testicle) resulting in increased mobility and twisting of the testicle on its vascular pedicle. This anatomic abnormality can be bilateral. Two thirds of all cases occur between the ages of 12 and 18 years in conjunction with maximal hormone stimulation at puberty, but testicular torsion may occur at any age. There is also a small peak occurrence in the neonatal period. If detorsion and orchiopexy (surgical fixation of testicle to scrotal wall) are performed within 6 hours, the testicular salvage rate is 80–100%. If more than 12 hours have elapsed, the salvage rate drops to near 0% and necessitates orchiectomy (removal of the ischemic testicle). Contralateral hemiscrotum is typically explored during surgery because the congenital bell clapper deformity is usually bilateral. Exploration allows for the fixation of the contralateral testicle so the future torsion is prevented. Diagnosis is made by clinical findings and Doppler sonography to differentiate testicular torsion from epididymitis.

1. Assessment
   a. Subjective data collection
      1) History of present illness/chief complaint
         a) Pain (see Chapter 8): testicular
            (1) Rapid onset, severe scrotal or testicular pain, usually <12 hours in duration
            (2) May radiate to lower abdomen and inguinal canal
            (3) Unrelieved by elevation or ice
            (4) May occur during exertion, be related to trauma, or develop during sleep
         b) Nausea and vomiting
         c) Low-grade fever
      2) Past medical history
         a) Current or preexisting diseases/illness
         b) Previous episode that spontaneously resolved is reported in up to 40% of patients
         c) Medications
         d) Allergies
   b. Objective data collection
      1) Physical examination
         a) General appearance
            (1) Possible tachycardia
            (2) Normal to low-grade temperature elevation
            (3) Moderate to severe distress/discomfort
         b) Inspection
            (1) Variable amount of scrotal enlargement
            (2) Edema, redness of scrotum
            (3) Pallor
         c) Palpation
            (1) Elevated testicle on affected side
            (2) Horizontal (versus vertical) lie of testicle with epididymis displaced anteriorly as testicle twists and elevates
            (3) Absence of cremasteric reflex on affected side
            (4) Firmness and tenderness of affected testicle
      2) Diagnostic procedures
         a) Urinalysis
            (1) Usually absent of significant pyuria (inflammatory versus infectious event)
            (2) May be present in approximately 30% of patients
         b) CBC with differential
         c) C-reactive protein: elevated
         d) Doppler sonography flow study
            (1) Color Doppler more accurate than plain Doppler

2. Analysis: differential nursing diagnoses/collaborative problems
   a. Ineffective tissue perfusion: testicular
   b. Acute pain
   c. Anxiety/fear
3. Planning and implementation/interventions
   a. Establish IV access for administration of crystalloid fluids/medications
   b. Prepare for/assist with medical interventions
      1) Manual detorsion: procedural sedation may be required
      2) Assist with obtaining urologic consultation
      3) Assist with hospital admission and surgery
   c. Administer pharmacologic therapy as ordered
      1) Procedural sedation medications
      2) Nonnarcotic analgesics
      3) Narcotics
      4) Sedatives
      5) Preoperative antibiotics
4. Evaluation and ongoing monitoring
   a. Testicular perfusion
   b. Pain relief

H. URINARY CALCULI

Urinary calculi are one of the most common urinary tract diseases seen in the emergency department. A urinary calculus, or stone, is the abnormal collection of one or more substances, including calcium, struvite, uric acid, or cystine, in the urinary system. Calculi vary in size and can occur anywhere along the genitourinary tract, with the renal pelvis the most common site. Acute pain is frequently described as excruciating, and it develops as the calculus descends from the renal pelvis through the ureter. The severity of pain is dependent on the degree of ureteral obstruction and ureteral spasm and on the presence of an associated infection. Approximately 80–85% of calculi pass through the urinary system and exit spontaneously. Risk factors for developing urinary calculi include the following: sedentary lifestyle; history of gout; previous calculi; frequent UTIs; large intake of protein, calcium, or fruit juices; pregnancy; and dehydration. A ureteral calculus causing obstruction and associated pyelonephritis is a true urologic emergency. Complications that can result include perinephric abscess, urosepsis, and death.

1. Assessment
   a. Subjective data collection
      1) History of present illness/chief complaint
         a) Pain (see Chapter 8)
            (1) Sudden onset severe, colicky flank pain with a constant, dull underlying pain
            (2) May radiate to abdomen, groin, scrotum, or labia as stone migrates
            (3) May worsen with voiding
            (4) No relieving factors, unable to find a comfortable position; restless and irritable
         b) Dysuria
         c) Nausea and vomiting

2) Past medical history
  a) Current or preexisting diseases/illness
    (1) Renal disease or surgery
    (2) Previous calculi, history of gout or UTIs
    (3) Pregnancy
  b) Diet high in proteins, calcium, or fruit juices
  c) Last normal menstrual period in female patients of childbearing age
  d) Family history of renal calculi
  e) Medications
  f) Allergies
b. Objective data collection
  1) Physical examination
    a) General appearance
      (1) Level of consciousness, behavior, affect: restlessness, irritability, writhing in pain
      (2) Elevated temperature if infection present
      (3) Tachycardia, hypertension
      (4) Moderate to severe distress/discomfort
    b) Inspection
      (1) Pallor, diaphoresis
    c) Palpation/percussion
      (1) CVA tenderness
  2) Diagnostic procedures
    a) Urine dipstick (for microscopic hematuria)
    b) Urinalysis
      (1) Degree of hematuria not predictive of stone size
      (2) pH >7 suggests struvite stone
      (3) pH <5 suggests uric acid stone
    c) Urine culture and sensitivity
    d) Urine pregnancy test in female patients of childbearing age
    e) CBC with differential
    f) Serum chemistries including BUN, creatinine
      (1) If creatinine >2 mg/dL, do not use diagnostic testing requiring contrast
    g) Serum uric acid
    h) Renal CT helical scan without contrast: test of choice
    i) Renal sonography
      (1) Poor visualization of nondilated ureters
      (2) Useful in pregnant female patients
      (3) Helpful in determining presence/absence of abdominal aneurysm in patients 60 years or older with first or atypical presentation of calculi
    j) IVP
      (1) Anaphylaxis occurs in 1–2 per 1,000 patients
      (2) Contraindicated in patients with history of severe contrast-induced reaction
    k) Abdominal KUB radiograph
      (1) Low sensitivity and specificity for presence of calculi
      (2) Helpful in establishing baseline for follow-up studies
    l) MRI with T2-weighted sequences
      (1) Useful in pregnant patients
2. Analysis: differential nursing diagnoses/collaborative problems
  a. Acute pain
  b. Impaired urinary elimination
  c. Risk for infection
  d. Anxiety/fear
  e. Deficient knowledge
3. Planning and implementation/interventions
  a. Establish IV access for administration of crystalloid fluid/medications as needed
  b. Prepare for/assist with medical interventions
    1) Assist with hospital admission if
      a) Continued pain
      b) Infection
      c) Inability to take oral fluids
      d) Solitary kidney
      e) Presence of ileus
      f) High-grade obstruction
      g) Underlying renal insufficiency
      h) Stones larger than 5 mm in diameter with obstruction or severe hydronephrosis
      i) Follow-up within 24 hours not available
  c. Administer pharmacologic therapy as ordered
    1) Nonnarcotic analgesics
    2) Narcotics
    3) Antiemetics
    4) Antiinflammatory agents
    5) Antibiotics
    6) Antipyretics
  d. Educate patient/significant others
    1) Increased risk for majority of patients with previous calculi
    2) Dietary changes depending on analysis of calculus
      a) Calcium: avoid spinach, rhubarb, parsley, chocolate, cocoa, instant coffee, tea, large amounts of milk
      b) Uric acid: avoid sardines, herring, liver, kidney, goose
    3) Increase fluid intake
    4) Strain urine for up to 72 hours after pain relief to retrieve stones for chemical analysis
4. Evaluation and ongoing monitoring
  a. Hemodynamic status
  b. Pain relief
  c. Intake and output

I. URINARY TRACT INFECTION

Urinary tract infection (UTI) is defined as symptomatic bacteriuria that occurs anywhere along the urinary tract, including the urethra, bladder, ureters, and kidney. Cystitis refers to infection of the lower urinary tract (bladder) and pyelonephritis refers to infection in the upper urinary tract (kidney). The urinary tract is normally sterile. Infection is caused by bacterial invasion of the mucosa and periurethral area that subsequently ascends into the bladder. An uncomplicated infection of the lower urinary tract is termed cystitis. The causative organism for 75–95% of UTIs is *E. coli*, but other organisms may cause cystitis. Populations at risk include neonates, prepubertal girls, sexually active young women, and elderly men and women. In the neonatal population, UTIs are more prevalent in boys than in girls and may manifest as a gram-negative sepsis syndrome. Circumcision reduces the risk of UTI in this population. The prevalence of UTI is highest in boys younger than 1 year and girls younger than 4 years.

In the school-age population, the incidence of UTI in girls increases to 5%; however, UTIs are rare in school-age boys. Predisposing factors in the pediatric population include lack of circumcision, vesicoureteral reflux, poor hygiene, the short urethra in girls, infrequent voiding, constipation, diabetes, and sexual activity or abuse. The largest group of patients with UTI is women, and the incidence increases with age and sexual activity. The symptoms of dysuria and/or urinary frequency in male patients younger than 50 years of age are usually related to STI-related urethritis. UTIs in men in this age group are often the result of urethral or prostatic infection. The incidence of UTI rises in older male patients because of obstruction or instrumentation. Susceptibility for frequent infections may have a genetic basis that involves the presence of epithelial cells that promote colonization of *E. coli*.

1. Assessment
   a. Subjective data collection
      1) History of present illness/chief complaint
         a) Dysuria: the most frequent complaint
         b) Other urinary symptoms: frequency, urgency, hematuria, nocturia, oliguria, voiding in small amounts or dribbling, feeling of incomplete emptying of the bladder, difficulty initiating urinary stream, night enuresis or daytime incontinence in children, or any change in color/consistency of the urine (cloudiness of urine most often the result of protein or crystals in the urine)
         c) Suprapubic abdominal discomfort or bladder fullness; CVA tenderness may be present in the absence of pyelonephritis as a result of referred pain pathways
         d) Fever, chills, and/or malaise (more frequently associated with pyelonephritis)
         e) Neonates and infants: feeding difficulties, irritability, elevated or above normal temperature, hypothermia or hyperthermia, manifestations of sepsis
      2) Past medical history
         a) Current or preexisting diseases/illness
         b) Previous UTI
         c) Recent surgery or urethral instrumentation
         d) Sexual activity, history of STIs, multiple current sexual partners
         e) Vaginal discharge, lesions
         f) Last normal menstrual period: female patients of childbearing age
         g) Medications
         h) Allergies
   b. Objective data collection
      1) Physical examination
         a) General appearance
            (1) Possible orthostasis: may be dehydrated secondary to a decreased oral intake to avoid urination
            (2) Possible temperature elevation
            (3) Mild to moderate distress/discomfort
         b) Palpation/percussion
            (1) Suprapubic tenderness or distention on palpation from retention or bladder spasms
            (2) CVA tenderness
      2) Diagnostic procedures
         a) Urine dipstick
         b) Urinalysis: may require catheterization or suprapubic bladder aspiration, if unable to obtain clean catch specimen, with menstruation, infants, and the elderly; midstream-voided technique is as accurate as catheterization if proper technique is followed
            (1) Nitrites, leukocyte esterases, and blood may be present
            (2) 100,000 colony-forming units of single organism in a clean-catch specimen: diagnostic of UTI
         c) Urine culture and sensitivity
         d) Urine pregnancy test in female patients of childbearing age
         e) CBC with differential
         f) Blood cultures
         g) BUN if suspicious of renal disease
         h) C-reactive protein (CRP)
2. Analysis: differential nursing diagnoses/collaborative problems
   a. Impaired urinary elimination
   b. Acute pain
   c. Deficient knowledge
3. Planning and implementation/interventions
   a. Establish IV access for administration of crystalloid fluids/medications as needed
   b. Prepare for/assist with medical interventions
      1) Possible pelvic examination in female patients
      2) Insert urinary catheter for specimen collection
      3) Suprapubic bladder aspiration
   c. Administer pharmacologic agents as ordered
      1) Antibiotics
      2) Analgesics

      3) Antipyretics

      4) Antispasmotics

  d. Educate patient/significant others

      1) Complete entire course of antibiotics

      2) Clean front to back in female perineal area

      3) Void frequently and completely

      4) Avoid bubble baths and perfumed soaps

      5) Void immediately after sexual intercourse

      6) Clean under foreskin in uncircumcised boys and men

      7) Encourage fruit juices and protein to increase acidification of urine

      8) Increase fluid intake

      9) Return for flank pain, fever, or persistent symptoms, which may indicate pyelonephritis

     10) Follow-up urine culture

4. Evaluation and ongoing monitoring

  a. Pain relief

Bibliography

Brenner J, Ojo A: Causes of scrotal pain in children and adolescents. Retrieved from http://www.uptodate.com/contents/causes-of-scrotal-pain-in-children-and-adolescents, 2015.

Deveci S: Priapism. Retrieved from http://uptodate.com/contents/prispism, 2015.

KDIGO: (n.d.). Clinical practice guideline for acute kidney injury. Retrieved from http://www.kidney-international.

Levey AS, Levin A, Kellum J: Definition and classification of kidney disease, *American Journal of Kidney Diseases* 686–688, 2013.

Marx J, Hockberger R: *Rosen's emergency medicine concepts and clinical practice*, Philadelphia, PA, 2014, Elsevier.

McInerny T: *AAP textbook of pediatrics*, Elk Grove Village, IL, 2009, American Academy of Pediatrics.

Palevsky P: Definition of acute kidney injury (acute renal failure). Retrieved from http://www.uptodate.com/home/index.html, 2015.

Tintinalli JE, Kelen GD, Stapczynski JS, editors: *Emergency medicine: A comprehensive study guide*, ed 7, New York, 2010, McGraw-Hill.

CHAPTER 19

Hematologic/Oncologic Emergencies

Nancy Zeller Smith, MS, RN, OCN
Kristine Kenney Powell, MSN, RN, CEN, NEA-BC, FAEN

MAJOR TOPICS
General Strategy
Assessment
Analysis: Differential Nursing Diagnoses/Collaborative
  Problems
Planning and Implementation/Interventions
Evaluation and Ongoing Monitoring
Documentation of Interventions and Patient Response
Age-Related Considerations
Specific Hematologic/Oncologic Emergencies
Disseminated Intravascular Coagulation
Hemophilia

Immune Compromise
Increased Intracranial Pressure
Neoplastic Cardiac Tamponade
Sickle Cell Crisis
Spinal Cord Compression
Superior Vena Cava Syndrome
Thrombocytopenia Purpura
Tumor Lysis Syndrome
Hematologic/Oncologic Complications
Sepsis
Syndrome of Inappropriate Antidiuretic Hormone
Hypersensitivity Reactions

I. General Strategy

A. ASSESSMENT

1. Primary and secondary assessment/resuscitation (see Chapter 1)
2. Focused assessment
   a. Subjective data collection
      1) History of present illness/chief complaint
         a) Fever
         b) Pain: PQRST (see Chapter 8)
         c) Fatigue, malaise
         d) Nausea, vomiting, diarrhea
         e) Weakness
         f) Bleeding from any site
         g) Rash
         h) Excessive bruising
         i) Dizziness
         j) Anorexia
         k) Altered mental status or decreased level of consciousness
         l) Current treatment plan/regimen
         m) Efforts to relieve symptoms
            (1) Home remedies
            (2) Alternative therapies
            (3) Medications
               (a) Prescription
               (b) OTC/herbal

      2) Medical/surgical history
         a) Current or preexisting diseases/illness
            (1) Clotting abnormalities
            (2) Blood dyscrasias
            (3) Cancer
               (a) Chemotherapy—date of last treatment
               (b) Radiation—date of last treatment
            (4) Cardiac disease
            (5) Splenectomy: alters immune response
            (6) Infection: viral, bacterial, fungal, rickett-sial, or parasitic
         b) Previous similar episodes
         c) Smoking history
         d) Substance and/or alcohol use/abuse
         e) Last normal menstrual period: female patients of childbearing age
         f) Current medications
            (1) Prescription
            (2) OTC/herbal
         g) Allergies
         h) Immunization status
      3) Psychological/social/environmental factors
         a) Age: illness may be more severe in very young
         b) Family history

c) Gender: some disorders are gender linked
d) Race: may determine increased incidence
e) Lifestyle
    (1) Sedentary or active lifestyle
    (2) Nutritional status: obesity and dietary excess or deficit
f) Inadequately treated disease process
g) Exposure to illness
h) Stressors: surgery, trauma, illness, psychosocial factors
    (1) Possible/actual assault, abuse, or intimate partner violence situations
i) Vitamin deficiency
j) Home environment
  b. Objective data collection
    1) General appearance
      a) Level of consciousness, behavior, affect
      b) Vital signs, including orthostatic blood pressure and pulse
      c) Odors
      d) Gait
      e) Hygiene
      f) Level of distress/discomfort
    2) Inspection
      a) Rash or urticaria
      b) Neck veins: distended, flattened
      c) Mucous membranes: moisture
      d) Evidence of trauma
      e) Erythema
      f) Skin color
    3) Auscultation
      a) Heart sounds: S_1 and S_2, other sounds (e.g., murmurs), dysrhythmias
      b) Breath sounds: clear, wheezes, crackles, rhonchi
      c) Bowel sounds: normal, hyperactive, hypoactive, absent
    4) Palpation
      a) Tenderness
      b) Edema
      c) Hyperthermia
      d) Arteries: equality of peripheral pulses
      e) Veins: venous filling
      f) Lymph nodes: enlarged
      g) Skin temperature, moisture
      h) Motor and sensory changes
3. Diagnostic procedures
  a. Laboratory studies
    1) Complete blood count (CBC) with differential
    2) Serum chemistries including glucose, BUN, creatinine
    3) Urinalysis: cultures if indicated
    4) Pregnancy test in female patients of childbearing age
    5) Arterial blood gas (ABG)

    6) Erythrocyte sedimentation rate (ESR)
    7) Creatine kinase (CK) and isoenzymes, lactate dehydrogenase (LDH), and aspartate aminotransferase (AST)
    8) Thyroid function tests
    9) Serum and urine toxicology screen: therapeutic and toxic ingestion
    10) Coagulation profile: partial thromboplastin time (PTT), prothrombin time (PT), fibrin degradation products (FDPs)
    11) Type and crossmatch
    12) Serum ammonia level
    13) Liver enzyme screen
    14) Sickle cell screen
    15) Serum ketone level
    16) Cerebrospinal fluid (CSF): cell count, glucose and protein counts, culture
    17) Blood cultures
  b. Imaging studies
    1) Chest radiograph
    2) Joint radiograph
    3) Computed tomography (CT) scan
    4) Magnetic resonance imaging (MRI) scan
    5) Sonography
  c. Other
    1) 12- to 15-lead electrocardiogram (ECG)
    2) Echocardiography
    3) Ultrasound

B. ANALYSIS: DIFFERENTIAL NURSING DIAGNOSES/COLLABORATIVE PROBLEMS

1. Impaired gas exchange
2. Decreased cardiac output
3. Deficient/excess fluid volume
4. Ineffective tissue perfusion
5. Fatigue
6. Impaired skin integrity
7. Deficient knowledge
8. Pain
9. Anxiety/fear
10. Risk for infection
11. Risk for injury

C. PLANNING AND IMPLEMENTATION/ INTERVENTIONS

1. Determine priorities of care
  a. Maintain airway, breathing, circulation
  b. Provide supplemental oxygen as indicated
  c. Establish intravenous (IV) access for administration of crystalloid fluids and blood products/medications
  d. Obtain and set up equipment and supplies
  e. Prepare for/assist with medical interventions
  f. Administer pharmacologic therapy as ordered
2. Relieve anxiety/apprehension

3. Allow significant others to remain with patient if supportive
4. Educate patient/significant others

D. EVALUATION AND ONGOING MONITORING

1. Continuously monitor and treat as indicated
2. Monitor patient response/outcomes, and modify nursing care plan as appropriate
3. If positive patient outcomes are not demonstrated, reevaluate assessment and/or plan of care

E. DOCUMENTATION OF INTERVENTIONS AND PATIENT RESPONSE

F. AGE-RELATED CONSIDERATIONS

1. Pediatrics
   a. Growth or development related
      1) According to 2014 estimates, over 15,000 new cases of cancer and almost 2,000 deaths occur annually from cancer among children and adolescents from birth to 19 years of age
      2) Communicate with patient, as appropriate, and parents regarding treatment plan, progress, and delays
         a) Shared decision making among the family, child, and medical team is the standard of care, and decisions are goal directed
         b) For patients with terminal illness, aiding parents in obtaining accurate prognostic information and potential poor prognosis, if applicable, will generate an earlier discussion of palliative care and hospice, less use of cancer-specific therapies in the last months of life, and earlier do not resuscitate (DNR) orders. Earlier acceptance of patient's prognosis may elevate comfort to the primary therapeutic goal
         c) Adolescents who have been involved and understand their medical conditions, when given the opportunity, can communicate their preferences
   b. "Pearls"
      1) Pediatric oncology patients account for a high proportion of severe sepsis in children presenting to the emergency department
      2) Antiemetic use to treat nausea and vomiting among pediatric patients continues to be evaluated by the American Academy of Pediatrics. IV fluid therapy followed by oral rehydration therapy is suggested. Overall side effects of antiemetic medications are of concern during reevaluation
         a) Promethazine (Phenergan) results in drowsiness, which interferes with the oral hydration process and assessment of lethargy
         b) Metoclopramide (Reglan) results in somnolence, nervousness, irritability, and dystonic reactions
         c) Ondansetron (Zofran) is still being evaluated for its sedative effects and no cases of extrapyramidal reactions have been noted

2. Geriatrics
   a. Aging-related
      1) By 80 years of age, only 10% of women and 19% of men are free of chronic illnesses. Cancer in this population may be a chronic condition. Recent advances in oncology care are improving survival of patients with cancer and more elderly patients are being treated and living longer with cancer
      2) About 50% of cancer diagnoses are in patients 70 years and older
      3) In 2011, cancer was the leading cause of death for people 60–79 years of age. For those above 80, it was the second leading cause of death behind heart disease
      4) Complicated family and social structures subsequent to elderly patients' being widowed, fewer siblings remaining, and children not in the vicinity may lead to lack of emotional and financial support
      5) Identifying and treating the underlying cause of symptoms is vital, primarily in the following areas: pain, dyspnea, constipation, oranorexia-cachexia
         a) Older adults may report fewer side effects or symptoms due to years of coping, especially in the long-term presence of symptoms
         b) Polypharmacy has been shown to be a leading cause of side effects and altered behavior. Obtaining a list of medications and dosages should be completed promptly and addressed by the physician or pharmacy before treatment begins
      6) Allow patient, if able, to maintain independence and assist in treatment plan decisions. Understand and respect patient's values and goals, including end-of-life decisions
   b. "Pearls"
      1) Pain control in older patients, especially older women, has been found to be inadequate
      2) Assessing quality of life is important from early cancer diagnosis to further progression of the disease. Many techniques such as surgery, chemotherapy, and radiation therapy (RT) can relieve cancer symptoms. However, if the disease progresses, the risk of morbidity and diminished quality of life versus potential benefits of therapeutic intervention must be evaluated

II. Specific Hematologic/ Oncologic Emergencies

It is estimated that in 2015 there will be approximately 1,658,370 new diagnoses of cancer and 589,430 deaths in the United States. It is important to identify and manage underlying hematologic and oncologic conditions in patients experiencing a life-threatening emergency. With accurate assessment, swift intervention, and proper management of hematologic/oncologic emergencies, dramatic improvement in quality of life may be attained. When immunocompromised patients present to the emergency department, prompt assessment of their medical history in relation to chief complaints will expedite care. Isolation from others with infectious conditions is a priority so as not to complicate or worsen their condition. Some patients with a compromised immune system may communicate their condition, may present wearing a facemask, or may ask to be placed in a separate area. Being responsive to their needs will decrease potential complications and convey compassion toward their condition.

A. DISSEMINATED INTRAVASCULAR COAGULATION

Disseminated intravascular coagulation (DIC) is a complex, consumptive, systemic, thrombohemorrhagic disorder involving the inappropriate and accelerated activation of the coagulation cascade resulting in thrombosis and subsequent hemorrhage. It is manifested by microvascular clots, depletion of platelets, clotting factors, and impaired hemostasis. Normal hemostasis is maintained through a balanced system of coagulation (clot formation) and fibrinolysis (clot breakdown) (Fig. 19.1). The process of thrombosis (abnormal clotting within a blood vessel) is initiated through disruption of the endothelial membrane and/or tissue. Fibrinolysis is the process that breaks down stable fibrin clots. As clots are rapidly lysed, fibrin degradation (split) products (FDP) are released and act as anticoagulants. During this time, the blood's clotting factors are depleted causing abnormal bleeding. DIC occurs as a complication of, or in association with, other conditions such as sepsis. The overall management goal is to locate and treat the underlying disorder.

1. Assessment
   a. Subjective data collection
      1) History of present illness/chief complaint
         a) Bleeding from any site
         b) Dizziness
         c) Weakness
         d) Rash
         e) Excessive bruising
         f) Nausea, vomiting, diarrhea
         g) Shortness of breath
         h) Joint pain
         i) Headache

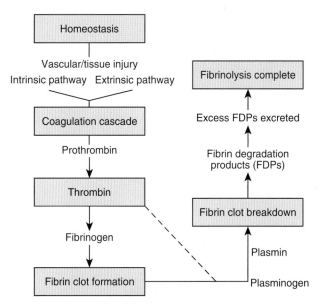

FIG. 19.1 Normal hemostasis. (From Itano, J., & Taoka, K. [Eds.]. *Core curriculum for oncology nursing* [4th ed.]. Philadelphia, PA: Elsevier Saunders, in collaboration with Oncology Nursing Society.)

      2) Medical history
         a) Current or preexisting diseases/illness
            (1) Cancer: acute leukemias or solid tumors (mucin-producing adenocarcinomas), such as lung, breast, prostate, pancreas, ovarian, and biliary tract malignancies
            (2) Infections and sepsis
            (3) Liver disease, both as primary liver disease and secondary metastasis from malignancy
            (4) Malaria
         b) Presence of peritoneovenous shunts for ascites fluid containing a number of procoagulant substances
         c) Massive blood transfusions, especially those with hemolytic transfusion reactions
         d) Transplant rejection
         e) Pregnancy and obstetrical complications in female patients of childbearing age
         f) Trauma: blunt or penetrating forces
         g) Snakebite
         h) Respiratory distress syndrome
         i) Prolonged extracorporeal circulation
         j) Last normal menstrual period: female patients of childbearing age
         k) Medications including aspirin, anticoagulants, oral contraceptives, estrogen replacement
         l) Allergies
         m) Immunization status
   b. Objective data collection
      1) Physical examination
         a) General appearance

          (1) Level of consciousness, behavior, affect: restlessness, confusion, lethargy, obtundation, seizure, coma

          (2) Tachypnea, tachycardia

          (3) Severe distress, critically ill

       b) Inspection

          (1) Jaundice, pallor, cyanosis

          (2) Bleeding

            (a) Overt: invasive sites, hematemesis, hematuria, and stools

            (b) Occult bleeding

          (3) Petechiae, ecchymosis

          (4) Hematomas

          (5) Abdominal distension

       c) Palpation

          (1) Abdominal tenderness

          (2) Diminished peripheral pulses

          (3) Extremity coolness

          (4) Joint tenderness

   2) Diagnostic procedures

       a) Coagulation profile

          (1) Prolonged PT and PTT

          (2) Presence of FDPs; titers increased

       b) CBC with differential

          (1) Platelet count: decreased (thrombocytopenia)

          (2) Hemoglobin/hematocrit: decreased

       c) Fibrinogen level: decreased

       d) BUN/creatinine levels: elevated

       e) Antithrombin III level: decreased

       f) D-dimer

       g) Bleeding time

          (1) Indicates presence of thrombin and plasmin

          (2) Greatest specificity and reliability for DIC diagnosis

       h) Urinalysis: presence of blood or hemoglobin in urine; pregnancy test in female patients of childbearing age

       i) Stool, emesis: heme positive

       j) Chest radiograph

       k) CT scan specific to potential bleeding site (i.e., head CT for altered level of consciousness; chest CT for hemoptysis; abdominal/pelvic CT for distension)

2. Analysis: differential nursing diagnoses/collaborative problems

   a. Ineffective tissue perfusion: renal, cerebral, peripheral, cardiopulmonary, and gastrointestinal

   b. Risk for deficient fluid volume

   c. Decreased cardiac output

   d. Impaired gas exchange

   e. Risk for injury

   f. Anxiety/fear

   g. Acute pain

3. Planning and implementation/interventions

   a. Maintain airway, breathing, circulation

   b. Provide supplemental oxygen

   c. Establish IV access for administration of crystalloid fluid, blood products, and/or medications

      1) Warmed packed red blood cell transfusion: washed cells

      2) Platelet concentrates

      3) Fresh frozen plasma (FFP)

      4) Cryoprecipitate

   d. Prepare for/assist with medical interventions

      1) Limit number of venipunctures

      2) Institute cardiac and pulse oximetry monitoring

      3) Apply pressure dressings to sites of active bleeding

      4) Insert gastric tube and attach to suction

      5) Insert indwelling urinary catheter

      6) Maintain normothermic body temperature

      7) Handle patient gently

      8) Assist with hospital admission

   e. Administer pharmacologic therapy as ordered

      1) Heparin

         a) Inhibits thrombin and Xa factor

         b) May accelerate bleeding

      2) Recombinant human activated protein C (rhAPC)

         a) Inhibits factors Va and VIIIa of coagulation cascade

         b) Inhibits plasminogen activator inhibitor

      3) Reversal agents for heparin-induced bleeding

      4) Nonnarcotic analgesics—do not use nonsteroidal antiinflammatory drugs (NSAIDs) or aspirin-containing medications

      5) Narcotics

4. Evaluation and ongoing monitoring

   a. Level of consciousness

   b. Hemodynamic status

   c. Breath sounds and pulse oximetry

   d. Cardiac rate and rhythm

   e. Intake and output, including overt and covert bleeding

   f. Serial laboratory changes: clotting time, platelet count, hematocrit, and hemoglobin

   g. Measure abdominal girth every 4 hours if bleeding present

   h. Pain relief

B. HEMOPHILIA

Hemophilia is an inherited, sex-linked disorder that occurs most frequently in boys and men. Female family members carry the gene and pass it to their children. There are four types of hemophilia: hemophilia A, hemophilia B, hemophilia C, and von Willebrand disease. Hemophilia A (classic hemophilia) is a coagulation disorder caused by a variant form of factor VIII. Severity of the disease is directly related to activity level of factor VIII. Activity level <1% is severe and accompanied by spontaneous bleeding. Activity level of 1–5% is moderately severe; there is rare spontaneous bleeding but difficulty during surgery or with trauma. Patients with 5–10% or greater activity of factor VIII have mild disease with little risk of spontaneous bleeding, but the PTT is prolonged. Bleeding may occur anywhere but characteristically affects joints, deep muscles, urinary tract, and cranial vault (Table 19.1). Immediately following injury, bleeding is usually absent because the initial coagulation step of platelet-plug formation is not affected by hemophilia. Hemophilia B (Christmas disease) results from absence or deficiency of factor IX. The condition is relatively rare, occurring in 1 in 100,000 persons in the United States, and is clinically indistinguishable from type A, except for treatment. Hemophilia C (Rosenthal syndrome) is caused by a deficiency of factor XI. Clinically, it is similar to hemophilia A, but usually has less severe bleeding. Von Willebrand disease (angiohemophilia) occurs in male and female patients and is less acute than hemophilia A or B. This type of hemophilia is characterized by defective platelet adherence and decreased factor VIII levels.

1. Assessment
   a. Subjective data collection
      1) History of present illness/chief complaint
         a) Prolonged bleeding after trauma or dental extraction
         b) Spontaneous hemorrhage
         c) Hemarthrosis with decreased movement
         d) Melena
      2) Medical history
         a) Current or preexisting disease/illness
            (1) Hemophilia
            (2) Hepatitis
            (3) Human immunodeficiency virus (HIV)
         b) Previous blood transfusions
         c) Trauma: blunt or penetrating forces
         d) Medications
         e) Allergies
         f) Immunization status
   b. Objective data collection
      1) Physical examination
         a) General appearance
            (1) Gait
            (2) Possible postural hypotension
            (3) Moderate to severe distress/discomfort
         b) Inspection
            (1) Uncontrolled bleeding from any sites
            (2) Skin pallor
            (3) Ecchymosis
            (4) Hematomas
            (5) Hemarthrosis
         c) Palpation
            (1) Joints
               (a) Decreased range of motion
               (b) Tenderness, pain
               (c) Pulses in extremities may be abnormal
            (2) Skin temperature
      2) Diagnostic procedures
         a) CBC: normal hematocrit, normal platelet counts
         b) Coagulation profile: PT and PTT normal to slightly prolonged
         c) Factor VIII activity level: decreased in hemophilia A and von Willebrand disease
         d) Factor IX activity level: decreased in hemophilia B
         e) Factor XI level: decreased in hemophilia C
         f) Urinalysis; pregnancy test in female patients of childbearing age
         g) Affected joint radiograph
            (1) May have synovial hypertrophy, fibrosis, and cartilage damage from recurrent episodes with inadequate treatment
         h) Affected joint sonography: acute or chronic effusion
         i) Head CT scan if neurologic symptoms or trauma
2. Analysis: differential nursing diagnoses/collaborative problems
   a. Risk for deficient fluid volume
   b. Deficient knowledge
3. Planning and implementation/interventions
   a. Maintain airway, breathing, circulation
   b. Provide supplemental oxygen as indicated
   c. Establish IV access for administration of crystalloid fluids, blood products, and/or medications
      1) Administer warmed ABO type-specific blood if warranted

Table 19.1

Common Bleeding Manifestations in Patients with Hemophilia

Site	Examples
Central nervous system	Intracranial bleeding, most common cause of hemorrhagic death; subdural hematomas occur spontaneously or with minimal trauma
Hemarthroses	Joints, leading to chronic atrophy if not treated aggressively
Hematomas	Soft tissue or muscles, most serious near the neck (airway compromise), extremities (massive blood loss)
Hematuria	Common, but not serious, and source is usually not located
Mucocutaneous tissues	Uncommon, but can be spontaneous from oropharynx, gastrointestinal, epistaxis, or hemoptysis; delayed bleeding after dental extraction can be common
Pseudotumor	Bone cysts that result from unresolved hematomas; usually surgically removed

Modified from Tintinalli, J. E., Kelen, G. D., & Stapczynski, J. S. (2004). *Emergency medicine: A comprehensive study guide* (6th ed., p. 1331). New York, NY: McGraw-Hill.

    2) FFP for hemophilia A and von Willebrand disease

    3) Factor VIII for severe cases: cryoprecipitate or recombinant factor VIII is preferred over commercial factor VIIIc because of greater risk for infection by hepatitis B virus and HIV

      a) Follow hospital policy for transfusion of blood products

    4) For severe hemorrhage, treat for shock. Anticipate use of cryoprecipitate

    5) For hemophilia B, use commercial factor IX or FFP

  d. Prepare for/assist with medical interventions

    1) Apply firm pressure to venipucture sites for a minimum of 5 minutes

    2) Hemarthrosis or hematoma

      a) Apply ice packs to area

      b) Immobilize area

      c) Elevate extremity

      d) Apply mild compressive pressure dressing

    3) Lacerations from injury

      a) Apply local pressure to wound

      b) Observe for 4 hours after suturing

  e. Administer pharmacologic therapy as ordered

    1) Minimize intramuscular injections

    2) Topical thrombin for minor wounds and epistaxis

    3) Wound repair anesthesia with epinephrine

    4) Desmopressin acetate (DDAVP) for mild to moderate disease severity: increases levels of factor VIIIc

    5) Nonnarcotic analgesics: avoid aspirin and nonsteroidal antiinflammatory drugs (NSAIDs)

    6) Narcotics

    7) Tetanus immunization: intramuscular injection is acceptable

  f. Educate patient/significant others

    1) Avoid bleeding episodes

      a) Safety measures

      b) Avoid rigorous activities (e.g., contact sports)

    2) Use medical alert (MedicAlert) tag

    3) Need for prophylactic dental care

    4) Avoid OTC medications containing aspirin and NSAIDs

    5) Use of factor VIII therapy at home to terminate early bleeding episode, decreasing complications

4. Evaluation and ongoing monitoring

  a. Level of consciousness

  b. Hemodynamic status

  c. Amount of continued bleeding or bleeding into central nervous system, neck, pharynx, retropharynx, retroperitoneum, or potential compartment syndrome

  d. Allergic reactions: urticaria, pruritis, fever

  e. Transfusion reactions

C. IMMUNE COMPROMISE

Disease, drugs, or nutritional deficits may adversely affect the immune system. Typically, the immunocompromised patient seen in the emergency department is receiving treatment for cancer or is currently receiving immunosuppressive therapy after organ transplantation. The immunocompromised patient experiences neutropenia (a decrease in neutrophils) and leukopenia (a decrease in total white cell count). A decreased neutrophil count places the patient at higher risk for infection from normal body flora as well as from opportunistic organisms. Classic signs of infection such as redness, heat, and swelling do not occur because the body's phagocytic response is impaired. Pus formation is also absent because white blood cells are the major component of pus. Consequently, the most significant indicator of infection in the patient with neutropenia is fever. Immunocompromised patients are instructed to call the physician any time the temperature is >100.4°F (38°C). Febrile neutropenia is defined as a temperature of 100.4°F (38°C)or greater with an absolute neutrophil count of 1,000/mm^3 or less and is considered a medical emergency. A patient who presents to triage with complaint of fever and recent history of chemotherapy administration or other cause of immunosuppression should be immediately placed in a treatment room with the door closed and should not be placed in the waiting room. Care of the immunocompromised patient in the emergency department focuses on protecting the patient, identifying the source of infection, and initiating antibiotic therapy rapidly.

1. Assessment

  a. Subjective data collection

    1) History of present illness/chief complaint

      a) Fever

      b) Cough, sore throat, dysphagia

      c) Dysuria, urinary frequency

      d) Pain

      e) Weakness, dizziness, fainting

      f) Confusion

      g) Redness or swelling

      h) Nausea, vomiting, diarrhea, anorexia

      i) Rectal tenderness

      j) Vaginal itching or discharge

    2) Medical history

      a) Current or preexisting diseases/illness

        (1) Cancer

        (2) Acquired immunodeficiency syndrome (AIDS)

        (3) Organ transplantation

        (4) Other immune diseases, infection, sepsis

      b) Chemotherapy, biologic therapy

      c) Radiation therapy

      d) Recent surgery

      e) Recent travel to developing country

      f) Medications

      g) Allergies

      h) Immunization history

b. Objective data collection
   1) Physical examination
      a) General appearance
         (1) Elevated temperature: 100.4°F (38°C) or greater
         (2) Tachypnea, tachycardia, normotension/hypotension
         (3) Moderate distress/discomfort, critically ill
      b) Inspection
         (1) Oral ulcerations: aphthous or herpetic stomatitis, xerostomia (dry mouth), mucositis
      c) Palpation
         (1) Areas of tenderness
   2) Diagnostic procedures
      a) CBC with differential
         (1) Total WBC count <5,000/mm³ of blood
         (2) Absolute neutrophil count 1,000/mm³ places patient at greater risk for infection
      b) Peripheral blood smear
      c) Hematocrit level, reticulocyte count, and platelet count: to evaluate general bone marrow function
      d) Cultures: blood, urine, stool, wounds, sputum, CSF if indicated
      e) Chest radiograph
      f) ECG if indicated
2. Analysis: differential nursing diagnoses/collaborative problems
   a. Risk for infection
3. Planning and implementation/interventions
   a. Maintain airway, breathing, circulation
   b. Provide supplemental oxygen
   c. Place patient in private room as soon as possible
   d. Establish IV access for administration of crystalloid fluids, and medications
   e. Prepare for/assist with medical interventions
      1) Institute cardiac and pulse oximetry monitoring
      2) Implement nursing care measures for immunosuppressed patients
         a) Follow hospital policy for neutropenia precautions
         b) Have patient wear a mask if being transported to another department/room
         c) Exemplary handwashing and equipment cleaning processes
         d) Limit number of personnel in room
      3) Avoid use of indwelling catheter
      4) Assist with hospital admission
      5) Evaluate primary nurse–patient assignments and adjust as needed to reduce risk of cross-contamination from other patient infections
   f. Administer pharmacologic therapy as ordered
      1) Antipyretics
         a) Use NSAIDs with caution in patients with thrombocytopenia

      2) Dilute all IV medications and administer carefully to minimize vein irritation
      3) Nonnarcotic analgesics
      4) Narcotics
      5) Antibiotics should be given within 1 hour of presentation
   g. Educate patient/significant others
      1) Avoid use of douches and tampons
      2) Encourage patient to eat well-balanced meals and increase fluid intake
      3) Signs and symptoms of potential infection
      4) Avoid persons with signs and symptoms of viral syndromes or infections
4. Evaluation and ongoing monitoring
   a. Hemodynamic status
   b. Breath sounds and pulse oximetry
   c. Cardiac rate and rhythm
   d. Intake and output
   e. Pain relief

D. INCREASED INTRACRANIAL PRESSURE

Patients with a diagnosis of leukemia or neuroblastoma; primary tumors of the brain or spinal cord; cancer of the lung, breast, testes, thyroid, stomach, kidney, melanoma; and thrombocytopenia or platelet dysfunction are all at high risk for developing increased intracranial pressure (ICP) due to metastases.

1. Planning and implementation/interventions
   a. Maintain airway, breathing, circulation
   b. Provide supplemental oxygen
   c. Establish IV access for administration of crystalloid fluids and medications
   d. Prepare for/assist with medical interventions
      1) Institute cardiac and pulse oximetry monitoring
      2) Assist with medical decompression of cranial vault to decrease ICP
         a) Increase venous outflow through elevation of head of bed, midline head and neck positioning, and avoidance of extreme hip flexion
      3) Decrease metabolic demands of the brain by
         a) Maintaining normothermia
         b) Preventing seizures
      4) Assist with hospital admission
         a) Radiation therapy (RT) for brain metastases
   e. Administer pharmacologic therapy as ordered
      1) Corticosteroids: used to decrease inflammation; given before radiation therapy (RT) but may require maintenance doses for residual tumor

E. NEOPLASTIC CARDIAC TAMPONADE

Cardiac tamponade occurs because of excess accumulation of fluid in the pericardial sac and results in decreased cardiac output and compromised cardiac function. It can be a life-threatening complication of cancer. The pericardial sac is normally filled with approximately 10–50 mL of fluid, which allows the heart to contract and relax without friction. Increased intrapericardial pressure can be caused by fluid accumulation in the pericardial sac, direct or metastatic tumor invasion to the pericardial sac, or fibrosis of the pericardial sac related to radiation therapy (RT). As pressure increases in the pericardium, there is decreased left ventricular filling, decreased pumping ability of the heart, decreased cardiac output, and impaired systemic perfusion.

1. Assessment
   a. Subjective data collection
      1) History of present illness/chief complaint
         a) Retrosternal chest pain: relieved by leaning forward or lying supine
         b) Dyspnea
         c) Cough
         d) Hiccoughs
      2) Medical history
         a) Current or preexisting diseases/illness
            (1) Primary tumors of the heart, including mesothelioma and sarcomas
            (2) Metastatic tumors to the pericardium: lung, breast, gastrointestinal tract, leukemia, Hodgkin or non-Hodgkin lymphoma, sarcoma, melanoma
            (3) Radiation therapy (RT) to a field in which the heart was included
            (4) AIDS-related Kaposi sarcoma
            (5) Cardiac disease
            (6) Chronic pulmonary illnesses
         b) Medications
         c) Allergies
   b. Objective data collection
      1) Physical examination
         a) General appearance
            (1) Level of consciousness, behavior, affect: anxiety
            (2) Hypotension
            (3) Moderate to severe distress/discomfort
         b) Inspection
            (1) Body position (sitting and leaning forward or lying supine)
            (2) Peripheral edema
               (a) Jugular vein distension (JVD)
            (3) Signs of trauma
            (4) Electrical alternans via Lewis lead (modified lead II, which highlights atrial activity) on ECG
         c) Auscultation
            (1) Heart sounds: distant or muffled
      2) Diagnostic procedures
         a) ABG if patient has respiratory distress
         b) CBC with differential
         c) Serum chemistries including glucose, BUN, creatinine
         d) ESR: elevated
         e) CK and isoenzymes: troponin I may be elevated
         f) LDH, AST: elevated
         g) Thyroid function tests
         h) Chest radiograph: enlarged pericardial silhouette and cardiomegaly occur with slow fluid accumulation
         i) Chest CT scan: may show pleural effusion, masses, or pericardial thickening
         j) Echocardiogram: most precise diagnostic test
            (1) Small effusions located posterior and inferior to left ventricle
            (2) Moderate effusions extend toward apex of the heart
            (3) Large effusions circumscribe the heart
         k) ECG
            (1) Alternating levels of ECG voltage of P wave, QRS complex, T wave
            (2) PR interval depression
            (3) Four-stage evolution
               (a) Stage 1: ST-segment elevation with concave configuration in all leads except V_1. Occurs within hours of chest pain and lasts for days
               (b) Stage 2: ST segment returns to baseline, T wave flattens
               (c) Stage 3: T-wave inversion without Q-wave formation
               (d) Stage 4: ECG normalization
         l) Cytology studies of pericardial fluid
2. Analysis: differential nursing diagnoses/collaborative problems
   a. Ineffective breathing pattern
   b. Decreased cardiac output
   c. Ineffective tissue perfusion: cardiopulmonary and cerebral
   d. Acute pain
   e. Anxiety
   f. Deficient knowledge
   g. Fatigue
3. Planning and implementation/interventions
   a. Maintain airway, breathing, circulation (see Chapter 1)
   b. Provide supplemental oxygen
   c. Establish IV access for administration of crystalloid fluid and medications
   d. Prepare for/assist with medical interventions
      1) Elevate head of bed in position of comfort to minimize shortness of breath and chest pain
      2) Institute cardiac and pulse oximetry monitoring
      3) Pericardiocentesis, pericardial window
      4) Possible thoracotomy
      5) Assist with hospital admission

e. Administer pharmacologic therapy as ordered
  1) Corticosteroids: temporary reduction of inflammation
  2) Anxiolytics
  3) Nonnarcotic analgesics
  4) Narcotics
4. Evaluation and ongoing monitoring
  a. Hemodynamic status
  b. Breath sounds and pulse oximetry
  c. Cardiac rate and rhythm
  d. Extremities for peripheral edema

F. SICKLE CELL CRISIS

Sickle cell disease is an inherited genetic disorder affecting primarily the African-American population. The abnormal hemoglobin S makes up 35% of total hemoglobin, whereas normal hemoglobin A accounts for 65%. Fully oxygenated hemoglobin S does not differ from hemoglobin A, so there are few clinical manifestations. A crisis arises from microcirculation obstruction (vasoocclusive crisis), a drop in hemoglobin levels (hematologic crisis), or the presence of infection (infectious crisis). Severe hypoxia, stress, exposure to cold temperature or water, or dehydration may precipitate a sickling crisis. When deoxygenation occurs, red blood cells containing hemoglobin S change from biconcave disks to crescents. These crescent-shaped cells become rigid and are incapable of traversing the microcirculation, thereby obstructing capillary blood flow. Obstruction leads to tissue hypoxia, which promotes deoxygenation and further sickling. The increased obstruction results in infarcted tissues and organs. Occasionally, there is splenic infarction caused by clumping of abnormally shaped cells. Oxygenation reverses the sickling process in about 80% of the cells; the remainder are irreversibly sickled and contribute to severe hemolytic anemia.

1. Assessment
  a. Subjective data collection
    1) History of present illness/chief complaint
      a) Pain (see Chapter 8)
        (1) Location: abdomen, chest, back, and joints
        (2) Onset: sudden
        (3) Frequency: cluster attacks are common
      b) Impaired growth patterns
        (1) Impaired growth and development
        (2) General failure to thrive
      c) Infection
        (1) Increased susceptibility, especially to *Streptococcus pneumoniae*
        (2) Impaired splenic function causes ineffective clearance of bacteria
    2) Medical history
      a) Current or preexisting diseases/illness
        (1) Sickle cell disease
        (2) Heart failure: secondary to chronic anemia and hypoxia
        (3) Chronic organ damage
      b) Genetic family history
      c) Increased tendency for gallstones
      d) Medications
      e) Allergies
  b. Objective data collection
    1) Physical examination
      a) General appearance
        (1) Level of consciousness, behavior, affect: 25% chance of significant neurologic event
        (2) Tachypnea, tachycardia
        (3) Possible positive orthostatic signs
        (4) Possible elevated temperature
        (5) Moderate to severe distress/discomfort
      b) Inspection
        (1) Jaundice
        (2) Possible chronic ulcers of lower extremities
        (3) Youthful appearance and long, thin extremities
        (4) Priapism
        (5) Eyes: vitreous hemorrhage, retinal detachment, and infarction
      c) Auscultation
        (1) Breath sounds
        (2) Heart sounds: systolic ejection murmur
        (3) Bowel sounds
      d) Palpation
        (1) Decreased peripheral blood flow
        (2) Capillary blanch test: delayed
    2) Diagnostic procedures
      a) CBC with differential
        (1) Hemolytic anemia: hematocrit 20–30%
        (2) Elevated reticulocytes
        (3) Peripheral smear: sickled erythrocytes
      b) Hemoglobin electrophoresis: sickle cell hemoglobin (hemoglobin S)
      c) ABGs: lowered partial pressure of arterial oxygen (PaO_2)
      d) Bilirubin: elevated secondary to hemolysis
      e) Liver function tests
      f) Serum chemistries including BUN and creatinine
      g) Urinalysis; pregnancy test in female patients of childbearing age
      h) Chest/abdomen radiograph: rules out infection or acute abdomen
      i) Abdominal sonography: useful to document spleen size and presence of biliary stones
      j) MRI: identifies avascular necrosis of femoral or humeral head
      k) Transcranial Doppler sonography: aids in identifying patients at risk for stroke; children should be tested
      l) ECG: rules out cardiac complication

2. Analysis: differential nursing diagnoses/collaborative problems
   a. Ineffective tissue perfusion: cerebral, cardiopulmonary, renal, hepatic, and splenic
   b. Risk for deficient fluid volume deficit
   c. Acute/chronic pain
   d. Deficient knowledge
3. Planning and implementation/interventions
   a. Maintain airway, breathing, circulation
   b. Provide supplemental oxygen as indicated
   c. Establish IV access for administration of crystalloid fluids, blood products, and medications
      1) Transfuse warmed packed red blood cells, as necessary
   d. Prepare for/assist with medical interventions
      1) Institute cardiac and pulse oximetry monitoring
      2) Provide support of extremities with pillows
      3) Aid patient to assume position of comfort
      4) Assist with hospital admission, as needed
   e. Administer pharmacologic therapy as ordered
      1) Nonnarcotic analgesics
      2) Narcotics: dosing individualized
         a) Morphine sulfate
         b) Hydromorphone (Dilaudid)
         c) Nalbuphine hydrochloride (Nubain)
         d) Codeine, hydrocodone
      3) Oral hydroxyurea: impedes the sickling of red blood cells and stimulates production of fetal hemoglobin (hemoglobin F), which has a high affinity for oxygen
      4) IV sodium bicarbonate, if severe metabolic acidosis present
   f. Educate patient/significant others
      1) Refer to social service agency or local support group for sickle cell disease
      2) Suggest alternative coping mechanisms for patient/significant others
      3) Provide preventive suggestions
         a) Ensure adequate fluid intake
         b) Avoid high altitudes
         c) Avoid stressful situations
         d) Avoid cold weather
         e) Avoid infection and trauma
         f) Elevate legs
      4) Instruct patient in use of prescribed medications
      5) Instruct patient regarding signs and symptoms that indicate need for emergency care, including recurrence of symptoms, severe abdominal pain, and illness with signs of dehydration
4. Evaluation and ongoing monitoring
   a. Level of consciousness
   b. Hemodynamic status
   c. Breath sounds and pulse oximetry
   d. Cardiac rate and rhythm
   e. Intake and output
   f. Pain relief

G. SPINAL CORD COMPRESSION

Spinal cord compression occurs when primary tumors within the cord or vertebral metastases compress neural tissues and their blood supply, resulting in compromised neurologic function. This can become a neurologic emergency if it is not treated properly. The spinal cord occupies the upper two thirds of the vertebral canal. Compression results when tumor invasion of the vertebrae collapses onto the spinal cord or pushes against it, causing pressure. Minor changes in motor, sensory, and autonomic function are early signs but can cascade into complete paralysis. Motor and autonomic function deterioration will occur if emergent treatment is delayed.

1. Assessment
   a. Subjective data collection
      1) History of present illness/chief complaint
         a) Diagnosis of ependymoma, astrocytoma, glioma, lymphoma, seminoma, neuroblastoma, breast, lung, prostate, renal, melanoma, or myeloma cancer
         b) Onset of symptoms: helps determine level of degree of compression
         c) Pain increases when supine, coughing, straining, or flexion of the neck
         d) Motor weakness or dysfunction
         e) Constipation
         f) Loss of bladder or bowel patterns (cauda equina)
         g) Paralysis
         h) Sensory loss for touch, pain, or temperature
         i) Sexual impotence
         j) Muscle atrophy
         k) Fatigue
      2) Medical history
         a) Current or preexisting diseases/illness
         b) Type of primary tumor
         c) Prior radiation therapy (RT) and/or chemotherapy
         d) Medications
         e) Allergies
   b. Objective data collection
      1) Physical examination
         a) General appearance
            (1) Gait
            (2) Moderate to severe distress/discomfort
         b) Palpation
            (1) Specific area that patient can pinpoint pain
            (2) Motor response: weakness, ataxia, and loss of coordination
            (3) Sensory changes to touch, pain, cold, or heat
      2) Diagnostic procedures
         a) CBC with differential
         b) Serum chemistries including glucose, BUN, creatinine

   c) Coagulation profile

   d) Any additional laboratory work needed prior to surgical intervention per facilities policies and procedures

   e) Spinal radiographs: show bone abnormalities, level of deformity, collapse, and soft tissue masses

   f) MRI: diagnostic procedure of choice for evaluating spinal cord compression

   g) CT scan: exceeds MRI in evaluation of vertebral stability and bone destruction

   h) Bone scan: identifies metastases to vertebral bodies

   i) Myelogram: used with or without CT scan when MRI is nondiagnostic

2. Analysis: differential nursing diagnoses/collaborative problems
   a. Acute pain
   b. Impaired physical mobility
   c. Risk of injury
   d. Disturbed sensory perception: tactile
   e. Impaired bladder and bowel elimination
   f. Sexual dysfunction
   g. Ineffective role performance
3. Planning and implementation/interventions
   a. Maintain airway, breathing, circulation
   b. Provide supplemental oxygen
   c. Establish IV access for administration of crystalloid fluid/medications
   d. Prepare for/assist with medical interventions
      1) Institute cardiac and pulse oximetry monitoring
      2) Mobilize patient according to finding of stable or unstable spine
      3) Maintain immobilization and instruct patient to utilize assistance with moving to ensure proper body alignment
      4) Assist with hospital admission
         a) Radiation therapy (RT): most common treatment for epidural metastases and cord compression when no spinal instability is present and tumor is radiosensitive
         b) Surgery: used if tumor is not responsive to RT, previous RT has been already used in the areas to the maximum dose, or decompression of tumor by laminectomy or resection of the vertebral body is needed
   e. Administer pharmacologic therapy as ordered
      1) Corticosteroids: reduce spinal cord edema and pain
      2) Chemotherapy: used as an adjuvant treatment to RT or recurrence of tumor at a site of previous surgery or radiation therapy (RT)
      3) Nonnarcotic analgesics
      4) Narcotics
      5) Anticonvulsants if indicated
      6) Antidepressants if indicated
      7) Physical therapy

Table 19.2

Common Toxicity Criteria—Neutrophils

Grade 1	>1,500 – <2,000/mm^3
Grade 2	>1,000 – <1,500/mm^3
Grade 3	>500 – <1,000/mm^3
Grade 4	<500/mm^3

(Data from Cancer Therapy Evaluation Program. [1999]. Common Toxicity Criteria, Version 2.0. Available at http://ctep.cancer.gov/protocolDevelopment/electronic _applications/docs/ctcv20_4-30-992.pdf)

4. Evaluation and ongoing monitoring
   a. Hemodynamic status
   b. Progression of motor or sensory deficits every 4–8 hours (Table 19.2)
   c. Breath sounds and pulse oximetry
   d. Cardiac rate and rhythm
   e. Intake and output
   f. Pain relief

H. SUPERIOR VENA CAVA SYNDROME

Superior vena cava (SVC) syndrome is the result of compromised venous drainage of the head, neck, upper extremities, and thorax through the SVC because of compression or obstruction of the vessel by a tumor, enlarged lymph nodes, or thrombus. The SVC is a low-pressure vessel that can easily become compressed, resulting in impaired venous return to the heart from the head, neck, thorax, and upper extremities. This compression causes an increase in venous pressure and a decrease in cardiac output. The diagnosis is frequently made on clinical presentation and history of thoracic malignant disease.

1. Assessment
   a. Subjective data collection
      1) History of present illness/chief complaint
         a) Shortness of breath: primarily when supine
         b) Chest pain
         c) Dizziness, syncope
         d) Headache
         e) Visual disturbances, blurred vision
         f) Irritability
         g) Edema to face and arms
         h) Head congestion and fullness sensation to face/neck
         i) Hemoptysis
      2) Medical history
         a) Current or preexisting diseases/illness
            (1) Lymphoma involving the mediastinum, germ cell tumor, cancers of the lung and breast, and Kaposi sarcoma
            (2) Aortic aneurysm
         b) Presence of central venous catheters and pacemakers
         c) Previous RT to mediastinum
         d) Medications
         e) Allergies

b. Objective data collection
  1) Physical examination
    a) General appearance
      (1) Hypotension
      (2) Moderate to severe distress/discomfort, critically ill
    b) Inspection
      (1) Upper torso cyanosis
      (2) Facial swelling (increased in morning)
      (3) Redness and edema to conjunctivae and around the eyes
      (4) Neck and thoracic vein distension
      (5) Facial erythema
      (6) Visible collateral veins on the chest and/or breast; women may experience swelling of the breasts
      (7) Telangiectasis: lesion formed by a dilated capillary or terminal artery
    c) Auscultation
      (1) Breath sounds: crackles
    d) Palpation
      (1) Chest wall mass or tenderness
  2) Diagnostic procedures
    a) CBC with differential
    b) Serum chemistries including glucose, BUN, creatinine
    c) Coagulation profile
    d) Chest radiograph: presence of mediastinal mass
    e) CT scan with contrast
    f) MRI: may be difficult to obtain because longer supine positioning is required

2. Analysis: differential nursing diagnoses/collaborative problems
  a. Ineffective airway clearance
  b. Decreased cardiac output
  c. Ineffective tissue perfusion: cardiopulmonary and cerebral
  d. Anxiety
  e. Deficient knowledge
  f. Disturbed body image

3. Planning and implementation/interventions
  a. Maintain airway, breathing, circulation
  b. Provide supplemental oxygen
  c. Establish IV access for administration of crystalloid fluids and medications
    1) Avoid IV fluid administration in upper extremities
  d. Prepare for/assist with medical interventions
    1) Avoid additional venipunctures or measurement of blood pressure in the upper extremities
    2) Elevate head of bed to decrease dyspnea
    3) Instruct the patient to avoid Valsalva maneuver or other activities that increase intrathoracic pressure
    4) Maintain lower extremities in a dependent position
    5) Remove rings and restrictive clothing

    6) Minimize ambulation and assist as needed
    7) Apply pressure to sites of invasive procedures in upper body
    8) Institute cardiac and pulse oximetry monitoring
    9) Assist with hospital admission
  e. Administer pharmacologic therapy as ordered
    1) Anticoagulation therapy
    2) Diuretics
    3) Glucocorticoids

4. Evaluation and ongoing monitoring
  a. Level of consciousness
    1) Possible disorientation to person, place, time
    2) Increased confusion
    3) Increased dizziness or blurred vision
    4) Presence of lethargy
    5) Increase in severity of headaches
  b. Hemodynamic status
  c. Breath sounds and pulse oximetry
  d. Progressive respiratory distress
    1) Increased respiratory rate with or without stridor
    2) Increased anxiety
    3) Presence of adventitious breath sounds
    4) Increased subjective complaints of difficulty breathing
  e. Cardiac rate and rhythm
  f. Signs of progressive edema
    1) Increased swelling in face, arms, or neck
    2) Increased venous distension of neck and thorax
  g. Changes in tissue perfusion
    1) Decreased or absent peripheral pulses
    2) Decrease in blood pressure: systolic pressure <90 mm Hg
    3) Pale or cyanotic skin of the face, extremities, or nail beds
  h. Signs and symptoms of anticoagulant therapy side effects
    1) Hematuria
    2) Epistaxis

I. THROMBOCYTOPENIA PURPURA

Congenital or acquired disorders such as decreased production of platelets in the bone marrow, increased splenic sequestration, or accelerated platelet destruction can lead to thrombocytopenia, a low platelet count. A normal platelet count is between 150,000 and 450,000/μL of blood. The most common form of thrombocytopenia is idiopathic thrombocytopenic purpura (ITP), and occurs acutely in children several weeks after a viral condition such as rubella or chickenpox. Chronic ITP is seen most often in women 20–40 years of age.

1. Assessment
  a. Subjective data collection
    1) History of present illness/chief complaint
      a) Bleeding
      b) Bruising
      c) Rash
      d) Abdominal pain and tenderness

e) Confusion
2) Medical history
   a) Current or preexisting diseases/illness
      (1) Existing coagulation disease
      (2) Nutrition status
      (3) Recent viral illness, infection, sepsis
      (4) Tumors
   b) Previous episodes of unexplained bleeding
   c) Medications
   d) Allergies
b. Objective data collection
   1) Physical examination
      a) General appearance
         (1) Moderate to severe distress/discomfort
      b) Inspection
         (1) Ecchymotic areas
         (2) Petechiae
         (3) Epistaxis, bleeding gums
         (4) Hematuria
         (5) Gastrointestinal bleeding, actual or occult
         (6) Retinal hemorrhage
      c) Palpation
         (1) Abdominal tenderness
   2) Diagnostic procedures
      a) CBC with differential: hemoglobin and white blood cell (WBC) count normal unless severe hemorrhage or infection present
      b) Platelet count <150,000/μL of blood
      c) Coagulation profile
         (1) Bleeding time: normal to slightly prolonged, not useful
         (2) PT, PTT: normal
      d) Radiographs, CT scans, and ECG as indicated
2. Analysis: differential nursing diagnoses/collaborative problems
   a. Risk for ineffective tissue perfusion: cardiopulmonary, cerebral, or renal
3. Planning and implementation/interventions
   a. Maintain airway, breathing, circulation (see Chapter 1)
   b. Provide supplemental oxygen as indicated

c. Establish IV access for administration of crystalloid fluid, blood products, medications
   1) Platelet transfusions
d. Prepare for/assist with medical interventions
   1) Institute cardiac and pulse oximetry monitoring
   2) Handle patient gently
   3) Apply firm pressure to venipuncture sites for minimum 5 minutes
   4) Apply ice to injured areas
   5) Do not use rectal thermometer for obtaining temperature
   6) Assist with hospital admission as needed
e. Administer pharmacologic therapy as ordered
   1) Avoid intramuscular injections or venipunctures; if necessary, use small-gauge needle
4. Evaluation and ongoing monitoring
   a. Level of consciousness
   b. Hemodynamic status
   c. Cardiac rate and rhythm
   d. Continued or new bleeding sites

J. TUMOR LYSIS SYNDROME

Occurs due to a rapid release of intracellular potassium, phosphorus, and nucleic acid into the blood as the result of a high rate of tumor cell kill. Tumor lysis syndrome (TLS) is a potentially life-threatening electrolyte and metabolic imbalance (Fig. 19.2). The syndrome includes hyperkalemia, hyperuricemia, hyperphosphatemia, and hypocalcemia. The effects of TLS include cardiac dysrhythmias, renal failure, and multisystem organ dysfunction.

1. Assessment
   a. Subjective data collection
      1) History of present illness/chief complaint
         a) Cardiac complaints: irregular heart beat, pain
         b) Dizziness/lightheadedness
         c) Nausea, vomiting, diarrhea
         d) Muscle weakness, cramps, tingling, twitching, paresthesia, paralysis
         e) Edema
         f) Seizures
         g) Altered mental status/lethargy/somnolence

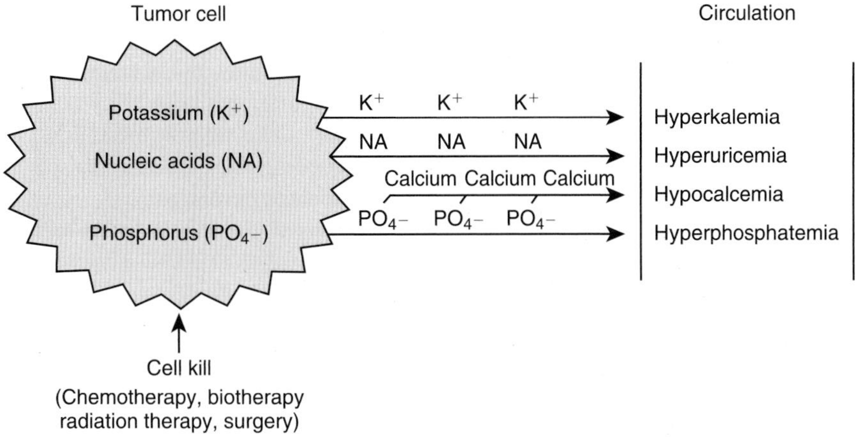

FIG. 19.2 **Metabolic consequences of cell death.** (From Itano, J., & Taoka, K. [Eds.]. *Core curriculum for oncology nursing* [4th ed.]. Philadelphia, PA: Elsevier Saunders, in collaboration with Oncology Nursing Society.)

    2) Medical history
      a) Current or preexisting diseases/illness
        (1) Cardiac disease
        (2) Renal disease
        (3) Hematologic tumors
          (a) Leukemia
          (b) Lymphoma
        (4) Solid tumors: small cell lung cancer, breast cancer, neuroblastoma
        (5) Current or recent chemotherapy
        (6) Current or recent RT, surgery, or spontaneous tumor lysis syndrome
      b) Medications
      c) Allergies
  b. Objective data collection
    1) Physical examination
    2) Diagnostic procedures
      a) CBC with differential: leukocyte and platelet counts
      b) Serum chemistries: potassium, phosphorus, calcium, ionized calcium, bicarbonate; compare with baseline testing prior to cytotoxic therapy
      c) Serum magnesium and phosphorus: possible hypomagnesemia
      d) Serum albumin: differentiates between hypocalcemia and pseudohypocalcemia
        (1) Decrease in serum albumin by 10 g/L lowers serum calcium by 0.2 mmol/L
        (2) Serum albumin does not affect ionized calcium
      e) Serum uric acid: compare with baseline testing prior to cytotoxic therapy
      f) Liver function: LDH—indication of tumor burden
      g) BUN and creatinine
      h) Urinalysis: pH and uric acid crystals
      i) Chest radiograph, CT scan: determine extent and invasion of lesion
      j) Abdominal sonography or CT scan if abdominal lesions or renal failure present
      k) ECG in clients identified with hyperkalemia, hypocalcemia
        (1) Hyperkalemia: tall peaked T waves, QRS widening
        (2) Hypocalcemia: prolonged QT interval
2. Analysis: differential nursing diagnoses/collaborative problems
  a. Decreased cardiac output
  b. Excess fluid volume
  c. Impaired urinary elimination
  d. Ineffective protection
  e. Risk for injury
  f. Self-care deficit
3. Planning and implementation/interventions
  a. Maintain airway, breathing, circulation
  b. Provide supplemental oxygen

  c. Establish IV access for administration of crystalloid fluids and medications
    1) Ensure adequate hydration of patient to maintain urine flow >150–200 mL/hour in adults and minimum 3 mL/kg/hour in children
  d. Prepare for/assist with medical interventions
    1) Institute cardiac and pulse oximetry monitoring
    2) Assist with hospital admission
  e. Administer pharmacologic therapy as ordered
    1) Sodium bicarbonate: alkalinize the urine to maintain a pH >7 and to decrease the solubility of uric acid
    2) Allopurinol (Zyloprim, Aloprim): decreases the production of uric acid
      a) Should never be given concurrently with Rasburicase
    3) Rasburicase (Elitek): converts circulating uric acid to a by-product excreted by the kidneys
      a) Should never be given concurrently with Allopurinol
      b) Labs drawn after Rasburicase is infused should be placed on ice; Rasburicase continues to work in vivo and will alter lab values
      c) Alkalinization of urine not recommended with use of Rasburicase
    4) Loop diuretics: maintain urinary output if urine flow is not achieved by hydration
    5) Mannitol (Osmitrol): maintains urinary output if urine flow is not achieved with loop diuretics
    6) Phosphate-binding, aluminum-containing antacids: correction of hyperphosphatemia will usually self-correct hypocalcemia
    7) Hypertonic glucose and insulin if potassium levels need to be addressed
    8) Sodium polystyrene sulfonate (Kayexalate) to treat mild hyperkalemia
    9) Calcium gluconate for severe hyperkalemia
    10) Avoid nephrotoxic medications
  f. Educate patient/significant others
    1) Avoid exogenous sources of potassium and phosphorus
      a) Oral supplements
      b) Enteral/parenteral nutrition
      c) Dietary sources of potassium: bananas, oranges, orange juice, tomatoes
      d) Dietary sources of phosphorus: meat, fish, poultry, eggs, cheese, nuts, bread, cereals, legumes, carbonated beverages
    2) Signs and symptoms of tumor lysis syndrome
    3) Medication compliance
    4) Oral hydration
4. Evaluation and ongoing monitoring
  a. Hemodynamic status
  b. Cardiac rate and rhythm
  c. Strict intake and output

III. Hematologic/Oncologic Complications

A. SEPSIS

Sepsis is defined as the systemic inflammatory response to pathogenic microorganisms and associated endotoxins in the blood. Untreated bacteremia in patients who are already immunocompromised can be fatal, especially in patients with hematologic malignant diseases. The incidence of sepsis in patients with malignant diseases is 15 times greater than in patients without malignant diseases. In addition, patients with cancer who have recently undergone treatment with chemotherapy and/or radiation therapy (RT) and who have other comorbid conditions are at greater risk for sepsis. Patients with cancer who have an established central venous catheter have another potential source of infection.

B. SYNDROME OF INAPPROPRIATE ANTIDIURETIC HORMONE

Syndrome of inappropriate antidiuretic hormone (SIADH) secretion is a serious endocrine emergency that alters the body's fluid and electrolyte balance. Neuroendocrine malignancies, particularly small cell lung cancer (SCLC), is a common cause. Other malignant diseases, including neuroendocrine tumors of the pancreas, duodenum, colon, bladder, prostate, as well as lymphomas, thymomas, and primary brain tumors may also develop SIADH secretion. This syndrome is seen in patients with neuroendocrine cancer because malignant cells synthesize, store, and release antidiuretic hormone (ADH), thus leading to water retention, hyponatremia, and increased extracellular volume.

C. HYPERSENSITIVITY REACTIONS

Certain classes of chemotherapy agents, like other foreign agents to the body, can trigger hypersensitivity reactions. For example, patients receiving paclitaxel may experience a reaction to the cremaphor, which is the solvent for the actual drug. Reactions typically occur in the first or second infusion and are not IgE-mediated reactions. Reactions to carboplatin and other agents in the platinum family are true IgE-mediated reactions and typically occur after the fifth or sixth infusion. Biotherapy agents, such as rituximab, may result in a reaction due to cytokine release. All chemotherapy and biotherapy agents have the potential to cause hypersensitivity reactions.

Bibliography

Anton M, Baratti P, Barsevick A, et al.: In Brunner D, Haas M, Gosselin-Acomb T, editors: *Manual for radiation oncology nursing practice and education*, ed 3, Pittsburgh, PA, 2005, Oncology Nursing Society.

Camp-Sorrell D: Myelosuppression. In Itano J, Taoka K, editors: *Core curriculum for oncology nursing*, ed 4, Philadelphia, 2005, Elsevier Saunders, in collaboration with Oncology Nursing Society.

Clancey J: Syndrome of inappropriate antidiuretic hormone secretion. In Kaplan M, editor: *Understanding and managing oncologic emergencies: a resource for nurses*, Pittsburgh, PA, 2006, Oncology Nursing Society.

Curler K, Thompson L: Managing chemotherapy side effects: tumor lysis syndrome, *Oncology Nurse Advisor*, 2013, January/February.

De Pauw B: Evolution in the treatment of hematologic malignancies, *Current Opinion in Oncology* 17(6):593–595, 2005.

Himelstein B: Palliative care in pediatrics, *Anesthesiology Clinics of North America* 23:837–856, 2005.

Holmes-Gobel B: Metabolic emergencies. In Itano J, Taoka K, editors: *Core curriculum for oncology nursing*, ed 4, Philadelphia, PA, 2005, Elsevier Saunders, in collaboration with Oncology Nursing Society.

Holmes-Gobel B: Tumor lysis syndrome. In Kaplan M, editor: *Understanding and managing oncologic emergencies: a resource for nurses*, Pittsburgh, PA, 2006, Oncology Nursing Society.

Holmes-Gobel B, Peterson G: Sepsis and septic shock. In Kaplan M, editor: *Understanding and managing oncologic emergencies: a resource for nurses*, Pittsburgh, PA, 2006, Oncology Nursing Society.

Hunter J: Structural emergencies. In Itano J, Taoka K, editors: *Core curriculum for oncology nursing*, ed 4, Philadelphia, PA, 2005, Elsevier Saunders, in collaboration with Oncology Nursing Society.

Koonz SE: A review of tumor lysis syndrome, *U.S. Pharmacist* 33:1, 2008.

Kyricou DN, Jovanovic B, Frankfort O: Timing of initial antibiotic treatment for febrile neutropenia in the emergency department: the need for evidence based guidelines, *Journal of the National Comprehensive Cancer Network* 12:1569–1573, 2014.

Owolabi DK, Rowland R, King L, Miller R, Gajanan GH, Venkat A: A comparison of ED and direct admission care of cancer patients with febrile neutropenia, *American Journal of Emergency Medicine* 33:966–969, 2015.

Polovich M, Olsen M, LeFebvre KB: *Chemotherapy and biotherapy guidelines and recommendations for practice*, ed 4, Pittsburgh, PA, 2014, Oncology Nursing Society.

Remick DG: Biological perspectives: pathophysiology of sepsis, *American Society for Investigative Pathology* 170:5, 2007.

Siegel RL, Miller KD, Jemal A: Cancer statistics, 2015, *CA: a Cancer Journal for Clinicians* 65:5–29, 2015.

Soares M, Salluh JI, Carvalho MS, Darmon M, Rocco JR, Spector N: Effect of age on survival of critically ill patients with cancer, *Critical Care Medicine* 34(3):715–721, 2006.

Taillibert S, Delattre J: Palliative care in patients with brain metastases, *Current Opinion in Oncology* 17(6):588–592, 2005.

Tamburro R: Pediatric cancer patients in clinical trials of sepsis: factors that predispose to sepsis and stratify outcome, *Pediatric Critical Care Medicine* 6(3):87–91, 2005.

Turner-Story K: Cardiac tamponade. In Kaplan M, editor: *Understanding and managing oncologic emergencies: a resource for nurses*, Pittsburgh, PA, 2006, Oncology Nursing Society.

Tzimenatos L, Geis G: Emergency department management of the immunosuppressed host, *Clinics of Pediatric Emergency Medicine* 6:173–183, 2005.

CHAPTER 20
Communicable and Infectious Disease Emergencies

Sharon Vanairsdale, MS, APRN, ACNS-BC, NP-C, CEN

I. General Strategy

A. ASSESSMENT

1. Primary and secondary assessment/resuscitation (see Chapter 1)
2. Focused assessment
   a. Subjective data collection
      1) History of present illness/chief complaint
         a) Pain: PQRST (see Chapter 8)
         b) Fatigue, malaise
         c) Vomiting
         d) Altered mental status or decreased level of consciousness
         e) Fever
         f) Shortness of breath
         g) Rash
         h) Edema: location and type
         i) Weakness
         j) Weight loss
         k) Cough
         l) Sore throat

         m) Other symptoms that match the pathogen: anorexia, pruritus, diarrhea, swollen lymph nodes, bleeding, headache
         n) Efforts to relieve symptoms
            (1) Home remedies
            (2) Alternative therapies
            (3) Medications
               (a) Prescription
               (b) OTC/herbal
      2) Past medical history
         a) Current or preexisting diseases/illness
            (1) Human immunodeficiency virus (HIV) infection
            (2) Diabetes
            (3) Alcoholism
            (4) Renal disease
            (5) Cardiovascular: hypertension
            (6) Cancer
            (7) Tuberculosis (TB) or exposure
         b) Recent major injury
         c) Surgical procedures (i.e., splenectomy)

d) History of similar episodes
e) Recent animal, vector, or tick bites
f) Blood transfusions, hemodialysis
g) Recent out-of-country travel
h) Previous measles, mumps, varicella
i) Vaccine failure in high school and college students
j) Smoking history
k) Substance and/or alcohol use/abuse
l) Last normal menstrual period: female patients of childbearing age
m) Current medications
    (1) Prescription
        (a) Anticoagulants
        (b) Insulin or oral hypoglycemic agents
        (c) Thyroid hormone
        (d) Diuretics
        (e) Oral contraceptives
        (f) Antiretroviral agents and protease inhibitors
        (g) Steroids or cancer-treating drugs
    (2) OTC/herbal
n) Allergies
o) Immunization status (for most current schedule, see Centers for Disease Control website at cdc.gov)
3) Psychological/social/environmental factors
    a) Age: illness may be more severe in very young and elderly
    b) Family history
    c) Race, culture, and socioeconomic status: may determine increased incidence
    d) Possible/actual abuse, assault, intimate partner violence situations (see Chapters 3 and 40)
    e) Lifestyle
        (1) Alcohol and street drug, especially IV use
        (2) Homosexually or bisexually active men
        (3) IV drug user sexual partner
        (4) Multiple sexual partners
        (5) Body piercing or tattooing
        (6) Intrauterine exposure of fetus
        (7) Prostitution: male or female
        (8) High-risk occupation for disease contact
        (9) Day care center utilization
        (10) Military camp residence
        (11) Homelessness, institutional residence
        (12) Crowded living conditions
        (13) Personal hygiene: handwashing, sharing bed/clothes/utensils
    f) Emigration from country with high incidence of specific pathogen
    g) Climate or environment
b. Objective data collection
    1) General appearance
        a) Level of consciousness, behavior, affect
        b) Vital signs, including orthostatic blood pressure/pulse
        c) Odors
        d) Gait
        e) Hygiene
        f) Level of distress/discomfort
    2) Inspection
        a) Neck veins
        b) Skin rash/lesions/petechiae
        c) Skin color
        d) Edema
        e) Eyes
        f) Meningeal signs
        g) Voice sounds: muffled, hoarse
        h) Mucous membranes
        i) Evidence of trauma
        j) Areas of erythema
        k) Head and pubic hair for nits (lice eggs)
    3) Auscultation
        a) Breath sounds: clear, wheezes, crackles, other sounds
        b) Bowel sounds: normal, hyperactive, hypoactive, absent
        c) Heart sounds: S_1 and S_2, other sounds (e.g., murmurs)
    4) Palpation/percussion
        a) Sinus tenderness
        b) Areas of tenderness
        c) Areas of edema
        d) Abdominal distention
        e) Organomegaly
        f) Areas of hyperthermia
        g) Lymph nodes
        h) Chest and abdomen: note tone
3. Diagnostic procedures
    a. Laboratory studies
        1) CBC with differential
        2) Serum chemistries including glucose, BUN, creatinine
        3) Arterial blood gas (ABG)
        4) Urinalysis; pregnancy test in female patients of childbearing age
        5) Alcohol level, if altered mental status
        6) Serum and urine toxicology screen: therapeutic level and toxic ingestions, if altered mental status
        7) Coagulation profile: clotting studies, partial thromboplastin time (PTT), and prothrombin time/international normalized ratio (PT/INR)
        8) Blood type and crossmatch
        9) Liver function tests
        10) Heterophile antibody titer (Monospot)
        11) TB skin test and sputum culture may be initiated in ED
        12) Hepatitis screen
        13) Viral serology

14) Cerebrospinal fluid: cell count, glucose and protein content, lactic acid, culture, Gram stain
15) Cultures: blood, sputum, wound, throat, nasopharyngeal, viral
16) HIV
   a) Enzyme-linked immunosorbent assay (ELISA): initial screening test
   b) Simple/rapid (S/R) assays: initial screening test, used more in mass screenings
   c) Western blot: confirmatory test, expensive
   d) Indirect immunofluorescent antibody (IFA): confirmatory test, expensive
   e) Line immunoassays (LIAs): confirmatory tests, less expensive than Western blot or IFA
17) Cluster of differentiation 4 ($CD4^+$) cell count
18) Skin scrapings
   b. Imaging studies
      1) Chest radiograph
      2) Skull and cervical spine radiographs, as indicated
      3) CT scan
      4) MRI scan
   c. Other
      1) 12- to 15-lead electrocardiogram (ECG)
      2) Electroencephalogram (EEG)

B. ANALYSIS: DIFFERENTIAL NURSING DIAGNOSES/COLLABORATIVE PROBLEMS

1. Ineffective airway clearance
2. Ineffective breathing pattern
3. Impaired gas exchange
4. Decreased cardiac output
5. Deficient fluid volume
6. Ineffective tissue perfusion
7. Impaired skin integrity
8. Impaired verbal communication
9. Knowledge deficit
10. Acute pain
11. Anxiety/fear
12. Risk for aspiration
13. Risk for injury
14. Risk for infection

C. PLANNING AND IMPLEMENTATION/ INTERVENTIONS

1. Determine priorities of care
   a. Maintain airway, breathing, circulation (see Chapter 1)
   b. Provide supplemental oxygen as indicated
   c. Establish IV access for administration of crystalloid fluid/blood products/medications as needed
   d. Obtain and set up equipment and supplies
   e. Prepare for/assist with medical interventions
   f. Administer pharmacologic therapy as ordered
2. Relieve anxiety/apprehension
3. Allow significant others to remain with patient if supportive
4. Educate patient/significant others

D. EVALUATION AND ONGOING MONITORING

1. Continuously monitor and treat as indicated
2. Monitor patient's responses/outcomes, and modify nursing care plan as appropriate
3. If positive outcomes are not demonstrated, reevaluate assessment and/or plan of care

E. DOCUMENTATION OF INTERVENTIONS AND PATIENT RESPONSE

F. AGE-RELATED CONSIDERATIONS

1. Pediatrics
   a. Growth or development related
      1) Neonates, infants, and toddlers are more susceptible to illness and injury but also have more recuperative capacity
      2) Immune systems are not completely developed
      3) At birth, newborns possess varying degrees of nonspecific and specific immunity, which lasts from 1–8 months of age
      4) Brain development is not complete until about age 21–25; therefore, this age group is more susceptible to injury
      5) Children may be exposed to illness more frequently in settings with other children such as school, day care, and recreational programs and activities; education related to hygiene and infection control may be lacking
      6) Fluid and electrolyte composition is an important factor; 75–80% of body weight in infants is fluid, thus making them more susceptible to dehydration
   b. "Pearls"
      1) Pediatric patients of certain ages are developmentally unable to care for themselves during illness (e.g., maintaining adequate fluid intake)
      2) Parents know their children better than anyone: listen to them
      3) Often the most therapeutic intervention is reassurance
2. Geriatric
   a. Aging related
      1) In healthy elderly adults, physiologic decreases in function are usually apparent only under stress
      2) Reserve capacity for responding to stress decreases
      3) Immune system is compromised
      4) Reduced ability to metabolize and clear medications leads to frequent occurrence of toxicity and adverse reactions

5) Neurologic system: loss of nonreplicating cells (neurons) may lead to permanent deficit
    a) Dopaminergic neurons are lost, impairing gait and balance and increasing susceptibility to side effects of medication
    b) Loss of other neurotransmitter systems leads to autonomic dysfunction and alterations in neuroendocrine control and mental function
6) Cardiovascular system
    a) Decreases in heart rate are accompanied by increased end-diastolic and end-systolic volumes; reserve mechanisms to increase cardiac output are used routinely and may be overwhelmed by illness
    b) Baroreceptor reflex sensitivity decreases, altering the response of system to changes in intravascular volume; orthostasis is more prevalent
7) Pulmonary system: elasticity of small airways is lost with increased tendency for alveoli to collapse
8) Endocrine system
    a) Glucose intolerance, insulin resistance, and abnormal regulation of insulin secretion occur
    b) Metabolic clearance of thyroid hormone decreases; in thyroid disease, the dose of exogenous thyroxine (thyroid medication) is usually decreased
    c) Decreased estrogen level alters bone metabolism, which can lead to osteoporosis
9) Fluid and electrolytes: adaptive mechanisms are impaired, although balance of volume and number of solutes is unchanged
    a) Nephron loss and decrease in renin and aldosterone levels contribute to increased sodium loss before compensatory mechanisms can be fully activated
    b) Decreased glomerular filtration rate, baroreceptor reflex sensitivity, and insulin and beta-adrenergic responsiveness increase the risk of hyperkalemia
    c) Water conservation and urine-concentrating ability, as well as thirst mechanism, are impaired, resulting in increased susceptibility to dehydration
    d) Increased osmoreceptor sensitivity with higher set point for vasopressin (antidiuretic hormone) increases the risk of syndrome of inappropriate antidiuretic hormone (SIADH) in patients taking certain drugs and in pulmonary and neurologic diseases
10) Renal system: renal blood flow, glomerular filtration rate, and creatinine clearance are decreased

11) Vision and hearing
    a) Decreased visual acuity, changes in refractive power, loss of accommodation, cataracts, and decreased tear secretion influence ability to see adequately
    b) Hearing loss occurs as a result of changes in peripheral auditory system and cerebral cortex
  b. "Pearls"
    1) Decreased activity and less emotional involvement in activity or roles occur
    2) Elderly patients have increased concern with immediate environment, health, and factors affecting them directly

II. Specific Communicable and Infectious Disease Emergencies

A. DIPHTHERIA

Diphtheria is an acute, highly contagious disease caused by a gram-negative bacillus, *Corynebacterium diphtheriae,* which produces a systemic toxin and usually causes membranous nasopharyngitis or obstructive laryngotracheitis. Cutaneous lesions may also occur. Diphtheria is spread by airborne respiratory droplets or by direct contact with respiratory secretions or skin lesion exudate. The exotoxin of this rapidly progressive illness can result in widespread organ damage and complications, including myocarditis, thrombocytopenia, vocal cord paralysis, acute tubular necrosis, and an ascending paralysis similar to Guillain-Barré syndrome. Diphtheria is rare in the United States and seen most often in the tropical countries among urban and rural poor populations. It may occur in both immunized and nonimmunized persons, and the severity of illness is directly related to immunization status. The only effective control of this disease is universal immunization. The incidence is greatest in fall and winter; transmission occurs by intimate contact, typically in crowded living conditions. The incubation period is 2–5 days. Treated illness is communicable for up to 4 days; untreated illness can be spread for up to 2–4 weeks. Occurrence of active disease may not confer immunity. Pseudomembranous inflammation develops on mucosal surfaces of the throat, which may lead to airway obstruction. Death usually results from respiratory (asphyxia) or cardiac (myocarditis) complications. Death is most common in the very young and elderly, usually within 3–4 days of illness onset.
1. Assessment
  a. Subjective data collection
    1) History of present illness/chief complaint
      a) Onset lasting 1–2 days
      b) Sore throat
      c) Difficulty in swallowing or breathing

d) Fever: low grade or high (rarely >103°F [39.4°C]), chills
e) Headache
f) Nausea
g) Malaise
h) Travel to endemic areas in previous week
i) Crowded living conditions
2) Past medical history
  a) Current or preexisting diseases/illness
  b) Childhood diseases
  c) Medications
  d) Allergies
  e) Immunization status
b. Objective data collection
1) Physical examination
  a) General appearance
    (1) Alteration in neurologic functions
      (a) Level of consciousness, behavior, affect: lethargy, withdrawal, confusion
      (b) Cranial nerve neuropathies
    (2) Tachycardia, tachypnea
    (3) Elevated temperature: fever >101°F (38.3°C)
    (4) Stridor
    (5) Severe distress/discomfort, critically ill
  b) Inspection
    (1) Dirty, gray-white, rubbery membrane covering structures of pharynx and larynx (removal of membrane leaves a bleeding surface)
    (2) Swelling of structures of pharynx
    (3) Cyanosis
    (4) Use of accessory muscles
    (5) Nasal flaring
    (6) Cardiac dysrhythmias on monitor
      (a) First-degree atrioventricular block
      (b) ST-segment and T-wave changes
  c) Palpation
    (1) Cervical lymphadenopathy
2) Diagnostic procedures
  a) Throat culture: specimen swabbed from beneath membrane or piece of membrane; notify laboratory that *C. diphtheriae* is suspected: requires special media and handling
    (1) Nasal and pharyngeal swabs of close contacts
  b) CBC with differential: mild leukocytosis, thrombocytopenia
  c) Serum antibodies to diphtheria toxin
  d) Cardiac, liver enzymes: elevated aspartate aminotransferase (AST) parallels myocarditis severity
  e) Urinalysis; pregnancy test in female patients of childbearing age
  f) Chest radiograph: subglottic narrowing
  g) ECG: ST-segment, T-wave changes; heart block, dysrhythmias with cardiac involvement

2. Analysis: differential nursing diagnosis/collaborative problems
  a. Ineffective airway clearance
  b. Pain
  c. Anxiety/fear
  d. Risk for aspiration
3. Planning and implementation/interventions
  a. Maintain airway, breathing, circulation (see Chapter 1)
  b. Provide supplemental oxygen
    1) Rapid sequence intubation (RSI) and ventilatory support in patients with airway compromise
    2) High-flow oxygen
  c. Establish IV access for administration of crystalloid fluid/medications
  d. Prepare for/assist with medical interventions
    1) Advanced airway management
      a) Nasal or oral intubation
      b) Supraglottic airway (e.g., King, Combitube, laryngeal mask airway)
      c) Surgical airway (e.g., cricothyrotomy)
    2) Maintain strict droplet precautions (per Centers for Disease Control and Prevention [CDC])
    3) Institute cardiac and pulse oximetry monitoring
    4) Assist with hospital admission
    5) Report to appropriate health department officials
  e. Administer pharmacologic therapy as ordered
    1) RSI premedications: sedatives, analgesics, neuromuscular blocking agents
    2) Diphtheria antitoxin
      a) Equine serum
      b) Test for sensitivity (intradermal or mucous membrane) before administration
      c) Often administered before diagnosis is confirmed because of virulence of disease
    3) Antibiotic: erythromycin or penicillin G
    4) Antitussives
    5) Antipyretics
    6) Topical anesthetic agents
  f. Educate patient/significant others
    1) Identify close contacts
    2) Culture and prophylactic antibiotics
    3) Booster of tetanus and diphtheria toxoid if none within 5 years
    4) Active immunization for nonimmunized persons (series of three doses)
4. Evaluation and ongoing monitoring
  a. Airway patency
  b. Hemodynamic status
  c. Breath sounds and pulse oximetry
  d. Cardiac rate and rhythm

B. GLOBAL/PANDEMIC ILLNESSES

A pandemic illness occurs when a new or previously eradicated disease appears, reappears, or emerges in the human population, spreading from person-to-person contact. These illnesses are frequently caused by viral agents; however, there is growing concern that pandemic illnesses may arise from outbreaks related to the use of weapons of mass destruction.

Influenza type A viral infection (Spanish flu) became a pandemic illness in 1918. The virus originated in the United States and was then rapidly transmitted worldwide by U.S. soldiers. Typical symptoms of these viral illnesses may not always be present in persons with chronic illnesses. Therefore, the diagnosis should be considered in any person who has traveled to countries where the virus is known to exist and who has a change in health that triggers fever or cough.

SEVERE ACUTE RESPIRATORY SYNDROME.

Severe acute respiratory syndrome (SARS) is a viral respiratory disease of zoonotic origin caused by a coronavirus called SARS-CoV. The previously unrecognized coronavirus was first reported in China in 2002 and later spread to more than two dozen countries before the outbreak was contained. Between November 2002 and July 2003, there were over 8,000 reported cases and almost 800 deaths. The virus is spread mostly by respiratory droplets through direct or indirect contact (e.g., touching a surface that had droplets on it). The incubation time is typically between 2 and 7 days but may be as long as 10–14 days. According to the CDC, known data suggests that a person with SARS is likely to be infectious only when symptomatic. The illness usually begins with a high fever, and up to 20% of patients with SARS will require mechanical ventilation. The majority of patients will develop pneumonia.

1. Assessment
   a. Subjective data collection
      1) History of present illness/chief complaint
         a) Fever and chills
         b) Sore throat
         c) Cough
         d) Headache
         e) Myalgias
         f) Shortness of breath
         g) Lethargy
         h) Diarrhea (seen in approximately 10–20% of patients)
      2) Past medical history
         a) Current or preexisting diseases/illness
         b) Medications
         c) Allergies
         d) Immunization status
   b. Objective data collection
      1) Physical examination
         a) General appearance
            (1) Elevated temperature
            (2) Moderate to severe distress/discomfort
         b) Auscultation
            (1) Cough
            (2) Breath sounds: wheezes, crackles
      2) Diagnostic procedures
         a) CBC with differential
         b) Serum chemistries

c) Blood cultures
         d) Sputum Gram stain/cultures
         e) Viral cultures
         f) ABGs
         g) SARS-CoV testing
         h) Chest radiograph: consolidation and ground-glass opacification (SARS)
2. Analysis: differential nursing diagnoses/collaborative problems
   a. Impaired gas exchange
   b. Anxiety/fear
   c. Deficient knowledge
3. Planning and implementation/interventions
   a. Maintain airway, breathing, circulation (see Chapter 1)
   b. Provide supplemental oxygen
   c. Establish IV access for administration of crystalloid fluid/medications
   d. Prepare for/assist with medical interventions
      1) Strict isolation utilizing a negative-pressure room
      2) Initiate airborne and droplet precautions
      3) Institute cardiac and pulse oximetry monitoring
      4) Assist with hospital admission and possible initiation of surge capacity guidelines per institutional protocols
      5) Notify CDC
   e. Administer pharmacologic therapy as ordered
      1) Antivirals—there is no specific antiviral treatment recommended for SARS; additional research is needed
         a) Oseltamir (Tamiflu): although used in the 2003 outbreak, its use is generally not recommended
         b) Ribavirin: widely chosen during the 2003 outbreak because of its broad-spectrum antiviral activity
      2) Antibiotics—empirical antibiotics until SARS can be confirmed
      3) Steroids
      4) Antipyretics
4. Evaluation and ongoing monitoring
   a. Hemodynamic status
   b. Breath sounds and pulse oximetry
   c. Cardiac rate and rhythm
   d. Fever control

MIDDLE EASTERN RESPIRATORY SYNDROME.

Middle Eastern respiratory syndrome is caused by a recently identified coronavirus, MERS-CoV. The zoonotic virus was initially isolated in Saudi Arabia in June 2012. In addition to humans, the virus has been found in camels. The virus is spread mostly by respiratory droplets through direct or indirect contact (e.g., touching a surface that had droplets on it). Based on current information, the incubation period for MERS ranges from 2–14 days but is usually about 5–6 days. The most common presentation is fever with respiratory illness. Hospitalization is required for the majority of patients. Severe illness is more common in patients with chronic illness and comorbidities including diabetes mellitus, chronic renal failure, chronic heart or lung disease, hypertension, and obesity. A major complication of MERS is acute respiratory distress syndrome (ARDS). Currently, the mortality rate is approximately 35% but may be higher in patients with preexisting illnesses. Shedding of the virus has also been reported in the urine and feces of the infected person. Patients who are asymptomatic are at low risk of transmission.

1. Assessment
   a. Subjective data collection
      1) History of present illness/chief complaint
         a) Fever and chills
         b) Sore throat
         c) Chest discomfort
         d) Headache
         e) Myalgias
         f) Shortness of breath
         g) Vomiting
         h) Diarrhea
         i) Recent direct contact with infected persons or camels
         j) Recent foreign travel to endemic countries
      2) Past medical history
         a) Current or preexisting diseases/illness
         b) Medications
         c) Allergies
         d) Immunization status
   b. Objective data collection
      1) Physical examination
         a) General appearance
            (1) Elevated temperature
            (2) Moderate to severe distress/discomfort
         b) Auscultation
            (1) Cough
            (2) Breath sounds: wheezes, crackles
      2) Diagnostic procedures
         a) CBC with differential: lymphopenia, leukopenia, and thrombocytopenia
         b) Serum chemistries: hyponatremia and hypokalemia
         c) Blood cultures
         d) Sputum Gram stain/cultures
         e) Viral cultures
         f) ABGs
         g) MERS-CoV testing
         h) Chest radiograph: unilateral or bilateral patchy densities, interstitial infiltrates, consolidations, and pleural effusions
2. Analysis: differential nursing diagnoses/collaborative problems
   a. Impaired gas exchange
   b. Anxiety/fear
   c. Deficient knowledge

3. Planning and implementation/interventions
   a. Maintain airway, breathing, circulation (see Chapter 1)
   b. Provide supplemental oxygen
   c. Establish IV access for administration of crystalloid fluid/medications
   d. Prepare for/assist with medical interventions
      1) Utilize a negative-pressure room
      2) Initiate airborne, contact, standard precautions
      3) Institute cardiac and pulse oximetry monitoring
      4) Assist with hospital admission
      5) Notify CDC
   e. No known treatment; supportive care as necessary; administer pharmacologic therapy as ordered
      1) Antivirals—there is no specific antiviral treatment recommended for MERS; additional research is needed
      2) Antibiotics—empirical antibiotics until MERS can be confirmed
      3) Steroids
      4) Antipyretics
4. Evaluation and ongoing monitoring
   a. Hemodynamic status
   b. Breath sounds and pulse oximetry
   c. Cardiac rate and rhythm
   d. Fever control

AVIAN INFLUENZA. There has been growing concern that a new avian virus will become pandemic. The pathogen, also known as bird flu virus, is a naturally occurring virus found in poultry. Although avian flu viruses do not typically infect humans, several cases of human infection have occurred since 1997 throughout Asia. Because of the possibility that avian influenza viruses could change and gain the ability to spread easily between people, monitoring for human infection and person-to-person transmission is extremely important for public health. Reported signs and symptoms of low pathogenic avian influenza (LPAI) A virus in humans range from conjunctivitis to flulike symptoms, including fever, cough, sore throat, and myalgias. In some cases, pneumonia requiring hospitalization has been seen. Highly pathogenic avian influenza (HPAI) A virus has been associated with conjunctivitis, flulike symptoms, and severe respiratory illness with multiorgan disease.

1. Assessment
   a. Subjective data collection
      1) History of present illness/chief complaint
         a) Fever and chills
         b) Sore throat
         c) Chest discomfort
         d) Headache
         e) Myalgias
         f) Shortness of breath

g) Vomiting/diarrhea

h) Neurological changes

i) Recent direct contact with infected poultry

j) Recent foreign travel to endemic countries

2) Past medical history

   a) Current or preexisting diseases/illness

   b) Medications

   c) Allergies

   d) Immunization status

b. Objective data collection

  1) Physical examination

    a) General appearance

      (1) Elevated temperature

      (2) Moderate to severe distress/discomfort

    b) Auscultation

      (1) Cough

      (2) Breath sounds: wheezes, crackles

  2) Diagnostic procedures

    a) CBC with differential: lymphopenia, leukopenia, and thrombocytopenia

    b) Serum chemistries: hyponatremia and hypokalemia

    c) Blood cultures

    d) Sputum Gram stain/cultures

    e) Viral cultures

    f) ABGs

    g) Avian influenza A testing

    h) Chest radiograph: consolidation and ground-glass opacification (SARS)

2. Analysis: differential nursing diagnoses/collaborative problems

a. Impaired gas exchange

b. Anxiety/fear

c. Deficient knowledge

3. Planning and implementation/interventions

a. Maintain airway, breathing, circulation (see Chapter 1)

b. Provide supplemental oxygen

c. Establish IV access for administration of crystalloid fluid/medications

d. Prepare for/assist with medical interventions

  1) Institute cardiac and pulse oximetry monitoring

  2) Assist with hospital admission and possible initiation of surge capacity guidelines per institutional protocols

  3) Notify CDC

e. Administer pharmacologic therapy as ordered

  1) Antivirals

    a) Oseltamir (Tamiflu), peramivir, and zanamivir are often used

  2) Antipyretics

  3) Supportive care—treat symptoms

4. Evaluation and ongoing monitoring

a. Hemodynamic status

b. Breath sounds and pulse oximetry

c. Cardiac rate and rhythm

d. Fever control

C. HEMORRHAGIC FEVERS

Ebola virus disease (EVD), Lassa fever, Marburg disease, and yellow fever are examples of viral hemorrhagic diseases that often produce high fevers with copious amounts of vomiting and diarrhea. As these diseases progress, the viral load increases and the symptoms typically become more intense and may lead to multisystem organ failure, sepsis, and death. Hemorrhaging may be seen as the patient develops thrombocytopenia caused by the disease process. The mortality rate is alarmingly high.

1. Assessment

a. Subjective data collection

  1) History of present illness/chief complaint

    a) Fever and chills

    b) Nausea

    c) Vomiting—may or may not be bloody

    d) Headache

    e) Myalgias

    f) Shortness of breath

    g) Diarrhea—may or may not be bloody

    h) Bleeding gums, bloodshot eyes

    i) Rash—petchiae may be seen

    j) Recent direct contact with infected persons

    k) Recent foreign travel to endemic countries

  2) Past medical history

    a) Current or preexisting diseases/illness

    b) Medications

    c) Allergies

    d) Immunization status

b. Objective data collection

  1) Physical examination

    a) General appearance

      (1) Elevated temperature

      (2) Moderate to severe distress/discomfort

    b) Auscultation

      (1) Cough

      (2) Breath sounds: crackles, wheezes

  2) Diagnostic procedures

    a) CBC with differential: lymphopenia, leukopenia, and thrombocytopenia

    b) Serum chemistries: hyponatremia and hypokalemia

    c) Coagulation function

    d) Virus testing specific to the pathogen including EVD, both serum and urine; individual health care facilities should confirm with local and state public health department officials to identify closest testing location

    e) ABGs

    f) Malaria smear—should be ruled out, because malaria may more frequently be the pathogen and requires immediate medical interventions

g) Blood cultures may be considered as necessary

h) Chest radiograph: may be required as patient becomes more ill; fluid may be noted; health care facilities need to develop protocols to ensure x-rays can be performed safely under stringent isolation precautions

2. Analysis: differential nursing diagnoses/collaborative problems
   a. Impaired gas exchange
   b. Anxiety/fear
   c. Deficient knowledge

3. Planning and implementation/interventions
   a. Maintain airway, breathing, circulation (see Chapter 1)
   b. Provide supplemental oxygen
   c. Establish IV access for administration of crystalloid fluid/medications; consider central line placement for confirmed patients who require critical care interventions
   d. Prepare for/assist with medical interventions
      1) Utilize a negative-pressure room if available; however, airborne precautions are not necessary unless a procedure that may produce aerosolized fluids is performed
      2) Initiate droplet, contact, and standard precautions
      3) Institute cardiac and pulse oximetry monitoring
      4) Assist with hospital admission
      5) Notify CDC
      6) CDC recommends that for symptomatic patients, health care workers should don personal protective equipment that covers all skin and mucous membranes (Chapter 9)
      7) Health care facilities need to develop protocols to safely manage patients with EVD or other highly infectious diseases; such protocols should include PPE, waste management, laboratory use, etc.; they also need to ensure that only health care workers trained in those protocols provide direct patient care
   e. No known treatment; supportive care as necessary; administer pharmacologic therapy as ordered
      1) Antivirals—at this time, there is no specific antiviral treatment recommended for Ebola or other hemorrhagic fevers; additional research is needed
      2) Antibiotics—empirical antibiotics until EVD or other hemorrhagic fever can be confirmed
      3) Electrolyte and fluid replacement therapy as needed
      4) Antipyretics

4. Evaluation and ongoing monitoring
   a. Hemodynamic status
   b. Breath sounds and pulse oximetry
   c. Cardiac rate and rhythm
   d. Fever control
   e. Input and output

D. HEPATITIS

Hepatitis is a viral syndrome involving the hepatic triad (bile duct, hepatic venule, and arteriole) and the central vein area. Cellular inflammation leads to disruption of the hepatic architecture. Types of hepatitis viruses are identified by letters and vary in incubation and duration periods. Hepatitis A virus (Table 20.1) is transmitted primarily through the fecal-oral route through person-to-person contact or consuming contaminated food or water. It is found in serum and stool and is infectious 2 weeks before and 1–2 weeks after symptoms appear. Hepatitis B virus (HBV) (see Table 20.1) is transmitted most commonly by IV drug use, sexual contact, and less frequently through blood transfusions since testing of the blood supply began. Hepatitis B surface antigen (HBsAg) appears early in the disease process. Hepatitis B e antigen (HBeAg), thought to be a degradation product of the hepatitis B core antigen (HBcAg), is a marker of hepatitis B replication and appears about the same time. Antibodies are produced for each antigen. Persistence of core antibodies indicates chronic infection. Persistence of surface antibodies indicates immunity to reinfection. HBsAg in the serum without symptoms is indicative of a carrier state. Hepatitis C virus (see Table 20.1) is transmitted mostly through IV drug use and blood transfusions and is identified by the presence of antihepatitis C virus antibodies. As many as 75–85% of hepatitis C infections become chronic, and there is no immunity or vaccine available. Hepatitis D, also known as "delta hepatitis," is found only in patients with acute or chronic HBV infection, because hepatitis D is an incomplete virus that requires the hepatitis B virus to replicate. It is transmitted most commonly by IV drug use and sexual contact. Hepatitis E is an endemic, enterically transmitted infection caused by eating or drinking contaminated food or water and is similar to hepatitis A. Hepatitis E is a self-limiting disease with no FDA-approved vaccine. Patients with all forms of hepatitis may present with the same clinical features; laboratory testing determines the specific origin. Hepatitis A usually resolves in 4–8 weeks and hepatitis E in 6–9 months, although new evidence suggests that hepatitis E can progress to chronic hepatitis in individuals on immunosuppressive treatment post solid organ transplant. The remaining types can all continue in a chronic state, which may result in cirrhosis and liver cancer. At this time, there is no cure; however, treatments using interferons, ribavirin, and several new direct acting antivirals are showing success in management of the diseases.

1. Assessment
   a. Subjective data collection
      1) History of present illness/chief complaint
         a) Prodrome: preicteric phase, occurs 1 week before jaundice
            (1) Low-grade fever

Table 20.1			
Comparison of Hepatitis A, B, and C			
	Hepatitis A	**Hepatitis B**	**Hepatitis C**
Incubation period	15–45 days; average, 28 days	30–180 days; average, 120 days	15–150 days; average, 45 days
Illness duration	4 to 8 wks	A few weeks—chronic, lifelong	A few weeks—chronic, lifelong
People at risk	Household and sexual contacts Travelers to or immigrants from endemic areas (everywhere except Western Europe, Japan, Australia, New Zealand, and Canada) Illegal drug use, injected or not Clotting-factor disorders such as hemophilia	Sexual contacts of infected persons People with multiple sexual partners, same sex partners (males) and/or diagnosed with sexually transmitted diseases Intravenous drug use Infants born to infected mothers Household contacts of chronically infected persons Immigrants from endemic area Health care workers Long-term hemodialysis recipients	Sexual contacts of infected persons People with multiple sexual partners Intravenous drug use Hemodialysis recipients Blood or solid organ recipients prior to 1992 Health care workers

(2) Malaise: earliest, most common symptom

(3) Arthralgias

(4) Headache

(5) Pharyngitis

(6) Nausea, vomiting

(7) Rash, with hepatitis B usually

(8) May or may not progress to icteric phase

(9) Incubation and duration

  b) Icteric phase

    (1) Disappearance of other symptoms

    (2) Anorexia

    (3) Abdominal pain

    (4) Dark urine

    (5) Pruritus

    (6) Jaundice

    (7) Clay-colored stool

 2) Past medical history

  a) Current or preexisting diseases/illness

    (1) Hemophilia or hemodialysis

  b) Alcohol consumption

  c) Blood transfusions

  d) Travel

  e) Living in institution

  f) IV drug use

  g) Living in area of recent floods or other natural disasters

  h) Occupation: blood exposures/needle sticks

  i) Medications: all medications are significant because they pass through liver

  j) Allergies

  k) Immunization status

 b. Objective data collection

  1) Physical examination

    a) General appearance

     (1) Elevated temperature

     (2) Moderate distress/discomfort

    b) Inspection

     (1) Jaundice

     (2) Scleral icterus

     (3) Rash

    c) Palpation

     (1) Posterior cervical lymph node enlargement

     (2) Enlarged, tender liver

     (3) Splenomegaly in 20% of cases

 2) Diagnostic procedures

  a) Liver enzymes: aspartate aminotransferase (AST) and alanine aminotransferase (ALT) levels: elevated

  b) Direct and indirect, bilirubin levels: elevated

  c) Alkaline phosphatase and gamma-glutamyl transpeptidase levels: elevated

  d) CBC with differential: leukopenia with lymphocytosis, atypical lymphocytes

  e) Serum chemistries

  f) Hepatitis antibody/antigen

    (1) Hepatitis A antibody

    (2) Hepatitis B antibody and HBsAg

    (3) Hepatitis C antibody

  g) Coagulation profile: prolonged PT

  h) Abdominal radiographs

  i) Urinalysis: elevated bilirubin level; pregnancy test in female patients of childbearing age

2. Analysis: differential nursing diagnoses/collaborative problems

  a. Deficient fluid volume

  b. Deficient knowledge

  c. Anxiety/fear

3. Planning and implementation/interventions

  a. Establish IV access for administration of crystalloid fluids/medications as needed

b. Prepare for/assist with medical interventions
   1) Limit exposure of medical personnel to blood, secretions, and feces
   2) Institute cardiac and pulse oximetry monitoring
   3) Insert gastric tube and attach to suction as indicated
   4) Assist with hospital admission if
      a) PT >15 seconds
      b) Unable to care for self
   5) Report to appropriate health department officials
c. Administer pharmacologic therapy as ordered
   1) Prophylaxis
      a) Type A
         (1) Immune serum globulin 80–90% effective if given within 7–14 days after exposure (family members and close personal contacts); use if exposed to fecal-oral secretions and contaminated food, water, or shellfish
         (2) Vaccine administered in two doses: given to high-risk population: foreign travel, endemic areas (e.g., Alaska), military, immunocompromised or at risk for HIV, chronic liver disease, hepatitis C
      b) Type B: hepatitis B immune globulin plus vaccination, for exposure to serum, saliva, semen, vaginal secretions, breast milk
      c) Type B: vaccination with HBV vaccine inactivated (Recombivax HB)
   2) Vaccinate high-risk persons
      a) Health care and public safety workers who have exposure to blood in workplace
      b) Clients and staff at institutions for developmentally disabled and extended care facilities
      c) Hemodialysis recipients
      d) Recipients of clotting factor concentrates
      e) Household contacts and sexual partners of HBV carriers
      f) Adoptees from countries where HBV infection is endemic: Pacific Islands and Asia
      g) IV drug users
      h) Sexually active homosexual and bisexual men
      i) Sexually active men and women with multiple partners
      j) Inmates of long-term correctional facilities
   3) Vaccinate all infants (universally) regardless of HBsAg status of mother (administer first dose in newborn period, preferably before leaving hospital)
d. Educate patient/significant others
   1) Increase calorie intake
   2) Strict hygiene
   3) Private bathroom at home, if possible
   4) Diet of small, frequent feedings low in fat, high in carbohydrates; patient should avoid handling food to be consumed by others

   5) Signs and symptoms that necessitate return to emergency care setting: bleeding, vomiting, increased pain
   6) Take medications as prescribed
   7) Weekly or biweekly follow-up with health care provider
   8) Activity as tolerated
   9) Avoid intake of alcohol during acute illness
   10) Take medications only if absolutely necessary
   11) Avoid steroids: they delay long-term healing
4. Evaluation and ongoing monitoring
   a. Hemodynamic status
   b. Breath sounds and pulse oximetry
   c. Cardiac rate and rhythm
   d. Intake and output

E. HERPES: DISSEMINATED

Herpes simplex virus (HSV) infection is a relatively benign disease when confined to cutaneous regions. However, it has the capability of disseminating and invading all body systems, leading to serious illness and death. Primary viremia occurs from spillover of the virus at its site of entry, thus infecting the susceptible organ. During the second stage, HSV disappears from the blood but grows within cells of infected organs. Secondary viremia results from increasing virus production, causing seeding to other organ systems. The organ systems involved and the extent of damage are variable. Dissemination occurs in susceptible persons: newborns, malnourished children, children with measles and other illnesses, people with skin disorders such as burns and eczema, immunosuppression, and immunodeficiency, especially HIV infection. HSV seems to have a predilection for the temporal lobe of the brain. Encephalitis is the most common manifestation of herpes infection of the brain and has a 70% mortality rate without treatment. Even with treatment, one half of survivors have residual neurologic deficits. The virus may have a latency period within sensory nerve ganglion sites that results in mild to life-threatening infection years later.

1. Assessment
   a. Subjective data collection
      1) History of present illness/chief complaint
         a) Onset: usually acute
            (1) After other illness
            (2) After outbreak of cutaneous infection
            (3) After any stressor
         b) Symptoms depend on organ system affected
            (1) Neurologic system: headache, confusion, seizures, coma, olfactory hallucinations
            (2) Liver: abdominal pain, vomiting
            (3) Lung: cough, fever
            (4) Esophagus: dysphagia, substernal pain, weight loss
      2) Past medical history
         a) Current or preexisting diseases/illness
            (1) HSV infection
            (2) Cancer

(3) HIV infection
  b) Medications: immunosuppressants
  c) Allergies
  d) Immunization status
b. Objective data collection
  1) Physical examination
    a) General appearance
      (1) Level of consciousness, behavior, affect: focal neurologic signs
        (a) Anosmia (loss or impairment of the sense of smell)
        (b) Aphasia
        (c) Seizures
        (d) Confusion, altered mental status, coma
      (2) Fever
      (3) Severe distress/discomfort, critically ill
    b) Auscultation
      (1) Breath sounds: crackles
  2) Diagnostic procedures
    a) Viral cultures: blood and skin
    b) CBC with differential
    c) Biopsy of target organ, especially brain
    d) Clotting profile for disseminated intravascular coagulation (DIC)
    e) Liver function tests
    f) Urinalysis; pregnancy test in female patients of childbearing age
    g) Lumbar puncture: cerebrospinal fluid for culture
    h) Brain CT scan, MRI: differentiation of encephalitis
    i) Fluorescein stain and slit-lamp examination if ocular involvement: possible dendritic lesions
2. Analysis: differential nursing diagnoses/collaborative problems
  a. Ineffective airway
  b. Ineffective breathing pattern
  c. Risk for injury
  d. Anxiety/fear
3. Planning and implementation/interventions
  a. Maintain airway, breathing, circulation (see Chapter 1)
  b. Provide supplemental oxygen as indicated
    1) RSI and ventilatory support in patient with compromised airway
    2) High-flow oxygen
  c. Establish IV access for administration of crystalloid fluid/medications
  d. Prepare for/assist with medical interventions
    1) Advanced airway management
      a) Nasal or oral intubation
      b) Supraglottic airway (e.g., King, Combitube, laryngeal mask airway)
      c) Surgical airway (e.g., cricothyrotomy)

2) Institute seizure precautions and restrain confused patients per institutional protocols
3) Institute cardiac and pulse oximetry monitoring
4) Insert gastric tube and attach to suction as indicated
5) Insert indwelling urinary catheter as indicated
6) Assist with hospital admission
  e. Administer pharmacologic therapy as ordered
    1) RSI premedications: sedatives, analgesics, neuromuscular blocking agents
    2) Antivirals
4. Evaluation and ongoing monitoring
  a. Airway patency
  b. Level of consciousness
  c. Hemodynamic status
  d. Breath sounds and pulse oximetry
  e. Cardiac rate and rhythm
  f. Intake and output

F. HUMAN IMMUNODEFICIENCY VIRUS/ACQUIRED IMMUNODEFICIENCY SYNDROME

Human immunodeficiency virus (HIV) results from infection by a retrovirus. Acquired immunodeficiency syndrome (AIDS) is a life-threatening disease, which is the late stage of HIV infection and the addition of opportunistic infections. Transmission occurs by direct contact of a person's blood or body secretions with the blood, or body secretions of a person infected with HIV. Antibody seroconversion usually takes place within 45 days of exposure but may not occur for up to 6 months after infection. Acute HIV infection is characterized by a mononucleosis-like or other viral-like syndrome occurring 2–6 weeks after exposure. This is followed by a clinically asymptomatic period lasting months to years, during which time the virus replicates, mutates, and destroys the immune system. Then development of persistent generalized lymphadenopathy occurs, and finally the opportunistic diseases develop, including constitutional disorders, neurologic disorders, secondary infections, secondary cancers, and other infections such as pneumonia. Development of these problems signals the beginning of AIDS. Almost all HIV infection will at some point result in AIDS. Without treatment or medications, the mean length of time between exposure to HIV and development of AIDS is about 10 years or sooner. For those on antiretroviral therapy (ART), individuals with HIV may live for several decades. The sooner treatment begins after infection, the better a person's long-term survival will be.

HIV infection causes a defect in cell-mediated immunity and results in decreased resistance to other opportunistic infections. Specifically, it attacks the CD4 cell, which is the cornerstone of the immune system that identifies everyday infections and starts an immune response. All patients are profoundly immunodeficient at the onset of AIDS. There is aberration in the number and function of T lymphocytes, with a decrease in T-helper cells, B lymphocytes, and macrophages. The prevalence of extrapulmonary

TB is increased in HIV-infected patients, particularly TB affecting the meninges, bones, joints, and urinary tract. Opportunistic infections, commonly *Pneumocystis carinii* pneumonia (PCP), cytomegalovirus (CMV) infection, and Kaposi sarcoma, are the common causes of death.

1. Assessment
   a. Subjective data collection
      1) History of present illness/chief complaint
         a) Generalized lymphadenopathy, persistent
         b) Fever for longer than 2–4 weeks
            (1) Episodic spiking
            (2) Persistent low-grade fever
         c) Diarrhea for longer than 2–4 weeks
         d) Weight loss
         e) Anorexia
         f) Dyspnea
         g) Night sweats
         h) Malaise or fatigue, arthralgias, myalgias
         i) Mild opportunistic infections
            (1) Oral candidiasis
            (2) Herpes zoster
            (3) Tinea
         j) Skin lesions, rashes
         k) Cough
         l) Broad range of neurologic complaints, both local and global, including dementia
      2) Past medical history
         a) Current or preexisting diseases/illness
            (1) HIV diagnosis
            (2) Blood transfusions, especially before 1985
            (3) Hemophilia
            (4) Tissue transplantation
            (5) Infant with HIV-positive mother
         b) Occupational needle sticks, blood exposure
         c) IV drug use
         d) Sexual contact
            (1) History of sexually transmitted infections (STIs)
            (2) Sexual contact with IV drug user
            (3) Sexual contact with HIV-positive partner
            (4) Sexual practices including multiple partners, anal sex, oral-anal sex, local repetitive trauma
         e) Recent TB exposure
         f) Medications
            (1) Antiretroviral therapy (ART)
            (2) Antibiotics
            (3) Antifungals
            (4) Protease inhibitors
         g) Allergies
         h) Immunization status
   b. Objective data collection
      1) Physical examination
         a) General appearance
            (1) Level of consciousness, behavior, affect: withdrawn, irritable, apathetic, depressed, dementia
            (2) Chronically ill appearance, wasting syndrome; signs of volume depletion
            (3) Gait: slow, unsteady; weakness; poor coordination
            (4) Possible elevated temperature
            (5) Mild to acute distress/discomfort
         b) Inspection: Kaposi sarcoma skin lesions
         c) Palpation: lymphadenopathy
         d) Auscultation: breath sounds: crackles and wheezes
      2) Diagnostic procedures
         a) CBC with differential
            (1) Anemia: blood loss or bone marrow infection
            (2) Lymphopenia
            (3) Thrombocytopenia
         b) ABGs
         c) Serum chemistries, liver function tests
         d) Determination of HIV antibodies (e.g., via ELISA and Western blot confirmatory analysis)
         e) CD4+ cell count: decreased
         f) Immunologic studies
         g) Blood cultures: if recurrent fever without source
         h) Urinalysis; pregnancy test in female patients of childbearing age
         i) Stool culture, ova and parasites
         j) Lumbar puncture if neurologic deficits or headache present
         k) Chest radiograph
         l) Head CT scan if neurologic deficits or headache present
2. Analysis: differential nursing diagnoses/collaborative problems
   a. Impaired gas exchange
   b. Risk for infection
   c. Deficient knowledge
   d. Anxiety/fear
3. Planning and implementation/interventions
   a. Maintain airway, breathing, circulation (see Chapter 1)
   b. Provide supplemental oxygen
      1) Rapid-sequence intubation (RSI) and ventilatory support in patients with respiratory distress
      2) High-flow oxygen
   c. Establish IV access for administration of crystalloid fluid/medications
   d. Prepare for/assist with medical interventions
      1) Advanced airway management
         a) Nasal or oral intubation
         b) Supraglottic airway (e.g., King, Combitube, laryngeal mask airway)
         c) Surgical airway (e.g., cricothyrotomy)
      2) Minimize contact with blood and body secretions: use standard precautions with every patient

3) Wear appropriately sized respiratory mask if patient is coughing
4) Institute cardiac and pulse oximetry monitoring
5) Anticipate hospital admission
   e. Administer pharmacologic therapy as ordered
1) RSI premedications if advanced airway is indicated: sedatives, analgesics, neuromuscular blocking agents
2) Antipyretics
3) Antibiotics
4) Other medications as needed
   f. Educate patient/significant others
1) Adhere to safer health and sex practices
   a) Know your sexual partner
   b) Engage in mutually monogamous sexual relationship
   c) Use condoms if sexually active
   d) Do not share drug paraphernalia
   e) Do not share razors, toothbrushes
   f) Avoid pregnancy to prevent fetal transmission
   g) Avoid high-risk sexual practices
2) Report any fever, cough, or unusual fatigue immediately to health care provider
3) Avoid contact with persons who are ill
4) Take medications correctly and at the same time every day
5) Drink adequate oral fluids and eat a healthy diet
6) Encourage smoking cessation and minimizing/stopping other types of substance abuse (alcohol, recreational drug use)
4. Evaluation and ongoing monitoring
   a. Hemodynamic status
   b. Breath sounds and pulse oximetry
   c. Cardiac rate and rhythm
   d. Intake and output

G. MEASLES

Measles (rubeola) is an acute, highly contagious viral illness caused by rubeola virus and occurring in late winter and early spring. It is transmitted by direct contact with infectious droplets or through airborne droplets. Health care workers should implement airborne precautions in the health care setting. The incubation period ranges from 7–21 days. The patient is considered to be contagious 4 days before to 4 days after the rash appears. The maculopapular rash first appears on the face on the third to seventh day. It then becomes more generalized, occurring on the extremities last, and progresses to a confluent rash of 4–7 days' duration.

Most persons experience fever, rash, cough, coryza, and/or conjunctivitis, and they recover uneventfully. However, there can be a significant incidence of complications such as otitis media, diarrhea, pneumonia, bronchiolitis, and encephalitis. Permanent brain damage may result from encephalitis. The disease is more serious in infants, malnourished children, immunocompromised

individuals, and pregnant women, with an increase in spontaneous abortion and preterm delivery. Most persons born before 1957 had the illness and are permanently immune. Compliance with childhood immunizations provides protection from contracting this disease. In addition, all high school or college-age persons should be revaccinated unless they had the active disease or two immunizations in childhood.

1. Assessment
   a. Subjective data collection
1) History of present illness/chief complaint
   a) Known exposure to measles
   b) Prodrome
      (1) Fever
      (2) Cough
      (3) Coryza (rhinitis)
      (4) Photophobia
      (5) Anorexia
      (6) Headache
      (7) Rarely seizures
   c) Rash
2) Past medical history
   a) Current or preexisting diseases/illness
   b) History of measles
   c) Current age: born before 1957
   d) Medications
   e) Allergies
   f) Immunization status
   b. Objective data collection
1) Physical examination
   a) General appearance
      (1) Level of consciousness, behavior, affect: irritability, nuchal rigidity, meningeal signs
      (2) Elevated temperature
      (3) Moderate to severe distress/discomfort
   b) Inspection
      (1) Koplik spots on buccal mucosa (bluish-gray specks on red base), appear 2–3 days after symptoms begin and 1–2 days before the rash appears
      (2) Conjunctivitis
      (3) Dull tympanic membrane: otitis media
      (4) Red, blotchy rash
   c) Auscultation
      (1) Harsh cough
      (2) Breath sounds: decreased, wheezes, crackles
2) Diagnostic procedures
   a) Viral cultures
   b) Immunoglobulin M (IgM) antibodies: measles specific
   c) CBC with differential: leukopenia in late stages
   d) Urinalysis; pregnancy test in female patients of childbearing age
   e) Nasopharyngeal swab

f) Lumbar puncture: if suspected encephalitis

g) Chest radiograph: if suspected pneumonia

2. Analysis: differential nursing diagnoses/collaborative problems

   a. Risk for injury

   b. Deficient knowledge

   c. Impaired skin integrity

3. Planning and implementation/interventions

   a. Prepare for/assist with medical interventions

   1) Provide respiratory isolation

   2) Isolate patient/significant others from other people in waiting room

   b. Administer pharmacologic therapy as ordered

   1) Acetaminophen (Tylenol)

   2) Postexposure prophylaxis for high-risk contacts who cannot show evidence of immunity against measles

   a) MMR: should be administered within 72 hours; monitor for signs and symptoms of the disease for one incubation period; for infants younger than 12 months of age, revaccination should occur at 12–15 months of age and again between 4 and 6 years of age.

   b) Immune globulin: should be used for people who are at high risk for severe illness or complication, including pregnant women without evidence of measles vaccination, immunocompromised individuals, and infants younger than 12 months of age within 6 days of exposure

   3) Immunocompromised persons should receive immune globulin even if previously immunized

   c. Educate patient/significant others

   1) Advise patient to avoid school, day care centers, and people outside immediate family until after contagious period

   2) Encourage rest in darkened room

   3) Encourage parents to have children immunized at appropriate times

   4) Signs/symptoms of serious illness or complications

   a) Persistent fever or cough

   b) Change in mental status or seizures

   c) Difficulty in hearing

4. Evaluation and ongoing monitoring

   a. Fever control

H. MENINGITIS

Meningitis is a bacterial, viral, or fungal infection that causes inflammation of the meningeal layers around the brain. Fungal infections usually occur in autoimmune-compromised patients and are caused by *Cryptococcus* and *Candida*. Noninfectious meningitis can also develop from certain drugs, toxic exposures, and neoplasms. Viral infections are usually mild and short lived, whereas bacterial infections can be severe and life threatening.

Streptococcus pneumoniae, Haemophilus influenzae (H. flu), *Neisseria meningitides,* and *Listeria monocytogenes* are the more common bacterial agents that cause meningitis. Bacteria enter through the blood, basilar skull fracture, infected facial structures, and brain abscesses. Bacteria initially colonize in the nasopharynx. In bacterial disease, the subarachnoid space is filled with pus, which may obstruct cerebrospinal fluid circulation and result in hydrocephalus and increased intracranial pressure (ICP). Infants and elderly patients often do not exhibit classic signs of meningeal irritation and fever. Death is most common within a few hours after diagnosis, especially in children. Up to one third of pediatric survivors are left with some type of permanent neurologic dysfunction. Any infant younger than 2 months old with fever or subnormal temperature must be evaluated for meningitis.

1. Assessment

   a. Subjective data collection

   1) History of present illness/chief complaint

   a) Antecedent illness or exposure

   b) Onset: sudden

   c) Headache, especially occipital

   d) Photophobia

   e) Fever and chills

   f) Anorexia or poor feeding

   g) Vomiting and diarrhea

   h) Malaise, weakness

   i) Pain (see Chapter 8: neck and back)

   j) Restlessness, lethargy, altered mental status

   k) Disinclination to be held: infants

   l) Seizures

   2) Past medical history

   a) Current or preexisting diseases/illness

   (1) Liver or renal disease

   (2) Diabetes mellitus

   (3) Multiple myeloma

   (4) Alcoholism

   (5) Malnutrition

   (6) Recurrent sinusitis, pneumonia, otitis media, mastoiditis

   b) Recent basilar skull fracture

   c) Asplenic

   d) Medications

   e) Allergies

   f) Immunization status if child

   b. Objective data collection

   1) Physical examination

   a) General appearance

   (1) Level of consciousness, behavior, affect

   (a) Confusion, delirium, decreased level of consciousness

   (b) Lethargy and confusion may be the only signs in elderly patients

   (c) Irritability

   (i) Paroxysmal irritability: infants with meningeal irritation cry when held and are quieter when left in crib

  (d) High-pitched cry in infants
  (e) Bulging fontanels in infants

(2) Focal neurologic signs, cranial nerve palsies

(3) Elevated temperature: >101°F (38.3°C) or <96°F (35.6°C)

(4) Tachycardia, hypotension, tachypnea

(5) Bradycardia in neonates

(6) Severe distress/discomfort, critically ill

b) Inspection

(1) Petechiae that do not blanch: 1–2 mm on trunk and lower portion of body; also mouth, palpebral, and ocular conjunctiva

(2) Purpura

(3) Cyanosis, mottled skin, and pallor

(4) Meningeal irritation: persons older than 12 months

  (a) Contraction and pain of hamstring muscles occur after flexion and extension of leg: Kernig's sign

  (b) Bending of neck produces flexion of knee and hip; passive flexion of lower limb on one side produces similar movement on other side: Brudzinski sign

  (c) Nuchal rigidity

  (d) Opisthotonos (abnormal posturing typically found in infants and young children; it is a condition in which the individual is rigid and arches the back with the head tilting backwards)

(5) Papilledema: unusual

c) Palpation

(1) Bulging fontanels

(2) Hyperreflexia

2) Diagnostic procedures

a) Serum glucose level: infants younger than 6 months old are prone to hypoglycemia

b) Serum chemistries: hyponatremia

c) BUN and creatinine levels

d) Serum osmolality: may be decreased or elevated

(1) Decreased because of inappropriate vasopressin secretion

(2) Elevated because of dehydration

e) CBC with differential

(1) Bacterial: elevated white blood cell (WBC) count

(2) Viral: normal or decreased WBC count

(3) Meningococcal: WBC count tends to be <10,000

f) Blood cultures: prior to lumbar puncture and imaging studies

g) ABGs: if severely ill

h) Coagulation profile (e.g., PT, PTT, fibrinogen, fibrin split products)

i) Lumbar puncture: cerebrospinal fluid (Table 20.2)

(1) Tube no. 1: glucose and protein

(2) Tube no. 2: cell count with differential

(3) Tube no. 3: Gram stain, cultures

(4) Tube no. 4: hold for repeat cell count with differential or other studies

  (a) Bacterial infection: cloudy appearance; elevated pressure; WBC count, 2,000–20,000 with increased polymorphonuclear (PMN) cells; glucose level decreased; protein level elevated; bacteria present on Gram stain

  (b) Viral infection: clear appearance; WBC count, usually <500 but may be higher; normal pressure; glucose level normal; protein level normal to mildly increased; no bacteria present on Gram stain

j) Latex agglutination

k) Urinalysis; pregnancy test in female patients of childbearing age

l) Chest radiograph

m) Head CT scan

2. Analysis: differential nursing diagnoses/collaborative problems

a. Acute pain

b. Deficient fluid volume

c. Ineffective tissue perfusion: cerebral

d. Risk for injury

e. Anxiety/fear

3. Planning and implementation/interventions

a. Maintain airway, breathing, circulation (see Chapter 1)

b. Provide supplemental oxygen

c. Establish IV access for administration of crystalloid fluid/medications

1) Consider intraosseous route

d. Prepare for/assist with medical interventions

1) Ensure that patient is placed in isolation, preferably negative pressure, and that health care providers wear masks if infection with meningococcus is suspected

2) Elevate head of bed to reduce ICP

3) Institute cardiac and pulse oximetry monitoring

4) Insert gastric tube and attach to suction as indicated

5) Insert indwelling urinary catheter as indicated

6) Protect seizing patient from physical injury (raise side rails)

7) Assist with hospital admission

e. Administer pharmacologic therapy as ordered

1) Antiemetics

Table 20.2

Cerebrospinal Fluid Analysis

CSF	Bacterial Meningitis	Viral Meningitis*	Fungal Meningitis†
Normal opening pressure 5–15 cm H_2O	Increased	Normal or mildly increased	Normal or mildly increased with TB May be increased in fungal
WBC count Normal: <5 WBCs/mm³ in children and adults Preterm infants: average count 9 WBCs/mm³, <61% PMNs Term infants: average count 8.2 WBCs/mm³, <57% PMNs	No cell count result can exclude bacterial meningitis Classic: cell counts 1,000 WBCs/mm³ >1,000 WBCs/mm³ with >50% PMNs	May be >1,000 with PMN percentage approximately 60%, but may be as high as 100%	Cryptococcal: range from 49–400 WBCs/mm³
Stained smears	Positive Gram stain Inadequate decolorization may mistake Haemophilus influenzae for gram-positive cocci Previous treatment with antibiotics can alter stain uptake and can cause gram-positive organisms to appear gram negative	Negative Gram stain	India ink 80–90% effective for fungi; AFB stain 40% effective for TB (increase yield by staining supernate from at least 5 mL CSF)
Glucose level Euglycemia: >50% serum Hyperglycemia: >30% serum; wait 4 hours after glucose load	Decreased	Normal	Sometimes decreased Aside from fulminant bacterial meningitis, the lowest levels of CSF glucose are seen in TB, primary amebic meningoencephalitis, neurocysticercosis
Total protein Normal: 15–45 mg/dL in children and adults Preterm infants: 65–150 mg/dL Term infants: 20–170 mg/dL	Usually >150 mg/dL, may be as high as 1,000 mg/dL	Mildly increased	Increased; >1,000 mg/dL with relatively benign clinical presentation

AFB, acid-fast bacillus; *CSF*, cerebrospinal fluid; *PMN*, polymorphonuclear leukocyte; *TB*, tuberculosis; *WBC*, white blood cell.
*Some bacteria (e.g., *Mycoplasma, Listeria, Leptospira* species, *Borrelia burgdorferi* [Lyme], spirochetes) may produce spinal fluid alterations resembling a viral profile.
†TB and parasitic meningitis closely approximate the fungal profile.

2) Antibiotics (usually ampicillins, aminoglycosides, cephalosporins) by IV or intraosseous route; administer as soon as possible
3) Benzodiazepines
4) Corticosteroids
5) Antipyretics
6) Barbiturates and diuretics to control ICP
f. Educate patient/significant others
1) Administer prescribed chemoprophylaxis (e.g., rifampin [Rifadin], ceftriaxone [Rocephin]) within 24 hours of disease identification to household contacts, day care center contacts, and health care providers if bacterial disease (anyone exposed directly to oral secretions, e.g., kissing, mouth-to-mouth resuscitation, endotracheal intubation, suctioning)
a) Side effects include gastrointestinal (GI) disturbance, lethargy, ataxia, chills, fever, and red-orange discoloration of urine, feces, sputum, tears, sweat
b) Soft contact lenses may be permanently stained with rifampin use
c) Medication may need to be taken with food for GI intolerance, although it is best absorbed on empty stomach
d) Oral contraceptives may not be effective in preventing pregnancy while taking rifampin: secondary birth control methods should be recommended
e) Do not give to pregnant women
2) Educate parents to have infants immunized against *H. influenzae* type B
4. Evaluation and ongoing monitoring
a. Level of consciousness
b. Hemodynamic status
c. Breath sounds and pulse oximetry
d. Cardiac rate and rhythm
e. Intake and output

I. MONONUCLEOSIS

Infectious mononucleosis is an acute viral illness with a broad range of signs and symptoms lasting 3–4 weeks. The main causal agent is EBV, a member of the herpes virus family. CMV has been found to be a causative agent as well. The usual transmission is person to person by the oropharyngeal route through saliva. Incubation period is 30–50 days. Symptoms usually begin 4–6 weeks after the individual is exposed. Peak incidence is in the 15- to 24-year age group; illness in older adults is uncommon because of prior immunity. Mononucleosis occurs 30 times more frequently in whites and in higher socioeconomic groups. Most people who become ill do not recall anyone who recently had mononucleosis because it can be transmitted by a non-symptomatic carrier of the EBV. Complications most often occur in patients under 10 years or greater than 50 years of age. These complications include spleen enlargement, glomerulonephritis, pericarditis, hepatitis, Guillain-Barré syndrome, meningitis, encephalitis, erythema multiforme, and pneumonia. Rare complications include splenic rupture, thrombocytopenia, hemolytic anemia, or airway obstruction as a result of tonsillar hypertrophy.

1. Assessment
   a. Subjective data collection
      1) History of present illness/chief complaint
         a) Prodrome lasting 3–5 days: malaise, anorexia, nausea and vomiting, chills/diaphoresis, distaste for cigarettes, headache, myalgias
         b) Subsequent development of fever 100.4–104°F (38–40°C) lasting 10–14 days, sore throat, diarrhea, earache
         c) Classic triage of fever, pharyngitis, and lymphadenopathy (most often posterior cervical) is seen in 80% of patients
      2) Past medical history
         a) Current or preexisting diseases/illness
         b) Exposure to mononucleosis, usually not known
         c) Medications
         d) Allergies
         e) Immunization status
   b. Objective data collection
      1) Physical examination
         a) General appearance
            (1) Elevated temperature
            (2) Mild to moderate distress/discomfort
         b) Inspection
            (1) Red throat with grey exudate; tonsils may be hypertrophied
            (2) Petechiae on palate
            (3) Fine red macular rash
            (4) Genital ulcers are rare but have been reported; periorbital edema—uncommon finding
         c) Palpation
            (1) Tender lymphadenopathy, particularly posterior cervical nodes
            (2) Abdominal tenderness with hepatomegaly
            (3) Splenomegaly in 50% of patients
      2) Diagnostic procedures
         a) Heterophile antibody titer (Monospot or Monolatex): may not be positive until second week of illness; may be less sensitive in very young children and older adults
         b) Throat culture for *Streptococcus* group A
         c) CBC with differential: neutropenia, thrombocytopenia, lymphocytosis with atypical lymphs, leukocytosis
         d) Liver function tests: may be elevated
         e) Urinalysis; pregnancy test in female patients of childbearing age
         f) Chest radiograph if pneumonia suspected
2. Analysis: differential nursing diagnoses/collaborative problems
   a. Pain
   b. Risk for deficient fluid volume
   c. Deficient knowledge
3. Planning and implementation/interventions
   a. Administer pharmacologic therapy as ordered
      1) Antipyretics: avoid aspirin in children
      2) Analgesics
      3) Corticosteroids and antiviral therapy are not routinely recommended but may be considered for severe symptoms
   b. Educate patient/significant others
      1) Isolation not necessary
      2) Avoid kissing on mouth
      3) No sharing of eating or drinking utensils
      4) Activity as tolerated but generally restricted to avoid splenic rupture
         a) Extra rest early in illness
      5) Warm saltwater gargles for sore throat
      6) Encourage fluids to avoid dehydration
      7) Avoid alcohol intake for at least a month to decrease work of liver
      8) Diet as tolerated
         a) Liquids initially
         b) Soft foods
      9) Do not donate blood until fully recovered
      10) Signs/symptoms of serious illness or complications
         a) Increasing fever
         b) Cough, chest pain
         c) Progression of illness
         d) Difficulty in breathing
         e) Signs of dehydration
         f) Increasing abdominal pain
4. Evaluation and ongoing monitoring
   a. Fever control

J. MUMPS

Mumps is an acute generalized, usually benign, viral infection caused by a virus of the Paramyxoviridae family that causes nonsuppurative swelling and tenderness of salivary glands and one or both parotid glands. It is transmitted through direct contact, droplet nuclei, or fomites, which enter through the nose or mouth. Incubation averages 14–18 days (range 2–4 weeks). Peak incidence is January–May. The infectious period typically occurs 3 days before to 4 days after illness; however, the virus may be present in saliva 7 days before to 9 days after parotitis onset and is most contagious prior to swelling of the parotid gland. Up to one third of cases are asymptomatic. Mumps occurs primarily in school-age children and adolescents and is uncommon in infants younger than 1 year. It is usually a more severe illness in the postpubertal age group; 20–30% of adult men experience epididymoorchitis. Testicular atrophy may develop, but sterility is rare. Other complications include viral meningitis, myocarditis, arthritis, arthralgias, pancreatitis, and deafness.

1. Assessment
   a. Subjective data collection
      1) History of present illness/chief complaint
         a) Known exposure to mumps
         b) Travel history
         c) Prodrome: fever (<104°F [40°C]), anorexia, malaise, headache within 24 hours
         d) Pain (see Chapter 8)
            (1) Earache and tenderness of ipsilateral parotid gland
            (2) Increased pain with ingestion of citrus fruits or juices
            (3) Testicular pain: orchitis
            (4) Abdominal pain: pancreatitis
         e) Fever, chills, headache, vomiting if meningitis
      2) Past medical history
         a) Current or preexisting diseases/illness
         b) Previous episode of mumps
         c) Medications
         d) Allergies
         e) Immunization status
   b. Objective data collection
      1) Physical examination
         a) General appearance
            (1) Trismus with difficulty in pronunciation and chewing
            (2) Elevated temperature (usually low-grade fever)
            (3) Moderate distress/discomfort
         b) Inspection
            (1) Swelling of parotid gland, maximal over 2–3 days, with earlobe lifted up and out and mandible obscured by swelling
            (2) Parotid duct (Stensen duct) opening: red and swollen
            (3) Testicle/scrotum: swollen, erythematous
         c) Palpation
            (1) Testicle/scrotum: warm and tender
            (2) Parotid gland: unilateral or bilateral edema with tenderness on palpation of jaw line
      2) Diagnostic procedures
         a) CBC with differential: WBC and differential normal or mild leukopenia
         b) Serum amylase: may be elevated for 2–3 weeks
         c) Urinalysis: pregnancy test in female patients of childbearing age
         d) Diagnosis can be made clinically but laboratory testing is necessary for confirmation
            (1) Antibody testing through blood specimen
            (2) Viral isolation using buccal and oral swab samples
            (3) Reverse transcriptase-polymerase chain reaction using buccal and oral swab samples
2. Analysis: differential nursing diagnoses/collaborative problems
   a. Deficient knowledge
   b. Acute pain
3. Planning and implementation/interventions
   a. Prepare for/assist with medical interventions
      1) Use droplet precautions in the health care setting
      2) Isolate patient/significant others from other people in waiting room
   b. Administer pharmacologic therapy as ordered
      1) Acetaminophen (Tylenol): avoid aspirin in children
      2) Nonnarcotic analgesics
   c. Educate patient/significant others
      1) Advise patient to avoid contact with others from the time of the diagnosis until at least 5 days after the onset of parotitis
      2) Encourage rest until feeling better
      3) Encourage fluids and avoid citrus and other foods that increase discomfort
      4) Warm or cold packs to face
      5) For orchitis
         a) Bed rest
         b) Scrotal elevation
         c) Ice packs
         d) Pain medicine as prescribed
      6) Public health authorities may give a third dose of measles/mumps/rubella (MMR) vaccine to target populations during an outbreak
4. Evaluation and ongoing monitoring
   a. Fever control
   b. Pain relief

K. PERTUSSIS

Pertussis (whooping cough) is an acute, widespread, highly contagious bacterial disease of the throat and bronchi caused by the gram-negative coccobacillus *Bordetella pertussis* and spread by direct contact of airborne droplets from sneezing and coughing. Infants and children up to 4 years of age who have not been immunized against pertussis are six times more likely to be infected than immunized children. Partially immunized children have a less severe illness. Adults usually have only minor respiratory symptoms and persistent cough. The incubation period is approximately 7–10 days but can vary from 6–21 days. Persons are contagious for 3 weeks but are most contagious up to about 2 weeks after the cough begins. The peak incidence is during spring and summer. The pertussis bacteria invade the mucosa of the upper respiratory tract and produce symptoms similar to those of the common cold, but progressively worsen. Symptoms include fever, hypoxia, and a paroxysmal whoop-type cough caused by spasm of the epiglottis. Petechial-type rash above the nipple line, otitis, and vomiting may also occur. Complications include pneumonia (a common cause of death), atelectasis, pneumothorax, seizures, and encephalitis. Children may experience laceration of the lingual frenulum and epistaxis.

1. Assessment
   a. Subjective data collection
      1) History of present illness/chief complaint
         a) Known exposure to pertussis
         b) Three stages but symptoms vary depending on patient's age and immunization status
            (1) Catarrhal stage lasts up to 2 weeks; "classic pertussis"
               (a) Conjunctivitis and tearing
               (b) Fever/chills
               (c) Rhinorrhea, sneezing
               (d) Irritability
               (e) Fatigue
               (f) Dry nonproductive cough, often worse at night
            (2) Paroxysmal stage lasts 4–6 weeks in children and up to 3 months in adults
               (a) Severe cough with hypoxia, unremitting paroxysms, and clear, tenacious mucus; patient appears well between paroxysms of coughing; cough often triggered by eating and drinking
               (b) Apnea can occur in rare cases
               (c) Vomiting follows cough
               (d) Anorexia
            (3) Convalescent stage typically lasts 1–2 weeks
               (a) Gradual decrease in cough frequency and severity
      2) Past medical history
         a) Current or preexisting diseases/illness
         b) Medications (especially angiotensin-converting enzyme inhibitors)
         c) Allergies
         d) Immunization status
   b. Objective data collection
      1) Physical examination
         a) General appearance
            (1) Level of consciousness, behavior, affect: restlessness
            (2) Elevated temperature >101°F (38.3°C)
            (3) Paroxysmal explosive coughing ending in prolonged high-pitched crowing inspiration
            (4) Moderate to severe distress/discomfort
         b) Inspection
            (1) Coryza (rhinitis)
            (2) Clear, tenacious mucus in large amounts
            (3) Periorbital/eyelid edema and subconjunctival hemorrhage
            (4) Rectal prolapse, especially in children
         c) Auscultation—assess breath sounds suggestive of pneumonia
         d) Palpation
            (1) Crepitus from subcutaneous emphysema
            (2) Pain with palpation of ribs—assess for fractures especially in adults
      2) Diagnostic procedures
         a) Culture, PCR, or serology may be used to confirm diagnosis of pertussis—culture is gold standard
            (1) Perform deep aspiration of posterior nasopharynx for 15–30 seconds
            (2) Negative results: common in immunized patients
         b) IFA staining of nasopharyngeal specimens
         c) CBC with differential: lymphocytosis
         d) Urinalysis; pregnancy test in female patients of childbearing age
2. Analysis: differential nursing diagnoses/collaborative problems
   a. Ineffective breathing pattern
   b. Ineffective airway clearance
   c. Acute pain
3. Planning and implementation/interventions
   a. Maintain airway, breathing, circulation (see Chapter 1)
   b. Provide supplemental oxygen
      1) RSI and ventilatory support in respiratory distress patients
      2) High-flow oxygen
   c. Establish IV access for administration of crystalloid fluid/medications as needed
   d. Prepare for/assist with medical interventions
      1) Maintain droplet precautions
      2) Advanced airway management
         a) Nasal or oral intubation
         b) Supraglottic airway (e.g., King, Combitube, laryngeal mask airway)
         c) Surgical airway (e.g., cricothyrotomy)

3) Minimize or prevent excitement, crying because this exacerbates the cough paroxysms
4) Institute cardiac and pulse oximetry monitoring
5) Assist with hospital admission if patient younger than 1 year
   e. Administer pharmacologic therapy as ordered
   1) RSI premedications: sedatives, analgesics, neuromuscular blocking agents
   2) Antibiotics: erythromycin, azithromycin (Zithromax), or clarithromycin (Biaxin)
   3) Antitussive although no evidence shows a reduction in severity of paroxysmal cough
   4) Nonnarcotic analgesics
   5) Antipyretics
   f. Educate patient/significant others
   1) Isolate patients with active disease from school or work for 5 days after starting antibiotics
   2) Educate parents about the importance of complete immunization
   3) All household and other contacts: prophylactic antibiotics may abort the disease or render the patient noncommunicable
      a) Erythromycin for 14 days or
      b) Azithromycin for 5 days or
      c) Clarithromycin for 7 days
   4) Immunization recommendations: Tdap (tetanus toxoid, reduced diphtheria toxoid, and acellular pertussis vaccine)
   5) Corticosteroids and beta$_2$-adrenergic bronchodilators: limited evidence
   6) Signs and symptoms that necessitate return to emergency care setting
      a) Difficulty in breathing recurs or worsens
      b) Blue color of lips or skin occurs
      c) Restlessness or sleeplessness develops
      d) Medicines are not tolerated
      e) Fluid intake decreases
4. Evaluation and ongoing monitoring
   a. Airway patency
   b. Level of consciousness
   c. Hemodynamic status
   d. Breath sounds and pulse oximetry
   e. Cardiac rate and rhythm

L. SHINGLES (HERPES ZOSTER)

Shingles is an acute localized infection caused by VZV. During an episode of chickenpox, VZV travels from skin lesions to sensory nerve ganglia, where it lies dormant. It is postulated that when immunity to VZV wanes, the virus replicates. The virus moves down the sensory nerve and causes dermatomal pain and skin lesions, which may last 2–4 weeks. The exact triggers are unknown, but normal aging and immunosuppression are primary risk factors. Shingles may occur at any age in persons previously infected with varicella but is most common in adults over age 60. Fluid from lesions is contagious, but the likelihood of transmission is low. Susceptible, exposed persons may develop varicella (chickenpox). The diagnosis is primarily made based on clinical presentation; however, in immunocompromised patients, the presentation may be atypical. Complications include postherpetic neuralgia, a debilitating pain syndrome that may last several months, blindness, disseminated disease, and occasionally death.

1. Assessment
   a. Subjective data collection
   1) History of present illness/chief complaint
      a) Prodromal: tingling, burning, itching, and hyperesthesia often precedes onset of rash by 1–5 days at involved dermatome
      b) Other symptoms that may precede outbreak include headache, photophobia, and malaise
   2) Past medical history
      a) Current or preexisting diseases/illness
         (1) HIV infection
         (2) Cancer
         (3) Blood dyscrasias
      b) History of chickenpox
      c) Chronic steroid use
      d) Medications
      e) Allergies
      f) Immunization status
   b. Objective data collection
   1) Physical examination
      a) General appearance
         (1) Elevated temperature: low grade if present
         (2) Change in visual acuity, if eye involved
            (a) Ophthalmic or trigeminal nerve branch involvement; can cause significant severe/permanent ocular damage
            (b) Vesicles on tip of the nose (Hutchinson sign) may precede ophthalmic symptoms
            (c) Lesions in the ear, mouth, or pharynx may indicate involvement of trigeminal nerve
         (3) Moderate to acute distress/discomfort
      b) Inspection
         (1) Rash
            (a) Unilateral; usually does not cross midline
            (b) Usually thoracic or lumbar dermatome
            (c) Small fluid-filled vesicle on red base
            (d) May become hemorrhagic
            (e) Successive crops of lesions occur for about 1 week
      c) Palpation
         (1) Tenderness over involved dermatome
            (a) Cervical and thoracic dermatomes most commonly affected

2) Diagnostic procedures
   a) Viral culture
   b) CBC with differential
   c) Lumbar puncture for patient with neurologic involvement
2. Analysis: differential nursing diagnoses/collaborative problems
   a. Acute pain
   b. Risk for infection
   c. Deficient knowledge
   d. Impaired skin integrity
3. Planning and implementation/interventions
   a. Establish IV access for administration of crystalloid fluids/medications as needed
   b. Prepare for/assist with medical interventions
      1) Infection control measures depend on whether patient is immunocompromised or immunocompetent and if rash is localized or disseminated
         a) Immunocompetent
            (1) Localized: standard precautions and lesions should be completely covered
            (2) Disseminated: contact plus airborne precautions until lesions are dry and crusted
         b) Immunocompromised
            (1) Localized: contact plus airborne precautions should be followed until disseminated infection is ruled out; then, standard precautions
            (2) Disseminated: contact plus airborne precautions until lesions are dry and crusted
      2) Ophthalmologic consult if facial/eye involvement
   c. Administer pharmacologic therapy as ordered
      1) Nonnarcotic analgesics
      2) Narcotics
      3) Antihistamines: use with caution in elderly patients; many topical antiitch medications include an antihistamine (e.g., diphenhydramine [Benadryl]): do not overuse
      4) Antivirals (acyclovir [Zovirax], famciclovir [Famvir], valacycolovir [Valtrex]) will lessen disease severity, pain, and incidence of postherpetic neuralgia if administered within 72 hours of onset of rash
   d. Educate patient/significant others
      1) Advise patient to avoid school/work until all lesions are crusted over
      2) Recommend immunization of high-risk contacts
         a) VZIG
            (1) Postexposure prophylaxis
            (2) Immunocompromised persons (HIV infection, AIDS, cancer, steroid therapy)
            (3) Effective up to 96 hours after exposure, but the sooner given the better
      3) Susceptible health care workers should be vaccinated

4) Cut fingernails short to prevent infection of lesions
5) Topical baking soda paste or baths and calamine lotion may help with itching
6) Topical capsaicin cream to area of healed outbreak may help control pain
7) Signs/symptoms of serious illness or complications
   a) Increased fever
   b) Cough
   c) Worsening illness
   d) Signs of skin infection
4. Evaluation and ongoing monitoring
   a. Pain relief

M. SKIN INFESTATIONS

LICE. Three types of lice infest humans: *Pediculus humanus* var *corporis* (human louse, body lice); *P. humanus* var *capitis* (human head louse); and *Pthirus pubis* (pubic or crab louse). Head and body lice are 2–4 mm grayish-white, flattened, wingless, and elongated insects with pointed heads. Pubic lice are wider and shorter and resemble a crab. Eggs (nits) laid by the female adhere firmly to body hairs or clothing fibers and look like white protrusions, which may be mistaken for dandruff. This problem is important because lice can cause significant cutaneous disease and may serve as vectors for infectious diseases such as typhus, relapsing fever, and trench fever. The head louse infects all socioeconomic groups and is more common among whites, women, and children. It is transferred by close personal contact and possibly by sharing hats, combs, and brushes. The body louse is seen with overcrowding and poor sanitation. The louse lays its eggs and resides in seams of clothing rather than on skin; it leaves clothing only to feed on a blood meal from its host. Nits are viable in clothing for up to 1 month. The pubic louse is transmitted by sexual or close body contact. It resides primarily in pubic hair, but it can also be seen in eyebrows, eyelashes, axillary hair, and coarse hair on the back and chest of men. It may also occasionally infest hair on the head. Up to one third of persons with pubic lice may have another sexually transmitted infection (STI).

1. Assessment
   a. Subjective data collection
      1) History of present illness/chief complaint
         a) Itching in infected area; may be severe on scalp
         b) Fever, malaise in severe infection
         c) Known exposure to lice
         d) Recent sharing of clothing, beds, combs/brushes
         e) Previous treatment for current infestation, including OTC medications
         f) Symptoms of concurrent STIs
      2) Past medical history
         a) Current or preexisting diseases/illness

b) Previous infestations
c) Medications
d) Allergies
e) Immunization status
   b. Objective data collection
      1) Physical examination
         a) General appearance
            (1) Mild distress/discomfort
         b) Inspection
            (1) Excoriation of scalp and skin
            (2) Secondary bacterial infection, especially of scalp
            (3) Weeping and crusting of skin
            (4) Small, red macules, papules on trunk
            (5) Small, gray to bluish macules measuring <1 cm on trunk (maculae ceruleae) from anti-coagulant injected into skin by biting louse
            (6) Nits or mature lice on hairs
            (7) Thick, dry skin; brownish pigmentation on neck, shoulder, back from chronic infection
            (8) Signs of concurrent STIs: genital discharge, lesions
         c) Palpation
            (1) Lymphadenopathy
      2) Diagnostic procedures: studies appropriate for possible STIs
2. Analysis: differential nursing diagnoses/collaborative problems
   a. Risk for impaired skin integrity
   b. Risk for infection
   c. Deficient knowledge
3. Planning and implementation/interventions
   a. Prepare for/assist with medical interventions
      1) Contact isolation
   b. Administer pharmacologic therapy as ordered
      1) Nonnarcotic analgesics
      2) Antihistamines
      3) Antibiotics
      4) Pediculicides
   c. Educate patient/significant others
      1) Advise patient/parent to avoid school/work until one treatment completed
      2) Use pediculicides as prescribed
      3) Treat sexual contacts
      4) Itching may continue after treatment: do not retreat without physician order
      5) Remove nits from hair
         a) Soak hair with equal parts warm vinegar and water
         b) Mechanically remove nits with fine-toothed comb
         c) If nits in eyelashes or eyebrows, apply layer of petroleum jelly; repeat two times a day for 10 days; do not have parents mechanically remove nits from eyelashes

d) Soak combs and brushes in pediculicide for 1 hour
      6) Launder clothing/bedding in hot water; dry in hot dryer if possible; discard clothing and linen if practical
      7) Iron seams of clothing if body lice
      8) Put socks over hands of small children at bedtime to decrease scratching
      9) Cut fingernails short
     10) Put hats, coats, other nonlaunderable items in plastic bags for 2–4 weeks to kill off any remaining lice
     11) Avoid sharing hats, combs, brushes
     12) Instruct patient/parent about signs/symptoms of serious illness or complications: signs of infection
4. Evaluation and ongoing monitoring

SCABIES. Scabies is a highly contagious infestation of the skin caused by the itch mite *Sarcoptes scabiei* var *hominis*. Eggs are laid in burrows several millimeters in length at the base of the stratum corneum layer of the epidermis. The mite causes significant cutaneous disease but is not a vector for other infectious diseases. Scabies is usually transmitted by intimate personal or sexual contact; however, it may be spread to health care workers by even casual contact. The most common complaint of persons infected with scabies is the unrelenting pruritus that is usually worse at night.
1. Assessment
   a. Subjective data collection
      1) History of current illness/chief complaint
         a) Intense itching, worse at night
         b) Rash
         c) Previous treatment for current problem
         d) Known exposure to scabies
      2) Past medical history
         a) Current or preexisting diseases/illness
         b) Previous infestations
         c) Medications
         d) Allergies
         e) Immunization status
   b. Objective data collection
      1) Physical examination
         a) General appearance
            (1) Hygiene: possibly poor
            (2) Mild to moderate distress/discomfort
         b) Inspection
            (1) Rash
               (a) Linear red papules, excoriations, and occasionally vesicles and visible threadlike burrows
               (b) More common in interdigit web spaces, wrists, anterior axillary folds, periumbilical skin, pelvic girdle, penis, ankles

(c) For infants and small children, soles, palms, face, neck, and scalp are often involved
(d) Patient scratching
(e) Signs of infection of lesions
2) Diagnostic procedures: skin scrapings for mite
2. Analysis: differential nursing diagnoses/collaborative problems
   a. Risk for impaired skin integrity
   b. Risk for infection
   c. Deficient knowledge
3. Planning and implementation/interventions
   a. Prepare for/assist with medical interventions
      1) Contact isolation
   b. Administer pharmacologic therapy as ordered
      1) Nonnarcotic analgesics
      2) Antihistamines
      3) Antibiotics
      4) Pediculicides
   c. Educate patient/significant others
      1) Advise patient/parent to avoid school/work until one treatment completed
      2) Use pediculicides as prescribed
      3) Itching may continue for up to 1 week after treatment; do not retreat without physician order
      4) Launder clothing/bedding in hot water; dry in hot dryer if possible; discard clothing and linen if practical
      5) Put socks over hands of small children at bedtime to decrease scratching
      6) Cut fingernails short
      7) Put hats, coats, and other nonlaunderable items in plastic bags for at least 1–2 weeks to kill off any remaining mites
      8) Signs/symptoms of serious illness or complications: signs of infection
4. Evaluation and ongoing monitoring

N. TUBERCULOSIS

Tuberculosis (TB), one of the world's deadliest diseases, is caused by the bacteria *Mycobacterium tuberculosis*, an acid-fast bacillus (AFB) that commonly invades the lung but can attack any part of the body. It is spread from the respiratory tract through exhaled air, by coughing, sneezing, speaking, or singing, as droplets small enough to be inhaled directly into the alveoli and bronchioles. Latent TB infection is asymptomatic and noninfectious, but PPD results are positive. Two to 12 weeks after infection, the body develops an immunologic response, which allows healing and results in a positive PPD test result. Active TB disease occurs when the patient becomes symptomatic and is infectious. The lung is the primary site of disease; however, 15% of cases are extrapulmonary. Most commonly affected sites are the kidney, lymphatic system, pleura, bones or joints, and blood (disseminated or miliary TB). Diagnosis is made by one of two groups of criteria: (1) culture of the bacteria from sputum or other body fluid and (2) positive tuberculin test result, signs and symptoms of TB, and chest radiographic findings. Noncompliance with medication regimens is the main difficulty in treating TB, and it has resulted in a growing number of drug-resistant cases.

1. Assessment
   a. Subjective data collection
      1) History of present illness/chief complaint
         a) Known exposure to TB
         b) Prolonged productive cough
            (1) Longer than 2 weeks
            (2) Becoming progressively worse
         c) Fever and chills
         d) Night sweats
         e) Easy fatigability and malaise
         f) Anorexia
         g) Weight loss
         h) Hemoptysis
         i) Recent tuberculin test conversion
         j) Foreign-born status, travel from or to high-prevalence country and high burden countries: Bangladesh, India, Indonesia, Nigeria, and Pakistan (see CDC or World Health Organization websites for most current information)
         k) Resident or staff member of nursing home, prison, or homeless shelter
         l) Alcoholic or other substance abuser
         m) Racial/ethnic minority: African-American, Hispanic, and Asians
      2) Past medical history
         a) Current or preexisting diseases/illness
            (1) Diabetes
            (2) Malignant disease
            (3) Silicosis
            (4) Chronic renal failure
            (5) Immunosuppression
            (6) HIV infection or AIDS
         b) Bacille Calmette-Guérin (BCG) vaccination (person usually from another country)
         c) Medications, especially prolonged steroid therapy
         d) Allergies
         e) Immunization status
   b. Objective data collection
      1) Physical examination
         a) General appearance
            (1) Elevated temperature
            (2) Moderate distress/discomfort
         b) Inspection
            (1) Thin appearing
            (2) Possible hemoptysis
         c) Auscultation
            (1) Breath sounds: decreased
      2) Diagnostic procedures

a) Tuberculin skin testing, may be initiated in the ED
  (1) PPD: induration of 5 mm or greater is considered positive if patient has HIV infection, is in close contact with person with newly diagnosed TB, or has abnormal radiograph with old healed TB scar; induration of 10 mm or greater is considered positive in all other persons (redness not a factor)
  (2) May repeat PPD immediately if first attempt went subcutaneous: place second one at least 2 inches away; if second attempt fails, wait 1 month to repeat
  (3) Only contraindication to PPD is previous positive test
  (4) Mono-Vacc Test: same criteria as for PPD; when administering, press hard enough to leave impression of points and base of device on forearm; use for mass screening only, never diagnosis; any palpable erythema is positive, even 1–2 mm, and warrants PPD
b) TB blood tests: interferon-gamma release assay (IGRA)
  (1) Positive: person has been infected with TB bacteria; additional testing is required to determine if latent TB or TB diseases
  (2) Negative: blood did not react to the test; latent TB and TB disease is unlikely
  (3) Preferred testing for the following groups: previous BCG vaccination and those who may not present for second appointment to evaluate skin reaction
c) AST level: obtain before starting isoniazid (INH) in persons older than 35 years or who have increased hepatotoxicity risk
d) Chest radiograph: infiltrates, especially of posterior upper lobe
e) Sputum for AFB and culture: three successive early-morning specimens
f) Gastric aspiration for obtaining swallowed sputum in young children
g) ECG

2. Analysis: differential nursing diagnoses/collaborative problems
   a. Impaired gas exchange
   b. Deficient knowledge
3. Planning and implementation/interventions
   a. Provide supplemental oxygen
   b. Establish IV access for administration of crystalloid fluids/medications
   c. Prepare for/assist with medical interventions
      1) Decrease transmission of disease
         a) Isolate coughing patient from waiting room, preferably in negative-pressure treatment room, and needs to wear appropriate mask when traveling outside the room
         b) Teach patient to cover nose and mouth with tissue when coughing or sneezing: reduces droplet nuclei
      2) Institute cardiac and pulse oximetry monitoring
      3) Tuberculin testing
      4) Assist with possible hospital admission
      5) Report patient and contacts to proper public health authorities
   d. Administer pharmacologic therapy as ordered
      1) INH
      2) Rifampin (Rifadin)
      3) Ethambutol (Myambutol)
      4) Pyrazinamide (PZA)
   e. Educate patient/significant others
      1) Isolate patient at home for first 2 weeks of therapy for active disease; patient is considered infectious until
         a) After 14 days of directly observed therapy
         b) Decrease in cough and afebrile
         c) Three consecutive negative AFB smears
      2) Surgical masks are helpful for patient to wear; not effective for health care staff or family; need special TB mask (N95 mask or particulate respirator)
      3) Ventilate living quarters (e.g., house and apartment) with fresh air and exhaust old air to outside: need about 20 air changes per day
      4) Encourage patient/significant others to return for reading of TB test
      5) Encourage compliance with medication regimen through education about disease and its transmission
      6) Education about medications
         a) All patients with active disease should be considered for directly observed therapy (DOT) but especially those with drug-resistant TB or patients at high risk for nonadherence, such as homeless persons, individuals who abuse alcohol or drugs, and children/adolescents.
         b) Preventive therapy given for 6 months and recommended for
            (1) Patients with HIV infection or suspected HIV infection with PPD induration of 5 mm or greater: treat for 12 months
            (2) Household members and close contacts of newly diagnosed patient
            (3) Recent tuberculin test converter
            (4) IV drug users known to be HIV negative with PPD induration of 10 mm or greater
            (5) Persons with past TB not treated
            (6) Persons with chronic medical conditions known to pose increased risk of TB who have PPD induration of 10 mm or greater

(e.g., diabetes, renal failure, leukemia, underweight, malnourishment)
    (7) Persons younger than 35 years with PPD induration of 10 mm or greater and no other risk factors
  c) Medications: both preventive and therapeutic; generally a four-drug regimen
    (1) INH
    (2) Pyridoxine (vitamin B_6): to prevent peripheral neuropathy from INH
    (3) Rifampin (Rifadin): discolors body fluid and permanently stains soft contact lenses
    (4) PZA
    (5) Ethambutol (Myambutol)
    (6) Avoid alcohol and acetaminophen intake
    (7) Continue to take the medications as directed—take it at the same time every day and don't discontinue even if feeling better
  7) Encourage testing for HIV
  8) Provide social service referral as indicated
4. Evaluation and ongoing monitoring
  a. Respiratory effort
  b. Breath sounds and pulse oximetry
  c. Cardiac rate and rhythm

O. VARICELLA (CHICKENPOX)

Chickenpox is a highly contagious disease caused by the varicella zoster virus (VZV). It is transmitted by direct contact with infected persons, through exposure of airborne droplets from respiratory tract secretions, or by contact with fluid from the vesicles. Incubation range is from 10–21 days, with the average onset of disease at 14–16 days. The contagious period starts 1–2 days before the rash and ends when all the lesions are crusted over, usually 4–5 days after the onset of the rash. Most cases in the United States occur in children less than 10 years of age. Adolescents, adults, and immunocompromised persons are at risk for more severe disease and complications. Complications include bacterial infection of lesions, pneumonia, thrombocytopenia, renal failure, encephalitis, and Reye syndrome. Congenital varicella syndrome may occur from infection during the first half of pregnancy, and there is a 31% mortality rate among neonates born to infected mothers. Compliance with childhood immunizations can provide protection from contracting this disease. Susceptible health care workers exposed to varicella should not work days 10–21 after exposure, to prevent inadvertent spread of disease.
1. Assessment
  a. Subjective data collection
    1) History of present illness/chief complaint
      a) Known exposure to chickenpox
      b) Prodrome (48 hours before rash): fever, cough, malaise, headache, rash often with itching

    2) Past medical history
      a) Current or preexisting diseases/illness
        (1) HIV infection
        (2) Cancer
        (3) Blood dyscrasias
        (4) Other immunocompromised state
      b) Pregnant or trying to become pregnant
      c) Medications
      d) Allergies
      e) Immunization status
  b. Objective data collection
    1) Physical examination
      a) General appearance
        (1) Level of consciousness, behavior, affect: restless, irritability, confusion
        (2) Elevated temperature: fever, low grade
        (3) Mild to moderate distress/discomfort; if other complications, may appear critically ill
      b) Inspection
        (1) Rash, typically 250–500 lesions
          (a) Starts on trunk as faint, red macules
          (b) Becomes teardrop vesicles on a red base, which dry and crust over
          (c) New crops appear over several days at various stages
          (d) Palms and soles are spared
          (e) Vesicles may occur on any mucous membranes, rupture, and become shallow ulcers
        (2) Skin excoriations from scratching
        (3) Signs of lesion infection: red, swollen, tender
      c) Auscultation
        (1) Cough
        (2) Breath sounds: possible wheezes, rhonchi
    2) Diagnostic procedures
      a) Generally none: diagnosis made clinically
      b) Urinalysis; pregnancy test in female patients of childbearing age
      c) If diagnosis in doubt, Tzanck smear, serology, PCR or indirect immunofluorescence may be used
      d) Liver function tests may indicate illness severity
      e) Lumbar puncture: if focal neurologic findings
      f) Chest radiograph: varicella pneumonia
2. Analysis: differential nursing diagnoses/collaborative problems
  a. Pain
  b. Risk for deficient fluid volume
  c. Deficient knowledge
  d. Risk for infection
  e. Impaired skin integrity
3. Planning and implementation/interventions
  a. Prepare for/assist with medical interventions

1) Provide airborne (respiratory) and contact precautions
2) Isolate patient/significant others from other people in waiting room
   b. Administer pharmacologic therapy as ordered
1) Acetaminophen (Tylenol): avoid aspirin because of the risk of Reye syndrome
2) Antihistamines
3) Antivirals, IV or oral, to older children and adults will lessen disease severity
   c. Educate patient/significant others
1) Advise patient to avoid school/work until all lesions are crusted over
2) Recommend immunization of high-risk contacts
   a) Varicella-zoster immune globulin (VZIG)
      (1) Postexposure prophylaxis
      (2) Immunocompromised persons (HIV infection, AIDS, cancer, steroid therapy)
      (3) Administer within 96 hours after exposure, but the sooner given, the better
      (4) Susceptible health care workers should have titers checked and be vaccinated if needed
3) Prevention of infection of lesions
   a) Suggest putting socks over small children's hands at bedtime to decrease scratching and excoriation
   b) Cut fingernails short to prevent injury from scratching
   c) Apply topical baking soda paste and calamine lotion to help with itching
   d) Use cool wet compresses or give bath in lukewarm to cool water every 3–4 hours for the first few days; pat the body dry—do not rub
4) Many topical antiitch medications include an antihistamine (e.g., diphenhydramine [Benadryl]): do not overuse
5) Serve foods that are cold, soft, and bland especially when vesicles are in the mouth
6) Encourage parents to have children immunized at appropriate times
7) Signs/symptoms of serious illness or complications
   a) Increased fever
   b) Cough
   c) Worsening illness
   d) Signs of skin infection
4. Evaluation and ongoing monitoring
   a. Fever control

P. VIRAL ENCEPHALITIS

Encephalitis is an infection of the brain that causes an inflammatory response of brain tissue. It often coexists with meningitis and has a broad range of signs and symptoms, ranging from unrecognized mild cases to profound neurologic involvement. Most cases in North America are viral in nature caused by arboviruses, herpes simplex virus (HSV) type 1, varicella-zoster virus (VZV), and Epstein-Barr virus (EBV). Transmission may be by animal bites or may occur seasonally from vectors (e.g., mosquitoes, ticks, and midges carry arboviruses, Lyme disease, Rocky Mountain spotted fever, and so on). The more common human viruses are transmitted via droplet or lesion exudate to the person, in whom replication takes place. The virus then enters the nervous system through the blood. In the brain, the virus enters the neuron, where it causes inflammation, neurologic dysfunction, and damage. Encephalitis occurs in all age groups, and mortality ranges from 5–10% from arbovirus infection to nearly 100% for rabies.

1. Assessment
   a. Subjective data collection
1) History of present illness/chief complaint
   a) Fever
   b) Headache
   c) Photophobia
   d) Nausea, vomiting
   e) Confusion, lethargy, coma, other alterations in sensorium
   f) New psychiatric symptoms
2) Past medical history
   a) Current or preexisting diseases/illness
      (1) Recent viral illness or herpes zoster
      (2) Immune disorders
   b) Recent animal or tick bite
   c) Travel history; season of year
   d) Medications
   e) Allergies
   f) Immunization status
   b. Objective data collection
1) Physical examination
   a) General appearance
      (1) Level of consciousness, behavior, affect: confusion, seizures, comatose
      (2) Elevated temperature
      (3) Moderate to severe distress, critically ill
   b) Inspection
      (1) Rash specific to cause
      (2) Abnormal muscle movements
      (3) Meningismus
      (4) Focal neurologic findings
   c) Palpation/percussion
      (1) Altered reflexes
2) Diagnostic procedures
   a) CBC with differential: results variable, depending on cause
   b) Blood cultures
   c) Serum chemistries
   d) Viral serology: aid in identifying arbovirus
   e) Coagulation profile
   f) Urinalysis; pregnancy test in female patients of childbearing age

Part 2

g) Lumbar puncture
h) Head CT scan, MRI
i) EEG
j) ECG

2. Analysis: differential nursing diagnoses/collaborative problems
   a. Risk for injury
   b. Risk for ineffective airway clearance
   c. Impaired verbal communication
3. Planning and implementation/interventions
   a. Maintain airway, breathing, circulation (see Chapter 1)
   b. Provide supplemental oxygen
      1) RSI and ventilatory support in patient with compromised airway
      2) High-flow oxygen
   c. Establish IV access for administration of medications/crystalloid fluid
      1) Minimize fluid overload to avoid cerebral edema
   d. Prepare for/assist with medical interventions
      1) Institute standard precautions and isolation until causative agent identified
      2) Advanced airway management
         a) Nasal or oral intubation
         b) Supraglottic airway (e.g., King, Combitube, laryngeal mask airway)
         c) Surgical airway (e.g., cricothyrotomy)
      3) Elevate head of bed 30 degrees
      4) Institute seizure precautions
      5) Institute cardiac and pulse oximetry monitoring
      6) Insert gastric tube as indicated
      7) Insert indwelling urinary catheter as indicated
      8) Maintain normothermic body temperature
      9) Assist with hospital admission
   e. Administer pharmacologic therapy as ordered
      1) RSI premedications: sedatives, analgesics, neuromuscular blocking agents
      2) Antibiotics
      3) Antivirals
      4) Steroids
      5) Diuretics
4. Evaluation and ongoing monitoring
   a. Airway patency
   b. Level of consciousness
   c. Hemodynamic status
   d. Breath sounds and pulse oximetry
   e. Cardiac rate and rhythm
   f. Intake and output

Bibliography

Bess M, Prevatte ED: Diagnosing and treating scabies, *Emergency Medicine* 35(3):52–56, 2003.

Bickley LS: *Bates' guide to physical examination and history taking*, ed 11, Philadelphia, PA, 2013, Lippincott.

Centers for Disease Control and Prevention: Adult and pediatric immunization schedule, 2015.

Centers for Disease Control and Prevention: Ebola virus disease. Retrieved from http://www.cdc.gov/vhf/ebola/about.html, 2015.

Centers for Disease Control and Prevention: Mumps. Retrieved from http://www.cdc.gov/mumps/index.html, 2015.

Centers for Disease Control and Prevention: Pertussis (whooping cough). Retrieved from http://www.cdc.gov/pertussis/index.html, 2015.

Centers for Disease Control and Prevention: Severe acute respiratory syndrome. Retrieved from http://www.cdc.gov/sars/index.html, 2015.

Cunha BA: Update on SARS, *Emergency Medicine* 35(5):23–28, 2003.

EBSCO DynaMed [online database]. Retrieved from http://www.ebscohost.com/dynamed, Accessed November 1.

Fleisher GR, Ludoig S: *Textbook of pediatric emergency medicine*, ed 4, Philadelphia, PA, 2000, Lippincott.

Kamps BS, Hoffman C: *SARS reference.* Retrieved from http://www.sarsreference.com, 2003.

Kasper DL, Braunwald E, Fauci AS, Hauser SL, Lango DL, Jameson JL: In *Harrison's principles of internal medicine*, ed 16, New York, NY, 2005, McGraw-Hill.

Mumps. (n.d.): EBSCO DynaMed [online database]. Retrieved from http://www.ebscohost.com/dynamed.

Newberry LN: *Sheehy's emergency nursing principles and practice*, ed 5, St. Louis, MO, 2003, Mosby.

Rosen R, Barkin RM: *Emergency medicine: concepts and clinical practice*, ed 4, St. Louis, MO, 2002, Mosby.

Tintinalli JE, Krome RL, Ruiz E: *Emergency medicine: a comprehensive study guide*, ed 4, New York, NY, 2004, McGraw-Hill.

Varicella-zoster virus: EBSCO DynaMed [online database]. Retrieved from http://www.ebscohost.com/dynamed.

World Health Organization: (n.d.). Clinical management of severe acute respiratory infections when novel coronavirus is suspected: what to do and what not to do. Retrieved from http://www.who.int/csr/disease/coronavirus_infections/InterimGuidance_ClinicalManagement_NovelCoronavirus_11Feb13u.pdf.

World Health Organization: (n.d.). Middle East respiratory syndrome coronavirus (MERS-CoV): summary of current situation, literature update and risk assessment. Retrieved from http://www.who.int/emergencies/mers-cov/en/.

CHAPTER 21

Medical Emergencies

Teri Arruda, DNP, FNP-BC, CEN

I. General Strategy

A. ASSESSMENT

1. Primary and secondary assessment/resuscitation (see Chapter 1)
2. Focused survey
   a. Subjective data collection
      1) History of present illness/chief complaint
         a) Pain: PQRST (see Chapter 8)
         b) Injury: mechanism (see Chapter 31) and time
         c) Fatigue, malaise, appetite changes
         d) Joint pain, muscle ache, weakness
         e) Nausea, vomiting, diarrhea, anorexia
         f) Altered mental status or decreased level of consciousness
         g) Fever
         h) Cough, dyspnea
         i) Rash, urticaria, pruritus
         j) Edema: location and type
         k) Sore throat
         l) Efforts to relieve symptoms
            (1) Home remedies or OTC medications
            (2) Alternative therapies/homeopathic remedies
            (3) Prescribed medications
               (a) Prescriptions
               (b) OTC/herbal
      2) Past medical history
         a) Current or preexisting diseases/illness
            (1) Cardiovascular disease
            (2) Diabetes

            (3) History of substance abuse or alcoholism
            (4) Sickle cell anemia
            (5) Hemophilia
            (6) Splenectomy: alters immune response
            (7) Recent or past history of infectious process such as a viral, bacterial, fungal, rickettsial, or parasitic infection
            (8) Current medications
            (9) Last menstrual period for women of childbearing years
      3) Psychological/social/environmental factors
         a) Age: illness more severe in very young and elderly
         b) Family history
         c) Gender: some disorders are gender linked
         d) Race: may determine increased incidence
         e) Lifestyle
      4) Nutritional status: under- or overnourished
      5) Assault, abuse, or intimate partner violence situations (see Chapters 3 and 40)
   b. Objective data collection
      1) General appearance
         a) Level of consciousness, behavior, affect
         b) Vital signs
         c) Odors
         d) Gait
         e) Hygiene
         f) Weight
         g) Level of distress/discomfort
      2) Inspection
         a) Neck veins

b) Skin: color
c) Rash or urticaria
d) Mucous membranes
e) Evidence of injury
f) Areas of erythema
g) Cardiac dysrhythmias on monitor
3) Auscultation
a) Breath sounds: clear, wheezes, crackles
b) Bowel sounds: normal, hyperactive, hypoactive, absent
c) Heart sounds: S_1 and S_2, other sounds (e.g., murmurs)
4) Palpation/percussion
a) Sinus: tenderness
b) Areas of tenderness
c) Skin: temperature, moisture, turgor
d) Areas of hyperthermia
e) Arteries: equality of peripheral pulses
f) Veins: venous filling and varicosities
g) Lymph nodes
h) Chest: note tone of percussion
i) Abdomen: areas of dullness
3. Diagnostic procedures
a. Laboratory studies
1) Complete blood count (CBC) with differential
2) Serum chemistries including glucose, BUN, creatinine
3) Urinalysis; pregnancy test in female patients of childbearing age
4) Arterial blood gases (ABGs)
5) Erythrocyte sedimentation rate (ESR)
6) Serum and urine toxicology screen: therapeutic drug levels and toxic ingestion
7) Clotting profile: partial thromboplastin time (PTT), prothrombin time (PT)
8) Type and crossmatch
9) Serum ammonia level
10) Carboxyhemoglobin level
11) Serum uric acid level
12) Liver enzyme levels
13) Sickle cell screen
14) Hepatitis screen
15) Serum ketone levels
16) Thyroid function tests
17) Cerebrospinal fluid (CSF): cell count, glucose and protein count, culture
b. Imaging studies
1) Chest radiograph
2) Computed tomography (CT) scan
3) Magnetic resonance imaging (MRI)
c. Other
1) 12- to 15-lead electrocardiogram (ECG)
2) Electroencephalogram (EEG)
3) Arthrocentesis

B. ANALYSIS: DIFFERENTIAL NURSING DIAGNOSES/COLLABORATIVE PROBLEMS

1. Ineffective airway clearance
2. Impaired gas exchange
3. Decreased cardiac output
4. Deficient/excess fluid volume
5. Ineffective tissue perfusion
6. Anxiety/fear
7. Fatigue
8. Impaired skin integrity
9. Deficient knowledge
10. Impaired memory
11. Ineffective coping
12. Acute/chronic pain
13. Risk for infection
14. Risk for injury
15. Disturbed sleep patterns

C. PLANNING AND IMPLEMENTATION/INTERVENTIONS

1. Determine priorities of care
a. Maintain airway, breathing, circulation (see Chapter 1)
b. Provide supplemental oxygen as indicated
c. Establish intravenous (IV) access for administration of crystalloid fluid/medications as needed
d. Obtain and set up equipment and supplies
e. Prepare for/assist with medical procedures
f. Administer pharmacologic therapy as ordered
2. Relieve anxiety/apprehension
3. Allow significant others to remain with patient if supportive
4. Educate patient/significant others

D. EVALUATION AND ONGOING MONITORING

1. Continuously monitor and treat as indicated
2. Monitor patient's responses/outcomes, and modify nursing care plan as appropriate
3. If positive patient outcomes are not demonstrated, reevaluate assessment and/or plan of care

E. DOCUMENTATION OF INTERVENTIONS AND PATIENT RESPONSE

F. AGE-RELATED CONSIDERATIONS

1. Pediatric
a. Growth or development related
1) Dehydration occurs rapidly because of a smaller volume of fluid, large body surface area, and increased metabolic rate
2) Higher metabolic rate increases the use of glucose/glycogen stores

3) Neonates, infants, and toddlers are more susceptible to illness because of their immature immune system

b. "Pearls"

1) Lack of social smile is the single most significant indicator for a potentially ill child
2) Pediatric patients are unable to care for themselves during illness
3) Inspect neonates before touching them to diminish the startle response
4) Degree of fever does not reflect severity of illness
5) Administer medication dosages based on child's weight

2. Geriatric

a. Aging related

1) Increased incidence of osteoporosis, osteoarthritis, joint cartilage atrophy, gout
2) Immune system is compromised, leading to an increased risk of infection
3) Reserve capacity for responding to stress decreases

b. "Pearls"

1) Infections may manifest with a fall or generalized weakness, rather than with fever or elevated white blood cell (WBC) count
2) Subtle changes in orientation, appetite, or mood can indicate a medical problem

II. Specific Medical Emergencies

A. ALLERGIC REACTION/ ANAPHYLAXIS

The true incidence of anaphylaxis is unknown, partly because of the lack of a precise definition of the syndrome. The frequency of anaphylaxis is increasing, and this has been attributed to the increased number of potential allergens to which people are exposed. As many as 500–1,000 fatal cases of anaphylaxis per year are estimated to occur in the United States.

Minor allergic reactions are frequently associated with the onset of skin manifestations such as urticaria (hives) and pruritus. Often, the offending allergen is not identified, and the cutaneous reactions are usually self-limiting. The more serious reaction of anaphylaxis refers to a life-threatening condition in which prominent dermal and systemic signs and symptoms manifest. The full-blown syndrome includes urticaria and/or angioedema with hypotension and bronchospasm. More than 90% of patients have some combination of urticaria, erythema, pruritus, or angioedema. The classic form, described in 1902, involves prior sensitization to an allergen with later reexposure producing symptoms by an immunologic mechanism. An anaphylactoid reaction produces a very similar clinical syndrome but is not immune mediated. Anaphylaxis presents a true medical emergency and must be rapidly assessed and treated.

In anaphylaxis, there is a rapid onset of increased secretion from mucous membranes, increased bronchial smooth muscle tone, decreased vascular smooth muscle tone, and increased capillary permeability occurring after exposure to an inciting substance. These effects are produced by the release of mediators, which include histamine, leukotriene C_4, prostaglandin D_2, and tryptase. In the classic form, mediator release occurs almost immediately when the antigen (allergen) binds to antigen-specific immunoglobulin E (IgE) attached to previously sensitized basophils and mast cells. In an anaphylactoid reaction, exposure to an inciting substance causes direct release of mediators, a process that is not mediated by IgE. Increased mucous secretion, increased bronchial smooth muscle tone, and airway edema contribute to the respiratory symptoms observed in anaphylaxis. Cardiovascular effects result from decreased vascular tone and capillary leakage. Histamine release in skin causes urticarial skin lesions. Itchy eyes with tearing and conjunctival injection are common.

The most common inciting agents in anaphylaxis are parenteral antibiotics (especially penicillins), IV contrast materials, Hymenoptera stings (wasps, hornets, yellow jackets, and fire ants), and certain foods (most notably, peanuts). Oral medications and many other types of exposures also have been implicated. Anaphylaxis may occur in a patient with no prior history of drug exposure. Anaphylaxis also may be idiopathic. Parenteral exposures tend to result in faster and more severe reactions. The faster a reaction develops, the more severe it is likely to be. Although most reactions occur within hours, symptoms may not occur for as long as 3–4 days after exposure.

1. Assessment

a. Subjective data collection

1) History of present illness/chief complaint

a) Description of precipitating event if known (i.e., sting, ingestion, or contact with allergen)
b) Location of allergen contact
c) Elapsed time since contact
d) Patient/family allergy history
e) Shortness of breath
f) Vomiting
g) Abdominal cramping; diarrhea
h) Pruritus
i) Irritated areas
j) Prehospital care

2) Past medical history

a) Current or preexisting diseases/illness
b) Medications
c) Common allergens to consider

(1) Medications

(a) Penicillin and cephalosporin antibiotics are the most commonly reported medical agents in anaphylaxis. However, history of penicillin or cephalosporin allergy often is unreliable and not predictive of future reactions

    (b) Aspirin and other NSAIDs are commonly implicated in allergic reactions and anaphylaxis

  (2) IV radiocontrast media

    (a) Shellfish or "iodine allergy" is not a contraindication to use IV contrast and does not mandate a pretreatment regimen

    (b) Term "iodine allergy" is a misnomer. Iodine is an essential trace element present throughout the body. No one is allergic to iodine. Patients who report iodine allergy usually have had either a prior contrast reaction or a shellfish allergy

    (c) Approximately 1–3% of patients who receive hyperosmolar IV contrast experience a reaction. Use of LMW contrast decreases the incidence of reactions to approximately 0.5%

  (3) Hymenoptera stings (see Chapter 14)

    (a) Hymenoptera stings: common cause of allergic reaction and anaphylaxis

  (4) Other allergens

    (a) Common food allergens: nuts (especially peanuts), legumes, fish, shellfish, milk, eggs

    (b) Latex

b. Objective data collection

  1) Physical examination

    a) General appearance

      (1) Level of consciousness, behavior, affect: dizziness, anxiety, restlessness, disorientation, seizure, coma

      (2) Tachypnea, stridor, hypotension, tachycardia, bradycardia, cyanosis

      (3) Mild to severe distress/discomfort

    b) Inspection

      (1) Angioedema: marked edema of the tongue and lips

      (2) Reddened skin areas

      (3) Localized erythema and edema

      (4) Urticaria

      (5) Conjunctivitis

    c) Auscultation

      (1) Adventitious breath sounds such as wheezing

      (2) Vocal hoarseness

2. Analysis: differential nursing diagnoses/collaborative problems

  a. Risk for ineffective airway clearance

  b. Pain

  c. Anxiety/fear

  d. Deficient knowledge

3. Planning and implementation/interventions

  a. If anaphylaxis

    1) Maintain airway, breathing, circulation (see Chapter 1)

      a) Initiate or continue Basic Life Support (BLS) and Advanced Life Support (ALS) per protocols if respiratory/cardiac compromise is present

    2) Provide supplemental oxygen

      a) RSI and ventilatory support in airway-compromised patients

      b) High-flow oxygen

    3) Establish large-bore IV access for administration of ACLS crystalloid fluids/medications

    4) Prepare for/assist with medical procedures

      a) Advanced airway management

        (1) Nasal or oral intubation

        (2) Supraglottic airway (e.g., King, Combitube, laryngeal mask airway)

        (3) Surgical airway (e.g., cricothyrotomy)

      b) Institute cardiac and pulse oximetry monitoring

      c) Insert gastric tube and attach to suction

      d) Insert indwelling urinary catheter

      e) Maintain normothermic body temperature

      f) Assist with hospital admission

    5) Administer pharmacologic therapy as ordered, which may include the following

      a) RSI premedications: sedatives, analgesics, neuromuscular blocking agents if intubation required

      b) Epinephrine: subcutaneous for allergic responses; may be given intravenous for life-threatening anaphylaxis

      c) ACLS medications per protocols

      d) Antihistamine diphenhydramine (Benadryl)

      e) Histamine-$_2$ blockers (e.g., ranitidine [Zantac], cimetidine [Tagamet])

      f) Corticosteroids (e.g., methylprednisolone [Solu-Medrol]) especially useful to treat refractory bronchospasm; onset of action is delayed for several hours

      g) Inhaled beta-agonists for bronchospasm (e.g., albuterol [Proventil, Ventolin])

      h) Glucagon is useful in patients taking beta blockers who have hypotension refractory to fluids and in patients taking epinephrine because it increases intracellular cyclic adenosine monophosphate (cAMP) levels

      i) If severe bronchospasm continues after therapy with epinephrine and bronchodilators, administer aminophylline

Part 2

j) Vasopressors with alpha-adrenergic activity such as levarterenol (Levophed) or dopamine (Intropin) may be considered in patients with refractory hypotension

b. Minor reaction with cutaneous involvement
   1) Administer pharmacologic therapy as ordered
      a) Diphenhydramine (Benadryl)
      b) Epinephrine: subcutaneous injection
      c) Cimetidine (Tagamet)
      d) Hydroxyzine (Atarax, Vistaril)
   2) Educate patient/significant others
      a) Avoid allergic stimulus, if known
c. If localized reaction: treat site of contact (see Chapter 15)
   1) Prepare for/assist with medical procedures
      a) Keep affected part at rest
      b) Remove insect stinger, if present, by scraping action; avoid pinching to minimize releases of additional venom
      c) Apply cool packs to area
      d) Wash site with mild antiseptic soap and water
   2) Administer pharmacologic therapy as ordered
      a) Apply paste of papain using meat tenderizer to inactivate venom
      b) Tetanus immunization
   3) Educate patient/significant others
      a) Apply cold, as needed
      b) Observe for signs of infection
      c) Situations to avoid
         (1) Use of perfumes, sprays, brightly colored clothing, and sweet, sticky substances because these attract insects
         (2) Extensive skin exposure, especially around the neck
         (3) Lying down or sitting in areas with many flowers, trees, and bushes
         (4) Going barefoot
      d) Obtain and familiarize self with emergency insect bite kit and administration of Epi-pen
      e) Encourage patient to wear Medic-Alert bracelet
      f) May benefit from carrying Epi-pen on person, vehicle, and school/work settings
4. Evaluation and ongoing monitoring
   a. Airway patency
   b. Level of consciousness
   c. Hemodynamic status
   d. Breath sounds and pulse oximetry
   e. Cardiac rate and rhythm
   f. Intake and output
   g. Urticaria changes

B. CHRONIC FATIGUE SYNDROME

Chronic fatigue syndrome (CFS) or systemic exertion intolerance disease (SEID) is a disease of unknown origin, although an infectious viral disease has been implicated. The patient presents with a history of fatigue of more than 6 months' duration despite being well rested. Also there must be the presence of four or more of the following symptoms: substantial impairment in short-term memory or concentration; sore throat; low-grade fever; tender lymph nodes; muscle pain; multiple-joint pain without swelling or redness; headaches of a new type, pattern, or severity; insomnia or hypersomnia; and postexertional malaise lasting more than 24 hours. Verbal dyslexia may be present; patients are unable to find the correct words and express themselves as they desire. CFS is more common in the United States than in other countries and is seen most commonly in young to middle-aged women. Persons presenting with symptoms need to rule out other chronic conditions such as malignancy, autoimmune disease, endocrinopathy, or chronic psychiatric disorders. Excluding other life-threatening illnesses becomes the focus of emergency department care; once accomplished, referral to appropriate subspecialties is critical for patient follow-up and support.

1. Assessment
   a. Subjective data collection
      1) History of present illness/chief complaint
         a) Fatigue longer than 6 months
         b) Occurs despite rest and sleep
      2) Cognitive difficulties
         a) Short-term memory problems
         b) Verbal dyslexia
         c) Frustration with the inability to accomplish everyday tasks
      3) Past medical history
         a) Current or preexisting diseases/ illness
            (1) Depression
         b) Active infection may have preceded the onset
            (1) Possible history of EBV infection or infectious mononucleosis
            (2) Patients may not remember this antecedent infection
         c) Medications
         d) Allergies
   b. Objective data collection
      1) Physical examination
         a) General appearance
            (1) Level of consciousness, behavior, affect: subdued behavior, depressed
            (2) Mild to moderate distress/discomfort
         b) Inspection
            (1) Crimson crescents on anterior pillars of tonsils
         c) Palpation
            (1) Small, movable nontender lymph nodes in neck, axilla, inguinal areas
      2) Diagnostic procedures
         a) Antibody titers
            (1) IgG VCA EBV titer and *Chlamydia pneumoniae* titer: may be elevated; not diagnostic for CFS
         b) CBC, chemistry, ESR

      c) Thyroid and adrenal function tests to rule out causative disease

      d) Head CT scan may demonstrate hypoperfusion of frontoparietal areas of brain

2. Analysis: differential nursing diagnoses/collaborative problems
   a. Fatigue
   b. Risk of infection
3. Planning and implementation/interventions
   a. Prepare for/assist with medical procedures
      1) Rule out organic diseases
         a) Hypothyroidism, adrenal insufficiency, malignant disease, Lyme disease, acquired immunodeficiency syndrome, liver and/or renal disease
      2) Initiate consultation with infectious disease specialists
   b. Educate patient/significant others
      1) Provide support for emotional impact of disease
      2) Inform patient that exacerbations are precipitated by stress, exercise
      3) Encourage rest
      4) Trials of antiviral agents and beta-carotene may be initiated by subspecialists
4. Evaluation and ongoing monitoring
   a. Level of consciousness
   b. Hemodynamic status

C. FEVER

Fever may accompany bacterial, viral, rickettsial, and parasitic infections, as well as neoplasms, diseases of the immune system, vascular inflammation, acute metabolic disorders, tissue infarction, and trauma. Infection is possible when fever is associated with abrupt onset of respiratory symptoms, nausea, vomiting and diarrhea, severe malaise, myalgias, arthralgias, acute enlargement of lymph nodes and spleen, meningeal signs, leukocyte count >12,000/mm^3 or <5,000/mm^3, dysuria or flank pain, rash, or cellulitis.

Tissue inflammation in response to bacteria causes release of histamine, bradykinin, and serotonin, which increases the local blood flow and permeability of capillaries. Large quantities of leaked fluid, protein, and fibrinogen form a clot around injured tissue and isolate the area. Some bacteria are walled off quickly because of extreme tissue toxicity. Others migrate throughout the body before isolation can occur. Neutrophilia (leukocytosis) occurs within a few hours as a result of release from inflamed tissue of leukocytosis-inducing factor, which stimulates increased bone marrow production of neutrophils. Infants between 1 and 28 days old, elderly persons, and immunosuppressed patients with either a fever or a subnormal temperature should be presumed to have a serious bacterial infection.

Fever is present in a child when the rectal temperature is >100.4°F (38°C). A child's core temperature normally varies by as much as 1–1.5°F (0.5–0.8°C) throughout the day, and increases may occur with or without pathologic processes.

Prostaglandins mediate the set point for heat regulation in the human body. Their effects are seen in the hypothalamus and affect the body's response to heat by altering vascular constriction and other heat production and/or release mechanisms. Pyrogens release prostaglandin E$_1$ and D$_2$. Pyrogens are low-molecular-weight (LMW) proteins produced by leukocytes. Of the pediatric visits to a general emergency department, fever appears to be a complaint of almost one half of the patients examined. An occult life-threatening event occurs in approximately 1% of children presenting to an acute care setting with fever. Serious bacterial infections include meningitis, bacteremia or sepsis, enteritis, pneumonia, pericarditis, osteomyelitis, septic arthritis, or cellulitis. Febrile patients may present with other common bacterial illnesses, such as otitis media, pharyngitis, sinusitis, urinary tract infections, enteritis, and appendicitis, or with viral illnesses, such as upper respiratory infections, bronchiolitis, enteroviral exanthems, gastroenteritis, and flulike illnesses.

Fevers may occur in any age group. Neonates (<28 days old) and young infants (<60 days old) have traditionally been grouped as one subset of pediatric febrile patients. Children younger than 24 months of age are another subset of febrile patients. The evaluation of any neonate should include documentation of the presence or absence of rectal temperature changes. Ear-probe thermometer readings may not be as accurate as rectal thermometer readings in the neonate. Some studies suggest that operator error is the main reason for inaccuracy with the ear-probe thermometer. A rectal-probe thermometer is recommended for obtaining an accurate assessment of a younger pediatric patient's temperature.

When presenting with fever, neonates and infants are considered at risk for sepsis until proven otherwise. This age group has been traditionally described as being at greater risk than older children for two reasons. First, their bacterial pathogens may be different from those in older children. Second, their immune systems are less able than those of older children to compartmentalize infection. Not all septic neonates present with fever and may even be hypothermic on presentation. Other potential signs and symptoms of sepsis unique to infancy should also be assessed, such as poor feeding, irritability, and lethargy. A physical finding of an isolated bacterial illness, such as otitis media or pneumonia, should not preclude pursuing a more extensive workup to exclude sepsis in the neonate.

Guidelines have been applied to neonatal emergency medicine. Traditionally, a febrile neonate (temperature >100.4°F [>38.0°C]) undergoes a full sepsis workup, such as CBC, one blood culture, chest radiography, urinalysis, and urine culture (obtained by catheter or suprapubic bladder aspiration), and diagnostic lumbar puncture (LP) for CSF analysis.

Occult bacteremia, elevated temperature with no identifiable signs or symptoms, occurred in approximately 3–5% of children younger than 24 months during the 1980s and 1990s. Since the 1990s, there has been a decline in those rates as a result of pneumococcal and *Haemophilus influenzae B* vaccinations.

Some pediatric patients may have had a subjective determination of an elevated temperature by their caregivers before coming to the hospital but are afebrile when they present to the emergency department. Parents may report a temperature elevation in their child without having actually recorded the temperature with a thermometer. Parental reporting of fever on the basis of subjective information (e.g., touching the child's torso or extremities or feeling his or her forehead) is a reliable indicator that a fever was present. Studies have shown that parental assessment of fever in this situation is usually accurate.

Evaluation of appropriate weight-based administration of antipyretics provides a valuable parental teaching opportunity. Over-the-counter medications do not always list the correct weight-based dose for children younger than 2 years. Some simply state, "call physician" or "seek medical care." Parents should be educated that the frequent weight changes of their child will result in a need to recalculate dosages to ensure appropriate dosing of antipyretics.

Noninfectious causes of fever include environmental factors such as high external temperature, overbundling of children, malignant diseases, rheumatoid diseases, and recent immunization administration. Anecdotal evidence suggests that teething may be associated with random temperature elevations, although some authors may disagree.

Febrile seizures generally occur between 5 months and 5 years; peak incidence is between 8 and 20 months. Fever increases the irritability of neurons and makes young patients more sensitive to seizures because of their immature nervous systems. Seizures result from the rapidity with which the temperature rises, rather than from the actual temperature level.

1. Assessment
   a. Subjective data collection
      1) History of present illness/chief complaint
         a) Onset of fever and associated symptoms
            (1) Rapid
            (2) Slow
         b) Prodrome
         c) Previous similar episode
         d) Pain (see Chapter 8)
            (1) Ear and throat
            (2) Chest or pleuritic
            (3) Abdomen
            (4) Headache
            (5) Dysuria
            (6) Myalgias and arthralgias
         e) Seizure
         f) Nausea or vomiting and diarrhea
         g) Rash
         h) Illness of other family members or friends
         i) In children, question level of activity, social overtures, eye contact, reaction to strangers, fluid intake, stool patterns, sleep pattern changes, and birth history if appropriate
         j) Recent travel to another country
         k) Recent immunizations
            (1) Administration of the diphtheria, tetanus, pertussis (DTP) vaccine may cause fever within a few hours and may persist up to 48 hours
            (2) Administration of live virus vaccinations such as the measles, mumps, rubella (MMR) vaccine may result in temperature elevations up to 7–10 days after administration of the vaccine
         l) Recent surgical or other invasive procedure
         m) Ingestion of untreated water
      2) Past medical history
         a) Current or preexisting diseases/illness
         b) Recent exposure to illness/communicable disease
         c) Last normal menstrual period: female patients of childbearing age
         d) Medications
         e) Allergies
         f) Immunization status
   b. Objective data collection
      1) Physical examination
         a) General appearance
            (1) Level of consciousness, behavior, affect
               (a) Lethargy: defined as a decrease in the level of consciousness; characterized by failure of the child to recognize parents or caregivers, absent eye contact with the examiner, and failure to interact with the environment at an age-appropriate level
               (b) Seizure or postictal
            (2) Cyanosis or other signs of respiratory distress
            (3) Tachycardia, tachypnea, dyspnea, grunting, nasal flaring or retractions: tachypnea remains the most sensitive indicator of lower respiratory tract infection and may indicate underlying acidosis
            (4) Elevated or subnormal temperature
            (5) Mild to severe distress/discomfort, possibly critically ill
         b) Inspection
            (1) Level of hydration: exhibited by dry mucous membranes, sunken fontanels, absence of tears when crying, and/or lack of urine output
            (2) Meningeal signs: Kernig sign (pain in lower back and inability to completely straighten leg while supine) or Brudzinski sign (involuntary flexion of the arm, hip, and knee with passive flexion of the neck)

(3) Local skin infections or lesions with secondary infection

(4) Rash: petechial or nonpetechial; hemorrhagic rash is classically described as the result of an overwhelming systemic bacterial infection caused by meningococcemia

(5) Inflammation of ears and pharynx

(6) Genital discharge

  c) Auscultation

(1) Breath sounds: crackles, decreased and/or abnormal breath sounds, wheezing

(2) Bowel sounds

  d) Palpation/percussion

(1) Poor perfusion as evidenced by delayed capillary refill; rapid, early assessment of hypoperfusion. A delay in capillary refill time of greater than 3 seconds indicates hypoperfusion

(2) Abdominal tenderness or guarding of the abdomen

(3) Nuchal rigidity

(4) Local hyperthermia, tenderness

(5) Tender cervix and adnexa

(6) Flank tenderness

 2) Diagnostic procedures

  a) CBC with differential: WBC elevated

  b) Urinalysis; pregnancy test in female patients of childbearing age

  c) Serum chemistries including glucose, BUN, creatinine

  d) Cultures: blood, urine, wound, cervical, sputum, nasopharyngeal, joint fluid

  e) Chest and abdominal radiographs; in the neonate and young infant, chest radiograph is a routine part of a septic workup

  f) Lumbar puncture as indicated

(1) Performed with first-time seizure before 12 months of age or temperature 106°F (41°C) or higher

(2) Indicated for adults with nuchal rigidity, headache, and fever of unknown origin

(3) Child who remains irritable and lethargic after aggressive antipyretic therapy

2. Analysis: differential nursing diagnoses/collaborative problems

  a. Risk for infection

  b. Risk for deficient fluid volume

  c. Risk for injury

  d. Deficient knowledge

3. Planning and implementation/interventions

  a. Maintain airway, breathing, circulation (see Chapter 1)

  b. Provide supplemental oxygen as indicated

  c. Establish IV access to administer crystalloid fluids/medications as needed

  d. Prepare for/assist with medical procedures

    1) Institute cardiac and pulse oximetry monitoring

    2) Insert indwelling urinary catheter as indicated

    3) Maintain normothermic body temperature: initiate cooling measures such as undressing child

    4) Pelvic examination

    5) Lumbar puncture

    6) Elevate and immobilize cellulitic extremity

    7) Protect patient from physical injury (e.g., side rails up and locked)

    8) Assist with hospital admission of infants and elderly patients if no definitive source of fever or infection is identified

  e. Administer pharmacologic therapy as prescribed such as

    1) Acetaminophen (Tylenol) or ibuprofen (Advil, Motrin) to control temperature >101°F (>38.3°C)

    2) Antibiotics

    3) IV dextrose for treatment of hypoglycemia

    4) IV anticonvulsants for status epilepticus: diazepam (Valium), lorazepam (Ativan), phenobarbital, phenytoin (Dilantin), or fosphenytoin (Cerebyx)

  f. Educate patient/significant others

    1) Fever control measures

    2) Temperature elevations may occur without infectious cause: antibiotics not always required

    3) Medications prescribed may include antipyretics, antibiotics, anticonvulsants, antiemetics

    4) Need for adequate fluid replacement to prevent dehydration

    5) Signs and symptoms that necessitate return to emergency care setting

      a) Inability to control fever

      b) Recurrence of seizures

      c) Change in mental status

      d) Illness does not improve or increases in severity

4. Evaluation and ongoing monitoring

  a. Level of consciousness

  b. Hemodynamic status

  c. Temperature control

  d. Breath sounds and pulse oximetry

  e. Cardiac rate and rhythm

  f. Intake and output

  g. Seizure activity

D. FIBROMYALGIA

Fibromyalgia is characterized by chronic widespread pain, fatigue, and multiple somatic symptoms and is more common in women 20–50 years of age. Biochemical changes are seen in the central nervous system that leads to hypersensitivity to pain and abnormal processing of painful stimuli. The cause remains unknown; however, there are many theories. Often patients present to the emergency department in acute pain with complaints of cognitive difficulties. Determining the diagnosis and best management course is recommended in a nonemergency setting, in which consistent follow-up and continuity of care can be maintained.

1. Assessment
   a. Subjective data collection
      1) History of present illness/chief complaint
         a) Pain (see Chapter 8)
            (1) Often described as burning, exhausting
            (2) Covers large muscle areas
            (3) Multiple tender points when tested
            (4) Onset: recent or ongoing (longer than 3 months)
            (5) Location: regional or generalized
         b) Fatigue
            (1) Often associated with poor sleep
      2) Past medical history
         a) Current or preexisting diseases/illness
         b) Memory problems
         c) Medications
         d) Allergies
   b. Objective data collection
      1) Physical examination
         a) Pain in more than 11 of 18 tender points as tested with dolorimeter
      2) Diagnostic procedures
         a) Appropriate laboratory studies to rule out other disease processes (e.g., hypothyroidism, rheumatoid arthritis [RA])
         b) Serotonin levels: abnormally low
2. Analysis: differential nursing diagnoses/collaborative problems
   a. Activity intolerance
   b. Chronic pain
   c. Impaired physical mobility
   d. Self-care deficit
3. Planning and implementation/interventions
   a. Administer pharmacologic therapy as ordered
      1) Antidepressants: amitriptyline (Elavil)
      2) Analgesics: NSAIDs, tramadol (Ultram)
      3) Skeletal muscle relaxants
      4) Anticonvulsants: gabapentin (Neurontin for pain)
      5) Dextromethorphan
   b. Educate patient/significant others
      1) Encourage physical therapies: massage, exercise, heat
      2) Teach patient about control of disease
         a) Symptoms may be triggered by stressors
         b) Avoid changes in diet
         c) Exercise as directed
         d) Patient should pace activities and know limits
         e) Lack of sleep or poor sleep will worsen symptoms

4. Referral to appropriate subspecialties: rheumatologist, psychologist, psychiatrist, neurologist
5. Evaluation and ongoing monitoring
   a. Pain relief

E. GOUT/PSEUDOGOUT

Gout and pseudogout can be debilitating conditions from the joint pain and inflammation that results from the overproduction or reduced secretion of uric acid. The goal of therapy is to intervene early and prevent permanent damage to the joints. This leads to the formation of crystals in the joint spaces. Gout and pseudogout are often indistinguishable in their presentations. They both can be caused by several factors which include lead poisoning, hemoproliferative disorders, and renal disease. Often the initial treatment for either condition is the same. Antiinflammatory agents are key.

Gout has been associated with a large number of different autoimmune and metabolic disorders. Three stages of gout typically occur: first is the asymptomatic hyperuricemia, then the acute gout, followed by the tophaceous gout. The most common first presentation of gout or gouty arthritis is typically seen at the first metatarsophalangeal joint (great toe). Males often present with gout 9 to 1 over females. It is common to recognize tophi or extra-articular deposits of MSU along the Achilles tendon, the ear helix, olecranon bursa, or repealer bursa. Treating the underlying disorders is key.

Pseudogout is joint inflammation that is caused by calcium pyrophosphate crystals. It has been associated with aging, trauma, and metabolic abnormalities such as hyperparathyroidism and hemochromatosis. Often the presentation is clinically indistinguishable from gout. Several other conditions can also present in similar ways such as acute monoarticular arthritis and septic arthritis (see Table 21.1). Unfortunately, there are no specific therapeutic regimens to treat the underlying causes of pseudogout.

1. Assessment
   a. Subjective data collection
      1) History of present illness/chief complaint
         a) Pain (see Chapter 8)
            (1) Location
               (a) First episode: spontaneous onset of pain, edema, and inflammation; monoarticular, usually first metatarsophalangeal joint
               (b) Recurrent episodes: polyarticular, can affect insteps
               (c) Ankles, heels, knees, wrists, fingers, and elbows
               (d) Other joints rarely involved except in established disease
            (2) Timing/onset of pain: often at night
            (3) Characteristics of pain
               (a) Intolerable pain
               (b) Any clothing, movement, or weight bearing is intolerable

b) Fever
  (1) Low-grade fever is not uncommon with the first episode
2) Past medical history
  a) Current or preexisting diseases/illness
    (1) Hypertension
    (2) Hypertriglyceridemia
  b) Risk factors for cellulitis or septic arthritis versus gout such as gonorrhea, recent puncture wound over a joint, or systemic signs of infection
  c) Current medications
  d) Allergies
b. Objective data collection
  1) Physical examination
    a) General appearance
      (1) Elevated temperature
      (2) Gait: altered, reluctant to use extremity
      (3) Moderate distress/discomfort
    b) Inspection
      (1) Affected joint erythema
      (2) Affected joint edema
    c) Palpation
      (1) Hyperthermic area
      (2) Affected joint tenderness
  2) Diagnostic procedures
    a) Uric acid: normal to elevated as demonstrated
      (1) As >7 mg/dL in male patients
      (2) As >6 mg/dL in female patients
    b) Serum chemistries to include glucose, BUN, creatinine
    c) Thyroid function tests

d) Arthrocentesis: affected joint aspiration of synovial fluid may demonstrate the following results
  (1) Monosodium urate crystals in WBCs: WBC count in the joint fluid is usually 50,000–100,000 in crystal-induced arthritis
  (2) Joint fluid: analyzed for cell count and differential, Gram stain, culture and sensitivity, microscopic analysis for crystals in addition to WBCs; if crystals are seen, their shape and appearance under polarized light can aid in diagnosis
    (a) Gout: crystals of MSU appear as needle-shaped intracellular and extracellular crystals; they are yellow when aligned parallel to the axis of the red compensator, but turn blue when aligned across the direction of polarization
    (b) Pseudogout: CPP crystals do not change color depending on their alignment relative to the direction of the red compensator
e) Joint radiograph
  (1) Chronic gout: lesions may appear as rat-bitten, sclerotic regions on the joint surfaces with overhanging margins
  (2) New-onset acute gout: usually shows no radiographic findings
  (3) Pseudogout: degenerative joint changes and calcifications in the soft tissues, tendons, or bursa

Table 21.1

Comparison of Gout, Pseudogout, Monoarticular Arthritis, and Septic Arthritis

Gout	Pseudogout	Monoarticular Arthritis	Septic Arthritis
Spontaneous onset of pain Edema and inflammation in the metatarsophalangeal joint of the great toe are the most common presentations of gout Other common sites include the ankle, wrist, and knee Symptoms tend to develop rapidly over a few hours Patients with gout most often present with a single joint that is hot, erythematous, tender, and affected with asymmetrical edema Although uncommon, acute gout may present with signs of carpal tunnel syndrome	The most common sites of pseudogout arthritis are the knee, wrist, and shoulder There have been reports of documented carpal tunnel syndrome as the initial presentation of pseudogout The onset of symptoms in pseudogout is usually more insidious and may occur over several days	Consider this diagnosis in any patient with acute monarticular arthritis of any peripheral joint except the glenohumeral joint of the shoulder, in which crystal-induced arthritis is more likely to be the result of pseudogout Crystal-induced arthritis is most commonly monarticular; however, polyarticular acute flare-ups are not rare, and many different joints may be involved simultaneously or in rapid succession Multiple joints in the same limb are often involved, as when inflammation begins in the great toe and then progresses to involve the midfoot and ankle	Consider septic arthritis in patients presenting with fever, chills, and malaise who have a history of risk factors for cellulitis or septic arthritis Possible exposure to gonorrhea, a recent puncture wound over the joint, or systemic signs of disseminated infection are examples Even when a patient has a history of crystal-induced arthritis, the possibility of septic arthritis must always be considered Septic arthritis must be diagnosed and treated promptly; irreversible damage can occur within 4–6 hours, and the joint can be completely destroyed within 24–48 hours

f) Bone scan: increased nuclide concentration at affected sites

g) MRI: may be very useful in determining extent of the disease

(1) Used with gadolinium to evaluate tendon sheath involvement or, if possible, osteomyelitis

2. Analysis: differential nursing diagnoses/collaborative problems

a. Pain

b. Anxiety/fear

c. Deficient knowledge

3. Planning and implementation/interventions

a. Provider will consider medications with consideration of comorbidities, response to past treatments, and patient preferences

1) Initial treatment is a nonsteroidal antiinflammatory agent (NSAID)

2) Colchicine is an alternative for patients who cannot tolerate NSAIDs

3) Corticosteroids

4) Glucocorticoid intraarticular steroid injection

5) Oral glucocorticoids when injections are not an option secondary to polyarticular disease such as prednisone

6) IV glucocorticoids are generally used for those hospitalized patients who cannot tolerate oral medications or are not candidates for intraarticular injections

b. Educate patient/significant others

1) Explain disease process

2) Avoid precipitating factors: empower with each patient about education of disease control

a) Low-purine diet: suggest dietary consultation to reinforce education regarding common foods high in purine (e.g., heart, herring, mussels, yeast, salmon, sardines, anchovies, veal, bacon)

b) Stress importance of lifestyle changes: avoid alcohol consumption, healthy weight

3) Discuss signs and symptoms that require intervention such as exacerbation of disease with uncontrollable pain or concerning medication side effects

4) Encourage follow-up appointment with their health care provider

4. Evaluation and ongoing monitoring

a. Pain relief

F. REYE SYNDROME

Reye syndrome is an acute noninflammatory encephalopathy characterized by the triad of hepatic, metabolic, and neurologic dysfunction often following clinical symptom improvement after viral syndrome such as varicella or influenza A or B. Prevalence is more typical in the winter or spring. The peak ages of developing Reye syndrome

are 6 and 11 years. Six-year-old children are more likely to develop Reye syndrome following a varicella illness, whereas 11-year-old patients tend to develop the syndrome following influenza B illnesses. Cases have dramatically decreased since 1980 after aspirin was identified as a risk factor and advice was given not to use in febrile children with varicella or influenza.

The primary defect is mitochondrial injury. Glycogen stores are depleted as a result of starvation from prolonged vomiting and dysfunction of gluconeogenesis enzyme pathways. An alternative energy source is not available because fatty acid breakdown does not occur normally. Consequently, acids build up because the body cannot eliminate waste products effectively. The liver enzyme system that converts ammonia to urea is damaged, so ammonia also accumulates. Additionally, the liver and renal tubules become edematous and infiltrated with fat droplets. Fatty infiltrates develop in the heart, with petechiae throughout the epicardium. Hyperammonemia, hypoglycemia, and acidosis contribute to neurologic dysfunction, cerebral edema, and coma.

The manifestations of Reye syndrome are not unique to this syndrome. There is no test specific for Reye syndrome; therefore, diagnosis must be one of exclusion. Signs and symptoms of Reye syndrome correlate with illness stages and include protracted vomiting with or without clinically significant dehydration, encephalopathy in afebrile patients with minimal or absent jaundice, and hepatomegaly in 50% of patients (Table 21.2). Some authorities postulate that antiemetics mask

Table 21.2	
Stages of Reye Syndrome	
Stage	**Signs and Symptoms**
Stage 0	Awake and alert
Stage I	Vomiting and lethargy or sleepiness
	Ability to obey commands
	Hepatic dysfunction
	EEG changes
Stage II	Delirium, combativeness, hyperreflexia, dilated pupils with sluggish response, tachycardia, appropriate response to noxious stimuli, hepatic dysfunction, EEG abnormalities
Stage III	Hyperventilation, obtunded, coma, decorticate posturing, normal pupillary and oculovestibular responses, continued hepatic changes, EEG changes
Stage IV	Deeper coma, decerebrate rigidity, fixed and dilated pupils, loss of oculocephalic reflex, abnormal oculovestibular reflex, minimal liver dysfunction, abnormal EEG findings
Stage V	Seizure, flaccidity, areflexia, dilated, nonreactive pupils, apnea, isoelectric EEG findings
Stage VI	Patients who cannot be classified because they have been treated with medication that alters level of consciousness

EEG, Electroencephalogram.

early symptoms, whereas others propose that antiemetics may further predispose the individual to the disease. Although it is rare, Reye syndrome needs to be considered in any child presenting with altered mental status and vomiting. An appropriate history should be obtained for all children presenting with symptoms similar to those of Reye syndrome to determine whether an inborn error of metabolism (IEM) should be considered. Diarrhea and hyperventilation may be the first signs in children younger than 2 years of age.

1. Assessment
   a. Subjective data collection
      1) History of present illness/chief complaint
         a) Onset
            (1) Viral illness in the first 3 weeks prior to onset of prolonged vomiting with abrupt onset of pernicious vomiting occurring 12 hours to 3 weeks after viral illness; the mean onset is 3 days along with subtle changes in mental status/behavior, irritability, restlessness, delirium, seizures, and coma; neurologic symptoms usually occur 24–48 hours after onset of vomiting; lethargy is usually the first neurologic manifestation
      2) Past medical history
         a) Current or preexisting disease/illness
         b) Medications
            (1) Salicylate (detectable in the blood of 82% of patients), phenothiazine, decongestant use
         c) Allergies
         d) Immunization status
   b. Objective data collection
      1) Physical examination
         a) General appearance
            (1) Level of consciousness, behavior, affect: lethargy, restlessness, delirium, seizures, combativeness
            (2) Slurred speech
            (3) Severe distress/discomfort, critically ill
         b) Inspection
            (1) Dilated and sluggish pupils
            (2) Engorged retinal veins with loss of venous pulsation
            (3) Persistent vomiting: gastrointestinal (GI) bleeding is a late finding
         c) Palpation/percussion
            (1) Hepatomegaly
            (2) Hypertonic to hypotonic muscle tone with abnormal flexion or extension
      2) Diagnostic procedures
         a) Serum ammonia level: may be elevated as much as 1.5 times normal (up to 1,200 mcg/dL)
         b) Liver enzyme levels: may be elevated with
            (1) Alanine aminotransferase (ALT), and aspartate aminotransferase (AST) increase to three times normal but may return to the reference ranges by stage IV or V
         c) Skeletal and cardiac isoenzymes: elevated (CK, CKMB)
         d) Coagulation profile: PT and PTT altered
         e) Serum chemistries including glucose, BUN, creatinine
            (1) Glucose decreased; hypoglycemia present in children younger than 1 year of age because of their higher metabolism and lower glycogen stores
            (2) Creatinine and BUN levels: mild to moderate elevation reflecting dehydration and acidosis
         f) Amino and free fatty acid levels (e.g., glutamine, alanine, lysine): elevated
         g) Factor assays: decreased factors II, VII, IX, X and fibrinogen because of the disruption of synthetic activities in the liver
         h) ABGs
            (1) Metabolic acidosis: increased anion gap
            (2) Respiratory alkalosis
         i) Serum bicarbonate: decreased secondary to vomiting
         j) Lactate dehydrogenase (LDH): may be high or low
         k) Bilirubin: >2 mg/dL (usually <3 mg/dL) in 10–15% of patients; if direct bilirubin is >15% of total or if total is >3 mg/dL, consider other diagnoses
         l) Urine specific gravity: increased; 80% of patients have ketonuria
         m) EEG: may reveal slow-wave activity in the early stages and flattened waves in advanced stages
         n) Cerebral spinal fluid (CSF) evaluation: opening pressure may or may not be increased; WBCs, usually lymphocytes, may be 9×10^9/L (<9/mm^3)
         o) Head CT scan: may reveal cerebral edema, but results are usually normal
2. Analysis: differential nursing diagnoses/collaborative problems
   a. Risk for ineffective airway clearance
   b. Impaired gas exchange
   c. Risk for deficient fluid volume
   d. Ineffective tissue perfusion: cerebral
   e. Ineffective family coping
3. Planning and implementation/interventions
   a. Maintain airway, breathing, circulation per ACLS guidelines (see Chapter 1)
   b. Provide supplemental oxygen as indicated
      1) Rapid-sequence intubation (RSI) and ventilatory support in obtunded patients
      2) High-flow oxygen
   c. Establish IV access for administration of crystalloid fluids/medications as needed
      1) Fluid challenge with 0.9% normal saline solution may be necessary

2) Avoid fluid overload in presence of cerebral edema: consider hypoosmotic fluids
3) Colloid (e.g., albumin) solutions as necessary to maintain intravascular volume

d. Prepare for/assist with medical interventions
   1) Advanced airway management
      a) Nasal or oral intubation
      b) Supraglottic airway (e.g., King, Combitube, laryngeal mask airway)
      c) Surgical airway (e.g., cricothyrotomy)
   2) Institute cardiac and pulse oximetry monitoring
   3) Insert gastric tube and attach to suction
   4) Insert indwelling urinary catheter
   5) Catheter placement and monitoring of arterial pressure (see Chapter 6)
   6) Catheter placement and monitoring of intracranial pressure (see Chapter 6)
   7) Maintain normothermic or slightly hypothermic body temperature
   8) Protect patient from injury (e.g., protective devices may be necessary if patient is combative, side rails up and locked)
   9) Assist with hospital admission
   10) Consider the following for adjunctive treatment that may be prescribed for clinical presentation
      a) Dextrose to counteract hypoglycemia
         (1) If patient is initially hypoglycemic, administer dextrose 25% as an IV bolus at a dose of 1–2 mL/kg
         (2) If initial pH is <7.2, consider the administration of bicarbonate (somewhat controversial) up to 1 mEq/kg per hour; avoid rapid correction or overcorrection
      b) Furosemide (Lasix) to control fluid overload
      c) Insulin to maintain euglycemia
      d) Sodium phenylacetate/sodium benzoate (Ammonul) for hyperammonemia; if the ammonia level is >500 mcg/dL or if the patient's condition fails to respond to the initial dose of sodium phenylacetate/sodium benzoate, start dialysis, preferably hemodialysis
      e) Ondansetron (Zofran), 0.15 mg/kg (not to exceed 8 mg every 8 hours), during the first 15 minutes of initial dose of sodium phenylacetate/sodium benzoate: aids in offsetting GI effects of sodium phenylacetate/sodium benzoate
      f) Phenytoin (Dilantin), 10–20 mg/kg IV for seizures as a loading dose, followed by 5 mg/kg IV per day in divided doses every 6 hours; or fosphenytoin (Cerebyx), dosed as 10–20 mg/kg phenytoin equivalents (PEs)
      g) Osmotic diuretic: mannitol (Osmitrol)
      h) Steroids as indicated
      i) Antipyretics (i.e., acetaminophen [Tylenol]); *do not* administer salicylates
   11) Refer to National Reye Syndrome Foundation if diagnosis is confirmed

4. Evaluation and ongoing monitoring
   a. Airway patency
   b. Level of consciousness
   c. Hemodynamic status
   d. Breath sounds and pulse oximetry
   e. Cardiac rate and rhythm
   f. Intake and output
   g. Serum electrolyte levels

G. RHEUMATOID ARTHRITIS

Rheumatoid arthritis (RA) is a symmetric, inflammatory disease characterized by swelling, warmth, and tenderness of the joints. It is a chronic inflammatory disease of unknown origin that involves the synovial membranes. Patients often present to the emergency department with complaints of pain without previous diagnosis of RA or during a rheumatoid flare (exacerbation). Those patients with suspected RA need immediate referral to rheumatology for definitive diagnosis and management with disease-modifying antirheumatic drugs to prevent deterioration of the joint spaces and long-term disability. Patients with rheumatoid flare require supportive therapies and measures to ensure appropriate drug therapy. Various inflammatory disorders of remote organ systems may be present and may contribute to the presenting problem. Organ systems that may be affected include cardiac (carditis, pericarditis), pulmonary (pleuritis, interstitial fibrosis, intrapulmonary nodules), hepatic (hepatitis), ocular (scleritis, episcleritis, eye dryness), and vascular (vasculitis).

1. Assessment
   a. Subjective data collection
      1) History of present illness/chief complaint
         a) Pain (see Chapter 8): insidious or abrupt
            (1) Joint stiffness/pain in peripheral joints lasting for more than 30 minutes in the morning
      2) Past medical history
         a) Current or preexisting diseases/illness
         b) Medications
         c) Allergies
   b. Objective data collection
      1) Physical examination
         a) General appearance
         b) Synovitis
         c) Swollen or tender joints and limited joint motion; extraarticular disease manifestations such as rheumatoid nodules
      2) Diagnostic procedures
         a) Rheumatoid factor and anti-CCP antibodies for initial testing
         b) CBC with differential, metabolic panel, and urinalysis

c) ESR and C-reactive protein levels which are typically elevated

d) ANA which is typically elevated in a third of patients

e) Exclude gout, pseudogout, infectious arthritis if there is a joint effusion. Synovial fluid testing for asymmetrical joint swelling should be considered

f) Joint radiographs for asymmetrical joint swelling should be considered

g) Cervical spine radiograph to be considered to determine inflammation and/or destruction of cartilage, bone, ligaments

2. Analysis: differential nursing diagnoses/collaborative problems
   a. Activity intolerance
   b. Chronic pain
   c. Impaired physical mobility
   d. Self-care deficit

3. Planning and implementation/interventions
   a. Prepare for/assist with medical procedures
      1) Joint space aspiration: rule out septic joint
      2) Rule out complications: pericarditis, pleuritis, vasculitis
   b. Administer pharmacologic therapy as ordered
      1) Disease-modifying antirheumatologic drugs (DMARDs)
      2) During flare, short-term narcotics may be required
   c. Educate patient/significant others
      1) Encourage physical therapies (e.g., massage, exercise, heat)
      2) Teach patient about control of disease
         a) Proper nutrition
         b) Exercise with low-impact exercises to increase flexibility
         c) Stress reduction
      3) Referral to appropriate subspecialties (e.g., rheumatology)

4. Evaluation and ongoing monitoring
   a. Pain relief

H. SYSTEMIC LUPUS ERYTHEMATOSUS

Systemic lupus erythematosus (SLE) is a multisystem autoimmune disorder most commonly seen in women of childbearing years. The disease stimulates an autoimmune response in which the patient's body generates autoantibodies but is unable to suppress them. Emergency department presentation occurs when the disease process becomes exacerbated and causes cardiac, respiratory, abdominal, neurologic, or renal disorders. Management of these disorders must take precedent when the patient exhibits life-threatening complications.

1. Assessment
   a. Subjective data collection
      1) History of present illness/chief complaint
         a) Pain (see Chapter 8)
            (1) Pleuritic pain with coughing
            (2) Abdominal pain, cramping, diarrhea
            (3) Intractable headaches; photosensitivity
         b) Onset of symptoms
            (1) Acute versus chronic
         c) Nausea, vomiting, associated weight loss
      2) Past medical history
         a) Current or preexisting diseases/illness
         b) Arthralgias, commonly accompanied by joint effusions
         c) Painful or painless oral, nasal, or vaginal ulcers
         d) Butterfly (malar) rash; discoid rash
         e) Fatigue
         f) Medications
         g) Allergies
   b. Objective data collection
      1) Physical examination
         a) General appearance
            (1) Level of consciousness, behavior, affect: confusion, dementia, psychosis, seizure
            (2) Elevated temperature
            (3) Tachypnea
            (4) Moderate distress/discomfort
         b) Inspection
            (1) Diffuse facial erythema: butterfly pattern
            (2) Hemoptysis
         c) Auscultation
            (1) Heart sounds: murmur
         d) Palpation
            (1) Abdominal tenderness
      2) Diagnostic procedures
         a) CBC with differential: anemia is common
         b) PTT
         c) Urinalysis: may show proteinuria or hematuria; pregnancy test in females of childbearing age
         d) BUN and creatinine
         e) Antinuclear antibody (ANA): higher titers are diagnostic for SLE
         f) Chest radiograph
         g) Echocardiogram: effusion
         h) Head CT/MRI scan

2. Analysis: differential nursing diagnoses/collaborative problems
   a. Acute pain
   b. Fatigue

3. Planning and implementation/interventions
   a. Acute exacerbation
      1) Pleurisy
      2) Pericarditis
      3) Intestinal perforation
      4) Renal failure
      5) Stroke
      6) Fever (see Section C [Fever])

   b. Prepare for/assist with medical procedures
      1) Refer to appropriate subspecialists including rheumatologist, infectious disease specialists, neurologist, cardiologist, gastroenterologist, pulmonologist, nephrologist, and dermatologist
      2) Rule out other disease processes: malignant disease, fever of unknown origin, drug-induced lupus, infective endocarditis
   c. Administer pharmacologic therapy as ordered
      1) NSAIDs
      2) Corticosteroids
      3) Antimalarials
      4) Immunosuppressants
4. Evaluation and ongoing monitoring
   a. Level of consciousness
   b. Hemodynamic status

Bibliography

American College of Emergency Physicians Clinical Policies Committee; American College of Emergency Physicians Clinical Policies Subcommittee on Pediatric Fever: Clinical policy for children younger than three years presenting to the emergency department with fever, *Annals of Emergency Medicine* 42(4):530–545, 2003.

Baumann R: Fever. Retrieved from http://www.emedicine.com/neuro/topic134.htm, 2005.

Cunha B: Chronic fatigue syndrome. Retrieved from http://www.emedicine.com/med/topic3392.htm, 2004.

Egland A: Fever. Retrieved from http://www.emedicine.com/ped/topic2700.htm, 2005.

Gilliland R: Fibromyalgia. Retrieved from http://www.emedicine.com/pmr/topic47.htm, 2005.

Goldenberg D, Burckhardt C, Crofford L: Management of fibromyalgia syndrome, *JAMA* 292(19):2388–2395, 2004.

Grisolia J: Systemic lupus erythematosus. Retrieved from http://www.emedicine.com/neuro/topic360.htm, 2005.

Hildebrand J, Muller D: Systemic lupus erythematosus. Retrieved from http://www.emedicine.com/med/topic2228.htm, 2005.

IOM (Institutes of Medicine): *Beyond myalgic encephalomyelitis/chronic fatigue syndrome: Redefining an illness*, Washington, DC, 2015, The National Academies Press. http://www.iom.edu/mecfs.

Kaplan J: Gout. Retrieved from http://www.emedicine.com/emerg/topic221.htm, 2005.

King R, Worthington R: Arthritis, rheumatoid. Retrieved from http://www.emedicine.com/emerg/topic48.htm, 2005.

Krause R: Allergic reaction. Retrieved from http://www.emedicine.com/emerg/topic25.htm, 2005.

Lamont D, Lai M: Systemic lupus erythematosus. Retrieved from http://www.emedicine.com/emerg/topic564.htm, 2006.

Nafari A, Buchwald D: Chronic fatigue syndrome: A review, *American Journal of Psychiatry* 160:221–236, 2003.

Newberry LN: *Sheehy's emergency nursing principles and practice*, 5th ed., St. Louis, MO, 2003, Mosby.

O'Dell J: Therapeutic strategies for rheumatoid arthritis, *New England Journal of Medicine* 350(25):2591–2602, 2004.

Tintinalli JE, Kelen GD, Stapczynski JS: *Emergency medicine: A comprehensive study guide*, 5th ed., New York, NY, 2000, McGraw-Hill.

Weiner D: Reye's syndrome. Retrieved from http://www.emedicine.com/emerg/topic399.htm, 2005.

Winfield J: Fibromyalgia. (2005). Retrieved from http://www.emedicine.com/med/topic790.htm, 2005.

CHAPTER 22

Neurologic Emergencies

Cynthia S. Baxter, RN, DNP, ACNS-BC, NEA-BC, VHA-CM

I. General Strategy

A. ASSESSMENT

1. Primary and secondary assessment/resuscitation (see Chapter 1)
2. Focused assessment
   a. Subjective data collection
      1) History of present illness/chief complaint
         a) Chronologic sequence of onset and development of neurologic symptoms
         b) Consciousness
            (1) Loss of consciousness: time of occurrence and duration
            (2) Alterations in consciousness: fluctuating, steady decline, or improvement
         c) Mentation
            (1) Memory: recent and remote
            (2) Changes in cognitive ability (e.g., problem solving)
            (3) Episodes of getting lost, forgetting everyday information (e.g., names, dates, locations)
         d) Alteration in personality
         e) Emotional lability or mood swings, irritability
         f) Alteration in health or personal habits, activities of daily living (ADLs)
         g) Alteration in communication
            (1) Speech changes: slurred, expressive aphasia
            (2) Comprehension difficulties: receptive aphasia
         h) Alteration in motor ability
            (1) Weakness (paresis)
            (2) Paralysis (plegia)
            (3) Loss of coordination
            (4) Tremors, twitching, or fasciculations
         i) Alteration in sensation
         j) Alteration in sexual performance
         k) Alteration in vision
            (1) Loss of vision, clouding or decrease in acuity or visual fields
            (2) Unilateral or bilateral diplopia
         l) Injury or fall
            (1) Mechanism
            (2) Time elapsed since occurrence
            (3) Changes in clinical status
         m) Pain (PQRST) (see Chapter 8)
         n) Headache
         o) Seizures
         p) Vomiting
         q) Incontinence
         r) Efforts to relieve symptoms
            (1) Home remedies
            (2) Complementary/alternative therapies
            (3) Medications
               (a) Prescription
               (b) OTC/herbal
      2) Past medical history
         a) Current or preexisting diseases/illness and treatment plan
         b) Any past surgical intervention
            (1) Cardiovascular disease

    (2) Neurologic disorders
- c) Tobacco use history
- d) Substance and/or alcohol use/abuse
- e) Last normal menstrual period: female patients of childbearing age
- f) Current medications
  - (1) Prescription
  - (2) OTC/herbal
- g) Allergies: food or drug
- h) Immunization status
3) Psychological/social/environmental factors related to neurologic emergencies
   - a) Stress factors
   - b) Living arrangements, caregiver
     - (1) Lifestyle
     - (2) Coping style
     - (3) Precipitating event
     - (4) Possible/actual assault, abuse, or intimate partner violence situations (see Chapters 3 and 40)
   - c) Personal habits/grooming changes
- b. Objective data collection
  1) General appearance
     - a) Level of consciousness, behavior, affect
     - b) Vital signs
     - c) Odors
     - d) Gait: balance and coordination, abnormal step motions
     - e) Hygiene
     - f) Level of distress/discomfort
  2) Inspection
     - a) Surface trauma
     - b) Symmetry of movements: facial, extremities
     - c) Cerebrospinal fluid (CSF) leaks: otorrhea and/or rhinorrhea
     - d) Seizure activity
     - e) Abnormal positioning: flexion/extension, abnormal movements (tremors)
  3) Auscultation
     - a) Heart sounds
     - b) Breath sounds
     - c) Carotid bruits: present or absent
  4) Palpation/percussion
     - a) Areas of tenderness
     - b) Deep tendon reflexes
     - c) Muscle strength and sensation
  5) Neurologic examinations
     - a) Cranial nerve assessment (Table 22.1)
     - b) Glasgow Coma Scale (GCS): adult or pediatric version (see Appendix A)
     - c) National Institutes of Health Stroke Scale (NIHSS)
       - (1) Standardized scale used to score stroke severity, determine suitability for recombinant tissue plasminogen activator (rt-PA [Alteplase]) administration,

or determine inclusion or exclusion into clinical trials for stroke
- d) FOUR Score Coma Scale (Fig. 22.1)
- e) Oculocephalic reflex (doll's eyes)
  - (1) Present when eyes move in the direction opposite that which the head is moving
  - (2) Occurs with an intact brainstem but damaged cerebral cortex
  - (3) Failure of the eyes to make the movement indicates severe brainstem damage
  - (4) Should not be performed if neck injury suspected
- f) Oculovestibular reflex (caloric testing)
  - (1) Present when eyes move toward the ear stimulated with cold water
  - (2) Occurs with intact brainstem but damaged cerebral hemispheres
  - (3) Absent caloric reflex indicates severe brainstem damage

Table 22.1

Cranial Nerve Assessment

Cranial Nerves	Assessment
Eye Signs/Movement	
CN II: Optic	Visual acuity (CN II)
CN III: Oculomotor	Visual fields (central, peripheral, temporal) (CN III, CN IV, and CN VI)
CN IV: Trochlear	Extraocular movements (CN III, CN IV, and CN VI)
CN VI: Abducens	
Speech Musculature	
CN VII: Facial	Lips (CN VII): "me, me, me"
CN IX: Glossopharyngeal	Palate (CN IX and X): "ga-ga, ka-ka"
CN X: Vagus	
CN XII: Hypoglossal	Tongue (CN XII): "la, la, la"
Protective Reflexes	
CN V: Trigeminal	Corneal (CN V and VII)
CN VII: Facial	
CN IX: Glossopharyngeal	Gag/swallow (CN IX and X)
CN X: Vagus	
Other	
CN I: Olfactory	Smell (CN I): rarely tested
CN V: Trigeminal	Sensory response to cotton wisp over forehead, cheek, and chin (CN V)
CN VII: Facial	Facial movement and expression (pucker, raise brow, smile) (CN VII)
CN VIII: Vestibulocochlear	Hearing (CN VIII)
CN XI: Accessory	Head turning, shoulder shrugging (CN XI)

CN, Cranial nerve.

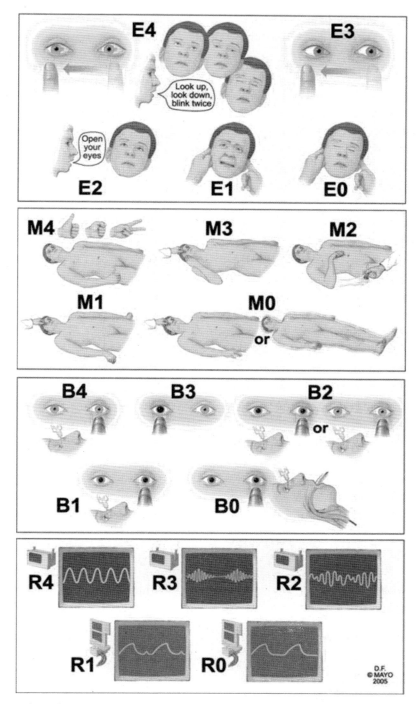

FIG. 22.1 FOUR Score Coma Scale (From Iyer, V. N., Mandrekar, J. N., Danielson, R. D., Zubkov, A. Y., Elmer, J. L., & Wijdicks, E. F. M. (2009). Validity of the FOUR Score Coma Scale in the Medical Intensive Care Unit. *Mayo Clinic Proceedings, 84,* 694–701. Retrieved from http://www.sciencedirect.com/science/article/pii/S0025619611605193.)

(4) Usually preserved longer than the oculo-cephalic reflex

g) Apnea test: allow carbon dioxide (CO_2) to build up to stimulate the respiratory system, and then determine whether patient will breathe spontaneously

h) Loss of brainstem reflexes (pupils, gag, cough, corneal reflexes)

6) Meningeal signs

a) Stiff neck, photophobia, pain on neck flexion

b) Positive Brudzinski sign (involuntary flexion of knees/hips when neck is flexed)

c) Positive Kernig sign (supine patient cannot completely straighten leg when hip is fully flexed to a 90-degree angle)
3. Diagnostic procedures
   a. Laboratory studies
      1) Complete blood count (CBC) with differential
      2) Erythrocyte sedimentation rate (ESR)
      3) Serum chemistries including glucose, BUN, creatinine
      4) Serum and urine toxicology screen
      5) Coagulation profile
      6) Arterial blood gases (ABGs)
      7) Urinalysis; pregnancy test in female patients of childbearing age
      8) Specific drug level testing
      9) CSF analysis
   b. Imaging studies
      1) Head CT scan without contrast, CT angiogram
      2) Cervical spine films (anteroposterior, lateral, odontoid)
      3) Cervical spine CT scan: depending on mechanism of injury
      4) Spinal radiograph or CT scan
      5) Chest radiograph
      6) MRI
      7) Magnetic resonance angiogram (MRA)
   c. Other studies
      1) Cerebral angiograms
      2) Carotid duplex studies
      3) Electroencephalogram (EEG)
      4) 12- to 15-lead electrocardiogram (ECG)
      5) Lumbar puncture: contraindicated with increased intracranial pressure (ICP)

B. ANALYSIS: DIFFERENTIAL NURSING DIAGNOSES/COLLABORATIVE PROBLEMS

1. Risk for ineffective airway clearance
2. Impaired gas exchange
3. Decreased cardiac output
4. Ineffective tissue perfusion: cerebral
5. Acute/chronic pain
6. Anxiety/fear
7. Impaired verbal communication
8. Risk for injury
9. Deficient knowledge
10. Noncompliance

C. PLANNING AND IMPLEMENTATION/ INTERVENTIONS

1. Determine priorities of care
   a. Maintain airway, breathing, circulation (see Chapter 1)
   b. Provide supplemental oxygen as indicated
   c. Establish IV access for administration of crystalloid fluid/medications as needed
   d. Obtain and set up equipment and supplies
   e. Prepare for/assist with medical interventions
   f. Administer pharmacologic therapy as ordered
2. Relieve anxiety/apprehension
3. Allow significant others to remain with patient if supportive
4. Educate patient/significant others

D. EVALUATION AND ONGOING MONITORING

1. Continuously monitor and treat as indicated
2. Monitor patient response/outcomes, and modify nursing care plan as appropriate
3. If positive patient outcomes are not demonstrated, reevaluate assessment and/or plan of care

E. DOCUMENTATION OF INTERVENTIONS AND PATIENT RESPONSE

F. AGE-RELATED CONSIDERATIONS

1. Pediatric
   a. Growth or development related
      1) Children have a higher metabolic rate and lack of kidney reserves
      2) Babinski reflex is normal up to age 2 years
      3) Fontanel closure: anterior fontanel closes between 9 and 18 months of age; posterior fontanel closes by 2 months of age
      4) Infants have flexion posture normally; floppy extended posture is abnormal
      5) Infants may not have tonic-clonic seizures but may posture with neck hyperextension and stiffened extremities (opisthotonos positioning)
   b. "Pearls"
      1) Avoid restraining the child as much as possible
      2) Monitor respiratory status carefully during lumbar puncture positioning
      3) Assess muscle tone by noting resting position of the child
      4) Meningeal irritation may manifest as sharp, shrill cry, irritability, and loss of appetite in infants
      5) Use pediatric GCS for children aged 2–5 years (see Appendix A)
      6) History of developmental delays, unusual behavior for age, clumsiness or progressive weakness, or learning difficulties may be indicative of neurologic abnormalities
2. Geriatric
   a. Aging related
      1) Approximately 75% of people older than 65 years have some degree of impaired cognitive function
      2) Gradual slowing of the conscious and reflex reaction time
      3) Impairment of fine discrimination abilities

4) Decreased corneal sensitivity, slower visual reflexes, decreased visual acuity and depth perception, decreased upward gaze, and smaller pupils

5) Diminished hearing abilities

6) Altered drug tolerance and response

b. "Pearls"

1) Use stronger stimuli, and allow more time to respond

2) Use sharper contrasts for testing sensory stimuli

3) Ensure a protected environment

4) Face patient directly, and use lower and louder voice tones

5) Ask one question at a time, and avoid overstimulation while patient answers

II. Specific Neurologic Emergencies

A. DEMENTIA

Dementia is an organic disorder characterized by significant deterioration from baseline of cognitive function in two or more domains without impaired consciousness that interferes with daily function and independence.[1] The most common cognitive ability lost is memory. Alzheimers disease accounts for 60–80% of dementia. Other dementia syndromes include dementia with Lewy bodies, frontotemporal dementia, vascular dementia, and Parkinson disease with dementia. Dementia affects more than 5 million persons in the United States and increases each year. Increasing age is the strongest risk factor for dementia, particularly Alzheimer disease, and doubles for every 10 years of age after age 60.

Associated risk factors for dementia are ischemic stroke, cardiovascular risk factors of hypertension, tobacco use, hypercholesterolemia, obesity, diabetes, and possibly hyperhomocysteinemia. There is some genetic and/or familial link in Alzheimer disease and involves complicated pathways. The pathologic process of Alzheimer disease involves disturbed neurotransmitters, especially the cholinergic system, and beta-amyloid proteins causing plaques and disruption of brain function.

1. Assessment

a. Subjective data collection

1) History of present illness/chief complaint, significant decline in one of the following cognitive domains interfering with independent living (generally relayed by significant others)

a) Learning and memory

b) Language

c) Executive function

d) Complex attention

e) Perceptual-motor function

f) Social cognition

(1) Onset: acute in addition to chronic cognitive loss may indicate delirium or another cause

(2) Duration: often difficult to pinpoint due to the insidious nature of dementia onset

g) Difficulty in performing ADLs or performing familiar tasks

h) Agitation or withdrawal

i) Mood swings

j) Baseline neurologic status

k) Repetitive behaviors or movements

l) Personality changes

m) Loss of initiative

n) Problems with language

o) Poor or decreased judgment

p) Misplaced objects

q) Disorientation to person, place, or time

r) Sleep disturbances

s) Gait disturbances

2) Past medical history

a) Current or preexisting diseases/illness

(1) Senile dementia: Alzheimer disease type

(2) Cardiovascular disease, previous stroke

(3) Parkinson disease

(4) Psychiatric disorder, depression

b) Head injury

c) Chronic substance and/or alcohol use/abuse

d) Medications: any new additions that may be interacting or causing a change or acceleration in symptoms such as analgesics, antidepressants, or antihistamines

e) Allergies

b. Objective data collection

1) Physical examination

a) General appearance

(1) Level of consciousness, behavior, affect: may not be engaged with surroundings

(2) Grooming: possibly unkempt

(3) Moderate to severe distress/discomfort

b) Complete neurologic exam

(1) Criteria for diagnosis (Box 22.1)

(2) Mini-Mental State Examination: a brief, quantitative measure of cognitive function in adults that can be used to follow the course of cognitive function over time and their response to treatment (decreasing use due to patent protection). Scores of zero in any category should be evaluated, and an overall score of 22 or less is suggestive of a dementia or delirium (87% sensitivity, 82% specificity)[1]

(3) Mini-cog uses a clock-drawing test (CDT) and uncued recall of three unrelated words, recall of zero words indicates dementia, recall of three words indicates nondemented, CDT is used with intermediate recall of

Box 22.1

Criteria for Dementia and Alzheimer Diagnosis from the Fourth Revised Edition of the Diagnostic and Statistical Manual of Mental Disorders

Multiple cognitive deficits demonstrating:

1. Memory impairment (impaired ability to learn new information or recall previously learned information)
2. At least one of the following
   - Aphasia (language disturbance)
   - Apraxia (impaired ability to perform motor activities despite intact motor function)
   - Agnosia (failure to recognize or identify objects despite intact sensory function)
   - Disturbances in executive functioning (i.e., planning, organizing, sequencing, abstracting)
3. Cognitive deficits interfere significantly with work or social activities, present major decline
4. Gradual onset and continuing cognitive decline
5. Cognitive deficits not due to other CNS conditions (cerebrovascular disease, Parkinson, Huntington, subdural hematoma, tumor, etc.) or systemic conditions known to cause dementia (e.g., hypothyroidism; vitamin B_{12}, folic acid, or niacin deficiency; neurosyphilis; human immunodeficiency virus infection)
6. Deficits do not occur only during episodes of delirium
7. Disturbance cannot be accounted for by any nonorganic mental disorder (i.e., schizophrenia, major depressive disorder)

Modified from Dynamed. (2006). Dementia. Retrieved from http://dynamed101.epnet.com/Detail.aspx?id=115618; Dynamed. (2006). Alzheimer's disease. Retrieved from http://dynamed101.epnet.com/Detail.aspx?id=114193.

words to determine dementia (comparison to MMSE with cut-off of 25, Mini-cog had similar sensitivity (76%) and specificity (89%) for dementia[1]

    2) Diagnostic procedures
      a) CBC with differential
      b) Serum chemistries including glucose
      c) Vitamin B_{12} levels
      d) Syphilis, Lyme disease, and HIV infection, when appropriate
      e) Thyroid function studies
      f) Urinalysis
      g) Chest radiograph
      h) Head CT scan or MRI
        (1) Single-photon emission CT (SPECT) and positron emission tomography (PET) may be able to identify pathologic features of dementia

      (2) May provide a baseline for future comparison
2. Analysis: differential nursing diagnoses/collaborative problems
  a. Anxiety
  b. Risk for injury
  c. Ineffective coping
  d. Risk for caregiver role strain
  e. Risk for hopelessness
  f. Risk for deficient knowledge
3. Planning and implementation/interventions
  a. Provide supplemental oxygen as indicated
  b. Establish IV access for administration of crystalloid fluid/medications as needed
  c. Prepare for/assist with medical procedures
    1) Protect patient from injury and provide a safe environment
    2) Assist with hospital admission as needed
  d. Administer pharmacologic therapy as ordered
  e. Educate patient/significant others
    1) Provide appropriate referrals as needed
4. Evaluation and ongoing assessment
  a. Level of consciousness
  b. Cognitive ability

B. GUILLAIN-BARRÉ SYNDROME

Guillain-Barré syndrome is an acute peripheral neuropathy causing ascending weakness progressing over a short time and is considered to be an autoimmune disease preceded by a bacterial or viral illness. *Campylobacter jejuni,* cytomegalovirus (CMV), Epstein-Barr virus (EBV), and *Mycoplasma pneumoniae* are the most common pathogens associated with Guillain-Barré syndrome. Progressive weakness can continue for up to 4 weeks, and in 10–30% of cases, ventilatory support is required. Weakness usually starts in the legs, about half the time includes facial weakness, includes mild paresthesias of the hands and feet, and dysautonomia (tachycardia, urinary retention, hypertension alternating with hypotension, bradycardia, and loss of sweating).[2] Mortality rate is approximately 10%, and 20% of survivors are left with severe disability. The incidence is 1.3 cases per 100,000 population; men are more often affected than women, and the incidence is higher in young adults. There are three major forms of the disease: (1) acute motor axonal neuropathy (AMAN), (2) acute sensorimotor axonal neuropathy (AMSAN), and (3) acute inflammatory demyelinating polyneuropathy (AIDP). AIDP is more common in Europe and North America, whereas AMAN is more common in East Asian countries. AMAN is mainly a motor disease, and AIDP is a demyelinating disease that has both motor and sensory effects.

1. Assessment
  a. Subjective data collection
    1) History of present illness/chief complaint
      a) Sequence of events
        (1) Weakness generally beginning in the lower extremities and ascending

(2) Symptoms peak 1–4 weeks
- b) Neurologic symptoms without change in consciousness: changes in motor function
- c) Pain (see Chapter 8)
- d) Difficulty breathing

2) Past medical history
- a) Current or preexisting diseases/illness
  - (1) Neurologic disease or family history of neurologic disease
  - (2) Preceding upper respiratory infection or diarrhea-type illness
  - (3) Chronic medical conditions
- b) Medications
- c) Allergies
- d) Immunization status

b. Objective data collection
1) Physical examination
- a) General appearance
  - (1) Possible orthostasis
  - (2) Gait: possibly altered
  - (3) Moderate to severe distress/discomfort
- b) Inspection
  - (1) Possible lower extremity weakness
- c) Auscultation
  - (1) Breath sounds: normal, possible diminished
- d) Palpation/percussion
  - (1) Bladder distention
  - (2) Extremity weakness and sensory changes
  - (3) Deep tendon reflex involvement (more common to have decrease in AIDP, increase in AMAN)

2) Diagnostic procedures
- a) CBC with differential: exclude other causes of weakness
- b) Serum chemistries including glucose
- c) Serologic studies for CMV, EBV, or *Mycoplasma* may be helpful in establishing the cause of Guillain-Barré syndrome for epidemiologic purposes
- d) Antibodies to determine epidemiology
- e) Other blood tests as appropriate to rule out other causes
  - (1) Thyroid function tests
  - (2) Rheumatology profiles
  - (3) ESR
  - (4) Immunoelectrophoresis or serum protein and tests for heavy metals
- f) Lumbar puncture and CSF studies
  - (1) Elevated protein (>0.55 g/L) without elevation in white blood cells (<10 lymphocytes/mm^3)
- g) Nerve conduction studies: electromyography (EMG) studies, not performed in the emergency department
- h) Pulmonary function studies: can be performed at bedside
  - (1) Vital capacity (VC): measured to evaluate the ability to cough and clear secretions; <10 mL/kg may require intubation to maintain airway
  - (2) Negative inspiratory function (NIF): measured to assess muscle strength and ability to sustain effective ventilation, <-20 cm/H_2O may require intubation and mechanical ventilation (i.e., -30 cm/H_2O is better; -15 cm/H_2O is worse)
- i) Chest radiograph
- j) Brain CT scan or MRI to rule out other causes

2. Analysis: differential nursing diagnoses/collaborative problems
- a. Risk for ineffective airway clearance
- b. Risk for ineffective breathing pattern
- c. Anxiety/fear
- d. Risk for injury
- e. Deficient knowledge
- f. Risk for impaired skin integrity

3. Planning and implementation/interventions
- a. Maintain airway, breathing, circulation (see Chapter 1)
- b. Provide supplemental oxygen
  1) RSI and ventilatory support if respiratory compromise is present
  2) High-flow oxygen
- c. Establish IV access for administration of crystalloid fluid/medications
- d. Prepare for/assist with medical interventions
  1) Advanced airway management
    - a) Nasal or tracheal intubation
    - b) Supraglottic airway (e.g., King, Combitube, laryngeal mask airway)
    - c) Surgical airway (e.g., cricothyrotomy)
  2) Increase venous outflow through elevation of head of bed and proper head and neck positioning
  3) Institute cardiac and pulse oximetry monitoring
  4) Insert gastric tube and attach to suction
  5) Insert indwelling urinary catheter
  6) Assist with hospital admission
- e. Administer pharmacologic therapy as ordered
  1) RSI premedications: sedatives, analgesics, neuromuscular blocking agents
  2) Analgesics

4. Evaluation and ongoing monitoring
- a. Airway patency
- b. Level of consciousness
- c. Hemodynamic status
- d. Breath sounds and pulse oximetry
- e. Cardiac rate and rhythm
- f. Intake and output
- g. Motor and sensory changes

C. HEADACHES

Of emergency department visits, 4.5% are for patients experiencing headaches. The primary goal is to identify the small percentage of patients whose headache may indicate a life-threatening condition. Headache occurs when there is traction, pressure, displacement, inflammation, or dilation of pain receptors (nociceptors) in the brain or surrounding tissues. A primary headache is one for which no organic cause can be consistently identified (e.g., migraines, tension type, or cluster). Headache with associated sinus symptoms meet criteria for migraine headache in both adults and children 80–90% of the time and tension headache approximately 8% of the time[3,4] (Table 22.2).

A secondary headache is associated with an organic cause such as a tumor, aneurysm, meningitis, or temporal arteritis. Characteristics suggestive of a serious underlying cause of headache include sudden onset that peaks in intensity within 1 minute, absence of similar headaches in the past, concurrent infection with or without fever, altered mental status, headache with exertion, first headache or worse headache in age 50 years and older, immunosuppression, neurologic abnormalities in conjunction with headache, stiff neck, papilledema, and/or toxic appearance.

1. Assessment
   a. Subjective data collection
      1) History of present illness/chief complaint
         a) Pain (see Chapter 8)
            (1) Provocation
               (a) Emotional or stress
               (b) Metabolic (fever/menses)
               (c) Flickering or bright lights
               (d) Alcohol or caffeine withdrawal or abuse
               (e) Sleep deprivation
               (f) Menstrual cycle
               (g) Food related: chocolate, nitrates, monosodium glutamate (MSG), tyramines (wine, cheese)
               (h) Sexual activity/exertion
               (i) Position changes: low pressure, orthostatic pressure drop
               (j) Minor head trauma
               (k) Muscle spasm
            (2) Quality: throbbing, diffuse or focal
            (3) Region/radiation: frontal sinus, neck tension, bilateral or unilateral, occipital
            (4) Severity of symptoms: increase or decrease with associated symptoms
            (5) Time of onset, frequency, symptom-free durations
         b) Associated symptoms: lacrimation, nausea, vertigo
            (1) Aura (visual or somatosensory, mostly associated with migraine)
            (2) Nausea and vomiting
            (3) Photophobia or phonophobia
            (4) Visual changes
            (5) Difficulty concentrating
      2) Past medical history
         a) Current or preexisting diseases/illness
            (1) Previous headache history or family history of headaches; strong family history of migraines, lesser association with cluster headaches
               (a) Change in usual headache history or similar
            (2) Seizure disorder
            (3) Previous sinus infections; many patients with reported "sinus headaches" may actually meet criteria for migraine diagnosis
         b) Last normal menstrual period in female patients of childbearing age
         c) Medications
            (1) Use of oral contraceptives; unclear association or causation with migraines
            (2) Increasing use of analgesics can increase headache frequency
            (3) Analgesic withdrawal may trigger
            (4) Association with aspartame has not been proven
            (5) Any new medications recently started
            (6) Steroid therapy or withdrawal
            (7) Medications that improve symptoms
         d) Allergies
         e) Immunization status
   b. Objective data collection
      1) Physical examination
         a) General appearance
            (1) Level of consciousness, behavior, affect: alert to comatose, irritable, depression
            (2) Possible elevated temperature
            (3) Moderate to severe distress/discomfort, possibly critically ill
         b) Inspection
            (1) Skin: pale color
            (2) Rash: petechial or purpuric suggestive of bacterial meningitis
         c) Auscultation
            (1) Breath sounds: normal
            (2) Heart sounds: normal
         d) Palpation/percussion
            (1) Sinus tenderness
            (2) Skin: possible diaphoresis, fever
            (3) Ispsilateral autonomic findings: lacrimation, rhinorrhea, ophthalmic injection (cluster)
            (4) Red flags: mnemonic SNOOP[5]
               (a) Systemic symptoms, illness, or conditions
               (b) Neurologic abnormal signs
               (c) Onset is new
               (d) Other associated signs or conditions

Table 22.2

Primary Headache Symptom Clusters and Diagnostic Criteria

Type	Most Common Symptom Cluster	International Headache Diagnosis Criteria*
Migraine Without aura With aura Complicated	***Without Aura (Most Common)*** Recurring, attacks lasting 4–72 hr Unilateral location Pulsating quality Moderate to severe intensity Aggravated by physical activity Associated with nausea, photophobia, and phonophobia	***Without Aura*** Five or more attacks with: 4- to 72-hr duration in adults and 2- to 48-hr duration in children less than 15 yr old (with unsuccessful or no treatment) At least two attacks that are unilateral, pulsating, moderate/severe (inhibits daily activity), aggravated by physical activity At least one attack with nausea, vomiting, photophobia, and phonophobia
	With Aura Recurring, localized to cerebral cortex or brainstem Most commonly develops over 5–20 min and lasts <60 min Headache, nausea, and/or photophobia may follow aura symptoms directly or patient may have symptom-free interval that lasts <1 hr Headache may last 4–72 hr or may not occur	***With Aura*** At least two attacks following an aura Aura with three of four of the following: 1. One or more completely reversible aura symptom with focal cerebral cortical or brainstem dysfunction 2. One or more aura symptom over more than 4 min or two developing or more symptoms in succession 3. No aura symptom lasting longer than 60 min (if more than one aura symptom present, add time for each one) 4. Headache follows aura with <60 min aura/symptom-free interval
	Complicated Severe neurologic deficit outlasting headache Hemiplegic (result of severe vasospasm) Basilar (most common in young women 15 to 25 yr old, visual aura may occur) Vertebrobasilar symptoms: dysarthria (slurred speech), facial/tongue numbness, dysphagia (swallowing difficulty); difficulty chewing; visual field deficits; one-sided sensory loss; vertigo or dizziness; staggering gait; incoordination; paresthesias; occipital headache within 30 min; may have stupor and confusion; may last hours Dysphoric (migraine with confusion)	***Ophthalmoplegic*** At least two attacks of headache with paresis of cranial nerve II, IV, or VI ***Retinal*** At least two attacks with: fully reversible monocular scotoma or blindness lasting >60 min Headache follows (or before) visual symptoms, with symptom-free interval <60 min
Cluster	Burning, severe, and sharp Excruciating and exquisite pain Tearing and nasal congestion on one side with lid edema, red eye, sweating, and pallor Rarely seen during an attack, but patient may rub or hit the affected side, pace, and be frantic Periorbital (80%) and temporal locations Usually no aura (reported in 14%) Strictly unilateral, changes sides in 10–15% of patients Photophobia and phonophobia common during active period Lasts less than 1 hr in 54% of patients Cluster frequency: one to eight/day, typically 60–90 min after falling asleep, 15- to 180-min duration, last weeks to months and may recur for months to years later (may be seasonal—spring and fall) May be precipitated by alcohol, histamine, or nitroglycerin	At least five attacks with: 1. Severe unilateral orbital, supraorbital, or temporal pain lasting 15–180 min (untreated); attacks may be less severe, frequent, and shorter during part of the time course but no less than half the time 2. Accompanied by one or more: ipsilateral conjunctival injection or lacrimation, ipsilateral nasal congestion or rhinorrhea, ipsilateral eyelid edema, ipsilateral forehead and facial sweating, ipsilateral miosis or ptosis, sense of restlessness or agitation. Frequency of one every other day to eight/day Note: probable cluster headache fulfills all but one of the foregoing criteria

Continued

Part 2

	Table 22.2	

Primary Headache Symptom Clusters and Diagnostic Criteria—cont'd

Type	Most Common Symptom Cluster	International Headache Diagnosis Criteria*
Tension type Episodic Chronic	Dull, nonpulsating Usually starts at the occiput and moves around bilaterally to the frontal area in a tight band of pressure May last up to 7 days Recurrent, usually in same location Rarely associated with nausea or vomiting No photophobia, phonophobia, or aura May have tight and tender posterior and cervical muscles May be associated with depression, premenstrual syndrome, fibromyalgia, or other somatization disorders	**Episodic** At least 10 headache episodes with: Headache duration 30 min to 7 days At least two of the following: 1. Pressing/tight, nonpulsating quality 2. Mild/moderate (inhibits but does not prohibit activity) 3. Bilateral location 4. No aggravation by physical activity. No nausea or vomiting (may have decreased appetite) No occurrence of photophobia AND phonophobia (only one) Number of days with such headache <180/yr (<15/mo) **Chronic** Same criteria except frequency >15 days/mo (>180 days/yr) for >6 months

*Assumes that the history, physical, and neurologic examination do not indicate other disorders.

Data from Dynamed. (2006). Migraine. Retrieved from http://dynamed101.epnet.com/Detail.aspx?id=114718; Dynamed. (2006). Cluster headache. Retrieved from http://dynamed101.epnet.com/detial.aspx?id=116292; Dynamed. (2006). Tension headache. Retrieved from http://dynamed101.epnet.com/Detail.aspx?style=1&docid=/dynamed/4689fa8c501833e8852562d8005337df.

(e) Previous headache history: presentation is different than

2) Diagnostic procedures: if organic disease is suspected
   a) ESR: elevated if temporal arteritis
   b) CBC with differential: obtain if patient has fever or temporal arteritis suspected
   c) Skull/sinus radiograph
   d) Head CT scan and/or MRI: routine imaging not recommended in patients with migraine and normal neurologic examination; imaging considered for the following
      (1) Sudden onset with peak pain within 1 minute (associated with increased chance of serious central nervous system [CNS] disease such as subarachnoid hemorrhage [SAH])
      (2) Onset of headache with physical exertion, sexual activity, or cough
      (3) Change in neurologic examination with headache
      (4) Stiff neck
      (5) Worsening condition
      (6) New onset in patient with history of cancer
      (7) Immunosuppression status (i.e., new headache in patient infected with human immunodeficiency virus [HIV])
      (8) New onset in persons aged 55 years and older
      (9) Considered with change in usual headache pattern
   e) EEG
      (1) With associated seizure symptoms
   f) Lumbar puncture
      (1) If suspected meningitis or SAH with normal CT scan
      (2) Neuroimaging first to reduce risk of lumbar puncture
      (3) May be contraindicated if signs of ICP
      (4) Results suggestive of meningitis: high opening pressure (>200 mm H_2O), elevated cell count, decreased glucose
      (5) Results suggestive of intracranial hypertension: high opening pressure, normal cell count and protein level
      (6) Results suggestive of SAH: grossly bloody, after 8 hours, xanthochromia (yellow hue caused by bilirubin from blood cell breakdown)
      (7) Other: toxicological testing if suspected by history

2. Analysis: differential nursing diagnoses/collaborative problems
   a. Risk for ineffective airway clearance
   b. Acute/chronic pain
   c. Risk for acute confusion
   d. Risk for injury
   e. Knowledge deficit (self-care, headache)

Part 2

3. Planning and implementation/interventions
    a. Maintain airway, breathing, circulation (see Chapter 1)
    b. Provide supplemental oxygen as indicated
        1) Intubation and ventilation in comatose patients
    c. Establish IV access for administration of crystalloid fluid/medications as needed
    d. Prepare for/assist with medical interventions
        1) Advanced airway management
            a) Nasal or oral intubation
            b) Supraglottic airway (e.g., King, Combitube, laryngeal mask airway)
            c) Surgical airway (e.g., cricothyrotomy)
        2) Place patient in dark and quiet room
        3) Institute cardiac and pulse oximetry monitoring as indicated
        4) Insert gastric tube and attach to suction as indicated
        5) Insert indwelling urinary catheter as indicated
        6) Assist with possible hospital admission as indicated
    e. Administer pharmacologic medications as ordered
        1) Nonnarcotic analgesics: NSAIDs, dopamine antagonists
        2) Narcotics
    f. Educate patient/significant others
        1) Avoid trigger mechanisms if possible
4. Evaluation and ongoing monitoring
    a. Airway patency
    b. Level of consciousness
    c. Hemodynamic status
    d. Pain relief

D. SEIZURES

A seizure is a sudden, paroxysmal discharge of a group of neurons that results in transient impairment of movement, sensation, or memory. The seizure may or may not impair consciousness. A trigger causes an abnormal burst of electrical stimulus that disrupts the brain's normal nerve conduction. Seizures are caused by three classes of etiology: genetic, structural or metabolic, or unknown.[6] Genetic etiologies are known or presumed causes with seizure as the core symptom. Structural disorders may be genetic or acquired (stroke, tumor, infection, etc.). Metabolic conditions include ionic changes (e.g., pH, electrolyte imbalances, hyperventilation) as well as fever or hyperglycemia. Unknown etiology includes all seizures with normal imaging and no other cause can be found. Seizures, according to the International League Against Epilepsy (ILAE) Classification, are identified as generalized, focal, or unknown (Table 22.3). The risk of recurrent seizure for patients experiencing their first seizure is greatest in the next 2 years at 40–50%.[7] Treatment with antiepileptic drugs is based on individual risk benefit determination. Patients of driving age who experience a first-time seizure should have a report filed with the state Department of Motor Vehicles.

The greatest numbers of seizures occur in children younger than 2 years or in persons older than 65 years. Forty percent of all new-onset seizures occur in those younger than 18 years; most are fever-related convulsive seizures. Patients at risk for developing seizures include those with previous head trauma, stroke, CNS infections, and degenerative CNS disorders (e.g., multiple sclerosis, Alzheimer disease, and Huntington chorea). Status epilepticus is a medical emergency characterized by a series of seizures without recovery of baseline neurologic status between seizures. This condition can lead to mortality and morbidity from hypoxia, acidemia, hypoglycemia, autonomic dysfunction, and hypercalcemia.

Some general rules apply to distinguishing true epileptic events from pseudoseizures (psychogenic paroxysmal events). Those include interruption of seizure activity by vocal or tactile/painful stimulation, abrupt return of consciousness (lack of postictal state) and subsequent loss of consciousness, waxing and waning of clonic or tonic activity, sudden loss of tone with protective behavior such as outstretched arms during fall, eyes tightly closed, avoidance of painful stimuli or positive "arm on face" maneuver (where an apparently flaccid arm avoids hitting the face when dropped from approximately 12 inches above the face of the patient), and weeping during seizure activity.

Surgical interventions are available when antiepileptic drug therapy fails. Surgical ablation of the epileptogenic zone for certain seizure types is available in centers that specialize in these surgical interventions. Vagus nerve stimulation devices are available for partial epilepsy and have been shown to reduce seizure frequency by about 50% in half of patients. The stimulator, about 5 cm in diameter, is surgically implanted under the skin of the lateral chest wall and is connected to stimulating electrodes attached to the left vagus nerve.

1. Assessment
    a. Subjective data collection
        1) History of present illness/chief complaint
            a) Precipitating event: fever, illness
            b) Site of origin and spread of the seizure
            c) Motor activity
            d) Duration and frequency of seizure
            e) Loss of consciousness or change in level of arousal
            f) Postictal behavior
            g) Incontinence
        2) Past medical history
            a) Current or preexisting diseases/illness
                (1) Seizure history
                (2) Recent infection or illness
                (3) Diabetes or other metabolic disorder
                (4) Neurologic disease or congenital anomalies
            b) Previous head injury
            c) Substance and/or alcohol use/abuse

Table 22.3

International Classification of Epileptic Seizures and Antiepileptic Drug Management*

Classification	Antiepileptic Drug Management†
Partial Seizures (Focal, Local)	***Partial (including secondarily generalized)***
A. Simple partial seizures (consciousness unimpaired)	Carbamazepine (Tegretol)
1. With motor symptoms	Phenytoin (Dilantin)
2. With somatosensory or special sensory symptoms	Lamotrigine (Lamictal)
3. With autonomic symptoms (sweating, heart rate)	Oxcarbazepine (Trileptal)
4. With psychic symptoms	
B. Complex partial seizures (with impairment of consciousness)	
1. Beginning as simple partial seizures and progressing to impairment of consciousness	
a. With no other features	
b. With features as in simple partial (as above, 1 to 4)	
c. With automatisms (no knowledge or control over: plucking at clothes, smacking of lips, wandering)	
2. With impairment of consciousness at the start	
a. With no other features	
b. With features as in simple partial (as above, 1 to 4)	
c. With automatisms	
C. Partial seizures evolving to secondarily generalized seizures	
1. Simple partial seizures evolving to generalized seizures	
2. Complex partial seizures evolving to generalized seizures	
3. Simple partial seizures evolving to complex partial seizures to generalized seizures	
Generalized Seizures (Convulsive or Nonconvulsive)	***Primary Generalized***
A. Absence seizures (includes atypical absence seizures)	Valproate (Depakote)
B. Myoclonic seizures	Phenytoin (Dilantin)
C. Clonic seizures	Carbamazepine (Tegretol)
D. Tonic seizures	***Absence***
E. Tonic-clonic seizures	Ethosuximide
F. Atonic seizures	Valproate (Depakote)
	Atypical Absence
	Valproate (Depakote)
	Lamotrigine (Lamictal)
Unclassified Epileptic Seizures	
Includes all seizures that cannot be classified because of inadequate or incomplete data or that do not fit into any of the foregoing categories, including neonatal seizures (i.e., rhythmic eye movements, chewing, and swimming movements)	

*Note: New classifications are being developed based on clinical classification in response to the problems of international classification (poor interexaminer reliability, inclusion of rare syndromes, impractical). One new classification is based on provoked/unprovoked and partial versus generalized seizures.

†Treatment is started with a single drug (monotherapy), with a gradual increase to produce seizure control. Combination therapy (polytherapy) is attempted only if at least two adequate sequential trials of single-dose agents have failed. Treatment after a first seizure can prevent a second seizure, but delaying treatment until a second seizure does not affect long-term remission rates. Many antiepileptic drugs have interactions when used concomitantly; check prescribing information.

Data from International classifications of seizure. (1989). Retrieved from http://www.epilepsy.org.uk/info/classifications.html; Dynamed. (2006). Epilepsy in general. Retrieved from http://dynamed101.epnet.com/Detail.aspx?id=115086; Schachter, S. C. (2005). Overview of the management of epilepsy in adults. *UpToDate*. Retrieved from http://www.utdol.com/utd/content/topic.do?topicKey=epilepsy/4878&view=print.

---

    d) Medications (there are over 30 medications for baseline seizure control)
    e) Allergies
    f) Immunization status
  b. Objective data collection
    1) Physical examination
      a) General appearance
        (1) Level of consciousness, behavior, affect: active seizure activity, postictal status
        (2) Possible elevated temperature
        (3) Moderate to severe distress/discomfort
      b) Inspection
        (1) Urinary or bowel incontinence
      c) Auscultation
        (1) Breath sounds: normal
    2) Diagnostic procedures
      a) CBC with differential: elevated WBC if infection
      b) Serum chemistries including glucose
      c) Serum and urinary toxicology screen: serum concentrations of anticonvulsants are helpful in making clinical decisions, but the patient's individual response should be the main consideration

d) Head CT scan or MRI if no seizure history
   (1) MRI has been shown to be diagnostically superior to CT in detecting epileptogenic lesions
   (2) SPECT or MRI obtained with thin coronal sections by using fast spin-echo (FSE) or inversion-recovery (IR) sequences will be more specific in assessing lesions for possible surgical intervention
e) EEG should be performed as indicated: consult neurologist for specific type of EEG (e.g., sleep, provoked)
f) Lumbar puncture if indicated for fever or to rule out meningitis

2. Analysis: differential nursing diagnoses/collaborative problems
   a. Risk for ineffective airway clearance
   b. Risk for ineffective breathing pattern
   c. Risk for injury
   d. Risk for impaired gas exchange
   e. Anxiety
   f. Risk for deficient knowledge
3. Planning and implementation/interventions
   a. Maintain airway, breathing, circulation (see Chapter 1)
   b. Provide supplemental oxygen
   c. Establish IV access for administration of crystalloid fluid/medications as needed
   d. Prepare for/assist with medical therapy
      1) Turn patient to side and suction oropharynx as needed
      2) Protect from injury (pad rails, protect head)
      3) Undress patient for cooling: if febrile seizure
      4) Institute cardiac and pulse oximetry monitoring
      5) Assist with possible hospital admission
   e. Administer pharmacologic therapy as ordered for emergent seizure control
      1) Anticonvulsants: phenytoin (Dilantin), at an IV infusion rate of 50 mg/min or less; fosphenytoin (Cerebyx), administered in phenytoin equivalents (PE)/kg
      2) Phenobarbital
      3) Benzodiazepines: lorazepam (Ativan), diazepam (Valium)
      4) Dextrose 50% if hypoglycemia present
      5) Thiamine, nutritional supplements if nutritionally deficient
      6) Antipyretics if fever present
   f. Educate patient/significant others
      1) Follow-up care and specialist consultation
      2) Education about specific medications prescribed
4. Evaluation and ongoing monitoring
   a. Level of consciousness
   b. Hemodynamic status
   c. Seizure activity

d. Breath sounds and pulse oximetry
e. Cardiac rate and rhythm
f. Temperature control

E. STROKE

Stroke is a neurologic syndrome characterized by a rapid or gradual nonconvulsive neurologic deficit that affects a known vascular territory and results in a focal neurologic deficit. Stroke is caused by an interruption or change in blood supply to an area of the brain. There are two major types of strokes, ischemic and hemorrhagic. An ischemic stroke results from an occlusion of the cerebral circulation by atherosclerosis, atherosclerotic plaques, or emboli, thus creating a narrow lumen and preventing adequate cerebral blood flow. A hemorrhagic stroke results from pressure increases on the cerebral arteries that cause a weakened blood vessel to rupture and leak blood into the brain (intracerebral hemorrhage [ICH]) or subarachnoid space (SAH). In the United States, the etiologic distribution is 87% ischemic, 10% intercerebral hemorrhage, and 3% subarachnoid hemorrhage.[8] The clinical picture of a stroke depends on the vessel involved, the location and extent of the damage, and collateral flow. There are approximately 795,000 new or repeat cases of stroke each year (77% new onset, 23% repeat), and stroke is a leading cause of disability in the United States.[8] Those at greatest risk for stroke include patients with hyperlipidemia, heart failure, mitral valve disorders, atrial fibrillation, diabetes, and hypertension and those with a history of obesity, tobacco or substance abuse (e.g., cocaine). Stroke occurs more often in men under 75 years of age, women over 75 years of age, black or Hispanic populations, and in the southeast United States (stroke belt).[8]

At the cellular level, once blood supply has been interrupted to the brain tissue, the ischemic cascade and resultant inflammatory process lead to neuronal death and resultant infarction. Preventing, reversing, or limiting the interruption of blood supply or the resultant ischemic and inflammatory processes serves as the basis for treatment. Recently completed studies investigating the induction of a state of therapeutic hypothermia early in the treatment of stroke have not demonstrated sustained, improved outcomes and is currently not recommended outside of research protocols.[8,9]

1. Assessment
   a. Subjective data collection
      1) History of present illness/chief complaint
         a) Chronologic sequence of onset and development of neurologic symptoms
            (1) Time of onset of symptoms: important in determining whether patient is a candidate for fibrinolysis
               (a) Witnessed: time symptoms started
               (b) Unwitnessed: time last seen at patient's baseline neurologic status
            (2) Symptoms improving and returning to baseline

        (a) Transient ischemic attack (TIA): neurologic deficit lasts minutes to 24 hours

        (3) Maximization of symptoms without progression or improvement: completed stroke

    b) Associated symptoms prior to change (e.g., pain, headache [associated with bleeding])

    c) Paresis or weakness of one side: more common in anterior circulation stroke

    d) Sensory deficits: usually face, then arm, then leg

    e) Visual changes

        (1) Amaurosis fugax: gray shade slowly pulled over eye, painless

        (2) Diplopia or loss of visual fields

    f) Incontinence

    g) Vertigo, dizziness: more common in posterior circulation stroke

    h) Speech changes: dysarthia (slurred speech) and/or aphasia (expressive, cannot use words appropriately or is mute; receptive, cannot understand words; global, both receptive and expressive)

    i) Gait abnormalities: ataxia

    j) Nausea and vomiting: associated with intracranial bleed

    k) Stiff neck: may be associated with intracranial bleed

    l) Photophobia and/or phonophobia: may be associated with SAH

  2) Past medical history

    a) Current or preexisting diseases/illness

        (1) Diabetes

        (2) Cardiovascular disease

           (a) Atrial fibrillation

           (b) Hypertension

           (c) Rheumatic heart disease

           (d) Heart valve replacement

           (e) Coronary artery disease, acute myocardial infarction, coronary artery bypass graft surgery

           (f) Heart failure

        (3) Migraine headaches

        (4) Age: increased risk with increased age

        (5) Heavy alcohol use

    b) Medications

        (1) Cocaine or other stimulants increase risk of stroke

    c) Allergies

b. Objective data collection

  1) Physical examination

    a) General appearance

        (1) Level of consciousness, behavior, affect: confused to comatose; speech difficulties

        (2) Hypertension

        (3) Moderate to severe distress/discomfort, possibly critically ill

    b) Inspection

        (1) Unilateral facial droop

        (2) Unilateral pronator drift

        (3) Cranial nerve dysfunction on ipsilateral stroke side of brain

        (4) Nystagmus

    c) Auscultation

        (1) Possible carotid bruits

        (2) Breath sounds: normal

        (3) Heart sounds: murmur or click if valve replacement

    d) Palpation/percussion

        (1) Muscle weakness or hemiplegia on contralateral stroke side of brain

        (2) Deep tendon reflexes: diminished on ipsilateral side

        (3) Nuchal rigidity

    e) National Institutes of Health Stroke Scale (NIHSS)

2) Diagnostic procedures

  a) CBC with differential: possible polycythemia, thrombocytosis, thromocytopenia, leukemia, anemia

  b) Serum chemistries including glucose, BUN, creatinine

  c) Coagulation profile: may reveal coagulopathy; provides baseline for fibrinolytic or anticoagulant therapy

  d) Cardiac biomarkers: if suspected cardiac event with stroke

  e) Serum and urine toxicology screen in selected patients

  f) Emergent CT of head without contrast: American Heart Association/American Stroke Association goal is to perform the test within 25 minutes of arrival, with the result within 45 minutes of arrival

  g) Serum pregnancy test in women of childbearing age

    (1) Used to differentiate between ischemic and hemorrhagic, a distinction that determines treatment priorities (ischemic and hemorrhagic are treated differently)

    (2) Normal CT with ischemic stroke within 6 hours of event

    (3) Ischemic stroke >6–12 hours after event will show regional hypodensity

    (4) Hemorrhagic stroke evident as hyperdensity on CT

    (5) Of SAHs, 5% may have normal CT results and will require lumbar puncture for diagnosis

    (6) ICHs <1 cm may not be visualized by CT and require MRI

h) Carotid duplex scanning: utilized in patient with acute ischemic stroke to evaluate for carotid artery stenosis or occlusion

i) MRA: utilized to visualize vascular flow and abnormalities when angiography is not indicated

j) Echocardiography: evaluate for possible cardiac emboli as the cause of ischemic stroke

k) MRI: useful for ischemic stroke involving cerebellar or lacunar structures but is costly and may not be available in all centers

l) ECG: 60% of cardiogenic emboli causing stroke are associated with atrial fibrillation or acute myocardial infarction

m) Angiography: useful in acute ischemic stroke for identifying appropriate treatment such as rt-PA (Alteplase), vascular coiling, stenting, or possible surgical management

2. Analysis: differential nursing diagnoses/collaborative problems
   a. Risk for ineffective airway clearance
   b. Risk for ineffective breathing pattern
   c. Ineffective tissue perfusion, cerebral
   d. Risk for impaired gas exchange
   e. Risk for acute confusion
   f. Anxiety
   g. Risk for aspiration
   h. Risk for injury
   i. Potential for unilateral neglect
   j. Deficient knowledge
   k. Risk for impaired coping
   l. Grief

3. Planning and implementation/interventions
   a. Maintain airway, breathing, circulation (see Chapter 1)
   b. Provide supplemental oxygen
      1) Rapid-sequence intubation (RSI) and ventilatory support in patients with GCS <8 or impaired airway control
      2) High-flow oxygen
   c. Establish IV access for administration of crystalloid fluid/medications
      1) Insert two IV lines
      2) Cautiously administer fluids: overhydration may increase fluid accumulation in the area of cerebral ischemia
   d. Prepare for/assist with medical interventions
      1) Advanced airway management
         a) Nasal or oral intubation
         b) Supraglottic airway (e.g., King, Combitube, laryngeal mask airway)
         c) Surgical airway (e.g., cricothyrotomy)
      2) Increase venous outflow through elevation of head of bed and proper head and neck positioning for hemorrhagic strokes. Increase cerebral perfusion in the ischemic brain by keeping head of bed lowered

3) Institute cardiac and pulse oximetry monitoring
4) Assist with hospital admission or transfer to a stroke center

e. Administer pharmacologic therapy as ordered
   1) RSI premedications: sedatives, analgesics, neuromuscular blocking agents
   2) Antihypertensives: maintain systolic pressure at <185 mm Hg and diastolic pressure at <110 mm Hg
      a) Avoid hypotension
      b) Preferred regimen[10]
         (1) Labetalol (Normodyne, Trandate) 10–20 mg IV over 1–2 minutes, may repeat once OR
         (2) Nicardipine 5 mg/h IV (titrate up by 2.5 mg/h every 5–15 min; maximum 15 mg/h—titrate to desired blood pressure)
         (3) Consider use of IV sodium nitroprusside if above is not successful
      c) Calcium channel blockers may decrease or avoid vasospasm in SAH
         (1) Use of oral sublingual nifedipine (Procardia) is discouraged because it may cause extreme hypotension
   3) Fibrinolytics for ischemic stroke: rt-PA (Alteplase) if patient meets guidelines
      a) IV rt-PA administration must start within 3 hours of symptom onset or last time known well: 0.9 mg/kg, maximum 90 mg, 10% administered as bolus followed by infusion of remainder over 1 hour (there is limited use of rt-PA later than 3 hours). Under some circumstances, this window may be expanded to 4.5 hours from last time known well
      b) Intraarterial rt-PA administration must start within 6 hours of symptom onset; generally limited to 30 mg total
      c) Must meet inclusion and exclusion criteria per package insert and institutional protocol
         (1) Evaluate risks and benefits: risk of bleeding with other comorbidities, risk increases with time lapse
         (2) NIHSS score, sequential scoring (baseline, prior, during, and after rt-PA, post, ongoing)
   4) Consider endovascular intervention (mechanical thrombectomy)
   5) Anticonvulsants given only if patient experiences seizures
   6) Non rt-PA candidates: ASA, antiplatelet therapy, statins, antipyretics

4. Evaluation and ongoing monitoring
   a. Airway patency
   b. Level of consciousness: changes in NIHSS score
   c. Hemodynamic status
   d. Breath sounds and pulse oximetry

e. Cardiac rate and rhythm
f. Intake and output
g. Changes in motor strength and sensation

F. VENTRICULAR SHUNT

Ventricular shunts are placed to relieve increased ICP from hydrocephalus by diverting CSF from the lateral ventricle to a low-pressure space such as the atrium or body cavities (peritoneal).[11] This diversion relieves the pressure by creating alternative pathways for free circulation and/or absorption of CSF. The two most common complications of shunt insertion are infection and shunt malfunction. Infections may result from the shunt itself, from meningitis, or from ventriculitis. Malfunctions result from obstruction (plugging by the choroid plexus, blood clots, or debris) or mechanical failure (detachment or malpositioning of the two ends).

1. Assessment
   a. Subjective data collection
      1) History of present illness/chief complaint
         a) Type of shunt and date placed
         b) Reason for shunt placement
         c) Length of shunt, proximal and distal location
         d) Neurologic changes or trends
         e) Fever
         f) Abdominal pain or headache
         g) Wound infection changes if shunt recently placed
         h) Nausea/vomiting
      2) Past medical history
         a) Current or preexisting diseases/illness
         b) Previous shunt malfunctions or infections
         c) Risk factors for shunt malfunction (i.e., outgrown)
         d) Medications
         e) Allergies
         f) Immunization status
   b. Objective data collection
      1) Physical examination
         a) General appearance
            (1) Level of consciousness, behavior, affect: lethargy, shrill cry
            (2) Possible elevated temperature: if infection
         b) Inspection
            (1) Abdominal distention
         c) Palpation
            (1) Tense fontanels
            (2) Abdominal tenderness
      2) Diagnostic procedures
         a) CBC with differential: elevated WBC if infection present
         b) Serum chemistries including glucose
         c) Head and abdominal CT scan
         d) CSF analysis and culture, direct shunt aspiration or lumbar puncture

         e) Blood cultures
2. Analysis: differential nursing diagnoses/collaborative problems
   a. Risk for ineffective airway clearance
   b. Risk for ineffective breathing pattern
   c. Risk for acute confusion
   d. Risk for infection
   e. Risk for deficient knowledge
3. Planning and implementation/interventions
   a. Maintain airway, breathing, circulation (see Chapter 1)
   b. Provide supplemental oxygen as indicated
   c. Establish IV access for administration of crystalloid fluids/medications
      1) Administer IV fluids cautiously to prevent overhydration
   d. Prepare for/assist with medical interventions
      1) Institute cardiac and pulse oximetry monitoring
      2) Assist with hospital admission or appropriate transfer
   e. Administer pharmacologic therapy as ordered
      1) Antibiotics: if infection present
      2) Antiemetics
   f. Provide appropriate referrals for patient and family/caregiver
4. Evaluation and ongoing monitoring
   a. Airway patency
   b. Level of consciousness
   c. Hemodynamic status
   d. Breath sounds and pulse oximetry
   e. Cardiac rate and rhythm

References

1. Schreiber CP, Hutchinson S, Webster CJ, Ames M, Richardson MS, Powers C: Prevalence of migraine in patients with a history of self-reported or physician-diagnosed "sinus" headache, *Arch Intern Med* 164(16):1769, 2004.
2. Kan L, Nagelberg J, Maytal J: Headaches in a pediatric emergency department: Etiology, imaging, and treatment, *Headache* 40(1):25, 2000.
3. Torelli P, Campana V, Cervellin G, Manzoni GC: Management of primary headaches in adult emergency departments: A literature review, the Parma ED experience and a therapy flow chart proposal, *Neurological Sciences* 31(5):545, 2010.
4. Go AS, Mozaffarian D, Roger VL, Benjamin EJ, Berry JD, Blaha MJ, et al.: American Heart Association Statistics Committee and Stroke Statistics Subcommittee. Heart disease and stroke statistics—2014 update: A report from the American Heart Association, *Circulation* 129(3):e28, 2014.
5. Samaniego SA: Therapeutic hypothermia in brain injury (chap. 4). In *Neuroscience*, INTECH, 2013. http://dx.doi.org/10.5772/51071. Retrieved from http://www.intechopen.com/books/therapeutic-hypothermia-in-brain-injury/therapeutic-hypothermia-in-acute-stroke.

6. Jauch EC, Saver JL, Adams HP, Bruno A, Connors JJ, Demaerschalk BM, et al.: Guidelines for the early management of patients with acute ischemic stroke, *Stroke* 44:870–947, 2013. Retrieved from http://stroke.ahajournals.org/content/44/3/870.full.pdf+html.

7. Larson EB: Evaluation of cognitive impairment and dementia, *UpToDate*, 2015. Retrieved from http://www.uptodate.com/contents/evaluation-of-cognitive-impairment-and-dementia?source=machineLearning&search=dementia&selectedTitle=1%7E150&sectionRank=1&anchor=H6#H6.

8. Baddour LM, Flynn PM, Fekete T: Infections of central nervous system shunts and other devices, *UpToDate*, 2015. Retrieved from http://www.uptodate.com/contents/infections-of-central-nervous-system-shunts-and-otherdevices?source=machineLearning&search=ventricular+shunt&selectedTitle=1%7E52&sectionRank=1&anchor=H2#H1.

9. Korff CM, Wirrell E: ILAE classification of seizures and epilepsy, *UpToDate*, 2015. Retrieved from http://www.uptodate.com/contents/ilae-classification-of-seizures-and-epilepsy?source=machinelearning&search=classification+of+seizure&selectedtitle=1%7e150&sectionrank=1&anchor=h26939147#h26939147.

10. Karceski S: Initial treatment of epilepsy in adults, *UpToDate*, 2015. Retrieved from http://www.uptodate.com/contents/initial-treatment-of-epilepsy-in-adults?source=see_link&sectionName=WHEN+TO+START+ANTIEPILEPTIC+DRUG+THERAPY&anchor=H2#H2.

11. Vriesendorp F: Clinical features and diagnosis of Guillain-Barre syndrome in adults, *UpToDate*, 2015. Retrieved from http://www.uptodate.com/contents/clinical-features-and-diagnosis-of-guillain-barre-syndrome-in-adults?source=preview&language=en-US&anchor=H1&selectedTitle=1~150#H1.

CHAPTER 23

Obstetric and Gynecologic Emergencies

Kathleen Sanders Jordan, DNP, MS, RN, FNP-BC, ENP-BC, SANE-P

MAJOR TOPICS
General Strategy
Assessment
Analysis: Differential Nursing Diagnoses/Collaborative
    Problems
Planning and Implementation/Interventions
Evaluation and Ongoing Monitoring
Documentation of Interventions and Patient Response
Age-Related Considerations
Specific Obstetric Emergencies
Ectopic Pregnancy
Emergency Delivery
Gestational Hypertension: Preeclampsia, Eclampsia, and
    Hemolysis, Elevated Liver Enzymes, Low Platelets (HELLP)

Hyperemesis Gravidarum
Neonatal Resuscitation
Placenta Previa and Abruptio Placentae
Postpartum Hemorrhage
Spontaneous Abortion
Specific Gynecologic Emergencies
Pelvic Inflammatory Disease
Pelvic Pain
Sexually Transmitted Infections
Vaginal Bleeding/Dysfunctional Uterine Bleeding
Vaginitis

I. General Strategy

A. ASSESSMENT

1. Primary and secondary assessment/resuscitation (see Chapter 1)
2. Focused assessment
   a. Subjective data collection
      1) History of present illness/chief complaint
         a) Last normal menstrual period (LNMP): female patients of childbearing age
         b) Positive pregnancy test: date, place (to determine whether there were early complications such as bleeding) and method (serum or urine)
         c) Expected date of delivery (EDD)
         d) Vaginal bleeding: amount, color, presence of clots/tissue, number of full pads/tampons used (each holds approximately 30 mL of blood), any changes in color since bleeding started
         e) Vaginal discharge: amount, color, quality, odor, itching, burning, irritation, start, possible exposure to sexually transmitted infection, last sexual encounter, new medications
         f) Pain (see Chapter 8): abdominal/pelvic pain: provocation, quality, radiation, severity, timing

         g) Nausea and vomiting
         h) Fever/chills
         i) Visual disturbances, headache, sudden weight gain, dependent/generalized edema
         j) Change in fetal movement
         k) Rupture of membranes: time, color, and odor
         l) Uterine contractions: onset, frequency, severity
         m) Urinary frequency, dysuria, urgency, hematuria
         n) Trauma: mechanism of injury (see Chapter 31)
         o) Efforts to relieve symptoms
            (1) Home remedies
            (2) Alternative therapies
            (3) Medications
               (a) Prescription
               (b) OTC/herbal
      2) Past medical history
         a) Current or preexisting diseases/illness
            (1) Cardiovascular disease
            (2) Deep venous thrombosis
            (3) Pulmonary disease/emboli
            (4) Hypertension
            (5) Diabetes
            (6) Thyroid disease
            (7) Renal disease/urinary tract infections

(8) Immunosuppression disease

b) Reproductive history: all pregnancies with dates (include premature deliveries, spontaneous abortions/therapeutic abortions, full-term deliveries, living children)

c) Prenatal care if appropriate

d) Date and type of delivery, if postpartum and any complications during antepartum or postpartum before the current encounter

e) Abdominal/pelvic surgery

f) Sexual activity/preference: new sexual partner within last 3 months or multiple sexual partners within last 6 months, high-risk behavior

g) Contraceptive use: type and length of use

h) Sexually transmitted infections (STIs)/pelvic inflammatory disease (PID), hepatitis and human immunodeficiency virus (HIV) status

i) Smoking history

j) Substance and/or alcohol use/abuse

k) Current medications

(1) Prescription

(2) OTC/herbal

l) Allergies

m) Immunization status

3) Psychological, social, environmental factors

a) Age: consider possibility of pregnancy in women 11–55 years of age

b) Nationality/ethnicity

c) Occupation

d) Economic capabilities and resources

e) Social support system

f) Nutritional status

g) Genetic history

h) Possible/actual abuse, assault, or intimate partner violence situations (see Chapters 3 and 40)

b. Objective data collection

1) General appearance

a) Level of consciousness, behavior, affect, mood

b) Vital signs: orthostasis; left lateral position if patient is 20 weeks' gestation or greater to prevent supine hypotension syndrome

c) Odors

d) Gait

e) Hygiene

f) Level of distress/discomfort

2) Inspection

a) Edema: facial, peripheral or generalized

b) Skin: color

c) Abdominal or perineal wound site

d) Vaginal bleeding: color and amount, passage of clots or tissue

e) Amniotic fluid: color and pH (amniotic fluid is clear and pH neutral)

3) Auscultation

a) Bowel sounds

b) Fetal heart tones (FHTs) if gestational age >14 weeks (uterus becomes an abdominal organ at 14 weeks; some as early as 12 weeks. Heart rate should be 130–160 bpm)

4) Palpation

a) Abdominal tenderness, rebound tenderness

b) Uterine size, fundal height, irritability, contractility

c) Skin temperature, moisture

5) Pelvic examination

a) External genitalia inspection, noting excoriation, erythema, and vesicular lesions

b) Vaginal mucosa inspected for color, edema, discharge, lesions; urethra inspected, noting Bartholin and Skene glands for erythema, edema, and discharge, palpated for tenderness

c) Vagina and cervix inspected for lesions, erosions, ulcerations, bleeding, and discharge

d) Bimanual examination; uterus palpated for size, shape, consistency, cervical motion tenderness; adnexal tenderness, fullness, masses

3. Diagnostic procedures

a. Laboratory studies

1) Complete blood count (CBC) with differential

2) Coagulation profile: prothrombin time (PT), partial thromboplastin time (PTT), fibrinogen, fibrin split products

3) Serum chemistries including glucose, BUN, creatinine

4) Urinalysis; pregnancy test: serum and/or urine female patients of childbearing age to detect human chorionic gonadotropin (HCG)

5) Serum and urine toxicology screen

6) Erythrocyte sedimentation rate (ESR)

7) Type and crossmatch, Rh factor

8) Thyroid function tests

9) Liver enzymes and uric acid

10) Arterial/venous blood gas

11) Kleihauer-Betke test: to assess and measure presence of fetomaternal hemorrhage

12) C-reactive protein: nonspecific method for evaluating severity and course of inflammatory diseases; positive C-reactive protein indicates presence of active inflammation

13) STI screening: *Chlamydia* infection, gonorrhea, trichomoniasis, syphilis, hepatitis B, and HIV

14) Wet mount: normal saline and potassium hydroxide (KOH) preparations

b. Imaging studies

1) Chest radiograph

2) Sonography: pelvic and/or transvaginal

3) Computed tomography (CT) scan

c. Other
1) 12- to 15-lead electrocardiogram (ECG)
2) Culdocentesis: performed infrequently
3) Cardiotocographic (electronic) monitoring: uterine contractions and fetal heart rate
4) pH level for amniotic fluid

B. ANALYSIS: DIFFERENTIAL NURSING DIAGNOSES/COLLABORATIVE PROBLEMS

1. Acute pain
2. Deficient fluid volume
3. Ineffective tissue perfusion
4. Anxiety
5. Fear
6. Risk for infection
7. Deficient knowledge
8. Anticipatory grieving
9. Alteration of fluids and electrolytes

C. PLANNING AND IMPLEMENTATION/ INTERVENTIONS

1. Determine priorities of care
   a. Maintain airway, breathing, circulation (see Chapter 1)
   b. Provide supplemental oxygen as indicated
   c. Establish intravenous (IV) access for administration of crystalloid fluid/blood products/medication as needed
   d. Obtain and set up equipment and supplies
   e. Prepare for/assist with medical interventions
   f. Administer pharmacologic therapy as ordered
2. Relieve anxiety/apprehension
3. Allow significant others to remain with patient if supportive
4. Educate patient/significant others

D. EVALUATION AND ONGOING MONITORING

1. Continuously monitor and treat as indicated
2. Monitor patient response/outcomes, and modify nursing care plan as appropriate
3. If positive patient outcomes are not demonstrated, reevaluate assessment and/or plan of care

E. DOCUMENTATION OF INTERVENTIONS AND PATIENT RESPONSE

F. AGE-RELATED CONSIDERATIONS

1. Pediatric
   a. Growth or development related
      1) Breast development signals the onset of puberty and usually occurs between 8 and 11 years of age
      2) The average age of menarche is 13 years
      3) Estrogen and progesterone production increase with puberty
      4) At puberty, the uterus descends into the lower pelvis
   b. "Pearls"
      1) Child maltreatment must always be considered in the presence of gynecologic complaints; however, the physical examination in more than 90% of sexually abused children is normal. History is the most critical part of the evaluation, and a high index of suspicion must be maintained
      2) Vulvovaginitis and vaginal discharges are common problems in prepubertal and pubescent girls, although the causes vary with age. The incidence of STIs in prepubertal children is increasing and mandates investigation for the possibility of sexual abuse. Other causes include poor hygiene with perineal contamination, chemical irritation (e.g., soaps, bubble bath, and douches), infections, allergic reactions, foreign body, and congenital anomaly
      3) The highest rate of STIs is in sexually active adolescents; additionally, this group is also at high risk for PID and is least likely to experience or report symptoms. Developmental and psychosocial characteristics of adolescent female patients also increase risk of contracting PID
      4) Pelvic pain in postmenarchal adolescents usually has the same causes as in adults
      5) Teenagers have a high risk of complications during pregnancy, labor, and delivery
2. Geriatric
   a. Aging related
      1) Malignant disease should always be considered because it is the most important, although not the most common, cause of bleeding in this age group. Postmenopausal hormonal changes may be responsible for dysfunctional uterine bleeding (DUB)
   b. "Pearls"
      1) The amount of bleeding does not correlate with the severity of disease
      2) Patients in this age group with vaginal bleeding are at increased risk for uterine cancer

II. Specific Obstetric Emergencies

A. ECTOPIC PREGNANCY

An ectopic pregnancy (EP) is defined as the implantation of the fertilized ovum outside the normal uterine cavity. Approximately 98% of EPs are implanted in the fallopian tube, frequently on the maternal right side. The remaining EPs implant in the peritoneal cavity, uterine cornu, ovary, or cervix. If the EP invades the tubal wall too deeply or grows too large, it can rupture the tube. This rupture leads to severe pain, intraperitoneal hemorrhage, and hemorrhagic shock. EP is the leading cause of pregnancy-related maternal death in the first trimester. The incidence of EP has been increasing worldwide, and during the last few decades, the rate has nearly quadrupled in industrialized nations, due to the increased prevalence of pelvic inflammatory disease. In the United States, the incidence of EP is approximately 2%; however, complications from EP account for approximately 4–10% of maternal mortality. Causes of EPs are classified as mechanical, functional, and assisted reproduction. Mechanical obstruction results from narrowing of the fallopian tube, which prevents the normal passage of the ovum. Factors that can lead to mechanical obstruction, which delay the fertilized egg from reaching the uterus, include pelvic inflammatory infection (in PID), salpingitis, fallopian tube surgery, tubal ligation, previous EP, intrauterine device (IUD) use, tumor, or developmental abnormalities of the tube. Functional causes of EP include altered tubal motility from infection or hormonal changes. Reproductive assistance such as the use of ovulation induction agents and in vitro techniques increase the risk of EP. Women of advanced maternal age and women who are African-American are also at a higher risk. However, it has been estimated that up over 50% of women presenting with EP have none of these risk factors. The treatment approach has changed from salpingectomy to a conservative plan that attempts to save the fallopian tube.

1. Assessment
   a. Subjective data collection
      1) History of the present illness/chief complaint
         a) Pain (see Chapter 8)
            (1) Abdominal pain: character may be nonspecific; may be diffuse, unilateral, or bilateral; may begin as vague discomfort and progress to sharp and colicky; typically, the pain is located in the pelvic area; rupture of tube may result in sudden, sharp, severe pain and may radiate to the middle or upper abdomen
            (2) Referred shoulder pain resulting from phrenic nerve irritation
         b) Vaginal bleeding: irregular, mild, or absent
         c) Fatigue, dizziness, lightheadedness, syncope
         d) Symptoms of pregnancy
      2) Past medical history
         a) Current or preexisting diseases/illness
         b) LNMP: history of amenorrhea or abnormal menses
         c) Reproductive history (gravidity, parity, previous EPs)
         d) History of PID or STI
         e) IUD use
         f) Tubal surgery
         g) Infertility treatment
         h) Medications
         i) Allergies
         j) Substance abuse
   b. Objective data collection
      1) Physical examination
         a) General appearance
            (1) Possible positive orthostasis and tachycardia
            (2) Moderate to severe distress/discomfort
         b) Auscultation
            (1) FHTs
         c) Palpation: abdominal tenderness
         d) Pelvic examination: cervical motion tenderness; adnexal fullness, mass, or tenderness
      2) Diagnostic procedures
         a) Serum and urine pregnancy test: quantitative β-HCG: correlate level in conjunction with sonography findings
         b) CBC with differential
         c) Type, rH, and crossmatch
         d) Coagulation profile: PT/PTT
         e) Serum chemistries
         f) Pelvic/transvaginal sonography
         g) Culdocentesis: rarely performed
2. Analysis: differential nursing diagnoses/collaborative problems
   a. Deficient fluid volume
   b. Acute pain
   c. Grieving
3. Planning and implementation/interventions
   a. Maintain airway, breathing, circulation (see Chapter 1)
   b. Provide supplemental oxygen as indicated
   c. Establish IV access for administration of crystalloid fluid/blood products/medications as needed
   d. Prepare for/assist with medical interventions
      1) Pelvic examination
      2) Assist with possible hospital admission and operative intervention
   e. Administer pharmacologic therapy as ordered
      1) Methotrexate (Folex): antimetabolite used to terminate EP; close follow-up mandated. The optimal candidate is hemodynamically stable, willing to comply with posttreatment follow-up, has no fetal cardiac activity, and has a serum hCG <5,000 IU/L
4. Evaluation and ongoing monitoring
   a. Maternal hemodynamic status
   b. Pain relief

B. EMERGENCY DELIVERY

When a pregnant patient arrives in the emergency department and delivery appears imminent, it is essential to obtain a rapid obstetric history and physical assessment of the labor status. Contractions alone are not an indication of advanced labor. Uterine contractions must be present with sufficient duration (30 seconds), frequency (every 5 minutes), and intensity to produce progressive effacement and dilation of the cervix. Signs of imminent delivery include a fully effaced and dilated cervix (approximately 10 cm in a full-term infant), palpable fetal parts in the pelvic floor, bulging of the perineum, and widening of the vulvovaginal area. The first stage of labor is the time from the onset of regular contractions until complete cervical dilation. The second stage of labor is the time from complete dilation until delivery of the infant. During this stage, the mother will have the urge to push. The third stage of labor is from the delivery of the infant until the delivery of the placenta.

1. Assessment
   a. Subjective data collection
      1) History of present condition/chief complaint
         a) Contractions: frequency, intensity, duration
         b) Rupture of amniotic membranes: time, color, odor
         c) Increase in bloody show
         d) Rectal pressure or passage of feces
      2) Past medical history
         a) Current or preexisting diseases/illness
         b) Reproductive history: gravidity and parity, EDD
         c) Obstetric care received during this pregnancy
         d) Previous labor and delivery history, including complications
         e) Medications
         f) Allergies
   b. Objective data collection
      1) Physical examination
         a) General appearance
            (1) Obvious pregnancy
            (2) Moderate to severe distress/discomfort
         b) Inspection
            (1) Vaginal bleeding: amount, color
            (2) Perineal bulging, presentation of fetal parts
         c) Auscultation
            (1) FHTs
         d) Palpation
            (1) Uterine size/tone, irritability, contractility
         e) Pelvic examination
            (1) Effacement (thinning) of cervix
            (2) Dilation of cervix
            (3) Consistency (softness or firmness) of the cervix
            (4) Station of fetal head
            (5) Status of membranes and color of amniotic fluid if ruptured
      2) Diagnostic procedures
         a) pH test of amniotic fluid: amniotic fluid has a neutral pH
2. Analysis: differential nursing diagnoses/collaborative problems
   a. Pain

   b. Anxiety/fear
3. Planning and implementation/interventions
   a. Establish IV access for administration of crystalloid fluids/medications as needed
   b. Prepare for/assist with medical procedures
      1) Delivery process
         a) Position patient comfortably: lithotomy or modified Fowler position with legs supported
         b) Assist the mother with proper breathing. As the head emerges, encourage the mother to "pant like a puppy" to prevent uncontrolled delivery, predisposing to maternal and fetal trauma
         c) Extend the fingers of the dominant hand on the infant's head for control and allow the head to emerge slowly
         d) Once the head is delivered, a finger should be passed around the neck of the infant to ascertain whether it is encircled by umbilical cord; if the cord is felt, it should be slipped over the infant's head; if the cord is tight, it should be clamped in two places and cut
         e) Quickly wipe the infant's face, and suction the mouth first, then nares to minimize likelihood of aspiration of amniotic fluid and blood
         f) While supporting the infant's head, deliver shoulders: anterior followed by posterior; remainder of infant's body should follow rapidly
         g) While holding the infant in a head-dependent position at the level of the introitus, suction the mouth and nose as needed
         h) When the umbilical cord stops pulsating, clamp it with two clamps placed about 4 and 5 cm from the infant's abdomen; then cut the cord
      2) Dry and wrap the infant to minimize heat loss and place on mother's chest
      3) Perform an Apgar score (Table 23.1) at 1 minute and 5 minutes, repeat every 5 minutes if scores are <7.
      4) Do not perform uterine massage or manipulate umbilical cord until placenta is expelled (up to 30 minutes after delivery of infant)
      5) Allow for early breastfeeding or bonding between mother and infant
      6) Assist with hospital admission and transport to labor and delivery unit
   c. Administer pharmacologic therapy as ordered
      1) Oxytocin (Pitocin) to initiate and maintain uterine contractility after delivery
      2) For persistent postpartum bleeding, methylergonovine (Methergine) or IM prostaglandin

Table 23.1

Apgar Scoring

Objective Sign	0	1	2
		Score	
Heart rate	Absent	<100 beats/minute	100 beats/minute
Respiratory effort	Absent	Irregular, slow	Crying, good
Muscle tone	Flaccid	Some flexion	Active motion
Reflex irritability	No response	Grimace, weak cry	Sneeze, cough, cry
Color	Blue	Pink body, blue extremities	Completely pink

4. Evaluation and ongoing monitoring
   a. Maternal and infant hemodynamic status
   b. Vaginal bleeding

C. GESTATIONAL HYPERTENSION: PREECLAMPSIA, ECLAMPSIA, AND HEMOLYSIS, ELEVATED LIVER ENZYMES, LOW PLATELETS (HELLP)

Gestational hypertension, formerly known as pregnancy-induced hypertension (PIH), is a clinical diagnosis defined as a new onset of hypertension (systolic blood pressure >140 mm Hg and/or diastolic blood pressure >90 mm Hg) after the 20th week of pregnancy. Preeclampsia is the new onset of hypertension and either proteinuria or end-organ dysfunction, or both, after the 20th week of pregnancy in a usually normotensive woman. Eclampsia is an extension of preeclampsia characterized by convulsions, coma, or both; it can occur during pregnancy but also in the early postpartum period. A severe form of preeclampsia characterized by *hemolysis, elevated liver* enzymes, and *low platelets* is the HELLP syndrome.

The exact cause of preeclampsia remains unclear; however, the basic underlying pathologic process is related to placental dysfunction, which initiates systemic vasospasm resulting in an overall increase in peripheral vascular resistance. Vasospasm contracts the intravascular space; therefore, the preeclamptic patient is volume contracted and is at risk for complications resulting from any change in intravascular volume. This generalized vasospasm also decreases perfusion in the uteroplacental circulation, thus reducing the delivery of oxygen and nutrients to the fetus. Preeclampsia is the most common complication of pregnancy and involves 4–8% of pregnancies in the United States. It is primarily a disease of first pregnancies and is one of the leading causes of maternal death. Risk factors include first pregnancy, extremes of reproductive age, chronic hypertension, and history of preeclampsia, mother or sister with history of preeclampsia, multiple gestation, diabetes, connective tissue disease, and vascular disease.

1. Assessment
   a. Subjective data collection
      1) History of present illness/chief complaint
         a) Persistent and/or severe headache
         b) Epigastric or right upper quadrant (RUQ) tenderness; nausea and/or vomiting
         c) Swelling of extremities, face, or generalized edema
         d) Visual disturbances, including photophobia, blurred vision or temporary blindness
         e) Decreased urine output
         f) Shortness of breath and exertional dyspnea
         g) Anxiety and apprehension
      2) Past medical history
         a) Current or preexisting diseases/illness
            (1) Chronic hypertension
            (2) Diabetes
            (3) Connective tissue disease, vascular disease
         b) Gestational age: estimated date of delivery (EDD), LNMP
         c) Age: young adolescent or older than 35 years, primigravida
         d) Personal or family history of preeclampsia-eclampsia
         e) Multiple gestations
         f) Medications
         g) Allergies
   b. Objective data collection
      1) Physical examination
         a) General appearance
            (1) Level of consciousness, behavior, affect: alert to confusion, seizure, comatose
            (2) Blood pressure: stage 1 hypertension is defined as a blood pressure reading of 140/90 mm Hg after 20 weeks' gestation or a reading that represents an increase of 30 mm Hg systolic or 15 mm Hg diastolic higher than the patient's baseline measurement. To determine this, two blood pressure readings must be taken at least 6 hours apart with the patient lying on her left side
            (3) Moderate distress/discomfort, possibly critically ill
         b) Inspection

    (1) Nondependent edema and excessive
        weight gain
  c) Auscultation
    (1) FHTs
  d) Palpation
    (1) Epigastric and RUQ tenderness
    (2) Uterine size, tone
    (3) Hyperreflexia
2) Diagnostic procedures
  a) Urinalysis: proteinuria 1+
  b) CBC with differential: anemia and
     thrombocytopenia (HELLP)
    (1) Anemia resulting from microangiopathic
        hemolytic anemia and dilution of preg-
        nancy
    (2) Thrombocytopenia: platelet count
        <100,000
  c) Aspartate aminotransferase (AST): elevated
    (1) Creatinine: elevated as a result of
        decreased intravascular volume and de-
        creased glomerular filtration rate (GFR)
  d) Liver function tests: HELLP syndrome
    (1) Serum glutamic-oxaloacetic transami-
        nase (SGOT): >72 units/L
    (2) Lactate dehydrogenase (LDH): >600
        units/L
    (3) Total bilirubin: >1.2 mg/dL
  e) Coagulation profile: PT/PTT, fibrin split
     products, fibrinogen level
  f) Pelvic sonography
  g) Head CT scan
2. Analysis: differential nursing diagnoses/collaborative
   problems
  a. Ineffective tissue perfusion: maternal and fetal
  b. Risk for injury
  c. Anxiety/fear
3. Planning and implementation/interventions
  a. Maintain airway, breathing, circulation (see
     Chapter 1)
  b. Provide supplemental oxygen as indicated
  c. Establish IV access for administration of crystalloid
     fluid/medications as needed
  d. Place patient in left lateral decubitus position
  e. Prepare for/assist with medical procedures
    1) Institute cardiac and pulse oximetry monitoring
    2) Insert indwelling urinary catheter as indicated
    3) Institute seizure precautions
    4) Minimize external stimuli
    5) Prepare for emergency delivery if pregnancy 30
       weeks or greater: definitive treatment
    6) Assist with possible hospital admission
  f. Administer pharmacologic therapy as indicated
    1) IV or intramuscular (IM) magnesium sulfate for
       seizure prophylaxis
    2) Benzodiazepine for seizures resistant to
       magnesium sulfate

    3) Antihypertensive therapy: hydralazine, labetalol
       (Normodyne, Trandate) or nifedipine (Adalat,
       Procardia), or nitroprusside (Nipride) if labetalol
       or nifedipine ineffective; maintain diastolic
       blood pressure approximately 90–100 mm Hg
       to prevent inadequate utero-placental perfusion
       and fetal distress
  g. Educate patient/significant others
    1) Maintain reduced activity/bed rest as directed
    2) Take medications as directed
    3) Return to emergency department for headaches,
       visual disturbances, increased swelling of face
       or fingers, or generalized, epigastric or RUQ
       abdominal pain, tremors, uterine contractions,
       vaginal bleeding
    4) Follow-up with obstetrician as directed
4. Evaluation and ongoing monitoring
  a. Level of consciousness
  b. Maternal hemodynamic status
  c. Breath sounds and pulse oximetry
  d. Cardiac rate and rhythm
  e. FHTs
  f. Intake and output
  g. Signs of magnesium toxicity: decrease or loss of
     patellar reflex, respiratory depression, cardiac arrest
     (if toxicity present, administer antidote calcium
     gluconate)

D. HYPEREMESIS GRAVIDARUM

Hyperemesis gravidarum is the most severe form of nausea and vomiting in pregnancy, characterized by persistent
nausea, vomiting, ketosis, and weight loss (>5% prepreg-
nancy weight). The peak incidence is at 8–12 weeks of pregnancy. Hyperemesis gravidarum is rare and cases severe
enough to necessitate hospitalization occur in up to 2% of
all pregnancies. The diagnosis is not well defined because
the diagnostic criteria used vary from one geographic area
to another. This condition usually necessitates hospitalization because both maternal and fetal well-being are threatened. The exact cause of hyperemesis gravidarum remains
unclear; however, the following causative factors have been
suggested: vitamin B_6 deficiency resulting from a change
in protein metabolism, impaired function of the adrenal cortex, hyperthyroidism and excess human chorionic
gonadotropin secretion, psychological factors, alterations
in gastrointestinal physiology, a hypersensitivity reaction,
and poor nutrition. The primary clinical manifestation of
hyperemesis gravidarum is frequent, sustained vomiting,
often lasting 4–8 weeks. This results in significant weight
loss and dehydration. Signs of starvation gradually develop
including metabolic acidosis, ketonuria, hypokalemic
alkalosis, oliguria, hemoconcentration, and constipation.
Complications of hyperemesis gravidarum include gastrointestinal bleeding, Mallory-Weiss tears, and Boerhaave
esophageal disruptions. Rare cases of Wernicke encephalopathy resulting from thiamine deficiency caused by

prolonged hyperemesis have been documented. The population at risk includes the following: primiparous, young, nonsmoking women; women with multiple-gestation pregnancies; women with a history of hydatidiform mole pregnancy; and women weighing more than 25% of their ideal body weight.

1. Assessment
   a. Subjective data collection
      1) History of present illness/chief complaint
         a) Nausea and vomiting: severity and duration
         b) Weight loss
      2) Past medical history
         a) Current or preexisting diseases/illness
         b) Reproductive history
         c) Gestational age: estimated date of delivery (EDD), LNMP
         d) Medications
         e) Allergies
   b. Objective data collection
      1) Physical examination
         a) General appearance and volume status (e.g., mucous membrane condition, skin turgor, neck veins, and mental status)
            (1) Possible positive orthostasis
            (2) Moderate distress/discomfort
         b) Auscultation
            (1) FHTs
      2) Diagnostic procedures
         a) CBC with differential
         b) Serum chemistries including glucose, BUN, creatinine
         c) Liver enzymes, bilirubin, amylase and lipase levels
         d) Serum ketones
         e) Urinalysis: specific gravity and ketones
         f) Serum and/or urine pregnancy test
2. Analysis: differential nursing diagnoses/collaborative problems
   a. Deficient fluid volume
   b. Imbalanced nutrition: less than body requirements
   c. Deficient knowledge
   d. Imbalanced fluids and electrolytes
3. Planning and implementation/interventions
   a. Maintain airway, breathing, circulation (see Chapter 1)
   b. Establish IV access for administration of crystalloid fluid/medications as needed
      1) Rapid infusion 1–2 L normal saline or lactated Ringer solution
      2) Volume replacement is then followed by a slower infusion of a dextrose-containing solution, which helps break the cycle of ketosis
   c. Prepare for/assist with medical procedures
      1) Insert gastric tube and attach to suction as indicated
      2) Assist with hospital admission for continued vomiting

      3) Gradual oral rehydration as tolerated
   d. Administer pharmacologic therapy as ordered
      1) Antiemetics: diphenhydramine (Benadryl), meclizine (Antivert), metroclopramide (Reglan), promethazine (Phenergan). Avoid ondansetron (Zofran)
   e. Educate patient/significant others
      1) Oral fluids as tolerated; advance to small, frequent meals consisting of easily digested high-energy foods
      2) Take medications as directed
      3) Return to emergency department for persistent vomiting
      4) Moderate activity as tolerated
      5) Follow up with obstetrician as directed
4. Evaluation and ongoing monitoring
   a. Maternal hemodynamic status
   b. Intake and output

E. NEONATAL RESUSCITATION

Newborn resuscitation is required for infants born with any signs of cardiovascular or respiratory compromise. Infants at high risk include those born prematurely (before 37 weeks' gestation), breech presentation, multiple gestation, meconium identified before or after delivery, Apgar scores at 1 and 5 minutes lower than 7, or any signs of infant compromise before or after delivery. Neonatal asphyxia is the direct result of conditions that interfere with the placenta's ability to function as the fetal organ of respiration or with the infant's ability to establish extrauterine respiration despite adequate placental functioning. The end result in this setting is an infant who is hypoxic, hypercapnic, and acidotic; however, most infants are not born asphyxiated and should only require maintenance of temperature, suctioning of the airway, and mild stimulation. Six percent of all newborns require further resuscitation. All neonatal resuscitation efforts should proceed in an orderly and systematic manner, and reassessment should follow each intervention to prevent any further and often unnecessary actions.

1. Assessment
   a. Subjective data collection
      1) History of present condition/chief complaint
         a) Gestational age: EDD, LNMP
         b) Prolonged and/or complicated labor
         c) Prolonged rupture of the membranes
         d) Prolapsed umbilical cord
         e) Breech or other abnormal presentation
         f) Meconium-stained amniotic fluid
         g) Multiple gestations
         h) Precipitous delivery
         i) Operative delivery
         j) Medications received during labor and delivery
         k) Signs of fetal distress

2) Maternal past medical history
   a) Current or preexisting diseases/illness
      (1) PIH/Gestational Hypertension
      (2) Diabetes
      (3) Cardiovascular disease
      (4) Thyroid
   b) Reproductive history: gravidity and parity
   c) Obstetric care received during this pregnancy
   d) Maternal age younger than 16 years or older than 35 years
   e) Substance use/abuse
   f) Medications
   g) Allergies
   b. Objective data collection
   1) Physical examination
      a) General appearance
         (1) Depressed/unresponsive infant
         (2) Severe distress, critically ill
      b) Inspection
         (1) Apgar scores at 1 and 5 minutes: depressed
         (2) Meconium-stained amniotic fluid
      c) Birth weight
   2) Diagnostic procedures
      a) Serum glucose
      b) CBC with differential
      c) Venous blood pH/ABG
      d) ECG
      e) Chest and abdominal radiograph
2. Analysis: differential nursing diagnoses/collaborative problems
   a. Ineffective airway clearance
   b. Impaired gas exchange
   c. Decreased cardiac output
   d. Ineffective tissue perfusion
3. Planning and implementation/interventions
   a. Maintain airway, breathing, circulation of mother (see Chapter 1)
   b. Prepare for/assist with medical procedures
   1) Quickly dry off amniotic fluid covering infant, and place infant under a heat source to maintain infant's temperature
   2) Maintain infant on back or side with neck in neutral position; do not hyperextend neck, or airway obstruction may result; gently suction trachea only if infant has absent, slow, or difficult respirations
   3) Provide tactile stimulation if necessary by flicking soles of feet and rubbing infant's back
   4) Provide blow-by oxygen therapy to stimulate infant if respirations are shallow or slow
   5) Institute positive-pressure ventilation at a rate of 40–60 breaths/minute with 100% oxygen if respirations are inadequate or gasping is present

6) Initiate chest compression if heart rate is <60–80 beats/min and not increasing rapidly despite positive-pressure ventilation within a period of 30–60 seconds
7) Assist with intubation if necessary
8) Initiate vascular access via the umbilical vein or intraosseous route
   a) Administer volume expanders for a hypovolemic infant: normal saline or lactated Ringer solution; albumin/saline; or whole blood crossmatched with mother's blood
9) Institute cardiac and pulse oximetry monitoring
10) Assist with hospital admission and transfer to neonatal unit when stable for transfer
   c. Administer pharmacologic therapy as indicated
   1) Use neonatal preparations of medications
      a) Epinephrine
      b) Naloxone (Narcan)
      c) Glucose
      d) Sodium bicarbonate (for prolonged resuscitation)
   d. Maintain communication with family members regarding infant's status
   e. Initiate consultation with social service, chaplain, or other crisis intervention worker
   f. Allow family to see infant as soon as possible
4. Evaluation and ongoing monitoring
   a. Maternal hemodynamic status
   b. Newborn's airway patency
   c. Newborn's respiratory effort
   d. Newborn's cardiovascular status, especially heart rate
   e. Newborn's color of mucous membrane (compared with general color) and warmth of skin

F. PLACENTA PREVIA AND ABRUPTIO PLACENTAE

Placenta previa and abruptio placentae are the most serious causes of vaginal bleeding in the second and third trimesters of pregnancy. The end result of each of these conditions may be catastrophic for both mother and fetus. Placenta previa is a condition in which the placenta is abnormally implanted in the lower uterine segment and partially or completely obstructs the internal cervical os. It is estimated that approximately 45% of gravid women have a placenta previa during the second trimester of pregnancy; however, the incidence at term is less than 1%. This is because the lower uterine segment grows and stretches during the third trimester of pregnancy and causes the placental site to rise up the uterine wall away from the internal os. Softening of the lower uterine segment and effacement of the cervix in preparation for labor tear the implanted placenta previa, resulting in painless, bright red vaginal bleeding. Hemorrhage can result as the cervix continues to efface and dilate.

The cause of placenta previa remains unknown. Associated etiologic factors include multiparity, multiple gestation, advanced maternal age, previous uterine scarring resulting from prior cesarean section birth or myomectomy, previous placenta previa, smoking, and placental abnormalities.

Abruptio placentae is an emergent obstetric condition that occurs when the placenta separates from its normal site of implantation before delivery of the fetus. The incidence is less than 3% of all pregnancies, although it is related to 15% of all perinatal deaths. Partial or complete separation of the placenta may occur, resulting in minimal to copious bleeding that may be seen vaginally or concealed behind the placenta. Damage to the vascular placental bed can cause a significant amount of blood loss, resulting in maternal hypotension and hypovolemic shock. The loss of placental circulation causes fetal distress or demise. Consumptive coagulopathy and progression to disseminated intravascular coagulopathy (DIC) may occur. The hallmark of abruption is vaginal bleeding with uterine tenderness or pain. The primary cause of placental abruption is unknown, but the following conditions have been suggested as etiologic factors: maternal hypertension, advanced maternal age, trauma (see Chapter 37), illegal drug use (e.g., cocaine), premature rupture of the membranes, short umbilical cord, uterine anomaly or tumor, pressure by the enlarged uterus on the inferior vena cava, low socioeconomic status, and dietary deficiency.

1. Assessment
   a. Subjective data collection
      1) History of the present illness/chief complaint
         a) Bleeding: onset, duration, quantity, and character
            (1) Placenta previa: sudden onset of bright red vaginal bleeding; may be profuse
            (2) Abruptio placentae: dark red vaginal bleeding; amount variable because bleeding may be concealed
         b) Pain (see Chapter 8): abdominal, pelvic, and/or back
            (1) Placenta previa: usually absent
            (2) Abruptio placentae: variable intensity
         c) Gestational age (LNMP, EDD)
         d) Maternal age: risks increased with advanced age
         e) Recent trauma
         f) Recent sexual intercourse
         g) Decrease/loss of fetal movement
      2) Past medical history
         a) Current or preexisting diseases/illness
         b) Multiparity
         c) Premature rupture of membranes
         d) History of placenta previa, abruptio placentae, previous cesarean section
         e) Substance use/abuse
         f) Smoking
         g) Low socioeconomic status
         h) Medications
         i) Allergies
         j) Lack of prenatal care
   b. Objective data collection
      1) Physical examination
         a) General appearance
            (1) Possible positive orthostasis
            (2) Mild to moderate distress/discomfort, possibly critically ill
         b) Auscultation
            (1) FHTs
         c) Palpation
            (1) Abdominal tenderness, uterine tone, contractions
         d) Perineal examination: evidence of bleeding (speculum or manual pelvic examination is contraindicated in second- and third-trimester vaginal bleeding until location of placenta is confirmed by sonography and placenta previa is ruled out)
      2) Diagnostic procedures
         a) CBC with differential
         b) Coagulation profile: PT, PTT, fibrinogen level, fibrin split products
         c) Type and crossmatch (at least four units packed red blood cells in hemorrhaging patient)
         d) Kleihauer-Betke test
         e) Serum chemistries
         f) Pelvic sonography
         g) Cardiotocographic monitoring (fetal monitoring)
2. Analysis: differential nursing diagnoses/collaborative problems
   a. Deficient fluid volume
   b. Ineffective tissue perfusion: maternal and fetal
   c. Anxiety/fear
   d. Anticipatory grieving
3. Planning and implementation/interventions
   a. Maintain airway, breathing, circulation (see Chapters 1 and 32)
   b. Provide supplemental oxygen as indicated
   c. Establish IV access for administration of crystalloid fluid/blood products/medications as needed
      1) Infuse warmed normal saline solution fluid boluses
   d. Maintain patient in left lateral decubitus position
   e. Prepare for/assist with medical interventions
      1) Emergency cesarean section
      2) Emergency vaginal delivery and possible infant resuscitation
      3) Assist with hospital admission and transport to labor and delivery unit when hemodynamically stable
   f. Administer pharmacologic therapy as ordered
      1) Rh immune globulin (RhoGAM or Rhophylac) to all Rh-negative women

4. Evaluation and ongoing monitoring
   a. Maternal and infant hemodynamic status
   b. Vaginal bleeding: color and amount, passage of clots and tissue
   c. Abdominal pain/uterine contractions
   d. Fundal height (may rise with concealed intrauterine bleeding, measurement should be in centimeters, each week fundal height should correlate to the number of weeks pregnant unless obesity exists)
   e. FHTs
   f. Pain relief

G. POSTPARTUM HEMORRHAGE

Postpartum hemorrhage (PPH) is defined as any bleeding that results in signs and symptoms of hemodynamic instability following the expulsion or extraction of the placenta and membranes. PPH can be a complication of either vaginal delivery or cesarean section. It is the leading cause of maternal mortality. PPH is classified as early if it occurs during the first 24 hours after delivery and late if it occurs 24 hours to 6 weeks after delivery. Late PPH usually occurs 6–10 days after delivery. The most common cause of early PPH is uterine atony, which accounts for approximately 90% of all cases. Other causes include lacerations of the cervix and/or vagina, retained placental tissue, placenta accreta, uterine inversion, uterine rupture, and maternal coagulopathy. The most common reasons for late PPH are retained products of conception, postpartum endometritis, subinvolution of the placental site, episiotomy breakdown, hematoma, and coital trauma. The factors that place a woman at higher risk for PPH include the following: overdistention of the uterus as a result of hydramnios, multiple gestation, or a macrosomatic fetus; multiparity; prolonged, difficult labor, especially after oxytocin induction; history of PPH, preeclampsia, placenta previa; Asian or Hispanic ethnicity; mediolateral episiotomy; and coagulation abnormalities.

1. Assessment
   a. Subjective data collection
      1) History of present illness/chief complaint
         a) Recent delivery
         b) Vaginal bleeding: amount and character
         c) Easy bruising/bleeding
      2) Past medical history
         a) Current or preexisting diseases/illness
            (1) Preeclampsia
            (2) Placenta previa
            (3) Coagulopathy
         b) Reproductive history
         c) Prolonged/complicated labor and delivery
         d) Previous PPH
         e) Medications
         f) Allergies
   b. Objective data collection
      1) Physical examination
         a) General appearance
            (1) Possible positive orthostasis
            (2) Moderate distress/discomfort, possibly critically ill
         b) Inspection
            (1) Vaginal bleeding: amount, color
         c) Palpation
            (1) Uterine size/tone
         d) Pelvic examination: manual exploration for retained placental fragments
      2) Diagnostic procedures
         a) CBC with differential
         b) Coagulation profile, fibrinogen, fibrin split products
         c) Type and crossmatch
         d) Pelvic/vaginal sonography
2. Analysis: differential nursing diagnoses/collaborative problems
   a. Deficient fluid volume
   b. Ineffective tissue perfusion
3. Planning and implementation/interventions
   a. Maintain airway, breathing, circulation (see Chapter 1)
   b. Provide supplemental oxygen as indicated
   c. Establish IV access for administration of crystalloid fluid/blood products/medications as needed
   d. Prepare for/assist with medical procedures
      1) Institute cardiac and pulse oximetry monitoring
      2) Decrease uterine atony
         a) Perform firm manual or bimanual massage of uterus if fundus is palpated
         b) Manual removal/curettage to expel retained placental fragments
      3) Assist with hospital admission and transfer to the labor and delivery unit when hemodynamically stable
         a) Possible surgical repair of genital tract lacerations
         b) Surgical intervention may be required for persistent bleeding not responsive to medical management (ligation of the uterine, ovarian, or hypogastric arteries; total or subtotal hysterectomy)
   e. Administer pharmacologic therapy as ordered
      1) IV oxytocin (Pitocin) to initiate and maintain uterine contractility
      2) For persistent bleeding, methylergonovine (Methergine) or IM prostaglandin or vaginal suppository
4. Evaluation and ongoing monitoring
   a. Maternal hemodynamic status
   b. Vaginal bleeding, passage of clots, tissue, placental fragments

H. SPONTANEOUS ABORTION

Spontaneous abortion, the most common complication of early pregnancy, is the loss of pregnancy before viability of the fetus, defined as 20 weeks' gestation or a fetus weighing less than 500 g. Spontaneous abortion should be considered in any woman of childbearing age who presents to the emergency department with vaginal bleeding. The incidence of spontaneous abortion in the United States is estimated to be 8–20% of all recognized pregnancies and 13–26% of all unrecognized or subclinical pregnancies. Most occur before 8 weeks' gestation; however, the true incidence of spontaneous abortion is much higher because many pregnancies terminate before diagnosis. The cause of spontaneous abortion is unknown in the majority of cases. Etiologic factors that have been implicated include chromosomal abnormalities, endocrine dysfunction, maldevelopment of the embryo, and trauma. Additional factors that increase an individual's risk of spontaneous abortion include maternal infections, advanced maternal age, previous spontaneous abortion, malnutrition, substance abuse (heavy smoking, alcohol consumption, cocaine, etc.), NSAID use around the time of conception, low folate levels, extremes of maternal weight, immunologic incompatibility, surgery during pregnancy, and structural anomalies of the reproductive organs. Spontaneous abortions are commonly categorized as threatened, inevitable, incomplete, complete, missed, or septic (Table 23.2).

1. Assessment
   a. Subjective data collection
      1) History of present illness/chief complaint
         a) Pain (see Chapter 8)
            (1) Pelvic pain: crampy, severity variable; may also be dull, constant, or intermittent
            (2) Back pain, pelvic pressure
         b) Vaginal bleeding: color, amount (volume or pattern of bleeding is variable, and not a reliable predictor)
         c) Passage of clots or fetal tissue
         d) Positive pregnancy test or confirmation via sonography: date and method
         e) Fatigue, dizziness, lightheadedness, headache, nausea, vomiting, syncope
      2) Past medical history
         a) Current or preexisting diseases/illness
         b) Gestational age: LNMP, EDD
         c) Reproductive history
         d) Contraceptive history
         e) Prenatal care
         f) Substance use/abuse
         g) Medications
         h) Allergies
   b. Objective data collection
      1) Physical examination
         a) General appearance
            (1) Possible positive orthostasis or tachycardia
            (2) Mild to moderate distress/discomfort
         b) Auscultation
            (1) FHTs if gestational age >13 weeks
         c) A complete pelvic examination is mandatory to determine the amount and site of bleeding, presence of cervical dilation, and passage of tissue. A speculum exam to confirm the uterus is the source of bleeding and to observe for the presence of products of conception at the cervix or vagina. A bimanual exam is done to determine uterine size.
      2) Diagnostic procedures
         a) Serum and/or urine pregnancy test: including quantitative serum human chorionic gonadotropin (β-hCG) level
         b) CBC with differential
         c) Type, Rh, and crossmatch
         d) Urinalysis
         e) STI screening
         f) Pelvic sonography to rule out ectopic pregnancy (EP), assess viability of fetus and gestational age, and diagnose retained products of conception
         g) Send any passed products of conception to pathology
2. Analysis: differential nursing diagnoses/collaborative problems
   a. Acute pain
   b. Anticipatory grieving
   c. Deficient knowledge
   d. Deficient fluid volume
3. Planning and implementation/interventions
   a. Maintain airway, breathing, circulation (see Chapter 1)

Table 23.2

Classification of Spontaneous Abortion

Type	Description
Threatened	Slight vaginal bleeding and mild uterine cramping with a closed cervical os
Inevitable	Moderate vaginal bleeding and moderate uterine cramping with an open cervical os, gross rupture of membranes
Incomplete	Heavy vaginal bleeding and severe uterine cramping with an open cervical os and tissue in the cervix, incomplete expulsion of the products of conception
Complete	Slight vaginal bleeding with mild uterine cramping with a closed cervical os, complete expulsion of the products of conception
Missed	Slight vaginal bleeding and absent uterine contractions with a closed cervical os, prolonged retention of dead products of conception
Septic	Malodorous vaginal bleeding/discharge and absent uterine contractions with a closed cervical os, fever, intrauterine infection

b. Establish IV access for administration of crystalloid fluid/blood products/medication as needed
c. Prepare for/assist with medical interventions
   1) Pelvic examination
   2) Dilation and evacuation procedure
   3) Assist with possible hospital admission
d. Administer pharmacologic therapy as ordered
   1) Rh immune globulin (RhoGAM or Rhophylac) to all Rh-negative women
   2) Oxytocin (Pitocin) or methylergonovine (Methergine) to control hemorrhage
   3) Analgesics
   4) Antibiotics
e. Educate patient/significant others
   1) For threatened abortion, provide discharge instructions
      a) Maintain bed rest for 24–48 hours or until bleeding subsides
      b) Pelvic rest (no sexual intercourse) until bleeding and cramping stop
      c) Use sanitary pads only; avoid tampons
      d) Return to emergency department if bleeding or pain increases
      e) Save any clots or tissue that passes and bring to emergency department or follow-up physician
      f) Ensure appropriate follow-up care with obstetrician
   2) For complete abortion, provide discharge instructions
      a) Mild abdominal pain/cramping is commonly experienced for several days
      b) Use sanitary pads only; avoid tampons
      c) Take temperature four times per day
      d) Take medications as prescribed
         (1) Methylergonovine (Methergine)
         (2) Nonnarcotic analgesics
         (3) Nonsteroidal antiinflammatory drugs (NSAIDs)
         (4) Antibiotics
      e) Bleeding should change from red to pink in appearance (dark to light in color) and decrease in amount
      f) Pelvic rest
      g) Ensure appropriate follow-up care with obstetrician
      h) Activity as tolerated
      i) Return to emergency department if temperature is >100.4°F (>38.0°C) or heavier bleeding, worsening pain, or foul-smelling discharge occurs
4. Evaluation and ongoing monitoring
   a. Maternal hemodynamic status
   b. Vaginal bleeding, passage of clots, tissue, products of conception
   c. Pain relief

III. Specific Gynecologic Emergencies

A. PELVIC INFLAMMATORY DISEASE

Pelvic inflammatory disease (PID) is a nonspecific term used to describe infection of the endometrium, fallopian tubes, ovaries, pelvic peritoneum, or pelvic connective tissue. The infection may be acute, subacute, or chronic. *N. gonorrhoeae* and *C. trachomatis* are the two most common organisms that cause PID, and they frequently coexist; however, other aerobes and anaerobes may also cause PID. Most PID cases result from upward migration of genital infections; the remaining cases are caused by introduction of microorganisms through instrumentation. Several factors facilitate the spread of organisms to the upper genital tract, including menses-related loss of the cervical barrier, hormonal changes reducing the bacteriostatic properties of cervical mucus, gynecologic procedures, and IUD use. *N. gonorrhoeae* infection is frequently menstruation dependent; spread of the disease from the cervix to the endometrium usually occurs within 5–7 days of the onset of menses, with classic clinical manifestations. In contrast, *C. trachomatis* infection is usually unrelated to menses and may present atypically or insidiously. Severe tubal damage resulting in infertility can result from *C. trachomatis* infection despite the absence of impressive clinical manifestations. Acute PID is often difficult to diagnose because of the wide variation in the severity of signs and symptoms. No single historical, physical, or laboratory finding is both sensitive and specific for the diagnosis of PID. Because of this, a diagnosis of PID is usually based on clinical history and physical findings. PID can have significant long-term sequellae, including chronic pelvic pain, dyspareunia, infertility, and EP. Because the clinical presentation of PID may be insidious, it is essential that the factors associated with an increased risk of PID be identified. Adolescents are at particularly high risk for PID. Predisposing factors for this age group include immature immune systems, larger zones of cervical ectopy, thinner cervical mucus, and greater exposure to multiple sexual partners. The other most common risk factors include individuals with multiple sexual partners, high frequency of intercourse, recent exposure to STDs, nonbarrier contraception, presence of an IUD, recent gynecologic procedures, douching, smoking, and proximity to menses.

1. Assessment
   a. Subjective data collection
      1) History of present illness/chief complaint
         a) Abdominal pain (see Chapter 8)
            (1) Exacerbated by movement, intercourse, and Valsalva maneuver; onset or increase in severity during menstruation
            (2) Ranges from dull and aching to sharp and persistent
            (3) May have RUQ pain in PID-related perihepatitis (Fitz-Hugh-Curtis syndrome)

b) Vaginal discharge: mucopurulent, malodorous

c) Vaginal bleeding: increased menstrual flow, breakthrough bleeding

d) Dysuria

e) Fever and chills

f) Vomiting

2) Past medical history

  a) Current or preexisting diseases/illness

  b) LNMP: female patients of childbearing age

  c) Previous pelvic infection

  d) Sexual activity, new (<2 months) or multiple sexual partners, nonbarrier contraception

  e) Recent gynecologic procedures/instrumentation

  f) Medications

  g) Allergies

b. Objective data collection

1) Physical examination

  a) General appearance

    (1) Elevated temperature: >101.3°F (>38.5°C)

    (2) Tachycardia

    (3) Moderate distress/discomfort

  b) Palpation

    (1) Lower abdominal tenderness, rebound tenderness

  c) Pelvic examination: abnormal vaginal discharge, cervical motion tenderness, uterine and/or adnexal tenderness

2) Diagnostic procedures

  a) CBC with differential: leukocytosis with "left shift"

  b) ESR: elevated

  c) C-reactive protein: elevated

  d) Serum chemistries including BUN and creatinine

  e) Blood cultures

  f) Serum and/or urine pregnancy test in female patients of childbearing age

  g) Urinalysis

  h) Endocervical culture, Gram stain

  i) Urine NAAT for GC and chlamydia

  j) Wet mount (saline, KOH)

  k) Pelvic sonography

  l) Abdominal CT scan

  m) Diagnostic laparoscopy

2. Analysis: differential nursing diagnoses/collaborative problems

a. Risk for infection

b. Acute pain

c. Deficient knowledge

3. Planning and implementation/interventions

a. Establish IV access for administration of crystalloid fluid/medications as needed

b. Prepare for/assist with medical procedures

1) Pelvic examination

2) Institute cardiac and pulse oximetry monitoring

3) Assist with hospital admission if

  a) Temperature: >101.3°F (>38.5°C)

  b) Suspected pelvic or tuboovarian abscess

  c) Nausea and vomiting impeding oral antibiotic therapy

  d) Pregnancy

  e) Perihepatitis

  f) Adolescents, children, nulligravidae

  g) IUD use

  h) Immunocompromised patients

  i) Failure to respond to outpatient therapy of 48–72 hours

c. Administer pharmacologic therapy as ordered

1) Analgesics

2) Antibiotics

d. Educate patient/significant others

1) Medication for infection: purpose, dose, schedule, importance of completing course of antibiotics, side effects

2) Use of analgesics

3) Follow up within 72 hours

4) Need to return for persistent or worsening symptoms: fever, chills, abdominal pain, nausea, vomiting

5) Discuss methods to prevent recurrence

  a) Abstain from sexual activity until after posttreatment examination/cultures

  b) Facilitate partner's assessment and treatment

  c) Use of prophylactic risk-reducing behavior and methods

  d) Periodic STD examinations if patient is sexually active with multiple partners

  e) HIV counseling and testing if patient is at high risk

4. Evaluation and ongoing monitoring

a. Hemodynamic status

b. Cardiac and pulse oximetry monitoring

c. Pain relief

d. Intake and output

B. PELVIC PAIN

Pain in the lower abdomen or pelvis may have a variety of causes. The pain may originate from within the organs anatomically located within the lower abdomen/pelvis, or it may be referred from other adjacent body regions, including the urinary and gastrointestinal systems. Poorly localized visceral pain originates in organs and viscera innervated by autonomic nerves. This may be caused by distention of a hollow viscus (e.g., fallopian tube or distended bowel), distention of the capsule of a solid organ, or stretching of pelvic ligaments or adhesions. In contrast, pain that is well localized originates from somatic nerve irritation, such as irritation of the parietal peritoneum caused by an inflamed organ or the presence of blood or purulent fluid (e.g., ruptured EP or acute appendicitis). The causes of pelvic pain can be classified as acute, chronic, and recurrent. Recurrent temporal pelvic pain is related to the menstrual cycle. An accurate history is essential to determine the acuity because the condition causing the pain may be life-threatening (Table 23.3).

1. Assessment
   a. Subjective data collection
      1) History of present illness/chief complaint
         a) Pain (see Chapter 8)
         b) Fever and/or chills
         c) Nausea and/or vomiting
         d) Relationship with menses
         e) Vaginal discharge
         f) Changes in bowel or bladder function
      2) Past medical history
         a) Current or preexisting diseases/illness
         b) LNMP, menstrual history
         c) History of abdominal/pelvic pain
         d) Reproductive history
         e) Previous abdominal/pelvic surgery
         f) Trauma: blunt or penetrating forces
         g) Medications
         h) Allergies
   b. Objective data collection
      1) Physical examination
         a) General appearance
            (1) Possible positive orthostasis
            (2) Moderate distress/discomfort
         b) Auscultation
            (1) Bowel sounds
         c) Palpation
            (1) Abdominal tenderness
            (2) Abdominal guarding
            (3) Abdominal masses
         d) Pelvic examination: abnormal vaginal discharge, cervical motion tenderness, adnexal tenderness
      2) Diagnostic procedures
         a) CBC with differential
         b) ESR
         c) C-reactive protein
         d) Serum chemistries including glucose, BUN, creatinine
         e) Blood cultures
         f) Serum and/or urine pregnancy test in female patients of childbearing age
         g) Urinalysis
         h) STI screening
         i) Wet mount (saline, KOH)
         j) Pelvic/transvaginal sonography
         k) Abdominal CT scan
         l) Diagnostic laparoscopy
2. Analysis: differential nursing diagnoses/collaborative problems
   a. Acute/chronic pain
   b. Deficient knowledge

3. Planning and implementation/interventions (see specific diagnosis if known)
   a. Establish IV access for administration of crystalloid fluid/medications as needed
   b. Prepare for/assist with medical procedures
      1) Pelvic examination
      2) Assist with possible hospital admission
   c. Administer pharmacologic therapy as indicated
      1) Nonnarcotic analgesics
      2) Narcotics
      3) Antibiotics
4. Evaluation and ongoing monitoring
   a. Pain relief

C. SEXUALLY TRANSMITTED INFECTIONS

Emergency care providers play an essential role in the prevention and treatment of sexually transmitted infections (STIs). This group of infectious diseases is classified on the basis of their mode of transmission: sexual activity. The primary STIs and pathogens include *Neisseria gonorrhoeae, Chlamydia trachomatis, Treponema pallidum* (syphilis), bacterial vaginosis, condyloma acuminatum (venereal wart), herpes simplex virus, and HIV (Table 23.4).

Hepatitis A, hepatitis B, and hepatitis C are also considered to be sexually transmitted. Hepatitis A and hepatitis B are both preventable with vaccines. The major sequellae associated with STIs include vaginitis, cervicitis, PID, urethritis, epididymitis, pharyngitis, proctitis, skin and mucous membrane lesions, and acquired immunodeficiency syndrome (AIDS) associated with HIV infection. Assessment and treatment for STDs are summarized in Table 23.4.

D. VAGINAL BLEEDING/DYSFUNCTIONAL UTERINE BLEEDING

Vaginal bleeding in the nonpregnant patient can have a variety of causes, including uterine fibroids, menstrual cycle irregularities, trauma, infection, malignant disease, or coagulopathy. Dysfunctional uterine bleeding (DUB) is a common form of abnormal vaginal bleeding and results from hormonal imbalance. It often occurs secondary to anovulation, which is common at both the beginning and end of the reproductive years. Causes of DUB may include dysfunction of the hypothalamic-pituitary-ovarian axis, thyroid or adrenal disorders, hormone replacement therapy, or use of steroids, androgens, digitalis, and anticoagulants. Typically, steady, painless bleeding and the absence of clots or tissue characterize DUB.

1. Assessment
   a. Subjective data collection
      1) History of present illness/chief complaint
         a) Vaginal bleeding
            (1) Quantity: spotting versus steady flow; number and type (e.g., mini, maxi) of pads or tampons used per hour; amount compared with normal menses

Table 23.3

Causes of Pelvic Pain

	Nature of Pain	Fever (+/-)	Nausea and/or Vomiting	Origin (Onset)	Medical History (Contributing Factors)	Pregnancy Test (+/-)	Region (Location of Pain)	Surgical History	Timing	Undulation (Aggravating)	Vaginal Discharge
Gynecologic											
Degenerating tumor	Fullness to sudden sharp	–	No	Slow	Chronic pelvic vascular congestion, fibroids	–	Midline or generalized	Nonspecific	Constant	Menses, stress, anxiety	None
Ectopic pregnancy (ruptured)	Sharp	–	Nausea possible	Acute	PID, pelvic surgery previous ectopic pregnancy, infertility surgery, IUD, older first maternal age	+	Pelvis	Tubal, infertility, etc.	Constant	Movement	No, may have light bleeding
Incomplete, threatened, or septic abortion	Sharp or crampy	±	No	Acute	PID, previous abortion	±	Generalized pelvic area	IUD, abortion	Constant	Movement	±
Endometriosis	Sharp	+	No	2–7 days pre-menses	Familial inherited, delay in childbearing, Asian, congenital anomalies	–	Posterior pelvis, bilateral	Infertility or sterility	Constant during menses	Intercourse, defecation, adhesions	Vaginal bleeding
Mittelschmerz	Sharp	–	No	Acute	Ruptured graafian follicle	–	Generalized midline	Nonspecific	Midcycle	None	None
Ovarian cyst (ruptured)	Sharp	–	No	Acute	Usually occurs during intercourse	–	Pelvis	Nonspecific	Constant	Movement	None
PID*	Sharp	+	Nausea	Acute	Previous PID, STD, frequent sex, multiple partners	–	Bilateral pelvis, (+) CMT	Abortion, IUD	Constant	Intercourse, menses, movement	Yes
PMS	Crampy	–	Nausea possible	Acute	Previous history of PMS	–	Generalized midline	Nonspecific	1–6 days pre-menses	None	None
Primary dysmenorrhea	Crampy	–	No	Acute	History of primary dysmenorrhea	–	Generalized	Nonspecific	Onset of menses	Movement	None
Septic pelvic thrombosis	Sharp	+	No	Acute	Pregnancy or postpartum status	±	Pelvis	Nonspecific	Throbbing	Position	None
Torsion of ovary, pedicle, cyst, or tumor	Intense, sharp	±	Nausea and vomiting	Acute	Cyst, fibroid	–	Unilateral or bilateral pelvis	Nonspecific	Constant	Movement, position	None
Tubo-ovarian abscess	Sharp	+	Nausea possible	Acute	History of PID, especially if GC	–	Unilateral or bilateral	Nonspecific	Constant	Movement	Purulent
Nongynecologic											
Appendicitis	Dull, then sharp	Low grade	Nausea	Slow then acute	Noncontributory	–	Periumbilical then RLQ	Nonspecific	Constant	Movement	None
Diverticulitis	Crampy	±	No	Slow	Peanuts, etc., may obstruct a diverticulum	–	LLQ	Nonspecific	Intermittent	Dietary	None

Continued

Table 23.3

Causes of Pelvic Pain—cont'd

	Nature of Pain	Fever (+/-)	Nausea and/or Vomiting	Origin (Onset)	Medical History (Contributing Factors)	Pregnancy Test (+/-)	Region (Location of Pain)	Surgical History	Timing	Undulation (Aggravating)	Vaginal Discharge
DKA[†]	Severe, sharp	±	Nausea, vomiting	Acute	Diabetes mellitus	-	Diffuse	Nonspecific	Constant	Acidosis, hyperglycemia	None
Gastroenteritis	Crampy	±	Nausea, vomiting	Acute	Viral infection, dietary, diarrhea necessary	-	Diffuse	Nonspecific	Constant	Food, peristalsis	None
Hernia (strangulated)	Dull or sharp	+	Nausea and/or vomiting	Slow	A defect in fascia, muscle, or peritoneum to trap the bowel	-	Generalized peritonitis	Possible	Intermittent	Peristalsis	None
Intussusception	Crampy	±	Vomiting	Slow	Familial history	-	Lower abdomen	No	Intermittent	Eating	None
Leaking AAA	Severe	-	No	Acute	Hypertension, familial history of AAA	-	Site of aneurysm, or may be referred	Nonspecific	Constant	Hypertension hypoxia, bleeding	None
Peritonitis (from ruptured viscus)	Vague then sharp	+	Nausea	Slow or acute	Nonspecific	±	Variable	Nonspecific	Constant	Movement	None
Sickle cell crisis	Severe	+	Nausea, vomiting	Acute	Hypoxia, acidosis, dehydration, infection	-	Diffuse	Nonspecific	Constant	Position	None
Small bowel obstruction	Crampy bloated, severe	-	Nausea, vomiting later stage	Slow	Cancer, adhesions, hernia, fecal impaction, foreign body, volvulus, intussusception	-	Diffuse, may localize	History of surgery	Intermittent, then constant	Movement if perforation peristalsis, eating	None
Ureteral stone	Sharp	-	Possible	Acute	History of ureteral stones, family history	-	Unilateral flank to groin	Nonspecific	Intermittent	Peristaltic movement of ureter	None
Urinary tract infection	Burning	±	No	Acute	Poor hygiene, frequent coitus, esp. multiple partners	-	Pelvis	Nonspecific	Intermittent	Voiding	None
Volvulus	Sharp		Nausea, vomiting	Acute	Previous surgery		Previous surgery localized	History of surgery	Intermittent, then constant	Peristalsis	None

*This includes salpingitis, endometritis, and pelvic peritonitis.

[†]This is often seen as a result of an infection; therefore, a fever may be present.

AAA, Abdominal aortic aneurysm; *CMT,* cervical motion tenderness; *DKA,* diabetic ketoacidosis; *GC,* gonococcal; *IUD,* intrauterine device; *LLQ,* left lower quadrant; *PID,* pelvic inflammatory disease; *PMS,* premenstrual syndrome; *RLQ,* right lower quadrant; *STD,* sexually transmitted disease.

Modified from Howel, J., Altieri, M., Jagoda, A., Prescott, J., Scott, J., & Stair, T. (1998). *Emergency medicine.* Philadelphia, PA: WB Saunders.

Table 23.4

Sexually Transmitted Diseases: Assessment and Intervention

Disease or Pathogen	Incubation Period (Timing)	Discharge	Lesions	Pain	Associated Symptoms	ED Treatment	Home Treatment	Discharge Teaching	Special Instructions
Neisseria gonorrhoeae	3–5 days	Yellow, mucopurulent	None	Male patients: dysuria Female patients: may be asymptomatic or have symptoms of PID	Urinary frequency Abnormal vaginal bleeding	Cetriaxone (Rocephin) Cefixime (Suprax)	None	Abstinence from sexual activity until treatment completed Partner(s) need treatment Use of barrier method to prevent transmission of STD Need to return in 7–10 days for follow-up Consider risk of HIV infection, hepatitis B, syphilis	
Chlamydia trachomatis	5–10 days or longer	Mucopurulent	None	Male patients: burning on urination, urethral itching, symptoms of epididymitis Female patients: usually asymptomatic		Azithromycin (Zithromax), Doxycycline	Doxycycline (Vibramycin) or Erythromycin or Ofloxacin		
Treponema pallidum (syphilis)	3 wk	None	Indurated ulcer (chancre) found on genitalia, rectum, mouth, or lips	None	May have fever, lymphadenopathy	Benzathine PCN (Bicillin L-A)	Doxycycline Erythromycin (will be covered by doxycycline given for Chlamydia)		
Trichomonas vaginalis	1 wk Worse immediately after menses Most acute during pregnancy	Greenish gray; thin, frothy; profuse; malodorous	None	Severe pruritus	Genital edema Erythema of vaginal vault	Metrondazole (Flagyl)	Metronidazole		Avoid contact with lesion

Continued

Table 23.4

Sexually Transmitted Diseases: Assessment and Intervention—cont'd

Disease or Pathogen	Incubation Period (Timing)	Discharge	Lesions	Pain	Associated Symptoms	ED Treatment	Home Treatment	Discharge Teaching	Special Instructions
Condyloma acuminatum (venereal wart)	3–6 mo May flourish during pregnancy	None	Pink-gray soft lesions, taller than they are wide, occur singly or in clusters, may bleed	None	None	Apply Imiquimod cream; Podofilix 0.5% solution or gel; Sinecatechins ointment 10–25% podophyllin in tincture of benzoin (not in pregnancy) or 50% trichloro-acetic acid or liquid nitrogen			
Chancroid	3–14 days	None	Nonindurated ulcer with undetermined edges May also be found intrameatally	Very painful Increased pain on voiding	Enlarged, tender inguinal glands	Ceftriaxone Azithromycin Erythromycin	Ciprofloxacin, amoxicillin-clavulanate (Augmentin)		Lesions heal within weeks but are infectious during that time; avoid contact
Herpes simplex virus type 2	2–12 days	May have purulent vaginal discharge	Multiple shallow vesicles on genital area, buttocks, or thighs Female patients most common sites are cervix, vulva Male patients: most common sites are glans, prepuce	Very painful dysuria	May have inguinal lympha-denopathy May have urinary retention related to pain May have fever, headache, mal-aise, myalgias Waddling gait	Famcyclovir (Famvir) Vancyclovir (Valtrex) Acyclovir	Acyclovir (Zovi-rax) Warm baths Topical anesthetic ointment Mild analgesics Loose fitting clothing Antimicrobials for bacterial superin fection may be neces-sary		About half the patients have recur-rence every 2 mo Local hyperesthesia usually occurs 24 hours before eruption of vesicular lesions No sexual activity during infectious outbreaks, including 24-hour prodromal period, until lesions dry up

ED, emergency department; *HIV*, human immunodeficiency virus; *PID*, pelvic inflammatory disease; *STD*, sexually transmitted disease.

     (2) Duration: onset; number of hours or days, compared with normal menses
     (3) Quality: color—bright red versus brown; presence of clots/tissue
     (4) Association with sexual intercourse
   b) Pain (see Chapter 8): abdominal pain/cramping
   c) Fever/chills
   d) Fatigue, dizziness, lightheadedness, syncope
  2) Past medical history
   a) Current or preexisting diseases/illness
   b) LNMP: female patients of childbearing age
   c) Reproductive history
   d) Sexual history
   e) Age-related factors: menarche, precocious puberty, menopause
   f) Contraceptive history (e.g., IUD use, oral contraceptives)
   g) Recent trauma or surgery
   h) Medications
   i) Allergies
 b. Objective data collection
  1) Physical examination
   a) General appearance
    (1) Possible positive orthostasis
    (2) Moderate distress/discomfort
   b) Inspection
    (1) Vaginal bleeding
   c) Pelvic examination
  2) Diagnostic procedures
   a) Serum and/or urine pregnancy test in female patients of childbearing age
   b) CBC with differential
   c) Coagulation profile: PT, PTT, fibrin split products
   d) Thyroid function tests, liver function tests, follicle-stimulating hormone (FSH) and luteinizing hormone (LH) levels
   e) Type and screen/crossmatch
   f) Urinalysis
   g) STD screening
   h) Pelvic/transvaginal sonography
2. Analysis: differential nursing diagnoses/collaborative problems
 a. Deficient fluid volume
 b. Deficient knowledge
3. Planning and implementation/interventions
 a. Provide supplemental oxygen as indicated
 b. Establish IV access for administration of crystalloid fluid/blood products/medications as needed
 c. Prepare for/assist with medical interventions
  1) Pelvic examination
  2) Diagnostic/therapeutic dilation and curettage (D&C): possible procedural sedation (see Chapter 9)
  3) Assist with possible hospital admission

 d. Administer pharmacologic therapy as ordered
  1) Low-dose combination oral contraceptive therapy: progesterone, estrogen
  2) Procedural sedation medications
 e. Educate patient/significant others
  1) Ensure appropriate follow-up care
  2) Activity as tolerated
  3) Return to emergency department if temperature is elevated to >100.6°F (>38.1°C), if bleeding occurs, or if pain increases
4. Evaluation and ongoing monitoring
 a. Hemodynamic status
 b. Vaginal bleeding, passage of clots, tissue
 c. Pain relief

E. VAGINITIS

Vaginal discharge may be a normal physiologic phenomenon for women of all ages. However, vaginal infections are a common reason that women seek emergency care. The most common cause of abnormal vaginal discharge is infection with bacteria, yeasts or fungi, or parasites. Vaginitis is extremely prevalent and may result in considerable discomfort for the woman. The most common infections are caused by bacterial vaginosis (40–50%), *Candida albicans* (20–25%), and *Trichomonas vaginalis* (15–20%). Multiple infectious agents may occur simultaneously and may be sexually transmitted (Table 23.5). Noninfectious processes, including retained foreign bodies, chemicals, hormonal changes, and alteration in vaginal flora, may also cause vaginitis. Causes of disturbances in the normal vaginal flora include pregnancy, recent antibiotic use, diabetes, HIV infection, high-carbohydrate intake, poor hygiene practices, stress, and vaginal hypersensitivity/allergen response.

1. Assessment
 a. Subjective data collection
  1) History of present illness/chief complaint
   a) Vaginal discharge: color, odor, duration, quantity
   b) Vaginal itching/irritation
   c) Vaginal erythema, edema
   d) Dysuria, urinary frequency
   e) Dyspareunia (abnormal pain during sexual intercourse), bleeding with intercourse
  2) Past medical history
   a) Current or preexisting diseases/illness
    (1) Diabetes
    (2) HIV infection
   b) Previous episodes of similar symptoms
   c) LNMP: female patients of childbearing age
   d) Reproductive history, birth control methods
   e) Sexual activity
   f) Recent antibiotic use
   g) Medications
   h) Allergies
 b. Objective data collection
  1) Physical examination

Table 23.5

Differential Diagnosis of Vaginal Infections

Diagnostic Criteria	Normal	Condition		
		Bacterial Vaginosis	Trichomonas Vaginitis	Candida Vulvovaginitis
Vaginal pH	3.8	<4.5	>4.5	<4.5 (usually)
Discharge	White, clear	Thin, homogeneous, white; adheres to vaginal walls	Watery, yellow, gray or green, frothy, or bubbly	White, curdy, "cottage cheese like"; adheres to vaginal walls
Amine odor (KOH whiff test)	Absent	Present (fishy)	May be present (fishy)	Absent
Main patient complaint	None	Discharge, bad odor (possibly bad odor, worse after intercourse), possible itching	Frothy discharge, vulvar pruritus, dysuria	Itching/burning, discharge

KOH, Potassium hydroxide.

a) General appearance
  (1) Level of consciousness, behavior, affect
  (2) Mild to moderate distress/discomfort
b) Inspection
  (1) Vaginal discharge
  (2) Vaginal irritation, lesions
c) Palpation
  (1) Abdominal tenderness
d) Pelvic examination
2) Diagnostic procedures
  a) Vaginal pH: normal, 3.8–4.2
  b) Wet mount (saline and KOH)
  c) Amine odor (KOH whiff test)
  d) Endocervical culture and Gram stain
  e) Serum and/or urine pregnancy test in female patients of childbearing age
  f) Urinalysis and urine culture
  g) Urine NAAT for GC and chlamydia

2. Analysis: differential nursing diagnoses/collaborative problems
  a. Acute pain
  b. Deficient knowledge
3. Planning and implementation/interventions
  a. Prepare for/assist with medical interventions
    1) Pelvic examination
  b. Administer pharmacologic therapy as ordered
    1) Antibiotics
  c. Educate patient/significant others
    1) Medications
      a) Dosage, schedule, and compliance with complete regimen
      b) Side effects
    2) Provide instructions in personal hygiene as needed (e.g., cleanse perineum from front to back with mild soap and water; avoid use of sprays, scented soaps, and douches; wear cotton underwear; avoid tight-fitting clothes and pantyhose)

3) Discuss methods to prevent recurrence
  a) Abstain from sexual activity until treatment is complete and patient is asymptomatic
  b) Facilitate partner's assessment and treatment (e.g., *T. vaginalis*)
  c) Use of prophylactic risk-reducing behavior and methods
  d) Periodic STI examinations if patient is sexually active with multiple partners
  e) HIV counseling and testing if patient is at high risk
4. Evaluation and ongoing monitoring
  a. Pain relief

Bibliography

American College of Obstetricians and Gynecologists, Task Force on Hypertension in Pregnancy: Hypertension in pregnancy, *Obstetrics and Gynecology* 122:1122–1131, 2013.

Centers for Disease Control and Prevention: Sexually transmitted diseases, *Summary of 2015 treatment guidelines*, 2015. Retrieved from http://www.cdc.gov/std/tg2015/2015-pocket-guide.pdf.

Hahn S, Lavonas E, Mace S, Napoli A, Fesmire F: Clinical policy: Critical issues in the initial evaluation and management of patients presenting the emergency department in early pregnancy, *Annals of Emergency Medicine* 60:381–389, 2012.

Lykke J, Dideriksen JK, Kidegaard O, Langhoof-Roof J: First-trimester vaginal bleeding and complications later in pregnancy, *Obstetrics & Gynecology* 115:935–944, 2010.

Marx J, Hockberger R: *Rosen's emergency medicine concepts and clinical practice*, Philadelphia, PA, 2014, Elsevier.

Sommerkamp S, Wittels K: OB/GYN emergencies, *Emergency Medical Clinical of North America* 30:837–1028, 2012.

Tintinalli JE, Kelen GD, Stapczynski JS, editors: *Emergency medicine: A comprehensive study guide*, 7th ed., New York, NY, 2010, McGraw-Hill.

CHAPTER 24

Orthopedic Emergencies

Mary Jo Cerepani, DNP, FNP-BC, CEN

MAJOR TOPICS
General Strategy
Assessment
Analysis: Differential Nursing Diagnoses/Collaborative
  Problems
Planning and Implementation/Interventions
Evaluation and Ongoing Monitoring
Documentation of Interventions and Patient Response
Age-Related Considerations

Specific Soft Tissue Emergencies
Low Back Pain
Overuse/Cumulative Trauma Disorders
Bursitis
Nerve Entrapment Syndrome
Tendinitis
Specific Bony Skeleton Emergencies
Costochondritis
Joint Effusions
Osteoarthritis
Osteoporosis

I. General Strategy

The primary goal in caring for the patient with an orthopedic emergency is to restore and preserve function.

A. ASSESSMENT

1. Primary and secondary assessment/resuscitation (see Chapter 1)
2. Focused assessment
   a. Subjective data collection
      1) History of present illness/chief complaint
         a) Pain: PQRST (see Chapter 8)
         b) Associated symptoms
            (1) Changes in neurovascular function
            (2) Ability to bear weight
            (3) Range of motion
            (4) Weakness versus pain as presenting symptom
         c) Swollen areas
            (1) Onset
            (2) Size
            (3) Location
            (4) Symptoms: pain, tenderness, numbness, weakness
         d) Efforts to relieve symptoms
            (1) Home remedies
            (2) Alternative therapies
            (3) Medications
               (a) Prescription
               (b) OTC/herbal

2) Past medical history
   a) Current or preexisting diseases/illness
      (1) Anemia, bleeding, coagulation disorder
      (2) Cardiovascular disease: may indicate peripheral vascular disease
      (3) Diabetes mellitus: associated with peripheral neuropathies and decreased microcirculation
      (4) Arthritis: degenerative or rheumatoid
      (5) Acute inflammatory diseases
      (6) Paget's disease: localized areas of bone destruction followed by replacement with overdeveloped, light, soft, porous bone and associated with deformities such as thickening of portions of the skull and bending of weight-bearing bones; cause unknown
      (7) Use of medications that predispose to fractures: phenytoin sodium and corticosteroids
      (8) Disorders associated with peripheral nerve injury: alcoholism, sudden significant weight loss, carcinomatous neuropathy, or diabetic peripheral neuropathy
      (9) Prior injury or surgery of affected extremity
      (10) Preexisting disabilities
      (11) Osteopenia or osteoporosis

(12) Infections: possible cause of septic arthritis or osteomyelitis in children
    (a) Streptococcal infections
    (b) Urinary tract infections
    (c) Upper respiratory tract infections
    (d) Ear infections
    (e) Other infectious disorders

b) Current health status
  (1) Recent injury or problem of affected extremity
  (2) Pregnancy: swelling precipitates overuse syndromes; prone to falls as a result of pelvic ligament laxity
  (3) Vitamin deficiency

c) Last normal menstrual period: female patients of childbearing age

d) Smoking history

e) Substance and/or alcohol use/abuse

f) Current medications
  (1) Prescriptions
  (2) OTC/herbal

g) Allergies

h) Immunization status if break in skin integrity
  (1) Tetanus, diphtheria, and acellular pertussis

3) Psychological/social/environmental factors related to orthopedic emergencies
  a) For syndromes of overuse, history of
    (1) Repetitive actions
    (2) High velocity forces
    (3) Awkward joint posture or prolonged constrained position
    (4) Direct pressure (e.g., leaning on elbow, kneeling)
    (5) Vibration (e.g., use of power tools)
  b) Possible/actual assault, abuse, intimate partner violence situations (see Chapters 3 and 40)

b. Objective data collection
  1) General appearance
    a) Level of consciousness
    b) Vital signs
    c) Odors
    d) Gait: ask patient to walk, if tolerated, both away from and toward the examiner, to assess balance, control, posture, and movement of arms and legs
    e) Hygiene
    f) Level of distress/discomfort
  2) Inspection
    a) Compare both sides of body to visualize symmetry, contour, size, alignment
      (1) Valgus: deformity of the distal portion of a joint that is angulated away from midline of body (e.g., knock-knees, hallux valgus)
      (2) Varus: deformity of the distal portion of a joint that is angulated toward midline of body (e.g., bowleg and pigeon toe)

b) Skin and soft tissue
  (1) Color changes and hair loss associated with peripheral vascular disease
  (2) Soft tissue swelling or ecchymosis
  (3) Gross deformities: associated with arthritis, tumors, or swelling
  (4) Muscle mass: hypertrophy and atrophy
  (5) Scars indicative of previous injury, surgery, invasive procedures, or intravenous (IV) drug abuse

c) Joints
  (1) Deformity (e.g., nodules in fingers, toes, knees)
  (2) Swelling: caused by inflammation, infection, or trauma
  (3) Erythema: caused by inflammation associated with infection, cellulitis, or gouty arthritis
  (4) Range of motion: passive and active
  (5) Rotation: position of joint or extremity and the ability to rotate internally or externally
  (6) Temperature
  (7) Swelling and pitting edema
    (a) Muscle tone

3) Palpation
  a) Skin and soft tissue
    (1) Decreased: result of musculoskeletal, neurologic, metabolic, or infectious disorders, and/or fatigue
    (2) Increased: result of spasms, injury, cramps, or tremors that are associated with electrolyte disorders, neurologic conditions, or infections (tetanus)
  b) Muscle strength: assess range of motion before muscle strength, because muscular contraction may produce enough pain to inhibit further examination
    (1) Ask patient to resist movement or move against resistance
    (2) Strength is subjectively graded by examiner on scale ranging from 1 to 5.
All findings are recorded and used as a baseline
0: Paralysis, no muscular contraction detected
1: Only slight contractility and no joint motion
2: Active movement, full range of motion with gravity eliminated
3: Active movement, full range of motion against gravity
4: Active movement, full range of motion against gravity and some resistance
5: Active movement, full range of motion against full resistance

Table 24.1

Peripheral Nerve Assessment

Nerve	Motor	Sensory
Radial	Extend wrist or thumb	Feeling on dorsum of thumb
Median	Oppose thumb to base of small finger	Feeling on tip of index finger
Ulnar	Abduct (fan) fingers	Feeling on tip of small finger
Tibial	Plantar flex toes (curl down)	Feeling on bottom of foot
Superficial peroneal	Laterally evert foot	Feeling on lateral aspect of dorsum of foot
Deep peroneal	Dorsiflex toes (curl toes up)	Feeling in first toe web space (between first and second toes)

   c) Deep tendon reflexes (DTRs)
     (1) Assess major reflexes: biceps, brachioradialis, triceps, patellar knee jerk, and Achilles tendon
     (2) Grade of reflexes: 0, none; +1, below normal; +2, average; +3, stronger than average; +4, intense (clonus)
   d) Joints
     (1) Temperature
     (2) Pain or tenderness with palpation
     (3) Crepitation with movement
     (4) Passive range of motion (done by examiner)
     (5) Joint laxity and stability; varies with each joint
   e) Bones
     (1) Tenderness along length
     (2) Resistance to deforming forces
     (3) Deformity, crepitus, or tenderness
  4) Peripheral nerve assessment (Table 24.1)
  5) Peripheral vascular assessment
   a) Inspection
     (1) Skin: acute (pallor) and/or chronic (cyanosis, pigmentation) circulatory changes
     (2) Amount and distribution of hair
     (3) Skin ulcers
     (4) Inspection of veins for distention: unilateral versus bilateral
   b) Palpation/percussion
     (1) Temperature/texture of skin
     (2) Pitting edema
     (3) Quality of arterial pulses: brachial, radial, ulnar, femoral, popliteal, posterior tibial, and dorsalis pedis; presence of pulse does not rule out arterial injury

     (4) Grading of pulse quality
      0: No pulse
      1: Weak and easily obliterated with pressure
      2: Difficult to palpate but easy to feel once located
      3: Easily palpated and considered normal
      4: Strong and bounding
     (5) Capillary refill test
      (a) Used when unable to palpate pulses because of casts, splints, or dressings
      (b) Nonspecific measure of tissue perfusion, which can be affected by multiple factors
      (c) Normal time for color to return after blanching is 2 seconds or less
3. Diagnostic procedures
  a. Laboratory studies
   1) Complete blood count (CBC) with differential
   2) Erythrocyte sedimentation rate (ESR)
   3) Serum chemistries including glucose
   4) Urinalysis; pregnancy test in female patients of childbearing age
  b. Imaging studies
   1) Plain film radiographs: provide data on bone and joint changes; useful for diagnosing open joint injuries (air visible in joint space); standard for acute fractures and dislocations; does not show soft tissue disorders, except for swelling
     a) Comparison radiographs of joints for patients <16 years of age
      (1) WEAK mnemonic: wrist, elbow, ankle, knee joints
   2) Computed tomography (CT) scan used for definitive diagnosis
     a) Bony abnormalities
     b) Metastatic processes
   3) Angiography: used to diagnose and treat vascular injuries, prevent hemorrhage, and relieve ischemia; useful for recognizing and selectively embolizing major bleeding vessels and injuries of extremities with suspected vascular involvement (e.g., penetrating wounds) via an arterial catheter
   4) Magnetic resonance imaging (MRI): used for soft tissue disorders such as ligament injury, meniscal damage, tendon ruptures, muscle tears, tumors, hematomas, spinal structures, infection, and degenerative disorders
   5) Bone scans: used for occult fractures and metastatic disease
   6) Doppler sonography study
  c. Other
   1) 12- to15-lead electrocardiogram (ECG)
   2) Arthroscopy: used to evaluate injury to joint structures

B. ANALYSIS: DIFFERENTIAL NURSING DIAGNOSES/COLLABORATIVE PROBLEMS

1. Acute/chronic pain
2. Impaired skin integrity
3. Ineffective tissue perfusion
4. Activity intolerance
5. Risk for injury/falls
6. Risk for infection
7. Anxiety/fear
8. Deficient knowledge

C. PLANNING AND IMPLEMENTATION/ INTERVENTIONS

1. Determine priorities
   a. Maintain airway, breathing, circulation (see Chapter 1)
   b. Provide supplemental oxygen as indicated
   c. Establish IV access for administration of crystalloid fluid/blood products/medications as needed
   d. Obtain and set up equipment and supplies
   e. Prepare for/assist with medical interventions
   f. Administer pharmacologic therapy as ordered
2. Relieve anxiety/apprehension
3. Allow significant other to remain with patient if supportive
4. Educate patient/significant others

D. EVALUATION AND ONGOING MONITORING

1. Continuously monitor and treat as indicated
2. Monitor patient response/outcomes and modify nursing care plan as appropriate
3. If positive patient outcomes are not demonstrated, reevaluate assessment and/or plan of care

E. DOCUMENTATION OF INTERVENTIONS AND PATIENT RESPONSE

F. AGE-RELATED CONSIDERATIONS

1. Pediatric
   a. Growth or development related
      1) Children's bone structure is different from adults; children are considered skeletally immature
         a) Growth plates (epiphyseal plate or physis): area of growing tissue at the end of long bones in children and adolescents
      2) Skeleton of infant and young child is largely cartilaginous, and bones are narrow and flexible
      3) Periosteum is thicker and resists disruption
         a) Provides circulation and nutrients to bone
         b) Allows bone to be more elastic and to resist fracture
      4) General appearance
         a) Observe legs while child is walking
            (1) Infants have bowlegged (genu varum) appearance until age 2 or 3 years
            (2) Infants and toddlers tend to evert feet and walk on inner aspects of feet
            (3) At age 3, child may appear knock-kneed (genu valgum)
            (4) Normal leg configuration should be present at approximately 6–7 years
         b) Feet appear flatfooted
            (1) Medial longitudinal arch normally obscured by fat pads until approximately 2 years
            (2) Arch better visualized when child not weight bearing, such as when seated or on tiptoe
         c) Child may normally walk with in-toeing (pigeon toed)
            (1) Rotational alignment of legs changes as skeleton matures producing spontaneous correction
            (2) Pathologic changes may be produced by disorders of the feet, lower legs, or hips
   b. "Pearls"
      1) Pulling injury to the arm can result in subluxation of the radial head ("nursemaid's elbow") and is commonly seen between 2 and 3 years of age
      2) Limping in children is uncommon; suspect hip disorder if found
      3) Unwillingness to bear weight requires further investigation
2. Geriatric
   a. Aging-related
      1) Loss of bone minerals and mass
         a) Regeneration prolonged
         b) Bones become more brittle
         c) Loss of vertebral body height results from compression, which occurs with normal aging and can lead to kyphosis
      2) Muscles lose the ability to regenerate new fibers to replace ones lost because of age; the result is atrophy
         a) Decreased muscular strength, endurance, and shuffling gait
         b) Longer contraction time and tendency to fatigue more easily, which may cause muscle tremors, even at rest
   b. "Pearls"
      1) Joint stiffness and degenerative changes contribute to decreased mobility
      2) Posture affected by age-related changes
      3) Gait affected by posture, balance, strength, and flexibility
      4) Changes in feet common
         a) Foot size decreases because of loss of subcutaneous fat
         b) Skin is drier; corns and calluses form at pressure points; epidermis thins and loses natural moisture

c) Decreased circulation from peripheral vascular disease may delay healing; venous stasis or arterial occlusion produces ulceration

d) Toenails thicken, affecting shoe fit

e) Bunion and toe overlapping or underriding may occur

5) Osteoporosis promotes fractures, especially in vertebral bodies, ribs, proximal femur

6) Osteoarthritis (degeneration of movable joints) affects mostly weight-bearing joints of knees, vertebrae, and small joints of hand and feet

7) Rheumatoid arthritis (systemic disease of connective tissue resulting in joint inflammation) produces swelling, stiffness, ankylosis, redness, and warmth of joints

8) Paget's disease
   a) Metabolic disease that causes excessive bone resorption and deposits
   b) Middle-aged and elderly men primarily affected
   c) Affected bones tend to fracture easily

9) Predisposition to falls

10) Fall prevention strategies
    a) Ensure adequate lighting
    b) Eliminate loose rugs and electrical cords
    c) Use bath/shower seats and rails
    d) Use walking aids such as walker or cane
    e) Wear supportive shoes

II. Specific Soft Tissue Emergencies

The soft tissues of the extremities include the skin, muscles, tendons, ligaments, nerves, and blood vessels. Injuries may occur with or without a bony injury, and in some cases it is difficult to make the diagnosis. A careful clinical examination along with radiologic studies to rule out skeletal trauma is necessary to identify the problem. Certain disorders may result from chronic overuse, and patients may not have an acute history of injury.

A. LOW BACK PAIN

Low back pain is usually a benign problem that affects up to 60–80% of the population at some time. Intervertebral disk disease and disk herniation are common causes of back pain and are most prominent in otherwise healthy people between 30 and 40 years of age. Disk degeneration is a normal part of the aging process in adults. Pain is the primary presenting complaint and may be localized or radiate to the buttock or lower extremities. Symptoms vary, depending on the specific structure involved. Risk factors include obesity, poor body mechanics, lifting or moving heavy objects, prolonged sitting, poor office furniture design, and hard floor surfaces. Ninety percent of

low back pain is musculoskeletal, and yet it never receives a precise diagnosis. The lumbar spinal column provides weight bearing, spinal cord protection, and trunk movement.

1. Assessment
   a. Subjective data collection
      1) History of present illness/injury/chief complaint
         a) Pain (see Chapter 8)
         b) Recent trauma or chronic injury
         c) Time of occurrence
            (1) Acute: <7 days
            (2) Subacute: 7 days to 7 weeks
            (3) Chronic: >7 weeks
         d) Associated symptoms: paresthesia, radiation of pain, impaired function of bladder or bowel, or impaired sexual function
         e) Psychosocial stressors
         f) Success of past therapeutic measures
      2) Past medical history
         a) Current or preexisting diseases/illness
         b) Previous back injury or strain
         c) Obesity
         d) Occupation or profession
         e) Current pregnancy or other gynecologic problems; last normal menstrual period in female patients of childbearing age
         f) Previous treatments, surgical procedures, and medications
         g) Smoking: may relate to poor nutritional status and delayed healing
         h) Substance abuse: may relate to nutritional status and other associated medical problems
         i) Medications
         j) Allergies
   b. Objective data collection
      1) Physical examination
         a) General appearance
            (1) Gait and posture
                (a) Steppage, or footdrop, gait
                (b) Leaning to painful side when knee flexed on that side
                (c) Stiff, rigid trunk
            (2) Moderate to severe distress/discomfort
         b) Inspection
            (1) Abnormal spinal curvature; lordosis, kyphosis, or scoliosis
         c) Palpation
            (1) Point tenderness or general area of tenderness
            (2) Swelling
            (3) Muscle spasm
         d) Spinal range of motion
         e) Deep tendon reflexes (DTRs)
            (1) Grade: 0, none; +1, below normal; +2, average; +3, stronger than average; +4, intense (clonus)
         f) Motor function

(1) Decreased strength in heel/toe walk
(2) Footdrop; loss of full dorsiflexion
    (a) Difficulty climbing stairs
  g) Sensory testing
    (1) Sharp-dull discrimination
  h) Other examinations
    (1) Rectal examination (e.g., sphincter tone)
    (2) Sensation of inner thigh and perineum to assess for saddle anesthesia
    (3) Arterial pulses and abdominal examination (e.g., abdominal aortic aneurysm)
 2) Diagnostic procedures
  a) Selected patients
    (1) CBC with differential
    (2) ESR
    (3) Urinalysis; pregnancy test in female patients of childbearing age
    (4) Lumbar, sacral, and pelvic radiographs
    (5) Thoracic/spinal CT scan
    (6) MRI

2. Analysis: differential nursing diagnoses/collaborative problems
  a. Acute/chronic pain
  b. Activity intolerance
  c. Risk for injury/falls
  d. Anxiety/fear
  e. Deficient knowledge

3. Planning and implementation/interventions
  a. Prepare for/assist with medical interventions
   1) Position of comfort: pelvic tilt may reduce pain
   2) Assist with hospital admission for intractable pain
  b. Administer pharmacologic therapy as ordered
   1) Nonnarcotic analgesics
   2) Narcotics
   3) Nonsteroidal antiinflammatory medications (NSAIDs)
  c. Educate patient/significant others
   1) Instruct on use of physical assistive devices (e.g., walker, cane)
   2) Instruct on methods of proper body mechanics
   3) Instruct on home safety: install railings, remove loose floor mats
   4) Arrange for appropriate follow-up care

4. Evaluation and ongoing assessment
  a. Pain relief

B. OVERUSE/CUMULATIVE TRAUMA DISORDERS

Symptoms of overuse are typically the result of repetitive and forceful use of the extremities in a work setting or as part of leisure activities. Injuries can be attributed to a multitude of factors, including lack of conditioning, overuse, misuse, and trauma. The repetitive stress produces soft tissue microtears and inflammation, which can lead to tendon inflammation and synovitis, muscle tears (typically at musculotendinous junctions), ligamentous

disorders, degenerative joint disease, bursitis, and nerve entrapment.

BURSITIS. Bursitis is inflammation of a bursa, a saclike structure that covers the bony prominence among bones, muscles, and tendons. The bursa contains only a small amount of viscous fluid. Inflammation of a bursa is the result of trauma (e.g., a direct blow or a chronic injury associated with prolonged, repetitive use) or infection (bacterial or fungal). The more common sites of bursitis are the shoulder, elbow, hip, knee, and heel of the foot. It is important to determine whether the bursitis is the result of inflammation or infection, because definitive therapy differs.

1. Assessment
  a. Subjective data collection
   1) History of present illness/injury/chief complaint
    a) Recent acute injury
    b) Recent localized infection
    c) Repetitive use of area: participating in vigorous sports, leaning on elbows, kneeling, and pressure from shoe rubbing on back of foot
    d) Pain (see Chapter 8): may have sudden or gradual onset and may persist for several days and then diminish abruptly or gradually
    e) Decreased joint range of motion
   2) Past medical history
    a) Current or preexisting diseases/illness
     (1) Previous or current bursitis
     (2) Infections
     (3) Arthritis
    b) Medications
    c) Allergies
  b. Objective data collection
   1) Physical examination
    a) General appearance
     (1) Mild to moderate distress/discomfort
    b) Inspection
     (1) Redness and warmth over area
     (2) Swelling of area
     (3) Limited range of motion of extremity
     (4) Increased pain with activity; severe pain suggestive of infection
     (5) Shoulder (subacromial): pain to upper humerus and in subacromial area; pain may radiate up to neck and down to fingertips
     (6) Elbow (olecranon): swollen area caused by acute trauma
     (7) Heel (posterior calcaneal): inflamed and thickened area at back of heel
    c) Palpation
     (1) Warmth of area
     (2) Soft or firm area
     (3) Hip: tenderness over greater trochanter; best elicited with patient lying on side with affected hip uppermost and ipsilateral knee slightly flexed

(4) Knee: does not involve knee joint: localized, fluctuant mass in prepatellar area can usually be palpated; often referred to as "housemaid's knee"
2. Analysis: differential nursing diagnoses/collaborative problems
   a. Acute/chronic pain
   b. Activity intolerance
   c. Risk for injury
   d. Anxiety/fear
   e. Deficient knowledge
3. Planning and implementation/interventions
   a. Prepare for/assist with medical interventions
      1) Immobilize joint with splint
   b. Administer pharmacologic therapy as ordered
      1) NSAIDs
      2) Nonnarcotic analgesics
      3) Antibiotics: if bursa aspirated and infection noted
   c. Educate patient/significant others
      1) Rest affected area
      2) Use moleskin over heel; wear properly fitting shoes
      3) Apply ice over affected areas during acute stage
      4) Use immobilization device (e.g., splint, sling)
      5) Apply and remove compressive dressing
      6) Elevate injured extremity
      7) Indications/precautions for prescribed medications
      8) Arrange follow-up care for orthopedic evaluation and possible need for
         a) Bursal injection
         b) Bursal aspiration and possible incision or drainage, if infection present
         c) Physical therapy
4. Evaluation and ongoing assessment
   a. Pain relief

NERVE ENTRAPMENT SYNDROME. Nerve entrapment syndrome results from compression of a peripheral nerve as it traverses a closed compartment. Other structures contained within the compartment can swell and compress nerve fibers. Carpal tunnel syndrome, compression of the median nerve at the wrist, is the most common nerve entrapment syndrome. Cubital tunnel syndrome involves entrapment of the ulnar nerve at the elbow. Tarsal tunnel syndrome results from compression of the medial tibial nerve at the medial malleolus. More than 80% of patients are older than 40 years at diagnosis. Nerve entrapment syndromes occur twice as frequently in women as men. Pregnant women are at risk for carpal tunnel syndrome as a result of fluid retention. Patients involved in repetitive actions are prone to nerve entrapment syndrome.
1. Assessment
   a. Subjective data collection
      1) History of present illness/injury/chief complaint
         a) Overuse risk factors
         b) Pain (see Chapter 8): in muscle group, joint, tendon, or along distribution of affected nerve
         c) Paresthesia, tingling, or numbness
         d) Pregnancy
      2) Past medical history
         a) Current or preexisting diseases/illness
            (1) Rheumatoid arthritis
            (2) Osteoarthritis
            (3) Growth hormone abnormalities (e.g., acromegaly)
            (4) Connective tissue disorders (e.g., amyloidosis)
         b) Medications
         c) Allergies
   b. Objective data collection
      1) Physical examination
         a) General appearance
            (1) Mild to moderate distress/discomfort
         b) Inspection
            (1) Soft tissue swelling
            (2) Possible atrophy in surrounding muscles
            (3) Muscle weakness
      2) Diagnostic procedures
         a) Tinel sign: sensation of tingling felt in hand when median nerve is tapped on volar wrist; diagnostic of carpal tunnel syndrome
         b) Phalen test: forced flexion of wrist for a minimum of 1 minute causes exacerbation of paresthesia along distribution of median nerve; diagnostic of carpal tunnel syndrome
         c) Electromyography (EMG): referral to identify muscle disease or defects in transmission of electrical impulses across anatomic areas
2. Analysis: differential nursing diagnoses/collaborative problems
   a. Acute/chronic pain
   b. Activity intolerance
   c. Risk for injury/falls
   d. Anxiety/fear
   e. Deficient knowledge
3. Planning and implementation/interventions
   a. Prepare for/assist with medical procedures
      1) Apply ice if swelling present
      2) Elevate if swelling present
   b. Administer pharmacologic therapy as ordered
      1) NSAIDs
      2) Nonnarcotic analgesics
      3) Narcotics
   c. Educate patient/significant others
      1) Rest affected area with immobilization device (use of cock-up splint, especially at night; elbow splint)
      2) Use nonrigid orthotic shoe inserts
      3) Apply cold packs
      4) Use compressive dressing and remove twice daily
      5) Elevate affected area

6) Indications/precautions for prescribed medications
7) Arrange orthopedic referral for follow-up care
4. Evaluation and ongoing assessment
   a. Pain relief

TENDINITIS. Tendinitis is an inflammation of the tendons and tendon-muscle attachments. Inflammation is the result of excessive, unaccustomed repetitive stress. The inflammation may be acute or chronic. Tendinitis commonly occurs in the shoulder (rotator cuff tendinitis), elbow (lateral epicondylitis or "tennis elbow" and medial epicondylitis or "golfer's elbow"), knee (patellar tendinitis or "jumper's knee"), and heel (Achilles tendinitis).
1. Assessment
   a. Subjective data collection
      1) History of present illness/injury/chief complaint
         a) Repetitive motions with affected extremity
         b) Prolonged use of area, such as leaning on elbow while seated at desk
         c) Pain (see Chapter 8): localized pain described as deep ache; typically becomes worse with motion
      2) Past medical history
         a) Current or preexisting diseases/illness
         b) Previous occurrences of tendinitis
         c) Medications
         d) Allergies
   b. Objective data collection
      1) Physical examination
         a) General appearance
            (1) Mild to moderate distress/discomfort
         b) Inspection
            (1) Swelling of area
         c) Palpation
            (1) Tenderness when pressure applied in rolling motion over tendon
      2) Diagnostic procedures: radiographs to identify whether calcification has occurred; because tendons are less vascular than other structures, tendinitis can lead to calcific deposits
2. Analysis: differential nursing diagnoses/collaborative problems
   a. Acute/chronic pain
   b. Activity intolerance
   c. Risk for injury/falls
   d. Anxiety/fear
   e. Deficient knowledge
3. Planning and implementation/interventions
   a. Prepare for/assist with medical procedures
      1) Apply compressive dressing to support joint
      2) Elevate to decrease swelling
   b. Administer pharmacologic therapy as ordered
      1) Nonnarcotic analgesics
      2) NSAIDs

c. Educate patient/significant others
   1) Rest tendon by avoiding use: immobilization and elevation of affected area
   2) Apply and remove compressive dressing twice daily
   3) Indications/precautions for prescribed medications
   4) Arrange for follow-up care
      a) Orthopedic evaluation
      b) Physical therapy
4. Evaluation and ongoing assessment
   a. Pain relief

III. Specific Bony Skeleton Emergencies

A. COSTOCHONDRITIS

Costochondritis is an acute, self-limiting inflammation of the costal cartilage of the rib and sternal junctions and may involve one or several junctions. Inflammation may result from physical exertion or repetitive movements. Pain in this region is similar to that of a rib fracture or myocardial infarction. A patient presenting with chest pain who is at risk for myocardial ischemia must have a thorough cardiac evaluation before assuming the symptoms are musculoskeletal in origin. Costochondritis is most commonly seen in people older than 20 years.
1. Assessment
   a. Subjective data collection
      1) History of presenting illness/injury/chief complaint
         a) Pain (see Chapter 8)
            (1) Characteristics: described as sharp, pleuritic, unilateral, or peristernal
         b) Factors that worsen or alleviate symptoms: movement, deep inspiration
         c) Medications
      2) Past medical history
         a) Current or preexisting diseases/illness
            (1) Cardiac or inflammatory processes
            (2) Upper respiratory tract infection
         b) Recent injury or surgery
         c) Medications
         d) Allergies
   b. Objective data collection
      1) Physical examination
         a) General appearance
            (1) Moderate distress/discomfort with movement
         b) Inspection
            (1) Anterior thorax for swelling, ecchymosis, or deformity
            (2) Painful facial grimace with deep inspiration, movement of upper extremities, or coughing

c) Palpation
  (1) Reproducible pain (point tenderness to palpation of chest wall)
2) Diagnostic procedures
  a) CBC with differential
  b) ESR
  c) C-reactive protein
  d) Chest radiograph
  e) ECG to rule out cardiac disease
2. Analysis: differential nursing diagnoses/collaborative problems
  a. Acute/chronic pain
  b. Activity intolerance
  c. Anxiety/fear
  d. Deficient knowledge
3. Planning and implementation/interventions
  a. Administer pharmacologic therapy as ordered
    1) Nonnarcotic analgesics
    2) Narcotics
    3) NSAIDs
  b. Educate patient/significant others
    1) Rest
    2) Encourage deep breathing to prevent respiratory complications
    3) Instruct patient to avoid exertional activities that exacerbate symptoms
    4) Instruct patient to report any increased symptoms
    5) Follow-up care arrangements/instructions
4. Evaluation and ongoing assessment
  a. Pain relief

B. JOINT EFFUSIONS

Joint effusions involve the collection of fluid in a joint as a result of an inflammatory process, previous surgery, or trauma. Effusions most commonly occur in the knee joint. Extreme stretching of the knee ligaments may result in microscopic tears of the meniscus, with consequent synovial fluid collection. Patients with prior knee surgery and traumatic injuries to the area are at risk for joint effusions. Patients with hemophilia who sustain minimal blunt force to the knees are at risk for hemarthrosis (blood collection in the joint space).

1. Assessment
  a. Subjective data collection
    1) History of present illness/injury/chief complaint
     a) History of recent or past trauma
     b) Joint involved: isolated or multiple
     c) Recent surgical procedure
     d) Recent infection
     e) Substance abuse: risk of septic arthritis
     f) Medication: diuretics associated with hyperuricemia, which may lead to gouty arthritis
     g) Repetitive use of joint
     h) Onset and speed of fluid accumulation
     i) Inability to bear weight fully
     j) Fevers, chills
    2) Past medical history
     a) Current or previous diseases/illness
      (1) Arthritis
      (2) Gout
      (3) Joint surgery
      (4) Infectious processes
      (5) Sexually transmitted infection
      (6) Bleeding disorders
     b) Medications
     c) Allergies
  b. Objective data collection
    1) Physical examination
     a) General appearance
      (1) Moderate distress/discomfort
     b) Inspection
      (1) Swelling of area
      (2) Erythema
      (3) Skin changes
     c) Palpation
      (1) Tenderness of area
      (2) Limited range of motion
    2) Diagnostic procedures
     a) CBC with differential
     b) ESR
     c) Urinalysis
     d) Venereal Disease Research Laboratories (VDRL) test or rapid plasma reagin (RPR)
     e) Hepatitis B
     f) C-reactive protein
     g) Joint radiograph: comparison with other extremity
     h) Joint aspiration
2. Analysis: differential nursing diagnoses/collaborative problems
  a. Acute/chronic pain
  b. Activity intolerance
  c. Risk for injury/falls
  d. Risk for infection
  e. Impaired skin integrity
  f. Anxiety/fear
  g. Deficient knowledge
3. Planning and implementation/interventions
  a. Prepare for/assist with medical procedures
    1) Immobilize affected joint
    2) Arthrocentesis
     a) Differentiates between hemarthrosis and infectious or inflammatory processes
     b) White blood cell count: 20,000–60,000 associated with inflammatory process; 100,000 associated with infection
  b. Administer pharmacologic therapy as ordered
    1) Nonnarcotic analgesics
    2) Narcotics
    3) Steroids

4) NSAIDs
5) Antibiotics

c. Educate patient/significant others
   1) Instruct on self-care measures at home
   2) Instruct on specific signs and symptoms indicating a need for medical reevaluation
   3) Facilitate completion of paperwork for employment release

4. Evaluation and ongoing assessment
   a. Pain relief

C. OSTEOARTHRITIS

Also known as degenerative joint disease, osteoarthritis is the most common joint disease and results in the degeneration of the articular cartilage in joints. The cartilage, which is made of proteins, provides a cushion between the bones. As the articular cartilage becomes thin, bony spur formation at the edges of the joint surfaces may be seen. Although the exact underlying mechanism is not known, there appears to be a biochemical abnormality of the cartilage. It affects adults, men before age 45 and women after age 55.

1. Assessment
   a. Subjective data collection
      1) History of present illness/chief complaint
         a) Pain (see Chapter 8): worse later in the day
         b) Pain and stiffness after long periods of inactivity
         c) Pain in affected joints after repetitive use most often located in hips, knees, vertebrae, fingers
      2) Past medical history
         a) Current or preexisting diseases/illness
         b) Excessive joint use, abuse, or obesity
         c) Trauma (acute or repetitive)
         d) Genetic influences
         e) Medications
         f) Allergies
   b. Objective data collection
      1) Physical examination
         a) General appearance
            (1) Mild distress/discomfort
         b) Inspection
            (1) Pain and swelling in one, two, or more joints, particularly after activity
            (2) Stiffness occurs less frequently than in rheumatoid arthritis
            (3) Limitation of joint motion in weight-bearing and finger joints
            (4) Heberden nodes: nodular bony enlargements that occur on the distal joints of some or all fingers
            (5) Bouchard nodes: nodular bony enlargements that occur on the proximal joints of some or all fingers
         c) Palpation
            (1) Crepitus: audible, grating sound produced by bony irregularities within the joint
      2) Diagnostic procedures
         a) Radiograph: demonstrates bony hypertrophy, spur formation, and cartilage disruption
         b) Arthrocentesis: aspiration of joint fluid for analysis to exclude other disease, infection, gout, or other types of arthritis
         c) Arthroscopy: surgical procedure performed by placing a viewing tube into the joint space. If cartilage is damaged, the procedure for repair may be done at that time

2. Analysis: differential nursing diagnoses/collaborative problems
   a. Acute/chronic pain
   b. Activity intolerance
   c. Risk for injury/falls
   d. Anxiety/fear
   e. Deficient knowledge

3. Planning and implementation/interventions
   a. Prepare for/assist with medical procedures
      1) Arthrocentesis
   b. Administer pharmacologic therapy as ordered
      1) Nonnarcotic analgesics
      2) NSAIDs
   c. Educate patient/significant others
      1) Stress the importance of a weight reduction program, under medical supervision, to decrease stress on weight-bearing joints
      2) Avoid activities that precipitate pain
      3) Provide rest for involved joints; excessive use aggravates symptoms and accelerates degeneration
      4) Use splints, braces, or lumbosacral supports
      5) Teach patient to use correct posture and body mechanics
      6) Physical and occupational therapy
      7) Rest to decrease both intensity and frequency of activities
      8) Exercise program to strengthen the muscles that support the joints

4. Evaluation and ongoing assessment
   a. Pain relief

D. OSTEOPOROSIS

Osteoporosis results from inadequate production of bone, excessive removal of bone, or a combination of both. It results in thin bones. Populations at risk include postmenopausal women, persons who take steroids, and persons who use alcohol. Symptoms include pain, from microscopic or obvious fractures, and loss of height.

1. Assessment
   a. Subjective data collection
      1) History of present illness/chief complaint
         a) Pain

(1) Back pain, especially thoracolumbar area
  (a) Often begins after "pop" felt
  (b) Pain radiates around ribs or along iliac crest
(2) Hip pain
  (a) Suggests impending or actual hip or pelvic fracture
  (b) Limp associated with hip pain
  (c) Could be impending fracture even with normal radiograph
(3) Wrist pain
  (a) Wrist fractures common after fall

2) Past medical history
  a) Current or preexisting diseases/illness
  b) Injury or problems with joint
  c) Postmenopausal status
  d) Alcohol use
  e) Loss of height
  f) Medications
    (1) Steroid use
  g) Allergies

b. Objective data collection
  1) Physical examination
    a) General appearance
      (1) Mild to moderate distress/discomfort
    b) Inspection
      (1) Colles fracture of wrist after fall
        (a) Often first sign of osteoporosis in women younger than 65 years
        (b) Kyphosis (dowager's hump): collapse of spine produces appearance of shortened trunk
  2) Diagnostic procedures
    a) Radiographs to rule out fractures
    b) Special studies to rule out microscopic fractures
      (1) CT scan, MRI, and bone scan
      (2) Referral to primary care provider (PCP) for definitive studies (e.g., dual-energy radiograph absorptiometry scan)

2. Analysis: differential nursing diagnoses/collaborative problems
  a. Acute/chronic pain
  b. Activity intolerance

c. Risk for injury/falls
d. Anxiety/fear
e. Deficient knowledge

3. Planning and implementation/interventions
  a. Administer pharmacologic therapy as ordered
  b. Educate patient/significant others
    1) Referral to PCP or orthopedic physician for definitive testing
    2) Preserve bone mass with adequate calcium intake and regular exercise

4. Evaluation and ongoing assessment
  a. Pain relief
  b. Stabilization of fractures

Bibliography

Back Pain Fact Sheet. (2015). National Institute of Neurological Disorders.

Bone & Joint Initiative. (2013). The burden of musculoskeletal diseases in the United States: Facts in brief. Retrieved from http://www.boneandjointburden.org/facts-brief.

Emergency Nurses Association: *Emergency nursing core curriculum*, ed 6, Philadelphia, PA, 2007, Saunders.

Marcus R: *Osteoporosis*, ed 4, New York, NY, 2013, Elsevier.

Nelson HD, Haney EM, Chou R, Dana T, Fu R, Bougatsos C: *Screening for osteoporosis systematic review to update the 2002 U.S. Preventive Services Task Force recommendation*, Rockville, MD, 2010, Agency for Healthcare Research and Quality.

Sarwark JF: *Essentials of musculoskeletal care*, ed 6, Rosemont, IL, 2010, American Academy of Orthopedic Surgeons.

Singer A, Exudides A, Spangler L, et al.: Burden of illness for osteoporotic fractures compared with other serious diseases among postmenopausal women in the United States, *Mayo Clinic Proceedings* 901(1):53–62, 2015.

Tintinalli JE, Kelen GD, Stapczynski JS: *Emergency medicine: A comprehensive study guide*, ed 6, New York, NY, 2004, McGraw-Hill.

Wolfson A: *Hardwood-Nuss clinical practice of emergency medicine*, ed 6, Philadelphia, PA, 2015, Lippincott Williams & Wilkins.

Part 2

CHAPTER 25

Pre- and Post-Transplant Emergencies

Christine Trotter, CCRN, ACNP

MAJOR TOPICS
General Strategy
Assessment
Analysis: Differential Nursing Diagnoses/Collaborative
  Problem
Planning and Implementation/Interventions
Pre-Solid Organ Transplant Emergencies
Notification of Patient's Arrival
Special Considerations

Post-Solid Organ Transplant Emergencies
General Strategy
Solid Organ Transplant Rejection and Infection
Special Considerations

I. General Strategy

A. ASSESSMENT

1. Primary and secondary assessment/resuscitation (see Chapter 1)
2. Specific assessment dependent on presenting clinical condition

B. ANALYSIS: DIFFERENTIAL NURSING DIAGNOSES/COLLABORATIVE PROBLEM

1. Decrease cardiac output
2. Risk for deficient fluid volume
3. Ineffective tissue perfusion
4. Impaired gas exchange
5. Risk for hypothermia
6. Risk for infection
7. Deficient knowledge

C. PLANNING AND IMPLEMENTATION/ INTERVENTIONS

1. See Chapter 1 and relevant system-related chapters
2. Evaluation and ongoing monitoring
   a. Hemodynamic status
   b. Breath sounds and pulse oximetry
   c. Cardiac rate and rhythm
   d. Intake and output
   e. Serum electrolytes

II. Pre-Solid Organ Transplant Emergencies

Patients awaiting solid organ transplant can present to the emergency department for many reasons, often related to the failing organ they are waiting for. Refer to organ-specific chapters for these emergencies, but there are specific considerations to keep in mind when caring for these patients that are awaiting solid organ transplant.

A. NOTIFICATION OF PATIENT'S ARRIVAL

1. Notify transplant team of patient's arrival to emergency department
2. May affect eligibility for transplant
   a. Too sick
   b. Active infection
   c. Suspicion of new malignancy
   d. Active alcohol or drug use
   e. Pregnancy
3. May alter patient's status on organ waiting list
   a. Heart
      1) Worsening functional status
      2) Mechanical ventilation
      3) Requiring a mechanical assist device such as intraaortic balloon pump (IABP), ventricular assist device (VAD)
      4) Inotropes

   b. Lung
      1) Worsening functional status
      2) Mechanical ventilation
      3) Worsening kidney function
   c. Liver
      1) Increasing INR
      2) Increasing bilirubin
      3) Worsening kidney function
   d. Kidney
      1) Loss of options for dialysis access
   e. Pancreas
      1) None; based on wait time

B. SPECIAL CONSIDERATIONS

Consult with transplant team regarding blood product transfusions in stable patients, as this can affect antibody formation. New antibody formation could limit access to potential donor organs. In the case of an unstable, actively bleeding patient, that patient's life should take priority over potential sensitization issues.

III. Post-Solid Organ Transplant Emergencies

Patients presenting to the emergency department after organ transplant can present for reasons not related to transplant, but hypervigilance needs to be exercised when caring for the special needs of these patients. Two main reasons for presentation to the emergency department are rejection of the transplanted graft and infection. The presenting signs and symptoms can be similar and often require diagnostics to differentiate the two.

Rejection is a very real complication of solid organ transplantation. There is a delicate balance between obtaining adequate immunosuppression to prevent graft rejection and oversuppressing the immune system, which can put the patient at risk for infection, malignancies, and drug toxicities.

Infection is more frequent in this patient population given the patient's immunosuppressed state to prevent the transplanted graft from rejection. Patients are placed on prophylactic antimicrobials in the posttransplant period, as this is the period of most immunosuppression, though some prophylactics continue lifelong. These usually include antivirals, antifungals, and antibiotics.

Immunosuppressive therapy is comprised of a cocktail of drugs that vary by organ type, disease state, antibodies, and length of time posttransplant. Initial immunosuppressive therapy, known as induction therapy, often includes one or more of the following agents: antilymphocyte antibodies, including antithymocyte globulin and alemtuzumab; IL-2 receptor antagonists, including basiliximab; and anti-CD20 antibodies, such as rituximab. These are often used in combination with high-dose corticosteroids while introducing maintenance therapy of calcineurin inhibitors (CNIs), such

as tacrolimus or cyclosporine, and antiproliferatives, such as mycophenolate mofetil (MMF) or azithioprine. Belatacept is a newer agent, which is a costimulation blocker that is approved in kidney transplant patients, which is the first IV only agent for maintenance immunosuppression. This drug can take the place of CNIs in EBV-positive patients only. Very rarely, patients may be weaned completely off immunosuppressive therapy.

A. GENERAL STRATEGY

1. Chief complaint/history of present illness/review of systems
   a. Transplant rejection/infection workup
      1) Identify organ transplanted
      2) Date of transplantation
      3) History of rejection/infections
      4) Timing onset of symptoms
      5) Sick contacts
      6) Recent travel
      7) Fever
      8) Fatigue
      9) Weight gain
      10) Shortness of breath
      11) Graft tenderness
      12) Nausea/vomiting
      13) Ascites
      14) Dysuria
      15) Changes in urine amount or color
      16) Hyperglycemia
      17) Edema
      18) Pruritus
      19) Jaundice
      20) Medication compliance
   b. Past medical/surgical history
      1) Disease process necessitating organ transplant
      2) See Chapter 1
   c. Social history
      1) Tobacco history
      2) Alcohol history
      3) Other substance abuse history. In addition to the normal sequelae of using illicit drugs, immunosuppressed patients smoking marijuana can present with infectious complications including aspergillosis
   d. Current medications
      1) Regularly prescribed (e.g., antihypertensives, anticoagulants)
      2) Immunosuppressive medications often including calcineurin inhibitors, antimetabolites, steroids
         a) Ask about compliance
      3) Prophylactic antifungals, antivirals, and antibiotics
         a) Duration of prophylactic therapy based on organ transplanted and center-specific protocol, may be lifelong
   e. Allergies

f. Objective
1) Vital signs
a) Febrile, often low grade
b) Hyper- or hypotension
c) Tachycardia
d) Tachypnea
e) Weight changes
2) Physical exam
a) Standard assessment (refer to Table 25.1 for further organ-specific findings)
b) Examine for lesions that could be consistent with herpes simplex or zoster
3) Diagnostics: workup for infection and rejection are similar, it is important to exclude one or the other as they can mimic each other upon presentation to the emergency department
4) Labs: CBC, CMP, PT/INR, blood cultures, UA, urine culture, sputum culture, serum CMV, EBV, VZV. Serum and urine BK in the kidney transplant recipient. Send for C. diffocele testing if symptomatic. Consider obtaining drug level trough of tacrolimus or cyclosporine if appropriate timing, 12 hours post dosing
5) CXR
6) EKG
7) Ultrasound of liver or kidney
8) Pulmonary function tests in lung recipient
9) Consider thoracentesis and/or bronchoscopy with BAL in lung recipient
10) Echocardiogram in heart recipient
11) Consider spinal tap if high suspicion for neurological infection
12) Possible biopsy of transplanted organ

g. Assessment/nursing diagnosis
1) Ineffective breathing pattern
2) Decreased cardiac output
3) Risk for infection
4) Excess fluid volume
5) Acute pain
6) Activity intolerance
7) Altered tissue perfusion
h. Planning and implementation
1) Establish and maintain adequate airway, breathing, circulation
2) Establish IV access
3) If possible, place patient in private room; consider reverse isolation
4) Anticipate and implement diagnostics as ordered
a) Labs
b) Radiology
c) EKG
d) Possible biopsy. Biopsy is the gold standard for the diagnosis of rejection
(1) Liver: transjugular in interventional radiology or percutaneously at the bedside with or without ultrasound guidance based on center protocols
(2) Kidney: ultrasound guided at bedside or in interventional radiology
(3) Heart: prepare for cardiac catheterization laboratory
(4) Lung: transbronchial lung biopsy via bronchoscopy
5) Administer medications as ordered
a) Antibiotics as indicated
b) Antiemetics
c) Analgesics

TABLE 25.1

Signs and Symptoms of Rejection and Infection

Heart	Lung	Liver	Kidney	Pancreas
Fever	Fever	Fever	Fever	Fever
JVD	Cough	Pain over graft site	Pain over graft site	Pain over graft site
Hypotension	Dyspnea	Jaundice	Decreased urine output	Elevated amylase, lipase
Shortness of breath	Fatigue	Ascites	Elevated BUN/creatinine	Hyperglycemia
Edema	Pleural effusions	Dark-colored urine	Edema	
Pericardial rub	Hypoxemia	Clay-colored stools	Electrolyte abnormalities	
Dysrhythmias	Perihilar opacities	Pruritis	Volume overload	
Increased weight	PFTs with ↓ in FEV1 or ↓ in both FVC and FEV1	Fatigue		
Crackles		Elevated LFTs		
Low voltage EKG		Elevated INR		
Syncope		Hepatosplenomegaly		
Signs of hepatic congestion including nausea, vomiting, abdominal pain		Nausea, vomiting, abdominal pain		

d) Possible treatment for rejection that may include high-dose steroids, antithymocyte globulin

e) Ensure receives other immunosuppressants as ordered

   (1) CNIs: usually dosed every 12 hours. If unable to take orally, can consider liquid dosing via enteral access or sublingual. Do not give IV CNIs unless cleared by transplant team attending. They have high risks involved, including neurotoxicity, and are not 1:1 dosing with oral equivalent

   (2) Antimetabolites: usually dosed every 12 hours. Can be given IV with 1:1 conversion if unable to take orally

   (3) Steroids: may convert to IV dosing

6) Educate

  a) Educate patient and family

   (1) Diagnostics

   (2) Prepare for possible admission

   (3) Enforce good hand hygiene

   (4) Consider controlling or screening visitors if immunocompromised

7) Evaluation and continued monitoring

  a) Level of consciousness

b) Adequate airway maintained

c) Hemodynamic monitoring

d) Pulse oximetry

e) Strict intake and output

f) Pain management

g) Treat and prevention of nausea and vomiting

h) Monitoring of specified laboratory levels

B. SOLID ORGAN TRANSPLANT REJECTION AND INFECTION

When an organ is transplanted into its host, the body can recognize this tissue as a foreign invader. In an attempt to prevent this, organs may be matched based on blood type and/or HLA typing depending on organ type and likelihood of rejection. In addition to immunosuppression maintenance therapy, protocol biopsies of transplanted organs may take place to identify and treat early rejection, based on center protocol. There are three types of rejection: hyperacute, acute, and chronic (Table 25.2). When the host's immune system attacks the transplanted graft, patients can present to the emergency room with anywhere from mild to severe or life-threatening signs and symptoms. Infection in these patients can present with the same signs and symptoms as rejection.

TABLE 25.2

Rejection

	Occurrence	Time of onset
Hyperacute	Has become less common as advances have been made in immunosuppression regimens and HLA matching.	Immediate. Occurs in the operating room or in the hours following transplantation
Acute	Heart: Peaks at 1 month posttransplant, then low, constant rate by 1 year posttransplant. Risk factors include young, female African-American recipient, female donor, HLA mismatch Lung: Common, one third of patients treated in first year. Risk factors include HLA mismatch, genetic factors, young, vitamin D deficiency Liver: Common, one study shows 64% of recipients reject. Usually occurs in first 3 months after transplant. Risk factors include low levels of immunosuppression, younger recipient age, fewer HLA-DR matches, longer cold ischemic time, donor age of at least 30, autoimmune disease as transplant indication Kidney: Usually occurs within the first 6 months posttransplant. Later occurrence is usually associated with medication noncompliance. Risk factors include recipients with high PRA (panel reactive antibody), African-American, retransplant Pancreas: Common, 60–80% of transplants	Can occur anytime, but usually occurs in the first year posttransplant
Chronic	Heart: 25–60% incidence. Risk factors include HLA mismatch, racial and sex discrepancies, history of acute rejection Lung: Varying rates. Risk factors include infections, low levels of immunosuppression, history of acute rejection, gastroesophageal reflux Kidney: Risk factors include history of acute rejection (frequency, timing, severity), infection, and low levels of immunosuppression Liver: Declining incidence. Risk factors include CMV infection, indications for transplant including primary sclerosing cholangitis (PSC), primary biliary cirrhosis (PBC), and autoimmune hepatitis (AIH) Pancreas: Variable rates. Undefined risk factors	Can occur months to years after transplant

C. SPECIAL CONSIDERATIONS

1. Drug toxicities
   a. CNIs
      1) Tremor
      2) Mood swings
      3) Seizures
      4) HTN
      5) Hyperlipidemia
      6) Nephrotoxicity
      7) New onset diabetes
   b. Antiproliferatives
      1) Nausea
      2) Vomiting
      3) Diarrhea
      4) Abdominal pain
      5) Leukopenia
      6) Thrombocytopenia
   c. Drug interactions
      1) Be aware that starting new medications can interact with immunosuppressive drugs, specifically CNIs. This is not an all-inclusive list, but a list of more common medications that may be seen in the emergency department. Check with your pharmacist regarding interactions when initiating new medications.
         a) Drugs that increase blood levels of CNIs
            (1) Calcium channel blockers: Diltiazem, Verapamil
            (2) Antifungals: voriconazole, ketoconazole, fluconazole
            (3) Macrolides: clarithromycin, erythromycin
            (4) Amiodorone
            (5) Protease inhibitors
            (6) Grapefruit juice
         b) Drugs that decrease blood levels of CNIs
            (1) Anticonvulsants: carbamazepine, phenobarbital, phenytoin
            (2) Antimicrobials: isoniazid, rifampin
            (3) Herbals: St. John's wort
   d. Malignancies
      1) Posttransplant lymphoproliferative disorder (PTLD)
      2) Skin cancers
   e. Organ-specific considerations
      1) Heart
         a) Baseline tachycardia
         b) Atropine ineffective in treating bradycardia
         c) May not have angina with ischemia
         d) Use care when considering beta blockade
      2) Lung
         a) Airway issues
            (1) Stenosis
            (2) Bronchomalacia
         b) Difficulty managing secretions as the lung is denervated
      3) Liver
         a) Vascular complications
            (1) Hepatic artery thrombosis or stenosis
            (2) Portal vein thrombosis
         b) Bile duct complications
            (1) Anastamotic leak
            (2) Biliary strictures
            (3) Bile leak
      4) Kidney
         a) Urine leak
         b) Urinary retention
         c) Stricture
         d) Renal artery thrombosis
         e) Declining kidney function
      5) Pancreas
         a) Vascular thrombosis
         b) Note technique for pancreatic drainage that the patient has (bladder drained versus enteric drainage)
         c) Pancreatic fistula

Bibliography

Baker R, Jardine A, Andrews P: *Postoperative care of the kidney transplant recipient guidelines*, The Renal Association, 2011, February.

Bell L: Caring for acutely ill patients before transplant, *American Journal of Critical Care* 23(6):516, 2014.

Chaoyang L, et al.: New onset diabetes after liver transplantation and its impact on complications and patient survival, *Journal of Diabetes* 7(6):881–890, 2015.

Colvin M, et al.: Heart, *American Journal of Transplantation* 16(2):S115–S140, 2016.

Cupples S, Ohler L: *Transplantation nursing secrets*, 2003, Hanley & Belfus.

Ferrerira S, et al.: Nursing diagnoses among kidney transplant recipients: evidence from clinical practice, *International Journal of Nursing Knowledge* 25(1):49–53, 2014.

Foster B, et al.: High risk of graft failure in emerging adult heart transplant recipients, *American Journal of Transplantation* 15(12):3185–3193, 2015.

Gaglio P: *Liver transplantation in adults: long-term management of transplant recipients*. Retrieved from Uptodate.com, 2016.

Hoffman, Francis, et al.: Caring for transplant recipients in a nontransplant setting, *Critical Care Nurse* 26(2):53–73, 2006.

Israelsen M, Gluud L, Krag A: Acute kidney injury and hepatorenal syndrome in cirrhosis, *Journal of Gastroenterology and Hepatology* 30(2):236–243, 2015.

Kadambi P, et al.: (n.d.). Differential diagnosis in renal allograft dysfunction. Retrieved from Uptodate.com.

Kirk A, et al. (2014). Late infectious disease after organ transplant, *Textbook of Organ Transplantation (chap. 94)*. Retrieved from http://onlinelibrary.wiley.com/book/10.1002/9781118873434.

Lucey M, et al.: Long-term management of the successful adult liver transplant: 2012 Practice Guideline by the American Association for the Study of Liver Diseases and the American Society of Transplantation, *Liver Transplantation* 19(1):3–26, 2013.

Lyu D, Zamora M: Medical complications of lung transplantation, *Proceedings of American Thoracic Society* 6(1):101–107, 2009.

Martin-Gandul C, Mueller N, Manuel O: The impact of infection on chronic allograft dysfunction and allograft survival after solid organ transplant, *American Journal of Transplantation* 15(12):3024–3040, 2015.

Moten M, Doligalski C: Postoperative transplant immunosuppression in the critical care unit, *AACN Advanced Critical Care* 24(4):345–350, 2014.

Niederhaus S, et al.: Acute cellular and antibody-mediated rejection of the pancreas allograft: incidence, risk factors and outcomes, *American Journal of Transplantation* 13(11): 2945–2955, 2013.

Samstein B, et al.: Complications and their resolution in recipients of deceased and living donor liver transplants: findings from the A2ALL Cohort Study, American Journal of Transplantation 16(2):594–602, 2016.

Singh R, Sutherland D, Kadaswamy R: *Pancreas transplantation. Abdominal Organ Transplantation: State of the Art (chap. 5)*, 2012.

Part 2

CHAPTER 26

Toxicologic Emergencies

Michael De Laby, MSN, RN, CCRN, CFRN, NRP

Toxicologic emergencies include acute poisonings and intake of substances of abuse. These situations pose a unique challenge to the emergency department nurse. The American Association of Poison Control Centers' annual report for 2013 stated that 93% of cases occurred in the home, with 48% occurring in children younger than 6 years and 35.5% involving children younger than 3 years of age. In addition, it was noted that 87.9% of toxic exposures were acute and 79.9% were unintentional. Therapeutic medication errors, such as double dosing or taking the wrong medication, accounted for more than 12.5% of all poisonings.[1] Ingestion or coingestion of over-the-counter (OTC) drugs such as antihistamines, antidiarrheals, or indigestion remedies in potential poisoning situations may cloud or mask true symptoms of acute poisoning. In 2011, over 5 million emergency department visits were associated with drugs of abuse or misuse, including prescription and OTC drugs, inhalants, and illicit drugs.[2] Patients may also use more than one drug in combination, with resulting polysubstance abuse, or may ingest a substance in combination with alcohol, thus leading to fatalities.

Consideration must be given to organic causes such as thyroid disease, hypoglycemia, hypoxia, or the purposeful or accidental exposure to a toxin or chemical when dealing with patients with an altered level of consciousness.

Treatment is directed toward preventing or decreasing absorption of the toxic substance (Table 26.1). This can be accomplished using measures to enhance elimination of the substance (Table 26.2) or by administering specific antidotes to counteract the toxic substance (Table 26.3).

I. General Strategy

A. ASSESSMENT

1. Primary and secondary assessment/resuscitation (see Chapter 1)
2. Focused assessment
   a. Subjective data collection
      1) History of present illness/chief complaint
         a) Information regarding use/abuse/ingestion from patient, family, friends

Table 26.1

Measures to Prevent or Decrease Absorption of Drugs or Chemicals

	Procedure	Indications	Contraindications/ Precautions	Comments
Ocular Decontamination				
Irrigation	Irrigation with water or saline, using Morgan lens as needed		Alkali solutions require longer periods of irrigation Ensure pH is neutral before discontinuing	Refer to ophthalmology for alkali or continued irritation
Dermal Decontamination				
Irrigation	Remove all contaminated clothing Flush surfaces with water or saline, including hair and under nails	Organophosphate insecticides Gasoline, hydrocarbons Acids, alkali Any chemical that may burn skin	Ensure chemical is not combustible with use of water	Ensure protective gear is used
Gastrointestinal Decontamination in Oral Ingestions				
Gastric emptying with syrup of ipecac		See comments	Contraindicated use in drugs causing central nervous system depression, inducing seizures (e.g., tricyclic antidepressants), caustics or corrosives, or having a potential for aspiration	Use is controversial American Academy of Pediatrics Policy Statement (2003) and American Association of Poison Control Centers Guideline (2005) issued recommendations limiting or discouraging use in out-of-hospital situations No recommendations regarding emergency department use have been made
Gastric lavage	Use large-lumen (36–40F) orogastric tube Best initiated within 60 min of ingestion		Potential for aspiration Caution in ingestion of caustics or corrosives Contraindicated in coingestion of sharp objects and nontoxic ingestions	Benefit is controversial
Cathartic administration	Use magnesium sulfate, magnesium citrate, sorbitol Mix and administer with activated charcoal orally or via lavage/ nasogastric tube Use single doses, do not repeat	May be used to enhance elimination of activated charcoal	Contraindicated with absent bowel sounds and preexisting renal and cardiac failure	May cause vomiting or severe diarrhea
Whole bowel irrigation (controversial)	Use nonabsorbable evacuant solution via nasogastric tube/lavage (GoLYTELY, CoLyte)	Used in enteric-coated or sustained-release products, drugs that may form concretions (e.g., aspirin) body packers, drugs not adsorbed by activated charcoal (e.g., iron, lithium)	Contraindicated in preexisting gastrointestinal disease, presence or risk of ileus, perforation, obstruction Precaution in pediatric patients	May cause nausea, vomiting, abdominal cramping, risk of electrolyte imbalance
Prevent or Limit Absorption/Adsorption of Drugs or Chemicals in Oral Ingestions				
Activated charcoal	Adults: 1 g/kg body weight Pediatrics: 0.5 g/kg	Used to adsorb most chemicals ingested	Contraindicated in corrosive or caustic ingestions, decreased or absent bowel sounds, toxins not bound by activated charcoal (iron, lead, lithium)	Specific substances may require multiple doses (e.g., aspirin)

Data from Olson, K. (2004). *Poisoning and drug overdose* (4th ed.). East Norwalk, CT: Appleton & Lange; Dart, R. C. (Ed.). (2004). *Medical toxicology* (3rd ed.). Philadelphia. PA: Lippincott Williams & Wilkins; Flomenbaum, N. E., Goldfrank, L. R., Hoffman, R. S., Howland, M. A., Lewin, N. A., & Nelson L. S. (2006). *Goldfrank's toxicologic emergencies* (8th ed.). New York, NY: McGraw-Hill.

Part 2

Table 26.2

Measures to Enhance Elimination of Drugs or Chemicals

	Procedure	Indications	Contraindications/ Precautions	Comments
Urinary alkalinization using sodium bicarbonate	Use of intravenous sodium bicarbonate	Used with chemicals altering pH (e.g., aspirin)	Contraindicated in presence of pulmonary edema or renal failure, fluid overload possible	Frequent pH and electrolyte levels indicated, particularly potassium
Hemodialysis	Venous blood sent across membrane and treated with dialysate, toxins removed	Salicylates/aspirin, valproic acid, methanol, ethylene glycol, others Renal dysfunction with long-term drug use (e.g., lithium)	Caution in patients with bleeding disorders	Drugs with large volumes of distribution not always dialyzable
Hemoperfusion	Similar to hemodialysis, charcoal filter often used	Phenobarbital, theophylline, others	May cause thrombocytopenia	Although clearance rates are frequently higher, it is not the treatment of choice

Data from Olson, K. (2004). *Poisoning and drug overdose* (4th ed.). East Norwalk, CT: Appleton & Lange; Dart, R. C. (Ed.). (2004). *Medical toxicology* (3rd ed.). Philadelphia, PA: Lippincott Williams & Wilkins; Flomenbaum, N. E., Goldfrank, L. R., Hoffman, R. S., Howland, M. A., Lewin, N. A., & Nelson L. S. (2006). *Goldfrank's toxicologic emergencies* (8th ed.). New York, NY: McGraw-Hill.

Table 26.3

Specific Antidotes

Antidote	Poisoning	Antidote	Poisoning
N-acetylcysteine Mucomyst (oral formulation) Acetadote (intravenous formulation)	Acetaminophen (Tylenol)	Ethanol intravenously 10%	Ethylene glycol, methanol
		Flumazenil (Romazicon)	Benzodiazepine
		Folic acid	Methanol
Atropine	Organophosphate, carbamate insecticide Bradycardia caused by toxins	Fomepizole (4 MP) (Antizol)	Ethylene glycol, methanol
		Glucagon	Beta-blocker, calcium channel blocker
Antivenins Polyvalent equine	Rattlesnake, copperhead envenomation	Methylene blue	Methemoglobinemia
		Naloxone (Narcan)	Narcotic overdose
Polyvalent immune Fab-Ovine/Cro-Fab	Rattlesnake, copperhead envenomation	Oxygen, hyperbaric oxygen	Carbon monoxide
Black Widow Spider	Black widow spider bite	Octreotide (Sandostatin)	Oral sulfonylurea hypoglycemia
Dimercaprol (BAL in oil)	Heavy metal	Physostigmine/Antilirium	Anticholinergic
Botulinum antitoxin	Botulism	Pralidoxime (2-PAM) (Protopam)	Organophosphate
Calcium chloride or gluconate	Calcium channel blocker, hydrofluoric acid: skin exposure or poisoning, hypocalcemia	Protamine	Heparin
		Pyridoxine	Isonicotinic acid hydrazide (INH), ethylene glycol
Cyanide antidote kit	Cyanide	Prussian blue	Thallium, radioactive cesium
Deferoxamine	Iron	Sodium bicarbonate	Sodium channel blockers, alkalinization of urine or serum
Dextrose	Hypoglycemia caused by toxins		
Digoxin Fab	Digoxin, oleander	Sodium thiosulfate	Cyanide
DMSA (Succimer) (Chemet)	Heavy metal (especially lead, mercury)	Thiamine	Ethylene glycol, Wernicke's syndrome, *Gyromitra* mushrooms, hydrazine
Edetate disodium, D-Penicillamine	Heavy metal	Vitamin K	Warfarin (Coumadin), warfarin-based rodenticides

Data from Tintinalli, J. E., Stapczynski, J. S., Cline, D. M., Ma, O. J., Cydulka, R. K., & Meckler, G. D. (Eds.). (2011). *Emergency medicine: A comprehensive study guide* (7th ed.). New York, NY: McGraw-Hill; Olson, K. (2004). *Poisoning and drug overdose* (4th ed.). East Norwalk, CT: Appleton & Lange; Poisondex System (Internet database, updated periodically). Greenwood Village, CO: Thomson Micromedex. Retrieved from http://www.thomsonhc.com.

    (1) Specific name and amount of substance(s)

    (2) Time of use or poisoning

    (3) Acute vs. chronic use

    (4) Symptoms experienced, including emesis, shortness of breath, chest pain/ palpitations

    (5) Patient location when poisoning occurred

    (6) First aid measures instituted before emergency department arrival/prehospital care, including emesis induction, decontamination

  b) Route of exposure

    (1) Oral ingestion

    (2) Inhaled, snorted, or smoked

    (3) Dermal contact

    (4) Injected or parenteral

    (5) Ocular exposure

    (6) Rectal

    (7) Other

  c) Reason for exposure

    (1) Unintentional or accidental

    (2) Intentional: suicide attempt, substance abuse

    (3) Recreational use

    (4) Occupational

      (a) Chemical exposure

      (b) Pesticide use

      (c) Acid or heavy metal exposure: stained-glass worker (lead), auto plating (hydrofluoric acid)

      (d) Other: carbon monoxide

    (5) Bioterrorism or other environmental event (see Chapters 15 and 41)

  d) Efforts to relieve symptoms

    (1) Home remedies

    (2) Alternative therapies

    (3) Medications

      (a) Prescription

      (b) OTC/herbal

2) Past medical history

  a) Current or preexisting diseases/illness

    (1) Hepatitis

    (2) Tuberculosis

    (3) Endocarditis

    (4) Human immunodeficiency virus (HIV) infection or acquired immunodeficiency syndrome (AIDS)

    (5) Psychological

  b) Previous trauma including falls, head injury

  c) Previous hospitalizations

  d) Withdrawal history

  e) Substance and/or alcohol use/abuse: polysubstance use may lead to masking of symptoms

    (1) Prescription drugs (e.g., narcotics)

    (2) OTC medications and products (inhalants)

    (3) Drugs used to treat substance abuse (methadone, disulfiram [Antabuse])

  f) Last normal menstrual period: females of childbearing age

  g) Current medications

  h) Allergies

3) Psychological/social/environmental factors

  a) Psychological

    (1) Suicidal ideation/intent and prior attempts; prior overdose

    (2) Patient may not seek care for treatment of addiction or overdose but for related symptoms

    (3) Personality traits and history of psychiatric illness; increase in stress/guilt may lead to emergency

    (4) Developmental stage may be altered by addiction/overdose

    (5) Substance abuse may lead to failure to fulfill obligations at home, work, school

    (6) Age of patient

    (7) Current life situation: medical or psychiatric illness, traumatic event

    (8) Possible/actual assault, abuse, or intimate partner violence situations (see Chapters 3 and 40)

  b) Social

    (1) Support network

      (a) Family, significant others, friends

      (b) Social and legal agencies: check for involvement of protective services or legal system

      (c) Parental and family supervision: may be lacking in pediatric or elderly cases

    (2) Occupational exposure

    (3) Fiscal status: insurance may determine aftercare availability

    (4) Cultural and religious beliefs

  c) Environmental

    (1) Living arrangements: homeless, apartment, home; rural, urban

    (2) Other residents or participants

    (3) Availability of substances, medications, alcohol

    (4) Storage of substances: original containers, child-resistant caps

    (5) Mass-casualty disaster related to naturally occurring or bioterrorist event

  d) Risk factors

    (1) Family history of substance use/abuse/ poisoning

    (2) Use of gateway substances before addiction

      (a) Alcohol

      (b) Marijuana

      (c) Tobacco

(d) Inhalants

(3) Peer group abuse of substances

(4) Psychiatric disorders, especially depression or bipolar disorder

(5) Decreased supervision of elderly persons or young children

b. Objective data collection

1) General appearance

a) Level of consciousness, behavior, affect

b) Vital signs

c) Seizure activity

d) Odors

e) Gait

f) Hygiene

g) Level of distress/discomfort

2) Inspection

a) Skin: color, capillary refill, track marks, bruising, rashes, abscesses, cellulitis

b) Tremors, tic

c) Pupil size, reactivity, nystagmus

d) Nares: epistaxis, perforation of septum

3) Auscultation

a) Heart sounds: murmurs, dysrhythmias on monitor

b) Breath sounds: crackles, wheezes, rhonchi

c) Bowel sounds: motility

4) Palpation: universal precautions because drug paraphernalia or used needles may be hidden in clothing

a) Skin moisture

b) Pulses, quality and symmetry

c) Abdomen: size, pain, tenderness, ascites

d) Extremity deformity

3. Diagnostic procedures

a. Laboratory studies

1) Therapeutic drug levels, as indicated by history, clinical condition

2) Fingerstick glucose

3) Serum and urine toxicology screen

4) Serum alcohol or breathalyzer

5) Complete blood count (CBC) with differential

6) Serum chemistries including glucose, serum lactate, blood urea nitrogen (BUN), creatinine

7) Arterial blood gas (ABG)

8) Liver function tests (LFTs)

9) Coagulation profile (prothrombin time [PT], partial thromboplastin time [PTT], international normalized ratio [INR], fibrinogen)

10) Urinalysis: pregnancy test in females of childbearing age

11) Carboxyhemoglobin (COHb) level

b. Imaging studies

1) Chest radiograph

2) Abdominal radiographs

3) C-spine radiograph if trauma suspected

4) Computed tomography (CT) scan, magnetic resonance imaging (MRI) based on history

c. Other

1) 12- to 15-lead electrocardiogram (ECG)

2) Esophagoscopy

B. ANALYSIS: DIFFERENTIAL NURSING DIAGNOSES/COLLABORATIVE PROBLEMS

1. Anxiety/fear

2. Ineffective coping

3. Risk for injury/falls

4. Risk for poisoning

5. Risk for self/other-directed violence

6. Disturbed sensory/perception: visual, auditory, kinesthetic

7. Risk for decreased cardiac output

8. Risk for impaired gas exchange

9. Risk for ineffective airway clearance

10. Risk for ineffective breathing pattern

11. Risk for aspiration

12. Risk for seizures

13. Risk for trauma

C. PLANNING AND IMPLEMENTATION/INTERVENTIONS

1. Determine priorities of care

a. Maintain airway, breathing, circulation (see Chapter 1)

b. Provide supplemental oxygen as indicated

c. Establish intravenous (IV) access for administration of crystalloid fluid/medications as needed

d. Obtain and set up equipment and supplies

e. Prepare for/assist with medical interventions

f. Administer pharmacologic therapy as ordered

2. Relieve anxiety/apprehension

3. Allow significant others to remain with patient if supportive

4. Educate patient/significant others

D. EVALUATION AND ONGOING MONITORING

1. Continuously monitor and treat as indicated

2. Monitor patient response/outcomes, and modify nursing care plan as appropriate

3. If positive patient outcomes are not demonstrated, reevaluate assessment and/or plan of care

E. DOCUMENTATION OF INTERVENTIONS AND PATIENT RESPONSE

F. AGE-RELATED CONSIDERATIONS

1. Pediatrics

a. Growth or development related

1) Decreased renal clearance in children younger than 6 months of age has a direct effect on half-life and duration of drugs

2) Infants have fewer binding sites for drugs, thus leading to greater chance for toxic effects

3) Lower glycogen stores place children at higher risk for developing hypoglycemia with ingestions

b. "Pearls"

1) Most poisonings occur in children younger than 6 years and in the home

2) Poisonings are usually unintentional or accidental and may occur as children are exploring their environment or through incorrect dosing

3) Munchausen syndrome by proxy, a form of child maltreatment, may manifest as an intentional form of poisoning

4) Very young children are less likely to develop hepatotoxicity with acetaminophen overdoses

5) Adolescents are at higher risk for drug use because of peer group usage or use by significant adults

6) Adolescents using recreational drugs may display behavioral changes such as drop in school performance, change in clothing style, or change in peer group attachment

7) Suicide attempts are infrequently intended to result in death

2. Geriatrics

a. Aging-related

1) Medical conditions may cause the patient to have to manage larger numbers of medications, thus putting him or her at risk for therapeutic medication errors

2) Decreased renal clearance may result in toxicity

3) Slowed metabolism of medications leads to greater chance of toxicity

b. "Pearls"

1) Consider chronic salicylism (poisoning by salicylic acid) in confused older adults

2) Unusual behaviors, symptoms, or responses may be the result of drug toxicity

3) Evaluate for mental illness, substance abuse, or depression

4) Older adults frequently forget to take medications or accidentally take extra medications

II. Specific Toxicologic Emergencies

A. ACETAMINOPHEN POISONING

A common analgesic with antipyretic properties, acetaminophen is seen in many OTC products and in combination with narcotics. It is rapidly absorbed from the GI tract and is metabolized by the liver. It is widely used because it has few side effects and drug interactions. Toxicity produces delayed coagulopathies, hepatic necrosis, and elevated LFTs. Children can tolerate larger doses and tend to have less hepatotoxicity than adults because of their ability to better metabolize acetaminophen. Hepatotoxicity may occur through therapeutic medication errors, in patients concurrently using acetaminophen and abusing alcohol, or in persons taking other medications that are metabolized by the liver.

Common products containing acetaminophen include NyQuil, Percogesic, and Tylenol PM. Formulations may vary in concentration (drops vs. elixir, extended relief vs. standard). Parents should be instructed to read labels carefully.

1. Assessment

a. Subjective data collection

1) History of present illness/chief complaint

a) Acute vs. chronic exposure

b) Concomitant use of alcohol or other drugs (e.g., narcotic preparations with acetaminophen)

c) Reason for exposure (e.g., suicide, chronic pain)

d) Dose form: regular or extended-release product; affects absorption

e) Symptoms

(1) Early (within 24–48 hours postingestion): malaise, nausea, emesis

(2) Later: metabolic acidosis, right upper quadrant pain, decreased urine output, LFTs rise with resultant jaundice, hypoglycemia, coagulopathies (possibly disseminated intravascular coagulopathy [DIC]), and sepsis

2) Past medical history

a) Current or preexisting diseases/illness

(1) Psychiatric history

(2) Alcohol use/abuse history

(3) Preexisting liver disease

b) Medications

c) Allergies

b. Objective data collection

1) Physical examination

a) General appearance

(1) Level of consciousness, behavior, affect: awake to lethargy

(2) Mild to severe distress/discomfort

b) Inspection

(1) Jaundice in later stages of hepatic failure

c) Palpation

(1) Right upper quadrant abdominal tenderness

(2) Hepatomegaly

2) Diagnostic procedures

a) Serum acetaminophen level 4 hours after ingestion: important indicator of eventual hepatotoxicity; compare with nomogram for acute acetaminophen toxicity (nomogram invalid in long-term exposures)

b) LFTs

c) CBC with differential

d) Serum chemistries

e) Coagulation profile

f) Serum and urine toxicology screen

g) Urinalysis; pregnancy test in female patients of childbearing age

2. Analysis: differential nursing diagnoses/collaborative problems

a. Risk for poisoning

3. Planning and implementation/interventions

a. Maintain airway, breathing, circulation (see Chapter 1)

b. Provide supplemental oxygen as indicated

c. Establish IV access for administration of crystalloid fluid/medications

d. Prepare for/assist with medical interventions

1) Institute cardiac and pulse oximetry monitoring

2) Insert gastric tube as indicated

3) Assist with possible hospital admission

e. Administer pharmacologic therapy as ordered

1) Activated charcoal with or without cathartic

2) N-acetylcysteine (Mucomyst) orally, by gastric tube, or by the IV route (Acetadote)

f. Hemodialysis

4. Evaluation and ongoing monitoring

a. Hemodynamic status

b. Acetaminophen levels

c. Educate parents/caregivers about toxicity of acetaminophen and dosing

d. Refer patient/family to social/support services

B. ALCOHOL USE

Alcohol is one of the most commonly used drugs in the United States. Approximately 16.6 million U.S. adults had alcohol use disorders (AUD), defined when a patient's drinking causes distress or harm, in 2013, and 1.3 million received treatment for AUD in a specialized facility. Alcohol abuse is a component of roughly 70% of overdose cases in the emergency department. Alcoholism is a chronic illness characterized by impaired control over drinking that leads to physiologic, psychological, and/or social dysfunction. Alcohol affects all socioeconomic levels and slightly more male than female patients. Alcohol may be the primary drug of abuse or may be used concomitantly with other drugs. It is contained in beverages, perfumes, mouthwashes, and many OTC preparations (e.g., NyQuil).

Alcohol is metabolized in the liver and affects all body systems, including the central nervous system (CNS), gastrointestinal (GI), and cardiovascular systems. The effects of alcohol use can lead to motor impairment, confusion, risky or violent behavior, and accidental injuries and death. The development of subdural hematomas is not uncommon in patients with chronic alcoholism. Although alcohol initially causes a state of euphoria, it is actually a CNS depressant.

1. Assessment

a. Subjective data collection

1) History of present illness/chief complaint

a) Symptoms may or may not be related to alcohol intoxication

b) Trauma from falls/head injury

c) Description of drinking episode: how much consumed, time, percentage of alcohol content

d) Tremors

e) Changes in level of consciousness

2) Past medical history

a) Current or preexisting diseases/illness

(1) Seizures/epilepsy

(2) Liver disease

(3) GI bleeding or varices

(4) Traumatic injury or recent fractures

(5) History of suicide gestures, anxiety, or depression

b) Concurrent medication use

(1) Prescription and/or OTC drug

(2) Lithium or disulfiram (Antabuse) use

(3) Seizure medications

c) Patterns of alcohol use/abuse

(1) Consumption pattern and type of alcohol

(2) Time since last drink

(3) Blackout history

(4) Change in tolerance

(5) Previous attempts to discontinue drinking, types of programs, duration of abstinence

3) Risk factors

a) Family history of alcoholism

b) Heavy drinking: more than five drinks in one sitting

c) Use of other drugs (prescription, illicit, or OTC)

b. Objective data collection

1) Physical examination

a) General appearance

(1) Level of consciousness, behavior, affect: disorientated to obtunded

(2) Decreased or elevated temperature

(3) Gait: staggering, ataxia

(4) Odors: alcohol, breath mints, mouthwash

(5) Hygiene: clean, well groomed to disheveled

(6) Moderate to severe distress/discomfort

b) Inspection

(1) Nystagmus: intoxication

(2) Tremors, hallucinations, diaphoresis: withdrawal

(3) Spider angiomas

(4) Scars from previous falls

(5) Multiple bruises

(6) Recent or healing burns

(7) Gynecomastia

(8) Jaundice, icteric sclera

  c) Palpation

    (1) Abdominal tenderness, ascites

    (2) Hepatomegaly

  2) Diagnostic procedures

    a) Serum blood alcohol level and/or breathalyzer

    b) CBC with differential

    c) Serum chemistries including glucose and ammonia levels

    d) Serum and urine toxicology screens

    e) LFTs

    f) Coagulation profile

    g) Urinalysis; pregnancy test in female patients of childbearing age

    h) C-spine radiograph

    i) Chest radiograph

    j) Head CT scan and/or MRI

    k) ECG

2. Analysis: differential nursing diagnoses/collaborative problems

  a. Acute/chronic confusion

  b. Disturbed sensory perception

  c. Risk for poisoning

  d. Risk for injury

  e. Risk for ineffective airway clearance

  f. Risk for deficient fluid volume

  g. Risk for decreased cardiac output

  h. Dysfunctional family processes due to alcoholism

  i. Risk for self/other-directed violence

  j. Risk for trauma

3. Planning and implementation/interventions

  a. Maintain airway, breathing, circulation (see Chapter 1)

    1) Provide supplemental oxygen as indicated

      a) Ventilatory support in obtunded patients

      b) High-flow oxygen

  b. Establish IV access for administration of crystalloid fluids/medications

  c. Prepare for/assist with medical interventions

    1) Advanced airway management

      a) Rapid sequence intubation (RSI)

      b) Nasal or oral intubation

      c) Supraglottic airway (i.e., King, Combitube, laryngeal mask airway)

      d) Surgical airway (e.g., cricothyrotomy)

    2) Institute cardiac, blood pressure, pulse oximetry monitoring

    3) Minimize stimulation to decrease sensory alteration

      a) Use quiet environment

      b) Keep lights on to decrease shadows and visual hallucinations

    4) Minimize behavior escalation to decrease violence potential

      a) Decrease stimulation and noise as needed

      b) Closely monitor patient behavior to prevent escalation

      c) Use restraints per institutional protocols: chemical, soft, leather

    5) Prevent injury

      a) Limit patient ambulation to prevent falls

      b) Initiate seizure precautions per institutional protocols

      c) Encourage behaviors that prevent self-harm or harm to others

    6) Insert gastric tube as indicated

      a) Gastric lavage: controversial and potentially useful only if performed within 1–4 hours after ingestion

    7) Insert indwelling urinary catheter as indicated

    8) Assist with possible hospital admission

  d. Administer pharmacologic therapy as ordered

    1) RSI premedications: sedatives, analgesics, neuromuscular blocking agents

    2) Dextrose 50% (D50W) if patient is hypoglycemic

    3) Thiamine and multivitamins to combat Wernicke-Korsakoff syndrome and malnutrition

    4) Replace depleted electrolytes as needed: potassium, magnesium

    5) Benzodiazepines: chlordiazepoxide hydrochloride (Librium), lorazepam (Ativan), diazepam (Valium) for agitation and seizures resulting from overdose or withdrawal

    6) Antipsychotics: haloperidol (Haldol) for delirium and agitation

  e. Educate patient/significant others

    1) Initiate social service consultation or psychiatric evaluation as needed

    2) Review discharge medications with patient and family

    3) Refer patient/family to social services and/or support groups (e.g., Alcoholics Anonymous)

    4) Encourage consistent primary care follow-up to encourage sobriety

    5) Refer patient/family to rehabilitation/recovery resources

4. Evaluation and ongoing monitoring

  a. Airway patency

  b. Level of consciousness

  c. Hemodynamic status

  d. Seizure activity

  e. Breath sounds and pulse oximetry

  f. Cardiac rate and rhythm

  g. Intake and output

  h. Ambulation ability

  i. Continued presence or absence of hallucinations

  j. Drug levels

C. AMPHETAMINE USE

Amphetamines are synthetic sympathomimetic drugs that stimulate the CNS and produce a feeling of excess energy.

They are commonly used to suppress appetite, elevate mood, stay awake, and control symptoms of attention-deficit disorder. Amphetamines are available in oral, intranasal, or parenteral forms. Common amphetamines include crystal methamphetamine, dextroamphetamine, and methylphenidate (Ritalin). Methamphetamine (also known as meth, crystal, chalk, ice) is a potent and highly addictive stimulant with severe psychological, medical, and social consequences. It is smoked, inhaled, injected, or orally ingested. Crystalline rock forms such as "ice" are smoked. "Body packers" are seen in the emergency department as a result of swallowing packages, condoms, or rocks while either transporting the drugs or evading law enforcement detection. Other drugs associated with amphetamines include MDMA (also known as Ecstasy or Molly). MDMA is a synthetic psychoactive drug that has stimulant effects of amphetamine and hallucinogen effects of mescaline. MDMA is orally consumed to increase energy and create a sense of euphoria, emotional warmth, and empathy toward others.

1. Assessment
   a. Subjective data collection
      1) History of present illness/chief complaint
         a) Type of drug ingested
         b) Route: oral, smoked, snorted, intravenous, body packing
         c) Time of ingestion and quantity: if a body pack ruptures, a large quantity will be absorbed internally at one time
         d) Reason for use: suicidal, recreational, intentional, weight loss
         e) Presenting symptoms: same as cocaine but longer duration
      2) Past medical history
         a) Current or preexisting diseases/illness
            (1) Obesity
            (2) Attention-deficit disorder
            (3) Hyperactivity
            (4) Narcolepsy
            (5) Psychiatric
         b) Previous substance use/abuse
         c) Medications
         d) Allergies
   b. Objective data collection
      1) Physical examination
         a) General appearance
            (1) Level of consciousness, behavior, affect: anxious, restless, paranoia/delusions, hallucinations, seizure activity
            (2) Hygiene: possibly unkempt
            (3) Hypertension, tachycardia, dysrhythmias, hyperthermia
            (4) Moderate distress/discomfort
         b) Inspection
            (1) Pupillary response: mydriasis
            (2) Tremors
            (3) Thin, emaciated appearing
            (4) Oral effects: "meth mouth"—severe pattern of tooth decay
            (5) Skin lesions related to formication (type of paresthesia from sensation of ants/insects running on skin)
         c) Auscultation
            (1) Heart sounds: rhythm/regularity; murmurs
      2) Diagnostic procedures, in addition to standard testing
         a) Serum and urine toxicology screen
         b) Urinalysis; pregnancy test in female patients of childbearing age
         c) Abdominal radiograph: assess body packing
         d) ECG
         e) Echocardiogram
         f) CT scan
2. Analysis: differential nursing diagnoses/collaborative problems
   a. Decreased cardiac output
   b. Risk for poisoning
   c. Risk for hyperthermia
   d. Ineffective coping, hopelessness
   e. Risk for suicide and/or self/other-directed violence
   f. Risk for trauma
   g. Risk for infection
3. Planning and implementation/interventions
   a. Maintain airway, breathing, circulation (see Chapter 1)
   b. Provide supplemental oxygen as indicated
   c. Establish IV access for administration of crystalloid fluid/medications
   d. Prepare for/assist with medical interventions
      1) Institute cardiac and pulse oximetry monitoring
      2) Insert gastric tube as indicated
         a) Gastric lavage; controversial and potentially useful only if immediate life-threatening intoxication; emesis contraindicated because of potential for aspiration
         b) Whole bowel irrigation through a gastric tube may be indicated with body packers
      3) Maintain normothermic body temperature: cooling measures for hyperthermia
      4) Decrease risk for violence; protect patient and staff
         a) Decrease sensory stimulation by placing patient in quiet area
         b) Use consistent, nonjudgmental caregivers; set appropriate limits on behavior
         c) If other measures fail, consider restraints to prevent staff and patient injury: soft, leather, or chemical per policy and procedures
   e. Administer pharmacologic therapy as ordered
      1) Activated charcoal: prevents systemic absorption
      2) Benzodiazepines: provides sedation

3) Whole bowel irrigation with polyethylene glycol and electrolyte solution such as GoLYTELY for body packers
   f. Educate patient/significant others
      1) Refer patient/family to social services and/or support groups (e.g., Narcotics Anonymous)
      2) Effects of amphetamines on body
      3) Refer patient/family to rehabilitation/recovery resources
4. Evaluation and ongoing monitoring
   a. Hemodynamic status
   b. Cardiac rate and rhythm
   c. Seizure activity
   d. Intake and output
   e. Core temperature
   f. Continued presence or absence of hallucinations or agitation

D. BETA-BLOCKER TOXICITY

Beta-adrenergic receptor blocking agents inhibit the $beta_1$ receptors (cardiac muscle) and the $beta_2$ receptors (bronchial and vascular musculature), thereby causing a decreased heart rate, decreased cardiac output at rest and with exercise, and hypotension. These effects make the drugs useful in the treatment of angina, hypertension, and chronic heart failure. Recent literature promotes the use of beta blockers to enhance survival after a myocardial infarction. The cardioprotective effects are thought to prevent reinfarction. Beta blockers have also been used in the treatment of migraines. An overdose of beta blockers causes severe hypotension and bradycardia. Death results from asystole. Abrupt withdrawal causes rebound hyperactivity, leading to unstable angina and a myocardial infarction. Common agents include propranolol (Inderal), metoprolol (Lopressor, Toprol XL), and atenolol (Tenormin), many of which have been formulated into sustained-release formulations to increase compliance.

1. Assessment
   a. Subjective data collection
      1) History of present illness/chief complaint
         a) Circumstances of exposure: unintentional, intentional
         b) Concurrent therapy: calcium channel blockers
         c) Nausea/vomiting
         d) Weakness
      2) Past medical history
         a) Current or preexisting diseases/illness
            (1) Cardiovascular disease
            (2) Migraine history
            (3) Asthma
         b) Medications
         c) Allergies
   b. Objective data collection
      1) Physical examination
         a) General appearance
            (1) Level of consciousness, behavior, affect: delirium to coma, seizures (especially with propranolol)
            (2) Hypotension, bradycardia, asystole
            (3) Moderate to severe distress/discomfort
         b) Inspection
            (1) Cardiac dysrhythmia on monitor: AV blocks
         c) Auscultation
            (1) Breath sounds: crackles, wheezes
      2) Diagnostic procedures
         a) Serum chemistries including glucose: hypoglycemia
         b) ABGs
         c) Urinalysis; pregnancy test in female patients of childbearing age
         d) Chest radiograph
         e) ECG
2. Analysis: differential nursing diagnoses/collaborative problems
   a. Decreased cardiac output
   b. Risk for poisoning
   c. Deficient knowledge
3. Planning and implementation/interventions
   a. Maintain airway, breathing, circulation (see Chapter 1)
   b. Provide supplemental oxygen
   c. Establish IV access for administration of crystalloid fluid/medications
   d. Prepare for/assist with medical interventions
      1) Institute cardiac and pulse oximetry monitoring
      2) Possible external cardiac pacing and pacemaker insertion
      3) Insert gastric tube as indicated
         a) Gastric lavage
            (1) Controversial and potentially useful only if performed within 1–2 hours of ingestion
            (2) Insert with caution because vagal stimulation may cause further decreases in heart rate and conduction
      4) Possible catheter placement and monitoring of pulmonary and/or arterial pressures (see Chapter 7)
      5) Assist with hospital admission: if patient is asymptomatic following 12-hour observation and GI decontamination, may consider discharge
      6) Assist with psychiatric consultation
   e. Administer pharmacologic therapy as ordered
      1) Activated charcoal with or without cathartic
      2) Atropine or glucagon: increases heart rate and inotropic effects of the heart
      3) Phenytoin (Dilantin), lidocaine: dysrhythmias; avoid quinidine or procainamide (Pronestyl), which may further depress cardiac function

4) Isoproterenol (Isuprel), magnesium sulfate: torsades de pointes
5) Beta$_2$-stimulating agent (albuterol): bronchospasms
6) Vasopressor therapy (dopamine [Intropin], dobutamine [Dobutrex]): hypotension
7) Phenytoin (Dilantin), diazepam (Valium): seizure activity
8) Dextrose 50%: hypoglycemia
    f. Educate patient/significant others
       1) Need for close medication supervision because of narrow range of toxicity/therapeutics
4. Evaluation and ongoing monitoring
   a. Hemodynamic monitoring
   b. Breath sounds and pulse oximetry
   c. Cardiac rate and rhythm
   d. Intake and output

E. CALCIUM CHANNEL BLOCKER TOXICITY

Calcium channel blockers, also known as slow channel blockers or calcium antagonists, inhibit the movement of calcium across the cell membrane. Because calcium is needed for generating an action potential and contractility, inhibition of this process causes a decrease in contractility, automaticity (impulse formation), and conduction velocity. Calcium channel blockers dilate the coronary arteries and reduce arterial resting blood pressure but are known to cause reflex tachycardia. They also decrease coronary artery spasm and increase oxygen delivery. Common medications include verapamil (Calan), nifedipine (Procardia), and diltiazem (Cardizem), many of which are available in sustained-release formulations designed to increase compliance. The toxic-therapeutic margin is small; thus, toxicity results in severely decreased cardiac output and junctional rhythms or heart blocks, especially in overdose or therapeutic error.

1. Assessment
   a. Subjective data collection
      1) History of present illness/chief complaint
         a) Circumstances of exposure: unintentional, intentional
         b) Route: dermal, oral, parenteral
         c) Type of preparation: sustained release
         d) Shortness of breath
         e) Lightheadedness
         f) Nausea/vomiting
      2) Past medical history
         a) Current or preexisting diseases/illness
            (1) Renal disease
            (2) Liver disease
            (3) Psychiatric history
            (4) Cardiovascular disease
         b) Medications
            (1) Use of beta-adrenergic blocking agents: may slow heart rate
         c) Allergies

   b. Objective data collection
      1) Physical examination
         a) General appearance
            (1) Marked hypotension
            (2) Bradycardia
            (3) Moderate to severe distress/discomfort
         b) Inspection
            (1) Cardiac dysrhythmias on monitor: junctional rhythms, bradycardia, heart blocks
      2) Diagnostic procedures
         a) CBC with differential
         b) Serum chemistries including glucose: hyperglycemia resulting from blockage of insulin release
         c) ABGs
         d) Urinalysis; pregnancy test in female patients of childbearing age
         e) ECG
2. Analysis: differential nursing diagnoses/collaborative problems
   a. Decreased cardiac output
   b. Risk for poisoning
   c. Deficient knowledge
3. Planning and implementation/interventions
   a. Maintain airway, breathing, circulation (see Chapter 1)
   b. Provide supplemental oxygen as indicated
   c. Establish IV access for administration of crystalloid fluid/medications
   d. Prepare for/assist with medical interventions
      1) Institute cardiac and pulse oximetry monitoring
      2) Possible external cardiac pacing and pacemaker insertion
      3) Possible cardioversion for rapid ventricular rate
      4) Insert gastric tube as indicated
         a) Gastric lavage: controversial and potentially useful only if performed within 1–2 hours after ingestion
         b) Consider whole bowel irrigation
      5) Assist with hospital admission: if patient is asymptomatic following 12-hour observation and GI decontamination, may consider discharge
   e. Administer pharmacologic therapy as ordered
      1) Activated charcoal with or without cathartics: multidose charcoal if sustained-release preparations
      2) Atropine or glucagon for bradycardia
      3) Calcium chloride or calcium gluconate to reverse effects of decreased contractility
      4) Vasopressors (e.g., dopamine [Intropin], epinephrine, amrinone): to maintain blood pressure
      5) Lidocaine or procainamide (Pronestyl): for rapid ventricular rate
   f. Educate patient/significant others

1) Need for close medication supervision because of narrow range of toxicity/therapeutics
4. Evaluation and ongoing monitoring
   a. Hemodynamic status
   b. Cardiac rate and rhythm
   c. Intake and output

F. CARBON MONOXIDE POISONING

Carbon monoxide (CO) is a colorless, odorless, and taste-less gas that easily binds with hemoglobin to form COHb. This combination decreases the ability of the blood to carry oxygen and leads to severe hypoxia. CO is produced by the combustion of organic materials in the setting of an enclosed space or poor ventilation. Common sources of CO include auto exhaust systems, smoke from wood fires, pro-pane heaters, hibachi grills and barbecues, Sterno (canned heat) stoves, and faulty furnaces. Length of exposure to the gas contributes to the poisoning. Symptoms rarely correlate with the serum COHb levels, although patients with values <20% rarely become symptomatic, and smokers frequently have a COHb level of 10% as baseline. Pregnant patients are of particular concern because the fetus is potentially at greater risk, even in the presence of low COHb levels. Death is usually the result of dysrhythmias.

1. Assessment
   a. Subjective data collection
      1) History of present illness/chief complaint
         a) Ventilation: enclosed space
         b) Sleeping/intoxicated at time of exposure (higher risk)
            (1) Associated with burn injury (see Chapter 34)
         c) Degree of exposure: time, mechanism (e.g., fire)
         d) Occupational/purposeful exposure (e.g., suicidal)
         e) Pregnancy
         f) Symptoms
            (1) Headache: most common
            (2) Nausea and vomiting, dizziness
            (3) Chest pain
      2) Past medical history
         a) Current or preexisting diseases/illness
            (1) Cardiac disease, especially dysrhythmias
            (2) Pulmonary disease
            (3) Suicidal tendencies
         b) Recent crisis/trauma resulting in ineffective coping mechanisms
         c) Medications
         d) Allergies
   b. Objective data collection
      1) Physical examination
         a) General appearance
            (1) Level of consciousness, behavior, affect: alert to comatose
            (2) Hypotension
            (3) Seizure: at higher COHb levels
            (4) Moderate to severe distress/discomfort
         b) Inspection
            (1) "Cherry red" skin and mucous membranes: classically noted but considered terminal findings
            (2) Cardiac dysrhythmias on monitor: ST-segment and T-wave changes indicating ischemia or infarction
      2) Diagnostic procedures
         a) ABGs
         b) COHb level: half-life is 4–5 hours
         c) Cardiac enzymes
         d) Urinalysis: myoglobin; pregnancy test in female patients of childbearing age
         e) Chest radiograph: may develop pulmonary edema or acute respiratory distress syndrome
         f) Head CT scan/MRI
         g) ECG
            (1) ST-segment and T-wave changes indicating ischemia or infarction
2. Analysis: differential nursing diagnoses/collaborative problems
   a. Impaired gas exchange
   b. Decreased cardiac output
   c. Risk for poisoning
3. Planning and implementation/interventions
   a. Maintain airway, breathing, circulation (see Chapter 1)
   b. Provide supplemental oxygen as indicated
      a) Ventilatory support in obtunded patients or respiratory arrest
      b) High-flow oxygen: 100% oxygen decreases half-life of COHb
   c. Establish IV access for administration of crystalloid fluid/medications
   d. Prepare for/assist with medical interventions
      1) Advanced airway management
         a) Rapid sequence intubation (RSI)
         b) Nasal or oral intubation
         c) Supraglottic airway (e.g., King, Combitube, laryngeal mask airway)
         d) Surgical airway (e.g., cricothyrotomy)
      2) Institute cardiac and pulse oximetry monitoring
      3) Insert gastric tube and attach to suction as indicated
      4) Insert indwelling urinary catheter as indicated
      5) Consider psychiatric consultation as needed
      6) Assist with possible hospital admission or transfer to facility with hyperbaric oxygen (HBO) therapy
   e. Administer pharmacologic therapy as ordered
      1) RSI premedications: sedatives, analgesics, neuromuscular blocking agents
   f. Educate patient/significant others
      1) Provide referral to social support service to assist in coping with crisis/trauma

2) Sources of CO poisoning
3) Review symptoms of poisoning and provide education on prevention of exposure
4) Advise patient to keep areas with combustible products well ventilated
5) Advise regarding use of CO detectors in home/work environment
6) Yearly maintenance of stoves/furnaces

4. Evaluation and ongoing monitoring
   a. Airway patency
   b. Level of consciousness
   c. Hemodynamic status
   d. Breath sounds and pulse oximetry
   e. Cardiac rate and rhythm
   f. Intake and output
   g. COHb level

G. COCAINE USE

Cocaine is the second most trafficked illegal drug in the world and continues as a popular drug of abuse. "Snorting" or intranasal use is the most common route of administration; however, it can be smoked or injected. "Crack," "rocks," or free-based smokable cocaine is more purified, it gives the user a "rush" similar to IV use, and it has a higher addiction potential.

Cocaine stimulates the CNS and autonomic nervous system to increase the release of catecholamines from the adrenergic nerve terminals. It blocks the reuptake of dopamine and norepinephrine, thereby resulting in increased motor activity, insomnia, and euphoria. Cocaine is more dangerous when combined with other drugs or alcohol. For example, the combination of cocaine and heroin, known as a speedball, carries a high risk of fatal overdose. Patients seen in the emergency department for cocaine use are there predominantly for management of secondary complications. Treatment is aimed at supportive corrective measures. Medicinally, cocaine is used as an anesthetic and a vasoconstrictor in nasal surgery.

1. Assessment
   a. Subjective data collection
      1) History of present illness/chief complaint
         a) Route of ingestion
         b) Time and amount (if known) of ingestion: cocaine's effects are short lived compared with those of other CNS stimulants
         c) Polysubstance abuse: alcohol, downers (sedatives), or speedballs (heroin and cocaine combination) to potentiate its effects
         d) Body packing: ingestion of large amounts of cocaine-filled balloons/condoms to avoid law enforcement detection
         e) Symptoms
            (1) Mood changes: euphoria, decreased fatigue, increased energy, agitation, aggression
            (2) Cardiac: palpitations, chest pain
            (3) Pupils: dilated pupils are hallmark
            (4) Seizures
            (5) Other: restless, jittery, anxious, talkativeness, weight loss, drug craving for more cocaine, auditory or visual hallucinations, tactile hallucinations such as "cocaine bugs" (formication: feeling insects crawling under skin) with long-term use
            (6) Hyperthermia, diaphoresis
      2) Past medical history
         a) Current or preexisting diseases/illness
            (1) Cardiovascular disease
            (2) Stroke, seizures
         b) Psychiatric history: suicidal ideation, substance use/abuse history
         c) Antibody status: HIV infection, hepatitis, tuberculosis
         d) Family history of substance use/abuse
         e) Last normal menstrual period: female patients of childbearing age because cocaine causes increased incidence of spontaneous abortions
         f) Medications
         g) Allergies
   b. Objective data collection
      1) Physical examination
         a) General appearance
            (1) Level of consciousness, behavior, affect: may range from hypomania to euphoria to depression
            (2) Presence of trauma/injury
            (3) Seizure activity
            (4) Hypertension, tachycardia, hyperthermia
            (5) Moderate to severe distress/discomfort
         b) Inspection
            (1) Pupillary response: mydriasis, photophobia
            (2) Perforated nasal septum from snorting
            (3) Skin infections/abscesses
         c) Auscultation
            (1) Breath sounds: respiratory pattern; crackles, rhonchi
            (2) Heart sounds: rate/rhythm; rubs, murmurs
      2) Diagnostic procedures
         a) Serum and urine toxicology screen; ethanol level
         b) Blood count, chemistries, including serum lactate
         c) Urinalysis: myoglobin; pregnancy test in female patients of childbearing age
         d) Chest radiograph
         e) Head CT scan/MRI: intracranial hemorrhage, cerebrovascular accident (CVA)
         f) ECG
         g) Echocardiogram

2. Analysis: differential nursing diagnoses/collaborative problems
   a. Impaired gas exchange
   b. Impaired tissue perfusion
   c. Decreased cardiac output
   d. Hopelessness
   e. Risk for suicide
   f. Risk for self/other-directed violence
   g. Ineffective coping
   h. Risk for poisoning or injury
   i. Risk for trauma
   j. Risk for infection
3. Planning and implementation/interventions
   a. Maintain airway, breathing, circulation (see Chapter 1)
   b. Provide supplemental oxygen as indicated
   c. Establish IV access for administration of crystalloid fluid/medications
   d. Prepare for/assist with medical interventions
      1) Institute cardiac and pulse oximetry monitoring
      2) Insert gastric tube as indicated
         a) Whole bowel irrigation through a gastric tube may be indicated for body packers
   e. Administer pharmacologic therapy as ordered
      1) Consider benzodiazepines for cardiovascular and CNS effects
      2) Activated charcoal may be administered prior to whole bowel irrigation
      3) Whole bowel irrigation with a polyethylene glycol and electrolyte solution such as GoLYTELY may be indicated. Surgical consultation should be obtained for patients with signs of intoxication
   f. Educate patient/significant others
      1) Knowledge of effects of cocaine on body
      2) Cocaine addiction/dependence
      3) Refer to social services and/or support groups (e.g., Narcotics Anonymous)
      4) Provide information on detoxification procedures
      5) Refer patient/family to rehabilitation/recovery resources
4. Evaluation and ongoing monitoring
   a. Hemodynamic status
   b. Cardiac rate and rhythm

H. CYANIDE POISONING

Cyanide is a very lethal poison that causes death within 2 minutes when inhaled as a gas. It interferes with cellular respiration and causes decreased utilization of oxygen by the tissues. This effect causes bright-colored venous blood with normal to high oxyhemoglobin saturation. Cyanide may be ingested orally or inhaled and is found in industrial fumigants, insecticides, and metal plating. It is also present in the pits of stone fruits such as cherries, peaches, and apricots (laetrile) and is liberated as a result of burning of plastics. Medically, cyanide may be generated from the long-term use of nitroprusside.

1. Assessment
   a. Subjective data collection
      1) History of present illness/chief complaint
         a) Circumstances of exposure: occupational, intentional, accidental, medical, corporal punishment
         b) Route: oral, inhaled
         c) Time of exposure
      2) Past medical history
         a) Current or preexisting diseases/illness
            (1) Psychiatric history: suicidal ideation
         b) Medication use contributing to cause: laetrile, nitroprusside
         c) Occupational hazard
         d) Medications
         e) Allergies
   b. Objective data collection
      1) Physical examination
         a) General appearance
            (1) Level of consciousness, behavior, affect: seizure activity, comatose
            (2) Breath odor: characteristic odor of bitter almonds
            (3) Hypertension, bradycardia followed by hypotension and tachycardia, cardiac arrest
            (4) Tachypnea initially, then slow and labored followed by respiratory arrest
            (5) Severe distress/critically ill
      2) Diagnostic procedures
         a) Serum cyanide level
         b) Serum lactate level
         c) Serum chemistries
         d) CBC with differential
         e) Venous and blood gases and ABGs
         f) Urinalysis; pregnancy test in female patients of childbearing age
         g) ECG
2. Analysis: differential nursing diagnoses/collaborative problems
   a. Impaired gas exchange
   b. Risk for poisoning
3. Planning and implementation/interventions
   a. Maintain airway, breathing, circulation (see Chapter 1)
      1) Initiate or continue BLS and ALS per protocols if respiratory or cardiac arrest is present
      2) Do not perform mouth-to-mouth resuscitation, as cyanide vapors can be exhaled by patient
   b. Provide supplemental oxygen as indicated
      1) Ventilatory support in patients with airway compromise
      2) High-flow oxygen
   c. Establish IV access for administration of crystalloid fluid/medications

d. Prepare for/assist with medical interventions
 1) Advanced airway management
 a) Rapid sequence induction (RSI)
 b) Nasal or oral intubation
 c) Supraglottic airway (e.g., King, Combitube, laryngeal mask airway)
 d) Surgical airway (e.g., cricothyrotomy)
 2) Institute cardiac and pulse oximetry monitoring
 3) Insert gastric tube and attach to suction
 4) Insert indwelling urinary catheter
 5) Assist with hospital admission if patient recovers
e. Administer pharmacologic therapy as ordered
 1) Cyanide antidote kit induces methemoglobinemia
 a) Amyl nitrite: apply nasally or inside mask
 b) Sodium nitrite: IV infusion
 c) Sodium thiosulfate: IV infusion
 2) Vasopressors: hypotension
 3) Benzodiazepines: control seizures
 4) ALS medications per protocols
f. Educate patient/significant others
 1) Proper storage, handling, labeling, and disposal of cyanide in occupational setting
 2) Prevention measures: rubber gloves, respirator use, protective clothing
 3) Encourage worksite evaluations by county/state agencies if unsafe practices exist
4. Evaluation and ongoing monitoring
a. Hemodynamic status
b. Breath sounds and pulse oximetry
c. Cardiac rate and rhythm
d. Intake and output

I. DIGOXIN TOXICITY

Digitalis and digoxin are drugs commonly prescribed in the middle-age and elderly population to increase myocardial contractility. Digoxin enhances cardiac contractility and reduces cardiac rate. It may be used to treat atrial fibrillation and paroxysmal atrial tachycardia. Digoxin toxicity may result from an overdose, hypokalemia, advanced heart disease with conduction disturbances, or a combination of these. It may also result from decreased renal elimination of the drug. Medication management and therapeutic errors may be a cause of toxicity. In children, toxicity may be manifested as atrial dysrhythmias. Digoxin toxicity is common because the toxic level is only slightly higher than the therapeutic serum level.

1. Assessment
a. Subjective data collection
 1) History of present illness/chief complaint
 a) Circumstances of exposure: intentional, accidental, recent surgery
 b) Acute vs. chronic ingestion
 c) Diuretic therapy causing hypokalemia
 d) Recent myocardial infarction or cardiac event
 e) Nausea/vomiting
 f) Visual disturbances: yellow halos around objects
 g) Weakness
 2) Past medical history
 a) Current or preexisting diseases/illness
 (1) Renal failure
 (2) Psychiatric history
 (3) Electrolyte imbalance
 (4) Cardiovascular disease
 b) Medications
 c) Allergies
b. Objective data collection
 1) Physical examination
 a) General appearance
 (1) Level of consciousness, behavior, affect: disorientation
 (2) Hypotension; bradycardia in children
 (3) Moderate to severe distress/discomfort
 b) Inspection
 (1) Photophobia
 (2) Pupil mydriasis
 (3) Decreased visual acuity
 c) Palpation
 (1) Abdominal tenderness
 2) Diagnostic procedures
 a) Serum digoxin level
 b) Serum chemistries including potassium, calcium, magnesium, BUN, creatinine
 c) LFTs
 d) Urinalysis; pregnancy test in female patients of childbearing age
 e) ECG
2. Analysis: differential nursing diagnoses/collaborative problems
a. Risk for poisoning
b. Decreased cardiac output
c. Deficient knowledge
3. Planning and implementation/interventions
a. Maintain airway, breathing, circulation (see Chapter 1)
b. Provide supplemental oxygen as indicated
c. Establish IV access for administration of crystalloid fluid/medications
d. Prepare for/assist with medical interventions
 1) Institute cardiac and pulse oximetry monitoring
 2) Possible external cardiac pacing and pacemaker insertion
 3) Hemodialysis for severe acute toxicity
 4) Assist with hospital admission
 5) Assist with psychiatric consultation in suicide gestures
e. Administer pharmacologic therapy as ordered
 1) Activated charcoal: no cathartic because of potential for diarrhea and further electrolyte imbalance
 2) Replace potassium and magnesium as needed

3) Lidocaine or phenytoin (Dilantin): dysrhythmias
4) Avoid beta blockers and quinidine administration: effects will be additive with digoxin
5) Digoxin immune Fab (Digibind): treatment of life-threatening dysrhythmias; may be administered to symptomatic children
f. Educate patient/significant others
1) Safe storage and use of digoxin
2) Take digoxin daily as scheduled and do not discontinue medication without notifying care provider
4. Evaluation and ongoing monitoring
a. Hemodynamic status
b. Cardiac rate and rhythm
c. Intake and output
d. Drug and electrolyte levels

J. ETHYLENE GLYCOL AND METHANOL POISONING

Ethylene glycol, the primary ingredient in antifreeze, is a sweet, thick substance that may be appealing to children and pets. Methanol is found in products such as windshield washer fluid, paint removers, and other solvents. Both require extremely small amounts to cause toxicity and are occasionally ingested by alcoholic patients to substitute for or supplement ethanol. Both substances are slowly metabolized by alcohol dehydrogenase to produce formic acid (methanol) or oxalic acid and glycolic acid (ethylene glycol), and they subsequently cause metabolic acidosis, renal failure, and death if patients are left untreated in a timely manner.

1. Assessment
a. Subjective data collection
1) History of present illness/chief complaint
a) History of exposure to chemical in home or work
b) Assess for history of alcoholism, drinking
c) Level of consciousness changes
d) Visual changes: blindness (methanol)
e) Nausea/vomiting
2) Past medical history
a) Current or preexisting diseases/illness
(1) Alcoholism
(2) Renal failure
(3) Suicide gestures, anxiety or depression
(4) Seizures
(5) GI bleeding or disorders
b) Medications
c) Allergies
b. Objective data collection
1) Physical examination (also see "Alcohol Use")
a) General appearance
(1) Level of consciousness, behavior, affect: initially appears inebriated, progress to coma; irritability in children

(2) Abnormal gait: ataxia, staggering
(3) Slurred speech
(4) Severe distress/discomfort
b) Palpation
(1) Abdominal tenderness
(2) Ascites (alcoholism)
2) Diagnostic procedures
a) Ethylene glycol or methanol levels
b) Serum blood alcohol
c) BUN and creatinine
(1) Ethylene glycol renal effects: 6–12 hours after ingestion
(2) Methanol renal effects: 6–30 hours after ingestion
d) Serum chemistries
e) ABGs: metabolic acidosis, increased anion gap
f) CBC with differential
g) Coagulation profile
h) Serum osmolality
i) Urinalysis; pregnancy test in female patients of childbearing age
(1) Calcium oxalate crystals may be visible with use of ultraviolet light (ethylene glycol)
2. Analysis: differential nursing diagnoses/collaborative problems
a. Risk for poisoning
3. Planning and implementation/interventions
a. Maintain airway, breathing, circulation (see Chapter 1)
b. Provide supplemental oxygen as indicated
c. Establish IV access for administration of crystalloid fluid/medications
d. Prepare for/assist with medical interventions
1) Institute cardiac and pulse oximetry monitoring
2) Insert gastric tube
3) Assist with possible admission for hemodialysis
4) Assist with psychiatric consultation for suicide gesture
e. Administer pharmacologic therapy as ordered
1) Sodium bicarbonate for metabolic acidosis
2) Activated charcoal ineffective for absorption
3) Folate, pyridoxine (vitamin B_6), and thiamine as cofactors to enhance metabolism to nontoxic metabolites
4) IV ethanol 10% or fomepizole (Antizol) to prevent metabolism of ethylene glycol and methanol to its toxic metabolites
f. Educate patient/significant others
1) Educate patient and family about safe use and storage of chemicals
4. Evaluation and ongoing monitoring
a. Level of consciousness and seizure activity
b. Hemodynamic status
c. Breath sounds and pulse oximetry

d. Cardiac rate and rhythm
e. Intake and output
f. Drug levels

K. GAMMA-HYDROXYBUTYRATE USE

Like phencyclidine (PCP), gamma-hydroxybutyrate (GHB) was originally used as an anesthetic agent, but its use was discontinued because of the adverse reactions of myoclonus and agitation. It is considered in a class of "designer drugs" (i.e., drugs manufactured by modifying existing drugs), and along with Ecstasy and others, it is used extensively in the dance club or rave scene. GHB is touted as a muscle-building agent, diet aid, sedative-hypnotic, and sexual enhancer; and it is used as a date-rape drug and/or ingested with alcohol. Available on the Internet, it is marketed as items such as cleaning agents and plant growth hormones. GHB (liquid Ecstasy, grievous bodily harm) and its precursors gamma-butyrolactone (GBL) (Renewtrient, Blue Nitro) and 1, 4-butanediol (1, 4-BD) (cherry bomb, Amino Flex, Serenity) are regulated as Schedule 1 controlled substances, and the penalties for possession and use are harsh. Some GHB effects are sedation, amnesia, respiratory depression, and loss of consciousness. Other drugs in the class of "designer drugs" include Rohypnol (see "Sedative-Hypnotic and Barbiturate Poisoning" for discussion of benzodiazepine), Ketamine (see "Phencyclidine Use"), and MDMA/Ecstasy (see "Amphetamine Use").

1. Assessment
   a. Subjective data collection
      1) History of present illness/chief complaint
         a) Route of exposure: ingestion
         b) Circumstances of use: recreational or date rape
         c) Concomitant alcohol or other drug use
         d) Time of ingestion: onset of effects is rapid, often within 15 minutes of ingestion
         e) Amount ingested: effects seen in small amounts, especially in combination with alcohol or other drugs; unrecognizable if mixed in beverage
      2) Past medical history
         a) Current or preexisting diseases/illness
         b) Previous use of GHB or other recreational drugs
         c) Trauma: suspected rape or physical abuse
         d) Medications
         e) Allergies
   b. Objective data collection
      1) Physical examination
         a) General appearance
            (1) Level of consciousness, behavior, affect: lethargy to deep coma
            (2) Respiratory depression: apnea, labored respirations
            (3) Generalized or tonic clonic seizures
            (4) Hypertension, bradycardia
            (5) Moderate to severe distress/discomfort
         b) Inspection
            (1) Evidence of sexual or physical assault
            (2) Mouth and oral mucosa: burns if chemicals used in manufacturing substance
         c) Auscultation
            (1) Breath sounds: crackles
      2) Diagnostic procedures
         a) Serum and urine toxicology screen
         b) GHB levels not readily available, few laboratories perform
         c) ABGs
         d) Serum chemistries
         e) Urinalysis: myoglobin; pregnancy test in female patients of childbearing age
2. Analysis: differential nursing diagnoses/collaborative problems
   a. Ineffective breathing pattern
   b. Impaired gas exchange
   c. Risk for poisoning
   d. Rape/trauma syndrome
3. Planning and implementation/interventions
   a. Maintain airway, breathing, circulation (see Chapter 1)
   b. Provide supplemental oxygen
      1) RSI and ventilatory support if patient obtunded
      2) High-flow oxygen
   c. Establish IV access for administration of crystalloid fluid/medications
   d. Prepare for/assist with medical interventions
      1) Advanced airway management
         a) Nasal or oral intubation
         b) Supraglottic airway (e.g., King, Combitube, laryngeal mask airway)
         c) Surgical airway (e.g., cricothyrotomy)
      2) Institute cardiac and pulse oximetry monitoring
      3) Assist with collection and maintenance of physical and forensic evidence as indicated (see Chapters 3 and 44)
   e. Administer pharmacologic therapy as ordered
      1) RSI premedications: sedatives, analgesics, neuromuscular blocking agents
      2) No pharmacologic antidote is available
      3) Seizures: benzodiazepines (short acting)
   f. Educate patient/significant others
      1) Refer to rape or assault counseling services
4. Evaluation and ongoing monitoring
   a. Airway patency
   b. Level of consciousness and presence of seizures
   c. Hemodynamic status
   d. Breath sounds and pulse oximetry
   e. Cardiac rate and rhythm
   f. Intake and output

L. HEAVY METAL POISONING

Poisoning from heavy metals (e.g., zinc, lead, mercury, arsenic) may affect every body system, including the CNS, heart, lungs, liver, and kidneys. These metals deposit themselves in the body and are excreted slowly. Children often eat chipped paint, thus exposing themselves to lead. Other sources of heavy metals include occupational sources (zinc, lead, mercury) and environmental sources in food and water (mercury). Lithium carbonate, a drug used in the treatment of bipolar disorders, is also a heavy metal.

1. Assessment
    a. Subjective data collection
        1) History of present illness/chief complaint
            a) Reason for exposure: unintentional, intentional, occupational (plumber, steel welders, glass workers [metal fume fever]), psychiatric (bipolar disorder)
            b) Route of exposure: inhalation, oral (lead), dermal
            c) Type of product
            d) Insomnia
            e) Headaches
            f) Confusion
            g) Paresthesias around lips and mouth, seizures
            h) Anorexia, nausea and vomiting, metallic taste, thirst
            i) Palpitations, substernal chest pain
            j) Shortness of breath
            k) Fever, chills, malaise (metal fume fever)
        2) Past medical history
            a) Current or preexisting diseases/illness
                (1) Neurologic history: seizures, mental retardation
                (2) Renal disease
            b) Chronic exposure from occupation or pre-1960 residence with lead-painted surfaces
            c) Medications
            d) Allergies
    b. Objective data collection
        1) Physical examination
            a) General appearance
                (1) Level of consciousness, behavior, affect: irritability, lethargy
                (2) Ataxia
                (3) Elevated temperature
                (4) Moderate to severe distress/discomfort
            b) Inspection
                (1) Burns: zinc
                (2) Cardiac dysrhythmias on monitor: ventricular fibrillation or tachycardia
            c) Auscultation
                (1) Breath sounds: crackles
        2) Diagnostic procedures
            a) CBC with differential
            b) Serum chemistries including BUN and creatinine
            c) Urinalysis; pregnancy test in female patients of childbearing age
            d) LFTs
            e) Serum and urine lead, mercury, arsenate levels
            f) Erythrocyte protoporphyrin level
            g) Abdominal radiographs: lead particles are radiopaque
            h) ECG: T-wave changes
2. Analysis: differential nursing diagnoses/collaborative problems
    a. Risk for poisoning
    b. Deficient knowledge
3. Planning and implementation/interventions
    a. Maintain airway, breathing, circulation (see Chapter 1)
    b. Provide supplemental oxygen
    c. Establish IV access for administration of crystalloid fluid/medications
    d. Prepare for/assist with medical interventions
        1) Institute cardiac and pulse oximetry monitoring
        2) Assist with admission to hospital: hemodialysis if renal dysfunction
        3) Report lead exposure to public health department for case management and investigation of source
    e. Administer pharmacologic therapy as ordered
        1) Chelation therapy as indicated
            a) Lead: succimer (Chemet), dimercaprol (BAL in oil), or edetate disodium (EDTA)
            b) Arsenic and mercury: dimercaprol, penicillamine (D-penicillamine, Cuprimine)
            c) Zinc: EDTA, dimercaprol
        2) Benzodiazepines: seizure control
        3) Nonnarcotic analgesics
        4) Antipyretics
        5) Whole bowel irrigation for lithium carbonate ingestion
    f. Educate patient/significant others
        1) Prevent occupational exposure and reexposure with use of protective equipment and safe practices
        2) Identify possible occupational or recreational exposure sources, which may include dietary, medication, or environmental sources (i.e., residences with pre-1960 lead-based paint)
        3) Observe child or other children for pica (consuming inedible products) and frequent hand-to-mouth activity
4. Evaluation and ongoing monitoring
    a. Level of consciousness and seizure activity
    b. Hemodynamic status
    c. Breath sounds and pulse oximetry
    d. Cardiac rate and rhythm
    e. Intake and output
    f. Heavy metal levels

M. INHALANT USE

Inhaling vapors from volatile substances such as solvents and hydrocarbons is a common practice, particularly among adolescents. These substances offer a cheap high because they are easily obtained and uncontrolled. Toluene-containing products are the most commonly abused and include metallic spray paint, glues, and aerosols from spray cans. Metallic gold spray paint produces the most desired effect. Other commonly sniffed substances include cleaning fluids, paints, lacquer, room deodorizers, computer keyboard dusters/cleaners, and Freon from air-conditioning units. Hydrocarbons produce a floating or numbing sensation and euphoria when they are inhaled, and they induce a pleasurable sensation. The substances are generally poured into a paper or plastic bag and inhaled (bagging), poured on a rag and held over the nose (huffing), or inhaled from the container (sniffing). Inhaled vapors are readily absorbed into the bloodstream and cross the blood-brain barrier, reaching the brain in high concentrations. Long-term effects include neurologic, renal, and cardiac disorders.

1. Assessment
   a. Subjective data collection
      1) History of present illness/chief complaint
         a) Age of patient
         b) Type of substance inhaled/empty solvent cans
         c) Method of inhalation: sniffing, huffing, bagging
         d) Polysubstance abuse
         e) Symptoms
            (1) GI: nausea
            (2) Muscle weakness/paralysis, seizure activity
            (3) Neurologic: headache, slurred speech, dizziness, altered level of consciousness, coma
            (4) Intoxication: euphoria, incoordination, confusion, hallucinations, disorientation
      2) Past medical history
         a) Current or preexisting diseases/illness
            (1) Psychiatric history
         b) Head trauma
         c) Medications
         d) Allergies
   b. Objective data collection
      1) Physical examination
         a) General appearance
            (1) Level of consciousness, behavior, affect: ranges from euphoria to intoxicated appearance to comatose
            (2) Odor: solvent, room deodorizer scent
            (3) Gait: ataxia, wide-base gait
            (4) Moderate to severe distress/discomfort
         b) Inspection
            (1) Mouth and nose: circumoral red spots if using spray paint, correction fluid; nosebleeds, sores in the nose, thermal burns from Freon in air-conditioning units
            (2) Cardiac dysrhythmias on monitor: causing sudden death (sudden sniffing death)
            (3) Paint/glue on hands/face, bloodshot eyes
         c) Auscultation
            (1) Breath sounds: wheezing
         d) Palpation/percussion
            (1) Decreased sensation
            (2) Motor loss
            (3) Decreased reflexes peripherally
      2) Diagnostic procedures
         a) Serum chemistries including phosphorus
         b) LFTs
         c) BUN and creatinine
         d) Urinalysis: hematuria, proteinuria, myoglobinuria; pregnancy test in female patients of childbearing age
         e) ABGs
         f) ECG
2. Analysis: differential nursing diagnoses/collaborative problems
   a. Risk for poisoning
   b. Risk for ineffective breathing pattern
   c. Risk for decreased cardiac output
   d. Impaired tissue perfusion
3. Planning and implementation/interventions
   a. Maintain airway, breathing, circulation (see Chapter 1)
   b. Provide supplemental oxygen as indicated
   c. Establish IV access for administration of crystalloid fluid/medications
   d. Prepare for/assist with medical interventions
      1) Institute cardiac and pulse oximetry monitoring
   e. Administer pharmacologic therapy as ordered
      1) Sodium bicarbonate for metabolic acidosis
      2) Electrolyte replacements, especially potassium
   f. Educate patient/significant others
      1) Refer patient/family to social services and/or support groups (e.g., Narcotics Anonymous)
      2) Refer patient/family to rehabilitation/recovery resources
4. Evaluation and ongoing monitoring
   a. Level of consciousness
   b. Hemodynamic status
   c. Breath sounds and pulse oximetry
   d. Cardiac rate and rhythm

N. IRON POISONING

Iron toxicity is an important cause of morbidity and mortality in children. Most cases of poisoning involve the unintentional ingestion of prenatal vitamins or children's vitamins by toddlers. In recent years, the advent of blister packaging of prenatal vitamins has markedly reduced mortality in children. Toxicity depends on the amount of elemental iron found in the preparation. An iron overdose can produce GI hemorrhage and result in cardiovascular collapse.

Table 26.4

Phases of Iron Toxicity

Phase 1 Less than 6 hr after ingestion	Corrosive effects of iron on gastrointestinal tract: symptoms include vomiting, abdominal pain, bloody diarrhea, and lethargy
Phase 2 6–12 hr after ingestion	"Recovery phase": patient may seem to improve
Phase 3 12–48 hr after ingestion	Cardiovascular collapse, shock, metabolic acidosis, gastrointestinal bleeding, coagulopathy, hepatic injury, sepsis, and coma
Phase 4 After 48 hr	If patient survives previous phases, intestinal obstructions or pyloric strictures may be present

Data from Olson, K. (2004). *Poisoning and drug overdose* (4th ed.). East Norwalk, CT: Appleton & Lange; Poisondex System (Internet database, updated periodically). Greenwood Village, CO: Thomson Micromedex. Retrieved from http://www.thomsonhc.com.

1. Assessment
   a. Subjective data collection
      1) History of present illness/chief complaint
         a) Number and kind of tablets ingested (e.g., prenatal vitamins, children's tablets)
         b) Type of iron and amount in compound: 40–60 mg/kg elemental iron can lead to severe symptoms
         c) Time of exposure and reason for ingestion
         d) Concurrent ingestion
         e) Symptoms associated with toxicity phase (Table 26.4)
      2) Past medical history
         a) Current or preexisting diseases/illness
            (1) Pregnancy
            (2) Anemia
         b) Medications
         c) Allergies
   b. Objective data collection
      1) Physical examination
         a) General appearance
            (1) Level of consciousness, behavior, affect: lethargy
            (2) Hypotension, tachycardia
            (3) Severe distress/discomfort, critically ill
         b) Palpation
            (1) Abdominal tenderness
            (2) Occult or frank blood in stool or emesis
      2) Diagnostic procedures
         a) Serum iron peak is 3–5 hours after ingestion
         b) Serum total iron-binding capacity (TIBC)
         c) Occult blood studies: stool, emesis, urine
         d) LFTs
         e) Coagulation profile
         f) Type and crossmatch
         g) ABGs
         h) Urinalysis: pregnancy test in female patients of childbearing age
         i) Abdominal radiograph: tablets may be radiopaque
2. Analysis: differential nursing diagnoses/collaborative problems
   a. Deficient fluid volume
   b. Risk for poisoning
3. Planning and implementation/interventions
   a. Maintain airway, breathing, circulation (see Chapter 1)
      1) Initiate or continue Basic Life Support (BLS) and Advanced Life Support (ALS) per protocols if cardiac arrest is present
   b. Provide supplemental oxygen
      1) Ventilatory support in obtunded patients or respiratory arrest
      2) High-flow oxygen
   c. Establish IV access for administration of crystalloid fluid/medications
   d. Prepare for/assist with medical interventions
      1) Advanced airway management
         a) Rapid sequence intubation (RSI)
         b) Nasal or oral intubation
         c) Supraglottic airway (e.g., King, Combitube, laryngeal mask airway)
         d) Surgical airway (e.g., cricothyrotomy)
      2) Institute cardiac and pulse oximetry monitoring
      3) Insert gastric tube as indicated
         a) Gastric lavage: controversial, difficult to remove iron tablets because of their size, and potentially useful only if performed within 1–2 hours after ingestion
      4) Whole bowel irrigation may be indicated
      5) Assist with hospital admission
      6) Assist with psychiatric consultation in suicide gesture
   e. Administer pharmacologic therapy as ordered
      1) ALS medications per protocols
      2) Activated charcoal: contraindicated because it does not bind iron
      3) Deferoxamine (Desferal): chelator that binds with iron and increases its renal excretion; may produce pink or red ("vin rose") urine, but not conclusive
      4) Sodium bicarbonate: correct acidosis
      5) Whole bowel irrigation with a polyethylene glycol and electrolyte solution (e.g., GoLYTELY)
   f. Educate patient/significant others
      1) Instruct caregiver on the toxicity of iron and safe storage of medicines
4. Evaluation and ongoing monitoring

a. Airway patency
b. Level of consciousness
c. Hemodynamic status
d. Breath sounds and pulse oximetry
e. Cardiac rate and rhythm
f. Intake and output
g. Iron

O. LYSERGIC ACID DIETHYLAMIDE USE

Hallucinogens such as lysergic acid diethylamide (LSD) cause changes in thought, mood, perception, and consciousness. LSD is also known as acid, blotter, doses, hits, microdots, sugar cubes, tabs, or window panes. The hallucinogenic effects last 6–12 hours and may include visual illusions and alteration in both sound and color intensity. LSD is known to flood the user with stimuli. LSD is colorless, odorless, and tasteless and comes in liquid or tablet form. It may also be absorbed through the skin. Initial symptoms are sympathomimetic: tachycardia, tachypnea, and the "fight-or-flight" response. LSD may be "laced" with phencyclidine (PCP), strychnine, or cocaine. Unlike most substances, LSD has no withdrawal syndrome, nor does it cause physical dependence. Other hallucinogens producing effects similar to LSD include psilocybin (magic mushrooms, shrooms, boomers, and little smoke), peyote (buttons, cactus, mesc), DMT (Dimitri), and ayahuasca (hoasca, aya, yage). Another plant-based drug of abuse with hallucinogenic properties is salvia (*Salvia divinorum*), an herb native to southern Mexico. It is a dissociative hallucinogen causing a feeling of detachment from reality. Street names include Magic Mint, Maria Pastora, and Sally D.

1. Assessment
   a. Subjective data collection
      1) History of present illness/chief complaint
         a) Route of ingestion
         b) Time of use
         c) Reason for use: accidental, recreational
         d) Substance used to "lace" or mix with the drug
         e) Polysubstance use
         f) Symptoms
            (1) Paranoia
            (2) Hallucinations, especially visual changes such as intense colors, perception of flowing objects
            (3) Mood changes: poor judgment, short attention span
      2) Past medical history
         a) Current or preexisting diseases/illness
            (1) Psychiatric history
         b) Previous LSD use
         c) Medications
         d) Allergies
   b. Objective data collection
      1) Physical examination
         a) General appearance
            (1) Level of consciousness, behavior, affect: ranges from euphoria to fear, anxiety and panic, rapid emotional swings, hallucinations, paranoia, psychosis
            (2) Tachycardia, hypertension, hyperthermia
            (3) Moderate to severe distress/discomfort
         b) Inspection
            (1) Pupil response: dilation (mydriasis)
      2) Diagnostic procedures
         a) Serum and urine toxicology screen
         b) Urinalysis; pregnancy test in female patients of childbearing age
         c) Other tests in addition to standard laboratory studies
2. Analysis: differential nursing diagnoses/collaborative problems
   a. Acute/chronic confusion
   b. Disturbed sensory perception
   c. Risk for injury or self/other-directed violence
   d. Anxiety/fear
   e. Risk for trauma
   f. Risk for infection
3. Planning and implementation/interventions
   a. Maintain airway, breathing, circulation (see Chapter 1)
   b. Provide supplemental oxygen as indicated
   c. Establish IV access for administration of crystalloid fluid/medications
   d. Prepare for/assist with medical interventions
      1) Minimize sensory-perceptual alteration
         a) Reinforce to patient that effects of drug are time limited
         b) Assist patient in separating hallucinations from real-life events
         c) Reduce sensory stimulation
      2) Decrease risk for violence; protect patient and staff
         a) Attempt to deescalate an agitated and anxious patient
         b) Maintain calm, nonjudgmental attitude and offer reassurance
         c) Consider use of soft, leather, or chemical restraints, per institutional protocols, if all measures to provide patient and staff safety fail
   e. Administer pharmacologic therapy as ordered
      1) Benzodiazepines: agitation
      2) Antipsychotics: haloperidol (Haldol): psychosis
   f. Educate patient/significant others
      1) Refer patient/family to social services and/or support groups (e.g., Narcotics Anonymous)
      2) Refer patient/family to rehabilitation/recovery resources
4. Evaluation and ongoing monitoring
   a. Hemodynamic status
   b. Continued presence or absence of hallucinations

P. MARIJUANA

Marijuana or cannabis refers to dried leaves, flowers, stems, and seeds from the hemp plant *Cannabis sativa*. Marijuana is the most commonly used illicit drug in the United States. It is smoked or consumed orally in food. The marijuana plant contains tetrahydrocannabinol (THC), the principle psychoactive constituent in cannabis, which acts on specific brain cell receptors and alters sense of time, mood, memory, thinking, and coordination. The use of marijuana extracts—THC-rich resins extracted from the plant—is on the rise. Marijuana extracts come in the form of oils such as hash or honey oil, wax, or solids such as shatter and can have concentrations of up to 90% THC. The use of marijuana oils, wax, and solids has been associated with severe hallucinations and psychosis and has contributed to an increase in emergency department visits. Long-term use of marijuana has been associated with depression, anxiety, and suicidal thoughts among teens. Preparation of marijuana extracts involves the use of butane, which has led to serious burns from fires and explosions for those attempting to extract.

1. Assessment
   a. Subjective data collection
      1) History of present illness/chief complaint
         a) Route of exposure: smoked, ingestion
         b) Circumstances of use: recreational or medicinal
         c) Concomitant alcohol or other drug use
         d) Time of ingestion: onset of effects is rapid, within seconds to minutes after smoking
         e) Amount ingested
      2) Past medical history
         a) Current or preexisting diseases/illness
         b) Previous use of marijuana or other recreational drugs
         c) Trauma
         d) Medications
         e) Allergies
   b. Objective data collection
      1) Physical examination
         a) General appearance
            (1) Level of consciousness, behavior, affect, reaction time, dizziness
            (2) Respiratory, shallow respirations, rapid respirations
            (3) Eyes: red, dilated pupil
         b) Inspection
            (1) Mouth and oral mucosa: burns if chemicals used in manufacturing substance
         c) Auscultation
            (1) Breath sounds: crackles
      2) Diagnostic procedures
         a) Serum and urine toxicology screen
         b) ABGs
         c) Serum chemistries
2. Analysis: differential nursing diagnoses/collaborative problems

   a. Ineffective breathing pattern
   b. Impaired gas exchange
   c. Risk for poisoning
   d. Risk for trauma
3. Planning and implementation/interventions
   a. Maintain airway, breathing, circulation (see Chapter 1)
   b. Provide supplemental oxygen
      1) Ventilatory support if patient obtunded
      2) High-flow oxygen
   c. Establish IV access for administration of crystalloid fluid/medications
   d. Prepare for/assist with medical interventions
      1) Decrease sensory-perceptual alteration
         a) Use quiet, nonstimulating room if possible
         b) Do not leave patient unattended; consider security standby if needed
         c) Keep side rails up to prevent falls
      2) Decrease risk for violence
         a) Consider use of leather or chemical restraints if all measures to provide patient and staff safety fail per institutional protocols
            (1) Chemical: benzodiazepines, haloperidol (Haldol)
      3) Consider psychiatric consultation for anxiety/depression after acute therapy
      4) Institute cardiac, blood pressure, and pulse oximetry monitoring
   e. Administer pharmacologic therapy as ordered
      1) Benzodiazepines: agitation
      2) Antipsychotics: haloperidol (Haldol)
   f. Educate patient/significant others
      1) Refer patient/family to social services and/or support groups (e.g., Narcotics Anonymous)
      2) Refer patient/family to rehabilitation/recovery resources
4. Evaluation and ongoing monitoring
   a. Airway patency
   b. Level of consciousness and presence of seizures
   c. Hemodynamic status
   d. Breath sounds and pulse oximetry
   e. Cardiac rate and rhythm
   f. Intake and output

Q. OPIATE USE

Opiates are narcotics, substances derived from the opium poppy that interact with opioid receptors on nerve cells in the body and brain. Opiates can be obtained by prescription or in illegal forms and include natural opiates such as morphine sulfate, semisynthetic derivatives such as hydrocodone, oxycodone, heroin, and synthetic derivatives such as fentanyl (Sublimaze). Opiates are prescribed to decrease severe pain. They blunt the perception of pain and are also used for preoperative sedation and as a supplement to anesthesia. Opiates usually produce brief euphoria followed by a pleasant, dreamlike state.

Opiates are common drugs of abuse due to the euphoria and dreamlike state they produce. It is not uncommon to see polydrug use to potentiate and increase the duration of action. Frequent use of opioids may lead to dependence, addiction, and tolerance. Death occurs from the side effects of the drugs, most notably respiratory arrest and pulmonary edema.

1. Assessment
   a. Subjective data collection
      1) History of present illness/chief complaint
         a) Substance ingested and amount
         b) Route of ingestion: oral, IV, nasal inhalation, smoked, skin-popping, topical
         c) Time of ingestion: short-term vs. long-term use, tolerance
         d) Polysubstance abuse, including chemicals used to "cut" the drug or dilute it (e.g., quinine, sugar, starch) and other drugs to potentiate its effects
         e) Symptoms: classic triad of pinpoint pupils, decreased respirations, and coma
            (1) Decreased consciousness/coma
            (2) Respiratory depression/arrest: slow, deep respirations of three to four per minute
            (3) Seizures (associated with meperidine, tramadol)
            (4) Nausea/vomiting, constipation
      2) Past medical history
         a) Current or preexisting diseases/illness
            (1) HIV infection or AIDS
            (2) Hepatitis
            (3) Endocarditis
            (4) Tuberculosis
         b) Suicidal ideation/gesture
         c) Detoxification history, rehabilitation/recovery history
         d) Medications
         e) Allergies
   b. Objective data collection
      1) Physical examination
         a) General appearance
            (1) Level of consciousness, behavior, affect: apathy, drowsiness, lethargy, seizures
            (2) Respiratory: apnea or arrest
            (3) Hypotension, bradycardia
            (4) Moderate to severe distress/discomfort
         b) Inspection
            (1) Pupils: pinpoint pupils (miosis) are hallmark of narcotic abuse
            (2) Skin: track marks, lesions secondary to skin-popping, abscesses, cyanosis
         c) Auscultation
            (1) Breath sounds: adventitious breath sounds
      2) Diagnostic procedures
         a) Serum and urine toxicology screen
         b) Urinalysis: pregnancy test in female patients of childbearing age
         c) ABGs
         d) Chest radiograph
2. Analysis: differential nursing diagnoses/collaborative problems
   a. Risk for ineffective airway clearance
   b. Impaired gas exchange
   c. Ineffective breathing pattern
   d. Risk for poisoning
   e. Risk for ineffective coping, hopelessness, suicide
   f. Risk for self/other-directed violence
   g. Risk for trauma
   h. Risk for infection
3. Planning and implementation/interventions
   a. Maintain airway, breathing, circulation (see Chapter 1)
   b. Provide supplemental oxygen as indicated
      1) Bag-mask ventilation if respiratory depression or arrest
   c. Establish IV access for administration of crystalloid fluid/medications
   d. Prepare for/assist with medical interventions
      1) Institute cardiac, blood pressure, and pulse oximetry monitoring
      2) Insert gastric tube as indicated
         a) Gastric lavage: controversial and potentially useful only if performed within 1 hour after ingestion
   e. Administer pharmacologic therapy as ordered
      1) Naloxone (Narcan): short-acting narcotic antagonist
         a) Actions: opioid antagonist and will precipitate withdrawal
         b) Administer by the IV, intranasal, or intramuscular route; may need to repeat doses secondary to its short length of action
         c) Consider repeated naloxone therapy before disposition
         d) Children and neonates should receive naloxone if suspected overdose or maternal addiction
      2) Activated charcoal with or without cathartic
   f. Educate patient/significant others
      1) Refer to social services and/or support groups (e.g., Narcotics Anonymous)
      2) Provide information on detoxification procedures
      3) Refer patient/family to rehabilitation/recovery resources
4. Evaluation and ongoing monitoring
   a. Airway patency
   b. Level of consciousness
   c. Hemodynamic status
   d. Breath sounds and pulse oximetry
   e. Cardiac rate and rhythm
   f. Seizure activity

R. ORGANOPHOSPHATE POISONING

Organophosphate pesticides inhibit acetylcholinesterase and result in nicotinic, muscarinic, and CNS symptoms. These include excess diaphoresis, urination, lacrimation, salivation, diarrhea, miosis, fasciculations, seizures, tremors, and weakness and may result in hypovolemia, shock, or respiratory depression. Organophosphates are found in insecticides and in some chemical weapons of mass destruction (see Chapter 40), and they range in toxicity from highly toxic (e.g., parathion) to less toxic (e.g., malathion, diazinon). Pediatric and elderly patients are at greater risk of toxicity because of their lower levels of cholinesterase activity. Along with the organochlorate compound in the pesticide, hydrocarbons may also produce toxic effects. Recent fears of bioterrorism highlight the importance and danger of organophosphates.

1. Assessment
   a. Subjective data collection
      1) History of present illness/chief complaint
         a) Route of exposure: dermal, ocular, ingestion, inhalation
         b) Circumstances of exposure: unintentional, intentional, occupational
         c) Symptoms: MUDDLES
            (1) Miosis (pinpoint pupils)
            (2) Urination: increased
            (3) Defecation
            (4) Diaphoresis
            (5) Lacrimation
            (6) Excitation
            (7) Salivation
      2) Past medical history
         a) Current or preexisting diseases/illness
            (1) Pulmonary disease
            (2) Cardiovascular disease
         b) Chronic exposure
         c) Medications
         d) Allergies
   b. Objective data collection
      1) Physical examination
         a) General appearance
            (1) Level of consciousness, behavior, affect: confusion to coma, seizures
            (2) Hypotension, bradycardia
            (3) Moderate to severe distress/discomfort
         b) Inspection
            (1) Hypersecretion: lacrimation, salivation, urination, defecation, vomiting, diarrhea
         c) Auscultation
            (1) Breath sounds: crackles
         d) Palpation
            (1) Flaccid paralysis
      2) Diagnostic procedures
         a) CBC with differential
         b) Pseudocholinesterase levels
         c) Serum chemistries including BUN and creatinine
         d) LFTs
         e) ABGs
         f) Creatine phosphokinase (CPK)
         g) Urinalysis; pregnancy test in female patients of childbearing age
         h) Chest radiograph
         i) ECG
2. Analysis: differential nursing diagnoses/collaborative problems
   a. Risk for poisoning
   b. Ineffective airway clearance
   c. Ineffective breathing pattern
   d. Risk for injury
3. Planning and implementation/interventions
   a. Maintain airway, breathing, circulation (see Chapter 1)
   b. Provide supplemental oxygen
      1) Ventilatory support in obtunded patients or respiratory arrest
      2) High-flow oxygen
   c. Establish IV access for administration of crystalloid fluid/medications
   d. Prepare for/assist with medical interventions
      1) Ensure protection of health care workers
         a) Protective clothing must be worn to prevent secondary contamination
         b) Thoroughly decontaminate patient with soap and water on all body surfaces
      2) Advanced airway management
         a) Rapid sequence intubation (RSI)
         b) Nasal or oral intubation
         c) Supraglottic airway (e.g., King, Combitube, laryngeal mask airway)
         d) Surgical airway (e.g., cricothyrotomy)
      3) Institute cardiac and pulse oximetry monitoring
      4) Insert gastric tube and attach to suction
      5) Insert indwelling urinary catheter
      6) Initiate seizure precautions per hospital protocol
      7) Assist with hospital admission: if brief exposure, patient may be discharged after 8 hours if asymptomatic and thoroughly decontaminated
   e. Administer pharmacologic therapy as ordered
      1) RSI premedications: sedatives, analgesics, neuromuscular blocking agents
      2) Atropine and pralidoxime (2-PAM) as ordered; large doses may be required for extended periods of time
      3) Antibiotics: hydrocarbon pneumonitis as indicated
      4) Benzodiazepines: seizures
   f. Educate patient/significant others
      1) Proper use, handling, and storage of pesticides
      2) Wear protective clothing and respirator when in contact with organophosphates

4. Evaluation and ongoing monitoring
   a. Airway patency
   b. Level of consciousness
   c. Hemodynamic status
   d. Breath sounds and pulse oximetry
   e. Cardiac rate and rhythm
   f. Intake and output

S. PETROLEUM DISTILLATE POISONING

Also known as hydrocarbons, petroleum distillates include gasoline, kerosene, paint thinner, motor oil, and mineral seal oil (found in furniture polish). Some pesticides have a petroleum base. Highly viscous products such as motor oil and heavy greases have low toxicity, whereas low-viscosity products such as mineral seal oil are highly toxic because of the potential for aspiration. These products spread over lung surfaces, causing chemical pneumonitis. Some halogenated hydrocarbons, such as methylene chloride, have the ability to produce systemic effects such as dysrhythmias and seizures. When injected, they have the ability to cause necrosis.

1. Assessment
   a. Subjective data collection
      1) History of present illness/chief complaint
         a) Route: oral, inhalation, dermal
         b) Circumstances: unintentional, intentional, occupational
         c) Type of product: pure petroleum distillates or products mixed with heavy metal or pesticides
         d) Vertigo
         e) Cough, choking
      2) Past medical history
         a) Current or preexisting diseases/illness
            (1) Neurologic illness
            (2) Cardiac disease
            (3) GI illness
            (4) Respiratory disease
         b) Medications
         c) Allergies
   b. Objective data collection
      1) Physical examination
         a) General appearance
            (1) Level of consciousness, behavior, affect: euphoria, hallucinations, seizures
            (2) Ataxia
            (3) Petroleum odor
            (4) Elevated temperature, tachypnea
            (5) Moderate to severe distress/discomfort
         b) Auscultation
            (1) Breath sounds: crackles, rhonchi, wheezes
      2) Diagnostic procedures
         a) CBC with differential
         b) Serum chemistries including glucose
         c) LFTs
         d) ABGs
         e) Urinalysis; pregnancy test in female patients of childbearing age
         f) Chest radiograph
         g) ECG
2. Analysis: differential nursing diagnoses/collaborative problems
   a. Risk for aspiration
   b. Impaired gas exchange
   c. Impaired skin integrity
   d. Risk for poisoning
3. Planning and implementation/interventions
   a. Maintain airway, breathing, circulation (see Chapter 1)
   b. Provide supplemental oxygen
      1) Ventilatory support in obtunded patients or in respiratory arrest
      2) High-flow oxygen
   c. Establish IV access for administration of crystalloid fluid/medications
   d. Prepare for/assist with medical interventions
      1) Advanced airway management
         a) Rapid sequence intubation (RSI)
         b) Nasal or oral intubation
         c) Supraglottic airway (e.g., King, Combitube, laryngeal mask airway)
         d) Surgical airway (e.g., cricothyrotomy)
      2) Institute cardiac and pulse oximetry monitoring
      3) Prevent further chemical burns and maintain skin integrity
         a) Remove contaminated clothing
         b) Copiously wash skin with soapy water to remove residue
      4) Assist with possible hospital admission: may be discharged if no symptoms are present after 6 hours of observation
   e. Administer pharmacologic therapy as ordered
      1) RSI premedications: sedatives, analgesics, neuromuscular blocking agents
      2) Sympathomimetic drugs (e.g., albuterol): caution because of possibility of dysrhythmias
      3) Antibiotics: for pneumonitis as indicated
4. Evaluation and ongoing monitoring
   a. Hemodynamic status
   b. Breath sounds and pulse oximetry
   c. Cardiac rate and rhythm

T. PHENCYCLIDINE USE

Phencyclidine (PCP) is a widely used street drug known as a dissociative anesthetic that decreases awareness of one's surroundings. PCP has characteristics similar to those of ketamine and was initially used as a surgical anesthetic in veterinary and human medicine. PCP use was discontinued when patients experienced terrifying emergence reactions, such as delusions and paranoia, when the drug's effects diminished. PCP is consumed by dusting it on a cigarette and smoking it, taking it in pill form, snorting it, or absorbing it through skin contact. It is rapidly absorbed in the bloodstream, quickly distributed to tissues, and is highly lipophilic. PCP affects the CNS and causes stimulation or depression, as well as cholinergic-like effects, including muscular rigidity, thought disorganization, and violent, agitated behavior. Common street names include angel dust, Cadillac, CJ, killer weed, magic mist, and cyclones. Acute complications resulting from the increased muscle rigidity include rhabdomyolysis and renal failure. Other complications include respiratory depression, apnea, cerebral hemorrhage, and psychosis. Other dissociative drugs include Ketamine (K, special K, cat Valium), DXM-dextromethorphan (Robo), and *Salvia divinorum*.

1. Assessment
   a. Subjective data collection
      1) History of present illness/chief complaint
         a) Route of exposure
         b) Circumstances of use: accidental vs. recreational deliberate use
         c) Concomitant drug use
         d) Symptoms
            (1) Violent combative behavior, increased strength, lack of pain sensation
            (2) Pupil changes: bidirectional nystagmus in an awake patient is classic; pinpoint pupils (miosis)
            (3) Tremors/increased strength: "superhuman" strength as the result of decreased pain feedback mechanism
            (4) Nausea, vomiting, abdominal pain
      2) Past medical history
         a) Current or preexisting diseases/illness
            (1) HIV infection
            (2) Psychiatric history
            (3) Hepatitis
            (4) Tuberculosis
         b) Previous PCP use
         c) History of recent trauma: death usually occurs from associated trauma/injury
         d) Medications
         e) Allergies
   b. Objective data collection
      1) Physical examination
         a) General appearance
            (1) Level of consciousness, behavior, affect: varies from drowsiness to irritability, euphoria and extreme agitation, bizarre or combative behavior, paranoia, seizure activity
            (2) Tachycardia, hypertension
            (3) Gait: altered, ataxia
            (4) Moderate to severe distress/discomfort
         b) Inspection
            (1) Nystagmus: bidirectional (horizontal, vertical, rotary)
            (2) Tremors and hyperactivity
            (3) Myoclonus or muscle rigidity
            (4) Drooling
         c) Palpation
            (1) Anesthesia to painful stimuli
      2) Diagnostic procedures
         a) Serum and urine for toxicology screen
         b) Creatine kinase (CK)
         c) Serum chemistries including glucose: hypoglycemia
         d) Urinalysis: myoglobin; pregnancy test in female patients of childbearing age
2. Analysis: differential nursing diagnoses/collaborative problems
   a. Risk for injury and self/other-directed violence
   b. Decreased cardiac output
   c. Risk for poisoning
   d. Risk for hyperthermia
   e. Risk for trauma
   f. Risk for infection
3. Planning and implementation/interventions
   a. Maintain airway, breathing, circulation (see Chapter 1)
   b. Provide supplemental oxygen as indicated
   c. Establish IV access for administration of crystalloid fluid/medications
   d. Prepare for/assist with medical interventions
      1) Decrease sensory-perceptual alteration
         a) Use quiet, nonstimulating room if possible
         b) Do not leave patient unattended; consider security standby if needed
         c) Keep side rails up to prevent falls
      2) Decrease risk for violence: protect patient and staff; PCP-impaired patients have increased strength and do not feel pain because of anesthetic effects of drug; therefore, they may be strong enough to break leather restraints
         a) Do not attempt deescalation because patients quickly become agitated and forceful
         b) Consider use of leather or chemical restraints if all measures to provide patient and staff safety fail per institutional protocols
            (1) Leather (soft restraints are generally ineffective)
            (2) Chemical: benzodiazepines, haloperidol (Haldol); short-term paralysis
            (3) Handcuffs: police application
         c) Contact law enforcement for security backup as needed
         d) Wear gloves when approaching patient because PCP may be absorbed through skin
      3) Consider psychiatric consultation for anxiety/depression after acute therapy
   e. Administer pharmacologic therapy as ordered
      1) Diazepam (Valium), haloperidol (Haldol), lorazepam (Ativan): decrease hallucinations

2) Short-term paralysis: ensure airway and ventilation
3) Avoid phenothiazines; may increase seizures
f. Educate patient/significant others
  1) Refer patient/family to social services and/or support groups (e.g., Narcotics Anonymous)
  2) Refer patient/family to rehabilitation/recovery resources
4. Evaluation and ongoing monitoring
  a. Hemodynamic status
  b. Continued presence or absence of agitation, seizures, hallucinations

U. PLANT POISONING

Many kinds of plants are considered poisonous. Cardiac glycoside plants such as oleander, foxglove, and lily of the valley cause a loss of cardiac excitability and hyperkalemia. Plants with anticholinergic properties antagonize acetylcholine at the neuroreceptor site and cause a typical anticholinergic presentation of tachycardia, mydriasis, and fever. Plants in this category include jimsonweed, deadly nightshade, and potato leaves, some of which are used in recreational abuse. Plants that contain oxalic acids may form needlelike calcium oxalate crystals and produce severe pain when ingested. These plants include dieffenbachia, philodendron, and rhubarb.

1. Assessment
  a. Subjective data collection
    1) History of present illness/chief complaints
      a) Identity of plant ingested, part of plant (bulb, blossoms, leaves)
      b) Short-term vs. long-term exposure
      c) Symptoms
        (1) Cardiac glycosides: vomiting
        (2) Anticholinergic: agitation, delirium, disorientation, visual hallucinations
        (3) Oxalic acid: bloody emesis and diarrhea, pain, and burning sensation orally
    2) Past medical history
      a) Current or preexisting diseases/illness
        (1) Cardiac disease
        (2) GI illness
        (3) Psychiatric history
      b) Medications
      c) Allergies
  b. Objective data collection
    1) Physical examination
      a) General appearance
        (1) Level of consciousness, behavior, affect: hallucinations, seizures, agitation with anticholinergics
        (2) Bradycardia with cardiac glycosides; tachycardia with anticholinergics
        (3) Elevated temperature: anticholinergics
        (4) Hypertension: anticholinergics
        (5) Moderate to severe distress/discomfort

      b) Inspection
        (1) Pupil mydriasis: anticholinergics
        (2) Flushed, hot skin: anticholinergics
        (3) Dry mucous membranes: anticholinergics
        (4) Swollen mouth, tongue: oxalic acids
        (5) Salivation: oxalic acids
      c) Auscultation
        (1) Breath sounds: crackles with oxalic acids
        (2) Bowel sounds: decreased with anticholinergics
    2) Diagnostic procedures
      a) Serum chemistries (cardiac glycosides and oxalic acids)
      b) LFTs (anticholinergics)
      c) Urinalysis (oxalic acids); pregnancy test in female patients of childbearing age
      d) ECG: QRS complex widening with anticholinergics
2. Analysis: differential nursing diagnoses/collaborative problems
  a. Risk for poisoning
  b. Decreased cardiac output
3. Planning and implementation/interventions
  a. Maintain airway, breathing, circulation (see Chapter 1)
  b. Provide supplemental oxygen as indicated
  c. Establish IV access for administration of crystalloid fluid/medications
  d. Prepare for/assist with medical interventions
    1) Sweep mouth for foreign body/choking hazard
    2) Apply ice to lips and oral area to decrease swelling
    3) Oral rinses with water to flush out oxalic acid crystals
    4) Institute cardiac and pulse oximetry monitoring
    5) Possible external cardiac pacemaker
    6) Assist with possible hospital admission
    7) Psychiatric consultation for chronic plant ingestions
  e. Administer pharmacologic therapy as ordered
    1) Activated charcoal with or without cathartic
    2) Phenytoin (Dilantin): dysrhythmias
    3) Benzodiazepines: agitation or seizures
    4) Replace electrolytes
    5) Sodium bicarbonate: QRS complex widening
    6) Consider physostigmine (Antilirium) for anticholinergic effects
  f. Educate patient/significant others
    1) Keep plants out of reach
    2) Dangers of using plants for recreational abuse
4. Evaluation and ongoing monitoring
  a. Level of consciousness and seizure activity
  b. Hemodynamic status
  c. Breath sounds and pulse oximetry
  d. Cardiac rate and rhythm

V. SALICYLATE POISONING

Salicylates are very common antipyretic, analgesic, and antiinflammatory OTC products. More than 200 products contain aspirin or salicylates. Toxicity may result from short-term or long-term exposure, particularly in children and elderly persons. However, this condition has become less common than in the past because of increased use of acetaminophen for pain and fever control. As a result of the life-threatening complication of Reye syndrome, salicylate use after viral infection has decreased. However, in the elderly population, there is an increased risk of chronic toxicity as a result of decreased renal function and the use of aspirin for many medical problems. This puts the elderly population at risk for developing respiratory alkalosis and metabolic acidosis, increased bleeding, and ulcer formation.

Salicylate poisoning affects the GI mucosa, coagulation, neurologic system, and acid-base status. Metabolic acidosis is common in children, and respiratory alkalosis with stimulation of the CNS respiratory center is common in adults. Peak serum salicylate levels usually occur 6 hours after short-term ingestion, but this may vary depending on the type of pill ingested (i.e., enteric-coated tablets have a longer absorption time). Concretions (solid masses of particles) have been shown to form in the intestines as a result of large overdoses; they are slowly released over a longer period of time, or they erode the gut. A toxic dose is 150–200 mg/kg body weight, and >500 mg/kg is considered lethal. Long-term intoxication may occur with ingestion of >100 mg/kg/day for 2 or more days.[3] Hemodialysis may be indicated in patients with high or rising levels. Common salicylate-containing products include Pepto-Bismol, Excedrin, and Alka-Seltzer. Oil of wintergreen topical agent is a toxic preparation because of its high salicylate content.

Treatment of salicylate poisoning should be approached aggressively, and the patient should be monitored closely. Deaths have occurred within a few hours of admission to the emergency department because presenting symptoms have been minimized or misinterpreted.

1. Assessment
   a. Subjective data collection
      1) History of present illness/chief complaint
         a) Long-term vs. short-term exposure: long-term use may be seen more in the elderly
         b) Reason for use: suicide attempt, accidental exposure, child maltreatment
         c) Incremental chronic dosing risk
         d) Dosage form: effervescent, uncoated, enteric coated
            (1) Enteric-coated tablets disintegrate in intestines and decrease gastric mucosal effects
            (2) Peak serum salicylate levels after enteric-coated use should occur at 6–9 hours after ingestion; can be delayed up to 60 hours after ingestion in enteric-coated or modified-release salicylate overdose
         e) Nausea/vomiting
         f) Tinnitus
      2) Past medical history
         a) Current or preexisting diseases/illness
            (1) Psychiatric history, especially depression
            (2) Chronic pain
            (3) Liver disease
         b) Breastfeeding mothers using salicylate products
         c) Medications
         d) Allergies
   b. Objective data collection
      1) Physical examination
         a) General appearance
            (1) Level of consciousness, behavior, affect: coma/stupor (ominous sign), seizure
            (2) Tachypnea, hyperthermia, tachycardia, diaphoresis
            (3) Moderate to severe distress/discomfort
         b) Inspection
            (1) Ecchymosis of skin
         c) Auscultation
            (1) Breath sounds: crackles
      2) Diagnostic procedures
         a) Serum salicylate level: on arrival and 6 hours after ingestion; compare level with nomogram for toxicity, but optimally done serially to detect rising levels earlier
         b) CBC with differential
         c) Serum chemistries including glucose
         d) ABGs: acidosis, alkalosis
         e) Coagulation profile
         f) Urinalysis; pregnancy test in female patients of childbearing age
         g) Emesis, stool testing: occult blood
         h) Chest radiograph
         i) ECG
2. Analysis: differential nursing diagnoses/collaborative problems
   a. Ineffective breathing pattern
   b. Impaired gas exchange
   c. Risk for poisoning
3. Planning and implementation/interventions
   a. Maintain airway, breathing, circulation (see Chapter 1)
   b. Provide supplemental oxygen
      1) Hyperventilation may be required if acidosis present, hypoventilation may have disastrous effects
      2) Severe metabolic acidosis requires intubation and controlled ventilation in hospital; the acidotic state can markedly worsen unless the hyperventilation is maintained
   c. Establish IV access for administration of crystalloid fluid/medications
      1) Large amounts of normal saline solution infusions may be required for renal clearance and hydration

d. Prepare for/assist with medical interventions
  1) Institute cardiac, blood pressure, and pulse oximetry monitoring
  2) Prevent absorption
    a) Insert gastric tube as indicated
      (1) Gastric lavage: controversial, potentially useful only if performed within 1 hour after ingestion
      (2) Whole bowel irrigation may be indicated
  3) Assist with possible hospital admission for hemodialysis for severe short- or long-term ingestion
e. Administer pharmacologic therapy as ordered
  1) Activated charcoal with or without cathartic (rule out GI bleeding before administration)
  2) Sodium bicarbonate: correct acidosis and alkalinize urine
  3) Replace electrolytes: especially potassium
  4) Dextrose 50% if hypoglycemic
f. Educate patient/significant others
  1) Effects of short- and long-term aspirin use
  2) Use of aspirin in pediatric and geriatric populations
4. Evaluation and ongoing monitoring
  a. Level of consciousness and seizure activity
  b. Hemodynamic status
  c. Breath sounds and pulse oximetry
  d. Cardiac rate and rhythm
  e. Intake and output
  f. Salicylate level

W. SEDATIVE-HYPNOTIC AND BARBITURATE POISONING

Sedative-hypnotics are CNS depressants. Their chief effect is respiratory depression, which can be increased by the coingestion of alcohol or other depressant medications. Their addiction potential is high. These medications are commonly prescribed to induce sleep and allay anxiety. They are known to relax inhibitions and act as mood elevators, and they may also be used as anticonvulsants. Sedative-hypnotics include the following: barbiturates such as phenobarbital; nonbarbiturates such as the benzodiazepines diazepam (Valium), alprazolam (Xanax), flurazepam (Dalmane), and chlordiazepoxide (Librium); and antihistamines such as hydroxyzine (Atarax, Vistaril). Benzodiazepines have a low order of toxicity when ingested alone and rarely cause death, whereas the others may cause hypotension and deep coma. Barbiturates are highly toxic, have a high abuse potential because of their euphoric effects, and are classified according to their duration of action. They concentrate in adipose tissue, a property that renders their effects profound and removal difficult in overdose. Rohypnol, a benzodiazepine chemically similar to prescription sedatives such as Valium and Xanax, in the class of "designer drugs," is commonly used at raves, parties, and nightclubs among teens and young adults. Rohypnol, like gamma-hydroxybutyrate (GHB), has been associated with use to commit sexual assaults due to its ability to sedate and incapacitate victims.

Infants born to addicted mothers may also be physically dependent on the drugs. Within 72 hours of birth, the neonate may show signs of withdrawal, including vomiting, tremors, seizures, and a high-pitched cry.

1. Assessment
  a. Subjective data collection
    1) History of present illness/chief complaint
      a) Agent ingested: short or long acting
      b) Route: oral or parental
      c) Other drugs ingested: narcotics, hallucinogens, alcohol, tricyclic antidepressants—the combination of which can be lethal
    2) Past medical history
      a) Current or preexisting diseases/illness
        (1) Psychiatric (e.g., suicidal intent, anxiety)
        (2) Seizures
      b) Medications
      c) Allergies
  b. Objective data collection
    1) Physical examination
      a) General appearance
        (1) Level of consciousness, behavior, affect
          (a) Mild use: drowsiness, euphoria, impaired memory and judgment, slurred speech, ataxia
          (b) Excessive use: CNS depression
        (2) Hypotension: excessive use
        (3) Hypothermia
        (4) Moderate to severe distress/discomfort
      b) Inspection
        (1) "Coma blisters" or "barb blisters": hemorrhagic blisters over areas of pressure that develop at approximately 4 hours after ingestion
        (2) Cardiac dysrhythmias on monitor
        (3) Pupillary changes
      c) Auscultation
        (1) Decreased bowel sounds (barbiturates)
    2) Diagnostic procedures
      a) Serum and urine toxicology screen
      b) Serum glucose
      c) Serum muscle enzymes: creatine kinase
      d) Therapeutic medication levels
      e) ABGs
      f) Urinalysis: myoglobinuria, pregnancy test in female patients of childbearing age
      g) Chest radiograph: possible pulmonary edema/pneumonia
      h) ECG
2. Analysis: differential nursing diagnoses/collaborative problems
  a. Ineffective airway clearance

b. Ineffective breathing
c. Decreased cardiac output
d. Risk for poisoning
e. Risk for suicide
3. Planning and implementation/interventions
   a. Maintain airway, breathing, circulation (see Chapter 1)
   b. Provide supplemental oxygen
      1) Ventilatory support if patient obtunded
      2) High-flow oxygen
   c. Establish IV access for administration of crystalloid fluid/medications
      1) Infuse normal saline solution fluid challenge
   d. Prepare for/assist with medical interventions
      1) Advanced airway management
         a) Rapid sequence intubation (RSI)
         b) Nasal or oral intubation
         c) Supraglottic airway (e.g., King, Combitube, laryngeal mask airway)
         d) Surgical airway (e.g., cricothyrotomy)
      2) Institute cardiac, blood pressure, and pulse oximetry monitoring
      3) Possible catheter placement and monitoring of pulmonary artery and/or arterial pressures (see Chapter 7)
      4) Insert gastric tube as indicated
      5) Treat "barb blisters" as partial-thickness burns (see Chapter 34)
      6) Assist with possible hospital admission: hemodialysis, hemoperfusion for barbiturates
      7) Assist with psychiatric consultation in suicide gesture
   e. Administer pharmacologic therapy as ordered
      1) RSI medications: sedatives, analgesics, neuromuscular blocking agents
      2) Activated charcoal with or without cathartics: multiple doses may be required for barbiturates; syrup of ipecac contraindicated because of potential for seizure activity and respiratory depression
      3) Flumazenil (Romazicon): use cautiously in benzodiazepine overdose because of potential for seizure activity in presence of coingestants or chronic benzodiazepine use
      4) Sodium bicarbonate: for urine and serum alkalinization in barbiturate overdose
      5) Vasopressors (e.g., dopamine [Intropin]): hypotension
   f. Educate patient/significant others
      1) Refer for psychiatric evaluation
      2) Refer patient/family to social services and/or support groups (e.g., Narcotics Anonymous)
      3) Refer patient/family to rehabilitation/recovery resources
4. Evaluation and ongoing monitoring
   a. Level of consciousness

b. Hemodynamic status
c. Breath sounds and pulse oximetry
d. Cardiac rate and rhythm
e. Drug levels: barbiturates

X. SELECTIVE SEROTONIN REUPTAKE INHIBITOR AND ATYPICAL ANTIDEPRESSANT POISONING

In the past 20 years, selective serotonin reuptake inhibitors (SSRIs) and other atypical antidepressants have largely replaced TCAs as drugs of choice for depression because SSRIs have fewer side effects and relative safety in overdosage. Commonly prescribed forms are trazodone (Desyrel), fluoxetine (Prozac), paroxetine (Paxil), sertraline (Zoloft), venlafaxine (Effexor), escitalopram (Lexapro), and bupropion (Wellbutrin, Zyban), some of which are now available in sustained-release preparations. Their mechanism of action is unclear, but SSRIs appear to moderate the utilization and storage of dopamine and serotonin, both of which play a role in the origin of depression. SSRIs may interact with other medications, such as dextromethorphan and meperidine (Demerol), to produce a "serotonin syndrome," which is characterized by symptoms of hyperthermia, diaphoresis, agitation, confusion, tonic-clonic seizures, rigidity, tachycardia, and hypertension.[4]

1. Assessment
   a. Subjective data collection
      1) History of present illness/chief complaint
         a) Amount of drug ingested and time
         b) Type of medication
      2) Past medical history
         a) Current or preexisting diseases/illness
            (1) Cardiac disease
            (2) Neurologic illness: seizures
            (3) Psychiatric illness: depression, prior suicide attempt
         b) Medications
         c) Allergies
   b. Objective data collection
      1) Physical examination
         a) General appearance
            (1) Level of consciousness, behavior, affect: normally CNS depression, confusion, and agitation with serotonin syndrome, seizures
            (2) Respiratory depression: alone or in conjunction with ethanol
            (3) Tachycardia
            (4) Hyperthermia with serotonin syndrome
            (5) Moderate to severe distress/discomfort
         b) Inspection
            (1) Myoclonus or tonic-clonic seizures with serotonin syndrome
            (2) Priapism with trazodone
      2) Diagnostic procedures
         a) Serum and urine toxicology screen

b) Urinalysis; pregnancy test in female patients of childbearing age

c) No definitive drug levels available

2. Analysis: differential nursing diagnoses/collaborative problems
   a. Decreased cardiac output
   b. Risk for suicide
   c. Risk for poisoning

3. Planning and implementation/interventions
   a. Maintain airway, breathing, circulation (see Chapter 1)
   b. Provide supplemental oxygen
   c. Establish IV access for administration of crystalloid fluid/medications
   d. Prepare for/assist with medical interventions
      1) Initiate seizure precautions
      2) Institute cardiac and pulse oximetry monitoring
      3) Assist with psychiatric consultation if suicide gesture
   e. Administer pharmacologic therapy as ordered
      1) Activated charcoal with or without cathartic
      2) Whole bowel irrigation with sustained-release formulations
      3) Benzodiazepines: seizure control

4. Evaluation and ongoing monitoring
   a. Airway patency
   b. Level of consciousness and seizure activity
   c. Cardiac rate and rhythm

Y. SYNTHETIC DRUGS OF ABUSE

Synthetic drugs are composed of man-made chemicals intended to mimic various illicit drugs of abuse. Two of the most common synthetic drugs of abuse include bath salts and synthetic cannabis. Bath salts are an emerging family of drugs containing one or more synthetic chemicals related to cathinone, a stimulant naturally occurring in the Khat plant. Bath salts are consumed orally, injected, or inhaled for the effects of euphoria, increased sociability, and sex drive. Some experience severe reactions that include paranoia, agitation, hallucinations, delirium, psychotic and violent behavior. Bath salts take the form of white or brown crystalline powder and are sold in foil packages labeled "not for human consumption." Bath salts are often sold as plant food, jewelry cleaner, or phone screen cleaner. Bath salt street names include cloud nine, cosmic blast, ivory wave, scarface, and vanilla sky.

Synthetic cannabis (K2, spice) is found as a wide variety of herbal mixtures containing man-made cannabinoid chemicals related to THC in marijuana. The man-made chemical is sprayed on dried, shredded plant material for smoking or prepared as a liquid that can be vaporized and inhaled in e-cigarettes or other devices (liquid incense). Synthetic cannabinoids are sometimes marketed as synthetic marijuana and are included in a group of drugs called "new psychoactive substances" (NPS), a class of unregulated psychoactive substances. Effects include elevated mood, altered perception, psychosis, extreme anxiety, confusion,

paranoia, and hallucinations. Side effects include violent behavior and suicidal thoughts.

1. Assessment
   a. Subjective data collection
      1) History of present illness/chief complaint
         a) Route of exposure: ingestion, intravenous, smoke, vape
         b) Concomitant alcohol or other drug use
         c) Time of ingestion
         d) Amount ingested
      2) Past medical history
         a) Current or preexisting diseases/illness
         b) Previous use of other recreational drugs
         c) Trauma
         d) Medications
         e) Allergies
   b. Objective data collection
      1) Physical examination
         a) General appearance
            (1) Level of consciousness, behavior, affect, hallucinations, agitation, paranoia
            (2) Respiratory distress
            (3) Generalized or tonic-clonic seizures
            (4) Violent behavior, suicidal thoughts
            (5) Hypertension, bradycardia
            (6) Moderate to severe distress/discomfort
         b) Inspection
            (1) Mouth and oral mucosa: burns if chemicals used in manufacturing substance
         c) Auscultation
            (1) Breath sounds: crackles
      2) Diagnostic procedures
         a) Serum and urine toxicology screen
         b) ABGs
         c) Serum chemistries
         d) Urinalysis: myoglobin; pregnancy test in female patients of childbearing age

2. Analysis: differential nursing diagnoses/collaborative problems
   a. Ineffective breathing pattern
   b. Impaired gas exchange
   c. Risk for poisoning
   d. Rape/trauma syndrome

3. Planning and implementation/interventions
   a. Maintain airway, breathing, circulation (see Chapter 1)
   b. Provide supplemental oxygen
      1) RSI and ventilatory support if patient obtunded
      2) High-flow oxygen
   c. Establish IV access for administration of crystalloid fluid/medications
   d. Prepare for/assist with medical interventions
      1) Decrease sensory-perceptual alteration
         a) Use quiet, nonstimulating room if possible
         b) Do not leave patient unattended; consider security standby if needed

c) Keep side rails up to prevent falls
2) Decrease risk for violence
   a) Consider use of leather or chemical restraints if all measures to provide patient and staff safety fail per institutional protocols
      (1) Chemical: benzodiazepines, haloperidol (Haldol)
3) Consider psychiatric consultation for anxiety/depression after acute therapy
4) Institute cardiac, blood pressure, and pulse oximetry monitoring
   e. Administer pharmacologic therapy as ordered
      1) Benzodiazepines: agitation
      2) Antipsychotics: haloperidol (Haldol)
   f. Educate patient/significant others
      1) Refer patient/family to social services and/or support groups (e.g., Narcotics Anonymous)
      2) Refer patient/family to rehabilitation/recovery resources
4. Evaluation and ongoing monitoring
   a. Airway patency
   b. Level of consciousness and presence of seizures
   c. Hemodynamic status
   d. Breath sounds and pulse oximetry
   e. Cardiac rate and rhythm
   f. Intake and output

Z. TRICYCLIC ANTIDEPRESSANT POISONING

Tricyclic antidepressant (TCA) medication overdoses can be extremely lethal and should be managed aggressively. The lethality of these drugs is related to their very narrow therapeutic index. They are analogues of the phenothiazines and share anticholinergic and alpha-adrenergic blocking properties. These actions produce cardiotoxic effects and CNS depression, resulting in fatalities. TCAs are absorbed from the GI tract and are rapidly distributed. Once absorbed, they become highly bound to plasma proteins, a property that makes them difficult to remove from the body. Death results from cardiotoxic effects. Examples of TCAs include amitriptyline (Elavil), desipramine, doxepin (Sinequan), trazodone (Desyrel), and nortriptyline. Although prescribed less frequently for depression, they are occasionally used as an adjunct in pain management and enuresis in children.

1. Assessment
   a. Subjective data collection
      1) History of present illness/chief complaint
         a) Amount of drug ingested and time
         b) Type of medication
      2) Past medical history
         a) Current or preexisting diseases/illness
            (1) Cardiac disease
            (2) Neurologic disease
            (3) Substance abuse, rehabilitation, recovery history
            (4) Psychiatric illness: depression, prior suicide attempt, nocturnal enuresis
         b) Medications
         c) Allergies
   b. Objective data collection
      1) Physical examination
         a) General appearance
            (1) Level of consciousness, behavior, affect: ranges from alert to disoriented, lethargic to comatose; progression may be rapid, seizure activity from anticholinergic effects
            (2) Hypotension
            (3) Possible cardiac arrest
            (4) Severe distress/discomfort
         b) Inspection
            (1) Cardiac dysrhythmias on monitor
               (a) Sinus tachycardia: sensitive, early indicator of toxicity
               (b) Premature ventricular contractions (PVCs)
               (c) Supraventricular tachycardia (SVT)
               (d) Ventricular tachycardia (VT)
               (e) QRS complex widening
            (2) Fine tremors
         c) Auscultation
            (1) Bowel sounds: decreased
      2) Diagnostic procedures
         a) Serum and urine toxicology screen
         b) Cardiac enzymes
         c) Serum chemistries
         d) ABGs
         e) Urinalysis: myoglobin; pregnancy test in female patients of childbearing age
         f) ECG
            (1) Prolonged PR interval
            (2) Wide QRS complex
            (3) QT prolongation
            (4) ST-segment depression
            (5) Atrioventricular (AV) conduction disturbance
2. Analysis: differential nursing diagnoses/collaborative problems
   a. Risk for poisoning
   b. Risk for suicide
   c. Risk for ineffective airway clearance
   d. Risk for decreased cardiac output
3. Planning and implementation/interventions
   a. Maintain airway, breathing, circulation (see Chapter 1)
   b. Provide supplemental oxygen
      1) Ventilatory support for obtunded patients
      2) High-flow oxygen
   c. Establish IV access for administration of crystalloid fluid/medications
   d. Prepare for/assist with medical interventions

1) Advanced airway management
   a) Rapid sequence intubation (RSI)
   b) Nasal or oral intubation
   c) Supraglottic airway (e.g., King, Combitube, laryngeal mask airway)
   d) Surgical airway (e.g., cricothyrotomy)
2) Insert gastric tube as indicated
   a) Gastric lavage: controversial, potentially useful only if symptoms appear early and performed within 1.5–2 hours after ingestion
3) Institute cardiac and pulse oximetry monitoring
4) Initiate seizure precautions
5) Assist with possible hospital admission: cardiac monitoring must occur for a minimum of 6 hours
6) Psychiatric consultation for suicide gesture
   e. Administer pharmacologic therapy as ordered
1) RSI premedications: sedatives, analgesics, neuromuscular blocking agents
2) Activated charcoal with or without cathartic
3) Sodium bicarbonate: QRS complex widening, acidosis secondary to seizures
4) Benzodiazepines: seizure control
5) Norepinephrine (Levophed): hypotension
4. Evaluation and ongoing monitoring
   a. Airway patency
   b. Hemodynamic status
   c. Level of consciousness and presence of seizures
   d. Cardiac rate and rhythm
   e. Breath sounds and pulse oximetry
   f. Intake and output

References

1. Mowry DB, Spyker DA, Cantilena LR, McMillan N, Ford M: 2013 Annual Report of the American Association of Poison Control Centers' National Poison Data System (NPDS): 31st Annual Report, *Clinical Toxicology* 52:1032–1283, 2014.
2. Substance Abuse and Mental Health Services Administration: *Drug Abuse Warning Network*, 2011: National estimates of drug related emergency department visits, 2015. Retrieved from http://www.dawninfo.samhsa.gov.
3. Olson K: *Poisoning and drug overdose*, ed 4, East Norwalk, CT, 2004, Appleton & Lange.
4. Bartlett D: Serotonin syndrome: A subtle toxicity, *Journal of Emergency Nursing* 32(3):277–279, 2006.

Bibliography

American Academy of Pediatrics Committee on Injury, Violence and Poison Prevention: Poison treatment in the home (policy statement), *Pediatrics* 112(5):1182–1185, 2003.

Bartlett D: Dangerous in small amounts: Ten non drug substances that can cause harm, *Journal of Emergency Nursing* 29:377–379, 2003.

Bartlett D: Tricky toxic presentations at triage, *Journal of Emergency Nursing* 31(4):403–404, 2005.

Buykx P, Dietze P, Ritter A, Loxley W: Characteristics of medication overdose presentations to the ED: How do they differ from illicit drug overdose and self-harm cases? *Emergency Medicine Journal* 27(7):499–503, 2010.

Camp NE: Understanding the assessment and treatment of caustic ingestions and the resulting burns, *Journal of Emergency Nursing* 31(6):594–596, 2005.

Dart RC, editor: *Medical toxicology*, ed 3, Philadelphia, 2004, Lippincott Williams & Wilkins.

Flomenbaum NE, Goldfrank LR, Hoffman RS, Howland MA, Lewin NA, Nelson LS: *Goldfrank's toxicologic emergencies*, ed 8, New York, 2006, McGraw-Hill.

Jones CM, Paulozzi LJ, Mack KA: Alcohol involvement in opioid pain reliever and benzodiazepine drug abuse-related emergency department visits and drug related deaths. United States, 2010, *Morbidity and Mortality Weekly Report* 63(40):881–885, 2014.

Lorenc JD: Inhalant abuse in the pediatric population: A persistent challenge, *Pediatrics* 15:204–209, 2003.

Manoguerra AS, Cobaugh DJ, Members of the Guidelines for the Management of Poisonings Consensus Panel: Guideline on the use of syrup of ipecac in the out of hospital management of ingested poisons, *Clinical Toxicology* 1:1–10, 2005.

National Institute on Drug Abuse: *Commonly abused drug charts*, Bethesda, MD, 2015, National Institute on Drug Abuse.

Pourmand P, Armstrong P, Mazer-Amirshahi M, Shokoohi H: The evolving high: New designer drugs of abuse, *Human and Experimental Toxicology* 33(10):993–999, 2014.

Tintinalli JE, Stapczynski JS, Cline DM, Ma OJ, Cydulka RK, Meckler GD, editors: *Emergency medicine: A comprehensive study guide*, ed 7, New York, NY, 2011, McGraw-Hill.

Wilcox HC, Anthony JC: The development of suicide ideation and attempts: An epidemiologic study of first graders followed into young adulthood, *Drug and Alcohol Dependence* 76:S53–S67, 2004.

CHAPTER 27
Psychiatric/Psychosocial Emergencies

Jaime V. Pitner, MSN, RN, MICP, CEN, RHC

I. General Strategy

A. SAFETY

1. Provide environment for patient that is safe, monitored, and clear of items that could be used to harm self or others[1]
2. Ensure patient's medical needs are met prior to mental health screening

B. ASSESSMENT

1. Primary and secondary assessment/resuscitation (see Chapters 1 and 32)
2. Focused assessment
   a. Subjective data collection
      1) History of present illness/chief complaint: patient's perspective and that of significant others
         a) Behavioral changes
         b) Somatic symptoms
         c) Hallucinations or thought disturbances
         d) Thoughts of harming oneself or others
         e) Precipitating event
         f) Mechanism and time of injury (see Chapter 31)
            (1) Unintentional
            (2) Intentional
         g) Efforts to relieve symptoms
            (1) Medications
               (a) Prescription
               (b) Illicit or street drugs
               (c) Alcohol use
               (d) OTC/herbal
      2) Past medical history
         a) Current or preexisting diseases/illness (especially affecting neurologic function or mental status)
            (1) Diabetes
            (2) Alcoholism/drug dependency
               (a) Recent use
               (b) Recent/past withdrawal history: seizures or delirium tremens (DTs)
            (3) Central nervous system (CNS) disorders such as Guillain-Barré syndrome, multiple sclerosis, and amyotrophic lateral sclerosis
            (4) Mental illness history
         b) Head trauma
         c) Previous similar episodes
         d) Previous hospitalizations: determine chronicity and frequency of disturbances
         e) Substance and/or alcohol use/abuse
         f) Last normal menstrual period: female patients of childbearing age
         g) Current medications
            (1) Prescription
               (a) Psychotropic drugs
               (b) Anticonvulsants
               (c) Hypoglycemic agents

(2) OTC/herbal
h) Allergies
i) Immunization status
3) Psychological/social/environmental factors
a) Family history of mental illness
b) Biochemical imbalances
c) Recent personal difficulties
d) Lack of social support system
(1) Broken family relationships, recent relationship losses/crisis
(2) Gang membership
(3) Disintegration of social relationships
e) Lack of knowledge and availability of community support or rehabilitative services
f) Loss of control/violence
(1) Possible/actual assault, abuse, intimate partner violence situations (see Chapters 3 and 40)
g) Fear
h) Guilt or anger
i) Poor self-image or self-esteem
j) Unhealthy work life
k) Spiritual values
l) Cultural influences
b. Objective data collection
1) General appearance
a) Level of consciousness, behavior, affect
b) Vital signs
c) Gait
d) Hygiene, odors
e) Level of distress/discomfort, pain (facial expressions)
2) Inspection
a) Tics or tremors, which may be evidence of dystonic reaction
b) Pupils: size and reactivity
c) Coordination and movement
d) Obvious injuries
3) Auscultation
a) Breath sounds
b) Heart sounds
c) Bowel sounds
4) Palpation/percussion
a) Extremity range of motion
b) Deep tendon reflexes
c) Areas of tenderness
3. Diagnostic procedures
a. Laboratory studies
1) Complete blood count (CBC) with differential
2) Serum chemistries including glucose, BUN, creatinine
3) Serum and urine toxicology screen and therapeutic drug levels
4) Thyroid function tests
5) Liver function tests

6) Urinalysis; pregnancy test in female patients of childbearing age
b. Imaging studies
1) Head computed tomography (CT) scan
c. Other
1) 12-lead electrocardiogram (ECG)

C. ANALYSIS: DIFFERENTIAL NURSING DIAGNOSES/ COLLABORATIVE PROBLEMS

1. Anxiety
2. Impaired verbal communication
3. Ineffective coping
4. Chronic/situational low self-esteem
5. Interrupted family processes
6. Disturbed sleep patterns
7. Disturbed sensory perception
8. Disturbed thought processes
9. Imbalanced nutrition: less than body requirements
10. Dysfunctional grieving
11. Risk for suicide
12. Risk for other-directed/self-directed violence
13. Deficient knowledge

D. PLANNING AND IMPLEMENTATION/ INTERVENTIONS

1. Determine priorities of care
   a. Maintain airway, breathing, circulation (see Chapters 1 and 32)
   b. Provide supplemental oxygen as indicated
   c. Establish intravenous (IV) access for administration of crystalloid fluids/blood products/medications
   d. Obtain and set up equipment and supplies
   e. Prepare for/assist with medical interventions
   f. Administer pharmacologic therapy as ordered
2. Relieve anxiety/apprehension
   a. Provide instruction in deep breathing and progressive muscle relaxation[2]
3. Allow significant others to remain with patient if supportive
4. Educate patient/significant others

E. EVALUATION AND ONGOING MONITORING

1. Continuously monitor and treat as indicated
2. Monitor patient response/outcomes, and modify nursing care plan as appropriate
3. If positive patient outcomes are not demonstrated, reevaluate assessment and/or plan of care

F. DOCUMENTATION OF INTERVENTIONS AND PATIENT RESPONSE

G. AGE-RELATED CONSIDERATIONS

1. Pediatrics

a. Growth or development related
   1) Appropriate behavior varies with age
   2) Many disorders have age-specific onset; others cross all age groups or occur at various points along age continuum
b. "Pearls"
   1) It is often difficult to determine whether a child's behavior is abnormal or merely part of normal adjustment to life's developmental challenges. If behavior seriously interferes with personal, family, or social adjustment, it is most likely deviant and in need of attention
   2) Many children and adolescents rely on acting-out behaviors to express emotions. This situation may signify a problem when behaviors are socially or culturally unacceptable. These children or adolescents may come to the attention of emergency department personnel when they are brought in by police, school, or family
2. Geriatrics
   a. Aging related
      1) Declining health may be contributory
      2) Dementia and Alzheimer disease
      3) Most common problems include depression, suicide potential, suspiciousness and altered perceptions, anxiety, situational crisis, and sleep pattern disturbances
   b. "Pearls"
      1) Assessment should include determination of drug/alcohol abuse and suicide risk
      2) Thorough assessment of prescribed medication therapy and dosing schedules: certain drugs can cause depression (e.g., propranolol [Inderal], chloral hydrate, digitalis, corticosteroids, and sulfonamides)
      3) Evaluation must rule out organic cause of mental health manifestations
      4) Personal losses and socioeconomic stressors, frequently seen with the older adult, can precipitate emotional disorders

II. Specific Psychosocial Emergencies

A. ANXIETY AND PANIC REACTIONS

It should be assumed that all patients who arrive in an emergency department are experiencing some level of stress and anxiety. Stress reduction interventions should be employed as a standard of care to reduce symptoms and improve clinical outcomes. Anxiety can be brought on by a situational event or it may be a chronic response to ineffective coping skills. Anxiety initiates the fight-or-flight stress response. The stress related to medical emergencies, treatment, or health conditions is often associated with concomitant anxiety. Levels of anxiety range from mild to severe, including panic reactions with corresponding symptoms ranging from mild discomfort to a lack of functional capability.[2] Anxiety is a subjective individual experience ranging from vague discomfort to a feeling of impending disaster or death. Approximately 18% of U.S. adults have an anxiety disorder. General anxiety disorder (GAD) is defined by symptomatic and extreme worry for over 6 months. Anxiety occurs as a result of a threat to self, self-esteem, or identity and can be manifested as apprehension in response to known or imagined threats. Anxiety may heighten during developmental changes; when extreme effort is needed to cope with a situational crisis; or with use of stimulants, iatrogenic agents such as inhaled beta$_2$ agonists, amphetamines, alcohol, or narcotics. A panic disorder is exhibited with a sudden and chronic attack of fear known as a panic attack. A panic attack is a fear of losing control, death, or catastrophe when no real danger exists. Patients can have real physical reactions that can include an accelerated heart rate, shortness of breath, dizziness, weakness, paraesthesia, and chest or abdominal pain.[3]

1. Assessment
   a. Subjective data collection
      1) History of present illness/injury/chief complaint (Table 27.1)
         a) Previous episodes
         b) Precipitating event
         c) Measures already taken by patient that have helped
         d) Family history of organic disease and anxiety disorders
         e) Occurrence during developmental cycle
            (1) Children: separation from parents
            (2) Adolescents: extreme peer pressure, perceived loss of love, failure to achieve
            (3) Adults: midlife crisis, marriage, divorce, menopause, failure to achieve goals
            (4) Elderly: loss of significant other, loss of home, increased dependence, death of friends
         f) Physical ailments causing pain or impairment in function
         g) Impaired communication abilities resulting from stroke, hearing impairment, blindness, lack of language fluency
         h) Insufficiency of previously used coping patterns
         i) Acute changes in health
         j) Lack of knowledge regarding available resources
         k) Inadequate parenting patterns with maltreatment (see Chapter 3)
         l) Recent life change (e.g., occupation, relationships, responsibilities)
         m) Difficulty with sleep
         n) Events causing anger

Part 2

Table 27.1

Anxiety Levels and Characteristics

Level	Characteristics
Level I	Mild state: patient aware of multiple environmental stimuli; able to solve problems; can understand information; has insight; vital signs slightly elevated
Level II	Moderate state: patient aware of environmental stimuli but focuses on immediate problem; voices concern; cooperative with caregiver; follows directions or instructions; slight increase in physiological responses (e.g., facial twitches, trembling lips)
Level III	Severe anxiety state: patient focuses on minute details; does not grasp entire situation; responds to multiple stimuli; unable to focus on priority events; demonstrates startle reaction; exhibits regressive behaviors, agitation, restlessness, sleeplessness, increased pacing with no purpose; difficulty with following directions and asks repeatedly for directions; increased tone, pitch, rate of speech; difficulty with sustaining meaningful conversation; diminished ability to organize; dependent on others to solve problems; decreased eye contact
Level IV	Panic anxiety state: patient cannot solve problems or think logically; requires safety precautions because of disrupted perceptual fields; appears terrorized, withdrawn, detached; exhibits intense nervousness, apprehension, or purposeless behavior; disengaged from environmental situation; completely absorbed with self; may be noncommunicative; may misinterpret stimuli and conversation with others; short of breath; exhibits poor motor coordination; pale skin and mucous membranes; muscle cramping; may experience personality disorganization

o) Passivity in face of threats
p) Feeling of impending doom, including sensation of heart attack or choking
q) Reports of sexual difficulties, including impotence, lack of desire, dyspareunia (abnormal pain during sexual intercourse)
2) Past medical history
a) Current or preexisting diseases/illness
(1) Anxiety disorder
(2) Conversion disorder
(3) Posttraumatic stress disorder
b) Phobias
c) Hyperventilation syndrome
d) Substance use/abuse
e) Medications
f) Allergies
g) Immunization status
b. Objective data collection
1) Physical examination (see Table 27.1)
a) General appearance
(1) Level of consciousness, behavior, affect: agitation, hyperalertness

(2) Tachycardia, hypertension, hyperventilation
(3) Possible elevated temperature
(4) Moderate to severe distress/discomfort
b) Inspection
(1) Pupillary dilation
(2) Ptosis (drooping of upper eyelids) may be caused by muscle fatigue, oculomotor nerve dysfunction, chronic eyelid edema
(3) Skin hair erect
(4) Nystagmus: eye movements that result from stimulation of semicircular canals and reflect oculovestibular and cerebral cortex functioning
(5) Tremors: tense musculature
(6) Startle reaction
(7) Pacing
(8) Cardiac dysrhythmias on monitor: premature ectopy
c) Auscultation
(1) Breath sounds: normal
(2) Bowel sounds: normal to hyperactive
(3) Heart sounds: tachycardic
d) Palpation/percussion
(1) Increased reflex responses and clumsy movements
(2) Abdominal distention: sympathetic nervous system stimulation
(3) Skin cool and clammy
2) Diagnostic procedures
a) CBC with differential
b) Serum chemistries
c) Serum and urine toxicology screen
d) ECG
2. Analysis: differential nursing diagnoses/collaborative problems
a. Anxiety/fear
b. Impaired gas exchange
c. Impaired verbal communication
d. Ineffective individual or family coping
e. Risk for injury
f. Deficient knowledge
g. Disturbed thought processes
3. Planning and implementation/interventions
a. Maintain airway, breathing, circulation (see Chapter 1)
b. Provide supplemental oxygen as indicated
1) If patient is hyperventilating, encourage slow, diaphragmatic breathing and relaxation exercises, after ruling out organic cause. Never use techniques such as paper bag rebreathing or applying an oxygen facemask without oxygen supply. This has been associated in patient deaths with AMI, PE, or pneumothorax[4]
c. Establish IV access for administration of crystalloid fluids/medications as needed

d. Prepare for/assist with medical interventions
   1) Institute cardiac and pulse oximetry monitoring
   2) Build trusting-caring relationship
      a) Introduce self and explain role to patient
      b) Enhance acceptance and self-esteem by acknowledging patient's anxiety and offering reassurance
      c) Provide for safety and security needs
   3) Communicate in calm manner
      a) Explain all procedures in simple, understandable terms
      b) Convey attitude of acceptance
   4) Employ stress reduction techniques using therapeutic communication, instruction on deep breathing, muscle relation, and guided imagery[2]
   5) Assist patient in recognizing causes and effects of anxiety
   6) Direct patient to refocus attention to begin problem-solving process
      a) Facilitate patient's expression of feelings
      b) Emphasize realistic perceptions
   7) Assist patient with problem-solving activities
      a) Identify precipitating event
      b) Determine measures already taken to resolve problem
      c) Determine usual coping measures
   8) Determine options available
      a) Select most desirable option
      b) Offer direct assistance
      c) Verbally acknowledge and comment positively on appropriate problem solving by patient
   9) Assist patient in determining source of fear and identify means of allaying fear
   10) If there is potential for injury related to poisoning or trauma, refer for crisis evaluation and suicide risk assessment
   11) Place patient in area where he or she can be closely observed
   12) If thought processes are altered, orient patient to current reality; refer for psychiatric evaluation to determine whether judgment is impaired; help make appropriate and safe discharge disposition
   13) Work with health care team to determine whether discharge is appropriate or supportive environment is necessary until acute stage of anxiety abates
e. Administer pharmacologic therapy as ordered
   1) Antianxiety
      a) Diazepam (Valium): long acting
      b) Chlordiazepoxide (Librium): medium acting
      c) Lorazepam (Ativan): short acting
   2) Antipanic
      a) Clonazepam (Klonopin)

f. Educate patient/significant others
   1) If patient has altered health maintenance, identify type of impairment and refer for appropriate follow-up care
   2) Ascertain degree of knowledge deficit and provide up-to-date information
   3) Refer to community resources such as Alcoholics Anonymous, counseling services, social support services, community mental health centers, crisis intervention hotlines as appropriate, depending on patient's underlying problems
   4) If patient expresses distress in parenting, determine severity and make referral to appropriate service: family counseling center, community outreach service, governmental child protective services
   5) If sleep disturbance is present, teach sleep hygiene measures; consult with physician regarding prescribed medications
   6) Teach patient appropriate use of prescribed medication
4. Evaluation and ongoing monitoring
   a. Decrease in anxiety level
   b. Hemodynamic status
   c. Breath sounds and pulse oximetry
   d. Cardiac rate and rhythm

B. BIPOLAR DISORDER

Manic-depressive illness, or bipolar affective disorder, is characterized by alternating euphoric moods and depressed periods (see "Depression"). Affect can be unpredictable and labile, with mood changes occurring in minutes, hours, or days, or there may be lengthy periods of stability between episodes. When in a manic state, a patient can be euphoric, highly social, and/or sexually inappropriate. Impairment in thinking may be present with flight of ideas and grandiosity. Grandiose auditory hallucinations may also be present. Subtle impairment of thinking may be evidenced by poor social judgment, inflated self-esteem, and arrogance. The patient may be irritable, hostile, and paranoid when stressed. Bizarre behavior may be present with flamboyant actions, impulsive behavior, and disorganized activity. There is often a family history of manic-depressive disease and a history of repeated cycles. Antidepressant therapy, substance abuse, and organic problems may precipitate mania. Pregnant female patients with a bipolar history have an increased risk of developing postpartum psychosis. Patients experiencing bipolar disorder often return to premorbid functioning with medication and therapy.
1. Assessment
   a. Subjective data collection
      1) History of present illness/injury/chief complaint
         a) Previous manic and/or depressive episodes
         b) Sleep pattern disturbance, with patient frequently feeling he or she requires very little sleep

c) Rapid onset of symptoms, usually during 2-week period
d) Labile emotions; euphoria and depression
e) Noncompliance with prescribed medication regimen (e.g., lithium, divalproex sodium [Depakote], carbamazepine [Tegretol], clonazepam [Klonopin]) may be precipitant
2) Past medical history
   a) Current or preexisting diseases/illness
      (1) Repeated cycles of mania and depression
      (2) Infections
      (3) Endocrine disorders
      (4) Neoplastic disorders
   b) Substance and/or alcohol use/abuse
   c) Medications
   d) Allergies
   e) Immunization status
b. Objective data collection
   1) Physical examination
      a) General appearance
         (1) Level of consciousness, behavior, affect: hallucinations, flight of ideas; sadness
         (2) Hygiene: poor, unkempt appearance or grandiose and bright clothing
         (3) Moderate to severe distress/discomfort
      b) Inspection
         (1) Rapid and pressured speech, or low and depressed speech pattern
         (2) Grandiose context to speech or mono-tone voice
         (3) Intact intellect
         (4) Hyperactivity/hypoactivity
   2) Diagnostic procedures
      a) CBC with differential
      b) ESR
      c) Serum chemistries including glucose, BUN, creatinine
      d) Serum and urine toxicology screen and drug levels
      e) Serum alcohol level
      f) Thyroid function tests
      g) Urinalysis; pregnancy test in female patients of childbearing age
      h) ECG
2. Analysis: differential nursing diagnoses/collaborative problems
   a. Disturbed thought processes
   b. Risk for injury
   c. Disturbed sensory perception: visual or auditory
   d. Ineffective coping
   e. Noncompliance
3. Planning and implementation/interventions
   a. Maintain airway, breathing, circulation (see Chapters 1 and 32)
   b. Provide supplemental oxygen as indicated

c. Establish IV access for administration of crystalloid fluids/medications as needed
d. Prepare for/assist with medical interventions
   1) Institute cardiac and pulse oximetry monitoring as indicated
   2) If patient is delusional, acknowledge thought disorder and orient to reality
   3) Provide safety by restraints per institutional policy, as necessary, and by continuous observation
   4) Treat injuries sustained as result of psychotic behavior
   5) Calm patient by speaking softly and placing away from stimulating environment
   6) Remove all implements or objects that may cause harm to patient or others
   7) Treat medical problems caused by malnutrition if present (e.g., dehydration and electrolyte imbalance)
   8) If patient's judgment is affected secondary to mania or depression, protect from external stimuli by removing to area where there are fewer stimuli; patient must be observable at all times
   9) Work with health care team to make appropriate disposition to supportive environment
e. Administer pharmacologic therapy as ordered
   1) Lithium
   2) Anticonvulsants
   3) Antipsychotic agents
   4) Antianxiety agents
f. Educate patient/significant others
   1) Refer patient to crisis intervention nurse or psychiatrist for evaluation
   2) Instruct patient on importance of taking prescribed medication
4. Evaluation and ongoing monitoring
   a. Hemodynamic status
   b. Cardiac rate rhythm

C. DEPRESSION

Depression consists of specific alterations in mood, often accompanied by a negative self-concept, and physical changes, along with changes in activity and interest levels. Depression is suspected when at least five of the following characteristics last for 2 weeks: (1) loss of interest in usual activities, (2) depressed mood, (3) appetite increase or decrease with weight change, (4) insomnia or hypersomnia, (5) fatigue, (6) psychomotor agitation or retardation, (7) decreased ability to think, (8) recurrent thoughts of death, or (9) feelings of worthlessness. The symptoms of clinical depression are distinct from those that may occur in situational events such as in bereavement, medical conditions, or substance abuse.
1. Assessment
   a. Subjective data collection

1) History of present illness/injury/chief complaint
   a) Precipitating events
   b) Depressed affect and loss of interest in diversional activities and social relationships
   c) Fatigue and insomnia or hypersomnia
   d) Somatic complaints
      (1) Low back pain
      (2) Fatigue
      (3) Headaches
   e) Weight changes: loss or gain
   f) Psychomotor agitation or retardation
   g) Difficulty in concentrating
   h) Recurrent thoughts of death and suicidal ideation
   i) Feelings of worthlessness
   j) Increase in substance abuse, alcohol, prescription, or OTC medication use
   k) Situational crisis
      (1) Recent childbirth (postpartum depression)
      (2) Loss of significant other or support system
      (3) Acute health changes
      (4) Chronic illness resulting from perpetual strain of long-term treatment regimens
      (5) Changes in role performance, occupational status, and power base
      (6) Separation from spiritual or cultural background
   l) Occurrence during developmental cycle
      (1) Children may demonstrate hyperactivity, enuresis, or regressive behavior
      (2) Adolescents may present as the result of delinquency or injuries related to trauma; they may be cynical, detached, angry, hostile, disillusioned, and lonely; there may also be sexual promiscuity, acting-out behavior, alcohol and drug abuse
      (3) Adults, including elderly, may have symptoms similar to those of adolescents; they may have poor hygiene; and they may relay loss of interest in social life, decreased sexual activity, inability to concentrate
   m) Toxic ingestion (see Chapter 26)
2) Past medical history
   a) Current or preexisting diseases/illness
      (1) Depression, including family history of depression
      (2) Illness that necessitates prolonged and painful treatment regimens or that has no known cure
   b) Injury that has caused debilitation/chronic pain
   c) Medications
   d) Allergies
   e) Immunization status
b. Objective data collection

1) Physical examination
   a) General appearance
      (1) Level of consciousness, behavior, affect: quiet and withdrawn demeanor, restricted affect (limited emotional expression), dysphoric mood
      (2) Gait: slowed
      (3) Hygiene: poor, unkempt
      (4) Moderate to severe distress/discomfort
   b) Inspection
      (1) Crying
      (2) Increased/decreased verbalization
   c) Auscultation
      (1) Breath sounds: normal
      (2) Bowel sounds: decreased
2) Diagnostic procedures
   a) Thyroid function tests
   b) Serum and urine toxicology screen
   c) Serum alcohol level
   d) Urinalysis; pregnancy test in female patients of childbearing age
   e) Brain CT scan or MRI
   f) ECG
2. Analysis: differential nursing diagnosis/collaborative problems
   a. Impaired verbal communication
   b. Ineffective coping
   c. Risk for injury
   d. Deficient knowledge
   e. Disturbed thought processes
3. Planning and implementation/interventions
   a. Maintain airway, breathing, circulation (see Chapters 1 and 32)
   b. Provide supplemental oxygen as indicated
   c. Establish IV access for administration of crystalloid fluids/medications as needed
   d. Prepare for/assist with medical interventions
      1) Institute cardiac and pulse oximetry monitoring as indicated
      2) Convey attitude of acceptance
      3) Encourage patient to identify feelings
      4) Assist patient in recognizing causes and effects of depression
      5) Place patient in safe and observable area
      6) Determine whether poison ingestion has occurred and treat: gastric lavage, activated charcoal as indicated (see Chapter 26)
      7) Refer for crisis evaluation of suicidal risk (see "Suicide or Suicidal Behavior")
      8) For impaired overall health, help patient identify type of impairment and necessary modifications in lifestyle
      9) Inquire whether spiritual belief and support systems can be used to affect feelings
      10) If thought processes are altered, orient patient to current reality

11) Work with health care team to determine whether discharge is appropriate or supportive environment is necessary until acute stage of depression abates
   e. Administer pharmacologic therapy as ordered
   f. Educate patient/significant others
      1) If nutritional excess is present, refer to community program for weight control and behavior modification
      2) Ascertain degree of knowledge deficit and provide up-to-date information
      3) Refer to community resources such as Alcoholics Anonymous for alcohol dependency, family counseling services or governmental family protective services for difficulty in parenting, social support services for economic difficulties or social isolation, counseling for underlying disturbance in self-concept, and crisis intervention hotlines for use in case of acute distress
      4) Consult with psychiatrist/physician regarding prescribed medications, and teach patient appropriate use of prescribed medications
      5) Refer to religious counseling if desired by patient or cultural centers if patient is not in native culture
4. Evaluation and ongoing monitoring
   a. Improvement in depression
   b. Hemodynamic monitoring
   c. Breath sounds and pulse oximetry
   d. Cardiac rate and rhythm

D. EATING DISORDERS

Although not commonly thought of as an emergency, eating disorders have the highest mortality rate of any psychological disorders. Patients with eating disorders often reach an emergency condition before they are diagnosed. Females account for 88% of all eating disorder hospitalizations. Admitting diagnoses include eating disorder—unspecified (39%), anorexia nervosa (34%), bulimia nervosa (21%), pica (6%), and psychogenic vomiting (2%). Almost half of all eating disorder admissions occur in patient 19–45 years of age. Physical results of this disorder may include dehydration, nutritional deficiencies (47%), electrolyte imbalance (34%), and cardiac arrhythmias (24%). These patients may require admission to the intensive care unit (ICU). Secondary diagnoses may include acute liver or renal failure (4%). Any adolescent or young adult female patient presenting to the emergency department with low body weight, amenorrhea, yellow skin (hypercarotenemia), muscle weakening, constipation, cool skin on the extremities, and dehydration should be assessed for possible eating disorders. Mood disorders are a principle diagnosis in 36% of those hospitalized with an eating disorder. Immediate care in the emergency department is directed by the physiologic symptoms that brought them to the emergency department, but the plan of care should consider the eating disorder as the underlying cause.[5]

1. Assessment
   a. Subjective data collection
      1) History of present illness/chief complaint
         a) Appetite and weight changes
         b) Exercise patterns
         c) Pain (see Chapter 8)
         d) Vomiting, diarrhea
      2) Past medical history
         a) Current or preexisting diseases/illness
            (1) Psychological disorders
            (2) Anorexia/bulimia
         b) Substance and/or alcohol use/abuse
         c) Laxative and/or diet pill use
         d) Last normal menstrual period: female patients of childbearing age
         e) Current medications
            (1) Prescription
            (2) OTC/herbal
         f) Allergies
         g) Immunization status
   b. Objective data collection
      1) Physical examination
         a) General appearance
            (1) Level of consciousness, behavior, affect: possible depression
            (2) Possible hypotension, tachycardia, orthostasis
            (3) Moderate to severe distress/discomfort
         b) Inspection
            (1) Thinness
            (2) Dry, brittle hair
            (3) Yellow skin
            (4) Tooth enamel erosion
            (5) Cardiac dysrhythmias on monitor
         c) Palpation/percussion
            (1) Diminished deep tendon reflexes
            (2) Cool, dry skin
            (3) Poor skin turgor
      2) Diagnostic procedures
         a) CBC with differential
         b) Serum chemistries including glucose, BUN, creatinine
            (1) Hyponatremia
            (2) Hypoglycemia
            (3) Hypokalemia
            (4) Hypomagnesemia
            (5) BUN: possible elevation
         c) ABGs
            (1) Metabolic alkalosis with prolonged vomiting
            (2) Metabolic acidosis with laxative abuse
         d) ESR: if elevated, possible organic cause
         e) Serum and urine toxicology screen
         f) Urinalysis; pregnancy test in female patients of childbearing age

g) Thyroid function tests

h) ECG

2. Analysis: differential nursing diagnoses/collaborative problems

   a. Imbalanced nutrition: less than body requirements

   b. Situational/chronic low self-esteem

3. Planning and implementation/interventions

   a. Maintain airway, breathing, circulation (see Chapter 1)

   b. Provide supplemental oxygen as indicated

   c. Establish IV access for administration of crystalloid fluids/medications

   d. Prepare for/assist with medical interventions

     1) Institute cardiac and pulse oximetry monitoring

     2) Assist with obtaining psychological consultation

     3) Assist with possible hospital admission

   e. Administer pharmacologic therapy as ordered

     1) Electrolyte replacements

   f. Educate patient/significant others

     1) Importance of nutritionally balanced diet

4. Evaluation and ongoing monitoring

   a. Hemodynamic status

   b. Cardiac rate and rhythm

E. GRIEF

Acute grief is a normal emotional reaction to a loss. Although death may be the most significant type of loss, other types of loss include changes in health, body function, body parts, mental acuity, self-image, relationships, economic security, independence, material possessions, and home.

In the emergency care setting, grief may be experienced by a patient who has survived when others perished or by family members who must cope with the sudden loss of a loved one. Regardless of who is experiencing the grief reaction, acceptance, comprehension of the loss, and the painful process of emotionally detaching oneself often begins in the emergency care setting.

The stages of grief are denial or isolation, anger, bargaining, depression, and acceptance. People do not always experience the stages of grief in the order listed. It is best to use them as a guide to understand the grieving process. People may be very emotional and demonstrative or experience their grief more internally. Emergency nurses must be careful not to judge how they believe a patient should or should not express grief.[6]

1. Assessment

   a. Subjective data collection

     1) History of present illness/injury/chief complaint

       a) Identifies loss as real or threatened

       b) Describes measures or attempts to resolve situations that have been successful or unsuccessful

       c) Somatic complaints

         (1) Abdominal pain

         (2) Vague symptoms similar to now deceased family member, friend

       d) Syncope

     2) Past medical history

       a) Current or preexisting diseases/illness

         (1) Cardiovascular disease

         (2) Pulmonary disease

       b) Medications

       c) Allergies

   b. Objective data collection

     1) Physical examination

       a) General appearance

         (1) Level of consciousness, behavior, affect: agitation, withdrawn

         (2) Tachypnea, tachycardia

         (3) Mild to moderate distress/discomfort

     2) Diagnostic procedures

       a) Thyroid function tests

       b) Serum and urine toxicology screen

       c) Serum alcohol level

       d) Urinalysis; pregnancy test in female patients of childbearing age

       e) ECG

2. Analysis: differential nursing diagnoses/collaborative problems

   a. Anticipatory/dysfunctional grieving

3. Planning and implementation/interventions

   a. Maintain airway, breathing, circulation (see Chapters 1 and 32)

   b. Provide supplemental oxygen as indicated

   c. Establish IV access for administration of crystalloid fluids/medications as needed

   d. Prepare for/assist with medical interventions

     1) Institute cardiac and pulse oximetry monitoring

     2) Appear confident, establish trusting relationship, and allow for unhurried time

     3) Escort into private room

     4) Facilitate discussion of concerns, worries, feelings

     5) Provide periodic reports to update progress or lack of progress; all information should be honest and delivered in a caring fashion

     6) Use hospital health care team members (e.g., social workers, clergy, psychiatric clinical nurse specialists, and mental health care team members) as needed to assist, support, and stay with individual experiencing grief

     7) Call other persons in the social network (family, friends, and clergy or spiritual advisor) to provide ongoing support and to help survivor work through and prepare for anticipated loss

     8) Suggest "what if ...?" situations to help survivor work through and prepare for anticipated death or loss

     9) Encourage survivor to talk about impending loss and its meaning

     10) Actively listen to response

11) Accept all behavioral responses (e.g., denial, hope for improved status, and silence); do not insist on talking
12) Evaluate survivor's coping ability and express confidence in his or her ability to cope
13) When death has occurred
    a) With physician, inform survivors or significant others of death and refer to deceased by name
    b) Explain course of resuscitation/death in simple and understandable terms
    c) Provide emotional support to bereaved; be aware of religious and cultural needs
    d) Offer opportunity to view body (offer may need to be repeated)
       (1) Prepare survivors for alterations in physical appearance (e.g., those caused by trauma) of deceased
       (2) Accompany survivors, but remain unobtrusive to provide privacy
    e) Report death to legal authorities
    f) Help survivors to focus attention on decisions requiring immediate action
       (1) Organ and tissue donation (see Chapter 7)
       (2) Postmortem examination, if family has option
       (3) Signing for valuables, property, clothing of deceased
       (4) Tentative selection of funeral home
    g) Assist survivors to practice how to tell others, especially young children, about death; emphasize use of words "he is dead" or "she is dead"
    h) Help survivors "leave" when the time is right
  e. Administer pharmacologic therapy as ordered
  f. Educate patient/significant others
    1) Plan with survivor, if possible, or arrange for appropriate referral to initiate follow-up telephone call in 4–6 weeks
    2) Refer as needed to community agencies

F. HOMICIDAL OR VIOLENT BEHAVIOR

Violence is the acting out of the emotions of fear or anger to achieve desired goals. The causation of violence may be due to psychosis, antisocial behavior, or organic disease. Violence is described as an assault on a person or object with intent to harm or destroy. Homicidal behavior is violence with intent to kill directed at another person. During a violent or homicidal encounter, a high level of panic may be present, with a resultant loss of reasoning ability. Violence may also be used as a defense mechanism for self-protection or for the protection of loved ones when a person is feeling attacked either emotionally or physically. The patient may be either the attacker or the victim. Violent behavior in the emergency department has become increasingly prevalent,

and it is imperative that personnel take measures to protect themselves and their patients from harm.

1. Assessment
   a. Subjective data collection
      1) History of present illness/injury/chief complaint
         a) Precipitating events
         b) Substance and/or alcohol use/abuse
         c) Previous homicidal or violent behavior
         d) Suicidal thoughts
         e) Child maltreatment
         f) Preoccupation with sexual thoughts and fantasies
         g) Childhood history of enuresis, fire setting, cruelty to animals, fighting, school problems
      2) Past medical history
         a) Current or preexisting diseases/illness
            (1) Psychosis
            (2) Organic disease: temporal lobe epilepsy
            (3) Head injury
         b) Medications
         c) Allergies
         d) Immunization status
   b. Objective data collection
      1) Physical examination
         a) General appearance
            (1) Level of consciousness, behavior, affect: alert, agitation
            (2) Tachycardia, hypertension
            (3) Moderate to severe distress/discomfort
         b) Inspection
            (1) Possible obvious injuries
            (2) Skin color: pale
            (3) Cardiac dysrhythmias on monitor: premature atrial contractions
         c) Palpation
            (1) Skin diaphoretic
      2) Diagnostic procedures
         a) CBC with differential: white blood cell count may be slightly elevated secondary to injury
         b) Serum chemistries: potassium level may be elevated with injury
         c) Serum and urine toxicology screen
         d) Serum alcohol level
         e) ECG
2. Analysis: differential nursing diagnoses/collaborative problems
   a. Ineffective coping
   b. Disturbed thought processes
   c. Risk for self-directed or other-directed violence
   d. Risk for injury
   e. Anxiety/fear
3. Planning and implementation/interventions
   a. Maintain airway, breathing, circulation (see Chapters 1 and 32)
   b. Provide supplemental oxygen as indicated

c. Establish IV access for administration of crystalloid fluids/medications as needed
d. Prepare for/assist with medical interventions
   1) Institute cardiac and pulse oximetry monitoring as indicated
   2) Ensure safety of self and others before intervening with violent/homicidal patient
   3) Treat any patient injuries
   4) Encourage patient to identify feelings
   5) Help patient to determine cause, effect, possible solutions to ineffective coping
   6) Orient patient to current reality (time, place, person)
   7) If thought processes are altered to degree that patient or others may be harmed, work with health care team to place patient in supportive environment
   8) Remove guns, knives, matches, or other devices that could harm others; use security or police personnel to assist
   9) Restrain patient per institutional protocols, as necessary, with mechanical restraints
   10) Provide safe environment; patient should be placed away from others whenever possible, yet within observable area for ease in monitoring
   11) Keep door open to area where patient is being treated to reduce possibility of patient's feeling trapped
   12) If family processes are altered, report to governmental authorities for investigation
   13) Facilitate open communication by listening objectively
   14) Provide reality orientation regarding role performance, personal identity, self-esteem, body image, obstacles to improved health
   15) Help patient decide whether spiritual belief and support systems can be used in current situation
   16) Contact spiritual advisor if patient requests
e. Administer pharmacologic therapy as ordered
   1) Antipsychotic medications: haloperidol (Haldol)
f. Educate patient/significant others
   1) Refer to community resources, including psychiatric counselors, mental health centers, and crisis intervention hotlines
   2) If patient is in police custody, arrange psychiatric follow-up care
4. Expected outcomes/evaluation
   a. Level of consciousness
   b. Hemodynamic status
   c. Breath sounds and pulse oximetry
   d. Cardiac rate and rhythm

G. INEFFECTIVE COPING AND SITUATIONAL CRISIS

Ineffective coping occurs when an individual is unable to solve problems and deal with internal or external stressors.

The events may be unexpected or anticipated occurrences with unanticipated consequences. A situational crisis is often initiated by a period of shock with a heightened emotional response and followed by an inability to function.[3] This can result in a feeling of fatigue and exhaustion. The situational crisis may precipitate behavior that includes excessive alcohol intake, drug abuse, and suicidal, homicidal, or criminal behavior. The individual experiencing the crisis may be so overwhelmed by the situation that he or she is unable to use help effectively. Social isolation may be a result of an individual's attempt to cope with anxiety and is often evident in patients with a chronic disease during an exacerbation of the illness.

1. Assessment
   a. Subjective data collection
      1) History of present illness/injury/chief complaint
         a) Precipitating event or change in previous level of functioning
         b) Recent loss or change in body appearance
         c) Persistent stressor or sudden, recent stressors
            (1) New employment
            (2) Move to new geographic location
            (3) Frequent illness or accidents
            (4) Demands of school or job/family
         d) Maturational crisis of patient or family member (e.g., birth, marriage, retirement)
         e) Ingestion of substance to alter mood
         f) Reliance on ineffective or inappropriate coping strategies
         g) Natural disaster
      2) Past medical history
         a) Current or preexisting diseases/illness
            (1) Pulmonary disease
            (2) Diabetes
            (3) Cardiovascular disease
         b) Substance or alcohol use/abuse
         c) Medications
         d) Allergies
         e) Immunization status
   b. Objective data collection
      1) Physical examination
         a) General appearance
            (1) Level of consciousness, behavior, affect: agitation, tremors, tenseness, altered affect, altered thought process
            (2) Hygiene: unkempt appearance
            (3) Moderate to severe distress/discomfort
         b) Inspection
            (1) Tremors
            (2) Diminished impulse control
            (3) Evidence of physical violence or self-destructive behavior
      2) Diagnostic procedures
         a) CBC with differential
         b) Serum chemistries
         c) Serum and urine toxicology screen

2. Analysis: differential nursing diagnoses/collaborative problems
   a. Ineffective individual or family coping
   b. Situational low self-esteem
   c. Disturbed thought processes
   d. Dysfunctional grieving
   e. Anxiety/fear
   f. Ineffective health maintenance
3. Planning and implementation/interventions
   a. Maintain airway, breathing, circulation (see Chapters 1 and 32)
   b. Provide supplemental oxygen as indicated
   c. Establish IV access for administration of crystalloid fluids/medications as needed
   d. Prepare for/assist with medical interventions
      1) Institute cardiac and pulse oximetry monitoring
      2) Assist patient to identify precipitating event
      3) Assist patient to identify measures to resolve problem with usual method of coping
      4) Help patient to define and clarify realistic options
      5) Structure priorities for problem-solving interventions
      6) Provide time and opportunity for communication and support the patient in seeking assistance in the emergency department
      7) If thought processes are disturbed, protect patient from harm
   e. Administer pharmacologic therapy as ordered
   f. Educate patient/significant others
      1) Refer to community resources such as Alcoholics Anonymous, counseling service, social support service, and community or mental health center
      2) Refer frequently seen patients to social worker, mental health professional, or mental health care team to establish realistic care plan
4. Evaluation and ongoing monitoring
   a. Deceased agitation, tenseness
   b. Hemodynamic status
   c. Breath sounds and pulse oximetry
   d. Cardiac rate and rhythm

H. PSYCHOTIC, OR BRIEF PSYCHOTIC, BEHAVIOR

Psychotic behavior is the result of a pathologic process that may be acute or chronic, with resultant distorted perceptions, disorganized thinking, impaired judgment, impaired decision making, and regression. Manifestations occur in the areas of affect, behavior, perception, and thinking. The mood may range from flat affect to euphoria. Behaviors exhibited may include acting-out, impulsiveness, and psychomotor retardation or agitation. Psychotic behavior can also include changes in perception such as illusions, hallucinations, and depersonalization. Impaired thinking is exhibited by delusions, loose associations, and incoherence. Psychoses can be functional or organic. Functional types

include schizophrenia, mania, psychotic depression, and brief reactive psychosis. Organic psychoses include dementia, delirium, and toxic drug-induced psychosis (Table 27.2).
1. Assessment
   a. Subjective data collection
      1) History of present illness/injury/chief complaint
         a) Schizophrenia: familial history and onset before age 45 years
            (1) Bizarre behavior, including but not limited to reports of decreased ability to care for self or function in work or social environment
            (2) Delusions
            (3) Auditory hallucinations
            (4) Paranoia
         b) Mania
            (1) Previous episodes
            (2) Decreased need for sleep
            (3) Increased physical activity
            (4) Paranoia may be present
            (5) Impulsive and flamboyant behavior
            (6) Euphoria or elation
            (7) Unrealistic plans or thoughts
         c) Psychotic depression
            (1) Loss of energy and pleasure
            (2) Possible command hallucinations
            (3) Agitation
            (4) Lack of communication with others
            (5) Psychomotor retardation
            (6) Decreased ability or desire to care for self

Table 27.2

Psychotic Disorders

Disorder	Characteristics
Schizophrenia	Familial history; onset before 45 years of age; bizarre behavior including but not limited to reports of decreased ability to care for self or function in work or social environment
Mania	Delusions of grandeur; auditory hallucinations; labile and euphoric affect; rapid and fluent speech; sexual content of thought or speech often present
Psychotic depression	Psychomotor retardation; paucity of speech; auditory or olfactory hallucinations; disorganized thinking; preoccupation with death and morbid thoughts; possible impaired cognition
Delirium	Rapid onset/fluctuating course; tactile, visual, olfactory hallucinations; disorientation to time, place, person; memory impairment; blunted affect; confabulation (fictitious stories that fill in memory gaps); can have organic causes
Dementia	Repetitive speech; recent memory loss and disorientation; lack of awareness of problem; impaired intellectual cognition

d) Delirium (organic disorders must be ruled out)
(1) Rapid onset of symptoms, fluctuating course
(2) Restlessness, insomnia, nightmares
(3) Trouble with thinking clearly and without insight into problems
(4) Changes in temperament
e) Dementia
(1) Gradual onset of symptoms
(2) Noticeable personality changes
(3) Memory loss and disorientation
(4) Possible paranoid delusions
(5) "Sundowning": lucid in morning with worsening at night
2) Past medical history
a) Current or preexisting diseases/illness
(1) Known psychiatric disorder
b) Substance and/or alcohol use/abuse
c) Medications
d) Allergies
e) Immunization status
b. Objective data collection
1) Physical examination
a) General appearance
(1) Level of consciousness, behavior, affect: agitation, presence of hallucinations
(2) Possible tachycardia, hypertension, tachypnea
(3) Severe distress/discomfort
b) Inspection (see Table 27.2)
2) Diagnostic procedures
a) CBC with differential: elevated white blood cell count if infection present
b) Serum chemistries including glucose, BUN, creatinine
c) Serum and urine toxicology screen
d) Urinalysis: leukocytes present if infection; pregnancy test in female patients of childbearing age
e) Thyroid function tests
f) Venereal Disease Research Laboratories (VDRL) or rapid plasma reagin (RPR) test
g) ABGs
h) Stool for occult blood
i) Lumbar puncture: cerebral spinal fluid analysis
j) ECG
k) Head CT scan
2. Analysis: differential nursing diagnoses/collaborative problems
a. Disturbed sensory perception: visual or auditory
b. Impaired verbal communication
c. Risk for injury
d. Ineffective coping
3. Planning and implementation/interventions
a. Maintain airway, breathing, circulation (see Chapters 1 and 32)

b. Provide supplemental oxygen as indicated
c. Establish IV access for administration of crystalloid fluids/medications as needed
d. Prepare for/assist with medical interventions
1) Institute cardiac and pulse oximetry monitoring
2) Orient patient to reality (time, place, person)
3) Provide safety per institutional policy by mechanical restraints, as necessary, and by continuous observation; separate patient from heavy traffic areas to avoid escalation that may result from added stimuli
4) Orient patient with respect to hallucinations or delusions; reinforce absence of visual and auditory phenomena
5) Provide atmosphere for open and objective communication
6) Treat injuries sustained as result of psychotic behavior
7) If possibility of environmental exposure exists, treat patient (see Chapter 15)
8) Calm patient by speaking softly and placing away from stimulating environment
9) Remove all implements or objects that may cause harm to patient or others; ask security or police personnel for assistance
10) If patient exhibits delusions of grandeur or other manifestations of distortion in personal identity, orient to and acknowledge reality
11) Work with health care team to make appropriate disposition to protective environment; discharge to home with follow-up services if patient is mentally stable or admit to hospital for continuous supportive environment
e. Administer pharmacologic therapy as prescribed
1) Antipsychotic medications: haloperidol (Haldol), ziprasidone (Geodon), olanzapine (Zyprexa)
2) Antianxiety medications: lorazepam (Ativan)
f. Educate patient/significant others
1) If coping, family process, or health maintenance is identified as an issue, refer to appropriate health care provider for individual or family care; refer to counseling or psychiatric services or department of family services
4. Evaluation and ongoing monitoring
a. Decrease in hallucinations
b. Hemodynamic status
c. Breath sounds and pulse oximetry
d. Cardiac rate and rhythm

I. SUICIDE OR SUICIDAL BEHAVIOR

Suicidal behavior includes acts of self-harm, suicidal ideation or intention, attempted suicide, and thoughts or behaviors that indicate a risk of suicide.[1] Suicide is the tenth leading cause of death in the United States and suicide attempts are responsible for a significant number of mental health–related emergency department admissions. The highest numbers of suicides are committed among the following age groups, respectively: 45–64 years, 85 years and over, and 15–24 years. Eighty percent of all suicides are committed by males, whereas females account for a higher number of suicide attempts. Although female patients make more attempts, the ratio of men to women who die by suicide is 4:1. Veterans are now recognized as a high-risk group as they comprise 22% of all suicides. Suicide by firearms is the most common method of completed suicides for both men (56%) and women (30%). Risk for suicide includes mental disorders (depression being the most common), previous attempt, family history of suicide, serious medical conditions and pain, environmental stressors, suicide contagion, and access to lethal methods.[7]

The patient who presents for emergency care may require immediate intervention for life-threatening situations, depending on the methods used for self-harm. The patient who has exhibited suicidal behavior frequently experiences depression and/or anxiety.

1. Assessment
   a. Suicide screening tools should be used as part of the assessment process for emergency department patients who present with behavioral health complaints or disorders.[1]
   b. Subjective data collection
      1) History of present illness/injury/chief complaint
         a) Precipitating factors
         b) Family history of attempting or succeeding in suicide
         c) Newly diagnosed disease with body changes
         d) Substance and/or alcohol use/abuse
         e) Signs of depression
         f) Prior psychiatric history[1]
         g) Previous suicide attempts
            (1) If there is a history of suicide or suicide attempts (patient or family), assess for
               (a) Intent: probability of being discovered or not
               (b) Lethality: was method used highly lethal or less lethal?
               (c) Did patient suffer physical harm?
         h) Presence of impulsive, violent temperament
      2) Past medical history
         a) Current or preexisting diseases/illness
            (1) Debilitating disease, such as multiple sclerosis and amyotrophic lateral sclerosis
            (2) Chronic disease, such as cancer, acquired immunodeficiency syndrome, human immunodeficiency virus infection, or Parkinson disease
            (3) Depressive illness
            (4) Alcoholism
            (5) Schizophrenia
         b) Substance use/abuse
         c) Medications
         d) Allergies
         e) Immunization status
   c. Objective data collection
      1) Physical examination
         a) General appearance
            (1) Level of consciousness, behavior, affect; depressed, anxiety, seizures, comatose
            (2) Possible hypotension, hypoventilation, tachycardia
            (3) Moderate to severe distress/discomfort
         b) Inspection
            (1) Pupillary changes with substances ingested (see Chapter 26)
            (2) Possible obvious injuries
            (3) Cardiac dysrhythmias on monitor
         c) Palpation/percussion
            (1) Possible depressed deep tendon reflexes
      2) Diagnostic procedures
         a) Serum and urine toxicology screen
         b) Serum alcohol level
         c) Urinalysis; pregnancy test in female patients of childbearing age
         d) Cerebrospinal fluid 5-hydroxyindoleacetic acid: low levels have been associated with suicide attempts
         e) ECG
            (1) QRS complex and QT-interval prolongation
            (2) Conduction defects
            (3) Sinus tachycardia, atrial fibrillation, ventricular dysrhythmias
2. Analysis: differential nursing diagnoses/collaborative problems
   a. Ineffective coping
   b. Risk for violence: self-directed
   c. Disturbed thought processes
3. Planning and implementation/interventions
   a. Maintain airway, breathing, circulation (see Chapters 1 and 32)
   b. Provide supplemental oxygen as indicated
   c. Establish IV access for administration of crystalloid fluids/blood products/medications as needed
   d. Prepare for/assist with medical interventions
      1) Institute cardiac and pulse oximetry monitoring
      2) Encourage patient to identify feelings
      3) Help patient to determine cause, effect, potential solutions to ineffective coping and fear
      4) Orient patient to current reality
      5) Provide safe environment to protect patient (situate in observable area and remove patient medications, guns, knives, sharp objects, matches, or other devices that could harm patient)

6) Restrain patient, per institutional policy, with mechanical restraints for patient safety, if needed

7) Treat toxic ingestion (see Chapter 26)

8) Treat traumatic injuries (see specific chapters)

9) Refer for psychiatric consultation

10) Provide information to consultant regarding patient's suicide plan

    a) Is plan specific?

    b) Does patient have available means?

    c) How lethal are means?

    d) Is patient's behavior impulsive?

11) Ascertain degree of knowledge deficit and provide information

12) Provide reality orientation regarding role performance, personal identity, self-esteem, perceived obstacles to health

13) Inquire whether spiritual belief and support systems can be used to affect feelings and situation

14) Work with health care team to determine whether discharge is appropriate or inpatient admission is necessary for either medical or psychiatric stabilization

15) If discharged, ensure that

    a) Firearms, lethal medications are secured and inaccessible to patient

    b) A supportive person is available and understands follow-up observation and communication

    c) Scheduled follow-up appointment with mental health worker has been made

    d) Name and telephone number of clinician who can be called if emergency occurs have been provided

    e) Crisis service telephone number has been provided

e. Administer pharmacologic therapy as ordered

f. Educate patient/significant others

    1) If patient expresses difficulty with home maintenance management, determine severity and make referral to appropriate home health care service: family counseling, community outreach service, governmental agency for family protection

    2) Refer to appropriate community resources if discharge is appropriate

4. Expected outcomes/evaluation

a. Level of consciousness

b. Hemodynamic status

c. Breath sounds and pulse oximetry

d. Cardiac rate and rhythm

References

1. ENA Emergency Nursing Resources Development Committee: *Clinical practice guideline: suicide risk assessment*, Des Plaines, IL, 2012, Emergency Nurses Association.

2. Park E, Traeger L, Vranceanu A, Scult M, Lerner J, Benson H, Fricchione G: The development of a patient-centered program based on the relaxation response: the Relaxation Response Resiliency Program (3RP), *Psychosomatics* 54(2):165–174, 2013.

3. National Institute of Mental Health: *Panic disorder: when fear overwhelms. NIH Publication No. TR 10–4679*, Bethesda, MD, 2013, NIMH.

4. Kern B: Hyperventilation syndrome treatment & management, *Medscape*, 2014. Retrieved from http://emedicine.medscape.com/article/807277-treatment.

5. Zhao Y, Encinosa W: *An update on hospitalizations for eating disorders, 1999 to 2009. Statistical brief #120: Healthcare Cost and Utilization Project (HCUP) Statistical Briefs*, Rockville, MD, 2011, Agency for Health Care Policy and Research.

6. Axelrod J: The 5 stages of loss and grief, *Psych Central*, 2014. Retrieved from http://psychcentral.com/lib/the-5-stages-of-loss-and-grief.

7. American Foundation for Suicide Prevention: *Suicide: 2015 facts and figures*, New York, NY, 2014, American Foundation for Suicide Prevention.

Bibliography

American Psychiatric Association: *Assessing and treating suicidal behaviors: a quick reference guide*, Arlington, VA, 2004, American Psychiatric Association.

Russinoff I, Clark M: *Suicidal patients: assessing and managing patients presenting with suicidal attempts or ideation. Emergency Medicine Practice*, Alpharetta, GA, 2004, EB Practice.

Shea SC: The delicate art of eliciting suicidal ideation, *Psychiatric Annals* 34(5):386–400, 2004.

Varcarolis E: Psychiatric emergencies. In *Foundations of psychiatric mental health nursing: a clinical approach*, ed 4, Philadelphia, PA, 2002, Saunders, pp 610–720.

Xu J, Kochanek K, Murphy S, Tejada-Vera B: Deaths: final data for 2007, *National Vital Statistics Reports* 58(19), 2010. Hyattsville, MD: NCHS.

Part 2

CHAPTER 28

Respiratory Emergencies

Justin J. Milici, MSN, RN, CEN, CPEN, CFRN, CCRN

MAJOR TOPICS

General Strategies

Assessment

Analysis: Differential Nursing Diagnoses/Collaborative Problems

Planning and Implementation/Interventions

Evaluation and Ongoing Monitoring

Documentation of Interventions and Patient Response

Age-related Considerations

Specific Respiratory Emergencies

Acute Bronchitis

Acute Respiratory Distress Syndrome

Asthma

Bronchiolitis

Chronic Obstructive Pulmonary Disease

Croup (Laryngotracheobronchitis)

Hyperventilation Syndrome

Pleural Effusion

Pneumonia

Pneumothorax (Iatrogenic and Spontaneous) and Pneumomediastinum

Pulmonary Embolism

I. General Strategies

A. ASSESSMENT

1. Primary and secondary assessment/resuscitation (see Chapter 1)
2. Focused assessment
   a. Subjective data collection
      1) History of present illness/chief complaint
         a) Increased work of breathing, shortness of breath
         b) Pain: PQRST (see Chapter 8)
         c) Coughing, choking
         d) Hemoptysis
         e) Sputum production
         f) Skin color: pallor, cyanosis, flushed
         g) Diaphoresis
         h) Hoarseness
         i) Dysphagia
         j) Abnormal respiratory sounds (e.g., wheezing, rhonchi, crackles, stridor)
         k) Anxiety/restlessness
         l) Time of symptom onset
         m) Association with exertion
         n) Association with chest pain
         o) Fever, chills
         p) Nausea, vomiting, diarrhea
         q) Anorexia, weight loss
         r) Efforts to relieve symptoms
            (1) Home remedies, specific cultural practices
            (2) Alternative therapies
            (3) Medications
               (a) Prescription
               (b) OTC/herbal
      2) Past medical history
         a) Current or preexisting diseases/illness
            (1) Pulmonary disease
            (2) Cardiovascular disease
            (3) Renal disease
            (4) Autoimmune disorders
            (5) Postsurgical recovery or immobility
            (6) Metabolic disorders
            (7) Neuromuscular disorders
            (8) Malignancies
            (9) Immunodeficiency status: human immunodeficiency virus (HIV) infection, therapeutic immunosuppression, underlying disease impairing pulmonary defense system
            (10) History of disseminated intravascular coagulation (DIC)
            (11) Respiratory infections: recent respiratory infection may increase susceptibility to other respiratory infections

b) Recent aspiration
c) Smoking history
d) Substance and/or alcohol use/abuse
e) Inhalation of toxic or caustic substances such as gases, animal products, chemicals, dusts, metals, wood dust, pharmaceuticals, and other dusts, sprays, and plant substances
f) Recent travel
g) Last normal menstrual period: female patients of childbearing age
h) Current medications
   (1) Prescription
   (2) OTC/herbal
i) Allergies to substances or materials, atopy (tendency to experience immediate allergic reactions because of antigen presence)
j) Immunization status
b. Objective data collection
 1) General appearance
   a) Level of consciousness, behavior, affect
   b) Vital signs including pulsus paradoxus, oxygen saturation, pain level
   c) Ability to breathe and speak in sentences simultaneously
   d) Gait
   e) Odors
   f) Level of distress/discomfort
 2) Inspection
   a) Respiratory rhythm, depth, effort
   b) Positioning (tripod)
   c) Skin and nail bed color
   d) Pupillary size and reaction
   e) Neck or facial swelling
   f) Carpopedal spasms
   g) Nasal flaring
   h) Use of accessory muscles
   i) Tracheal position (late sign)
   j) Neck veins (late sign)
   k) Pharynx
   l) Thorax
     (1) Shape of chest: deformities, symmetry, anteroposterior diameter; barrel chest may be present in chronic obstructive pulmonary disease (COPD)
     (2) Wounds: surgical scars
     (3) Use of accessory muscles
     (4) Abnormal retraction or bulging of interspaces
  m) Use of accessory muscles
  n) Positioning (tripod)
  o) Neck/facial swelling
 3) Palpation/percussion
   a) Areas of tenderness, crepitus, deformity
   b) Respiratory excursion
   c) Fremitus (tremulous vibration of the chest wall)

d) Subcutaneous emphysema
e) Tracheal position, movement
f) Diaphragmatic level and excursion
g) Skin and mucosa: temperature, moisture
h) Location of percussion sounds
 4) Auscultation
   a) Breath sounds
     (1) Presence, equality, or absence
     (2) Distribution
   b) Adventitious breath sounds
     (1) Wheezing: musical sound
     (2) Crackles: small popping sounds produced by passage of air through secretions or slightly closed airways
     (3) Rhonchi: snoring, low-pitched sounds similar to wheezes, produced by air passing through narrowed air passages
     (4) Pleural friction rub: grating heard with inspiration and expiration as a result of inflammation of the pleural surfaces
   c) Voice sounds: sound of a spoken word may be increased, decreased, or modified by disease
   d) Heart sounds
 5) Physiological/social/environmental factors
   a) Heredity: tendency to develop certain respiratory diseases, such as asthma, can be inherited
   b) Obesity
   c) Environmental pollution
   d) Occupational exposure (e.g., firefighters, coal miners, cotton mill workers)
   e) Changes in weather: extremes of hot or cold; humidity changes
   f) Exercise induced
   g) Stress factors
     (1) Emotional distress: may precipitate asthma exacerbation
     (2) Possible/actual assault, abuse, or intimate partner violence situations (see Chapters 3 and 40)
3. Diagnostic procedures
 a. Laboratory studies
  1) Complete blood count (CBC) with differential
  2) Serum chemistries including glucose, BUN, creatinine
  3) Arterial blood gases (ABGs) (Tables 28.1 and 28.2); capillary gases, venous gases
  4) Urinalysis; pregnancy test in female patients of childbearing age
  5) Blood alcohol level: elevations may lead to respiratory depression, possible aspiration
  6) Serum and urine toxicology levels: may explain cause of increased or decreased respiratory rate or depth

Table 28.1

Blood Gas: Normal Values

Variable	Arterial	Capillary	Venous
pH	7.35–7.45	7.35–7.45	7.31–7.41
PaO_2	80–100	40–60	35–40
$PaCO_2$	35–45	35–45	41–51
HCO_3^-	22–26	22–26	22–26
BE	±2	±2	±2
Acid/base	pH 7.35–7.45	Increased pH = alkalosis >7.45 Decreased pH = acidosis <7.35	
Metabolic component	HCO_3^- 22–26 mEq	Increased HCO_3^- = metabolic alkalosis >26 mEq Decreased HCO_3^- = metabolic acidosis <22 mEq	
Respiratory component	$PaCO_2$ 35–40 mm Hg	Increased $PaCO_2$ = respiratory acidosis >40 mm Hg Decreased $PaCO_2$ = respiratory alkalosis <35 mm Hg	

BE, Base excess; HCO_3^-, bicarbonate radical; $PaCO_2$, partial pressure of arterial carbon dioxide; PaO_2, partial pressure of arterial oxygen.

From Tipsord-Klinkhammer, B., & Andreoni, C. P. (1998). *Quick reference for emergency nursing.* Philadelphia, PA: WB Saunders.

Table 28.2

Interpretation of Arterial Blood Gas Values

Variable	pH	PCO2	HCO3−
Respiratory acidosis	↓	↑	Normal
Respiratory acidosis with metabolic compensation	↓	↑	↑
Metabolic acidosis	↓	Normal	↓
Metabolic and respiratory acidosis	↓	↑	↓
Metabolic alkalosis	↑	Normal	↑
Metabolic alkalosis with respiratory compensation	↑	↑	↑
Respiratory alkalosis	↑	↓	Normal
Metabolic and respiratory alkalosis	↑	↓	↑

HCO_3^-, Bicarbonate radical; PCO_2, partial pressure of carbon dioxide.

7) Coagulation profile: prothrombin time (PT), partial thromboplastin time (PTT), PT-INR
8) Thoracentesis fluid analysis
9) D-dimer
10) Lactate
11) B-type natriuretic peptide (BNP) level
b. Imaging studies
1) Chest radiograph
2) Computed tomography (CT) scan
3) CT angiogram
4) Magnetic resonance imaging (MRI)
5) Esophagogram
6) Lung scan (ventilation-perfusion [V/Q] scan)
7) Doppler sonography
8) Pulmonary angiography
c. Other
1) 12- to 15-lead electrocardiogram (ECG)
2) Esophagoscopy
3) Bronchoscopy
4) Simple spirometry: to estimate patient's ability to exhale (significant in asthma)
5) Peak flow rate: measurement of choice in asthma; a decreasing peak flow should raise suspicion of narrowed airways
6) Forced expiratory volume (FEV_1): amount of air that can be forced from lungs in 1 second; FEV_1 of <80% of predicted tidal volume is indicative of obstructive lung disease

B. ANALYSIS: DIFFERENTIAL NURSING DIAGNOSES/COLLABORATIVE PROBLEMS

1. Ineffective airway clearance
2. Ineffective breathing pattern
3. Impaired gas exchange
4. Decreased cardiac output
5. Deficient/excess fluid volume
6. Ineffective tissue perfusion: cardiopulmonary
7. Acute pain
8. Risk for infection
9. Anxiety/fear
10. Deficient knowledge
11. Noncompliance

C. PLANNING AND IMPLEMENTATION/INTERVENTIONS

1. Determine priorities of care
   a. Maintain airway, breathing, circulation (see Chapter 1)
   b. Maintain adequate ventilation and oxygenation
   c. Provide supplemental oxygen as indicated
   d. Establish IV access for administration of crystalloid fluids/medications as needed
   e. Obtain and set up equipment and supplies
   f. Prepare for/assist with medical interventions
   g. Administer pharmacologic therapy as ordered
2. Relieve anxiety/apprehension
3. Allow significant others to remain with patient if supportive
4. Educate patient/significant others on disease processes and care

D. EVALUATION AND ONGOING MONITORING

1. Continuously monitor and treat as indicated
2. Monitor patient response/outcomes and modify nursing care plan as appropriate
3. If positive patient outcomes are not demonstrated, reevaluate assessments and/or plan of care

E. DOCUMENTATION OF INTERVENTIONS AND PATIENT RESPONSE

F. AGE-RELATED CONSIDERATIONS

1. Pediatric
   a. Growth or development related
      1) Ribs are more compliant; adult-level compliance reached by age 20 years
      2) Mediastinum thinner, more mobile
      3) Infants are preferential nose breathers; children depend on diaphragm for adequate chest expansion; may exhibit grunting or head bobbing with respiratory distress
      4) Airways are small in size and easily obstructed by edema or mucus
      5) Children's metabolic rate and oxygen consumption are much higher than those of adults
   b. "Pearls"
      1) Respiratory distress is a primary cause of cardiac arrest in infants and children
      2) Airway resistance in infants is 15 times greater than in adults
      3) Infants in respiratory distress tire quickly due to increased work of breathing, accessory muscle use, and decreased glycogen stores
      4) Greater body surface area and increased respiratory rate lead to rapid heat and insensible fluid loss with infection and fever
      5) Weak intercostal muscles result in observable retractions when respiratory effort is increased
   c. Assessment
      1) Evaluate work of breathing
         a) Tachypnea or bradypnea
         b) Respiratory effort
         c) Nasal flaring
         d) Abnormal airway sounds such as stridor, wheezing, grunting
         e) Tachycardia
         f) Skin signs: cool, pale, diaphoretic
2. Geriatric
   a. Aging related
      1) Decreased vital capacity, FEV_1, and maximum midexpiratory flow
      2) Increased residual volume and functional residual capacity
      3) Decreased static muscle strength and lung compliance
      4) Increased work of breathing
      5) Decreased diffusion capacity and arterial oxygenation
      6) Increased V/Q inequality, alveolar-arterial oxygen gradient
   b. "Pearls"
      1) Pulmonary defense mechanisms are reduced, making older adults more susceptible to infections

      2) Diminished ventilatory response to hypoxic and hypercapnic challenge
      3) Older adults may report dyspnea as breathlessness
      4) Causes of dyspnea in older adults include
         a) Functional impairment of pulmonary or cardiopulmonary system
         b) Impaired oxygen delivery secondary to hematologic dysfunction
      5) ECG is mandatory because acute coronary syndrome can present with dyspnea
      6) Aspiration mortality rate of 40–70%; significant cause of pulmonary morbidity
      7) Pneumonia is leading infectious disease cause of death in older adults; first sign may be deterioration in general health; nonpulmonary complaints, such as weakness and lethargy, are common. Pneumococcal vaccines do not necessarily prevent pneumococcal pneumonia. Older patients with concurrent rheumatoid arthritis, systemic lupus erythematosus (SLE), or alcoholism often remain susceptible to pneumococcal pneumonia because they may not develop an antibody response to the pneumococcal vaccine
      8) Normally patients older than 60 years can exhale 75% of vital capacity in 1 second
         a) 65–75%: mild obstruction
         b) 50–65%: moderate obstruction
         c) <50%: severe obstruction

II. Specific Respiratory Emergencies

A. ACUTE BRONCHITIS

Bronchitis is an inflammation of the bronchi and/or trachea believed to result from irritation of the bronchial mucosa by such elements as pollen, smoking, and inhalation of irritating substances. Acute bronchitis is commonly seen at the time of, or shortly after, an upper respiratory tract infection (URI) and is generally caused by influenza, parainfluenza, adenovirus, or rhinovirus. A secondary infection may also occur, but the acute episode generally clears without treatment unless a chronic disease is present. As a precursor to COPD, acute bronchitis often occurs in middle-aged persons, is more common in men than in women, and occurs most frequently during the winter. This condition may be referred to as chronic bronchitis if it is characterized by persistent production of excess bronchial mucus.

1. Assessment
   a. Subjective data collection
      1) History of present illness/chief complaint
         a) Dyspnea, wheezing
         b) Cough: initially dry, then productive
         c) Fever
         d) Pain (see Chapter 8): chest/back

e) Malaise
f) Repeated respiratory infections
g) Environmental history: smoking, occupational factors (e.g., coal miners, chemical workers)
2) Past medical history
a) Current or preexisting diseases/illness
(1) Recent URI
(2) Pulmonary disease
b) Smoking history
c) Medications
d) Allergies
e) Immunization status
b. Objective data collection
1) Physical examination collection
a) General appearance
(1) Slight tachypnea
(2) Moderate level of distress/discomfort
b) Inspection
(1) Use of accessory muscles for breathing
(2) Prolonged expiratory phase
(3) Sputum: thin and clear to thick and purulent
(4) Neck vein distention in chronic bronchitis secondary to cor pulmonale
c) Auscultation
(1) Breath sounds: rhonchi that may clear after cough
d) Percussion
(1) Resonant sounds
2) Diagnostic procedures
a) CBC with differential
b) Serum chemistries
c) Sputum examination: Gram stain, culture and sensitivity (C&S)
d) Chest radiograph: exclude pneumonia
e) Pulmonary function tests (PFTs)
2. Analysis: differential nursing diagnoses/collaborative problems
a. Risk for ineffective airway
b. Impaired gas exchange
c. Anxiety/fear
d. Deficient knowledge
3. Planning and implementation/interventions
a. Provide supplemental oxygen as indicated
b. Establish IV access for administration of crystalloid fluid/medications as needed
c. Prepare for/assist with medical interventions
1) Position patient to facilitate breathing
2) Provide heated aerosol treatments
3) Institute cardiac and pulse oximetry monitoring
4) Perform postural drainage as indicated
d. Administer pharmacologic therapy as ordered
1) Nonnarcotic analgesics
2) Antipyretics
3) Bronchodilators: nebulizer treatment
4) Expectorants and antitussives
5) Corticosteroids
6) Anxiolytics
7) Antivirals, influenza vaccinations
a) Provide greater protection for the appropriate populations because they offer coverage for influenza A and B
b) Amantadine (Symmetrel) and rimantadine (Flumadine) can be useful during epidemics of influenza A
8) Antibiotics: may be beneficial in patients with concurrent COPD or who have limited cardiopulmonary reserve
e. Educate patient/significant others
1) Remove environmental irritants (including smoking)
2) Increase oral fluids to liquefy secretions
4. Evaluation and ongoing monitoring
a. Hemodynamic status
b. Breath sounds and pulse oximetry
c. Cardiac rate and rhythm

B. ACUTE RESPIRATORY DISTRESS SYNDROME

Acute respiratory distress syndrome (ARDS) is a sudden, progressive, severe pulmonary disorder characterized by hypoxia, hypoxemia, and diffuse bilateral infiltrates. ARDS is also known as adult hyaline membrane disease, wet lung, posttraumatic pulmonary insufficiency, Da Nang lung, shock lung, and acute lung injury (ALI). ARDS is frequently considered a secondary lung injury caused by an acute illness or injury. It affects approximately 150,000 adults per year, with a mortality risk of 40–70%, although often it occurs in adults in the absence of chronic illness or lung disease. The syndrome may be caused by direct pulmonary injury or may result from systemic illness or trauma. Specific pulmonary insult occurs from pneumonia, embolism, aspiration, inhalation of smoke or toxins, prolonged exposure to oxygen, high-altitude pulmonary edema, and lung contusions. Indirect pulmonary assaults causing ARDS include sepsis, DIC, pancreatitis, uremia, anaphylaxis, drug overdose, eclampsia, radiation therapy, shock, multisystem trauma, and the administration of massive blood transfusions. The lung tissue responds to the assault with a diffuse inflammatory response in the microvasculature of the lungs. The release of chemical mediators, cytokines, alveolar macrophages, and vasoactive substances causes increased permeability of the capillary and alveolar membranes with resultant noncardiogenic pulmonary edema. Damage to the alveolar epithelium results in impaired gas exchange, decreased surfactant, and alveolar and interstitial edema, which contribute to decreased lung compliance. The resultant atelectasis causes severe respiratory distress, leading to respiratory failure. If the patient survives, the lungs are typically scarred. Investigational treatment modalities include pharmacologic therapies to inhibit the destructive activity of chemical mediators and alternative ventilation procedures.

1. Assessment
   a. Subjective data collection
      1) History of present illness/injury/chief complaint
         a) Sudden marked respiratory distress
         b) Recent injury
         c) Shock
         d) Multiple blood transfusions
         e) Fluid overload
         f) Pulmonary embolism
         g) Drug overdose
         h) Drowning incident
         i) Inhalation of caustic toxic materials
         j) Pulmonary contusion
         k) Burns
         l) Aspiration
         m) Radiation exposure
         n) Uremia
         o) Pregnancy-related hypertension
         p) Sepsis
         q) Multiple fractures
      2) Past medical history
         a) Current or preexisting diseases/illness
            (1) Cardiovascular disease
            (2) Pulmonary disease
            (3) Pancreatic disease
            (4) Central nervous system (CNS) disease
         b) Past surgical procedures
         c) Smoking history
         d) Substance use/abuse
         e) Last normal menstrual period: female patients of childbearing age
         f) Medications
         g) Allergies
   b. Objective data collection
      1) Physical examination
         a) General appearance
            (1) Level of consciousness, behavior, affect: restless, anxiety
            (2) Tachypnea: early sign
            (3) Hypoxia, increased work of breathing, respiratory distress
            (4) Hypotension (late sign), tachycardia
            (5) Severe distress, critically ill
         b) Inspection
            (1) Cyanosis (late sign)
            (2) Accessory muscle use
         c) Auscultation
            (1) Breath sounds: fine to coarse crackles
            (2) Diminished breath sounds
      2) Diagnostic procedures
         a) ABG/VBG: hypoxia
            (1) Respiratory alkalosis early in disease
            (2) Respiratory acidosis and hypercarbia occur as disease progresses
         b) CBC with differential
         c) Serum chemistries, including BUN, creatinine, glucose, electrolytes
         d) Blood cultures in cases of severe ARDS if infection is suspected: sepsis is the most common cause
         e) Urinalysis; pregnancy test in female patients of childbearing age
         f) Chest radiograph
         g) Chest CT
            (1) Possible absence of infiltrates early in disease
            (2) Bilateral, diffuse, white infiltrates without cardiomegaly
            (3) Complete whiteout of lung fields as disease progresses
         h) Respiratory function measures (FEV_1, forced vital capacity [FVC])
         i) Pulmonary shunting studies
2. Analysis: differential nursing diagnoses/collaborative problems
   a. Ineffective airway clearance
   b. Impaired gas exchange
   c. Ineffective tissue perfusion: cardiopulmonary
   d. Decreased cardiac output
   e. Excess fluid volume
   f. Anxiety/fear
3. Planning and implementation/interventions
   a. Maintain airway, breathing, circulation (see Chapters 1 and 3)
   b. Maintain adequate ventilation and oxygenation
   c. Provide supplemental oxygen
      1) Rapid sequence intubation (RSI) and ventilatory support in patients with respiratory compromise
      2) High-flow oxygen
   d. Establish IV access for administration of crystalloid fluids/medications
   e. Prepare for/assist with medical interventions
      1) Advanced airway management
         a) Nasal or oral intubation
         b) Supraglottic airway (e.g., King, Combitube, laryngeal mask airway)
         c) Surgical airway (e.g., cricothyrotomy)
      2) Position patient in way to maximize ventilation when possible
      3) Institute cardiac, pulse oximetry, and end-tidal CO_2 monitoring
      4) Suction as indicated
         a) Have patient cough and breathe deeply
         b) Use incentive spirometry to help loosen secretions and facilitate coughing; suction as indicated
      5) Catheter placement and monitoring of central venous, arterial, and pulmonary pressures (see Chapter 7)
      6) Assist with chest tube placement as needed
         a) High peak pressures (i.e., >50 cm of water) may indicate pneumothorax
      7) Insert indwelling urinary catheter
      8) Assist with hospital admission

f. Administer pharmacologic therapy as ordered
   1) RSI premedications: sedatives, analgesics, neuromuscular blocking agents
   2) Nonnarcotic analgesics
   3) Corticosteroids: if appropriate (asthma)
   4) Antibiotics (as appropriate): controversial because routine or prophylactic use may lead to development of multiple drug-resistant infections
4. Evaluation and ongoing monitoring
   a. Airway patency
   b. Level of consciousness
   c. Hemodynamic status
   d. Breath sounds, pulse oximetry, end-tidal CO_2
   e. Cardiac rate and rhythm
   f. Intake and output

C. ASTHMA

Asthma is a chronic, reversible obstructive pulmonary disease that is caused by airway inflammation, increased airway responsiveness (bronchospasm) to stimuli, and mucus plugging. Ten to 15 million persons in the United States have asthma. The disease affects more male than female patients, and it is the most common chronic childhood illness. Asthma affects approximately 5–10% of children and is more prevalent among lower-income, inner-city African-American children; children with low birth weight; children of young mothers; and those with genetic atopic disease. Two-thirds of patients with asthma are diagnosed by the age of 40 years. The morbidity and mortality of asthma are increasing, causing approximately 5,000 deaths per year in the United States. The death rate for asthma is greater for female patients and for African-Americans.

The typical presentation includes increased work of breathing, wheezing, and a cough. Multiple factors may be involved in an exacerbation, including biochemical, immunologic, endocrine, infectious, autonomic, and psychological precipitators. Typically, environmental factors trigger the response in those individuals with an inherited predisposition to the disease. An allergen or stimulant causes B lymphocytes to produce immunoglobulin E (IgE), which attaches to mast cells and basophils in the bronchial walls. These cells then release their chemical mediators: histamine, prostaglandins, bradykinins, slow-reacting substances of anaphylaxis (SRS-A), and leukotrienes. Steroids may interrupt the release of the chemical mediators that cause mucus secretion, inflammation, and bronchospasm. Chronic inflammation causes hyperresponsiveness of the airways, which can be stimulated by exercise or cold air.

The Global Initiative for Asthma has developed a stepwise therapy model with guidelines for the successful management of long-term outpatient management of asthma. Management involves four strategies: (1) objective measures of lung function, (2) environmental control measures and avoidance of risk factors, (3) comprehensive pharmacologic therapy, and (4) patient education. Other strategies include management of exacerbations and regular follow-up care. Prior to treatment, asthma severity based on symptom prevalence and measurement of lung function needs to be established (Table 28.3).

Status asthmaticus (acute, severe, and prolonged asthma exacerbation) is a life-threatening emergency. The bronchospasm does not respond to conventional therapy, thus leading to a worsening hypoxemia acid-base balance disturbance and eventual respiratory arrest, if uninterrupted.

1. Assessment
   a. Subjective data collection
      1) History of present illness/chief complaint
         a) Increased work of breathing, cough, wheezing
         b) Restlessness resulting from increased hypoxia
         c) Tightness in chest
         d) Symptoms of infection: productive cough, fever, general upper respiratory symptoms such as malaise, sore throat, "stuffy nose"
         e) Exposure to known allergens or triggers
         f) Emotional factors
         g) Environmental factors: exposure to extremes of heat/cold, humidity, dust, mold, smoke, pets
         h) Time of onset of symptoms
      2) Past medical history
         a) Current or preexisting diseases/illness
            (1) Cardiovascular disease
            (2) Pulmonary disease
         b) Previous asthma problems, including last emergency department visit, hospital admission, or intubation
         c) Hereditary asthma/allergy problems
         d) Medications

Table 28.3				
Classification of Asthma Severity				
	Days with Symptoms	**Nights with Symptoms**	**PEF or FEV₁***	**PEF Variability**
Step 1: Mild intermittent	Up to 2/wk	Up to 2/mo	80% or greater	<20%
Step 2: Mild persistent	3–6/wk	3–4/mo	80% or greater	20–30%
Step 3: Moderate persistent	Daily	5/mo or more	>60% to <80%	>30%
Step 4: Severe persistent	Continual	Frequent	Up to 60%	>30%

*Percentage of predicted values for forced expiratory volume in 1 second (FEV_1) and percentage of personal best for peak expiratory flow (PEF) (relevant for children 4 years old or older who can use these devices).

Part 2

- e) Allergies
- f) Immunization status
b. Objective data collection
  1) Physical examination
    a) General appearance
      (1) Level of consciousness, behavior, affect: restlessness; children with significant hypercarbia may demonstrate somnolence
      (2) Tachypnea, tachycardia: children with significant hypoxemia or hypercarbia may demonstrate decreased respiratory effort, bradycardia, and possible periodic apnea
      (3) Inability to speak complete sentences
      (4) Pulsus paradoxus: present in some patients
      (5) Orthopneic posturing
      (6) Moderate to severe distress/discomfort
    b) Inspection
      (1) Prolonged expiratory phase of respiratory cycle
      (2) Use of accessory muscles
      (3) Pallor and/or cyanosis (late sign)
      (4) Diaphoresis
      (5) Physical exhaustion
    c) Auscultation
      (1) Breath sounds: wheezing on expiration; as disease progresses, wheezing on inspiration; diminishing to absent breath sounds as air movement ceases
    d) Percussion
      (1) Hyperresonance
  2) Diagnostic procedures
    a) CBC with differential: leukocytosis, eosinophilia, increased hematocrit (if possible, obtain specimen before bronchodilator therapy and steroids)
    b) Serum chemistries: potassium and chloride may be decreased in long-standing respiratory acidosis
    c) ABGs: may initially be normal or demonstrate respiratory alkalosis, then reflective of hypoxemia, hypercarbia (an ominous sign), and resulting respiratory acidosis
    d) Sputum cultures
    e) Medication levels (e.g., theophylline level)
    f) Chest radiograph: hyperinflation; findings may help rule out other reactive airway causes (e.g., allergic bronchopulmonary aspergillosis or sarcoidosis)
    g) Sinus CT scan: useful in excluding acute or chronic sinusitis as a contributing factor
    h) Objective measurement of airflow obstruction: spirometry, peak flow meter
    i) ECG in adult patients

2. Analysis: differential nursing diagnoses/collaborative problems
   a. Risk for ineffective airway clearance
   b. Impaired gas exchange
   c. Ineffective breathing pattern
   d. Anxiety/fear
   e. Deficient knowledge
3. Planning and implementation/interventions
   a. Maintain airway, breathing, circulation (see Chapter 1)
   b. Maintain adequate ventilation and oxygenation
   c. Provide supplemental oxygen as indicated
     1) RSI and ventilatory support in patients with respiratory compromise or status asthmaticus
     2) High-flow oxygen
   d. Establish IV access for administration of crystalloid fluid/medications as needed
   e. Prepare for/assist with medical interventions
     1) Advanced airway management
       a) Nasal or oral intubation
       b) Supraglottic airway (e.g., King, Combitube, laryngeal mask airway)
       c) Surgical airway (e.g., cricothyrotomy)
     2) Position patient to facilitate maximum ventilation
     3) Assist patient in removal of secretions: coughing, deep-breathing exercises, suction as necessary
     4) Institute cardiac, pulse oximetry, and end-tidal CO_2 monitoring
     5) Assist with possible hospital admission
   f. Administer pharmacologic therapy as ordered
     1) RSI premedications: sedatives, analgesics, neuromuscular blocking agents
     2) Bronchodilators
       a) Short-acting beta agonists, handheld nebulizer treatment
       b) Magnesium sulfate: inhibits calcium influx into airway smooth muscle cells
     3) Rescue medications
       a) Short-acting beta agonists
       b) Anticholinergics: used for severe exacerbations
       c) Corticosteroids
     4) Oral or intravenous fluids
     5) Keep NPO if indicated
   g. Educate patient/significant others
     1) Reduce aggravating allergens and precipitating factors
     2) Medications: purpose, route, dose, and side effects
       a) Stress that corticosteroid therapy should never be stopped abruptly but should be tapered off as prescribed
       b) Use of home medications to prevent exacerbations

3) Importance of hydration
4) Use of home nebulizers and peak flow meters
5) Relaxation techniques and controlled breathing information
6) Importance of providing a smoke-free environment and instituting environmental control measures to reduce allergens, furred animal exposure, molds, dust mites, and other pests
7) Necessity for providing updated records, medications, and physical activity restrictions to child's school administration and health services

4. Evaluation and ongoing monitoring
   a. Airway patency
   b. Level of consciousness
   c. Hemodynamic status
   d. Breath sounds and pulse oximetry
   e. Cardiac rate and rhythm
   f. Respiratory effort

D. BRONCHIOLITIS

Bronchiolitis is a lower respiratory tract infection characterized by an inflammatory obstruction of the airway. This infection primarily affects children younger than 2 years, typically infants less than 1 year old. In adults, the symptoms are generally mild. Respiratory syncytial virus (RSV) causes 90% of bronchiolitis infections in children and occurs primarily during the winter months. Other causes include parainfluenza, influenza, adenovirus (causing very severe illness), rhinovirus, enterovirus, herpes simplex, and mycoplasma pneumonia. The causative virus initiates an inflammatory response with profuse respiratory secretions and a necrotic response producing cellular debris and fibrin that create obstruction of the bronchi and bronchioles (smaller airways) and contribute to upper airway reactivity. The airway obstruction leads to air trapping, high resistance, and atelectasis (patchy infiltrate on chest radiograph film). This results in a V/Q defect, hypoxemia, and eventual fatigue. At risk for serious illness or complications are very young children or premature infants and children with chronic lung disease or hemodynamically significant congenital heart disease, immunodeficiency, or those with a history of previous mechanical ventilation. Bronchiolitis/RSV is an important risk factor for the subsequent development of asthma.

1. Assessment
   a. Subjective data collection
      1) History of present illness/chief complaint
         a) Several days of mild/moderate URI symptoms of rhinorrhea, cough, and low-grade fever, progressing to increased dyspnea
         b) Increased cough
         c) Poor feeding, vomiting
         d) Irritability
         e) Decreased sleep

2) Past medical history
   a) Current or preexisting diseases/illness
      (1) Chronic pulmonary disease
      (2) Congenital heart disease with significant hemodynamic compromise
      (3) Immunodeficiency
   b) Medications
   c) Allergies
   d) Immunization status
b. Objective data collection
   1) Physical examination
      a) General appearance
         (1) Level of consciousness, behavior, affect: lethargy
         (2) Tachypnea, apnea possible in infants
         (3) Tachycardia
         (4) Elevated temperature
         (5) Moderate to severe distress/discomfort, possibly critically ill
      b) Inspection
         (1) Grunting, nasal flaring, intercostal and suprasternal retractions
         (2) Cyanosis
      c) Auscultation
         (1) Breath sounds: wheezing
      d) Palpation
         (1) Fontanel depression: if dehydration present
   2) Diagnostic procedures
      a) Capillary blood gases or ABGs if acutely ill or require mechanical ventilation
      b) CBC with differential: not useful because white blood cell (WBC) count is usually normal
      c) Urine specific gravity may provide useful information regarding fluid balance and possible dehydration
      d) Serum chemistries: not affected directly by the infection but helpful in determining dehydration severity
      e) Chest radiograph: hyperinflation, patchy infiltrates; may indicate alternative diagnoses (e.g., lobar pneumonia, heart failure, or foreign body aspiration)
2. Analysis: differential nursing diagnoses/collaborative problems
   a. Ineffective airway clearance
   b. Ineffective breathing pattern
   c. Impaired gas exchange
   d. Activity intolerance
   e. Deficient knowledge
3. Planning and implementation/interventions
   a. Maintain airway, breathing, circulation (see Chapter 1)
   b. Provide supplemental oxygen
      1) Blow-by oxygen: infants
      2) Humidified oxygen if oxygen saturation is <94% on room air

c. Establish IV access for administration of crystalloid fluid/medications as needed

d. Prepare for/assist with medical interventions
  1) Institute cardiac and pulse oximetry monitoring
  2) Assist with hospital admission if
    a) Respiratory fatigue or impending respiratory failure
    b) Continued oxygen saturation <90%
    c) Continued tachypnea >70 breaths/minute
    d) Apneic episodes

e. Administer pharmacologic therapy as ordered
  1) Anticholinergics: inhibit smooth muscle contraction, useful in patients with a significant bronchospasmodic component of illness
  2) Antibiotics: indicated if bacterial infection is suggested (e.g., toxic appearance, hyperpyrexia, consolidation or focal lobar infiltrates on chest radiograph, leukocytosis, positive bacterial cultures)
  3) Adrenergic agents: may relieve reversible bronchospasm by relaxing smooth muscles of the bronchi
  4) Corticosteroids: no benefit in the treatment of bronchiolitis but may be useful in patients with history of reactive airway disease
  5) Ribavirin (Virazole): nucleoside analogue that inhibits viral replication

f. Educate patient, parent, significant others
  1) Use of home nebulizer treatments
  2) Fever management
  3) Encourage small, frequent feedings
  4) Signs of increasing respiratory distress
  5) Physician follow-up
    a) Reevaluation within 24 hours
    b) Possible administration of prophylactic antiviral immunoglobulins (palivizumab [Synagis]) for high-risk patients (e.g., premature babies)

4. Evaluation and ongoing monitoring
  a. Level of consciousness
  b. Hemodynamic status
  c. Breath sounds and pulse oximetry
  d. Cardiac rate and rhythm
  e. Intake and output

E. CHRONIC OBSTRUCTIVE PULMONARY DISEASE

Chronic obstructive pulmonary disease (COPD) is characterized by chronic or recurrent airflow obstruction. Smoking, environmental pollution, occupational exposure to chemicals, tuberculosis, aging, and heredity are causative factors in the development of COPD. These irritants, diseases, and genetic factors cause bronchial mucosa edema and smooth muscle contraction (resulting in increased airway resistance) and decreased elastic recoil. The physiologic changes cause difficulty in exhaling and impaired alveolar gas exchange. The disease entities that comprise COPD include asthma (airway reaction) (see "Asthma"), chronic obstructive bronchitis (airway inflammation), and emphysema (airway collapse). Individuals generally have all three components present, but one type usually predominates. COPD affects approximately 1 in 10 people and is second only to heart disease in morbidity and mortality, causing more than 100,000 deaths per year. It typically affects men older than 45 years, but a greater number of women are developing the disease secondary to smoking.

Chronic obstructive bronchitis is characterized by inflammation of the bronchi that leads to increased mucus production and chronic cough (Table 28.4). It is diagnosed by the presence of symptoms for at least 3 months of the year for 2 consecutive years. Chronic irritation causes an increase in the number and size of mucous cells and leads to increased mucus production and impaired ciliary function. These physiologic changes also inhibit the normal defense mechanisms against infection. Because of the airway obstruction, airway collapse occurs, causing air trapping and chronic hypoxia with possible hypercapnia. Under normal physiologic circumstances, the respiratory drive is triggered by a high partial pressure of arterial carbon dioxide ($PaCO_2$). However, the patient with chronic obstructive bronchitis may have a chronically elevated $PaCO_2$ and may lose this drive as a respiratory stimulus. Hypoxia becomes the respiratory stimulus, and excessive oxygen administration may obliterate that drive. Polycythemia and pulmonary hypertension leading to cor

Table 28.4

Comparison of Symptoms of Chronic Obstructive Bronchitis and Emphysema

Chronic Obstructive Bronchitis	Emphysema
"Blue bloater"	"Pink puffer"
Productive cough	Cough uncommon
Stocky build	Thin
Onset 40–50 yr	Onset 50–75 yr
Normal respiratory rate	Tachypnea
Hypoxemia	PaO_2 normal or slightly decreased
Increased $PaCO_2$	$PaCO_2$ usually low or normal until end stage
Cyanosis	Barrel chest
Polycythemia	Accessory muscle use
Cor pulmonale	Leans forward while sitting
Peripheral edema	Pursed-lip breathing
Risk for pulmonary embolism	Hyperresonance on percussion
Radiograph film shows enlarged heart	Lung overinflation, diaphragm low

$PaCO_2$, Partial pressure of arterial carbon dioxide; PaO_2, partial pressure of arterial oxygen.

pulmonale may develop. Cor pulmonale is visibly evident in the classic "blue bloater" with symptoms of peripheral edema, anasarca (severe, generalized edema), and chronic neck vein distention.

Emphysema is a disorder of impeded exhalation caused by permanent overdistention of air spaces, alveolar wall destruction, partial airway collapse, and loss of elastic recoil of the lungs. Pockets of air that form between the alveoli and within the lung parenchyma cause increased ventilatory dead space and decreased functional lung tissue that lead to increased work of breathing. In addition, the pulmonary capillary bed is essentially obliterated by enzymatic activity, with consequent decreased oxygen perfusion and ventilation. The two enzymes, protease and elastase, appear to be involved in this tissue-destructive component of emphysema because of the breakdown in the lung's normal defense mechanism involving alpha1-antitrypsin. Symptoms of emphysema begin with dyspnea on exertion deteriorating to dyspnea at rest and accompanied by tachypnea (see Table 28.4). A cough is not typical, but respiratory infections are common because of alterations in normal respiratory defenses and immunity and may precipitate respiratory failure.

1. Assessment (see Table 28.4)
   a. Subjective data collection
      1) History of present illness/chief complaint
         a) Dyspnea
         b) Current URI
         c) Air pollution exposure
      2) Past medical history
         a) Current or preexisting diseases/illness
            (1) Pulmonary disease
            (2) Recent URI
            (3) Cardiac disease
         b) Cigarette smoking or exposure
         c) Medications
         d) Allergies
         e) Immunization status: pneumococcal immunization
   b. Objective data collection
      1) Physical examination
         a) General appearance
            (1) Level of consciousness, behavior, affect: confusion, agitation
            (2) Inability to speak in complete sentences without taking a breath
            (3) Tachycardia, cardiac dysrhythmias on monitor
            (4) Elevated temperature: if concurrent infection
            (5) Moderate to severe distress/discomfort
         b) Inspection
            (1) Pursed-lip breathing
         c) Auscultation
            (1) Breath sounds: crackles, rhonchi, expiratory wheezes

   2) Diagnostic procedures
      a) ABGs: hypoxemia, hypercarbia
      b) CBC with differential
         (1) Secondary polycythemia, resulting from chronic hypoxemia
         (2) Hematocrit of >52% in male patients and >47% in female patients indicates disease
         (3) Eosinophilia, increased WBC count
      c) BNP level: may aid in differentiating between COPD and heart failure
      d) Sputum: culture and sensitivity
         (1) Mucoid sputum in stable chronic bronchitis
         (2) Purulent sputum with an exacerbation
         (3) *Streptococcus pneumoniae* and *Haemophilus influenzae* most common pathogens during exacerbation
      e) Enzymes: α_1-antitrypsin (deficiency indicative of emphysema)
         (1) Measure in all patients younger than 40 years or in those with a family history of emphysema at an early age
         (2) If level is low, phenotyping should be obtained
      f) Chest radiograph: hyperinflation, flattened diaphragm, increased retrosternal air space, and long, narrow heart shadow
         (1) Emphysema: rapid tapering vascular shadows with hyperlucency
         (2) Complicating pulmonary hypertension: prominent hilar vascular shadows, possible right ventricular enlargement, and lower retrosternal air space opacity
      g) Chest CT scan: high-resolution CT (HRCT) scan more sensitive than standard chest radiograph
         (1) HRCT scan highly specific for diagnosing emphysema because the outlined bullae are not always visible on a radiograph
         (2) Not useful in routine care of patients with COPD because therapy is not altered
      h) PFT measurements
         (1) Essential for diagnosis and assessment of severity of disease
         (2) Spirometry: best method to determine borderline to mild airway obstruction
            (a) Measurement of FEV_1 and FVC
            (b) Most available and useful PFT
            (c) Should be performed in all smokers over the age of 45 years, to screen for COPD
         (3) Peak flow meter
2. Analysis: differential nursing diagnoses/collaborative problems
   a. Risk for ineffective airway clearance
   b. Impaired gas exchange

c. Anxiety/fear

d. Deficient knowledge

3. Planning and implementation/interventions

a. Maintain airway, breathing, circulation (see Chapter 1)

b. Provide supplemental oxygen

1) Possible continuous positive airway pressure (CPAP) or biphasic positive airway pressure (Bi-PAP) ventilation assistance

c. Establish IV access for administration of crystalloid fluids/medications as needed

d. Prepare for/assist with medical interventions

1) Position patient to facilitate breathing

2) Institute cardiac and pulse oximetry monitoring

3) Assist with hospital admission

e. Administer pharmacologic therapy as ordered

1) Beta-adrenergic agonist and anticholinergic agent combinations

2) Bronchodilators: long acting

3) Mucolytic agents

4) Antiinflammatory drugs, inhaled and oral steroids

5) Antibiotics

6) Helox: controversial, may provide short-acting relief

7) Antidepressants

8) Nicotine patches

f. Educate patient/significant others

1) Body positioning for optimal air exchange

2) Eat small, frequent meals as opposed to heavy traditional meals

3) Importance of exercise

4) Coughing and deep-breathing exercises

5) Maintain adequate hydration

6) Medication compliance: inhalers, nebulizers, possible need for pneumococcal and viral immunizations

7) Stop smoking

4. Evaluation and ongoing monitoring

a. Level of consciousness

b. Hemodynamic status

c. Breath sounds and pulse oximetry

d. Cardiac rate and rhythm

e. Intake and output

F. CROUP (LARYNGOTRACHEOBRONCHITIS)

Croup is an acute viral syndrome characterized by barking cough, hoarse voice, inspiratory stridor, and variable degrees of respiratory distress. It most commonly affects children ages 6–36 months (more often boys), and it peaks in late fall and early winter. The most common causative agent is the parainfluenza virus type I, which causes the yearly winter epidemic. Other causes include the parainfluenza virus type III, adenovirus, RSV, and influenza A virus (which may produce very severe cases). The initial portal of entry is the nasopharynx, then spreading to the larynx and trachea, where it causes erythema and edema of the tracheal walls. An inflammatory exudate is produced, and the vocal cords swell, causing the typical stridor, hoarseness, and barking cough. Symptoms typically occur or recur at night and usually resolve with humidified air. Total obstruction rarely occurs.

1. Assessment

a. Subjective data collection

1) History of present illness/chief complaint

a) "Barking" cough

b) Evidence of URI for 1–2 days

c) Low-grade to moderate fever, rarely exceeds 102.2°F (39°C)

d) Current medications

e) Physical exhaustion

2) Past medical history

a) Current or preexisting diseases/illness

(1) Recent infections of measles, adenovirus, influenza A and B, rhinovirus, parainfluenza

b) Medications

c) Allergies

d) Immunization status

b. Objective data collection

1) Physical examination

a) General appearance

(1) Level of consciousness, behavior, affect: restless to lethargy

(2) Croup cough: harsh, barking cough

(3) Minimal drooling

(4) Elevated temperature

(5) Tachypnea, tachycardia

(6) Stridor: inspiratory and expiratory

(7) Mild to severe distress/discomfort

b) Inspection

(1) Possible inflamed pharynx

(2) Suprasternal retractions

c) Auscultation

(1) Breath sounds: normal to diminished

2) Diagnostic studies

a) CBC with differential: WBC count generally within normal reference range; however, lymphocytosis or leukopenia may be present

b) ABGs or capillary blood gases if indicated

(1) Hypoxia present with severe episodes

c) Soft tissue radiograph of neck

(1) Rule out epiglottitis

(2) Possible subglottic narrowing resulting from edema in severe disease

(3) Possible distention of hypopharynx during inspiration

(4) Possible laryngeal air column narrowing below vocal cord (steeple sign)

d) Direct laryngoscopy in a stable child
   (1) Exclude other entities, such as peritonsillar abscess
   (2) Pale, boggy laryngeal mucosa
   (3) Bacterial tracheitis: abundant purulent exudate and pseudomembranes
   (4) Spasmodic croup: mucosa inflamed, erythematous with a velvety appearance
e) Chest radiograph: unnecessary unless the diagnosis is in question
2. Analysis: differential nursing diagnoses/collaborative problems
   a. Risk for ineffective airway clearance
   b. Anxiety/fear
   c. Deficient knowledge
3. Planning and implementation/interventions
   a. Provide supplemental oxygen
      1) Cool, humidified oxygen
   b. Prepare for/assist with medical interventions
      1) Position patient to facilitate breathing
      2) Institute pulse oximetry monitoring
      3) Assist with possible hospital admission
   c. Administer pharmacologic therapy as ordered
      1) Racemic epinephrine
         a) Decreases edema and dilates larynx
         b) Effective in reducing stridor
         c) Requires period of observation because patient may rebound in 1–1.5 hours
      2) Corticosteroids: decrease airway inflammation
         a) Routine use is controversial
         b) Administered for severe, moderate, and even mild croup
   d. Educate patient, parent, significant others
      1) Signs of respiratory distress
      2) Explain disease process
      3) Use of cool, humidified air, increased fluids, and follow-up
4. Evaluation and ongoing monitoring
   a. Level of consciousness
   b. Hemodynamic status
   c. Breath sounds and pulse oximetry

G. HYPERVENTILATION SYNDROME

Hyperventilation syndrome (HVS) is a manifestation of rapid breathing thereby increasing the amount of CO_2 blown off in ventilation. Anxiety (see Chapter 26) is a common precipitating factor; however, hyperventilation may be caused by disease processes, such as myocardial infarction, intracerebral bleeding, ketoacidosis, or salicylate overdose. The cause must be determined before treatment is initiated. Hyperventilation is accompanied by a fall in the partial pressure of CO_2 (PCO_2), which causes constriction of cerebral vasculature, respiratory alkalosis, and tetany. Diagnosis is dependent on recognizing the typical constellation of signs and symptoms and ruling out serious causes, such as coronary artery disease and pulmonary embolism (PE), which can cause similar presenting symptoms. With subsequent exacerbations, the diagnosis is made clinically, without repeating extensive workups on each occasion. The typical constellation of signs and symptoms includes dyspnea, agitation, dizziness, atypical chest pain, tachypnea and hyperpnea, paresthesias, and carpopedal spasm in a young, otherwise healthy patient. Once life-threatening conditions have been ruled out or eliminated, simple reassurance and an explanation in understandable terms of how hyperventilation produces the patient's symptoms are usually sufficient to terminate the episode.

Pulse oximetry may identify the occasional patient with PE or other primary pulmonary disease that is so severely hypoxemic that oxygen saturation cannot be maintained. A normal pulse oximetry reading is not always helpful, because hyperventilation can mask a severe defect in gas exchange. Some fraction of patients with chronic PE may have compensated chronic hyperventilation that can mimic primary chronic hyperventilation. Imaging studies are not indicated when the diagnosis of HVS is clear, because the findings are usually normal. Because PE can manifest with findings identical to those of HVS, a first-time episode of acute HVS may warrant a V/Q scan, CT scan, or pulmonary angiogram to rule out perfusion defects.

1. Assessment
   a. Subjective data collection
      1) History of present illness/chief complaint
         a) Shortness of breath or feeling of air hunger
         b) Tingling sensation or numbness of extremities, lips
         c) Light headedness
         d) Diaphoresis
         e) Headache
         f) Chest discomfort
         g) Recent anxiety-producing situation
         h) Pregnancy
         i) Exercise
         j) Fever
         k) Time of onset
      2) Past medical history
         a) Current or preexisting diseases/illness
            (1) Cardiac disease
            (2) Diabetes
            (3) Panic attacks (see Chapter 26)
         b) Possible toxicity
         c) Medications
         d) Allergies
   b. Objective data collection
      1) Physical examination
         a) General appearance
            (1) Level of consciousness, behavior, affect: anxious or panicky appearance
            (2) Tachypnea
            (3) Moderate level of distress/discomfort

b) Inspection
  (1) Carpopedal spasms (spasms of hands and feet sometimes seen in HVS)
  c) Auscultation
  (1) Breath sounds: clear
  2) Diagnostic procedures
  a) ABGs: if indicated
  (1) Question exists as to patient's underlying respiratory status
  (2) May be helpful when HVS-induced acidosis is suspected or when shunting or impaired pulmonary gas exchange is being considered
  (3) Compensated respiratory alkalosis in a majority of cases: pH normal, with a low PCO_2 and low bicarbonate (HCO_3)
  b) Serum and urine toxicology screen
  c) Quantitative enzyme-linked immunosorbent assay (ELISA) D-dimer assay: if acute PE is considered
  d) Chest radiograph: patients with high risk of cardiac or pulmonary pathology, or if diagnosis is unclear
  e) ECG: possible findings
  (1) Prolonged QT interval
  (2) ST-segment depression or elevation
  (3) T-wave inversion
  (4) Sinus tachycardia
2. Analysis: differential nursing diagnoses/collaborative problems
  a. Impaired gas exchange
  b. Anxiety/fear
  c. Deficient knowledge
3. Planning and implementation/interventions
  a. Prepare for/assist with medical interventions
  1) Position patient to facilitate breathing
  2) Instruct patient on decreasing hyperventilation
  a) Physically compressing the upper thorax and having the patient exhale maximally decreases hyperinflation of the lungs
  b) Instruct patient to breathe abdominally: use of the diaphragm rather than chest wall often improves subjective dyspnea and reverses associated symptoms
  c) Diaphragmatic breathing slows the respiratory rate
  3) Remain with patient during rebreathing process
  4) Institute cardiac and pulse oximetry monitoring
  5) Assist with interventions for metabolic causes of hyperventilation
  a) Diabetic ketoacidosis (see Chapter 13)
  b) Poisoning (see Chapter 25)
  c) Myocardial infarction (see Chapter 11)
  d) Intracerebral bleeding (see Chapters 21 and 34)
  b. Administer pharmacologic therapy as ordered
  1) Anxiolytics: benzodiazepines for stress relief and resetting the trigger for hyperventilation

c. Educate patient/significant others
  1) Early recognition of predisposing situations, rebreathing exercises
  2) Instruct patient in techniques of diaphragmatic breathing and refer to a specialist, such as a physical therapist, psychologist, psychiatrist, family physician, internist, or respiratory therapist who can reinforce this approach
4. Evaluation and ongoing monitoring
  a. Level of consciousness
  b. Hemodynamic status
  c. Breath sounds and pulse oximetry
  d. Resolution of carpopedal spasms

H. PLEURAL EFFUSION

Pleural effusion is the collection of excess fluid (>15 mL) in the pleural space. Under normal physiologic conditions, this fluid is formed by the parietal pleura and is absorbed by the visceral pleura. Increased fluid accumulation may result from (1) increased subpleural capillary pressure as in heart failure, (2) decreased capillary oncotic pressure as in liver and renal failure, (3) inflammatory conditions such as infections, or (4) impairment/obstruction of lymphatic flow. In descending order of frequency, the most common causes of pleural effusion are heart failure, pneumonia, malignant disease, and PE. Dyspnea and pain or dull ache may or may not be present. Dyspnea is caused by fluid accumulation that inhibits lung expansion. If the effusion is excessive, it can cause a mediastinal shift. Small effusions (250 mL) may be asymptomatic and detected only on radiograph. Thoracentesis is performed to remove excess fluid and for diagnostic fluid analysis. The appearance of the fluid may be hemorrhagic, chylous (white/thick), or purulent (empyema). Empyema must be drained and treated or it will solidify, becoming fibrous and constricted, requiring surgical intervention and possibly causing permanent lung damage. An effusion may be recurrent, requiring repeated drainage, and may even require therapeutic adhesion formation of the parietal and visceral pleura.
1. Assessment
  a. Subjective data collection
  1) History of present illness/chief complaint
  a) Shortness of breath
  b) Cough
  c) Hemoptysis
  d) Pleuritic pain
  2) Past medical history
  a) Current or preexisting diseases/illness
  (1) Cardiovascular disease
  (2) PE
  (3) Bacterial pneumonia
  (4) Malignant disease, especially of lung or breast
  (5) Tuberculosis
  (6) Pancreatitis
  (7) Abdominal surgery, subphrenic or hepatic abscess

b) Medications
c) Allergies
b. Objective data collection
1) Physical examination
a) General appearance
(1) Level of consciousness, behavior, affect: anxious to confusion
(2) Tachypnea
(3) Possible elevated temperature
(4) Moderate to severe distress/discomfort
b) Inspection
(1) Use of accessory muscles with respirations
(2) Decreased movement of chest wall
c) Auscultation
(1) Breath sounds: diminished or absent over effusion
(2) Egophony: "e-" sound heard as "ä" when auscultated over area of effusion
d) Percussion
(1) Increased fremitus above effusion, absent fremitus over effusion
(2) Dullness over effusion
2) Diagnostic procedures
a) CBC with differential: possible WBC elevation
b) Chest radiograph
(1) Possible diagnostic clues to cause of effusion
(2) Lateral decubitus film more reliably detects smaller pleural effusions
c) Sonography: identify area for thoracentesis
d) Chest CT scan, spiral CT
e) Thoracentesis for fluid analysis: amount, protein, lactate dehydrogenase (LDH), amylase, glucose, differential, pH, Gram stain with culture, cytology
f) ECG
2. Analysis: differential nursing diagnoses/collaborative problems
a. Impaired gas exchange
b. Pain
c. Anxiety/fear
d. Deficient knowledge
3. Planning and implementation/interventions
a. Maintain airway, breathing, circulation (see Chapter 1)
b. Provide supplemental oxygen as indicated
c. Establish IV access for administration of crystalloid fluids/medications as needed
d. Prepare for/assist with medical interventions
1) Institute cardiac and pulse oximetry monitoring
2) Assist with thoracentesis procedure/tube thoracostomy
3) Pleurodesis (pleural sclerosis)
4) Assist with possible hospital admission
e. Administer pharmacologic therapy as ordered
1) Nonnarcotic analgesics
2) Narcotics

3) Antibiotics
4. Evaluation and ongoing monitoring
a. Level of consciousness
b. Hemodynamic status
c. Cardiac rate and rhythm
d. Breath sounds and pulse oximetry
e. Pain relief

I. PNEUMONIA

Community-acquired pneumonia (CAP) is one of the most common infectious illnesses and a major cause of mortality and morbidity worldwide. Older individuals and those with COPD, such as patients with chronic bronchitis, are most frequently admitted to the hospital for treatment. CAP is usually acquired by either inhalation or aspiration of the pathogenic organisms into a lung segment or lobe. It may also result from secondary bacteremia, such as an Escherichia coli urinary tract infection and/or bacteremia. CAP resulting from aspiration of oropharyngeal contents is the only form of CAP with multiple pathogens. Nursing home–acquired pneumonia (NHAP) is common, and the list of pathogens associated with the illness closely resembles that for CAP. The severity of CAP is determined by impaired cardiopulmonary or splenic function.

An estimated 2–4 million cases of pneumonia occur annually in the United States. Pneumonia is an inflammation of the pulmonary parenchyma resulting from tissue invasion by inhaled, aspirated, or bloodborne pathogens. Once the pathogen reaches the alveoli and begins to replicate, fluids and antiinflammatory cells enter the alveolar spaces to attack the infection, thereby causing symptoms and radiographic signs of pneumonia.

The illness ranges in severity from mild to life threatening. The most common pneumonia pathogens are viral (60–90%), bacterial (which cause the majority of deaths), or mycoplasmal. Other causes include fungi, rickettsiae, parasites, and occasionally a noninfectious insult. Table 28.5 describes the most typical bacterial pneumonia infections associated with CAP; additional agents include Legionella pneumophila and Chlamydia. Viral causes include RSV, influenza, cytomegalovirus (CMV), herpes simplex, varicella, and Epstein-Barr virus.

Differentiating between viral and bacterial pneumonia can be difficult. Viral infections most commonly occur in winter and last approximately 2 weeks. Bacterial pneumonias typically develop more acutely and are associated with high temperature, coughing, and chest pain. The signs and symptoms of pneumonia in children depend on the age of the patient, the specific pathogen, and the severity of disease. Infants typically have less characteristic symptoms but are at greater risk for complications. RSV and influenza are the most common viral causes in children younger than 1 year. In older children, pneumonia is usually subacute, and presenting signs and symptoms include a nonproductive cough, moderate fever, headache, sore throat, and general fatigue.

Table 28.5

Pathogens in Community-Acquired Pneumonia

	Streptococcus pneumoniae	*Staphylococcus aureus*	*Klebsiella pneumoniae*	*Pseudomonas aeruginosa*	*Haemophilus influenzae*
Risk factors	Immunosuppression, alcoholism, cardiopulmonary disease, diabetes mellitus	Drug abuse, immunosuppression, complication of influenza epidemic	Male gender, alcoholism, age >50 yr, cardiopulmonary disease, diabetes mellitus, aspiration	Alcoholism, Nosocominal infection, immunosuppression, diabetes mellitus	Alcoholism, age >50 yr, cardiopulmonary disease, immunosuppression, diabetes mellitus
Signs/symptoms	Malaise, sore throat, chills/fever, cough, rust-colored sputum, chest pain, vomiting, abdominal pain, dyspnea, tachypnea, tachycardia, diminished breath sounds, rales	Fever, chills, cough, chest pain, purulent sputum, tachypnea, tachycardia, rales, rhonchi	Fever, cough, hemoptysis, dyspnea, tachypnea	Same as *Klebsiella*	Low-grade fever, dyspnea, slight tachycardia and tachypnea
Diagnostic findings	↑ White blood cell count with left shift, pleural infiltrates	↑ White blood cell count, lower lobe infiltrates, possible pleural effusion or abscess	↑ or ↓ White blood cell count, pleural infiltrates with consolidation, pleural abscess or effusion	↑ White blood cell count with left shift, lower pleural infiltrates	↑ White blood cell count, lower pleural infiltrates, pleural effusion
Treatment	Macrolides (azithromycin [Zithromax], clarithromycin [Biaxin], erythromycin); doxycycline (Vibramycin); fluoroquinolones (levofloxacin [Levaquin]) or amoxicillin-clavulanate (Augmentin) if patient received antibiotics within prior 3 mo; additional third-generation cephalosporins if cardiopulmonary disease or patient from nursing home	Fluroquinolones (levofloxacin [Levaquin]); vancomycin (Vancocin) if drug resistant	Third-generation cephalosporins plus aminoglycosides	Cefepime (Maxipime), imipenem-cilastatin (Primaxin), meropenem (Merrem), or piperacillin (Zosyn), plus ciprofloxacin (Cipro)	Macrolides (azithromycin [Zithromax], clarithromycin [Biaxin], erythromycin); second- or third-generation cephalosporins

In the older population, bacteremia and complications such as empyema and meningitis may develop with pneumonia. Pneumonia is the sixth leading cause of death in the United States; it causes approximately 80,000 deaths annually, and it is the leading cause of death in the geriatric population. Those at greatest risk include patients with chronic illness, congenital anomalies, pulmonary disease, and immunosuppression.

1. Assessment
   a. Subjective data collection
      1) History of present illness/chief complaint
         a) Dyspnea
         b) Cough
            (1) *Legionella:* productive or nonproductive cough
            (2) *Mycoplasma pneumoniae* or *Chlamydia pneumoniae:* nonproductive cough
         c) Pain (see Chapter 8)
            (1) Chest, back, abdominal
            (2) Chest pain frequently absent with CAP atypical pathogen but may be present with *Legionella* CAP
         d) Fever/chills
         e) Changes in sensorium: may be presenting symptom in elderly patients
         f) Recent URI or flu
         g) Diarrhea: mycoplasma, *Legionella*
         h) Abdominal pain: common in children and elderly
         i) Infants: vomiting, poor feeding, dehydration
      2) Past medical history
         a) Current or preexisting diseases/illness
            (1) Cardiovascular disease

Part 2

      (2) Pulmonary disease: COPD (pneumonia poses an immediate life-threatening situation to these patients)

      (3) Immunosuppression

      (4) High-risk category for human immunodeficiency virus (HIV) infection, known HIV infection, or acquired immunodeficiency syndrome (AIDS)

      (5) Congenital abnormalities

      (6) Cystic fibrosis, cerebral palsy

   b) Smoking history

   c) Previous episodes of pneumonia

   d) Medications

   e) Allergies

   f) Immunization status: pneumococcal, *Haemophilus*

  b. Objective data collection

   1) Physical examination

     a) General appearance

      (1) Level of consciousness, behavior, affect: alert to confusion, lethargy in infants

      (2) Elevated temperature: may be subnormal in infants and elderly patients

      (3) Tachypnea, tachycardia

      (4) Moderate to severe distress/discomfort

     b) Inspection

      (1) Possible cyanosis

      (2) Decreased respiratory excursion secondary to pain

      (3) Infant: retractions

      (4) Sputum

        (a) Purulent with bacterial pathogens

        (b) Blood-tinged with pneumococcal, *Klebsiella*, or *Legionella* infections

     c) Auscultation

      (1) Breath sounds: coarse crackles, bronchial sounds over affected area

      (2) Possible pleural friction rub

      (3) Grunting in infants

     d) Percussion/palpation

      (1) Dullness over consolidated area

      (2) Increased fremitus

   2) Diagnostic procedures

     a) CBC with differential: elevated WBC with bacterial origin

     b) Gram stain and culture of sputum

      (1) Direct fluorescent antibody (DFA) testing of the sputum: assists in making the diagnosis of *Legionella* if obtained early and before antimicrobial treatment

     c) Blood cultures: twice at least 15 minutes apart prior to antibiotic administration

      (1) *S. pneumoniae* and *H. influenzae*: frequently associated with positive blood cultures

      (2) *M. catarrhalis* bacteremia is unusual

     d) Cold hemagglutination: useful in mycoplasmal infection

     e) Urinalysis: pregnancy test in females of childbearing age

     f) ABGs

     g) Chest radiograph: confirm the presence of an infiltrate

      (1) May be negative in early CAP

      (2) Viral pneumonias: few or no infiltrates

      (3) Bacterial pneumonias: focal, segmental, or lobar infiltrate distribution

      (4) Legionnaires disease: rapidly progressive, asymmetric infiltrates, chest radiograph may also be useful for identifying alternative diagnosis and/or associated conditions

     h) Chest CT: if underlying bronchogenic carcinoma is suggested or any abnormalities are not consistent with the diagnosis

     i) ECG

2. Analysis: differential nursing diagnoses/collaborative problems

  a. Risk for ineffective airway clearance

  b. Impaired gas exchange

  c. Anxiety

3. Planning and implementation/interventions

  a. Maintain airway, breathing, circulation (see Chapter 1)

  b. Provide supplemental oxygen

   1) RSI and ventilatory support if impending respiratory failure

   2) CPAP or Bi-PAP ventilation support

   3) High-flow oxygen

  c. Establish IV access for administration of crystalloid fluid/medications as needed

  d. Prepare for/assist with medical interventions

   1) Advanced airway management

     a) Nasal or oral intubation

     b) Supraglottic airway (e.g., King, Combitube, laryngeal mask airway)

     c) Surgical airway (e.g., cricothyrotomy)

   2) Position patient to facilitate breathing

   3) Institute cardiac and pulse oximetry monitoring

   4) Insert indwelling urinary catheter as indicated

   5) Assist with possible hospital admission

  e. Administer pharmacologic therapy as ordered

   1) RSI premedications: sedatives, analgesics, neuromuscular blocking agents

   2) Antibiotics: must be administered within 4 hours of admission, including emergency department presentation time

     a) Tetracyclines should not be administered to patients who are pregnant or younger than 10 years of age

b) Short course of fluoroquinolones is safe for patients older than 6 years

c) Preferred monotherapy for CAP includes doxycycline (Dynapen) or levofloxacin (Levaquin)

3) Bronchodilators

4) Antipyretics

f. Educate patient/significant others

1) Importance of medication compliance

2) Increase fluid intake

3) Importance of follow-up

4. Evaluation and ongoing monitoring

a. Level of consciousness

b. Hemodynamic status

c. Cardiac rate and rhythm

d. Breath sounds and pulse oximetry

e. Intake and output

J. PNEUMOTHORAX (IATROGENIC AND SPONTANEOUS) AND PNEUMOMEDIASTINUM

Pneumothorax is defined as air in the intrapleural space. Different causes of pneumothoraces include (1) trauma (see Chapter 38), (2) primary spontaneous occurrence with no obvious underlying lung disease, (3) secondary spontaneous occurrence with underlying lung disease, and (4) iatrogenic occurrence. Spontaneous pneumothorax may occur because of a rupture of subpleural apical emphysematous blebs, smoking history, or increased body height because alveoli are subjected to a greater mean distending pressure, thereby leading to subpleural bleb formation and rupture. Iatrogenic pneumothoraces can be caused by transthoracic needle aspiration procedures, such as subclavian and supraclavicular needle insertions, thoracentesis, mechanical ventilation with increased peak airway pressures, bronchial and lung biopsies, cardiopulmonary resuscitation, and tracheostomy. Pneumothorax can also result from a pneumomediastinum caused by increased intrathoracic pressure, asthma, smoking marijuana, inhalation of cocaine, athletic competition, respiratory tract infection, parturition (giving birth), vomiting, severe cough, mechanical ventilation, trauma, or surgical disruption of the oropharyngeal, esophageal, or respiratory mucosa.

1. Assessment

a. Subjective data collection

1) History of present illness/chief complaint

a) Generalized malaise: especially with primary spontaneous pneumothorax

b) Dyspnea: often disproportional to size of pneumothorax with secondary spontaneous pneumothorax

c) Pain (see Chapter 8): chest

(1) Primary spontaneous pneumothorax: acute onset, ipsilateral pain

(2) Secondary spontaneous pneumothorax: ipsilateral pain

(3) Pneumomediastinum: substernal chest pain radiating to the neck, back, or shoulders and exacerbated by deep inspiration, coughing, or supine positioning

d) Vomiting

2) Past medical history

a) Current or preexisting diseases/illness

b) Smoking history

c) Substance use/abuse

d) Medications

e) Allergies

b. Objective data collection

1) Physical examination

a) General appearance

(1) Tachypnea: primary and secondary to spontaneous pneumothorax

(2) Tachycardia: secondary to spontaneous pneumothorax

(3) Hypoxia: primary and secondary to spontaneous pneumothorax

(4) Hypotension: secondary to spontaneous pneumothorax

(5) Moderate to severe distress/discomfort

b) Inspection

(1) Cyanosis: secondary to spontaneous pneumothorax (late sign)

c) Auscultation

(1) Breath sounds: decreased or absent on side of pneumothorax

(2) Hamman sign: precordial crunching noise synchronous with the heartbeat, often accentuated during expiration; occurs with pneumomediastinum

d) Percussion/palpation

(1) Hyperresonance over pneumothorax

(2) Subcutaneous emphysema: with pneumomediastinum; most consistent sign

2) Diagnostic procedures

a) Chest radiograph for evaluation of pneumothorax and/or pneumomediastinum

(1) Pneumothorax: clearly defined line paralleling chest wall, absence of lung markings between chest wall and lung edge

(2) Pneumomediastinum: thin, radiolucent line outlining cardiac silhouette; thin, vertical radiolucent steaks within the mediastinum; well-defined radiolucency around pulmonary artery; retrosternal air on lateral view

b) Contrast-enhanced esophagogram: if emesis precipitated event

2. Analysis: differential nursing diagnoses/collaborative problems

a. Impaired gas exchange

b. Decreased cardiac output

c. Pain

d. Anxiety/fear

e. Deficient knowledge

3. Planning and implementation/interventions

   a. Maintain airway, breathing, circulation (see Chapter 1)

   b. Provide supplemental oxygen as indicated

   c. Establish IV access for administration of crystalloid fluids/medications as needed

   d. Prepare for/assist with medical interventions

      1) Institute cardiac and pulse oximetry monitoring

      2) Assist with tube thoracostomy: if patient is hemodynamically stable, consider procedural sedation with careful titration of a short-acting narcotic and benzodiazepine (see Chapter 9)

      3) Needle or catheter aspiration: if pneumothorax <15%

         a) Obtain chest radiograph postinsertion to assess degree of success

         b) Obtain second chest radiograph in 4 hours to confirm absence of recurring accumulation of air

            (1) If no recurrence is present, remove catheter and discharge patient with appropriate return instructions

            (2) If pneumothorax persists, attach a Heimlich valve or a water seal and hospitalize patient

      4) Pleurodesis (surgical creation of a fibrous adhesion between the visceral and parietal pleura by the insertion of a sterile irritant into the pleural canal) with talc and tetracycline derivatives to decrease the risk of recurrence

      5) Assist with possible hospital admission

   e. Administer pharmacologic therapy as ordered

      1) Nonnarcotic analgesics

      2) Narcotics

      3) Antibiotics: following chest tube insertion to reduce risk of empyema

      4) Procedural sedation medications (see Chapter 9)

4. Evaluation and ongoing monitoring

   a. Level of consciousness

   b. Hemodynamic status

   c. Breath sounds and pulse oximetry

   d. Cardiac rate and rhythm

   e. Pain relief

K. PULMONARY EMBOLISM

Pulmonary embolism (PE) is caused by a free-floating thrombus from the venous system of the legs, pelvis, or right side of the heart. A PE may consist of fat, bone, or amniotic fluid but is most often clotted blood. The thrombus lodges in a branch of the pulmonary artery and causes total or partial occlusion and potential infarct. As a result, the affected area of the lung is ventilated but inadequately perfused. Histamine and prostaglandin are released, causing bronchoconstriction and pulmonary vasoconstriction and resulting in alveolar hypoventilation and intrapulmonary shunting. The decreased perfusion reduces surfactant, thereby contributing to additional atelectasis. PE is the third most common cardiovascular cause of death, after ischemic heart disease and stroke, in the United States (approximately 50,000 deaths per year). PE frequently is difficult to diagnose because of vague symptoms and specificity of the noninvasive diagnostic tests. On autopsy, 80–100% of patients with PE have deep venous thrombosis (DVT), whereas only 40% had clinical signs of DVT. Ten percent of patients with acute PE die within the first hour. Those who survive are at risk for recurrent PE, and up to 70% develop pulmonary hypertension. PE may develop in any patient population (although it is rare in children), but the risk increases with age. PE should always be considered in the geriatric patient with shortness of breath. The highest incidence of recognized PE occurs in hospitalized patients. At autopsy, 70–90% of elderly patients who died during hospitalization were found to have PE.

1. Assessment

   a. Subjective data collection

      1) History of present illness/chief complaint

         a) Dyspnea

         b) Pain (see Chapter 8): chest

         c) Cough

      2) Past medical history

         a) Current or preexisting diseases/illness

            (1) History of thrombosis

            (2) Immobility/prolonged seated position

            (3) Obesity

            (4) Pregnancy

         b) Recent trauma

         c) Recent long bone fracture/surgery

         d) Medications: oral contraceptives

         e) Allergies

   b. Objective data collection

      1) Physical examination

         a) General appearance

            (1) Level of consciousness, behavior, affect: anxiety, restlessness

            (2) Tachypnea, tachycardia most common findings

            (3) Hypotension if large PE

            (4) Moderate to severe distress/discomfort

         b) Inspection

            (1) Cyanosis: large PE

            (2) Petechiae: particular to a fat embolus

         c) Auscultation

            (1) Breath sounds: crackles

            (2) Pleural friction rub

            (3) Heart sounds: accentuated S_2

      2) Diagnostic procedures

         a) CBC with differential: normal or increased leukocytes

         b) Erythrocyte sedimentation rate: elevated

c) Fibrin split products: increased fibrin degradation products

d) ABGs

e) D-dimer: more specific test for fibrin split products; positive if the level is >500 ng/mL

f) Chest radiograph: initial radiograph usually normal

   (1) On rare occasions may show Westermark sign, a dilatation of the pulmonary vessels proximal to an embolism along with collapse of distal vessels, sometimes with a sharp cutoff

   (2) Initially normal, radiograph may begin to show atelectasis, which can progress to cause a small pleural effusion and an elevated hemidiaphragm

   (3) Focal infiltrates may develop after 24–72 hours

g) Venous-Doppler sonography

h) V/Q studies: important when multidetector CT angiography not available

i) Pulmonary angiography

j) Possible spiral CT with transesophageal echocardiogram (TEE) or MRI

   (1) High-resolution multidetector CT angiography (MDCTA) has sensitivity and specificity comparable to that of contrast pulmonary angiography

   (2) MDCTA: preferred primary diagnostic modality and criterion standard for making or excluding diagnosis of PE

k) Duplex sonography

l) ECG: nonspecific ST-segment and T-wave abnormalities most common findings

   (1) S1-Q3-T3 pattern: prominent S wave in lead I, Q wave in lead III, and slight S- and T-wave elevations and T-wave inversion in lead III

   (2) Tall peaked P waves, right axis deviation, right bundle branch block

2. Analysis: differential nursing diagnoses/collaborative problems

a. Impaired gas exchange

b. Ineffective tissue perfusion

c. Anxiety/fear

3. Planning and implementation/interventions

a. Maintain airway, breathing, circulation (see Chapter 1)

b. Provide supplemental oxygen

c. Establish IV access for administration of crystalloid fluids/medications

d. Prepare for/assist with medical interventions

   1) Institute cardiac and pulse oximetry monitoring

   2) Apply compression stockings

   3) Assist with hospital admission

e. Administer pharmacologic therapy as ordered

   1) Anticoagulants: heparin, low-molecular-weight heparin

   2) Fibrinolytics

   3) Analgesics

4. Evaluation and ongoing monitoring

a. Hemodynamic status

b. Level of consciousness

c. Cardiac rate and rhythm

d. Breath sounds and pulse oximetry

e. Intake and output

f. Pain relief

Bibliography

Bartlett J, Breiman R, Mandell L, File T: Community-acquired pneumonia in adults: Guidelines for management, *Guidelines from the Infectious Disease Society of America* 26:811–838, 1998.

Braithwaite S, Perina D: Dyspnea. In 6th ed., Marx JA, Hockberger R, Walls R, editors: *Rosen's emergency medicine: Concepts and clinical practice*, vol. 1. St. Louis, MO, 2006, Elsevier Mosby, pp 175–181.

Charose J: Respiratory emergencies. In Jordan KS, editor: *Emergency nursing core curriculum*, 5th ed., Philadelphia, PA, 2000, Saunders and Emergency Nurses Association, pp 551–591.

Edwards G: Respiratory emergencies. In Newberry LN, editor: *Sheehy's manual of emergency care*, 6th ed., St. Louis, MO, 2005, Mosby, pp 307–325.

Emergency Nurses Association: Respiratory distress and failure. In *Emergency nursing pediatric course*, Chicago, IL, 2004, Emergency Nurses Association, pp 69–80.

Kline J, Runyon M: Pulmonary embolism and deep vein thrombosis. In 6th ed., Marx JA, Hockberger R, Walls R, editors: *Rosen's emergency medicine: Concepts and clinical practice*, vol. 2. St. Louis, MO, 2006, Elsevier Mosby, pp 1371–1381.

Kosowsky J: Pleural disease. In 6th ed., Marx JA, Hockberger R, Walls R, editors: *Rosen's emergency medicine: Concepts and clinical practice*, vol. 2. St. Louis, MO, 2006, Elsevier Mosby, pp 1143–1154.

Mandavia D, Swadron S: Chronic obstructive pulmonary disease. In 6th ed., Marx JA, Hockberger R, Walls R, editors: *Rosen's emergency medicine: Concepts and clinical practice*, vol. 2. St. Louis, MO, 2006, Elsevier Mosby, pp 1097–1109.

Manno M: Pediatric respiratory emergencies: Upper airway obstruction and infections. In 6th ed., Marx JA, Hockberger R, Walls R, editors: *Rosen's emergency medicine: Concepts and clinical practice*, vol. 3. St. Louis, MO, 2006, Elsevier Mosby, pp 2519–2531.

Maxwell R, Campbell D, Fabian T, et al.: Use of presumptive antibiotics following tube thoracostomy for traumatic hemopneumothorax in the prevention of empyema and pneumonia: A multi-center trial, *Journal of Trauma* 57(4):742–748, 2004.

Melio F: Upper respiratory tract infections. In 6th ed., Marx JA, Hockberger R, Walls R, editors: *Rosen's emergency medicine: Concepts and clinical practice*, vol. 2. St. Louis, MO, 2006, Elsevier Mosby, pp 1109–1127.

Moran G, Talan D: Pneumonia. In 6th ed., Marx JA, Hockberger R, Walls R, editors: *Rosen's emergency medicine: Concepts and clinical practice*, vol. 2. St. Louis, MO, 2006, Elsevier Mosby, pp 1128–1141.

National Asthma Education and Prevention Program, National Heart, Lung and Blood Institute: *Expert Panel Report 2: Guidelines for the diagnosis and management of asthma*, NIH Publication No. 97–4051. Washington, DC, 1997, National Heart, Lung and Blood Institute.

National Heart, Lung and Blood Institute: *National asthma education and prevention program. Expert panel report 2: Guidelines for the diagnosis and management of asthma*, Bethesda, MD, 2002, National Heart, Lung and Blood Institute.

Nowak R, Tokarski G: Asthma. In 6th ed., Marx JA, Hockberger R, Walls R, editors: *Rosen's emergency medicine: Concepts and clinical practice*, vol. 2. St. Louis, MO, 2006, Elsevier Mosby, pp 1078–1096.

Rowe B, Bretzlaff J, Bourdon C, Bota G, Camargo C: Intravenous magnesium sulfate treatment for acute asthma in the emergency department: A systematic review of literature, *Annals of Emergency Medicine* 36(3):181–190, 2000.

Urden LD, Lough ME, Stacy KM: Pulmonary disorders. In *Thelan's critical care nursing, diagnosis and management*, 5th ed., St. Louis, MO, 2005, Elsevier Mosby, pp 617–656.

Venes D, editor: *Taber's encyclopedic medical dictionary*, 20th ed., Philadelphia, PA, 2005, FA Davis.

Williams J, Hutson H, Spears K: Dyspnea. In 4th ed., Barber B, Rosen P, editors: *Emergency medicine: Concepts and clinical practice*, vol. 2. 1998, p 1465.

CHAPTER 29

Shock Emergencies

Reneé Semonin Holleran, FNP-BC, PhD, CEN, CCRN (emeritus), CFRN, and CTRN (retired), FAEN

MAJOR TOPICS
General Strategy
Assessment
Analysis: Differential Nursing Diagnoses/Collaborative
  Problems
Planning and Implementation/Interventions
Evaluation and Ongoing Monitoring
Documentation of Interventions and Patient Response
Age-Related Considerations

Specific Shock Emergencies
Cardiogenic
Distributive
Hypovolemia
Obstructive

I. General Strategy

Shock is not a disease, but a clinical manifestation of the body's inability to perfuse its tissues adequately.[1] Shock is recognized as a systemic response to a clinical insult (illness or injury) resulting in inadequate tissue perfusion and decreased oxygen to the cells. Shock can occur from alterations in circulating volume (hypovolemic), alterations in cardiac pump function (cardiogenic), alterations in peripheral vascular resistance or redistribution of blood in the periphery (distributive), and alterations in the blood's ability to perfuse major organs such as the heart and lungs (obstructive). No matter what the cause of shock is, the final common pathway, when interventions fail, is multiple organ failure and eventual death.

The pathophysiologic alterations that occur during shock may be roughly divided into three stages: compensated, uncompensated, and irreversible.[1-4] These stages are summarized in Table 29.1.

A. ASSESSMENT

1. Primary and secondary assessment/resuscitation (see Chapters 1 and 32)
2. Focused assessment
   a. Subjective data collection
      1) History of present illness/injury/chief complaint
         a) Pain: PQRST (see Chapter 8)
         b) Injury
            (1) Mechanism (see Chapter 31)
            (2) Time
            (3) Use of protective devices

   c) Infection
      (1) Recent exposure
      (2) Presence of an invasive device (e.g., peripherally inserted central catheter [PICC] line, feeding tube, or indwelling urinary catheter)
      (3) Travel outside the country
   d) Symptoms
      (1) Fatigue and generalized weakness
      (2) Syncope and dizziness
      (3) Dyspnea and/or orthopnea
      (4) Palpitations
      (5) Vomiting and hematemesis
      (6) Diarrhea, melena, hematochezia
      (7) Headache
      (8) Alteration in mentation
      (9) Behavioral changes
      (10) Sense of impending doom, anxious, apprehensive
      (11) Vaginal bleeding
      (12) Abdominal cramping or pain
      (13) Epistaxis or hemoptysis
      (14) Thirst
      (15) Polyuria
      (16) Anuria
      (17) Sensation of feeling cold
      (18) Unexplained rash or bruising
      (19) Alteration in motor and sensory function
      (20) Urticaria

Table 29.1

Stages of Shock

Stage	Pathophysiology
Compensated (nonprogressive)	Various receptors sense the drop of systemic pressure, initiating a cascade of physiologic changes. Homeostatic compensatory mechanisms mediated by the sympathetic nervous system are activated to restore adequate tissue perfusion and preserve vital organ function in the brain and the heart. Oxygen delivery (DO_2) to nonvital organs is not sufficient to meet cellular demand (measured as oxygen consumption [VO_2]). To remain viable, the cell will convert from aerobic to anaerobic metabolism. Although initially beneficial, this conversion results in a drastic reduction in energy production and accumulation of lactic acid, the by-product of anaerobic metabolism. The resulting lactic acidemia begins to cause cellular damage. Preexisting conditions such as chronic obstructive pulmonary edema or cardiovascular disease as well as the age of the patient will cause additional stress during this process.
Uncompensated (progressive)	The compensatory mechanisms begin to fail to maintain adequate tissue perfusion in the vital organs. Mechanisms that were initially helpful become ineffective and cause additional tissue damage. Cellular derangement and death within all organ systems begin to occur at this point. Additional pathologic responses to the shock state (e.g., severe lactic acidemia and inflammatory/immune system activation) may lead to multiple system deterioration or failure. Even if DO_2 is sufficient, some cells may not be able to use the oxygen as a result of cellular damage.
Irreversible (refractory)	The final stage of shock is the critical point at which no treatment can reverse the process. Cellular destruction is so severe that death is inevitable. At this stage, specific causes of shock are indistinguishable. Each patient's shock state is unique, and its clinical progression may be altered by several factors. These include the cause of shock, patient age, severity and duration of hypoperfusion, and the presence of underlying disease.

e) Efforts to relieve symptoms
 (1) Home remedies
 (2) Alternative therapies
 (3) Medications
  (a) Prescription
  (b) OTC/herbal
2) Past medical history
 a) Current or preexisting diseases/illness
  (1) Immunocompromised
   (a) Human immunodeficiency virus (HIV) positive
   (b) Transplant recipient
   (c) Chemotherapy recipient
  (2) Diabetes
  (3) Cardiovascular disease
  (4) Pulmonary disease
  (5) Hematologic disorders
  (6) Gastrointestinal disorders
  (7) Cancer
 b) History of recent surgery
 c) History of a recent invasive procedure
  (1) Colonoscopy
  (2) Insertion of a feeding tube
  (3) Insertion of a PICC line
  (4) Indwelling urinary catheter
 d) Recent travel outside the country
 e) Previous splenectomy
 f) Exposure to others with infectious illness
 g) Smoking history
 h) Substance and/or alcohol use/abuse
 i) Last normal menstrual period: female patients of childbearing age
 j) Bioterrorism attack (see Chapter 41)

k) Current medications
 (1) Prescription
  (a) Corticosteroids
  (b) Antibiotics
  (c) Chemotherapy
  (d) Immunosuppressants
  (e) Insulin
 (2) OTC/herbal
l) Allergies to
 (1) Medications
 (2) Known environmental agents
 (3) Food
 (4) New items in environment
m) Immunization status
3) Psychological/social/environmental factors related to shock emergencies
 a) Stress factors
  (1) Lifestyle
  (2) Lack of knowledge, absence of injury prevention
  (3) Immobility/ General debilitation
  (4) Malnutrition
  (5) Possible/actual abuse, assault, intimate partner violence situations (see Chapters 3 and 40)
 b) Extremes of age (younger than 1 year; older than 65 years)
 c) Coping patterns
 d) Precipitating event
  (1) Noncompliance with medical regimen
b. Objective data collection
 1) General appearance
  a) Level of consciousness, behavior, affect

b) Vital signs
(1) Blood pressure: narrowing pulse pressure is an ominous sign in shock
(2) Orthostasis
c) Odors
d) Hygiene
e) Level of distress/discomfort
2) Inspection
a) Airway patency
b) Work of breathing (respiratory rate, use of accessory muscles)
c) Skin color
(1) Pink
(2) Pale
(3) Mottled
d) Obvious signs of external bleeding
e) Flattened or distended external jugular veins
f) Chest, abdomen, and extremities for signs of obvious bleeding or deformity, fractures, or major soft tissue injury
g) Bruising
h) Rash
i) Petechiae
j) Purpura
k) Appliances
(1) Tracheotomy tube
(2) Venous access devices
(3) Feeding tubes
(4) Indwelling urinary catheter
3) Auscultation
a) Breath sounds: crackles, wheezes, rhonchi
b) Heart sounds: distant or muffled
c) Bowel sounds: decreased or absent
4) Palpation/percussion
a) Peripheral and central pulses
b) Skin temperature
c) Skin moisture
d) Dullness indicating blood-filled cavities
e) Resonance indicating air-filled cavities
3. Diagnostic procedures
a. Laboratory studies
1) CBC with differential
2) Type and screen or crossmatch
3) Serum chemistries including glucose, BUN, creatinine
4) Liver function tests
5) Serum lactate level
6) Coagulation profile
7) Arterial blood gas (ABG)
8) Serum and urine toxicologic screen
9) Cardiac enzymes
10) Urinalysis; pregnancy test in female patients of childbearing age
11) Cultures: blood, catheters, wound, invasive devices

b. Imaging studies
1) Chest radiograph
2) Pelvic radiograph
3) Long bone radiographs
4) Computed tomography (CT) scan for selected areas of concern: head, neck, chest, abdomen
5) Magnetic resonance imaging (MRI) for selected areas of concern: head, neck, chest, abdomen
6) Focused Assessment Sonography for Trauma (FAST)
c. Other
1) 12- to 18-lead electrocardiogram (ECG)
2) Diagnostic peritoneal lavage (DPL)
3) Bronchoscopy
4) Paracentesis
5) Gastroscopy or endoscopy

B. ANALYSIS: DIFFERENTIAL NURSING DIAGNOSES/COLLABORATIVE PROBLEMS

1. Ineffective airway clearance
2. Ineffective breathing pattern
3. Impaired gas exchange
4. Ineffective tissue perfusion
5. Deficient fluid volume
6. Excess fluid volume
7. Anxiety/fear
8. Risk for injury
9. Acute pain
10. Impaired skin integrity

C. PLANNING AND IMPLEMENTATION/ INTERVENTIONS

1. Determine priorities of care
a. Maintain airway, breathing, circulation (see Chapters 1 and 32)
b. Provide supplemental oxygen as indicated
c. Establish IV access for administration of crystalloid fluids/blood products/medications
d. Obtain and set up equipment and supplies
e. Prepare for/assist with medical interventions
f. Administer pharmacologic therapy as ordered
2. Relieve anxiety/apprehension
3. Allow significant others to remain with patient if supportive
4. Educate patient/significant others

D. EVALUATION AND ONGOING MONITORING

1. Continuously monitor and treat as indicated
2. Monitor patient response/outcomes, and modify nursing care plan as appropriate
3. If positive patient outcomes are not demonstrated, reevaluate assessment and/or plan of care

E. DOCUMENTATION OF INTERVENTIONS AND PATIENT RESPONSE

F. AGE-RELATED CONSIDERATIONS

1. Pediatric
   a. Growth or development related
      1) A greater percentage of a child's body weight is water
      2) Pediatric myocardial fibers are shorter and less compliant. A child's heart rate must increase in order to increase cardiac output
      3) Infants have a higher cardiac output and less oxygen reserve
      4) An infant's circulating blood volume is 90 mL/kg, and a child's is 80 mL/kg. A small amount of blood loss can be significant in either the infant or child
      5) Hypotension is a late sign of circulatory compromise in an infant or child
   b. "Pearls"
      1) Children are at greater risk of becoming dehydrated with fluid loss
      2) Because young children need to increase their heart rate to increase their cardiac output, using heart rate to determine a child's level of shock may not be accurate
      3) Palpation of the child's central and peripheral pulses and observation of capillary refill time are better tools to assess the child's level of shock and to determine his or her response to interventions such as fluid resuscitation
      4) Accidental hypothermia may occur during shock resuscitation and can be very detrimental to young children and infants
      5) Infants and young children may become hypovolemic from blood loss that occurs from intracranial hemorrhage and scalp lacerations
2. Geriatric
   a. Aging related
      1) Cardiac function decreases by almost 50% with age
      2) Cardiac output and stroke volume decrease
      3) Decreased perfusion to end organs
      4) Less pulmonary reserve
      5) Preexisting chronic diseases and medications used for these conditions
   b. "Pearls"
      1) Preexisting cardiovascular disease may limit patient's ability to compensate in the shock state and may cause patient to become hypoxic with volume loss
      2) Geriatric patients are less able to tolerate changes in end-organ perfusion and develop multiple organ failure more quickly
      3) Changes related to age make it difficult to accurately assess the severity of shock and patient's response to interventions

      4) Medications interfere with patient's ability to compensate in shock
      5) Many elderly patients have advance directives that need to be considered before treatment

II. Specific Shock Emergencies

A. CARDIOGENIC

Cardiogenic shock occurs when there is an alteration in pump function. Ventricular ischemia, structural variations, myocardial infarction, cardiac contusion, and dysrhythmias are some of the causes of cardiac compromise that may lead to shock. Generally, patients who have suffered a myocardial infarction damaging 40% or more of the left ventricle are at risk of developing cardiogenic shock. Despite medications and mechanical assistance, the mortality related to this type of shock remains high.

1. Assessment
   a. Subjective data collection
      1) History of present illness/injury/chief complaint
         a) Pain (see Chapter 8): chest
            (1) Onset with or without exertion: severe
            (2) Dull, squeezing, "weight," "tightness," or "heaviness" on one's chest
            (3) Midsternal area, radiating to the jaw or back, down both arms
         b) Shortness of breath
         c) Nausea and vomiting
         d) Diaphoresis
      2) Past medical history
         a) Current or preexisting diseases/illness
            (1) Cardiovascular disease
               (a) Cardiomyopathy
               (b) Valvular disease
               (c) Previous myocardial infarctions
            (2) Pulmonary disease
         b) Recent chest trauma
         c) Medications
            (1) Blood pressure management
            (2) Beta blockers
            (3) Insulin or glycemic medications
            (4) Cholesterol lowering
            (5) Nitroglycerin
            (6) Anticoagulants
         d) Allergies
   b. Objective data collection
      1) Physical examination
         a) General appearance
            (1) Level of consciousness, behavior, affect: anxious, restless, confused, comatose
            (2) Tachycardia/bradycardia, hypotension, tachypnea
            (3) Severe distress/discomfort, critically ill

b) Inspection
    (1) Paleness
    (2) Jugular vein distention
    (3) Cardiac dysrhythmias on monitor
c) Auscultation
    (1) Breath sounds: bilateral crackles
    (2) Heart sounds: S_3, S_4 heart sounds, murmur
d) Palpation
    (1) Diaphoresis
    (2) Decreased or absent peripheral pulses
2) Diagnostic procedures
    a) ECG
    b) Cardiac enzymes
    c) Serum lactate level
    d) Serum chemistries
    e) ABGs
    f) Chest radiograph
2. Analysis: differential nursing diagnoses/collaborative problems
    a. Ineffective tissue perfusion: peripheral, cardiac
    b. Acute pain
    c. Anxiety/fear
3. Planning and implementation/interventions
    a. Maintain airway, breathing, circulation (see Chapters 1 and 32)
    b. Provide supplemental oxygen
        1) RSI and ventilatory support
        2) High-flow oxygen
    c. Establish IV access for administration of crystalloid fluids/medications
        1) Administer normal saline solution in small amounts to avoid fluid overload
    d. Prepare for/assist with medical interventions
        1) Advanced airway management
            a) Nasal or oral intubation
            b) Supraglottic airway (e.g., King, Combitube, laryngeal mask airway)
            c) Surgical airway (e.g., cricothyrotomy)
        2) Institute cardiac and pulse oximetry monitoring
        3) Insert gastric tube and attach to suction
        4) Insert indwelling urinary catheter
        5) Assist with hospital admission, possible reperfusion therapy (PCTA) or insertion of mechanical assist devices (e.g., intraaortic balloon pump [IABP])
    e. Administer pharmacologic therapy as ordered
        1) RSI premedications: sedatives, analgesics, neuromuscular blocking agents
        2) Decrease preload
            a) Furosemide (Lasix)
            b) Nitrates (nitroglycerin)
            c) Morphine sulfate (used for pain relief, reduces preload as a secondary effect)
        3) Increase contractility
            a) Dopamine (Intropin)
            b) Dobutamine (Dobutrex)

c) Inamrinone (Inocor)
d) Milrinone (Primacor)
4) Decrease afterload
    a) Nitroprusside (Nipride)
    b) Nitrates
    c) Angiotensin-converting enzyme inhibitors
5) Increase afterload
    a) Norepinephrine bitartrate (Levophed)
    b) Epinephrine
4. Evaluation and ongoing monitoring
    a. Airway patency
    b. Level of consciousness
    c. Hemodynamic status
    d. Breath sounds and pulse oximetry
    e. Cardiac rate and rhythm
    f. Pain relief
    g. Intake and output

B. DISTRIBUTIVE

The majority of the patient's systemic blood volume is in the venous capacitance system. The arterial system functions as a pressure system to maintain blood flow to the tissues. Distributive shock (Table 29.2) occurs because of either a maldistribution of volume resulting from vasodilation (sepsis or anaphylaxis [see Chapter 21]) or a loss of autonomic sympathetic functions (neurogenic). A national campaign represented by 11 international

Table 29.2
Causes of Distributive Shock

Sepsis
This results from an infectious agent or infection-induced mediators that cause systemic decompensation. There is a decrease in systemic vascular resistance as well as maldistribution of blood into the microcirculation causing altered tissue perfusion and cellular dysfunction. The mortality rate related to septic shock is 50%, and the risk of death increases in patients with additional comorbid risks such as extremes in age (younger than 1 year or older than 65 years). High cardiac output occurs in early sepsis, progressing to low cardiac output in later stages.

Anaphylaxis
This occurs when there is an antigen–antibody reaction. The body becomes hypersensitive to a specific agent such as the protein in shellfish. The reaction produces vasodilatation and pooling of blood in the periphery as well as vasoconstriction of the pulmonary vasculature resulting in respiratory distress and eventual respiratory arrest if no interventions are initiated.

Neurogenic
This results from an imbalance between the sympathetic and parasympathetic stimulation of vascular smooth muscle. This imbalance may be caused by medications such as spinal anesthesia or direct damage to the spinal cord. Because of this imbalance, clinical symptoms associated with shock such as tachycardia are different. The patient will be hypotensive, but bradycardic.

organizations and supported by evidence-based management has delineated surviving sepsis guidelines for the medical management of sepsis in the older adult (Table 29.3).

The loss of autonomic sympathetic function results in the following: (1) loss of vasomotor tone, which is regulated by the sympathetic nervous system and causes peripheral vasodilation and maldistribution of blood volume in the peripheral vessels, especially the veins, thus leading to hypotension; (2) loss of cutaneous control of sweat glands that results in an inability to sweat, loss of thermoregulatory control (poikilothermia), and warm, dry skin; and (3) increased parasympathetic control of heart rate that results in bradycardia.[5–7]

1. Assessment
   a. Subjective data collection
      1) History of present illness/injury/chief complaint
         a) Hyperthermia
         b) Hypothermia
         c) Shaking chills/fever
         d) Spinal cord injury
         e) Exposure to an infectious agent or antigen
         f) Incontinence of bowel and bladder
         g) Rash, urticaria
      2) Past medical history
         a) Current or preexisting diseases/illness
            (1) Immunosuppression
            (2) HIV positive status
            (3) Diabetes
         b) Recent surgery or invasive procedure or instrumentation
         c) Recent infection (e.g., pneumonia, urinary tract)
         d) Recent obstetric procedure or abortion
         e) Recent traumatic wound or thermal injury
         f) Presence of long-term invasive device
            (1) Venous access
            (2) Feeding tube
            (3) Urinary catheter
         g) Substance abuse
         h) Allergy to foods, medications, environmental triggers
         i) Medications: antibiotics, steroids, chemotherapy
         j) Immunization status
   b. Objective data collection
      1) Physical examination
         a) General appearance
            (1) Level of consciousness, behavior, affect: confusion to comatose
            (2) Stridor
            (3) Tachycardia/bradycardia, hypotension, tachypnea
            (4) Elevated or subnormal temperature: subnormal temperature is an indication of sepsis in neonatal infants, and elderly patients
            (5) Severe distress/discomfort, critically ill
         b) Inspection
            (1) Skin: pink/flushed; pale; mottled; rash; petechiae
            (2) Incontinence of bowel or bladder

Table 29.3
Surviving Sepsis Guidelines

Grade*	Recommendations
A	Initiate prophylactic measures against deep vein thrombosis, stress ulcer
B	Initial fluid resuscitation to maintain central venous pressure of 8–12 mm Hg Packed red blood cell transfusion to achieve hematocrit of 30% Mechanical ventilation for acute lung injury or acute respiratory distress syndrome via rapid-sequence induction and administration of premedications Administration of inotropic infusion Administration of recombinant human activated protein C in patients with multiple organ failure, sepsis induced, with no absolute contraindication related to bleeding risk Administration of blood products to maintain hemoglobin of 7–9 g/dL Treat acute renal failure with renal replacement
C	Enhance perfusion with fluid therapy Administration of steroids in patients with adrenal insufficiency
D	Diagnostics: Obtain cultures Minimum of two blood cultures: one obtained percutaneously and one obtained through each vascular device Urine, wounds Respiratory secretions prior to initiating antibiotic therapy Administration of glucose to maintain serum glucose at <150 mg/dL
E	Sonography: ultrasound, imaging studies Administration of empirical antibiotics Control source Remove potentially infected devices Drain abscess Débride infected necrotic tissue Enhance perfusion by administration of vasopressors, inotropic therapy Consider limitation of support: discuss end-of-life care for critically ill patients

*Grading system:

Grade A: Supported by a minimum of two level I investigations (large, randomized trials with confident results).

Grade B: Supported by one level I investigation.

Grade C: Supported by level II investigations only (small, randomized trials with uncertain results).

Grade D: Supported by a minimum of one level III investigation (nonrandomized study).

Grade E: Supported by level IV (nonrandomized, historical controls, and expert opinion) of level V evidence (case series, uncontrolled studies, and expert opinion).

(Retrieved from http://www.survivingsepsis.org/professional_resources/guidelines/index.asp.)

(3) Flaccid paralysis below level of injury: neurogenic shock
(4) Priapism: neurogenic shock
c) Auscultation
(1) Breath sounds: crackles, wheezes, "silent" chest
d) Palpation
(1) Skin: warm, hot, cool
(2) Pulses: bounding, decreased, absent
(3) Capillary refill: normal to delayed
(4) Decreased or absent sensation below level of injury
2) Diagnostic procedures
a) CBC with differential
b) Serum chemistries
c) Lactate level
d) Urinalysis; pregnancy test in female patients of childbearing age
e) ABGs
f) Cultures of blood, urine, wounds, any invasive devices that were removed
g) Lumbar puncture
h) ECG
i) Chest radiograph
j) Cervical spine radiograph series
k) Spine, chest, abdominal, head CT scan
2. Analysis: differential nursing diagnoses/collaborative problems
a. Ineffective tissue perfusion: peripheral
b. Impaired gas exchange
c. Risk for ineffective airway clearance
d. Risk for infection
e. Anxiety/fear
3. Planning and implementation/interventions
a. Maintain airway, breathing, circulation (see Chapters 1 and 32)
b. Provide supplemental oxygen
1) RSI and ventilatory support in obtunded patients or those with respiratory compromise
2) High-flow oxygen
c. Establish IV access for administration of crystalloid fluids/medications
d. Prepare for/assist with medical interventions
1) Advanced airway management
a) Nasal or oral intubation
b) Supraglottic airway (e.g., King, Combitube, laryngeal mask airway)
c) Surgical airway (e.g., cricothyrotomy)
2) Institute cardiac and pulse oximetry monitoring
3) Insert gastric tube and attach to suction
4) Insert indwelling urinary catheter
5) Assist with hospital admission
e. Administer pharmacologic therapy as ordered
1) RSI premedications: sedatives, analgesics, neuromuscular blocking agents
2) Epinephrine, bronchodilators, antihistamines, and steroids: for anaphylaxis
3) Vasopressors
4) Methylprednisolone (SoluMedrol): for spinal cord injury
5) Antibiotics, antithrombotics/anticoagulants: for sepsis
6) Antipyretics
7) Nonnarcotic analgesics
8) Narcotics
4. Evaluation and ongoing assessment
a. Airway patency
b. Level of consciousness
c. Hemodynamic status
d. Breath sounds and pulse oximetry
e. Cardiac rate and rhythm
f. Pain relief
g. Intake and output

C. HYPOVOLEMIA

Hypovolemic shock results from significant fluid loss including loss of blood, plasma, or other body fluids. Hypovolemic shock is the most common type of shock encountered in the emergency department. It is frequently associated with multiple trauma, but it can occur with gastrointestinal hemorrhage, epistaxis, dissecting aortic aneurysm, and vaginal hemorrhage. Significant volume loss can also occur with burn injuries, vomiting, and diarrhea. Volume loss leads to decreased venous return, diminished stroke volume, and reduced cardiac output, ultimately causing inadequate tissue perfusion and cellular oxygenation. As volume loss continues, arterial pressure drops, and tissue perfusion to vital organs becomes inadequate.
1. Assessment
a. Subjective data collection
1) History of present illness/injury/chief complaint
a) Mechanism of injury: blunt or penetrating forces (see Chapter 31)
(1) Chest
(2) Abdomen
(3) Pelvic
(4) Long bone(s)
(5) Multiple sources
b) Thermal injury (see Chapter 34)
c) Bleeding
(1) Vaginal
(2) Hematuria
(3) Melena or hematochezia
(4) Epistaxis, hemoptysis, aneurysm
(5) Wound
d) Protracted vomiting
e) Diarrhea
2) Past medical history
a) Current or preexisting diseases/illness
b) Recent surgery
c) Recent childbirth
d) Medications
e) Allergies
f) Immunization status

b. Objective data collection
  1) Physical examination
     a) General appearance
        (1) Level of consciousness, behavior, affect: slightly anxious to confused, comatose
        (2) Hypotension, tachycardia, tachypnea
        (3) Severe distress/discomfort, critically ill
     b) Inspection
        (1) Obvious external bleeding
        (2) Fractures/obvious deformity
        (3) Burn wounds
        (4) Pale, mottled skin
        (5) Flattened jugular veins
     c) Auscultation
        (1) Breath sounds: diminished with hemothorax
     d) Palpation/percussion
        (1) Decreased or absent peripheral pulses
        (2) Decreased central pulse
        (3) Decreased capillary refill
        (4) Skin cool, diaphoretic
        (5) Distention/swelling (e.g., abdomen or thigh)
        (6) Abdominal rigidity
        (7) Chest: abnormal dull sounds
        (8) Abdomen: abnormal dull sounds
  2) Diagnostic procedures
     a) CBC with differential
     b) Type and screen or crossmatch
     c) Serum chemistries
     d) Lactate level
     e) ABGs
     f) Urinalysis; pregnancy test in female patients of childbearing age
     g) Chest, pelvic, long bone radiographs
     h) FAST
     i) DPL
     j) Chest, abdominal CT scans
2. Analysis: differential nursing diagnoses/collaborative problems
   a. Deficient fluid volume
   b. Ineffective tissue perfusion
   c. Risk for impaired skin integrity
3. Planning and implementation/interventions
   a. Maintain airway, breathing, circulation (see Chapters 1 and 32)
   b. Provide supplemental oxygen as indicated
     1) Rapid sequence intubation (RSI) and ventilatory support in obtunded patients
     2) High-flow oxygen
   c. Control any uncontrolled external bleeding
   d. Stop further burning process if thermal injury present (see Chapter 34)
     1) Remove patient's clothing and jewelry
     2) Cover patient with dry sheet or blanket

e. Establish IV access for administration of crystalloid fluids/blood products/medications
  1) Insert minimum of two large-bore intravenous catheters in adults: largest size possible in children
  2) Initiate fluid resuscitation[8] with warmed isotonic crystalloid solution such as lactated Ringer's or normal saline solutions
     a) First bolus should be administered rapidly: 1–2 L in the adult patient and 20 mL/kg for the pediatric patient
     b) Fluid requirements should be based on assessment of the patient's response as evidenced by adequate end-organ perfusion and oxygenation as seen in improvement in the patient's level of consciousness, peripheral perfusion, and urinary output
     c) Administer warmed blood and blood products as indicated by the patient's condition
f. Prepare for/assist with medical interventions
  1) Advanced airway management
     a) Nasal or oral intubation
     b) Supraglottic airway (e.g., King, Combitube, laryngeal mask airway)
     c) Surgical airway (e.g., cricothyrotomy)
  2) Institute cardiac and pulse oximetry monitoring
  3) Consider application of a pneumatic antishock garment or pelvic binder to control hemorrhage with a pelvic fracture
  4) Insert gastric tube and attach to suction
  5) Insert indwelling urinary catheter
  6) Assist with hospital admission or transfer to an institution providing a higher level of care
g. Administer pharmacologic therapy as ordered
  1) RSI premedications: sedatives, analgesics, neuromuscular blocking agents
  2) Vasopressors: only after fluid resuscitation
  3) Antibiotics
  4) Nonnarcotic analgesics
  5) Narcotics
  6) Tetanus immunization
4. Evaluation and ongoing assessment
   a. Airway patency
   b. Level of consciousness
   c. Hemodynamic monitoring
   d. Breath sounds, pulse oximetry
   e. Cardiac rate and rhythm
   f. Pain relief
   g. Intake and output

D. OBSTRUCTIVE

Obstructive shock results from inadequate circulating blood volume because of an obstruction or compression of a vessel(s). Pulmonary embolus, pericardial tamponade, and tension pneumothorax can lead to obstructive shock. Air can obstruct the pulmonary artery and cause an obstruction to right ventricular blood outflow during systole, with resulting obstructive shock. Blood in the pericardial sac can compress the heart. When this occurs, the patient becomes hypotensive, bradycardic, and hypoxic despite an adequate blood supply. The cause of the obstruction needs to be quickly recognized and appropriate interventions initiated in order to prevent morbidity and mortality.

1. Assessment
   a. Subjective data collection
      1) History of present illness/injury/chief complaint
         a) Pain; chest (see Chapter 8)
            (1) Severe and continuous
            (2) Squeezing, sharp, "tearing," midsternal radiating to back
         b) Chest injury (see Chapter 39): blunt or penetrating forces
         c) Diving under pressure (see Chapter 15)
         d) Shortness of breath
         e) Rapid ascent to altitude (see Chapter 15)
      2) Past medical history
         a) Current or preexisting diseases/illness
            (1) Cardiovascular disease
            (2) Pulmonary disease
         b) Medications
         c) Allergies
         d) Immunization status
   b. Objective data collection
      1) Physical examination
         a) General appearance
            (1) Level of consciousness, behavior, affect: confusion to comatose
            (2) Tachycardia/bradycardia, tachypnea, hypotension
            (3) Severe distress/discomfort, critically ill
         b) Inspection
            (1) Diaphoresis
            (2) Jugular vein distention
            (3) Tracheal deviation: late finding with tension pneumothorax
            (4) Cyanotic upper chest and face
         c) Auscultation
            (1) Breath sounds: absent on affected side
            (2) Heart sounds: distant or muffled
      2) Diagnostic procedures
         a) ABGs
         b) D-dimer level
         c) Urinalysis; pregnancy test in female patients of childbearing age
         d) Chest radiograph
         e) Echocardiogram
         f) Pulmonary ventilation-perfusion scan
         g) Spiral CT scan with contrast
         h) ECG

2. Analysis: differential nursing diagnoses/collaborative problems
   a. Ineffective tissue perfusion
   b. Impaired gas exchange
   c. Anxiety/fear
3. Planning and implementation/interventions
   a. Maintain airway, breathing, circulation (see Chapters 1 and 32)
   b. Provide supplemental oxygen
      1) RSI and ventilatory support in obtunded patients or those with respiratory compromise
      2) High-flow oxygen
   c. Establish IV access for administration of crystalloid fluids/blood products/medications
   d. Prepare for/assist with medical interventions
      1) Needle decompression and chest tube insertion[9]
      2) Advanced airway management
         a) Nasal or oral intubation
         b) Supraglottic airway (e.g., King, Combitube, laryngeal mask airway)
         c) Surgical airway (e.g., Cricothyrotomy)
      3) Possible pericardiocentesis[10]
      4) Institute cardiac and pulse oximetry monitoring
      5) Insert gastric tube and attach to suction
      6) Insert indwelling urinary catheter
      7) Assist with hospital admission: operative interventions such as pericardial window
   e. Administer pharmacologic therapy as ordered
      1) RSI premedications: sedatives, analgesics, neuromuscular blocking agents
      2) Vasopressors
4. Evaluation and ongoing monitoring
   a. Airway patency
   b. Level of consciousness
   c. Hemodynamic status
   d. Breath sounds and pulse oximetry
   e. Cardiac rate and rhythm
   f. Pain relief
   g. Intake and output

References

1. McCance KL, Huether SE: *Pathophysiology: The biologic basis for disease in adults and children,* ed 7, St. Louis, MO, 2014, Mosby.
2. Emergency Nurses Association: *Emergency nursing pediatric course,* ed 4, Des Plaines, IL, 2014, Emergency Nurses Association.
3. Emergency Nurses Association: *Course for advanced trauma nursing,* Des Plaines, IL, 2015, Emergency Nurses Association.
4. Emergency Nurses Association: *Trauma nursing core course,* ed 7, Des Plaines, IL, 2014, Emergency Nurses Association.
5. Rogers WK, Todd M: Acute spinal cord injury, *Best Practice & Research Clinical Anaesthesiology,* 2015. http://dx.doi.org/10.1016/j.bpa.2015.11.003.

6. American College of Surgeons Committee on Trauma: Shock. In *Advanced trauma life support for doctors*, ed 9, Chicago, IL, 2012, American College of Surgeons, pp 62–93.

7. Micek S, Shah R, Kollef M: Management of severe sepsis: integration of multiple pharmacologic interventions, *Pharmacotherapy* 23(11):1486–1496, 2003.

8. Guyton A, Hall J: *Textbook of medical physiology*, ed 13, Philadelphia, PA, 2015, Elsevier.

9. Adler E, Blok B: Thoracentesis. In Roberts J, editor: *Roberts and Hedges' clinical procedures in emergency medicine*, ed 6, 2014, pp 173–188.

10. Mallemat H, Tewelde S: Pericardiocentesis. In Roberts J, editor: *Roberts and Hedges' clinical procedures in emergency medicine*, ed 6, 2014, pp 298–318.

Bibliography

Dellinger RP, Levy MM, Rhodes A, Annane D, Gerlach H, Opal SM, Moreno R, and the Surviving Sepsis Campaign Guidelines Committee including the Pediatric Subgroup. Surviving sepsis campaign: international guidelines for management of severe sepsis and septic shock: 2012; 2013. Retrieved from http://www.survivingsepsis.org/Guidelines/Pages/default.aspx.

CHAPTER 30

Wounds and Wound Management

Elda G. Ramirez, PhD, RN, FNP-BC, FAANP, FAEN

MAJOR TOPICS
General Strategy
Assessment
Analysis: Differential Nursing Diagnoses/Collaborative
 Problems
Planning and Implementation/Interventions
Evaluation and Ongoing Monitoring
Documentation of Interventions and Patient Response
Age-Related Considerations

Specific Wound Management Emergencies
Abrasions
Avulsions
Foreign Bodies
Human Bites
Lacerations
Missile Injuries
Puncture Wounds
Wound Complications

I. General Strategy

A. ASSESSMENT

1. Primary and secondary assessment/resuscitation (see Chapters 1 and 32)
2. Focused assessment
   a. Subjective data collection
      1) History of present injury/chief complaint
         a) Description and location of injury
         b) Cause of injury
         c) Mechanism of injury (see Chapter 31)
         d) Age of chronic wound
         e) Recent débridement/surgery to wound
            (1) Angle of blow
            (2) Direction of fall
            (3) Deceleration of vehicle
            (4) Compressive force injuries more suscep-
                tible to infection
         f) Time elapsed since injury
         g) Bleeding
            (1) Estimated amount of blood loss at time
                of assessment and since injury
            (2) Venous (dark and oozing) and/or arterial
                (bright red and pulsating)
            (3) Systemic responses (e.g., nausea)
         h) Pain: PQRST (see Chapter 8)
         i) Numbness/tingling in immediate area or in
            other parts of body
         j) Patient hand dominance and profession if
            hand involved
         k) Work related

         l) Efforts to relieve symptoms
            (1) Home remedies
            (2) Alternative therapies
            (3) Medications
               (a) Prescription
               (b) OTC/herbal
      2) Past medical history
         a) Current or preexisting diseases/illness:
            comorbidity factors affecting healing
            (1) Diabetes
            (2) Long-term steroid use
            (3) Host immunocompromise
            (4) Poor tissue perfusion
            (5) Predisposition to frequent infections or
                delayed healing
            (6) Extended time between injury and
                treatment
         b) History of injuries (frequent falls, self-
            mutilation)
         c) Discolorations on skin, both old and new
         d) Scars: location, type, and age
         e) Smoking history
         f) Substance and/or alcohol use/abuse
         g) Last normal menstrual period: female
            patients of childbearing age
         h) Current medications
            (1) Prescription
               (a) Steroids
               (b) Immunosuppressive drugs
               (c) Anticoagulants
            (2) OTC/herbal

i) Allergies
j) Immunization status
3) Psychological, social, environmental factors
   a) Exposure: or injury-prone activities
   b) Socioeconomic factors that may result in
      (1) Exposure to certain types of injuries (e.g., stab wounds)
      (2) Inadequate follow-up care
   c) Social history
      (1) Possible/actual abuse, assault, intimate partner violence situations (see Chapters 3 and 40)
      (2) Smoking
      (3) Living conditions (e.g., able to care for self, homeless)
   d) Nutritional status
      (1) General appearance and grooming
      (2) Obesity
      (3) Underweight
   e) Fear of disfigurement or scarring
b. Objective data collection
   1) Physical examination
      a) General appearance
         (1) Level of consciousness, behavior, affect
         (2) Vital signs
         (3) Odors
         (4) Body size, stage of growth
         (5) Gait
         (6) Hygiene
         (7) Level of distress/discomfort
      b) Inspection
         (1) Color: pallor, cyanosis, discoloration
         (2) Edema of surrounding tissues
         (3) Characteristics of wound
         (4) Location of wound or injury
         (5) Underlying structures
         (6) Effect on function of involved part
            (a) Blood vessel involvement
            (b) Arterial and venous flow
            (c) Lymphadenopathy
            (d) Nerve involvement
            (e) Tendon involvement
            (f) Bone injury (open fracture)
         (7) Extent of wound contamination
         (8) Presence of necrotic tissue
         (9) Presence of foreign bodies
      c) Palpation
         (1) Areas of tenderness
         (2) Bony deformity
         (3) Circulation: distal pulses and, if indicated, capillary refill
         (4) Sensation: absence or deficiencies in sensation
         (5) Tendon function: flexion/extension and movement of involved area
         (6) Temperature of affected area

3. Diagnostic procedures
   a. Laboratory studies
      1) Complete blood count (CBC) with differential: if wound infection present, determine leukocytosis, anemia, thrombocytopenia
      2) Wound culture and sensitivity: if infection present
      3) Coagulation profile: if bleeding is uncontrolled evaluate for coagulation abnormalities especially if deep wound excision required
      4) Serum glucose: patients with new onset diabetes may present with wound infection
   b. Imaging studies
      1) Diagnostic imaging of affected area to identify
         a) Underlying injury
         b) Foreign body
         c) Gas formation
         d) Possible osteomyelitis
         e) Abscess
      2) Fluoroscopy to identify location of foreign body
      3) Computed tomography (CT) scan to identify location of foreign body or underlying injury

B. ANALYSIS: DIFFERENTIAL NURSING DIAGNOSES/COLLABORATIVE PROBLEMS

1. Anxiety/fear
2. Body image disturbance
3. Impaired skin integrity
4. Deficient knowledge
5. Risk for deficient fluid volume
6. Risk for infection (Box 30.1)
7. Risk for injury
8. Acute pain

Box 30.1

Risk Factors for Wound Infection

Risk Factors for Wound Infection

1. Injury more than 8–12 hours old (varies depending on the following factors)
2. Location: leg and thigh, then arms, then feet, then chest, then back, then face, then scalp
3. Contamination with devitalized tissue, foreign matter, saliva, or stool
4. Blunt (crush) mechanism
5. Presence of subcutaneous sutures
6. Type of repair: risk greatest with sutures > staples > tape
7. Anesthesia with epinephrine
8. High-velocity missile injuries

(From Marx, J. A., Hockberger, R. S., & Walls, R. M. [Eds.]. [2012]. *Rosen's emergency medicine: Concepts and clinical practice* [8th ed.]. St. Louis, MO: Elsevier Mosby.)

C. PLANNING AND IMPLEMENTATION/ INTERVENTIONS

1. Determine priorities of care
   a. Maintain airway, breathing, circulation (see Chapters 1 and 32)
      1) Tourniquet
   b. Provide supplemental oxygen as indicated
   c. Establish IV access for administration of appropriate fluid/blood products/medications as needed
   d. Obtain and set up equipment and supplies
   e. Prepare for/assist with medical interventions (Box 30.2)
   f. Administer pharmacologic therapy as ordered
2. Relieve anxiety/apprehension
3. Allow significant others to remain with patient if supportive
4. Educate patient/significant others

D. EVALUATION AND ONGOING MONITORING

1. Continuously monitor and treat as indicated
2. Monitor patient response/outcomes and modify nursing care plan as appropriate
3. If positive patient outcomes are not demonstrated, reevaluate assessment and/or plan of care

---

Box 30.2

Wound Care Instructions

Wound Care Instructions

A. Elevate the injured extremity above the level of the heart. Wear a sling when appropriate.
B. Cleanse daily in a gentle manner to remove debris and crusting that develops. Use dilute hydrogen peroxide.
C. Immobilization should be maintained at least until suture removal.
D. Signs of infection
   1. Redness
   2. Increasing pain
   3. Swelling
   4. Fever
   5. Red streaks progressing up an extremity
E. Wound check
   1. As needed to check signs of infection
   2. Routine at 48 hours for high-risk wounds
F. Suture removal (*Note:* Suture may be removed earlier if Steri-Strips reinforce the wound.)
   1. Face: 3–5 days (always replace with Steri-Strips)
   2. Scalp: 7–10 days
   3. Trunk: 7–10 days
   4. Arms and legs: 10–14 days
   5. Joints: 14 days

(From Marx, J. A., Hockberger, R. S., & Walls, R. M. [Eds.]. [2012]. *Rosen's emergency medicine: Concepts and clinical practice* [8th ed.]. St. Louis, MO: Elsevier Mosby.)

E. DOCUMENTATION OF INTERVENTIONS AND PATIENT RESPONSE

F. AGE-RELATED CONSIDERATIONS

1. Pediatric
   a. Growth or development related
      1) Pediatric healing responses are more rapid than those of adults
      2) Close fluid monitoring is essential
      3) Major heat loss can occur in young children left unclothed for a period of time because of their large body surface area
      4) High metabolic rate and low glycogen stores in infants can lead to hypoglycemia during stress
      5) Calming techniques are based on developmental stage of child
   b. "Pearls"
      1) It is important to develop and maintain a relationship with family, along with child, because security for most children comes from parents
      2) It is essential to communicate at child's level of understanding when possible
      3) Child's need to remain covered should be respected
      4) Child maltreatment should always be considered because surface trauma is often associated with, or is the most evident sign of, nonaccidental injuries in children
2. Geriatric
   a. Aging-related
      1) Reduced elasticity of skin, decreased subcutaneous fat layer, and reduced perfusion
      2) Limited mobility and joint flexion as a result of osteoarthritis
      3) Capillary fragility, leading to large ecchymosis
      4) Adaptive responses take longer
      5) Poor tolerance for cold as result of peripheral vascular changes and diminished thermoregulatory ability
      6) Loss of visual acuity
      7) Hearing impairments
      8) Diminished temperature sensation
      9) Frequent chronic dysrhythmias
   b. "Pearls"
      1) Increased risk of infection owing to decreased healing ability
      2) Increased risk of skin breakdown owing to decreased subcutaneous tissue
      3) Skin tears easily making wound repair more difficult and leading to poor cosmetic outcomes

II. Specific Wound Management Emergencies

A. ABRASIONS

Abrasions are skin wounds caused by tangential trauma to the dermis and epidermis. This injury is similar to a burn. These common injuries are painful and can result from falls, scrapes, and cycling accidents. Meticulous wound care is essential to avoid a tattooing effect from imbedded debris.

1. Assessment
   a. Subjective data collection
      1) History of present injury/chief complaint
         a) Description of injury
         b) Time elapsed: dirt and debris should be removed within 4–6 hours from extremity wounds and within 8 hours from facial wounds
         c) Location of injury
         d) Pain (see Chapter 8)
      2) Past medical history
         a) Current or preexisting diseases/illness
         b) Medications
         c) Allergies
         d) Immunization status
   b. Objective data collection
      1) Physical examination
         a) General appearance
            (1) Mild to moderate distress/discomfort
         b) Inspection
            (1) Extent of denuded tissue
            (2) Depth of injury
            (3) Presence of embedded dirt and debris (tattooing or "road rash")
         c) Palpation
            (1) Pulses distal to injury
            (2) Flexion/extension against resistance if joint involvement
            (3) Areas of tenderness
            (4) Sensation surrounding and distal to injury
      2) Diagnostic procedures
         a) CBC with differential: if infection present
         b) Radiographs of affected part if indicated
2. Analysis: differential nursing diagnoses/collaborative problems
   a. Impaired skin integrity
   b. Risk for infection
   c. Acute pain
   d. Anxiety/fear
   e. Deficient knowledge
3. Planning and implementation/interventions
   a. Establish IV access for administration of crystalloid fluid/medications as needed
   b. Prepare for/assist with medical interventions

1) Place affected part in position of comfort
2) Cleanse abraded skin area: may require whirlpool therapy or procedural sedation (see Chapter 9) if area large
3) Apply; nonadhering dressing to area
   c. Administer pharmacologic therapy as ordered
   1) Possible procedural sedation medications
   2) Nonnarcotic analgesics
   3) Narcotics
   4) Tetanus immunization
   d. Educate patient/significant others
   1) Change dressing and apply ointment as indicated and recommended
   2) Wash facial area four times a day and reapply ointment
   3) Avoid direct sunlight to area for 6 months because of risk of pigmentary changes
   4) Take or use medication according to directions
   5) Return or make appointment for follow-up care, as indicated
4. Evaluation and ongoing monitoring
   a. Hemodynamic status
   b. Pain relief

B. AVULSIONS

Avulsions are characterized by full-thickness tissue loss that prevents wound edge approximation. This injury is commonly seen in fingertip and tip of the nose injuries. Hemostasis is the immediate problem. Small avulsions heal by secondary intention. Larger avulsed areas may require split-thickness grafting. A "degloving" injury is a severe avulsion, in which the full thickness of skin is peeled away from a finger, hand, foot, or area of a limb, with resulting devascularization of the skin and potential damage to underlying tissues. Flap replacement and grafting are frequently required.

1. Assessment
   a. Subjective data collection
      1) History of present injury/chief complaint
         a) Description of accident
         b) Time lapse since injury
         c) Location of injury
         d) Efforts made to preserve avulsed tissue
         e) If hand involvement: determine patient hand dominance
         f) Pain (see Chapter 8)
         g) Treatment of wound and avulsed tissue before arrival
      2) Past medical history
         a) Current or preexisting diseases/illness
         b) Medications
         c) Allergies
         d) Immunization status
   b. Objective data collection
      1) Physical examination
         a) General appearance
            (1) Moderate to severe distress/discomfort

b) Inspection
   (1) Amount of bleeding
   (2) Extent of injury: structures involved
c) Palpation
   (1) Pulses distal to injury
   (2) Flexion/extension against resistance if joint involvement
   (3) Areas of tenderness
   (4) Sensation surrounding and distal to injury
2) Diagnostic procedures
   a) CBC with differential: if infection present
   b) Radiographs as indicated: degloving injury associated with possible associated fracture
2. Analysis: differential nursing diagnoses/collaborative problems
   a. Impaired skin integrity
   b. Risk for infection
   c. Pain
   d. Anxiety/fear
   e. Deficient knowledge

3. Planning and implementation/interventions
a. Establish IV access for administration of appropriate fluid/medications
b. Prepare for/assist with medical interventions
   1) Elevate affected part
   2) Apply sterile, saline-soaked gauze to area
   3) Apply steady pressure to decrease blood loss
   4) Cleanse wound with antiseptic soap and irrigate thoroughly (Table 30.1)
   5) If small avulsion
      a) Apply petrolatum (Vaseline) or Xeroform gauze or other nonadhering material
      b) Apply pressure dressing
   6) If large avulsion
      a) Apply product for bleeding control (e.g., Gelfoam)
      b) Apply petrolatum (Vaseline) or Xeroform gauze or other nonadhering material to avulsed area and donor site
      c) Apply layered dressing
      d) Apply metal protector, if indicated

Table 30.1

Antiseptic Solutions

Agents	Antimicrobial Activity	Mechanisms of Action	Tissue Toxicity	Indications and Contraindications
Povidone-iodine solution (iodine complexes) (Betadine)	Available as a 10% solution with polyvinyl-pyrrolidone (povidone) containing 1% free iodine with broad rapid-onset antimicrobial activity	Potent germicide in low concentrations	Decreases PMN migration and lifespan at concentration >1% May cause systemic toxicity at higher concentrations; questionable toxicity at 1% concentration	Probably a safe and effective wound cleanser at a 1% concentration 10% solution is effective to prepare skin around the wound
Povidone-iodine surgical scrub	Same as the solution	Same	Toxic to open wounds	Appear to be effective, safe wound cleansers
Nonionic detergents Pluronic F-68 Shur-Clens	Ethylene oxide is 80% of their molecular weight No antimicrobial activity	Wound cleansers	No toxicity to open wounds, eyes, or intravenous solutions	Appear to be effective, safe wound cleansers
Hydrogen peroxide	3% solution in water has brief germicidal activity	Oxidizing agent that denatures protein	Toxic to open wounds	Should not be used on wounds after initial cleaning; may be used to clean intact skin
Hexachlorophene (polychlorinated bisphenol) (pHisoHex)	Bacteriostatic (2–5%) Greater activity against gram-positive organisms	Interruption of bacterial electron transport and disruption of membrane-bound enzymes	Little skin toxicity; the scrub form is damaging to open wounds	Never use scrub solution in open wounds Very good preoperative hand preparation
Alcohols	Low-potency antimicrobial most effective as a 70% ethyl and 70% isopropyl alcohol solution	Denatures protein	Kills irreversibly and functions as a fixative	No role in routine care
Phenols	Bacteriostatic >0.2% Bactericidal >1% Fungicidal 1.3%	Denatures protein	Extensive tissue necrosis and systemic toxicity	Never use >2% aqueous phenol or >4% phenol plus glycerol

(From Marx, J. A., Hockberger, R. S., & Walls, R. M. [Eds.]. [2012]. *Rosen's emergency medicine: Concepts and clinical practice* [8th ed.]. St. Louis, MO: Elsevier Mosby.)

7) If degloving injury
   a) Realign soft tissue to prevent further damage
   b) Cover with sterile dressing
   c) Assist with hospital admission for débridement and grafting
   c. Administer pharmacologic therapy as ordered
   1) Assist with administration of local or regional anesthetic
   2) Nonnarcotic analgesics
   3) Narcotics
   4) Antibiotics
   5) Tetanus immunization
   d. Educate patient/significant others
   1) Elevate part to reduce bleeding
   2) Apply ice as indicated
   3) Care for wound and dressing
   4) Observe for signs of infection
   5) Take medications, as ordered
   6) Return or make appointment for follow-up care
4. Evaluation and ongoing monitoring
   a. Hemodynamic status
   b. Bleeding control
   c. Pain relief

C. FOREIGN BODIES

Foreign bodies include wood and metal splinters, glass, clothing, fragments from gunshot wounds, pins and needles, rubber from tennis shoes, fishhooks, and many other items that become embedded in various parts of the body. Occasionally, objects that are difficult to find but are not likely to cause a tissue reaction will be left in place (e.g., glass, metal). Vegetative foreign bodies (e.g., thorns, wood) are highly reactive, lead to infection, and should be removed as quickly as possible. Unfortunately, vegetative foreign bodies are also more difficult to visualize on plain radiographs and may require CT scans, sonograms, fluoroscopy, or local wound exploration to aid in removal.

1. Assessment
   a. Subjective data collection
   1) History of present injury/chief complaint
      a) Description of injury
      b) Characteristics of suspected foreign body
      c) Location of injury
      d) Direction of entry
      e) Time elapsed since injury
      f) Extent of contamination by foreign body
      g) Pain and discomfort (see Chapter 8)
   2) Past medical history
      a) Current or preexisting diseases/illness
      b) Medications
      c) Allergies
      d) Immunization status
   b. Objective data collection
   1) Physical examination
      a) General appearance
         (1) Mild to moderate distress/discomfort

   b) Inspection
      (1) Open wound
      (2) Embedded or protruding foreign object
   c) Palpation
      (1) Pulses distal to injury
      (2) Flexion/extension against resistance if joint involvement
      (3) Areas of tenderness
      (4) Sensation surrounding and distal to injury
   2) Diagnostic procedures
      a) CBC with differential: if infection present
      b) Radiograph of involved area
         (1) Underlying injury
         (2) Not useful for visualizing pieces of clothing or natural wood splinters
         (3) Fluoroscopy may be required for foreign body removal
2. Analysis: differential nursing diagnoses/collaborative problems
   a. Impaired skin integrity
   b. Risk for infection
   c. Pain
   d. Anxiety/fear
   e. Deficient knowledge
3. Planning and implementation/interventions
   a. Prepare for/assist with medical interventions
   1) Thoroughly cleanse area around entry site with a mild antiseptic solution
      a) Do not soak part of body containing a wooden splinter because wood absorbs liquid and may disintegrate during removal
   2) Carefully, apply gentle traction with small forceps to remove objects that lie close to or protrude through skin
   3) Apply appropriate dressing
   b. Administer pharmacologic therapy as ordered
   1) Assist with administration of local or regional anesthetic
   2) Nonnarcotic analgesics
   3) Antibiotics
   4) Tetanus immunization
   c. Educate patient/significant others
   1) Soak wound in warm, soapy water two or three times a day for 2–4 days
   2) Watch for signs of infection
   3) Return or make appointment for follow-up care, if indicated
4. Evaluation and ongoing monitoring
   a. Pain relief

D. HUMAN BITES

All human bite wounds are at increased risk of becoming infected because of the multiple bacterial organisms located in the human mouth. The injuries may be self-inflicted or may result from person-to-person contact. Puncture wounds or deep lacerations that are inadequately cleaned are at particular risk of developing wound sepsis. Clenched-fist injuries (e.g., human bites over the metacarpophalangeal joint) typically occur during an altercation and are at an increased risk of developing an infection because of joint penetration. Other common sites of human bites involve the ears, nose, vagina, and penis.

1. Assessment
   a. Subjective data collection
      1) History of present injury/chief complaint
         a) Description of incident
         b) Time elapsed since injury
         c) Location of bite
         d) Extent of bleeding
         e) Pain or discomfort (see Chapter 8)
      2) Past medical history
         a) Current or preexisting diseases/illness
         b) Medications
         c) Allergies
         d) Immunization status
   b. Objective data collection
      1) Physical examination
         a) General appearance
            (1) Possible elevated temperature
            (2) Moderate distress/discomfort
         b) Inspection
            (1) Edema surrounding wound
            (2) Erythema surrounding wound
            (3) Presence of discharge, pus
            (4) Lymphangitis
            (5) Necrotic tissue
         c) Palpation
            (1) Pulses distal to injury
            (2) Flexion/extension against resistance if joint involvement
            (3) Areas of tenderness
            (4) Sensation surrounding and distal to injury
      2) Diagnostic procedures
         a) CBC with differential: if infection present
         b) Saliva residue samples (swabs)
         c) Wound discharge culture and sensitivity
         d) Radiograph of injury
            (1) Presence of foreign body
            (2) Underlying bony injury
2. Analysis: differential nursing diagnoses/collaborative problems
   a. Impaired skin integrity
   b. Risk for infection
   c. Pain
   d. Anxiety/fear
   e. Deficient knowledge
3. Planning and implementation/interventions
   a. Establish IV access for administration of crystalloid fluids/medications

   b. Prepare for/assist with medical interventions
      1) Place affected part in position of comfort
      2) Cleanse wound thoroughly with mild antiseptic solution and irrigate extensively with normal saline solution/tap water
         a) Consider taking photographs before cleaning if injury is associated with crime (see Chapter 44)
         b) Assist with collection and maintenance of physical and forensic evidence as indicated (see Chapter 44)
      3) Assist with wound débridement, as needed
      4) Assist with wound closure, if required; delayed closure is preferred
      5) Apply appropriate dressing
      6) Assist with possible hospital admission
   c. Administer pharmacologic therapy as ordered
      1) Assist with administration of local or regional anesthetic
      2) Antibiotics
      3) Nonnarcotic analgesics
      4) Narcotics
      5) Tetanus immunization
   d. Educate patient/significant others
      1) Specific wound care instructions based on situation
      2) Change dressings, as indicated
      3) Signs of infection and other complications
      4) Take antibiotic medication, as ordered
      5) Return or schedule appointment for follow-up care
4. Evaluation and ongoing monitoring
   a. Neurovascular and neuromuscular function of injured area
   b. Pain relief

E. LACERATIONS

The goals of wound management are to restore function, repair tissue integrity, and minimize risk of infection. Lacerations are open wounds that result from sharp or blunt trauma to the skin. The laceration may be superficial and may only penetrate the epidermis, or it may extend past the dermis into fascia and muscle involving the underlying structures. At the time of the injury, immediate vasospasm and clot formation occur; within 6 hours, the inflammatory phase takes place and continues for up to 3 days. A waterproof covering develops after the first 24 hours. Epithelial cell growth takes place within 6 hours to 1 month of injury. Repigmentation of the wound may take longer than a year. Because sutures or staples are left in for extended periods and epithelialization takes up to 1 month, reinforcement of the wound is necessary after removal of closure methods, especially in areas of flexion and extension.

1. Assessment
   a. Subjective data collection
      1) History of present injury/chief complaint

a) Description of what caused the injury (wood, metal, velocity)
b) Extent of instrument contamination (sewage pipe vs. tree limb)
c) Time elapsed since injury
d) Primary or secondary closure
e) Location of injury
f) Extent of bleeding
g) Pain (see Chapter 8)
h) Care measures before arrival (tourniquet)
2) Past medical history
a) Current or preexisting diseases/illness
b) Medications
c) Allergies
d) Immunization status
b. Objective data collection
1) Physical examination
a) General appearance
(1) Bleeding activity
(2) Mild to moderate distress/discomfort
b) Inspection
(1) Depth, length of laceration
(2) Surrounding and underlying structure involvement
(3) Presence of necrotic tissue
(4) Foreign body or wound contamination
c) Palpation
(1) Pulses distal to injury
(2) Flexion/extension against resistance if joint involvement
(3) Areas of tenderness
(4) Sensation surrounding and distal to injury
2) Diagnostic procedures
a) CBC with differential: if wound infection present—hemorrhage
b) Wound discharge culture and sensitivity: if wound infection present
c) Diagnostic imaging of affected area
(1) Possible associated bony injury/open fracture
(2) Foreign body in wound
2. Analysis: differential nursing diagnoses/collaborative problems
a. Risk for deficient fluid volume
b. Impaired skin integrity
c. Risk for infection
d. Acute pain
e. Anxiety/fear
f. Deficient knowledge deficit
3. Planning and implementation/interventions
a. Establish IV access for administration of crystalloid fluid/medications as needed
b. Prepare for/assist with medical interventions
1) Control local bleeding
a) Direct pressure
b) Elevation of part

2) Place affected part in position of comfort
3) Cleanse/irrigate skin around wound with normal saline solution/tap water and/or antiseptic agent (many agents are caustic to vascularized tissue)
4) Irrigate wound thoroughly with normal saline solution/tap water with a psi ≤15.
5) Assist with débridement of tissue
6) Assist with wound closure
a) Suture material
b) Staples
c) Skin glue (Dermabond®)
d) Tape (e.g., Steri-Strips)
7) Primary closure is when the wound is closed immediately; the provider may leave the wound open and packed for 3–4 days then close (primary delay closure) or may leave the wound open for secondary closure with close follow-up care. A facial wound may still be closed by primary intent after 24 hours
8) Apply appropriate dressing to wound
9) Apply splint if partial immobilization of part is indicated
10) Assist with hospital admission if extensive débridement, irrigation, or repair required, or other injuries present
c. Administer pharmacologic therapy as ordered
1) Assist with administration of local or regional anesthetic
2) Procedural sedation medications if extensive repair required
3) Nonnarcotic analgesics
4) Narcotics
5) Antibiotics
6) Tetanus immunization (Table 30.2)
d. Educate patient/significant others
1) Elevate affected part for 48 hours to minimize pain and swelling
2) Apply ice or heat, as directed
3) Wound care instructions: keep wound and dressing clean and dry; soap and water two times a day; keep covered for first 24 hours
4) Change dressing if wet and/or soiled
5) Observe for local redness, swelling, warmth, discharge, or development of fever
6) Take medications according to directions, if ordered
7) Return or make appointment for follow-up care as indicated
8) Sutures removed as directed by provider
9) Use sunblock over wound for at least 6 months (sun protection factor [SPF] of 15 or stronger)
4. Evaluation and ongoing monitoring
a. Hemodynamic status
b. Bleeding control
c. Pain relief

Table 30.2

CDC Tetanus Recommendation

Age/Status	Recommendations
Birth through 6 years	DTaP is routinely recommended at 2, 4, and 6 months, at 15 through 18 months, and at 4 through 6 years.
7 through 10 years	Tdap is recommended for children ages 7 through 10 years who are not fully vaccinated (see note 1) against pertussis: Single dose of Tdap for those not fully vaccinated (see note 1) **or** If additional doses of tetanus and diphtheria toxoid-containing vaccines are needed, then children aged 7 through 10 years should be vaccinated according to the catch-up schedule, with Tdap preferred as the first dose. **UPDATED JAN 2011**
11 through 18 years	Tdap is routinely recommended as a single dose for those 11 through 18 years of age with preferred administration at 11 through 12 years of age. If adolescent was not fully vaccinated (see note 1) as a child, check the ACIP recommendations and catch-up schedule to determine what's indicated. If adolescents (13 through 18 years) missed getting Tdap at 11 to 12 years of age, administer at the next patient encounter or sooner if adolescent will have close contact with infants.
19 years and older	Any adult 19 years of age and older who has not received a dose of Tdap should get one as soon as feasible—to protect themselves and infants. This Tdap booster dose can replace one of the 10-year Td booster doses. Tdap can be administered regardless of interval since the previous Td dose. Shorter intervals between Tdap and last Td may increase the risk of mild local reactogenicity but may be appropriate if your patient is at high risk for contracting pertussis, such as during an outbreak, or has close contact with infants. When feasible, Boostrix (GSK) should be used for adults 65 years and older; however, either vaccine product administered to a person 65 years or older provides protection and may be considered valid. Providers should not miss an opportunity to vaccinate persons aged 65 years and older with Tdap. Therefore, providers may administer the Tdap vaccine they have available. **UPDATED JUN 2012**
Pregnant women	Pregnant women should get a dose of Tdap during each pregnancy, preferably at 27 through 36 weeks gestation. By getting Tdap during pregnancy, maternal pertussis antibodies transfer to the newborn, likely providing protection against pertussis in early life, before the baby starts getting DTaP vaccines. Tdap will also help protect the mother at time of delivery, making her less likely to transmit pertussis to her infant. It is important that all family members and caregivers of the infant are up-to-date with their pertussis vaccines (DTaP or Tdap, depending on age) before coming into close contact with the infant. Tdap is recommended in the immediate postpartum period before discharge from the hospital or birthing center for new mothers who have never received Tdap before or whose vaccination status is unknown. **UPDATED AUG 2013**
Health care personnel (see note 2)	A single dose of Tdap is recommended for health care personnel who have not previously received Tdap as an adult and who have direct patient contact. Tdap vaccination can protect health care personnel against pertussis and help prevent them from spreading it to their patients. Priority should be given to vaccinating those who have direct contact with babies younger than 12 months of age. Tdap can be administered regardless of interval since the previous Td dose. However, shorter intervals between Tdap and last Td may increase the risk of mild local reactogenicity. For additional guidance, see Evaluating Revaccination of Healthcare Personnel. **NEW JUN 2015**

Abbreviation: ACIP, Advisory Committee on Immunization Practices

Note 1: Fully vaccinated is defined as 5 doses of DTaP or 4 doses of DTaP if the fourth dose was administered on or after the fourth birthday.

Note 2: Health care personnel include but are not limited to physicians, other primary care providers, nurses, aides, respiratory therapists, radiology technicians, students (e.g., medical, nursing, and pharmaceutical), dentists, social workers, chaplains, volunteers, and dietary and clerical workers.

(From Centers for Disease Control and Prevention. [2013]. Pertussis: Summary of vaccine recommendations. Retrieved from http://www.cdc.gov/vaccines/vpd-vac/pertussis/recs-summary.htm.)

F. MISSILE INJURIES

Missile injuries include stab wounds, gunshot wounds, and other high-pressure, penetrating wounds. Bullet wounds, especially those of high velocity, may cause bony, neurovascular, and soft tissue injuries remote from the projectile's path. Consider the potential for occult neurovascular injury, especially in high-velocity injuries of the arm and leg.

Forensic considerations include appropriate reporting to law enforcement agencies, careful documentation of patient's condition with accurate description of injury, careful removal of clothing (including not cutting through areas of "evidence"), and appropriate handling and disposition of bullets and weapons (see Chapter 44).

Patients experiencing high-pressure injection injuries generally require débridement and extensive irrigation under anesthesia because serious problems result from the injected material's spreading along fascial planes, neurovascular bundles, and tendon sheaths.

1. Assessment
   a. Subjective data collection
      1) History of present injury/chief complaint
         a) Mechanism of injury (see Chapter 31)
            (1) Bullets
            (2) Stabbing instrument

b) High-pressure injection: paint and grease guns, staple or nail guns
  (1) Location of wound: most commonly index finger of nondominant hand
  (2) Amount of pressure involved
  (3) Type of material in instrument
c) Projectile missile
  (1) Bolt from high-powered machine
  (2) Rock thrown by lawn mower
d) Extent of bleeding
e) Pain (see Chapter 8)
f) Time elapsed since injury
2) Past medical history
  a) Current or preexisting diseases/illness
  b) Medications
  c) Allergies
  d) Immunization status
b. Objective data collection
1) Physical examination
  a) General appearance
    (1) Moderate to severe distress/discomfort
  b) Inspection
    (1) Active bleeding: arterial or venous
    (2) Depth, length of wound
    (3) Structures involved
    (4) Extent of necrotic tissue
    (5) Wound contamination
  c) Palpation
    (1) Pulses distal to injury
    (2) Flexion/extension against resistance if joint involvement
    (3) Areas of tenderness
    (4) Sensation surrounding and distal to injury
2) Diagnostic procedures
  a) CBC with differential: if infection present
  b) Radiographs of affected area
    (1) Foreign body location
    (2) Underlying bony injury
2. Analysis: differential nursing diagnoses/collaborative problems
  a. Risk for deficient fluid volume
  b. Impaired skin integrity
  c. Risk for infection
  d. Acute pain
  e. Anxiety/fear
  f. Deficient knowledge
3. Planning and implementation/interventions
  a. Maintain airway, breathing, circulation (see Chapters 1 and 32)
  b. Provide supplemental oxygen as indicated
  c. Establish IV access for administration of crystalloid fluid/blood products/medications as needed
  d. Prepare for/assist with medical interventions
    1) Control local bleeding
      a) Direct pressure
      b) Elevation of part

c) Ligation of major bleeding points if other methods fail (avoid masses of ligatures)
2) Cleanse and irrigate skin around wound with mild antiseptic solution
  a) If injury is associated with crime, photographs before cleaning or destroying of evidence may be indicated
3) Assist with débriding, irrigating, removal of missile, packing, and closing procedures as needed
  a) Collect and maintain physical and forensic evidence as indicated (see Chapter 44)
4) Apply appropriate dressing
5) Assist with possible hospital admission
e. Administer pharmacologic therapy as ordered
1) Assist with administration of local or regional anesthetic
2) Antibiotics
3) Nonnarcotic analgesics
4) Narcotics
5) Tetanus immunization
f. Educate patient/significant others
1) Elevate affected part
2) Keep wound and dressing clean and dry
3) Change dressing if wet or soiled
4) Observe for redness, swelling, heat (fever), discharge
5) Take medications, if ordered, according to directions
6) Return or make appointment for follow-up care as indicated
4. Evaluation and ongoing monitoring
  a. Hemodynamic status
  b. Pain relief

G. PUNCTURE WOUNDS

Puncture wounds occur when tissue is penetrated by sharp or blunt objects. Such wounds most commonly result from stepping on nails, tacks, needles, or broken glass. Running into or being assaulted with sharp objects may also cause these injuries. Characteristically, puncture wounds bleed minimally and tend to seal off, thus creating a high infection potential.

Puncture wounds near joints carry a high risk for bacterial inoculation into the joint space and subsequent sepsis. A puncture wound on the plantar aspect of the foot increases the risk of developing cellulitis, chondritis, and osteomyelitis (0.4–0.6% of cases). Plantar puncture wounds that pierce the sole of a shoe are at an increased risk of transmitting *Pseudomonas* (prophylaxis treatment with Ciprofloxacin) into the tissue, thereby resulting in the development of infection and osteomyelitis.

1. Assessment
  a. Subjective data collection
    1) History of present injury/chief complaint
      a) Description of accident
      b) Location of injury

c) Type of injuring object
d) Length or depth of penetration
e) Degree of contamination
f) Time elapsed since injury
g) Pain/discomfort (see Chapter 8)
2) Past medical history
a) Current or preexisting diseases/illness
b) Medications
c) Allergies
d) Immunization status
b. Objective data collection
1) Physical examination
a) General appearance
(1) Mild to moderate distress/discomfort
b) Inspection
(1) Estimation of wound depth
(2) Possible presence of foreign body or material
(3) Extent of injury: structures involved
c) Palpation
(1) Pulses distal to injury
(2) Flexion/extension against resistance if joint involvement
(3) Areas of tenderness
(4) Sensation surrounding and distal to injury
2) Diagnostic procedures
a) CBC with differential: if infection present
b) Diagnostic imaging of area
(1) If embedded foreign body is suspected and cannot be easily located
(2) May involve use of soft tissue films with special composition giving clear images with marker placed near suspected entry site
c) Possible fluoroscopy to assist with removal of foreign object
2. Analysis: differential nursing diagnoses/collaborative problems
a. Impaired skin integrity
b. Risk for infection
c. Pain
d. Anxiety/fear
e. Deficient knowledge
3. Planning and implementation/interventions
a. Prepare for/assist with medical interventions
1) Removal of foreign body if present
2) Assist with opening, débriding, irrigating, and packing severely contaminated wound
3) Apply appropriate dressing
b. Administer pharmacologic therapy as ordered
1) Assist with administration of local or regional anesthetic
2) Nonnarcotic analgesics
3) Narcotics
4) Antibiotics
5) Tetanus immunization

c. Educate patient/significant others
1) Soak wound in warm, soapy water two or three times a day for 2–4 days, unless packing in place
2) Observe for signs of infection
3) Return or make appointment for follow-up care, if indicated
4. Evaluation and ongoing monitoring
a. Pain relief

H. WOUND COMPLICATIONS

Uncomplicated localized infections and abscesses are treated in the emergency setting. Infections associated with body jewelry/piercings often require removal of the object. Patients experiencing major systemic infections are admitted to the hospital for general support and definitive treatment.
1. Assessment
a. Subjective data collection
1) History of present injury/chief complaint
a) Circumstances of recent injury/wound/body piercing
b) Characteristics of common wound-related infections
(1) *Staphylococcus* infections
(a) *Staphylococcus aureus* (gram-positive bacteria)
(b) Associated with most skin infections
(c) Usually localized abscesses in superficial subcutaneous tissues
(d) Infection may become systemic
(e) Community-associated methicillin-resistant *S. aureus* (MRSA)
(2) Pasteurellosis
(a) *Pasteurella multocida*
(b) Necrotizing infection associated with animal bites, especially cats
(c) Progresses to cellulitis, osteomyelitis, sinusitis, pleuritis
(3) Cat-scratch fever
(a) Origin possibly *Afipia felos*, or *Bartonella henselae*
(b) Associated with cat or dog scratches
(c) Regional or local lymphadenitis, fever, self-limiting
(4) Wound botulism
(a) Anaerobic *Clostridium botulinum*
(b) Associated with crush injuries or major trauma
(c) Incubation period 4–14 days
(d) Symptoms
(i) Weakness
(ii) Blurred vision
(iii) Difficulty speaking/swallowing
(iv) Dry mucous membranes
(v) Dilated fixed pupils
(vi) Progressive muscular paralysis

(5) Gas gangrene
  (a) Anaerobic *Clostridium perfringens*
  (b) History of intestinal or gallbladder surgery or minor trauma to old scar containing spores
  (c) Incubation period 1 day to 6 weeks
  (d) Symptoms
      (i) Rapidly developing tense, hard edema, leading to hypoxia
      (ii) Thrombosis of local vessels
      (iii) Soft tissue crepitus (hydrogen sulfide and carbon dioxide in tissues)
      (iv) Severe pain
      (v) Thin, watery, brown or brown-gray drainage
      (vi) Elevated temperature: low-grade fever
      (vii) Increased pulse rate
      (viii) Anorexia
      (ix) Vomiting
      (x) Diarrhea
      (xi) Coma
(6) Tetanus
  (a) Anaerobic *Clostridium tetanii*
  (b) Organism found in soil and in human and animal intestines
  (c) Entry to body through break in skin
  (d) Incubation period 2 days to several months (mean, 6–14 days)
  (e) Prodromal symptoms
      (i) Restlessness
      (ii) Headache
      (iii) Muscle spasms
      (iv) Pain: initially in back, neck, or face
      (v) Low back pain
  (f) Progression of disease
      (i) Extreme stiffness
      (ii) Tonic spasms of voluntary muscles
      (iii) Exaggerated reflex activity
      (iv) Generalized convulsions
      (v) Respiratory depression
(7) Rabies
(8) Group A *Streptococcus* (GAS)
  (a) Found in throat and on skin
  (b) May cause life-threatening disease
  (c) Necrotizing fasciitis, streptococcal toxic shock syndrome
  c) Time elapsed since injury
  d) Pain (see Chapter 8)
2) Past medical history
  a) Current or preexisting diseases/illness
  b) Medications
  c) IV drug use

d) Allergies
e) Immunization status
b. Objective data collection
  1) Physical examination
    a) General appearance
      (1) Elevated temperature
      (2) Moderate distress/discomfort
    b) Inspection
      (1) Erythema surrounding wound
      (2) Lymphangitis
      (3) Lymphadenopathy
      (4) Edema
      (5) Raised, indurated abscess
      (6) Wound discharge, pus
      (7) Other findings specific to offending organism
    c) Palpation
      (1) Pulses distal to injury
      (2) Flexion/extension against resistance if joint involvement
      (3) Areas of tenderness
      (4) Warmth of area
      (5) Sensation surrounding and distal to injury
      (6) Other findings specific to offending organism
  2) Diagnostic procedures
    a) CBC with differential
    b) Serum electrolytes including glucose
    c) Wound discharge culture and sensitivity
2. Analysis: differential nursing diagnoses/collaborative problems
  a. Impaired skin integrity
  b. Acute pain
  c. Anxiety/fear
  d. Deficient knowledge
3. Planning and implementation/interventions
  a. Maintain airway, breathing, circulation (see Chapters 1 and 32)
  b. Provide supplemental oxygen as indicated
  c. Establish IV access for administration of crystalloid fluids/medications
  d. Prepare for/assist with medical interventions
    1) Institute cardiac and pulse oximetry monitoring
    2) Provide meticulous wound care
      a) Removal of body jewelry if required
        (1) Stud earring
          (a) Common site: ear lobe
          (b) Removal: grasp front of earring and pull the back straight off the stud; screw-on backs: rotate to left
        (2) Barbell stud
          (a) Straight, curved, or circular bar with threaded ball on each end
          (b) Common sites; tongue, navel, eyebrow, nipple, genitalia

(c) Removal: unscrew either ball, pull bar through soft tissues
(3) Labret stud
  (a) Straight bar with ball on one side and permanently fixed disc on opposite side
  (b) Common site: lip
  (c) Removal: unscrew ball and pull bar through soft tissues
(4) Captive bead ring
  (a) Partial ring with beads with small dimples on opposite sides held "captive" by tension from sides of ring
  (b) Removal: hold ring on either side of bead and release tension, or using small pliers, spread ring apart; bead will drop
(5) Segment ring
  (a) Ring with one bead permanently coupled at one end
  (b) Removal: remove free end of ring
(6) Circle or screwball ring
  (a) Screw holds ring in place
  (b) Removal: grasp segment or ball with forceps and rotate counter-clockwise
(7) Plugs
  (a) Secured in place with O-ring
  (b) Removal: slide O-ring off plug
(8) Tunnels
  (a) Flared outer edge: secured by surface tension of skin and removed using gentle traction
  (b) Two separate pieces: screw together; remove by grasping each half, front and back, and rotate counter-clockwise

3) Assist with incision and drainage to relieve pressure and provide for drainage: may require procedural sedation
4) Apply appropriate dressing
5) Assist with hospital admission if infection more than localized involvement

e. Administer pharmacologic therapy as ordered
  1) Procedural sedation medications for large abscess incision and drainage
  2) Assist with administration of local or regional anesthetic
  3) Antibiotics
  4) Nonnarcotic analgesics
  5) Narcotics
  6) Tetanus immunization (see Table 30.2)
    a) Tetanus toxoid, reduced diphtheria toxoid, and acellular pertussis (Tdap) booster currently recommended for persons up to age 64 years; tetanus, diphtheria (Td) may be substituted

    b) Human tetanus immune globulin (TIG), if patient not adequately immunized, to provide passive immunity for 1 month (may be repeated at end of month if needed)

f. Educate patient/significant others
  1) Encourage all individuals to maintain current diphtheria, pertussis, and tetanus (Tdap) immunization status according to current Recommendations of the Immunization Practices Advisory Committee, Centers for Disease Control and Prevention (CDC), and Committee on Infectious Diseases of the American Academy of Pediatrics
    a) Avoid overimmunization because of hypersensitivity reactions to tetanus when antibody titers are high; signs include
      (1) Rash
      (2) Serum sickness
      (3) Anaphylaxis
  2) Maintain adequate drainage through use of warm saline solution soaks
  3) Continue specific wound care measures as indicated
  4) Take mild analgesic, if needed
  5) Observe for signs of continuing infection
  6) Observe for side effects of administered vaccine
  7) Return or make an appointment for follow-up care; completion of immunization series

4. Evaluation and ongoing monitoring
  a. Hemodynamic status
  b. Pain relief
5. Non-healing wounds: diabetic foot is a common emergency care presentation.
There is evidence that the combination of honey and silver-coated bandages have better outcomes with malignant wounds. Topical antimicrobials are at risk for resistance
  a. Assessment for cellulitis, abscess, drainage
  b. Diagnostic imaging for gas, bone infection
  c. Management of underlying disease (diabetes, immunocompromised)
  d. What chromic management have they utilized?
    1) Honey
    2) Silver-impregnated dressing
    3) Oak bark extract
    4) Antibiotics (oral, topical)
  e. Maintain alert for necrotizing fasciitis

Bibliography

Centers for Disease Control and Prevention (CDC): *Cat-scratch disease*. Retrieved from http://www.cdc.gov/healthypets/diseases/cat-scratch.html, 2014.

Centers for Disease Control and Prevention (CDC): *Pertussis: Summary of vaccine recommendations.* Retrieved from http://www.cdc.gov/vaccines/vpd-vac/pertussis/recs-summary.htm, 2015.

Gottrup F, Apelqvist J, Bjansholt T, et al.: EWMA document: antimicrobials and non-healing wounds – Evidence, controversies and suggestions, *Journal of Wound Care* 22(5):S1–S92, 2013.

Kragh Jr JF, et al.: Practical use of emergency tourniquets to stop bleeding in major limb trauma, *The Journal of Trauma Injury, Infection, and Critical Care* 64(2):s38–s49, 2008.

Kragh Jr JF, Beebe DF, O'Neill ML, et al.: Performance improvement in emergency tourniquet use during the Baghdad surge, *American Journal of Emergency Medicine* 31(5):873–875, 2013.

Marx JA, Hockberger RS, Walls RM, editors: *Rosen's emergency medicine: Concepts and clinical practice,* ed 8, St. Louis, MO, 2012, Elsevier Mosby.

National Institute for Allergy and Infectious Disease (NIAID): *Methicillin-resistant Staphylococcus aureus (MRSA).* Retrieved from http://www.niaid.nih.gov/topics/antimicrobialresistance/examples/mrsa/Pages/default.aspx, 2015.

Trott AT: *Wounds and lacerations: Emergency care and closure,* ed 4, St. Louis, MO, 2012, Elsevier Saunders.

CHAPTER 31

Mechanism of Injury

Kyle Madigan, RN, MSN, CEN, CFRN, CCRN, CMTE

MAJOR TOPICS
Biomechanics and Kinematics
Definitions
Physics Laws and Application

Types of Injuries
Blast Forces
Blunt Forces
Penetrating Forces
Predictable Injuries

I. Biomechanics and Kinematics

Unintentional injury is the leading cause of death for persons between 1 and 44 years of age.[1] Understanding the laws and principles of the transfer of energy and their effect on the human body is key to providing timely and thorough care to the trauma patient. The tissues comprising the human body (connective, epithelial, nerve, muscle) have a specific tolerance and response to the effects of energy loading and transfer.

A. DEFINITIONS

1. Mechanism of injury (MOI)
   a. Circumstance in which an injury occurs, such as with sudden deceleration, wounding by a projectile, or explosion[2]
2. Kinematics
   a. Study of energy transfer as it applies to identifying actual or potential injuries[3]
   b. Kinetic energy (KE)
      1) Energy that a body possesses as a result of its motion
         a) The amount of energy to be transferred as related to weight (mass) and speed (velocity)
      2) Function of the relationship of body weight (mass) and speed (velocity): $KE = \frac{1}{2}mv^2$
      3) Standard metric unit of measurement (SI) for KE is the joule
      4) Production of KE is influenced by velocity more than mass
         a) Doubling the mass doubles the KE
            (1) Example: a 6,000-pound SUV strikes an object with twice the force of a 2,000-pound compact car

      b) Doubling the velocity quadruples the KE
         (1) Example: a car traveling at 40 mph has four times the impact of a car traveling at 20 mph
3. Biomechanics
   a. Study of forces and their effects on the body tissues[3]

B. PHYSICS LAWS AND APPLICATION

1. Newton's laws of motion
   a. First law
      1) A body at rest or a body in motion will remain in that state unless acted on by an outside force (energy)[3]
   b. Second law
      1) Acceleration of a body is parallel and directly proportional to the net force (F) acting on the body[3]
   c. Third law
      1) For every action (energy impact), there is an equal and opposite reaction resulting from the transfer of energy[3]
2. Law of conservation of energy
   a. Energy can be neither created nor destroyed, only changed in form
   b. As motion starts or stops, energy must be changed to another form
      1) Mechanical energy
         a) External forces: acceleration/deceleration
            (1) In motor vehicle collisions, the moving vehicle strikes an immovable object, causing a sudden deceleration of the vehicle, whereas the occupant accelerates until he or she strikes an immovable object (e.g., dashboard, steering wheel, restraint system)

    (2) Organs, and fixed structures, within the body go through the same acceleration/deceleration sequence, causing internal injuries

        (a) Brain: coup/contrecoup injuries: energy transfer causes acceleration/deceleration of the brain within the confined space of the skull. The brain travels within the skull causing "shearing." That sliding or oscillation of the brain further propels it in the opposite direction, resulting in a second and opposite impact against the skull

        (b) Heart: ligamentum arteriosum, aortic arch disruption: energy transfer causes acceleration/deceleration within the body with impact against fixed anatomic structures and hyperextension/hyperflexion of major vessels

        (c) Duodenum: ligament of Treitz, duodenal injury

  b) Internal forces: tissue strength

    (1) Stress: internal condition of any physical tissue structure, under any load, that does not exceed the elastic limit of that tissue structure

        (a) Tensile stress: when the length of a material (tissue) tends to increase in the tensile direction, thus causing the cells to separate

        (b) Compressive stress: the stress applied to materials (tissue) resulting in their compaction (decrease of volume)

        (c) Shearing stress: a state in which the shape of a material tends to change without particular volume change

    (2) Strain

        (a) Deformation (injury) caused by the action of stress on a physical body

        (b) Dependent on tissue type. Dependent on density, different structures (bones, muscles, tendons) have different ability to respond to stress

2) Thermal energy: transfer of heat from an area of higher temperature to an area of lower temperature

  a) Heat may be transferred between objects by radiation, conduction, or convection

  b) May be created by vibration and or friction

3) Electrical energy: transfer of energy when a body is exposed to an electrical source or current

  a) High versus low voltage

  b) Lightning

  c) Electrical currents

    (1) Alternating current (AC)

        (a) Considered more dangerous than direct current (DC)

        (b) May cause muscle tetany, resulting in longer exposure

        (c) Greater affinity for causing ventricular fibrillation when current travels from one hand to the other

    (2) Direct current

        (a) Often causes single convulsive contraction

        (b) May cause sudden cardiac arrest from asystole[4]

        (c) Throws victim away from source

  d) Entrance and exit wounds

4) Chemical energy: substances introduced to body tissues disrupt the chemical structure of the tissue. Tissue damage influenced by

  a) Length of time of contact

  b) Concentration of chemical

  c) Amount of chemical exposure

  d) Chemical makeup and toxicity of the substance

II. Types of Injuries

A. BLAST FORCES

Explosions cause varying degrees of injuries depending on the size of the explosion and the proximity of the victims. Explosive injuries are classified as primary, secondary, tertiary, quaternary, and quinary. Most patients involved in a blast exposure will have multiple categories of injuries.[5]

1. Injury classification

  a. Primary

    1) Caused by pressure wave from the blast: damages air-filled organs

      a) Ruptured tympanic membranes

      b) Pneumothoraces

      c) Gastric or intestinal rupture

  b. Secondary

    1) Occurs as a result of flying debris (shrapnel) from the blast

      a) Common cause of greatest number of casualties

    2) Causes penetrating trauma and lacerations

  c. Tertiary

    1) The pressure wave may cause the victim to be thrown a distance, thus causing blunt trauma

      a) Acceleration/deceleration-type injuries

  d. Quaternary

    1) Caused as a result of exposure to heat, flames, and smoke

      a) Thermal burn injuries

e. Quinary
  1) Injuries associated with exposure from biological, chemical, and radioactive materials of a blast[5]
    a) HAZMAT and decontamination should be considered

B. BLUNT FORCES

Blunt injury occurs when the KE from an object is transferred to the human body without penetration of the skin tissues. Blunt injuries are most commonly associated with motor vehicle collisions, automobile versus pedestrian collisions, motorcycle collisions, sports-related activities, and falls. Injury occurs from a multitude of factors including speed at impact (acceleration), stopping distance (deceleration), and body surface area affected.

1. Contributing factors
  a. Motor vehicle collision
    1) Location in vehicle: driver versus passenger, front seat versus back seat
    2) Restraints
      a) Seat belts, proper use of
      b) Airbags, location within vehicle
        (1) Secondary injuries
    3) Speed at impact
    4) Impact direction
      a) Frontal
      b) Rear
      c) Lateral
      d) Rotational
      e) Rollover
    5) Ejection
      a) Ejection from a vehicle greatly increases the risk of serious injury, or death
    6) Intrusion into vehicle space
    7) Condition of other occupants in vehicle, especially death or prolonged extrication
  b. Motorcycle collision
    1) Helmet and protective apparel
    2) Speed at impact
    3) Direction of impact
      a) Frontal
      b) Rear
      c) Lateral
      d) Rotational
    4) Ejection distance from motorcycle
    5) Loss of consciousness
  c. Falls
    1) Height: fall from 20 feet or greater is generally considered significant MOI
    2) Surface of impact
    3) Position of impact
      a) Feet first
      b) Head first
      c) Lateral
      d) Prone
      e) Supine

d. Sports-related activities
  1) Protective equipment, apparel, or helmet use
  2) Type of impact
  3) Force or speed of impact

C. PENETRATING FORCES

Penetrating force injury is commonly associated with firearm and stabbing injuries, but may also be caused by impalement on an object. Tissue damage or destruction occurs when the penetrating object transfers its energy into the tissue.

1. Wounding characteristics
  a. Velocity
    1) The velocity of the projectile is directly proportional to the amount of energy transfer[5]
    2) Low velocity
      a) Generally caused by hand-driven weapons, such as knives
      b) Lower KE transfer to the body, thereby creating smaller temporary cavity
    3) Medium velocity
      a) Handguns
      b) Shotguns
    4) High velocity
      a) Long guns and assault rifles
      b) High-velocity weapons create a significantly larger temporary cavity
  b. Cavitation
    1) Permanent cavity is formed as the projectile travels through the tissue
    2) Temporary cavity is created around the permanent cavity, by the dissipation of the KE as it is transferred to the surrounding tissues[6]
      a) Depending on the amount of energy transferred, area may extend beyond the permanent cavity
2. Stab wounds
  a. Commonly associated with knives; however, other impaling objects may cause stab-type injuries
  b. Tissue damage is caused by the velocity and length of the penetrating object
  c. Consideration should be given to underlying structures and anatomy
  d. Consideration should also be given to position of possible assailant to patient (e.g., large man stabbing small woman versus small assailant stabbing upward at larger victim)
3. Gunshot wounds
  a. Bullet characteristics
    1) Projectile profile
      a) Refers to size and shape of projectile as it enters the body
      b) Deformation of projectile
        (1) Increases the surface area creating additional tissue damage
        (2) Causes more tissue damage and injury

2) Projectile tumble
   a) Occurs as projectile deforms on impact
   b) Center of gravity is altered causing the projectile to turn end over end within the tissue
   c) Increases the energy transfer and size of both the permanent and temporary cavities
3) Projectile fragmentation
   a) Occurs with many soft-tip or hollow-tip bullets. Also occurs with improvised explosive devices (IEDs)
   b) Mass of fragments causes widespread tissue damage and energy transfer to a larger area
b. Entrance versus exit wounds
   1) Document anatomic location of wounds
   2) Avoid identifying wounds as either "entrance" or "exit"

D. PREDICTABLE INJURIES

Through the understanding of the biomechanics and kinematics associated with energy transfer, injury patterns may be anticipated.

1. Motor vehicle collision
   a. Dependent on direction of impact
   b. Acceleration/deceleration
      1) Head injuries
         a) Striking interior of vehicle, windshield
            (1) Contusions
            (2) Fractures
            (3) Intracranial bleeding, subdural hematoma, subarachnoid hematoma
         b) Shearing
            (1) Diffuse axonal injury
      2) Chest injuries
         a) Contusions, pulmonary, and/or cardiac
         b) Pneumothoraces
         c) Aorta
            (1) Aortic arch tear, ligamentum arteriosum
         d) Clavicle fracture
      3) Abdominal injuries
         a) Hollow organ disruption
            (1) Intestines
            (2) Gastric
         b) Solid organ fracture
            (1) Spleen
            (2) Liver
         c) Great vessel injury

      4) Musculoskeletal
         a) Long bone fractures
         b) Dislocations of the femur from striking the interior of the vehicle
         c) Pelvic fractures
2. Falls
   a. Acceleration/deceleration
   b. Injuries dependent on how body lands
      1) Musculoskeletal
         a) Spine fractures
            (1) Vertebral body compression, most commonly in lumbar spine
            (2) Wedge fractures
         b) Calcaneus fractures
         c) Wrist fractures
         d) Hip or pelvic fractures in geriatric population
3. Penetrating trauma
   a. Difficult to predict injuries as missile(s) may tumble or transfer energy to tissues
   b. Anatomical location of penetration is important in anticipating underlying injury
      1) Hollow organ
         a) Spillage of contents into surround tissue and space
      2) Solid organ
         a) Occult hemorrhage

References

1. Injury prevention & control: Data & statistics. (2015, September 30). Centers for Disease Control and Prevention. Retrieved from http://www.cdc.gov/injury/wisqars/overview/key_data.html.
2. Mechanism of injury: *Mosby's medical dictionary*, ed 9. Retrieved from http://medical-dictionary.thefreedictionary.com/mechanism+of+injury, 2012.
3. Emergency Nurses Association: *Trauma nursing core course: Provider manual*, ed 7, Des Plaines, IL, 2014, Emergency Nurses Association.
4. *Environmental and weapon-related electrical injuries.* UpToDate.com, 2014, May 20.
5. Trauma nursing core course (TNCC): *Provider manual*, Des Plaines, IL, 2014, Emergency Nurses Association, pp 25–37.
6. Hafertepen SC, Davis JW, Townsend RN, Sue LP, Kaups KL, Cagle KM: Myths and misinformation about gunshot wounds may adversely affect proper treatment, *World Journal of Surgery* 39(7):1840–1847, 2015.

CHAPTER 32

Nursing Assessment and Trauma Resuscitation

Reneé Semonin Holleran, FNP-BC, PhD, CEN, CCRN (emeritus), CFRN and CTRN (retired), FAEN

MAJOR TOPICS

Primary Assessment
Overview of Major Components
Individual Components of Primary Assessment

Resuscitation
Airway Management
Breathing Management
Circulation Management
Disability Management
Exposure and Environmental Management

Secondary Assessment
Major Components of Secondary Assessment
Reevaluation Adjuncts

Consider Need for Transfer
Indications
Emergency Medical Treatment and Active Labor Act (EMTALA) (see Chapter 45)

Analysis: Differential Nursing Diagnoses/Collaborative Problems
Risk for Ineffective Airway Clearance
Ineffective Breathing Pattern
Deficient Fluid Volume
Acute Pain
Risk for Infection
Anxiety/Fear

Planning and Implementation/Interventions
Determine Priorities of Care
Relieve Anxiety/Apprehension
Allow Significant Others to Remain with Patient if Supportive
Educate Patient and Significant Others

Evaluation and Ongoing Monitoring
Continuously Monitor and Treat as Indicated
Monitor Patient Response/Outcomes and Modify Nursing Care Plan as Appropriate
If Patient Outcomes Are Not Demonstrated, Reevaluate Assessment and/or Plan of Care

Documentation of Interventions and Patient Response
Subjective Data Collection
Objective Data Collection
Analysis: Differential Nursing Diagnoses/Collaborative Problems
Planning and Implementation/Interventions
Evaluation and Ongoing Monitoring

Age-Related Considerations
Pediatric
Geriatric

Note: Standard precautions should be observed and personal protective equipment worn as indicated.

I. Primary Assessment[1-6]

The goal of the primary assessment in the traumatically injured patient is to provide rapid identification of potentially life-threatening conditions that require immediate intervention. Treatment of life-threatening abnormalities found during the primary assessment takes place BEFORE the assessment process continues.

A. OVERVIEW OF MAJOR COMPONENTS

1. Subjective data collection
   a. Brief history of present injury/chief complaint
      1) Mechanism of injury (see Chapter 31)
      2) Pain: location (see Chapter 8)
   b. Brief past medical history
      1) Current or preexisting diseases, illnesses, surgical procedures, especially any conditions that may have contributed to the cause of the injury (e.g., hypoglycemia)
      2) Past/current substance and/or alcohol use/abuse

3) Last normal menstrual cycle: female patients of childbearing age
4) Current medications
   a) Prescription
   b) OTC/herbal
5) Allergies
6) Immunization status
2. Objective data collection
   a. Airway patency with simultaneous cervical spine protection
   b. Breathing effectiveness
   c. Circulation effectiveness
   d. Disability (brief neurologic assessment)
   e. Expose/environmental controls
3. Preparation and triage of injured patient[1]
   a. Preparation
      1) Notification of arrival of injured patient
      2) Severity of injury (number based on trauma designation); type of injury (head, abdomen, etc.); use of prehospital field triage guidelines
      3) Team activation
      4) Resuscitation room preparation
      5) Use of standard precautions

B. INDIVIDUAL COMPONENTS OF PRIMARY ASSESSMENT

1. Airway with simultaneous C-spine protection
   a. Open, clear, patent
      1) Vocalization present
      2) No tongue obstruction
      3) No loose teeth or foreign objects in oral cavity
      4) No bleeding, vomitus, or other secretions in oral cavity
      5) No facial/neck edema or wounds
   b. Partially obstructed or obstructed/unacceptable requiring immediate intervention
      1) Subjective data collection
         a) Trauma to face, mouth, pharynx, neck, or chest
      2) Objective data collection
         a) Absence of breathing
         b) Patient unable to speak or vocalize appropriate for age
         c) Substernal, intercostal retracting
         d) Decreased level of consciousness
         e) Inspiratory and/or expiratory stridor
         f) Pale, cyanotic, dusky-gray skin color, especially mucous membranes and nail beds
         g) Facial/neck injury compromising airway
   c. Planning and implementation/interventions (interventions for obstructed airway must be implemented before proceeding in the primary assessment; see "Resuscitation")
      1) If mechanism of injury, symptoms, or physical findings suggest a spinal cord injury, the cervical spine must be stabilized and protected

2) Verify that airway is established, open, and clear and patency is maintained
2. Cervical spine
   a. Acceptable, stable
      1) Subjective data collection
         a) No history of head, neck, chest injury
         b) No complaints of pain with movement or palpation of cervical spine
      2) Objective data collection
         a) Movement in all extremities without limitation or weakness
         b) Breathing effective: no intercostal retractions or abdominal breathing
         c) Active full range of motion of neck without limitation or tenderness with palpation
   b. Unacceptable or requiring immediate intervention/unstable
      1) Subjective data collection
         a) Mechanism of injury (see Chapter 31) with potential for cervical trauma (e.g., direct injury to head or neck, trauma involving sudden deceleration [motor vehicle crash or fall], high-voltage electrical shock)
         b) Symptoms: inability to move extremities
         c) Pain with movement of neck
      2) Objective data collection: possibility of no objective findings as nondisplaced fractures of cervical spine may not compromise neurologic system
         a) Tenderness in cervical spine with patient movement or palpation
         b) Paralysis or paresthesia
         c) Abdominal breathing indicating possible paralysis of diaphragm
         d) Decreased or absent movement/sensation below level of injury
         e) Weakness
         f) Bowel or bladder incontinence or retention
         g) Loss of sympathetic outflow
            (1) Hypotension
            (2) Bradycardia
         h) Flaccid paralysis
         i) Loss of sphincter tone
         j) Priapism
         k) Warm, dry skin
         l) Bounding peripheral pulses
         m) Poikilothermia: loss of temperature regulation; patient's body assumes temperature of external temperature
         n) Inability to shiver or sweat
      3) Planning and implementation/interventions (interventions for C-spine protection must be implemented before proceeding in the primary assessment; see "Resuscitation")
3. Breathing
   a. Effective
      1) Subjective data collection

a) No respiratory difficulty
b) No neck, chest, abdominal injury
  2) Objective data collection
    a) Spontaneous breathing
    b) Rate, pattern of breathing normal for patient's age
    c) Chest symmetry and no use of accessory muscles or diaphragmatic breathing
    d) Skin color: absence of paleness, duskiness
    e) Integrity of the soft tissue and bony structures of the chest wall
  b. Compromised or absent/unacceptable requiring immediate intervention will differ depending on whether breathing is compromised or absent
    1) Subjective data collection
      a) Blunt or penetrating injury to neck, chest, back, or abdomen
      b) Dyspnea
    2) Objective data collection
      a) Marked tachypnea
      b) Agonal breathing (fewer than 10 breaths/minute in adults)
      c) Shallow, weak, gasping respirations
      d) Marked increase in respiratory effort
      e) Cyanosis, diaphoresis
      f) Severe retractions
      g) Absent breath sounds, unilaterally or bilaterally
      h) Open or sucking chest wounds
      i) Paradoxical chest wall movement
      j) Apnea
    3) Planning and implementation/interventions (interventions for ineffective or absent breathing must be implemented before proceeding in the primary assessment; see "Resuscitation")
4. Circulation
  a. Acceptable or adequate
    1) Subjective data collection
      a) No report or suspicion of significant blood loss
    2) Objective data collection
      a) Radial pulse palpable
      b) Rate: approximately 60–100 beats/minute in uncompromised adults
      c) Pediatric heart rate: between 100 and 160 beats/minute in infants, 80 and 130 beats/minute in small children
      d) No external hemorrhage
  b. Compromised or absent/unacceptable requiring immediate intervention
    1) Subjective data collection
      a) Unconsciousness or significantly altered level of consciousness
      b) Reported or suspected significant blood loss
    2) Objective data collection
      a) Heart rate: <60 beats/minute or >100 beats/minute and weak in adults

b) Pediatric heart rate: <100 beats/minute in infants, <80 beats/minute in small children, or sustained tachycardia (see Appendix B)
c) Unresponsive or significantly altered level of consciousness
d) Gross swelling of injured extremities (e.g., thigh)
e) Distended, rigid abdomen
f) Carotid and/or femoral pulses not palpable
g) Auscultate blood pressure: if other members of the trauma team are available, blood pressure may be obtained. Systolic blood pressure <90 mm Hg in adults, rapid heart rate and thready, weak pulse indicate poor circulation. If no other trauma team members are available, continue with primary assessment and obtain blood pressure during secondary assessment
h) Positive FAST exam: Focused Assessment Sonography in Trauma used to evaluate for the presence of internal hemorrhage with blunt or penetrating trauma to the torso (see Chapter 33, Figure 33.1)
i) Positive diagnostic peritoneal lavage (DPL): may be used to diagnose hemoperitoneum or ruptured viscous. The American College of Surgeons recommends its use for patients who have a change in sensorium related to substance abuse,[2] changes in sensation from a spinal cord injury, injury to adjacent structures (e.g., lower rib, pelvis, and lumbar spine fractures), equivocal physical examination, and lap belt sign
5. Disability
  a. Acceptable
    1) Subjective data collection
      a) No history of loss of consciousness
      b) No history of neurologic trauma
    2) Objective data collection
      a) Determine gross level of consciousness using AVPU scale
        A = Alert, awake; responsive to voice; oriented to person, time, and place
        V = Verbal; responds to voice but not fully oriented to person, time, or place
        P = Pain; does not respond to voice but responds to painful stimuli
        U = Unresponsive; does not respond to voice or painful stimuli
      b) Pupil assessment: pupils equal and briskly reactive to light
      c) Glasgow Coma Scale scores 15
      d) Moves all four extremities
      e) No lateralizing signs (neurologic assessment findings on one side of the body)
  b. Unacceptable/requiring immediate intervention

1) Subjective data collection
   a) History of loss of consciousness or unconscious
   b) Neurologic injury
2) Objective data collection
   a) Altered level of consciousness
   b) Abnormal flexion/extension posturing
   c) Pupillary assessment: unequal, large and fixed or reaction to light slow or absent
   d) Lateralizing signs: unilateral deterioration in motor movements or unequal pupils, aid in locating the area of injury in the brain
3) Planning and implementation/interventions
   a) Continue to monitor for compromise to airway, breathing, circulation
   b) Consider limited hyperventilation if patient is exhibiting signs of herniation, or neurologic deterioration unresponsive to other resuscitative measures
   c) Measures to decrease intracranial pressure if suspected (avoid hip flexion, Head of Bed 15–30°, monitor I&O)
6. Exposure/environment controls
   a. Remove patient's clothing to identify life-threatening injuries quickly
      1) Cut clothing, without destroying physical or forensic evidence (see Chapter 44)
      2) Exercise caution for possible sharp objects (e.g., needles) or weapons in pockets or under patient
      3) Maintain body temperature
         a) Cover the patient with warm blankets
         b) Keep resuscitation room warm
         c) Administer warm resuscitation fluids
         d) Use radiant warming lights
         e) Use forced air warmers

II. Resuscitation[1-6]

The goal of resuscitation in the primary assessment is to correct all life-threatening deviations from normal. Resuscitation priorities follow the same A-B-C-D-E mnemonic because interventions occur simultaneously during the primary assessment.

A. AIRWAY MANAGEMENT[4]

1. Airway patent
   a. Apply/maintain cervical spine protection
      1) Any patient whose mechanism of injury, symptoms, or physical findings suggest a spinal injury must be immobilized and their cervical spine protected
      2) If the patient is awake and breathing, he or she may have assumed a position that maximizes the ability to breathe. Before proceeding

with cervical spine protection, be sure interventions do not compromise patient's breathing status
2. Airway totally or partially obstructed
   a. Place patient in supine position
   b. Logroll while maintaining C-spine protection
   c. Remove any headgear that may interfere with the airway, such as a football or motorcycle helmet
   d. Open and clear the airway
      1) Jaw thrust: angles of the lower jaw are grasped on each side with the index fingers and thumbs on the cheekbone to move the mandible forward. This method can be used with the bag-mask device to provide a good seal for ventilation
      2) Chin lift: place fingers of one hand under the mandible and gently lift upward to raise the chin while the thumb pulls the lower lip to open the mouth. Avoid hyperextending the neck when performing this maneuver
      3) Remove loose objects or foreign debris either manually or by suctioning
         a) Suction gently so as not to stimulate a gag reflex or induce vomiting
      4) Insert airway adjuncts to maintain patency
         a) Nasopharyngeal airway in a responsive or unresponsive patient: do not insert in a patient with facial trauma
         b) Oropharyngeal airway in an unresponsive patient
      5) Advanced airway management: requires tube placement into the trachea for the purpose of obtaining or maintaining airway patency
         a) Oral intubation: maintain C-spine protection during procedure; requires a second person to assist
         b) Blind nasal intubation: not indicated when patient is apneic or when there are signs of midface fractures or basilar skull fracture
         c) Medications to facilitate intubation: several medications may be administered to facilitate rapid sequence intubation; these may include premedication, sedation, analgesia, and neuromuscular blocking agents
      6) Alternative airways: may be used to manage trauma patient's airway when endotracheal intubation cannot be accomplished
         a) Laryngeal mask airway (LMA): designed to cover the supraglottic airway with an inflatable, elliptical, silicone rubber collar (laryngeal mask) at the distal end. LMAs are available in sizes for both pediatric and adult patients
         b) Intubating LMA (ILMA): allows for insertion of a specially designed endotracheal tube through the ILMA

c) CombiTube: a dual-lumen, dual-cuff airway placed blindly into the esophagus to establish an airway. If inadvertently inserted in the trachea, it can function as an endotracheal tube. Used only in an unresponsive patient whose airway protective reflexes are not intact. Use with caution in any patient with esophageal disease or upper airway trauma

d) King Airway: a single tube inserted into the esophagus that traps the glottal opening between the esophageal cuff and an oropharyngeal cuff. The device has two ports with separate cuffs that can be inflated. The distal cuff inflates in the esophagus and the proximal cuff inflates at the base of the tongue. This device does not provide protection from aspiration, is not recommended for pediatric patients, and is contraindicated in those with a gag reflex, esophageal disease, or suspected upper airway burns

e) Needle cricothyrotomy: involves the insertion of a large-bore needle through the cricoid membrane

f) Surgical cricothyrotomy: performed by making an incision into the cricothyroid membrane and placing a cuffed endotracheal or tracheostomy tube into the trachea. Indicated when other methods of airway management have failed to adequately ventilate and oxygenate patient. Only trained personnel should perform a surgical airway. Complications related to a cricothyrotomy include aspiration, hemorrhage, or hematoma formation, as well as lacerations of the trachea or esophagus

B. BREATHING MANAGEMENT

1. Breathing effective
   a. Administer 100% oxygen with appropriately fitting nonrebreather mask
2. Breathing ineffective
   a. Administer 100% oxygen with appropriately fitting nonrebreather mask
   b. Assist ventilations with a bag-mask ventilation device attached to 100% oxygen
   c. Prepare for definitive airway management if not previously performed
   d. Needle decompression as indicated
   e. Chest tube thoracostomy as indicated
3. Breathing absent
   a. Ventilate patient with bag-mask ventilation device attached to 100% oxygen
   b. Assist with definitive airway management, as needed, to support ventilations
   c. Needle decompression as indicated
   d. Chest tube thoracostomy as indicated

C. CIRCULATION MANAGEMENT

1. Circulation effective
   a. Establish IV fluids for administration of crystalloid solutions/blood products/medications
      1) Insert one or two large-bore IV catheters
      2) Infuse warmed isotonic crystalloid solutions as required by patient's condition
2. Circulation ineffective
   a. Control any uncontrolled bleeding
      1) Apply pressure over the bleeding site
      2) Elevate bleeding extremity
      3) Apply pressure over arterial pressure points
      4) Apply tourniquet only as a lifesaving procedure
   b. Establish IV access for administration of crystalloid fluids/blood products/medications
      1) Insert two large-bore IV catheters
      2) Infuse warmed isotonic crystalloid solutions at a rate required by patient's condition
      3) Use rapid infusion devices per institutional protocols
      4) Administer blood and blood products through 0.9% NS solution primed IV tubing, using a warmer as indicated by patient's condition
      5) Consider intraosseous access if unable to quickly obtain venous access
      6) Venous cannulation may require a surgical cutdown or insertion of a central line
      7) When obtaining IV access, obtain blood samples to determine blood type and Rh group and to facilitate any additional laboratory studies
      8) Initiate massive transfusion protocol (MTP) per institution
   c. Prepare patient for operative interventions as indicated
3. Circulation absent[5]
   a. Initiate or continue Basic Life Support (BLS) and Advanced Life Support (ALS) per protocols
   b. Establish IV access for administration of crystalloid fluids/blood products/medications
      1) Insert two large-bore IV catheters
      2) Infuse warmed crystalloid solutions, blood, and blood products
   c. Prepare to assist with emergency thoracotomy, as indicated
   d. Discuss when resuscitative efforts should be discontinued[5]

D. DISABILITY MANAGEMENT

1. Determine patient's level of consciousness
2. Ensure adequate oxygenation and perfusion (see "Breathing Management" and "Circulation Management")
3. Maintain head midline, position head of bed flat or elevated per institutional policy (if no C-spine injury)

as prescribed; do not place head lower than body because this may increase intracranial pressure
4. Prepare patient for further neurologic evaluation
   a. C-spine radiograph
   b. Computed tomography (CT) scans
   c. Magnetic resonance imaging (MRI)

E. EXPOSURE AND ENVIRONMENTAL MANAGEMENT

1. Ensure safety of health care providers
2. Decontaminate patients who may have been exposed to hazardous substances
3. Keep patient warm with blankets or heating lamps or by keeping the resuscitative room warm

III. Secondary Assessment[3]

A. MAJOR COMPONENTS OF SECONDARY ASSESSMENT

1. Full set of vital signs
   a. Blood pressure
   b. Pulse rate
   c. Respiratory rate
   d. Temperature
2. Facilitate family presence
   a. Assess patient and family diversity
   b. Assess family's desires and needs
   c. Facilitate and support family's involvement in the care
   d. Assign a health care professional to provide explanations about procedures and to be with the family in the emergency department
   e. Utilize resources to support family's emotional and spiritual needs
3. Get resuscitation adjuncts[1]
   a. LMNOP mnemonic
      1) L: laboratory studies
         a) Lactic acid
         b) CBC
         c) Type and crossmatch
         d) Electrolytes
         e) Urinalysis
      2) M: monitor cardiac rate and rhythm
      3) N: naso or orogastric tube insertion if indicated by patient's injury, altered mental status, airway protection
      4) O: oxygenation and ventilation assessment should be monitored using a pulse oximeter and $ETCO_2$ (capnography).
      5) P: pain assessment (see Chapter 8)
   b. Sources of pain
      1) Injuries
         a) Fractures
         b) Burns
         c) Lacerations
      2) Procedures
         a) IV cannulation
         b) Chest thoracostomy
         c) Intubation
         d) Fracture reduction
         e) Wound care
      3) Treatment environment
         a) Light
         b) Noise
   c. Physical signs of pain
      1) Tachypnea
      2) Shallow respirations
      3) Nausea and vomiting
      4) Diaphoresis
      5) Protective behaviors
      6) Pinched facial expressions
      7) Clenched fist or teeth
      8) Crying
      9) Diaphoresis
      10) Pain rating scale
4. History
   a. Prehospital information: MIST
      1) M: mechanism of injury (see Chapter 31)
      2) I: injuries sustained
      3) S: signs and symptoms (in the field)
      4) T: treatment initiated in the field and patient response
   b. Past medical history: not previously obtained
      1) Current or preexisting diseases/illness
      2) Previous hospitalizations and surgical procedures
      3) Recent substance and/or alcohol use/abuse
      4) Possible/actual assault, abuse, or intimate partner violence situations (see Chapters 3 and 40)
      5) Patient violence at scene (see Chapter 48)
      6) Medications
         a) Prescription
         b) Over the counter
      7) Allergies
      8) Immunization status
      9) Comorbid factors (Box 32.1)
5. Head-to-toe assessment
   a. General appearance
      1) Body position
      2) Guarding
      3) Self-protection movements
      4) Hygiene
      5) Unusual odors
      6) Level of distress/discomfort
   b. Head and face
      1) Inspection: lacerations, abrasions, contusions, avulsions, puncture wounds, impaled objects, ecchymosis, and edema
      2) Palpation: crackling associated with subcutaneous emphysema, depressions, angulation, and areas of tenderness
      3) Do not obstruct any suspected cerebrospinal drainage from nose or ears

Box 32.1

Comorbid Factors

- Smoking
- Substance abuse
- Age >55 years
- Age <5 years
- Cardiovascular disease
- Pulmonary disease
- Diabetes
- Blood disorders
- Morbid obesity
- Pregnancy
- Immunosuppression
- Use of anticoagulants

Box 32.2

Peripheral Pulses

Upper Extremities

- Brachial pulse
- Radial pulse

Lower Extremities

- Femoral
- Popliteal
- Dorsalis pedis
- Posterior tibialis

---

c. Chest
  1) Inspection: breathing, rate, depth and degree of effort; use of accessory muscles or abdominal muscles; paradoxical chest movement; abrasions, lacerations, puncture wounds, ecchymosis, or impaled objects
  2) Auscultation: breath sounds and heart sounds
  3) Palpation: depressions, areas of tenderness, crepitus
  4) Percussion: areas of hyperresonance, dullness
d. Abdomen/flanks
  1) Inspection: lacerations, abrasions, contusions, puncture wounds, impaled objects, ecchymosis, edema, and scars that may indicate previous surgical procedures
  2) Auscultation: bowel sounds
  3) Palpation: all four quadrants for rigidity, guarding, masses, areas of tenderness
  4) Percussion: areas of dullness
e. Pelvis/perineum
  1) Inspection: lacerations, abrasions, contusions, avulsions, puncture wounds, impaled objects, ecchymosis, edema and scars, blood at the meatus, priapism
  2) Palpation: areas of tenderness
  3) Assist with determining rectal tone, displacement of the prostate in the male patient
f. Extremities
  1) Inspection: color, active bleeding, lacerations, abrasions, contusions, avulsions, amputations, angulations, protruding bones, edema, ecchymosis, abnormal movement
  2) Palpation: crepitus, step-off, deformities, areas of tenderness, motor strength and range of motion, sensation, and pulses in all extremities (Box 32.2)
6. Inspect the posterior surfaces
  a. Maintain C-spine protection, support injured extremities, and logroll patient with appropriate number of assistants

  1) Avoid logrolling patients onto an injured side
  2) Logroll patient away from nurse when possible
  b. Inspection: back, flanks, buttocks, and posterior thighs for lacerations, abrasions, contusions, avulsions, puncture wounds, impaled objects, ecchymosis, or edema or scars and any rectal bleeding
  c. Palpation: vertebral column including the costovertebral column for deformity and areas of tenderness
  d. Palpate all posterior surfaces for deformity and areas of tenderness
  e. Assist with assessment of anal sphincter for presence or absence of tone

B. REEVALUATION ADJUNCTS[2]

1. Following the primary and secondary assessments and simultaneous interventions, additional tests to evaluate the injured patient may be performed. The following are examples of some these diagnostic tests
2. Additional diagnostic procedures
  a. Angiography
  b. 12- to 15-lead electrocardiogram (ECG)
  c. Bronchoscopy
  d. Esophagoscopy
  e. Echocardiogram
3. Additional radiologic tests
  a. Extremity radiographs
  b. CTA of chest
  c. MRI of head/cervical spine
4. Additional interventions
  a. Wound care (see Chapter 30)
  b. Restraints per institutional policy for patient's displaying violent behavior
  c. Application of traction devices
  d. Assist with collection and maintenance of physical and forensic evidence as indicated (see Chapter 48)
  e. Administration of pharmacologic therapy as ordered
    1) Antibiotics
    2) Nonnarcotic analgesics
    3) Narcotics

4) Sedation
5) Neuromuscular blocking agents
6) Alkalinization of urine to prevent rhabdomyolysis
7) Tetanus immunization
f. Assist with hospital admission, preparation for the operating suite, or transfer and transport to institution with higher level of care

IV. Consider Need for Transfer[2,3]

A. INDICATIONS

1. Central nervous system
   a. Head injury
      1) Penetrating injury or depressed skull fracture
      2) Open injury with or without cerebrospinal fluid leak
      3) Lateralizing signs
   b. Spinal cord injury
2. Chest
   a. Widened mediastinum
   b. Major chest wall injury or pulmonary contusion
   c. Cardiac injury
   d. Patient may require prolonged ventilation
3. Pelvis/abdomen
   a. Unstable pelvic ring disruption
   b. Pelvic ring disruption with shock and evidence of continued hemorrhage
   c. Open pelvic injury
   d. Solid organ injury
4. Extremity
   a. Severe open fractures
   b. Traumatic amputation with potential for replantation
   c. Complex auricular fractures
   d. Major crush injury
   e. Ischemia
5. Multisystem injury
   a. Head injury with face, chest, abdominal, and pelvic injury
   b. Injury to more than two body regions
   c. Major burns or burns with associated injuries
   d. Multiple, proximal long-bone fractures
6. Comorbid factors
   a. Age >55 years
   b. Age <5 years
   c. Cardiac or respiratory disease
   d. Insulin-dependent diabetes, morbid obesity
   e. Pregnancy
   f. Immunosuppression
7. Secondary deterioration
   a. Mechanical ventilation required
   b. Sepsis
   c. Single or multiple organ system failure
   d. Major tissue necrosis

B. EMERGENCY MEDICAL TREATMENT AND ACTIVE LABOR ACT (EMTALA)[1] (SEE CHAPTER 45)

1. Requirements
   a. Accepting physician at receiving facility
   b. Available bed and resources to care for patient at receiving facility
   c. Appropriate mode of transport used to transfer patient based on his or her injury and needs

V. Analysis: Differential Nursing Diagnoses/Collaborative Problems

A. RISK FOR INEFFECTIVE AIRWAY CLEARANCE

B. INEFFECTIVE BREATHING PATTERN

C. DEFICIENT FLUID VOLUME

D. ACUTE PAIN

E. RISK FOR INFECTION

F. ANXIETY/FEAR

VI. Planning and Implementation/Interventions

Planning is selecting appropriate interventions to manage identified health care problems and needs. These nursing actions include both collaborative and independent interventions. All interventions are patient oriented and goal directed.

A. DETERMINE PRIORITIES OF CARE

B. RELIEVE ANXIETY/APPREHENSION

C. ALLOW SIGNIFICANT OTHERS TO REMAIN WITH PATIENT IF SUPPORTIVE

D. EDUCATE PATIENT AND SIGNIFICANT OTHERS

VII. Evaluation and Ongoing Monitoring

This is the determination of whether the patient achieved the expected responses to interventions. Further assessment is necessary if the patient does not demonstrate positive outcomes with a reevaluation of the plan of care and the development of specific interventions.

A. CONTINUOUSLY MONITOR AND TREAT AS INDICATED

1. Airway patency
2. Level of consciousness
3. Hemodynamic status
4. Respiratory status, including breath sounds and pulse oximetry
5. Cardiac rate and rhythm
6. Pain relief
7. Intake and output

B. MONITOR PATIENT RESPONSE/ OUTCOMES, AND MODIFY NURSING CARE PLAN AS APPROPRIATE

C. IF POSITIVE PATIENT OUTCOMES ARE NOT DEMONSTRATED, REEVALUATE ASSESSMENT AND/ OR PLAN OF CARE

VIII. Documentation of Interventions and Patient Response

A. SUBJECTIVE DATA COLLECTION

B. OBJECTIVE DATA COLLECTION

C. ANALYSIS: DIFFERENTIAL NURSING DIAGNOSES/ COLLABORATIVE PROBLEMS

D. PLANNING AND IMPLEMENTATION/ INTERVENTIONS

E. EVALUATION AND ONGOING MONITORING

IX. Age-Related Considerations

A. PEDIATRIC

1. Growth or developmental related
   a. Pediatric airway is smaller and can become more easily compromised by the tongue, swelling, and foreign objects

b. Respiratory rates are faster and children are at greater risk of becoming hypoxic more quickly
   c. Because young children are normally tachycardic, capillary refill, level of consciousness, and urine output are better indicators of perfusion
   d. Children have proportionally greater body surface areas; they lose heat more quickly than adults do
2. "Pearls"
   a. It is important to know age-appropriate behaviors so that providers can determine whether the child is exhibiting normal mental status
   b. It is important to facilitate family presence as a primary part of the child's care throughout assessment and resuscitation

B. GERIATRIC

1. Age related
   a. Physiologic changes related to age make the geriatric patient more difficult to resuscitate adequately
   b. Many geriatric patients are taking medications, or have preexisting conditions that interfere with their physiologic response to a traumatic insult
2. "Pearls"
   a. The geriatric trauma patient may have advance directives and end-of-life issues that need to be considered during resuscitation

References

1. Gurney D, Westegard AM (DATE): Initial assessment. In *Trauma nursing core course* ed 7, Des Plains, IL, 2013, Emergency Nurses Association, pp 39–54.
2. American College of Surgeons Committee on Trauma: Initial assessment and management. In *Advanced trauma life support student course manual*, ed 9, Chicago, IL, 2012, American College of Surgeons, pp 2–28.
3. Thibeault SM, editor (DATE): *Transport professional advanced trauma course manual.* Aurora, CO: Air and Surface Transport Nurses Association.
4. Walls R: The emergency airway algorithms. In Walls R, Murphy M, editors: *Manual of emergency airway management*, ed 4, Philadelphia, PA, 2012, Lippincott Williams and Wilkins, pp 23–34.
5. Hazinski MF, Nolan JP, Aickin R, Bhanji F, Billi JE, Callaway CW, et al.: Part 1: Executive summary 2015 international consensus on cardiopulmonary resuscitation and emergency cardiovascular care science with treatment recommendations, *Circulation* 132:S2–S39, 2015.
6. Rodriguez L: Pathophysiology of pain: Implications for perioperative nursing, *AORN Journal* 101(3):338–344, 2015.

Part 3

CHAPTER 33
Abdominal and Urologic Trauma

Melody R. Campbell, DNP, RN, CEN, TCRN, CCRN, CCNS

MAJOR TOPICS
General Strategy
Assessment
Analysis: Differential Nursing Diagnoses/Collaborative
  Problems
Planning and Implementation/Interventions
Evaluation and Ongoing Monitoring
Documentation of Interventions and Patient Response
Age-Related Considerations

Specific Abdominal Injuries
Gastric
Liver

Pancreatic/Duodenal
Small Bowel/Large Bowel
Spleen
Specific Urologic Injuries
Bladder
Renal
Urethra

I. General Strategy

A. ASSESSMENT

1. Primary and secondary survey/resuscitation (see Chapters 1 and 32)
2. Focused assessment
   a. Subjective data collection
      1) History of present injury/chief complaint
         a) Mechanism of injury (see Chapter 31)
            (1) Blunt force: motor vehicle crash, fall, struck pedestrian, motorcycle crash
            (2) Penetrating force: gun shot or stab wounds
         b) Pain: PQRST (see Chapter 8)
         c) Efforts to relieve symptoms
            (1) Home remedies
            (2) Medications
               (a) Prescription
               (b) OTC/herbal
      2) Past medical history
         a) Current or preexisting diseases/illness
         b) Past surgical procedures
         c) Substance and/or alcohol use/abuse
         d) Last normal menstrual period: female patients of childbearing age
         e) Current medications—inquire about anticoagulant/antiplatelet medication use
            (1) Prescription
            (2) OTC/herbal
         f) Allergies
         g) Immunization status
      3) Psychological/social/environmental
         a) Stress factors
            (1) Lifestyle
            (2) Coping patterns
            (3) Precipitating event
            (4) Significant others involved in traumatic event
         b) Possible/actual victim of assault, abuse, or intimate partner violence situations (see Chapters 3 and 40)
   b. Objective data collection
      1) General appearance
         a) Level of consciousness, color, behavior, affect
         b) Vital signs
         c) Odors
         d) Gait
         e) Level of distress/discomfort
      2) Inspection
         a) Abdominal distention/flatness
         b) Symmetry
         c) Contour (flat, rounded, herniation)
         d) Abrasions, contusions, open wounds, lacerations
         e) Ecchymosis, "seat belt sign"

Table 33.1

Comparison of Diagnostic Tests

Procedure	Advantages	Disadvantages	Results
FAST	Noninvasive Provides rapid evaluation of hemo-peritoneum	Operator dependent Hollow organ injury rarely identified	Free fluid appears as black Sensitivity 86–97%
CT	Provides most detailed images Useful in determining nonoperative management of solid organ injuries Noninvasive	Expensive, time consuming Use only on hemodynamically stable patients May miss injuries to diaphragm and gastrointestinal tract Exposure to radiation Requires transport from one department to another—risk for dislodgement of devices/tubes	High specificity 92–98% sensitive
DPL	Provides rapid evaluation of intra-peritoneal blood Useful in unstable patients Detects bowel injury	Invasive procedure Complications include bleeding, possibility of infection	Specificity low Sensitivity high 98% Can have false-positive results leading to unnecessary laparotomy

CT, Computed tomography; *DPL*, diagnostic peritoneal lavage; *FAST*, Focused Assessment Sonography for Trauma.

3) Auscultation
   a) Breath sounds: normal, absent, crackles
   b) Bowel sounds: normal, decreased, or absent
4) Palpation/percussion: all four quadrants of the abdomen
   a) Abdominal tenderness
   b) Rigidity/guarding
   c) Peritoneal irritation
3. Diagnostic procedures
   a. Laboratory studies
      1) Complete blood count (CBC) with differential
      2) Serum chemistries including glucose, blood urea nitrogen (BUN), and creatinine
      3) Liver function tests (aspartate aminotransaminase [AST], alanine aminotransferase [ALT], lactate dehydrogenase [LDH], alkaline phosphatase)
      4) Serum amylase, lipase
      5) Type and crossmatch
      6) Serial hematocrits
      7) Coagulation profile: prothrombin time (PT), partial thromboplastin time (PTT), international normalized ratio (INR), thromboelastography (TEG or ROTEM)
      8) Urinalysis; pregnancy test in female patients of childbearing age
   b. Imaging studies
      1) Abdominal flat plate radiograph
      2) Chest radiograph
      3) Pelvis radiograph
      4) Focused Assessment Sonography for Trauma (FAST) (Table 33.1)
         a) Detects bleeding within chest or abdominal cavity
         b) Four areas of abdomen are examined
            (1) Hepatorenal fossa
            (2) Splenorenal fossa
            (3) Pericardial sac
            (4) Pelvis (Fig. 33.1)
            (5) As little as 100 mL of fluid can be detected, but examination is usually considered positive when there is at least 200–500 mL of fluid noted
            (6) Injuries of the small and large bowel as well as retro/retroperitoneal trauma are unable to be diagnosed with the use of FAST
      5) Cystography
      6) Retrograde urethrography
      7) Intravenous pyelogram (IVP)
      8) Angiography
         a) Identifies active bleeding
         b) Interventional radiologists may embolize, stent, or coil to treat the injury
      9) Abdominal/pelvic/thoracic computed tomography (CT) scan (see Table 33.1)
         a) Oral contrast is usually not administered in the resuscitative phase
         b) IV contrast assists in diagnosis of active bleeding; a blush on the CT is an indication of active bleeding with possible need for embolization or operative intervention
      10) Abdominal ultrasound—may be used in pediatrics to limit exposure to radiation
   c. Other
      1) 12- to 15-lead electrocardiogram (ECG)
      2) Gastroscopy or endoscopy
      3) Sigmoidoscopy/proctoscopy/colonoscopy

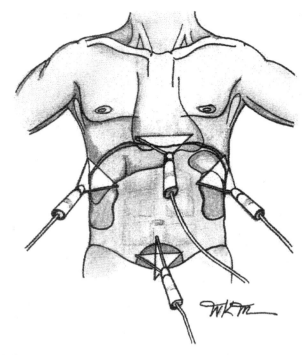

FIG. 33.1 The Focused Assessment Sonography for Trauma (FAST) examination consists of ultrasound views of four sites: pericardial, perihepatic (right upper quadrant), perisplenic (left upper quadrant), and pelvic. *(From Macdougall, D. B. [2005]. Abdominal trauma. In Emergency Nurses Association [Ed.], Sheehy's manual of emergency care (6th ed). St. Louis, MO: Mosby. Courtesy of William Mallon, MD.)*

    4) Diagnostic peritoneal lavage (DPL)/diagnostic peritoneal aspirate (DPA) (see Table 33.1)
       a) Identifies intraabdominal bleeding
       b) Following decompression of bladder and stomach, a peritoneal catheter is inserted into abdomen below umbilicus
       c) Aspiration of gross red blood is considered positive
       d) If gross blood is not noted, 1 L of isotonic crystalloid solution is infused through the catheter. The lavage fluid is then allowed to passively drain back out by gravity and is sent to laboratory for analysis
       e) Presence of red or white blood cells, bile, amylase, food fiber, or feces is noted. DPL/DPA may be performed in the unstable patient who has experienced blunt force injury.

B. ANALYSIS: DIFFERENTIAL NURSING DIAGNOSES/COLLABORATIVE PROBLEMS

1. Risk for deficient fluid volume
2. Ineffective tissue perfusion
3. Acute pain
4. Anxiety/fear
5. Risk for infection

C. PLANNING AND IMPLEMENTATION/INTERVENTIONS

1. Determine priorities of care
   a. Obtain and set up equipment and supplies, notify additional resources (in instances of prenotification)
   b. Maintain airway, breathing, circulation (see Chapters 1 and 32)
   c. Provide supplemental oxygen as indicated
   d. Establish IV access for administration of crystalloid fluids/blood products/medications
   e. Prepare for/assist with medical interventions
   f. Administer pharmacologic therapy as ordered
2. Relieve anxiety/apprehension
3. Allow significant others to remain with patient if supportive
4. Educate patient/significant others

D. EVALUATION AND ONGOING MONITORING

1. Continuously monitor and treat as indicated
2. Monitor patient response/outcomes, and modify nursing care plan as appropriate
3. If positive patient outcomes are not demonstrated, reevaluate assessment and/or plan of care

E. DOCUMENTATION OF INTERVENTIONS AND PATIENT RESPONSE

F. AGE-RELATED CONSIDERATIONS

1. Pediatrics
   a. Growth or development related
      1) Because of greater fluid needs related to body surface area, fluid, fluid/electrolyte, and acid-base balance are more precarious
      2) Acidosis develops more rapidly
      3) Children can compensate for a 25% blood loss by increasing their heart rate and peripheral vascular resistance, thereby maintaining normal systolic blood pressure. Blood pressure is an unreliable early indicator of shock in children
      4) The abdominal muscles are thinner, weaker, and less developed. The liver is more easily injured because it lies anteriorly and is less protected by the ribs. The kidneys are mobile and are not protected by fat
   b. "Pearls"
      1) The hollow and solid abdominal organs are more prone to injury than in adults
      2) Intraabdominal injury can result from airbag deployment
      3) Abdominal injuries may be the result of child maltreatment

2. Geriatrics
   a. Aging related
      1) There is a loss of pulmonary reserve with aging; the cardiovascular system is not as responsive
      2) The older adult has a decreased ability to adjust to extremes of temperature; care should be taken to minimize body exposure and maintain normothermia
      3) Peristalsis and gastric motility slow with aging. Older adults often have preexisting malnutrition and anemia
   b. "Pearls"
      1) Shock may be present in the presence of normal vital signs
      2) Urine output may not be a reliable indicator of overall tissue perfusion because the older adult has a decreased ability to concentrate urine
      3) Any degree of hypoxemia is detrimental in the older adult
      4) Common disorders often accompany the geriatric trauma patient's presentation to the hospital. These disorders include acute coronary syndrome, hypovolemia/dehydration, urinary tract infection, pneumonia, acute renal failure, cerebrovascular event, and syncope

II. Specific Abdominal Injuries

A. GASTRIC

Gastric injuries are usually associated with penetrating forces such as gunshot wounds. Blunt force injury is rare, but it is more common in children because of the greater elasticity of the anterior abdominal wall. Injury to the stomach interferes with peristalsis and digestion. If there is gastric perforation, severe peritonitis may result from chemical irritation.

1. Assessment
   a. Subjective data collection
      1) History of present injury/chief complaint
         a) Pain (see Chapter 8): in the epigastric area or LUQ
         b) Hematemesis
         c) Mechanism of injury (see Chapter 31)
      2) Past medical history
         a) Current or preexisting diseases/illness
            (1) Bleeding tendencies
         b) Medications
         c) Allergies
         d) Immunization status
   b. Objective data collection
      1) Physical examination
         a) General appearance
            (1) Possible hypotension, tachycardia
            (2) Moderate to severe distress/discomfort

b) Inspection
   (1) Abrasions, contusions, open wounds, lacerations
   (2) Ecchymosis over epigastric area/LUQ abdomen
   (3) Abdominal distention
c) Auscultation
   (1) Breath sounds: normal to decreased
   (2) Bowel sounds: normal to decreased or absent
d) Palpation
   (1) Abdominal tenderness
   (2) Rebound tenderness
   (3) Rigid abdomen specifically in epigastric area/LUQ
2) Diagnostic procedures
   a) CBC with differential
   b) Serum chemistries including glucose, BUN, creatinine
   c) Type and crossmatch blood
   d) Coagulation profile: PT, PTT, INR, thromboelastography
   e) Urinalysis; pregnancy test in female patients of childbearing age
   f) Abdominal radiograph: flat plate may demonstrate free air
   g) Chest radiograph
   h) FAST
   i) Abdominal CT scan
2. Analysis: differential nursing diagnoses/collaborative problems
   a. Deficient fluid volume
   b. Ineffective tissue perfusion: peripheral
   c. Acute pain
   d. Anxiety/fear
   e. Risk for infection
3. Planning and implementation/interventions
   a. Maintain airway, breathing, circulation (see Chapters 1 and 32)
   b. Provide supplemental oxygen
   c. Establish IV access for administration of crystalloid fluids/blood products/medications
      1) Insert two large-bore IV catheters
      2) Infuse warmed normal saline solution
      3) Infuse warmed blood products as needed
   d. Prepare for/assist with medical interventions
      1) Institute cardiac and pulse oximetry monitoring
      2) Insert gastric tube and attach to suction as indicated
      3) Insert indwelling urinary catheter as indicated
      4) Maintain normothermic body temperature
      5) Assist with collection and maintenance of physical and forensic evidence as indicated (see Chapter 43)
      6) Assist with hospital admission, preparation for the operating suite, or transfer to an institution providing a higher level of care

e. Administer pharmacologic therapy as ordered
1) Nonnarcotic analgesics
2) Narcotics
3) Antibiotics
4) Tetanus immunization
4. Evaluation and ongoing monitoring
a. Hemodynamic status
b. Breath sounds and pulse oximetry
c. Cardiac rate and rhythm
d. Pain relief
e. Intake and output

B. LIVER

The liver is one of the most commonly injured organs in the abdomen. Blunt force is more often the cause of liver injury. Penetrating injury can cause both minor lacerations and severe damage to the parenchyma resulting in rapid blood loss. Liver injuries are graded on a scale from 1 to 6, with type 1 being the least severe injury and type 6 being hepatic avulsion. Injury to the liver affects its functions, including blood storage (up to 500 mL) and filtration, secretion of bile, conversion of glucose into glycogen, synthesis and breakdown of fats and temporary storage of fatty acids, and synthesis of serum proteins (globulins, albumin) that aid in the regulation of blood volume and essential clotting factors (fibrinogen and prothrombin). Because blood flow through the liver at any one time is approximately 25% of the cardiac output, and blood is also stored within the liver, there is a great potential for significant blood loss with liver injuries. Liver injury should be suspected in any patient with lower chest or abdominal injury on the right side of the body.

1. Assessment
   a. Subjective data collection
      1) History of present injury/chief complaint
         a) Pain (see Chapter 8): in right upper quadrant (RUQ), hypochondriac, or epigastric region
         b) Mechanism of injury (see Chapter 31)
      2) Past medical history
         a) Current or preexisting diseases/illness
            (1) Bleeding tendencies
            (2) Liver disease or enlarged liver
         b) Medications
         c) Allergies
         d) Immunization status
   b. Objective data collection
      1) Physical examination
         a) General appearance
            (1) Level of consciousness, color, behavior, affect: alert to confusion, coma
            (2) Possible hypotension, tachycardia
            (3) Moderate to severe distress/discomfort
         b) Inspection
            (1) Abrasions, contusions, open wounds, lacerations
            (2) Ecchymosis over right lower chest wall/ RUQ abdomen
            (3) Abdominal distention
         c) Auscultation
            (1) Breath sounds: normal to decreased or absent on right side
            (2) Bowel sounds: normal to decreased or absent
         d) Palpation
            (1) Right lower chest wall tenderness
            (2) Abdominal tenderness
            (3) Rebound tenderness
            (4) Rigid abdomen specifically in RUQ
      2) Diagnostic procedures
         a) CBC with differential
         b) Serum chemistries including glucose, BUN, creatinine
         c) Serial hematocrits
         d) Type and crossmatch
         e) Coagulation profile: PT, PTT, INR, thromboelastography
         f) Urinalysis; pregnancy test in female patients of childbearing age
         g) Liver enzymes: elevated alkaline phosphate, ALT, AST
         h) Abdominal radiograph: flat plate (portable)
         i) Chest radiograph: may indicate right pneumothorax or fractured ribs
         j) FAST
         k) Abdominal CT scan with IV contrast
         l) Possible DPL/DPA: positive for blood
         m) Angiography
2. Analysis: differential nursing diagnoses/collaborative problems
   a. Deficient fluid volume
   b. Ineffective tissue perfusion: peripheral
   c. Acute pain
   d. Anxiety/fear
   e. Risk for infection
3. Planning and implementation/interventions
   a. Maintain airway, breathing, circulation (see Chapters 1 and 32)
   b. Provide supplemental oxygen
   c. Establish IV access for administration of crystalloid fluids/blood products/medications
      1) Insert two large-bore IV catheters
      2) Infuse warmed normal saline solutions
      3) Infuse warmed blood products as needed
   d. Prepare for/assist with medical interventions
      1) Institute cardiac and pulse oximetry monitoring
      2) Insert gastric tube and attach to suction as indicated
      3) Insert indwelling urinary catheter as indicated
      4) Maintain normothermic body temperature
      5) Assist with collection and maintenance of physical and forensic evidence as indicated (see Chapter 43)
      6) Assist with hospital admission, preparation for the operating suite/interventional radiology, or

transfer to an institution providing a higher level of care

e. Administer pharmacologic therapy as ordered
   1) Antifibrinolytics
   2) Nonnarcotic analgesics
   3) Narcotics
   4) Antibiotics
   5) Tetanus immunization
4. Evaluation and ongoing monitoring
   a. Level of consciousness
   b. Hemodynamic status
   c. Breath sounds and pulse oximetry
   d. Cardiac rate and rhythm
   e. Pain relief
   f. Intake and output

C. PANCREATIC/DUODENAL

Both the pancreas and the majority of the duodenum are retroperitoneal organs. Retroperitoneal symptoms may often be difficult to detect or may take 24–72 hours to manifest.

The pancreas is rarely injured. Direct blunt force to the epigastric area from the impact of a steering wheel during a motor vehicle crash may result in injury to the pancreas. Pancreatic injury is often associated with severe injuries to the liver, stomach, spleen, and great vessels with related high mortality rates. The pancreas produces enzymes, electrolytes, and bicarbonate to aid in digestion and nutrient absorption. Additionally, the pancreas regulates the secretion of insulin and glucagon, which aids in carbohydrate metabolism.

Duodenal injury is often associated with injuries to the pancreas, bile duct, or vena cava. A blunt injury, usually occurring in the second or third portion of the duodenum, may result in hematoma formation within the wall of the duodenum, thus decreasing the size of the lumen or causing obstruction. Duodenal perforation may result in retroperitoneal and peritoneal contamination with gastric secretions, bile, and digestive enzymes and requires emergent operative management. Of duodenal injuries, 75% are secondary to penetrating forces. A shearing-type injury can also occur adjacent to the ligament of Treitz.

1. Assessment
   a. Subjective data collection
      1) History of present injury/chief complaint
         a) Pain (see Chapter 8): in the epigastric area or back
         b) May be asymptomatic unless peritoneal irritation is present
         c) Mechanism of injury (see Chapter 31)
      2) Past medical history
         a) Current or preexisting diseases/illness
            (1) Bleeding tendencies
         b) Medications
         c) Allergies
         d) Immunization status
   b. Objective data collection
      1) Physical examination
         a) General appearance
            (1) Possible hypotension, tachycardia
            (2) Moderate to severe distress/discomfort
         b) Inspection
            (1) Abrasions, contusions, open wounds, lacerations
            (2) Ecchymosis over epigastric area
            (3) Abdominal distention
         c) Auscultation
            (1) Breath sounds: normal to decreased
            (2) Bowel sounds: normal to decreased or absent
         d) Palpation
            (1) Abdominal tenderness
            (2) Rebound tenderness
            (3) Rigid abdomen specifically in epigastric area
      2) Diagnostic procedures
         a) CBC with differential
         b) Serum chemistries including glucose, BUN, creatinine
         c) Serum amylase and lipase
         d) Type and crossmatch
         e) Coagulation profile: PT, PTT, INR, thromboelastography
         f) Urinalysis; pregnancy test in female patients of childbearing age
         g) Abdominal radiograph: flat plate
         h) Chest radiograph
         i) FAST
         j) Abdominal CT scan
         k) Possible DPL/DPA: positive for amylase
2. Analysis: differential nursing diagnoses/collaborative problems
   a. Deficient fluid volume
   b. Ineffective tissue perfusion: peripheral
   c. Acute pain
   d. Anxiety/fear
   e. Risk for infection
3. Planning and implementation/interventions
   a. Maintain airway, breathing, circulation (see Chapters 1 and 32)
   b. Provide supplemental oxygen
   c. Establish IV access for administration of crystalloid fluids/blood products/medications
      1) Insert two large-bore IV catheters
      2) Infuse warmed normal saline solution
      3) Infuse warmed blood products as needed
   d. Prepare for/assist with medical interventions
      1) Institute cardiac and pulse oximetry monitoring
      2) Insert gastric tube and attach to suction as indicated
      3) Insert indwelling urinary catheter as indicated
      4) Maintain normothermic body temperature

5) Assist with collection and maintenance of physical and forensic evidence as indicated (see Chapter 43)
6) Assist with hospital admission, preparation for the operating suite, or transfer to an institution providing a higher level of care
  e. Administer pharmacologic therapy as ordered
    1) Nonnarcotic analgesics
    2) Narcotics
    3) Antibiotics
    4) Tetanus immunization
4. Evaluation and ongoing monitoring
  a. Hemodynamic status
  b. Breath sounds and pulse oximetry
  c. Cardiac rate and rhythm
  d. Pain relief
  e. Intake and output

D. SMALL BOWEL/LARGE BOWEL

Both the small bowel and the large bowel are hollow structures. The small bowel, composed of the duodenum, jejunum, and ileum, is the organ most often injured by a direct blunt force to the abdominal wall. This causes the intestine to be crushed between the applied force and the spinal column. Transverse fractures of the spine in the lumbar region (Chance fractures) should increase suspicion for small bowel injury. Shearing of the small bowel can result from rapid deceleration in a motor vehicle crash. Penetrating injuries are most often caused by gunshots. Small bowel injuries may produce nonspecific symptoms that delay diagnosis until peritonitis is present.

The large bowel has four sections: (1) ascending colon, (2) transverse colon, (3) descending colon, and (4) sigmoid colon. Injury to the large bowel causes gross fecal contamination of the abdomen that can lead to sepsis. Blunt forces may result in injury to the transverse and sigmoid colon because of their more mobile state and location.

1. Assessment
  a. Subjective data collection
    1) History of present injury/chief complaint
      a) Pain (see Chapter 8): generalized abdominal pain
      b) Nausea and vomiting
      c) Mechanism of injury (see Chapter 31)
    2) Past medical history
      a) Current or preexisting diseases/illness
        (1) Bleeding tendencies
      b) Medications
      c) Allergies
      d) Immunization status
  b. Objective data collection
    1) Physical examination
      a) General appearance
        (1) Possible hypotension, tachycardia
        (2) Moderate to severe distress/discomfort
      b) Inspection
        (1) Abrasions, contusions, open wounds, lacerations
        (2) Ecchymosis over abdomen; "seat belt sign"
        (3) Abdominal distention
      c) Auscultation
        (1) Breath sounds: normal to decreased
        (2) Bowel sounds: normal to decreased or absent
      d) Palpation
        (1) Abdominal tenderness
        (2) Rebound tenderness
        (3) Rigid abdomen specifically in epigastric area/LUQ
    2) Diagnostic procedures
      a) CBC with differential
      b) Serum chemistries including glucose, BUN, creatinine
      c) Serum amylase
      d) Type and crossmatch
      e) Coagulation profile: PT, PTT, INR, thromboelastography
      f) Urinalysis; pregnancy test in female patients of childbearing age
      g) Abdominal radiograph: flat plate
        (1) May demonstrate presence of free air, fluid, or obliteration of psoas shadow
        (2) Not highly specific or sensitive for evaluation of bowel injury
        (3) Presence of pneumoperitoneum does not always correlate with bowel injury
      h) Chest radiograph
      i) FAST—limited to detecting free intraperitoneal fluid in unstable patients
      j) Abdominal CT scan
        (1) Preferred diagnostic test
        (2) Of limited value if DPL performed prior to CT scan
      k) Possible DPL/DPA: positive for amylase
      l) Angiography: useful only in identifying visceral bleeding site
2. Analysis: differential nursing diagnoses/collaborative problems
  a. Deficient fluid volume
  b. Ineffective tissue perfusion
  c. Acute pain
  d. Anxiety/fear
  e. Risk for infection
3. Planning and implementation/interventions
  a. Maintain airway, breathing, circulation (see Chapters 1 and 32)
  b. Provide supplemental oxygen
  c. Establish IV access for administration of crystalloid fluids/blood products/medications
    1) Insert two large-bore IV catheters
    2) Infuse warmed normal saline solution
    3) Infuse warmed blood products as needed

d. Prepare for/assist with medical interventions
  1) Institute cardiac and pulse oximetry monitoring
  2) Insert gastric tube and attach to suction as indicated
  3) Insert indwelling urinary catheter as indicated
  4) Maintain normothermic body temperature
  5) Assist with collection and maintenance of physical and forensic evidence as indicated (see Chapter 44)
  6) Assist with hospital admission, preparation for the operating suite, or transfer to an institution providing a higher level of care
e. Administer pharmacologic therapy as ordered
  1) Nonnarcotic analgesics
  2) Narcotics
  3) Antibiotics
  4) Tetanus immunization
4. Evaluation and ongoing monitoring
  a. Hemodynamic status
  b. Breath sounds and pulse oximetry
  c. Cardiac rate and rhythm
  d. Pain relief
  e. Intake and output

E. SPLEEN

The spleen is the abdominal organ most frequently injured by blunt force, and is associated with fractures of the left-side ribs 9 through 11. Penetrating forces may also cause injury to the spleen. An injury grading system similar to that developed for liver injuries, with a scale of 1–5, is used to describe injury to the spleen. Grades 1–3 are less severe, whereas grades 4–5 usually require operative intervention. Active bleeding may also be managed by interventional radiology procedures. The spleen plays a role in immune competence, filtration of blood, and removal of bloodborne bacteria. It also stores up to 200 mL of blood. Because of the spleen's important role in immunity, intervention is aimed at spleen or partial spleen salvage.

1. Assessment
  a. Subjective data collection
    1) History of present injury/chief complaint
      a) Pain (see Chapter 8)
        (1) Left upper quadrant (LUQ)
        (2) Referred to left shoulder (Kehr sign)
      b) Mechanism of injury (see Chapter 31)
    2) Past medical history
      a) Current or preexisting diseases/illness
        (1) Bleeding tendencies
      b) Medications
      c) Allergies
      d) Immunization status
  b. Objective data collection
    1) Physical examination
      a) General appearance
        (1) Level of consciousness, color, behavior, affect: alert to confusion, comatose
        (2) Possible hypotension, tachycardia
        (3) Moderate to severe distress/discomfort
      b) Inspection
        (1) Abrasions, contusions, open wounds, lacerations
        (2) Ecchymosis over left lower chest wall/LUQ abdomen
        (3) Abdominal distention
      c) Auscultation
        (1) Breath sounds: normal to decreased or absent on left side
        (2) Bowel sounds: normal to decreased or absent
      d) Palpation
        (1) Lower left chest wall tenderness
        (2) Abdominal tenderness
        (3) Rebound tenderness
        (4) Rigid abdomen specifically in LUQ
    2) Diagnostic procedures
      a) CBC with differential
      b) Serial hematocrits
      c) Type and crossmatch
      d) Serum chemistries including glucose, BUN, creatinine
      e) Coagulation profile: PT/PTT/INR, thromboelastography
      f) Urinalysis; pregnancy test in female patients of childbearing age
      g) Chest radiograph (portable): may indicate left pneumothorax or fractured left-side ribs 9–11
      h) Abdominal radiograph: flat plate (portable)
      i) FAST
      j) Abdominal CT scan with IV contrast
      k) Possible DPL/DPA: positive for blood
      l) Angiography
2. Analysis: differential nursing diagnoses/collaborative problems
  a. Deficient fluid volume
  b. Ineffective tissue perfusion: peripheral
  c. Acute pain
  d. Anxiety/fear
  e. Risk for infection
3. Planning and implementation/interventions
  a. Maintain airway, breathing, circulation (see Chapters 1 and 31)
  b. Provide supplemental oxygen
  c. Establish IV access for administration of crystalloid fluids/blood products/medications
    1) Insert two large-bore IV catheters
    2) Infuse warmed normal saline solution
    3) Infuse warmed blood products as needed
  d. Prepare for/assist with medical interventions
    1) Institute cardiac and pulse oximetry monitoring
    2) Insert gastric tube and attach to suction as indicated
    3) Insert indwelling urinary catheter as indicated
    4) Maintain normothermic body temperature

5) Assist with collection and maintenance of physical and forensic evidence as indicated (see Chapter 43)
6) Assist with hospital admission, prepare for the operating suite/interventional radiology, or transfer to an institution providing a higher level of care
  a) Nonoperative management
    (1) Hemodynamically stable patients
    (2) Stable hemoglobin levels
    (3) Minimal blood transfusion requirements (2 units or less)
  b) Operative management
    (1) Hemodynamically unstable patients
    (2) Signs of ongoing bleeding
e. Administer pharmacologic therapy as ordered
  1) Antifibrinolytics
  2) Nonnarcotic analgesics
  3) Narcotics
  4) Antibiotics
  5) Tetanus immunization
4. Evaluation and ongoing monitoring
  a. Level of consciousness
  b. Hemodynamic status
  c. Breath sounds and pulse oximetry
  d. Cardiac rate and rhythm
  e. Pain relief
  f. Intake and output

III. Specific Urologic Injuries

A. BLADDER

Most bladder injuries result from blunt forces. It is estimated that more than 80% of bladder ruptures are associated with a pelvic fracture. Penetrating mechanisms, such as stab or gunshot wounds, are frequently associated with concurrent bowel injuries and carry an associated mortality rate of approximately 60%. Ruptured bladder alone is an uncommon injury, occurring only 2% of the time with concomitant abdominal injury and 5–10% of the time with pelvic fractures. The rupture may be extraperitoneal, intraperitoneal, or a combination of the two (Table 33.2). Bladder contusion is a more common injury.

Table 33.2

Traumatic Bladder Ruptures

Perforation Type	Frequency	Significance
Extraperitoneal	50–71%	Usually managed safely with urethral or suprapubic catheter drainage
Intraperitoneal	25–43%	Higher incidence in children than adults Requires surgical exploration
Combined intraperitoneal	7–14%	Mortality rates approach 60% and extraperitoneal

Children are more susceptible to sustaining bladder injuries from direct forces because the bladder is an abdominal organ in the younger population. Moreover, in children, the bony pelvis is less rigid, and therefore injury transmits more force to adjacent structures. A distended bladder increases the risk of injury in all ages. Ruptures may involve extravasation of blood and urine into the abdomen or pelvis that can result in the complications of peritonitis and sepsis.

1. Assessment
  a. Subjective data collection
    1) History of present injury/chief complaint
      a) Pain (see Chapter 8): abdominal or pelvic pain; suprapubic, dull, constant, or sharp
      b) Difficulty or inability to void
      c) Hematuria
    2) Past medical history
      a) Current or preexisting diseases/illness
        (1) Renal disease
      b) Medications
      c) Allergies
      d) Immunization status
  b. Objective data collection
    1) Physical examination
      a) General appearance
        (1) Possible hypotension, tachycardia
        (2) Moderate to severe distress/discomfort
      b) Inspection
        (1) Lower abdominal or perineal hematoma
        (2) Abrasions or lacerations over suprapubic or perineal area
        (3) Abdominal distention
      c) Auscultation
        (1) Bowel sounds: normal to decreased or absent
      d) Palpation
        (1) Abdominal tenderness
        (2) Rebound tenderness
        (3) Rigid abdomen related to extravasation of urine or intraabdominal bleeding
        (4) Possible pelvic instability
    2) Diagnostic procedures
      a) CBC with differential, platelet count
      b) Serum chemistries including glucose, BUN, creatinine
      c) Coagulation profile: PT/PTT, INR, thromboelastography
      d) Type and crossmatch
      e) Urinalysis; pregnancy test in female patients of childbearing age
      f) Abdominal radiograph: kidneys, ureter, bladder (KUB)
      g) Pelvic CT scan
        (1) Replaces conventional cystography as most sensitive to determine bladder perforation
        (2) Urethral intactness first determined by retrograde urethrogram

(3) Diluted contrast medium passed through urethral catheter and CT scan performed

(4) Reveals subtle perforations

h) Cystography: criterion standard

(1) Preferably performed under fluoroscopy

(2) Static cystogram is satisfactory

i) Retrograde urethrogram

(1) Blood at urinary meatus is absolute indication

j) Pelvic sonography

2. Analysis: differential nursing diagnoses/collaborative problems

a. Deficient fluid volume

b. Ineffective tissue perfusion

c. Impaired urinary elimination

d. Acute pain

e. Anxiety/fear

f. Risk for infection

3. Planning and implementation/interventions

a. Maintain airway, breathing, circulation (see Chapters 1 and 32)

b. Provide supplemental oxygen

c. Establish IV access for administration of crystalloid fluids/blood products/medications

1) Insert two large-bore IV catheters

2) Infuse warmed normal saline solution

3) Infuse warmed blood products as needed

d. Prepare for/assist with medical interventions

1) Institute cardiac and pulse oximetry monitoring

2) Insert gastric tube and attach to suction as indicated

3) Insert indwelling urinary catheter if no blood at the urinary meatus, or assist with placement of suprapubic catheter

4) Maintain normothermic body temperature

5) Assist with collection and maintenance of physical and forensic evidence as indicated (see Chapter 44)

6) Assist with hospital admission, preparation for the operating suite, or transfer to an institution providing a higher level of care

e. Administer pharmacologic therapy as indicated

1) Nonnarcotic analgesics

2) Narcotics

3) Antibiotics

4) Tetanus immunization

4. Evaluation and ongoing monitoring

a. Hemodynamic status

b. Breath sounds and pulse oximetry

c. Cardiac rate and rhythm

d. Pain relief

e. Intake and output

B. RENAL

Renal injury seldom occurs in isolation, and it should be considered in any patient presenting with chest, abdominal, or back trauma. The most common cause of renal injury is blunt force, followed by penetrating force. Motor vehicle collisions and gunshot wounds account for 80% of renal injuries. In motor vehicle collisions, the sudden rapid deceleration force can lead to an avulsion injury; the left renal vein may often be involved. Renal injuries should be suspected if the patient has fractures of the posterior lower ribs and/or spinal processes or a history of sudden deceleration, fall from height, or lateral force. Renal injuries are graded on a 1–5 scale, with type 1 being minor and type 5 being severe. Of renal injuries, 85–90% are minor and do not require surgical intervention. When required, surgical repair must be performed within 12 hours to salvage the ischemic kidney. Regardless of the mechanism of injury, extrarenal or intrarenal bleeding can occur as well as urine extravasation, leading to hypovolemic shock, pain, and inflammation.

1. Assessment

a. Subjective data collection

1) History of present injury/chief complaint

a) Mechanism of injury (see Chapter 31)

b) Pain (see Chapter 8): costovertebral angle (CVA) or abdominal, with varying quality depending on severity and mechanism of injury

c) Hematuria

2) Past medical history

a) Current or preexisting diseases/illness

(1) Renal disease

(2) Hypertension

(3) Solitary kidney

(4) History of renal surgery

b) Medications

c) Allergies

d) Immunization status

b. Objective data collection

1) Physical examination

a) General appearance

(1) Possible hypotension, tachycardia

(2) Moderate to severe distress/discomfort

b) Inspection

(1) Flank mass or hematoma

(2) Contusions, abrasions, lacerations in area of injury

c) Auscultation

(1) Breath sounds: normal to decreased

(2) Bowel sounds: normal to decreased or absent

d) Palpation

(1) Flank tenderness

(2) Abdominal or back tenderness

2) Diagnostic procedures

a) CBC with differential

b) Serum chemistries including glucose, BUN, creatinine

c) Coagulation profile: PT/PTT, INR, thromboelastography

d) Urinalysis: gross blood; urine dipstick positive (absent in one-third of patients); pregnancy test in female patients of childbearing age
e) Type and crossmatch
f) Abdominal radiograph
g) Abdominal and pelvis CT scan (Table 33.3)
h) FAST (see Table 33.3)
i) IVP (see Table 33.3)
   (1) May use "one-shot" technique—rarely done
   (2) Traditional IVP not used in urgent evaluation of renal injury
j) Renal arteriogram (see Table 33.3)

2. Analysis: differential nursing diagnoses/collaborative problems
a. Deficient fluid volume
b. Impaired tissue perfusion
c. Acute pain
d. Risk for infection
e. Anxiety/fear

3. Planning and implementation/interventions
a. Maintain airway, breathing, circulation (see Chapters 1 and 32)
b. Provide supplemental oxygen
c. Establish IV access for administration of crystalloid fluids/blood products/medications
   1) Insert two large-bore IV catheters
   2) Infuse warmed normal saline solution
   3) Infuse warmed blood products as needed
d. Prepare for/assist with medical interventions
   1) Institute cardiac and pulse oximetry monitoring
   2) Insert gastric tube and attach to suction as indicated

   3) Insert indwelling urinary catheter as indicated
   4) Maintain normothermic body temperature
   5) Assist with collection and maintenance of physical and forensic evidence as indicated (see Chapter 44)
   6) Assist with hospital admission, prepare for the operating suite/interventional radiology, or transfer to an institution providing a higher level of care
e. Administer pharmacologic therapy as ordered
   1) Nonnarcotic analgesics
   2) Narcotics
   3) Antibiotics
   4) Tetanus immunization

4. Evaluation and ongoing monitoring
a. Hemodynamic status
b. Breath sounds and pulse oximetry
c. Cardiac rate and rhythm
d. Pain relief
e. Intake and output

C. URETHRA

Urethral injury occurs predominately in male patients. The male urethra is divided into posterior and anterior segments. Injuries to the posterior segment more commonly occur in association with pelvic fractures, whereas injuries to the anterior segment are more commonly the result of straddle injuries (e.g., bicycles) or a direct blow to the perineum. Urethral injuries can also result from mutilation or instrumentation. In female patients, urethral injury is rare because the urethra is short, unexposed, and less mobile. When injury does occur, it is usually at the site of the bladder neck. The mechanisms

Table 33.3

Radiography Tests Advantages and Disadvantages

Test	Advantages	Disadvantages
IVP	Provides detailed anatomic assessment of kidneys and ureters "One-shot" study can be performed in the emergency department	Requires administration of contrast Requires multiple images for maximal information Has relatively high radiation dose Findings may not reveal full extent of injury Complete study needs to be performed in radiology suite Ultrasound or CT may provide similar or more detailed information
CT scan	Provides best functional and anatomic assessment of kidneys and urinary tract Aids in diagnosis of concurrent injuries	Requires IV contrast to provide maximal information Patient must be hemodynamically stable
Angiography	Aids in both diagnosis and treatment of renal vascular injury Provides further diagnosis of injury in patients with IVP abnormalities	Invasive Requires use of contrast Time consuming Performed in radiology suite
Sonography	Noninvasive Performed along with resuscitation Performed in the emergency department May aid in defining traumatic anatomy	Injury definition requires experienced sonographer FAST does not define anatomy: only identifies free fluid Bladder injuries may be missed

FAST, Focused Assessment Sonography for Trauma; *IV*, intravenous; *IVP*, intravenous pyelography.

of injury include childbirth or vaginal surgery, straddle injuries, and associated pelvic fractures. Approximately 10–25% of patients with a pelvic fracture also have urethral trauma. Complete rupture of the urethra is more common in children because the urethra is less elastic. Urethral rupture should be considered early in the management of patients with pelvic trauma to avoid converting a partial urethral tear to a complete transection during the insertion of a urinary catheter. The insertion of foreign bodies into the urethra should also raise the suspicion of urethral injury.

1. Assessment
   a. Subjective data collection
      1) History of present injury/chief complaint
         a) History of injury
         b) Suprapubic, perineal, or genital pain related to voiding and/or bladder distention
         c) Feeling unable to void, or inability to void
         d) Hematuria
      2) Past medical history
         a) Current or preexisting diseases/illness
         b) Medications
         c) Allergies
         d) Immunization status
   b. Objective data collection
      1) Physical examination
         a) General appearance
            (1) Possible hypotension, tachycardia
            (2) Moderate to severe distress/discomfort
         b) Inspection
            (1) Blood at urinary meatus
            (2) Swelling of suprapubic area (bladder distention) or genitalia/perineum
            (3) Hematoma of lower abdomen or perineum: butterfly-shaped and resulting from straddle injury
            (4) Local abrasions or lacerations
         c) Auscultation
            (1) Bowel sounds: normal to decreased or absent
      2) Diagnostic procedures
         a) CBC with differential
         b) Serial hematocrits if suspicion of pelvic fracture
         c) Type and crossmatch if suspicion of pelvic fracture
         d) Urinalysis; pregnancy test in female patients of childbearing age
         e) Coagulation profile: PT/PTT, INR, thromboelastography
         f) Abdominal and pelvic radiographs
         g) Pelvis CT
         h) Retrograde urethrogram: standard imaging study to determine injury
         i) Cystography: to determine minor injury or patency

2. Analysis: differential nursing diagnoses/collaborative problems
   a. Impaired urinary elimination
   b. Acute pain
   c. Anxiety/fear
   d. Risk for infection
3. Planning and implementation/interventions
   a. Maintain airway, breathing, circulation (see Chapters 1 and 32)
   b. Provide supplemental oxygen
   c. Establish IV access for administration of crystalloid fluids/blood products/medications
      1) Insert two large-bore IV catheters
      2) Infuse warmed normal saline solution
      3) Infuse warmed blood products as needed
   d. Prepare for/assist with medical interventions
      1) Institute cardiac and pulse oximetry monitoring
      2) Insert gastric tube and attach to suction as indicated
      3) Assist with suprapubic catheter insertion as indicated
         a) Safest approach to establish urinary drainage
         b) Does not require urethral manipulation
      4) Maintain normothermic body temperature
      5) Assist with collection and maintenance of physical and forensic evidence as indicated (see Chapter 43)
      6) Assist with hospital admission, prepare for the operating suite, or transfer to an institution providing a higher level of care
   e. Administer pharmacologic therapy as ordered
      1) Nonnarcotic analgesics
      2) Narcotics
      3) Antibiotics
      4) Tetanus immunization
4. Evaluation and ongoing monitoring
   a. Hemodynamic status
   b. Breath sounds and pulse oximetry
   c. Cardiac rate and rhythm
   d. Pain relief
   e. Intake and output

Bibliography

ACEP Clinical Policies Committee: Clinical policy: Critical issues in the evaluation of adult patients presenting to the emergency department with acute blunt abdominal trauma, *Annals of Emergency Medicine* 57(4):387–404, 2011.

American College of Surgeons: Abdominal and pelvic trauma. In *Advanced trauma life support for doctors*, 9th ed., American College of Surgeons, 2012, pp 122–147.

American College of Surgeons Trauma Quality Improvement Program: Geriatric Trauma Management Guidelines. (2015). Retrieved from https://www.facs.org/~/media/files/qualityprograms/trauma/tqip/geriatricguidetqip.ashx.

Bokhari, F, Phelan, H, Holevar, M, Brautigam, R, Collier, B et al., Smith, L. (2009). EAST guidelines for the diagnosis and management of pancreatic trauma. Retrieved from https://www.east.org/education/practice-management-guidelines/pancreatic-trauma-diagnosis-and- -and-management-of.

Burlew CC, Moore EE: Severe pelvic fracture in the adult trauma patient. UpToDate. Retrieved from http://www.uptodate.com/contents/severe-pelvic-fracture-in-the-adult-trauma-patient, 2014.

Calland JF, Ingraham AM, Martin N, Marshall CT, Schulman CI, Barraco RD: Evaluation and management of geriatric trauma: An Eastern Association for the Surgery of Trauma practice management guideline, *Journal of Trauma and Acute Care Surgery* 73(5/4):S345–S350, 2012. Retrieved at https://www.east.org/education/practice-management-guidelines/geriatric-trauma-evaluation-and-management-of.

Chestovich PJ, Browder TD, Morrissey SL, Fraser DR, Ingalls NK, Fildes JJ: Minimally invasive is maximally effective: Diagnostic and therapeutic laparoscopy for penetrating abdominal injuries, *Journal of Trauma and Acute Care Surgery* 78(6):1076–1085, 2015.

Como JJ, Bokhari F, Chiu WC, Duane TM, Holevar MR, Scalea TM: Practice management guidelines for selective nonoperative management of penetrating abdominal trauma, *The Journal of Trauma Injury, Infection and Critical Care* 68(3):721–733, 2010. Retrieved from https://www.east.org/education/practice-management-guidelines/penetrating-abdominal-trauma-selective-non-operative-management-of.

Eckert K: Penetrating and blunt abdominal trauma, *Critical Care Nursing Quarterly* 28(1):41–59, 2005.

Emergency Nurses Association: Abdominal and pelvic trauma. In *Trauma nursing core course*, 7th ed., Des Plaines, IL, 2014, ENA Publications, pp 151–172.

Goldberg SR, Anand RJ, Como JJ, Dechert T, Dente C, Duane TM: Prophylactic antibiotic use in penetrating abdominal trauma: An Eastern Association for the Surgery of Trauma practice management guideline, *Journal of Trauma and Acute Care Surgery* 73(5/4):S321–S325, 2012. Retrieved from https://www.east.org/education/practice-management-guidelines/penetrating-abdominal-trauma-prophylactic-antibiotic-use-in.

Hoff WS, Holevar M, Nagy KK, Patterson L, Young JS, Valenziano CP: Practice management guidelines for the evaluation of blunt abdominal trauma: The EAST Practice Management Guidelines Work Group, *The Journal of Trauma, Injury, Infection and Critical Care* 53(3):602–615, 2002. Retrieved from https://www.east.org/education/practice-management-guidelines/blunt-abdominal-trauma-evaluation-of.

Kozar RA, Feliciano DV, Moore EE, Moore FA, Cocanour CS, McIntyre RC: Western Trauma Association critical decisions in trauma: Operative management of adult blunt hepatic trauma, *The Journal of Trauma, Injury, Infection, and Critical Care* 71(1):1–5, 2011.

Kozar RA, Moore FA, Moore EE, West M, Cocanour CS, McIntyre RC: Western Trauma Association critical decisions in trauma: Nonoperative management of adult blunt hepatic trauma, *The Journal of Trauma, Injury, Infection and Critical Care* 67(6):1144–1149, 2009.

Maxwell CA: Trauma in the geriatric population, *Critical Care Nursing Clinics of North America* 27(2):183–197, 2015.

Moore EE, Cogbill TH, Jurkovich GJ, Shackford SR, Malangoni MA, Champion MR: Organ injury scaling: Spleen and liver (1994 revision), *Journal of Trauma* 38(3):323–324, 1995.

Stassen NA, Bhullar I, Cheng JD, Crandall ML, Friese RS, Kerwin AJ: Nonoperative management of blunt hepatic injury: An Eastern Association for the Surgery of Trauma practice management guideline, *Journal of Trauma and Acute Care Surgery* 73(5/4):S288–S293, 2012. Retrieved from https://www.east.org/education/practice-management-guidelines/blunt-hepatic-injury-selective-nonoperative-management-of.

Stassen NA, Bhullar I, Cheng JD, Crandall ML, Friese RS, Kerwin AJ: Selective nonoperative management of blunt splenic injury: An Eastern Association for the Surgery of Trauma practice management guideline, *Journal of Trauma and Acute Care Surgery* 73(5/4):S294–S300, 2012. Retrieved from https://www.east.org/education/practice-management-guidelines/blunt-splenic-injury-selective-nonoperative-management-of.

Zacharias C, Robinson JD, Linnau KF, Mannelli L: Blunt urinary bladder trauma, *Current Problems in Diagnostic Radiology* 41(4):140–141, 2012.

CHAPTER 34

Burn Trauma

Cheryl Wraa, RN, MSN, FAEN

MAJOR TOPICS

General Strategy
Assessment
Analysis: Differential Nursing Diagnoses/Collaborative
  Problems
Planning and Implementation/Interventions
Evaluation and Ongoing Monitoring

Documentation of Interventions and Patient Response
Age-Related Considerations
Specific Burn Injuries
Chemical Burns
Electrical/Lightning Burns
Thermal and Inhalation Burns

Each year in the United States, approximately 1.25 million people seek medical attention for burn injuries. Of these patients, 63,000 have minor burns that are primarily treated in the emergency department; the remainder require acute hospital admission, with over 60% being admitted to burn centers. Annually, 3,240 people die of burns and related inhalation injuries. Most deaths occur from residential fires, followed by vehicle crash fires. Statistics from the American Burn Association National Burn Repository report that of those patients admitted to a burn unit:

Survival rate: 96.7%
Gender: 69% male, 31% female
Admission cause: 43% fire/flame, 34% scald, 9% con-
  tact, 4% electrical, 3% chemical, and 7% other
Place of occurrence: 73% home, 8% occupational, 5%
  street/highway, 5% recreational/sport, and 9% other

Advances in areas such as fluid resuscitation, management of inhalation, wound care practice with early débridement and excision, as well as a better understanding of the importance of increased nutritional support have contributed to a decrease in burn-related deaths. Very young and very old patients have a high risk of death because of their immature and stressed immunologic systems and preexisting medical conditions. Burns in combination with an inhalation injury significantly worsen a patient's prognosis.

A burn injury is defined as tissue injury that results from exposure to flames, hot liquids, hot objects, caustic chemicals, radiation, or electric current. Burn injury can cause a hypermetabolic response including physiologic, catabolic, and immune system effects. The injury initiates an inflammatory response, which includes heat, redness, and pain, with localized and systemic edema formation. The amount of edema is related to the extent and depth of the burn injury as well as the amount of fluid administered during fluid resuscitation. The combination of fluid shift, edema

formation, and evaporative water loss from the burn wound can lead to hypovolemia ("burn shock"). Loss of plasma is greatest during the first 4–6 hours after the burn injury, but may continue up to 24 hours after injury. The decreased circulating blood volume becomes thickened and sluggish, thereby diminishing tissue oxygenation and causing injury to end organs such as the kidneys. Hypovolemia reduces cardiac output and thus causes the sympathetic nervous system to respond by releasing catecholamines, a process that leads to increased peripheral vascular resistance, increased afterload, and increased heart rate. Fluid resuscitation can stabilize cardiac output during the resuscitative phase of burn injury. Because of the tissue damage that occurs with major burn injuries, hemolysis may occur resulting in hemoconcentration, thrombocytopenia, decreased platelets, and potential clotting abnormalities. Rhabdomyolysis can occur with significant injury to muscle tissue, causing hyperkalemia and renal failure. Post initial resuscitation, a hypermetabolic response occurs that includes an increase in cardiac output and resting energy expenditure. This response also includes accelerated gluconeogenesis, insulin resistance, and increased protein catabolism. Research is ongoing in this area of physiology.

Burn injuries are classified according to the depth and extent of the injury. Populations at risk for burn injury include children, the elderly, substance abusers (e.g., alcohol, tobacco, or drugs), and those with suicidal ideation.

I. General Strategy

A. ASSESSMENT

1. Primary and secondary assessment/resuscitation (see Chapters 1 and 32)
2. Focused assessment

a. Subjective data collection
  1) History of present injury/chief complaint
    a) Mechanism of injury (see Chapter 31)
    b) Pain (see Chapter 8)
    c) Length of time exposed to burn source
    d) Time of occurrence
    e) Body area involved and type of burn
      (1) Environment in which patient was found: enclosed space, industrial setting, presence of combustible substances (e.g., wood, petroleum products, plastics)
      (2) Electrical/lightning injury: amount of voltage, alternating current (AC) or direct current (DC), resistance, path of current
      (3) Chemical injury: type of chemical, concentration, mechanism of action, extent of tissue penetration, duration of contact, treatment prior to arrival
    f) Level of consciousness
    g) Related injuries: cervical spine, spine, leg, or arm fractures; thoracic or abdominal injury; evidence of maltreatment
    h) Cardiopulmonary resuscitation (CPR) at the scene
    i) Efforts to relieve symptoms
      (1) Home remedies
      (2) Alternative therapies
      (3) Medications
        (a) Prescription
        (b) OTC/herbal
  2) Past medical history
    a) Current preexisting diseases/illness
      (1) Cardiovascular disease
      (2) Pulmonary disease
      (3) Diabetes
    b) Previous surgical procedures
    c) Smoking history
    d) Substance and/or alcohol use/abuse
    e) Last normal menstrual period: female patients of childbearing age
    f) History of suicidal behavior
    g) Current medications
      (1) Prescription
      (2) OTC/herbal
    h) Allergies
    i) Immunization status
b. Objective data collection
  1) General appearance
    a) Level of consciousness, behavior, affect
    b) Vital signs
    c) Odors
    d) Gait
    e) Hygiene
    f) Level of distress/discomfort
  2) Inspection
    a) Airway: patent, maintainable, not maintainable
      (1) Carbonaceous sputum
      (2) Singed hair, nasal hairs/eyebrows
      (3) Face and/or neck burns
      (4) Carbon deposits and inflammation/blistering in the oropharynx
    b) Burned tissues
      (1) Erythema of area
      (2) Red or mottled appearance
      (3) Blister formation
      (4) Dark or leathery appearance
      (5) Waxy white appearance
    c) Cardiac rhythm on monitor
    d) Sternal retractions
  3) Auscultation
    a) Breath sounds: wheezing, rhonchi
    b) Heart sounds
    c) Bowel sounds
  4) Palpation
    a) Peripheral and central pulses
    b) Deformities
    c) Sensory perception surrounding burned tissue
3. Psychological/social/environmental factors
  a. Occupational risk factors
    1) Firefighters, emergency medical service, and rescue personnel
    2) Occupation involving exposure to excessive heat, electricity, or chemicals
    3) Military
  b. Alterations in ability to perceive environmental threats
    1) Age of the patient
      a) Pediatric: decision making and recognition of threat limited to developmental level
      b) Elderly: reduced mobility, changes in vision, and decreased sensation in the feet and hands
  c. Social risk factors
    1) Possible/actual assault, abuse, or intimate partner violence situations (see Chapters 3 and 40)
    2) Homelessness
    3) Depression: suicide ideation
  d. Environmental risk factors
    1) Contact with flame, hot object, water, or chemicals
    2) Enclosed area
    3) Contact with electricity or lightning
4. Diagnostic procedures
  a. Laboratory studies
    1) Complete blood count (CBC) with differential
    2) Serum chemistries including glucose, CPK, BUN, creatinine
    3) Carboxyhemoglobin (HbCO) level
    4) Type and crossmatch
    5) Coagulation profile
    6) Urinalysis; pregnancy test in female patients of childbearing age

7) Arterial blood gas (ABG) determinations

8) Serum and urine toxicology screens

  b. Imaging studies

    1) Chest radiograph

    2) Cervical spine, extremity radiographs as indicated for associated injuries

    3) Computed tomography (CT) scan for associated injury

    4) Focused Assessment Sonography for Trauma (FAST) as indicated for associated abdominal trauma (see Chapter 32)

  c. Other

    1) Possible peritoneal lavage for associated trauma (see Chapter 32)

    2) 12- to 15-lead electrocardiogram (ECG) if electrical or lightning injury

B. ANALYSIS: DIFFERENTIAL NURSING DIAGNOSES/ COLLABORATIVE PROBLEMS

1. Risk for ineffective airway clearance
2. Risk for impaired gas exchange
3. Risk for ineffective breathing pattern
4. Risk for deficient fluid volume
5. Risk for hypothermia
6. Acute pain
7. Risk for ineffective tissue perfusion
8. Risk for infection
9. Impaired skin integrity
10. Anxiety related to fear

C. PLANNING AND IMPLEMENTATION/ INTERVENTIONS

1. Determine priorities of care
   a. Maintain airway, breathing, circulation (see Chapters 1 and 32)
   b. Provide supplemental oxygen as indicated
   c. Stop the burning process; remove clothing and jewelry as indicated
   d. Establish IV access for administration of crystalloid fluids/blood products
   e. Obtain and set up equipment and supplies
   f. Prepare for/assist with medical interventions
   g. Administer pharmacologic therapy as ordered
   h. Prevent hypothermia
2. Relieve anxiety/apprehension
3. Allow significant others to remain with patient if supportive
4. Educate patient/significant others

D. EVALUATION AND ONGOING MONITORING

1. Continuously monitor and treat as indicated
2. Monitor patient response/outcomes, and modify nursing care plans as appropriate

3. If positive patient outcomes are not demonstrated, reevaluate assessment and/or plan of care
4. Prepare for admission or transfer to burn center

E. DOCUMENTATION OF INTERVENTIONS AND PATIENT RESPONSE

F. AGE-RELATED CONSIDERATIONS

1. Pediatric
   a. Growth or developmental related
      1) Death from burns is among the leading causes of death in children
      2) Infants and children have small airways that are more easily obstructed by edema from inhalation injury
      3) Children's high ratio of total body surface area (TBSA) to body mass increases heat exchange with the environment and directly affects their ability to regulate core temperature
      4) Lack of substantial subcutaneous tissue and thin skin contribute to increased evaporative heat loss and caloric expenditure
      5) Children are dependent on caregivers to educate and protect them about environmental hazards
      6) The potential for maltreatment should be considered
      7) Children's healing responses are more rapid than those of adults
   b. "Pearls"
      1) Children are curious about their environment and may not be afraid to touch flame or a hot object
      2) Burns occur in 6–20% of maltreated children. Findings associated with inflicted burns include burns to both hands or both legs, brands/contact burns (imprint of a hot object), cigarette burns (circular and of uniform depth), and immersion burns, usually seen on the buttocks or legs or in a stocking or glove distribution on the extremities (sparing of the palms, soles, and skin folds where knees and hips are flexed is common)
      3) Hypothermia may render an injured child refractory to treatment, prolonged coagulation times, and adversely affect central nervous system (CNS) function. During resuscitation, if exposed, overhead heat lamps or heaters may be necessary to maintain body temperature. IV fluids, blood products, and inhaled gases should be warmed
      4) Children have poor glycogen storage, so glucose levels should be closely monitored
2. Geriatric
   a. Aging related
      1) Loss of subcutaneous tissue and thinning of the dermis the elderly predispose to a deep injury from thermal burn

2) Decreased touch receptors with corresponding slowing of reflexes and pain sensation

3) Decreased proliferative potential of skin delays wound healing and vitamin D production

4) Decreased airway clearance, decreased cough and laryngeal reflexes

5) Stiffening of elastin and the collagen connective tissue supporting the lungs

6) Decreased alveolar surface area available for gas exchange

7) Decreased ciliary action can contribute to higher risk of inhalation injury

8) Increased chest wall stiffness with declining strength in chest muscles

b. "Pearls"

1) Older adults with altered mental status are dependent on caregivers to protect them from danger in the surrounding environment

2) Slowing of reflexes and decreased sensation increase the risk for burn injury; scalds and flames are the leading causes. Also, these changes make it difficult for elderly persons to extinguish the fire or remove themselves from the burn source

3) Older adults are more likely to have chronic illnesses that decrease the ability to withstand the multisystem stresses imposed by burn injury

II. Specific Burn Injuries

A. CHEMICAL BURNS

A chemical burn results from contact with any one of the three types of chemicals: acids, alkali, and organic compounds. Acids are found in cleaning products such as drain cleaners. Alkalis are found in such products as rust removers and swimming pool cleaners. Organic compounds include phenols or petroleum products such as gasoline and creosote.

Chemicals cause a denaturing of protein within the tissues or a desiccation of cells. The extent of the burn is dependent on the concentration of the chemical and the time of exposure. Alkali products cause more tissue damage than acids.

Dry substances should be brushed off the skin before flushing the area. Wet chemicals should be removed as soon as possible by flushing with copious amounts of water. Care must be taken by the caregiver to not become exposed to the chemical. Contaminated clothing should be removed and bagged as soon as possible. All fluids used to flush the patient should be collected and contained and not allowed to drain into the general drainage system.

Chemical burn depth can be deceiving until the tissue begins to slough days later. For that reason, all chemical burns should be considered deep partial-thickness or full-thickness burns until proven otherwise.

1. Assessment
   a. Subjective data collection
      1) History of present injury/chief complaint
         a) Type of chemical injury: type of chemical, concentration, chemical's mechanism of action, extent of tissue penetration, duration of contact, treatment prior to arrival
         b) History of associated trauma
         c) Length of time exposed to the chemical source
         d) Level of consciousness
         e) Pain (see Chapter 8)
            (1) Pain out of proportion to skin involvement with hydrofluoric acid burns
      2) Past medical history
         a) Current or preexisting diseases/illness
            (1) Cardiovascular disease
            (2) Pulmonary disease
            (3) Diabetes
         b) Smoking history
         c) Alcohol or substance abuse
         d) Medications
         e) Allergies
         f) Immunization status
   b. Objective data collection
      1) Physical examination
         a) General appearance
            (1) Odors: chemical
            (2) Mild to severe distress/discomfort
         b) Inspection
            (1) Location of burned tissue
            (2) Color of involved tissue
            (3) Tissue blistering: open or intact
         c) Auscultation
            (1) Breath sounds: wheezing if inhaled chemicals
      2) Diagnostic procedures
         a) Serum chemistries: hypocalcemia, hyperkalemia with hydrofluoric acid
         b) Chest radiograph: if chemical inhaled
         c) ECG: hydrofluoric acid exposure
            (1) Prolonged QT interval
            (2) Peaked T waves
            (3) Ventricular dysrhythmias
2. Analysis: differential nursing diagnoses/collaborative problems
   a. Risk for ineffective breathing pattern
   b. Risk for impaired gas exchange
   c. Acute pain
   d. Impaired skin integrity
   e. Risk for infection
3. Planning and implementation/interventions
   a. Stop the burning process
      1) Decontaminate patient as indicated: flush area with warm water medially to laterally
      2) Personnel may be required to wear chemical-resistant jumpsuits, rubber aprons, latex gloves, or face and eye shields

b. Maintain airway, breathing, circulation (see Chapters 1 and 32)

c. Provide supplemental oxygen as indicated

d. Establish IV access for administration of crystalloid fluid/medications as needed

e. Prepare for/assist with medical interventions
   1) Clean open wounds gently with mild soap solution or normal saline
   2) Institute cardiac monitoring if hydrofluoric acid burn

f. Administer pharmacologic therapy as ordered
   1) Nonnarcotic analgesics
   2) Narcotics
   3) Topical burn wound medications for open wounds
      a) Silver sulfadiazine (Silvadene)
      b) Mafenide acetate (Sulfamylon)
      c) Water-based ointment to face, ears, neck, and perineum (e.g., bacitracin)
   4) Calcium gluconate for hydrofluoric acid burn
      a) Apply 2.5% calcium gluconate gel to burn area
      b) Subcutaneous infiltration: 0.5 mL of 10% calcium gluconate/cm^2 of burn, extending 0.5 cm beyond margin of involved tissue
      c) IV regional: dilute 10–15 mL of 10% calcium gluconate in 5,000 units heparin, then dilute in 40 mL dextrose 5% in water (D$_5$W)
      d) Inhalation hydrofluoric acid burn administer 2.5% calcium gluconate by nebulizer with 100% oxygen
   5) Tetanus immunization

g. Educate patient/significant others
   1) Wound care
   2) Signs and symptoms of infection
   3) Medications
   4) Nutrition
   5) When to return for follow-up care

4. Evaluation and ongoing monitoring
   a. Pain relief

B. ELECTRICAL/LIGHTNING BURNS

Electrical current can either be alternating (most household current) or direct (car battery). As electricity passes through the body and meets resistance from tissues, it converts to heat in direct proportion to the amperage and the body's electrical resistance. This pass of electrical current through the skin causes an external burn at both entry and exit sites. Extensive damage occurs internally between these sites. Nerves, blood vessels, and muscle are less resistant and more easily damaged than bone or fat. The nervous system is particularly sensitive to electrical burns, which can cause damage to the brain, spinal cord, and myelin-producing cells. The smaller the body part through which the electricity passes, the more intense the heat and the less it is dissipated. If the path is near the heart, damage to the electrical conduction system can cause spontaneous ventricular fibrillation or other dysrhythmias. AC is more likely to induce fibrillation than DC.

Lightning injuries usually do not traverse the body but flow around it. This flow can create a shock wave capable of causing fractures and dislocations. Approximately 70% of lightning strike survivors complain of paresthesia and/or paralysis, which are usually temporary.

Lightning strikes account for about 23 deaths and many more injuries annually in the United States. A lightning strike can cause immediate cardiac and respiratory arrest; 89% of patients present with burns, though only 5% have deep burns. A person may be injured by a direct hit, splash effect, step voltage, or concussive injury. A lightning strike results in a massive DC of 10,000–20,000 amperes, lasting only a few microseconds. The path of the bolt and the amount of resistance determine the type of injury that may result. Additionally, shock waves of up to 20 atmospheres may result in trauma to lungs and viscera. Tympanic membrane rupture occurs in 50% of patients. Those at risk for lightning strike include hikers, campers, farmers, and golfers.

1. Assessment
   a. Subjective data collection
      1) History of present injury/chief complaint
         a) Mechanism of injury (see Chapter 30)
            (1) Patient found down after electrical current exposure or a storm
            (2) Electrical injury: amount of voltage, AC or DC, path of current
         b) Witnessed strike
         c) Unsafe electrical exposure
         d) Cardiac arrest during exposure or during a storm
         e) Chest pain (see Chapter 8)
         f) Deafness
         g) Blindness
         h) Muscle aches
      2) Past medical history
         a) Current or preexisting diseases/illness
         b) History of being struck by lightning
         c) Lack of preparation for outside activity
         d) Medications
         e) Allergies
         f) Immunization status
   b. Objective data collection
      1) Physical examination
         a) General appearance
            (1) Level of consciousness, behavior, affect: awake, confused, amnesic, seizures, comatose
            (2) Possible cardiac/respiratory arrest
            (3) Moderate to severe distress/discomfort, critically ill
         b) Inspection

(1) Ventricular fibrillation or asystole on monitor
(2) Contusions from shock wave
(3) Tympanic membrane rupture
(4) Cutaneous burns

2) Diagnostic procedures
  a) CBC with differential
  b) Serum chemistries including BUN and creatinine
  c) Hepatic and renal profiles
  d) Cardiac enzymes: CPK
  e) Coagulation profile
  f) Urinalysis: presence of myoglobin; pregnancy test in female patients of childbearing age
  g) ECG
  h) Radiographs, CT scan as indicated by injury

2. Analysis: differential nursing diagnoses/collaborative problems
  a. Ineffective breathing pattern
  b. Deficient fluid volume
  c. Ineffective tissue perfusion
  d. Acute pain
  e. Impaired skin integrity

3. Planning and implementation/interventions
  a. Maintain airway, breathing, circulation (see Chapters 1 and 32)
    1) Initiate or continue Basic Life Support (BLS) and Advanced Life Support (ALS) per protocols if respiratory/cardiac arrest is present
  b. Provide supplemental oxygen
    1) Intubation and ventilatory support in arrest patients
    2) High-flow oxygen
  c. Establish IV access for administration of crystalloid fluids/medications
  d. Prepare for/assist with medical interventions
    1) Advanced airway management
      a) Nasal or oral intubation
      b) Supraglottic airway (e.g., King, Combitube, laryngeal mask airway)
      c) Surgical airway (e.g., cricothyrotomy)
    2) Institute continuous cardiac and pulse oximetry monitoring
    3) Insert gastric tube and attach to suction
    4) Insert indwelling urinary catheter
    5) Perform burn wound care as indicated
    6) Assist with hospital admission or transfer to burn center
  e. Administer pharmacologic therapy as ordered
    1) ALS medications per protocols
    2) Narcotics
    3) Tetanus immunization

4. Evaluation and ongoing monitoring
  a. Airway patency
  b. Level of consciousness
  c. Hemodynamic monitoring
  d. Breath sounds and pulse oximetry
  e. Cardiac rate and rhythm
  f. Pain relief
  g. Intake and output

C. THERMAL AND INHALATION BURNS

Thermal burns are the most common type of burn injury. These burns are caused by ultraviolet light exposure or by contact with flame, flash, steam, or scalding liquid (Table 34.1). The majority of burn injuries are caused by thermal sources. Most burns from flame are caused by careless smoking, motor vehicle crashes, clothing ignited from a stove or heater, and gasoline or kerosene placed on a charcoal or wood fire. Contact with a hot object such as coals, glass, or metal will cause a burn that is usually not extensive, but tends to be deep.

Scalds and hot surface burns are the most common cause of serious burns to children younger than 2 years and older adults. Exposure to heat source including liquids, at 140°F (60°C) for 3 seconds can cause a deep partial-thickness or full-thickness burn. Freshly brewed coffee is approximately 180°F (82°C).

Flash burns are the result of an explosion from a flammable liquid such as propane or gasoline. The explosion causes intense heat for a brief time and usually results in partial-thickness burns. Flash burns can be large and are often associated with thermal upper airway damage.

An inhalation burn results from the inhalation of superheated air or steam or of toxic substances that cause cellular hypoxia. Although smoke from a fire in an enclosed space has a high temperature, it is usually dry and therefore has a low specific heat. Because the upper airways have excellent heat-exchanging properties, thermal injuries tend to be limited to the supraglottic airways. Thermal injury of the lower airways may occur when there is inhalation of superheated particles or steam. Heat produces immediate injury to the mucosa that results in edema. If significant edema develops, the upper airway may become obstructed. The presence of external neck or facial burns may cause anatomic distortion of the upper airway, further impairing gas flow.

Smoke inhalation may lead to the absorption of carbon monoxide (CO), an odorless, tasteless, nonirritating gas formed by the incomplete combustion of carbon-containing compounds. CO impairs the delivery and/or utilization of oxygen, which eventually results in systemic tissue hypoxia and death. Diagnosis of CO poisoning is based on history, physical examination, and an elevated HbCO level. Failure to diagnose CO poisoning can result from reliance on pulse oximetry. Most two-channel pulse oximeters cannot reliably differentiate between oxyhemoglobin (HbO_2) and carboxyhemoglobin (HbCO).

Soot contains elemental carbon and can absorb toxins from burning materials that are toxic to the bronchial mucosa and alveoli because of their pH and the ability to form free radicals. These compounds may cause acute neutrophilic airway inflammation. Physiologic changes

Table 34.1

Common Burn Injuries

Type	Cause	Body Areas Involved	Other Considerations
Sunburn	Direct ultraviolet radiation exposure	Any exposed skin area	Sunscreen aids in prevention; sunscreen with sun protection factor (SPF) of 30 usually sufficient
Flame	Contact with open flame	Direct tissue injury	May ignite clothing; natural fibers burn; synthetic fibers melt
Contact	Direct contact with hot object	Confined to point of contact	Examples: cooking appliances, irons, cigarettes
Scald	Contact with hot liquids	Accidental: splash pattern Intentional: may involve whole extremity, circumferential pattern	More viscous the liquid, longer the skin contact, greater the damage
Steam	Industry, automobile radiator accidents	Face, exposed upper body, may cause injury to distal airways of lungs	Extensive injury from high heat-carrying capacity and dispersion of pressurized steam
Gasoline	Inhalation of hot gas	Upper airway at risk from heat and edema	Distal airway involvement from products of combustion on mucosa and alveoli
Electrical, lightning	Heat produced as it passes through tissue	Injury deep into the skin and muscle	
Flash	Rapid ignition of flammable gas or liquid	Exposed areas when ignition occurs	Face may be involved, but inhalation risk is low
Tar	Liquid tar: roofing	Point of contact	Asphalt boils at 284°F (140°C), asphalt roofing tar at 450°F (232°C); tar cools rapidly to 199–219°F (93–104°C)

include disruption of mucociliary transport, increased alveolocapillary permeability, impaired lymphatic flow, worsened ventilation/perfusion (V/Q) matching, and an increased susceptibility to respiratory infections.

1. Assessment
   a. Subjective data collection
      1) History of present injury/chief complaint
         a) Mechanism of injury (see Chapter 31)
            (1) Time of occurrence
            (2) Length of exposure time, history of confined space
         b) History of associated trauma, evidence of maltreatment
         c) Level of consciousness
         d) Environment in which patient was found: enclosed space
         e) Pain (see Chapter 8)
      2) Past medical history
         a) Current or preexisting diseases/illness
            (1) Cardiac disease
            (2) Pulmonary disease
            (3) Diabetes
         b) Smoking history
         c) Alcohol or substance abuse
         d) Medications
         e) Allergies
         f) Immunization status

   b. Objective data collection
      1) Physical examination
         a) General appearance
            (1) Level of consciousness, behavior, affect: alert to comatose
            (2) Hypotension, tachycardia
            (3) Inspiratory/expiratory stridor
            (4) Moderate to severe distress/discomfort
         b) Inspection
            (1) Location of burned tissue
               (a) Face, hands, feet, genitalia, perineum, overlying major joints
               (b) Circumferential burns that encompass an entire extremity or area such as the thorax; skin inelasticity and edema cause tissue ischemia and death
            (2) Depth of burned tissue (Table 34.2): superficial, partial thickness, full thickness
            (3) Extent of burn: determined by estimation of TBSA involved
               (a) Rule of nines (Fig. 34.1)
               (b) Lund and Browder chart (Fig. 34.2)
            (4) Singed hair, nasal hair, eyebrows
            (5) Carbonaceous sputum
            (6) Blistering around or in mouth
            (7) Skin erythema
            (8) Blistering: intact or open

Table 34.2

Depth of Burn Injury

Description	Depth	Characteristics	Healing Period
Superficial	First two or three of the five layers of the epidermis	Erythema and mild discomfort	2–7 days
Partial-thickness or superficial dermal burn	Upper third of the dermis	Light to bright red or mottled May appear wet, may blister Very painful and sensitive to air currents	7–21 days
Deep-dermal partial-thickness	Entire epidermal layer and part of the dermis	Red with patchy white areas that blanch with pressure	4–6 wk
Full-thickness	Destruction of all the layers of the skin down to and including the subcutaneous	White or charred, red or brown, and leathery Painless at the full-thickness tissue	Skin grafting required burn

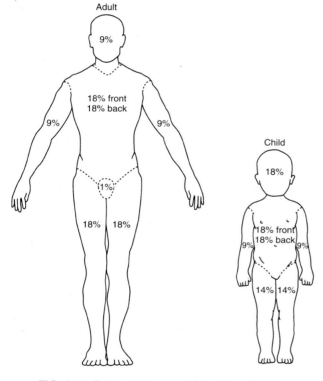

FIG. 34.1 Rule of nines, adult and pediatric.

c) Auscultation
  (1) Breath sounds: wheezing with inhalation injury
d) Palpation
  (1) Quality of peripheral pulses
  (2) Sensation surrounding and distal to burned tissue
2) Diagnostic data and procedures
  a) CBC with differential
  b) Serum chemistries including glucose, BUN, creatinine
  c) HbCO level
  d) Type and crossmatch/screen blood
  e) Urinalysis; pregnancy test in female patients of childbearing age
  f) ABGs
  g) Coagulation profile, creatine phosphokinase (CPK), urine myoglobin in patients with full-thickness burns
  h) Serum and urine toxicology: patients with loss of consciousness or in cardiac arrest
  i) Chest radiograph: any possibility of smoke inhalation
  j) Other radiographs as indicated for appraisal of associated injuries
  k) Fiberoptic bronchoscopy: suspected inhalation burn
2. Analysis: differential nursing diagnoses/collaborative problems
  a. Risk for ineffective airway clearance
  b. Risk for ineffective breathing pattern
  c. Risk for impaired gas exchange
  d. Risk for deficient fluid volume
  e. Risk for ineffective tissue perfusion
  f. Acute pain
  g. Impaired skin integrity
  h. Risk for infection
3. Planning and implementation/interventions
  a. Stop burning process
    1) Remove all of patient's clothing
    2) Remove all jewelry
  b. Maintain airway, breathing, circulation (see Chapters 1 and 32)
  c. Provide supplemental oxygen
    1) Rapid-sequence intubation (RSI) and ventilatory support in patients with inhalation injury, oropharyngeal burns
    2) High-flow oxygen
  d. Establish IV access for administration of crystalloid fluid/medications
    1) Fluid replacement formula
      a) Infuse warmed crystalloid solution, 0.9% normal saline or lactated Ringer
      b) Adults: 2–4 mL × body weight in kilograms × % TBSA burned

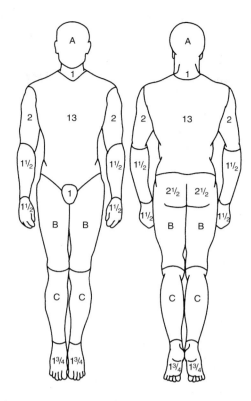

Relative percentage of body surface area affected by growth

Area	Age 0	1	5	10	15	Adult
A = ½ of head	9½	8½	6½	5½	4½	3½
B = ½ of one thigh	2¾	3¼	4	4½	4½	4¾
C = ½ of one leg	2½	2½	2¾	3	3¼	3½

FIG. 34.2 Lund and Browder chart.

c) Children: 3–4 mL × body weight in kilograms × % TBSA burned

d) Administer one-half of fluid in the first 8 hours from time of burn injury

e) Remaining fluid is administered over the next 16 hours

2) In infants and young children: infuse fluid with D_5W at a maintenance rate in addition to the resuscitation fluid noted earlier. Maintenance rate is calculated as

a) For the first 10 kg of body weight: 100 mL/kg over 24 hours

b) For the second 10 kg of body weight: 50 mL/kg over 24 hours

c) For each kilogram of body weight >20 kg: 20 mL/kg over 24 hours

e. Prepare for/assist with medical interventions

1) Advanced airway management

a) Nasal or oral intubation

b) Supraglottic airway (e.g., King, Combitube, laryngeal mask airway)

c) Surgical airway (e.g., cricothyrotomy)

2) Institute cardiac and pulse oximetry monitoring

a) Pulse oximetry: use with caution when inhalation suspected; reading may be falsely elevated by CO

3) Escharotomy for circumferential burns

4) Catheter placement and invasive monitoring (see Chapter 6)

5) Compartment pressure monitoring: extremity circumferential burns

6) Insert gastric tube and attach to suction

7) Insert indwelling urinary catheter

8) Apply cool, moistened dressings to burns <10% TBSA

a) Do not use ice

b) Do not use antibiotic or chemical solutions

c) Keep patient warm

9) Maintain normothermic body temperature by keeping patient covered with clean sheets/blankets

10) Assist with collection and maintenance of physical and forensic evidence as indicated (see Chapter 43)

Table 34.3

Burn Center Transfer Criteria

Percentage of Body Surface Area Involved	Specific Body Areas	Injury Types	Additional Considerations
Combination partial- and full-thickness burns of 10% or more: children less than 10 years old or adults more than 50 years old Combination partial- and full-thickness burns of greater than 20% in other age groups Full-thickness burns of greater than 5% in any age group	Partial- and full-thickness burns involving face, eyes, ears, hands, feet, genitalia, perineum, or major joints	Inhalation injury; high-voltage electricity; lightning; significant chemical burns	Any preexisting illness that may complicate recovery In combination with other traumatic injury Require special social, emotional services; require long-term rehabilitation; suspected child maltreatment Children initially treated in hospital without qualified personnel or necessary equipment

Modified from American College of Surgeons Committee on Trauma. (2004). *Advanced trauma life support for doctors* (7th ed.). Chicago, IL: American College of Surgeons.

11) Provide burn wound care: may not be initiated in emergency department for severely burned patient; consider procedural sedation
    a) Clean wound gently with chlorhexidine gluconate
    b) Assist with débridement of nonviable epidermis
    c) Treat blisters as prescribed by burn surgeon
12) Assist with possible hospital admission or transfer to burn center (Table 34.3)
  f. Administer pharmacologic therapy as prescribed
    1) RSI premedications; sedatives, analgesics, neuromuscular blocking agents
    2) Narcotics: administer pain medication before beginning treatment
    3) Procedural sedation medications as needed (see Chapter 9)
    4) Topical burn wound medications
       a) Silver sulfadiazine (Silvadene)
       b) Mafenide acetate (Sulfamylon)
       c) Water-based ointment to face, ears, neck, and perineum (e.g., bacitracin)
    5) Other pharmacological interventions as indicated
       a) Antibiotics, if evidence of infection
       b) Tetanus immunization
  g. Educate patient/significant others
    1) Wound care
    2) Signs and symptoms of infection
    3) Medications
    4) Nutrition
    5) When to return for follow-up care
4. Evaluation and ongoing monitoring
  a. Airway patency
  b. Level of consciousness
  c. Hemodynamic status
  d. Breath sounds and pulse oximetry
  e. Cardiac rate and rhythm
  f. Pain relief
  g. Intake and output
  h. Extremity edema

Bibliography

American Burn Association. (2015). Burn incidence and treatment in the United States. Retrieved from http://www.ameriburn.org.

Cooper MA (2014). Lightning injuries clinical presentation: History, physical examination. Retrieved from http://www.emedicine.medscape.com.

Harbin KR, Norris TE: Anesthetic management of patients with major burn injury, *American Association of Nurse Anesthetists Journal* 80(6):430–439, 2012.

Hospenthal DR, & Fonseca JA (2014). Burn wound infections medication. Retrieved from http://www.emedicine.medscape.com.

Jenkins JA (2014). Emergent management of thermal burns. Retrieved from http://www.emedicine.medscape.com.

Oliver RI (2014). Burn resuscitation and early management. Retrieved from http://www.emedicine.medscape.com.

Sheridan RL (2013). Initial evaluation and management of the burn patient. Retrieved from http://www.emedicine.medscape.com.

Snell JA, Loh NW, Mahambrey T, Shokrollahi K: Clinical review: The critical care management of the burn patient, *Critical Care* 17:241, 2013.

Toon MH, Maybauer DM, Arceneaux LL, Fraser JF, Meyer W, Runge A, Maybauer MO: Child abuse and burn injury, *Journal of Injury and Violence Resuscitation* 3(2):98–110, 2011.

Wilkes G (2014). Hydrofluric acid burns. Retrieved from http://www.emedicine.medscape.com.

CHAPTER 35
Neurologic Trauma

Anne C. Albers, RN, MSN, CPNP-PC

I. General Strategy

A. ASSESSMENT

1. Primary and secondary assessment /resuscitation (see
   Chapters 1 and 32)
2. Focused assessment
   a. Subjective data collection
      1) History of present injury/chief complaint
         a) Mechanism of injury (see Chapter 31)
         b) Level of consciousness
            (1) Loss of consciousness: time of occur-
                rence, duration, severity
            (2) Alterations: fluctuating, steady decline
         c) Mentation
            (1) Memory: recent and remote
            (2) Changes in cognitive ability (e.g., prob-
                lem solving)
         d) Alteration in communication
         e) Alteration in motor ability
         f) Alterations in sensation
         g) Alteration in vision
         h) Pain: PQRST (see Chapter 8)
         i) Headache
         j) Seizures
         k) Vomiting
         l) Effort to relieve symptoms
            (1) Home remedies
            (2) Alternative therapies
            (3) Medications
                (a) Prescription

                (b) OTC/herbal
      2) Past medical history
         a) Current or preexisting diseases/illness
         b) Previous trauma
         c) Fainting, dizziness
         d) Substance and/or alcohol use/abuse
         e) Last normal menstrual period: female
            patients of childbearing age
         f) Current medications
            (1) Prescription
                (a) Anticonvulsants
                (b) Anticoagulants, antiplatelet agents
            (2) OTC/herbal
                (a) Antiinflammatory agents, analgesics,
                    aspirin
         g) Allergies
         h) Immunization status
      3) Psychological, social, environmental risk
         factors
         a) Stress factors/personal habits
            (1) Possible/actual assault, abuse, or intimate
                partner violence situations (see Chapters
                3 and 40)
            (2) Use of protective equipment: seat belts/
                helmets
         b) Extremes of age
   b. Objective data collection
      1) General appearance
         a) Level of consciousness, behavior, affect
            (1) Wakefulness/response

(2) Glasgow Coma Scale (GCS) (see Appendix A)

(3) Awareness: ability to interact with and interpret the environment
  (a) Orientation: person, place, time, event
  (b) Memory: short and long term
  (c) Judgment and reasoning
  (d) Communication: verbalization and comprehension
  (e) Attention span

(4) Tremors/seizure

b) Vital signs
  (1) Blood pressure: include pulse pressure and mean arterial pressure (MAP)
  (2) Pulse: rate and rhythm
  (3) Respirations: rate, depth, pattern, muscles used
  (4) Evaluate for Cushing triad: seen as a *very* late sign with increased intracranial pressure (ICP) and signifies an extreme attempt to perfuse the brain
    (a) Increased systolic blood pressure, widened pulse pressure
    (b) Profound bradycardia
    (c) Abnormal respirations
  (5) Temperature: core preferred

c) Odors

d) Hygiene

e) Level of distress/discomfort

2) Inspection
  a) Surface trauma
  b) Bony symmetry
  c) Pupillary response
    (1) Size and equality
    (2) Reaction: direct and consensual
  d) Coordination/motor response
    (1) Movement
      (a) Normal: follows commands, localizes/purposeful
      (b) Abnormal: withdrawal from stimulus, posturing, rigid flexion (decortication), rigid extension (decerebration), no response
  e) Cranial nerves (Table 35.1)
  f) Cerebrospinal fluid leaks: otorrhea and/or rhinorrhea
  g) Meningeal signs

3) Palpation/percussion
  a) Muscle tone: increased, decreased
  b) Muscle strength
    (1) Symmetry: upper and lower extremity comparison as well as between right and left
    (2) Grading scale (Table 35.2)
  c) Reflexes
    (1) Deep tendon

(2) A positive Babinski reflex (upgoing or fanning toe response) is considered abnormal in patients older than 2 years of age

d) Sensory response
  (1) Pain perception: use the point of a sharp object, such as a pin
  (2) Touch and pressure: use the head of a pin
  (3) Proprioception: Is the toe up or down?

4) Brainstem integrity (Table 35.3): cervical spine and tympanic membrane must be intact before performing these tests

3. Diagnostic procedures
  a. Laboratory studies
    1) Complete blood count (CBC) with differential
    2) Serum chemistries including glucose, BUN, creatinine
    3) Serum and urine toxicology screen
    4) Coagulation profile
    5) Arterial blood gases (ABGs)
    6) Urinalysis; pregnancy test in female patients of childbearing age

Table 35.1

Cranial Nerve Assessment

Cranial Nerve	Assessment
I: Olfactory	Not routinely tested
II: Optic	Visual acuity: read or see printed material, count fingers, see light
III: Oculomotor	Extraocular movements (EOMs) Pupil assessment: constriction/dilation
IV: Trochlear	Extraocular movement
V: Trigeminal	Corneal reflex Facial sensation
VI: Abducens	Extraocular movements
VII: Facial	Speech musculature Taste (not routinely tested) Raise eyebrows, smile
VIII: Vestibulocochlear	Hearing
IX: Glossopharyngeal	Swallowing, gag reflex
X: Vagus	Speech musculature
XI: Spinal accessory	Shoulder shrug
XII: Hypoglossal	Speech musculature

Table 35.2

Muscle Strength Grading

0	No detectable movement
1	Flicker of muscle movement
2	Joint movement with gravity eliminated
3	Moves against gravity, not resistance
4	Moves weakly against resistance
5	Full strength against resistance

b. Imaging studies
   1) Spinal radiograph: all seven vertebrae of the cervical spine
   2) Chest radiograph
   3) Head, spinal computed tomography (CT) scan
   4) Magnetic resonance imaging (MRI)
c. Other
   1) 12- to 15-lead electrocardiogram (ECG)

B. ANALYSIS: DIFFERENTIAL NURSING DIAGNOSES/COLLABORATIVE PROBLEMS

1. Ineffective airway clearance
2. Impaired gas exchange
3. Decreased cardiac output
4. Ineffective tissue perfusion: cerebral
5. Pain
6. Anxiety/fear
7. Impaired verbal communication
8. Risk for injury
9. Deficient knowledge

C. PLANNING AND IMPLEMENTATION/INTERVENTIONS

1. Determine priorities of care
   a. Maintain airway, breathing, circulation (see Chapters 1 and 32)
   b. Provide supplemental oxygen as indicated
   c. Establish IV access for administration of crystalloid fluids/blood products/medications as needed
   d. Obtain and set up equipment and supplies
   e. Prepare for/assist with medical interventions
   f. Administer pharmacologic therapy as ordered
2. Relief of anxiety/apprehension

Table 35.3

Brainstem Integrity Tests

Test	Description
Doll's eyes (oculocephalic reflex)	Present when eyes move in the direction opposite in which the head is moving (found with an intact brainstem but damaged cerebral cortex)
Caloric testing (oculovestibular reflex)	Present when eyes move toward the ear stimulated with cold water (found with an intact brainstem but damaged cerebral hemispheres; with a brainstem lesion, caloric reflex will be absent or ocular movement will be disconjugate)
Apnea test	Allowing carbon dioxide to build up to stimulate the respiratory system in order to determine whether or not patients will breathe on their own
Brainstem reflexes	Pupils Gag Cough Corneal

3. Allow significant others to remain with patient if supportive
4. Educate patient/significant others

D. EVALUATION AND ONGOING MONITORING

1. Continuously monitor and treat as indicated
2. Monitor patient response/outcomes, and modify nursing care plan as appropriate
3. If positive outcomes are not demonstrated, reevaluate assessment and/or plan of care

E. DOCUMENTATION OF INTERVENTIONS AND PATIENT RESPONSE

F. AGE-RELATED CONSIDERATIONS

1. Pediatric
   a. Growth and development related
      1) Perinatal problems may affect neurologic status
      2) Babinski reflex is normal up to 2 years of age
      3) Fontanel closure: anterior fontanel closes between 9 and 18 months of age; posterior fontanel closes by 2 months of age
      4) Large occiput causes flexion of neck when in supine position
      5) Ligamentous and muscular laxity of spine predisposes child to spinal cord injury (SCI) without radiographic abnormality (SCIWORA)
   b. "Pearls"
      1) Assess tone by noting resting position of the infant
      2) Meningeal irritation may present as a sharp, shrill cry, with irritability and loss of appetite in infants
      3) Adaptation of the GCS for infants and children (see Appendix A)
      4) History that indicates possible abnormalities: delay or regression in developmental milestones, unusual behavior for age, clumsiness or progressive weakness, changes in learning or school performance
      5) Consider maltreatment in unusual situations
2. Geriatric
   a. Aging related
      1) Gradual slowing of the conscious and reflex reaction time
      2) Impairment of fine discrimination abilities
      3) Decreased corneal sensitivity, slower visual reflexes, decreased visual acuity and depth perception, decreased upward gaze, and smaller pupils
      4) Altered drug response and tolerance
      5) Cortical atrophy stretches subdural bridging veins and increases the risk of subdural hematoma (SDH)
      6) Consider abuse or neglect in unusual situations

b. "Pearls"
  1) Use stronger stimuli and allow more time to respond
  2) Use sharper contrasts with sensory stimuli

II. Specific Traumatic Neurologic Injuries

A. AUTONOMIC DYSREFLEXIA IN SPINAL CORD INJURY

Autonomic dysreflexia or hyperreflexia is a syndrome that sometimes occurs after the acute phase of SCI in patients with lesions at or above T6. It is more commonly seen in patients with complete SCIs than in those with incomplete spinal cord syndromes. It is seen only after recovery from spinal shock when reflex activity has returned. Noxious stimuli (e.g., bladder or intestinal distention, pressure on glans penis, renal calculi, cystitis, acute abdomen, pressure sores) may produce a sympathetic discharge that causes reflex vasoconstriction of blood vessels in the skin and splanchnic bed below the level of the injury. Vasoconstriction of splanchnic bed distends baroreceptors in the carotid sinus and aortic arch, and the body attempts to lower hypertension by superficial dilation of vessels above the level of the injury resulting in sweating and flushing.

1. Assessment
  a. Subjective data collection
    1) History of present injury/chief complaint
     a) Onset
     b) Current bowel/bladder program
     c) Visual changes (blurred vision or spots in visual fields)
     d) Headache
     e) Anxiety
    2) Past medical history
     a) Current or preexisting diseases/illness
      (1) SCI at or above T6
     b) Medications
     c) Allergies
  b. Objective data collection
    1) Physical examination
     a) General appearance
      (1) Severe hypertension
      (2) Bradycardia
      (3) Severe distress/discomfort, critically ill
     b) Inspection
      (1) Vasomotor changes: flushed head and neck, pale lower extremities
      (2) Nasal congestion: common
      (3) Pupil dilation
      (4) Sweating above level of lesion
      (5) Goose bumps above or below level of lesions
     c) Palpation
      (1) Bladder distention
2. Analysis: differential nursing diagnoses/collaborative problems

  a. Ineffective tissue perfusion
  b. Deficient knowledge
3. Planning and implementation/interventions
  a. Elevate head of bed
  b. Establish IV access for administration of crystalloid fluids/medications as needed
  c. Prepare for/assist with medical interventions
    1) Relieve trigger mechanism
     a) Check patency of urinary drainage system or insert urinary catheter
     b) Check for fecal impaction, lubricate rectum, or use local anesthetic
     c) Eliminate pressure from skin
    2) Institute cardiac and pulse oximetry monitoring
    3) Assist with hospital admission
  d. Administer pharmacologic therapy as ordered
    1) Ganglionic blocking agents for hypertension
4. Evaluation and ongoing monitoring
  a. Hemodynamic status
  b. Urinary output, bowel elimination
  c. Cardiac rate and rhythm
  d. Breath sounds and pulse oximetry

B. CONCUSSION—MILD TRAUMATIC BRAIN INJURY

A trauma-induced transient impairment of mental status with or without loss of consciousness, concussion is usually caused by a strong rapid rotational acceleration of the brain. It can be caused by a direct blow to the head or elsewhere on the body with force transmitted to the head. The trauma causes complex biomechanical forces that affect the brain. It results in rapid short-lived neurologic impairment resulting in a clinical symptom but may have no structural abnormality. The concussion may be classified as mild, moderate, or severe on the clinical symptoms. If the concussion occurred from participation in contact sports, the patient should not be allowed to return to the sport until all symptoms such as headache, dizziness, amnesia, blunted affect, and delayed verbal or ocular responses have completely disappeared. Postconcussion syndrome is present when symptoms remain for a prolonged period of time. Concussion severity does not predict which patients will develop this syndrome. Other, more serious conditions that must be considered following minor traumatic brain injury (TBI) include SDH, subarachnoid bleeding, cerebral contusion, or parenchymal injury.

1. Assessment
  a. Subjective data collection
    1) History of present injury/chief complaint
     a) Mechanism of injury (see Chapter 31)
     b) Level of consciousness change if any
     c) Duration of loss of consciousness
     d) Changes in neurologic status since the event
      (1) Dizziness
      (2) Headache
      (3) Nausea or vomiting

(4) Memory or recall, concentration, or feeling foggy

(5) Unsteadiness of gait

2) Past medical history

    a) Current or preexisting diseases/illnesses

       (1) Neurologic disease or injury

    b) Recent fall or trauma

    c) Medications

    d) Allergies

b. Objective data collection

  1) Physical examination

    a) General appearance

       (1) Level of consciousness, behavior, affect

          (a) Memory changes

             (i) Retrograde or antegrade amnesia

             (ii) Ability to learn new information is present despite amnesia of the event

          (b) Impaired attention, vacant stare

       (2) Mild to moderate distress/discomfort

    b) Inspection

       (1) Incoordination—unsteady gait or balance

       (2) Slow speech

  2) Diagnostic procedures

    a) Clinical presentation and history are frequently diagnostic

    b) Head CT scan if

       (1) Focal neurologic findings

       (2) GCS score <15

       (3) Presence of seizures

    c) Head MRI if

       (1) Persistent symptoms: for more than 7 days

       (2) Late changes in neurologic findings

2. Analysis: differential nursing diagnoses/collaborative problems

  a. Risk for injury

  b. Deficient knowledge

3. Planning and implementation/interventions

  a. Maintain bed rest and raise side rails

  b. Educate patient/significant others

    1) Postconcussion syndrome

      a) Clinical presentation

        (1) Headache

        (2) Dizziness (usually positional)

        (3) Tinnitus

        (4) Diplopia (usually transient)

        (5) Inability to concentrate

        (6) Memory disturbance

        (7) Personality changes

        (8) Decreased energy level

        (9) Changes in sleep pattern

        (10) Changes in sense of taste/smell

      b) Duration: days to years

      c) Social/occupational consequences

        (1) Difficulty with performance in school/work

        (2) Behavioral/emotional changes

    2) Provide community resources available for help (e.g., support groups)

    3) Avoid medications that may worsen signs and symptoms

4. Evaluation and ongoing monitoring

  a. Level of functional return

  b. Changes in headache intensity, amnesia of events, GCS, resolution of symptoms

C. INCREASED INTRACRANIAL PRESSURE

Increased intracranial pressure (ICP) is a reflection of three relatively fixed volumes: (1) brain, (2) cerebrospinal fluid, and (3) blood. As the level of any one of these increases, the levels of the other two components must decrease to provide compensation and keep the ICP within normal limits, despite increasing pathologic processes. As a result, in early stages, the brain will demonstrate only slight increases in pressure despite a wide range of volume expansion. However, as the disorder progresses, compensatory mechanisms are depleted, resulting in a rapid increase in ICP even though there may only be a small concurrent increase in volume. This produces a shift of the brain tissue with eventual herniation of the brain through the tentorial opening that results in pressure on the brainstem and produces a clinical picture of altered level of consciousness as well as pupillary, motor, and vital sign changes. As ICP rises, cerebral perfusion pressure (CPP) decreases, leading to cerebral ischemia and the potential for hypoxia with secondary insult. Cerebral ischemia can lead to increased concentrations of carbon dioxide and decreased concentrations of oxygen in cerebral vessels. Carbon dioxide causes vasodilation of blood vessels that further contributes to the problem. Underlying causes of an increase in ICP include conditions that (1) increase brain volume, (2) increase cerebral blood volume, or (3) increase cerebrospinal fluid volume. CPP is the blood pressure gradient needed to perfuse the brain and is normally in the range of 70–100 mm Hg. It reflects a balance between the incoming blood (MAP) and the opposing pressure existing in the brain (ICP) and is determined by the following equation: MAP – ICP = CPP. Either a decrease in the MAP or an increase in the ICP can lead to insufficient CPP (Table 35.4).

1. Assessment

  a. Subjective data collection

    1) History of present injury/chief complaint

      a) Chronologic sequence of onset and development of neurologic symptoms

      b) Consciousness

        (1) Alterations in consciousness

        (2) Loss of consciousness

      c) Alterations in mentation

      d) Alterations in personality

      e) Alterations in communication

      f) Alterations in motor ability

        (1) Weakness (paresis)

        (2) Paralysis (plegia)

Table 35.4

Insufficient Cerebral Perfusion Pressure

Mean Arterial Pressure	Intracranial Pressure	Cerebral Perfusion Pressure
Unchanged	Increased (↑ in intracranial volume)	Insufficient to perfuse brain
Decreased (hypovolemic or distributive shock)	Unchanged	Insufficient to perfuse brain

     g) Alterations in sensation
     h) Alterations in vision
     i) Injury or fall
       (1) Mechanism (see Chapter 31)
       (2) Time elapsed since occurrence
       (3) Treatment received prior to arrival
       (4) Changes in clinical status
     j) Pain (see Chapter 8)
     k) Headache
     l) Seizures
     m) Vomiting (especially in children)
  2) Past medical history
     a) Current or preexisting diseases/illness
       (1) Neurologic diseases
     b) Trauma
     c) Substance and/or alcohol use/abuse
     d) Medications
     e) Allergies
 b. Objective data collection
  1) Physical examination
     a) General appearance
       (1) Early increased ICP findings
         (a) Level of consciousness, behavior, affect: anxiety, restlessness, agitation, slower response to stimulation required to achieve the same response, loss of finer detail in orientation response, speech less distinct, memory alterations, sudden quietness in a very restless patient
         (b) Pupils: sluggish response to light; usually unilateral and ipsilateral to the lesion
         (c) Motor function: usually contralateral to the lesion, pronator drift, loss of one or more grades on the strength scale, increased tone
         (d) Vital signs: occasionally tachycardic, occasionally hypertensive swings
       (2) Late increased ICP findings (herniation)
         (a) Level of consciousness alteration: arousable only with deep pain or unarousable

         (b) Pupils: fixed and/or dilated
         (c) Motor response to stimuli: dense hemiparesis, abnormal flexion/extension, no response
         (d) Vital signs (Cushing response): elevated systolic blood pressure, profound bradycardia, abnormal respirations, widening pulse pressure
       (3) Moderate to severe distress/discomfort, critically ill with variations in any or all systems
  2) Diagnostic procedures
     a) CBC with differential
     b) Serum chemistries including glucose, BUN, creatinine
     c) Coagulation profile
     d) ABGs, specifically partial arterial pressure of carbon dioxide ($PaCO_2$)
     e) Urinalysis; pregnancy test in female patients of childbearing age
     f) Head CT scan or MRI
2. Analysis: differential nursing diagnoses/collaborative problems
 a. Ineffective tissue perfusion: cerebral
 b. Impaired gas exchange
 c. Disturbed sensory perception
 d. Risk for ineffective airway clearance
3. Planning and implementation/interventions
 a. Maintain airway, breathing, circulation (see Chapters 1 and 32)
 b. Provide supplemental oxygen as indicated
  1) Rapid sequence intubation (RSI) and ventilatory support in patients with airway compromise; hyperventilation is controversial because it constricts cerebral arteries and thereby decreases cerebral blood flow
  2) High-flow oxygen
 c. Establish IV access for administration of crystalloid fluids/medications as needed
  1) Cautious administration of IV solutions (depending on cause of decreased blood pressure)
 d. Prepare for/assist with medical interventions
  1) Advanced airway management
     a) Nasal or oral intubation
     b) Supraglottic airway (e.g., King, Combitube, laryngeal mask airway)
     c) Surgical airway (e.g., cricothyrotomy)
  2) Assist with medical decompression of cranial vault to decrease the ICP
     a) Increase venous outflow through elevation of head of bed, midline head and neck positioning, and avoidance of extreme hip flexion
  3) Decrease metabolic demands of the brain
     a) Maintaining normothermia
     b) Controlling seizures if present
  4) Institute cardiac and pulse oximetry monitoring

5) Catheter placement and monitoring of ICP recommended if GCS score <8
6) Insert gastric tube and attach to intermittent suction
7) Insert indwelling urinary catheter
8) Assist with collection and maintenance of physical and forensic evidence as indicated (see Chapter 43)
9) Assist with hospital admission or transfer to an institution providing a higher level of care
   e. Administer pharmacologic therapy as ordered
   1) RSI premedications: sedatives, analgesics, neuromuscular blocking agents
   2) Diuretics to decrease water content in the brain
   3) Vasopressor agents to maintain blood pressure
   4) Continued neuromuscular blockade with sedation and analgesia to control agitation and pain
   5) Lidocaine to decrease response to suctioning
   6) Anticonvulsants
   7) Antiinflammatory agents (steroids)
4. Evaluation and ongoing monitoring
   a. Airway patency
   b. Level of consciousness, neurologic changes; ICP readings
   c. Hemodynamic status: maintain adequate CPP
   d. Breath sounds and pulse oximetry
   e. Cardiac rate and rhythm
   f. Maintain normoglycemia
   g. Intake and output

D. SKULL FRACTURES

The most common area of skull fracture is the parietal bone. The most common type of fracture is the linear fracture. A temporal bone fracture has the potential for sequelae such as extraaxial bleeding. A depressed skull fracture damages the underlying cerebral tissue by compression or laceration. Retained bony fragments may lacerate the dura or set up a focus for seizures. Basilar skull fractures occur in any of the five bones of the skull base but are most common in the temporal bone. The overall complications of skull fractures include infections, hematoma, cerebrospinal fluid leaks, loss of smell (anosmia), loss of hearing, seizures, and pneumocephalus. In children, maltreatment must be considered as an underlying cause of injury.

1. Assessment
   a. Subjective data collection
   1) History of present injury/chief complaint
      a) Recent injury
      b) Time elapsed from event to present
      c) Complaint of tasting something sweet or salty in the back of the throat because of cerebrospinal fluid leakage
      d) Complaint of "postnasal drip"
      e) Vertigo
      f) Hearing impairment
   2) Past medical history
      a) Current or preexisting diseases/illness
         (1) Malignant disease
      b) Medications
      c) Allergies
   b. Objective data collection
   1) Physical examination
      a) General appearance
         (1) Level of consciousness, behavior, affect: alert, lethargic, comatose
         (2) Mild to severe distress/discomfort
      b) Inspection
         (1) Surface trauma (scalp lacerations may lead to significant blood loss, especially in children)
         (2) Altered pupillary or motor responses
         (3) Cerebrospinal fluid leak (otorrhea or rhinorrhea)
         (4) Periorbital ecchymosis (raccoon eyes)
         (5) Mastoid bruising (Battle sign) usually seen after 24 hours
         (6) Hemotympanum
   2) Diagnostic procedures
      a) Possible ABGs
      b) Possible urinalysis; pregnancy test in female patients of childbearing age
      c) Head CT scan (if underlying injury suspected)
      d) Test for glucose in the watery nasal discharge
      e) Cerebrospinal fluid "halo" test with otorrhea/rhinorrhea
2. Analysis: differential nursing diagnoses/collaborative problems
   a. Risk for ineffective airway clearance
   b. Risk for infection
   c. Risk for ineffective tissue perfusion: cerebral
3. Planning and implementation/interventions
   a. Maintain airway, breathing, circulation (see Chapters 1 and 32)
   b. Provide supplemental oxygen as indicated
   1) RSI and ventilatory support in patients with airway compromise; avoid nasal intubation if basilar skull fracture present or suspected
   2) High-flow oxygen
   c. Establish IV access for administration of crystalloid fluids/medications
   d. Prepare for/assist with medical interventions
   1) Advanced airway management
      a) Oral intubation
      b) Supraglottic airway (e.g., King, Combitube, laryngeal mask airway)
      c) Surgical airway (e.g., cricothyrotomy)
   2) Instruct patient to avoid nose blowing or sneezing if basilar skull fracture present
   3) Provide drip pads if cerebrospinal fluid rhinorrhea present

Table 35.5

Classification of Spinal Cord Injuries

		Clinical Presentation of Symptoms (below the level of the injury)
Complete		Transection of the cord with no preservation of sensorimotor function
Incomplete	Central cord syndrome	Motor and sensory deficits more pronounced in the upper extremities than in the lower extremities
	Anterior cord syndrome	Loss of motor function
		Loss of pain and temperature perception
		Vibration, light touch, and position perception intact
	Brown-Séquard syndrome	Ipsilateral paralysis or paresis
		Ipsilateral loss of pressure, touch, and vibration perception
		Contralateral loss of pain and temperature perception

4) Cleanse the outer ear if otorrhea present (*never* put anything in the ear)
5) Institute cardiac and pulse oximetry monitoring
6) Insert gastric tube attached to suction as indicated
   a) Avoid nasogastric tube if basilar skull fracture present: insert orogastric tube
7) Insert indwelling urinary catheter as indicated
8) Assist with collection and maintenance of physical and forensic evidence as indicated (see Chapter 44)
9) Assist with possible hospital admission or transfer to an institution providing a higher level of care: possible surgical intervention (depressed skull fracture, especially with a dural tear)

e. Administer pharmacologic therapy as ordered
   1) RSI medications: sedatives, analgesics, neuromuscular blocking agents
   2) Anticonvulsants
   3) Antibiotics

4. Evaluation and ongoing monitoring
   a. Airway patency
   b. Level of consciousness
   c. Hemodynamic status
   d. Breath sounds and pulse oximetry
   e. Cardiac rate and rhythm
   f. Intake and output

E. SPINAL CORD INJURIES

Spinal cord injuries (SCIs) involve bruising or tearing of spinal cord substance from penetrating trauma or a fracture/dislocation of the spinal column. SCIs almost always are the result of trauma (vehicular, falls, personal violence) and are caused by a variety of mechanisms, including axial loading, hyperflexion, and hyperextension. Damage to the spinal cord occurs from extrinsic (bony and soft tissue injury) or intrinsic (hemorrhage, edema, hypoxia, or biochemical changes) sources. SCIs may be classified as complete or incomplete (Table 35.5) and can result in spinal or neurogenic shock (Table 35.6).

Respiratory complications become evident when the diaphragm, innervated by the phrenic nerve, which exits from

Table 35.6

Spinal/Neurogenic Shock

Spinal Shock	Neurogenic Shock
Loss of all neurologic function below the level of injury	Loss of sympathetic function below the level of injury: unopposed vagal (parasympathetic) influence causes
Flaccid paralysis	
Loss of spinal reflexes	Vasodilation
Loss of sensation	Pooling of blood in extremities
Loss of autonomic function	Hypotension
Spinal reflexes return in 4–6 wk	Bradycardia

the cervical cord at the level of C3, C4, and C5, is damaged. This results in a compromised ability to breathe. Even with the phrenic nerve intact, a low cervical spine injury causes loss of innervation of the intercostal muscles (T1–T12) that allow one to take a deep breath, cough, and sigh.

1. Assessment
   a. Subjective data collection
      1) History of present injury/chief complaint
         a) Mechanism of injury (see Chapter 31)
         b) Neurologic ability at the scene
         c) Stabilization provided at the scene
      2) Past medical history
         a) Current or preexisting diseases/illness
         b) Medications
         c) Allergies
   b. Objective data collection
      1) Physical examination
         a) General appearance
            (1) Respiratory ability
               (a) Muscles used: diaphragm, intercostals, accessory
               (b) Depth of respiration: shallow, deep
            (2) Possible hypotension, bradycardia
            (3) Moderate to severe distress/discomfort
         b) Inspection
            (1) Surface trauma

(2) Priapism

c) Auscultation

(1) Bowel sounds: decreased, ileus

d) Palpation

(1) Guarding, pain, or tenderness over the spine

(2) Paraparesis/paraplegia or quadriparesis/quadriplegia

(3) Rectal tone

(4) Sensory perception

(a) Examine distal to proximal

(b) Response to pain: use the point of a pin

(c) Response to pressure: use the head of a pin

(d) Proprioception: Is the toe up or down?

(e) Atonic bladder

e) Neurogenic shock

(1) Hypotension: blood pressure usually <90 mm Hg systolic

(2) Profound bradycardia

(3) Warm, dry skin (resulting from loss of sympathetic response)

(4) Decreased reflexes or areflexia

(5) Loss of motor ability and sensation below level of the lesion

(6) Poikilothermy

2) Diagnostic procedures

a) CBC with differential

b) Serum chemistries including glucose, BUN, creatinine

c) Coagulation profile

d) Type and screen/crossmatch

e) Urinalysis; pregnancy test in female patients of childbearing age

f) Spinal radiograph (lateral and oblique)

g) Odontoid view radiograph

h) Head, spine CT scan or MRI

2. Analysis: differential nursing diagnoses/collaborative problems

a. Ineffective airway clearance

b. Impaired gas exchange

c. Decreased cardiac

d. Risk for injury

e. Ineffective individual or family coping

3. Planning and implementation/interventions

a. Maintain airway, breathing, circulation (see Chapters 1 and 32)

1) Prevent head and neck manipulation during the establishment of an airway

2) Stabilize cervical spine, regardless of examination findings, until cervical films are taken and read as negative (C1–C7)

b. Provide supplemental oxygen

1) RSI and ventilatory support in obtunded patients or patients with respiratory fatigue

2) High-flow oxygen

c. Establish IV access for administration of crystalloid fluids/medications

d. Prepare for/assist with medical interventions

1) Advanced airway management

a) Nasal or oral intubation

b) Supraglottic airway (e.g., King, Combitube, laryngeal mask airway)

c) Surgical airway (e.g., cricothyrotomy)

2) Enhance venous return to the heart

a) Elastic (Ace) wrap, antiembolic hose

b) Elevate lower extremities

3) Remove patient from backboard as soon as possible to prevent skin breakdown

4) Normalize room temperature to reduce severity of poikilothermy

5) Prepare for and assist with realignment of the spine (tong insertion)

6) Institute cardiac and pulse oximetry monitoring

7) Insert gastric tube and attach to suction

8) Insert indwelling urinary catheter

9) Assist with collection and maintenance of physical and forensic evidence as indicated (see Chapter 44)

10) Assist with hospital admission or transport to an SCI center, if applicable

e. Administer pharmacologic therapy as ordered

1) RSI medications: sedatives, analgesics, neuromuscular blocking agents

2) Atropine to elevate heart rate if symptomatic bradycardia occurs

3) Medications to preserve, protect, and possibly restore remaining spinal cord: high-dose steroids (controversial) over a 24- to 48-hour period begun within 8 hours after the event

4. Evaluation and ongoing monitoring

a. Airway patency

b. Hemodynamic status

c. Changes in movement, sensation; documentation on a dermatome flowsheet is extremely important in patients with SCI

d. Breath sounds and pulse oximetry

e. Cardiac rate and rhythm

f. Intake and output

F. TRAUMATIC BRAIN INJURY: CEREBRAL CONTUSION

A cerebral contusion is an actual brain tissue. It is characterized by petechial hemorrhages and extravasation of fluid from the vessels. This results in focal ischemia and edema with the potential for infarction, necrosis, and/or increased ICP. Trauma, acceleration or deceleration, high-velocity blows, or the rotation of the brain following such a blow can cause cerebral contusions. Frequently, the brain has a rebound of its contents following such a blow that results in an injury opposite the point of impact (contre-coup injury). Cerebral contusions are often associated with traumatic subarachnoid hemorrhage (tSAH). Gliding contusions result in tearing and stretching of veins, the arachnoid membrane, and the cerebrum and frequently are accompanied by diffuse axonal injuries. Contusions may also progress over time. The clinical presentation depends on the area involved and the extent of the damage.

1. Assessment
   a. Subjective data collection
      1) History of present injury/chief complaint
         a) Mechanism of injury (see Chapter 31)
         b) Changes in neurologic status since the event
      2) Past medical history
         a) Current or preexisting diseases/illness
            (1) Neurologic diseases or injury
         b) Substance and/or alcohol use/abuse
         c) Medications
         d) Allergies
   b. Objective data collection
      1) Physical examination
         a) General appearance
            (1) Level of consciousness, behavior, affect: altered for more than several hours
            (2) Brainstem contusion
               (a) Loss of brainstem reflexes
               (b) Unconsciousness
               (c) Posturing
            (3) Moderate to severe distress/discomfort
         b) Inspection
            (1) Presence of surface trauma (occasional)
      2) Diagnostic procedures
         a) CBC with differential
         b) Serum chemistries including glucose, BUN, creatinine
         c) Coagulation profile
         d) ABGs
         e) Serum and urine toxicology screen
         f) Urinalysis; pregnancy test in female patients of childbearing age
         g) Head CT scan
            (1) May not be evident on initial CT scan
            (2) Becomes obvious on follow-up scans
         h) Head MRI
            (1) Present from onset of injury
            (2) Sensitive to hyperacute hemorrhagic contusions
2. Analysis: differential nursing diagnoses/collaborative problems
   a. Ineffective tissue perfusion: cerebral
   b. Risk for ineffective airway clearance
3. Planning and implementation/interventions
   a. Maintain airway, breathing, circulation (see Chapters 1 and 32)
   b. Provide supplemental oxygen as indicated

   1) RSI and ventilatory support in patients with airway compromise; hyperventilation is controversial because it constricts cerebral arteries and thereby decreases cerebral blood flow
   2) High-flow oxygen
   c. Establish IV access for administration of crystalloid fluids/medications as needed
      1) Cautious administration of IV fluid
   d. Prepare for/assist with medical interventions
      1) Advanced airway management
         a) Nasal or oral intubation
         b) Supraglottic airway (e.g., King, Combitube, laryngeal mask airway)
         c) Surgical airway (e.g., cricothyrotomy)
      2) Assist with medical decompression of cranial vault to decrease the ICP
         a) Increase venous outflow through elevation of head of bed, midline head and neck positioning, and avoidance of extreme hip flexion
      3) Decrease metabolic demands of the brain by
         a) Maintaining normothermia
         b) Preventing seizures
      4) Institute cardiac and pulse oximetry monitoring
      5) Catheter placement and monitoring of ICP recommended if GCS score <8
      6) Insert gastric tube and attach to suction
      7) Insert indwelling urinary catheter
      8) Assist with collection and maintenance of physical and forensic evidence as indicated (see Chapter 43)
      9) Assist with hospital admission or transfer to an institution providing a higher level of care
   e. Administer pharmacologic therapy as ordered
      1) RSI medications: sedatives, analgesics, neuromuscular blocking agents
      2) Diuretics to decrease water content in brain
4. Evaluation and ongoing monitoring
   a. Airway patency
   b. Level of consciousness changes; ICP readings
   c. Hemodynamic status
   d. Cardiac rate and rhythm
   e. Breath sounds and pulse oximetry
   f. Intake and output

G. TRAUMATIC BRAIN INJURY: DIFFUSE AXONAL INJURY (MODERATE TO SEVERE)

This type of injury results from the widespread disruption of neurologic function without any focal lesions noted most likely due to shearing. It is characterized by microscopic damage to axons, diffuse white matter degeneration, global neurologic dysfunction, and diffuse cerebral swelling. The outcome of this injury is a gray-white matter junction. Axonal injury may involve different areas of the brain and develop over the course of hours to days. The patient may not have elevated ICP.

1. Assessment
    a. Subjective data collection
        1) History of present injury /chief complaint
            a) Mechanism of injury (see Chapter 31)
            b) Onset of loss of consciousness
            c) Duration of loss of consciousness
        2) Past medical history
            a) Current or preexisting diseases/illness
                (1) Neurologic disease or injury
            b) Substance and/or alcohol use/abuse
            c) Medications
            d) Allergies
    b. Objective data collection
        1) Physical examination
            a) General appearance
                (1) Level of consciousness, behavior, affect: immediate loss of consciousness lasts days to months
                (2) Brainstem dysfunction
                    (a) Rigid flexion (decorticate posturing) or rigid extension (decerebrate posturing)
                    (b) Loss of brainstem reflexes (e.g., cough, gag)
                    (c) Hypertension
                    (d) Hyperthermia
                    (e) Excessive sweating
                (3) Moderate to severe distress/discomfort
        2) Diagnostic procedures
            a) CBC with differential
            b) Serum chemistries including glucose, BUN, creatinine
            c) Coagulation profile
            d) ABGs
            e) Urinalysis; pregnancy test in female patients of childbearing age
            f) Head CT scan
                (1) May be normal at presentation
                (2) Edema and atrophy are late findings
            g) Head MRI: more sensitive for subtle soft tissue abnormalities
2. Analysis: differential nursing diagnoses/collaborative problems
    a. Ineffective tissue perfusion: cerebral
    b. Risk for ineffective airway clearance
    c. Risk for injury
3. Planning and implementation/interventions
    a. Maintain airway, breathing, circulation (see Chapters 1 and 32)
    b. Provide supplemental oxygen as indicated
        1) RSI and ventilatory support in patients with airway compromise; hyperventilation is controversial because it constricts cerebral

arteries and thereby decreases cerebral blood flow
        2) High-flow oxygen
    c. Establish IV access for administration of crystalloid fluids/medications as needed.
    d. Prepare for/assist with medical interventions
        1) Advanced airway management
            a) Nasal or oral intubation
            b) Supraglottic airway (e.g., King, Combitube, laryngeal mask airway)
            c) Surgical airway (e.g., cricothyrotomy)
        2) Assist with medical decompression of cranial vault to decrease the ICP
            a) Increase venous outflow through elevation of head of bed, midline head and neck positioning, and avoidance of extreme hip flexion
        3) Decrease metabolic demands of the brain by
            a) Maintaining normothermia
            b) Preventing seizures
        4) Institute cardiac and pulse oximetry monitoring
        5) Catheter placement and monitoring of ICP recommended if GCS <8
        6) Insert gastric tube and attach to suction
        7) Insert indwelling urinary catheter
        8) Assist with collection and maintenance of physical and forensic evidence as indicated (see Chapter 44)
        9) Assist with hospital admission or transfer to an institution providing a higher level of care
    e. Administer pharmacologic therapy as ordered
        1) RSI premedication: sedatives, analgesics, neuromuscular blocking agents
        2) Antipyretics
        3) Diuretics to decrease water content in brain
4. Evaluation and ongoing monitoring
    a. Airway patency
    b. Level of consciousness changes; ICP readings
    c. Hemodynamic status
    d. Breath sounds and pulse oximetry
    e. Cardiac rate and rhythm
    f. Intake and output

H. TRAUMATIC BRAIN INJURY: EPIDURAL HEMATOMA

An epidural hematoma is a collection of blood between the skull and dura. It is usually the result of a laceration of the middle meningeal artery associated with a temporal skull fracture; the fracture crosses the middle meningeal arterial groove in the temporal bone, lacerates the artery, and allows bleeding into the epidural space. Because the arterial bleed is under high pressure, it does not tamponade but instead rapidly progresses to become a mass lesion causing increased ICP, brain shift, and uncal herniation (a forcing of the medial portion of the temporal lobe, the uncus, to herniate down through the tentorial opening). The mortality for epidural hematomas is approximately 50%. Other associated lesions include cerebral contusions, SDHs, and intracerebral hematomas.

1. Assessment
   a. Subjective data collection
      1) History of present injury/chief complaint
         a) Mechanism of injury (see Chapter 31)
         b) Pattern of unconsciousness following injury (occurs approximately 30% of the time)
            (1) Initial unconsciousness
            (2) Lucid interval: 5 minutes to 6 hours
            (3) Rapid unconsciousness
      2) Past medical history
         a) Current or preexisting diseases/illness
         b) Previous head injury
         c) Medications
         d) Allergies
   b. Objective data collection
      1) Physical examination
         a) General appearance
            (1) Level of consciousness, behavior, affect: comatose
            (2) Vital signs: Cushing response (late)
            (3) Severe level of distress/discomfort, critically ill
         b) Inspection
            (1) Pupils: unilateral, fixed, and/or dilated
            (2) Motor: contralateral paresis or paralysis progressing to posturing
      2) Diagnostic procedures
         a) CBC with differential
         b) Serum chemistries including glucose, BUN, creatinine
         c) Coagulation profile including platelet count
         d) Urinalysis; pregnancy test in female patients of childbearing age
         e) Head CT scan
            (1) Most accurate and sensitive for diagnosis
2. Analysis: differential nursing diagnoses/collaborative problems
   a. Impaired gas exchange
   b. Ineffective tissue perfusion: cerebral
   c. Risk for ineffective airway clearance
3. Planning and implementation/interventions
   a. Maintain airway, breathing, circulation (see Chapters 1 and 32)
   b. Provide supplemental oxygen
      1) RSI and ventilatory support in patients with airway compromise; hyperventilation is controversial because it constricts cerebral arteries and thereby decreases cerebral blood flow
      2) High-flow oxygen
   c. Establish IV access for administration of crystalloid fluids/medications
   d. Prepare for/assist with medical interventions
      1) Advanced airway management
         a) Nasal or oral intubation
         b) Supraglottic airway (e.g., King, Combitube, laryngeal mask airway)
         c) Surgical airway (e.g., cricothyrotomy)
      2) Assist with medical decompression of cranial vault to decrease the ICP
         a) Increase venous outflow through elevation of head of bed, midline head and neck positioning, and avoidance of extreme hip flexion
      3) Decrease metabolic demands of the brain by
         a) Maintaining normothermia
         b) Preventing seizures
      4) Institute cardiac and pulse oximetry monitoring
      5) Insert gastric tube and attach to suction
      6) Insert indwelling urinary catheter
      7) Assist with collection and maintenance of physical and forensic evidence as indicated (see Chapter 44)
      8) Assist with hospital admission or transfer to an institution providing a higher level of care: emergency surgery for clot evacuation
4. Evaluation and ongoing monitoring
   a. Airway clearance
   b. Level of consciousness changes
   c. Hemodynamic status
   d. Breath sounds and pulse oximetry
   e. Cardiac rate and rhythm
   f. Intake and output

I. TRAUMATIC BRAIN INJURY: PENETRATING HEAD INJURY

Penetrating head injury occurs when any object enters the cranial vault forcibly. The force damages scalp, skull, meninges, cerebral blood vessels, and cerebral parenchyma. The most common cause of high-velocity penetrating head trauma is gunshot wounds (GSWs). Causes of lower-velocity injuries include stab injuries and impaled objects. In GSWs, the damage results not only from the bullet itself but also from a major transfer of energy from the bullet to the brain. The passage of the bullet through the brain tissue creates a cavity three to four times the actual diameter of the bullet. Penetrating trauma is associated with an overall mortality rate >60%. The GCS score is predictive of the outcome of GSWs. Patients with penetrating head wounds are at risk for developing the following complications: disseminated intravascular coagulopathy, increased ICP, associated intracranial hematomas, seizures, infection, and hydrocephalus.

1. Assessment
   a. Subjective data collection
      1) History of present injury/chief complaint
         a) Mechanism of injury (see Chapter 31)
            (1) High- or low-velocity projectile or agent
            (2) Character of GSW
               (a) Gauge

(b) Bullet type

(c) Distance

b) Trends in neurologic status

2) Past medical history

a) Current or preexisting diseases/illness

(1) Neurologic disease or injury

b) Substance and/or alcohol use/abuse

c) Medications

(1) Anticoagulants or antiplatelet agents

d) Allergies

e) Immunization status

b. Objective data collection

1) Physical examination

a) General appearance

(1) Level of consciousness, behavior, affect: alert to comatose

(2) Moderate to severe distress/discomfort

b) Inspection

(1) Open wounds

(2) Pupil reaction: brisk to nonreactive

(3) Focal neurologic findings

2) Diagnostic procedures

a) Head CT scan

b) Angiography

c) Head MRI: may be contraindicated if wounding agent is metallic

2. Analysis: differential nursing diagnoses/collaborative problems

a. Ineffective tissue perfusion: cerebral

b. Risk for infection

c. Risk for ineffective airway clearance

3. Planning and implementation/interventions

a. Maintain airway, breathing, circulation (see Chapters 1 and 32)

b. Provide supplemental oxygen

1) RSI and ventilatory support in patients with airway compromise or decreasing level of consciousness; hyperventilation is controversial because it constricts cerebral arteries and thereby decreases cerebral blood flow

2) High-flow oxygen

c. Establish IV access to administer crystalloid fluid/medications/blood products

d. Prepare for/assist with medical interventions

1) Advanced airway management

a) Nasal or oral intubation

b) Supraglottic airway (e.g., King, Combitube, laryngeal mask airway)

c) Surgical airway (e.g., cricothyrotomy)

2) Assist with medical decompression of cranial vault to decrease the ICP

a) Increase venous outflow through elevation of head of bed, midline head and neck positioning, and avoidance of extreme hip flexion

3) Stabilize impaled objects until definitive treatment is available

4) Insert gastric tube and attach to suction

5) Insert indwelling urinary catheter

6) Assist with collection and maintenance of physical and forensic evidence as indicated (see Chapter 44)

7) Assist with hospital admission for surgical intervention or transfer to an institution providing higher level of care

e. Administer pharmacologic therapy as ordered

1) RSI medications: sedatives, analgesics, neuromuscular blocking agents

2) Osmotic diuretic (e.g., Mannitol [Osmitrol]) for increasing ICP: hypertension, bradycardia, and widening pulse pressure (an increase in the difference between systolic and diastolic pressure over time)

3) Antibiotics

4) Antiepileptics if seizure activity

5) Tetanus immunization

4. Evaluation and ongoing monitoring

a. Airway patency

b. Level of consciousness

c. Hemodynamic status

1) Maintain systolic blood pressure >90 mm Hg

d. Breath sounds and pulse oximetry

e. Cardiac rate and rhythm

f. Intake and output

J. TRAUMATIC BRAIN INJURY: SUBDURAL HEMATOMA

Subdural hematoma (SDH) is a collection of blood between the dura mater and the subarachnoid layer of the meninges, usually caused by trauma or as the extension of an intracerebral hematoma into the subdural space. Veins that bridge the subdural space are torn, and this allows venous blood to collect beneath the dura. SDHs are classified based on the onset of clinical signs and symptoms: (1) acute (within 48 hours), (2) subacute (2–14 days), and (3) chronic (>14 days). The elder adult and persons with chronic alcoholism are at an increased risk for sustaining SDHs because as the brain atrophies, a space is created where venous blood may accumulate without causing initial pressure effects on the brain. In infants and very young children, maltreatment must be considered as a causative factor.

1. Assessment

a. Subjective data collection

1) History of present injury/chief complaint

a) Mechanism of injury (see Chapter 31)

b) Time interval

c) Trends in neurologic status

2) Past medical history

a) Current or preexisting diseases/illness

(1) Chronic alcoholism

(2) Coagulopathy

b) Medications: anticoagulants, antiplatelet therapy
c) Allergies
b. Objective data collection
1) Physical examination
a) General appearance/inspection
(1) Acute subdural
(a) Level of consciousness, behavior, affect: steady decline in alertness
(b) Ipsilateral, unilateral pupillary dilation with lack of response to light
(c) Contralateral motor changes (hemiparesis)
(d) Gait disturbance, ataxia
(2) Chronic and subacute subdural
(a) Level of consciousness, behavior, affect: gradual and nonspecific changes
(b) Alteration in mentation
(c) Alteration in motor ability (ipsilateral or contralateral hemiparesis)
(d) Papilledema
(e) Dilated, ipsilateral pupil sluggish to light
(3) Moderate to severe distress/discomfort, critically ill
2) Diagnostic procedures
a) CBC with differential
b) Serum chemistries including glucose, BUN, creatinine
c) Serum and urine toxicology screen
d) Coagulation profile
e) Urinalysis; pregnancy test in female patients of childbearing age
f) Type and screen/crossmatch
g) Head CT scan
(1) Midline shift present with moderate or large hematomas
(2) Contralateral mass may account for absent midline shift
h) Head MRI
i) Angiography
2. Analysis: differential nursing diagnoses/collaborative problems
a. Impaired gas exchange
b. Ineffective tissue perfusion: cerebral
c. Risk for ineffective airway clearance
3. Planning and implementation/interventions
a. Maintain airway, breathing, circulation (see Chapters 1 and 32)
b. Provide supplemental oxygen as indicated
1) RSI and ventilatory support in patients with airway compromise; hyperventilation is

controversial because it constricts cerebral arteries and thereby decreases cerebral blood flow
2) High-flow oxygen
c. Establish IV access for administration of crystalloid fluids/medications as needed
d. Prepare for/assist with medical interventions
1) Acute
a) Advanced airway management
(1) Nasal or oral intubation
(2) Supraglottic airway (e.g., King, Combitube, laryngeal mask airway)
(3) Surgical airway (e.g., cricothyrotomy)
b) Assist with medical decompression of cranial vault to decrease the ICP
(1) Increase venous outflow through elevation of head of bed, midline head and neck positioning, and avoidance of extreme hip flexion
c) Decrease metabolic demands of the brain by
(1) Maintaining normothermia
(2) Preventing seizures
d) Institute cardiac and pulse oximetry monitoring
e) Insert gastric tube and attach to suction
f) Insert indwelling urinary catheter
g) Assist with collection and maintenance of physical and forensic evidence as indicated (see Chapter 44)
h) Assist with hospital admission or transfer to an institution providing a higher level of care
2) Nonacute
a) Elevate head of bed
b) Assist with hospital admission, possible surgery
e. Administer pharmacologic therapy as ordered
1) RSI medications: sedatives, analgesics, neuromuscular blocking agents
2) Diuretics to decrease the water content in the brain
3) Anticonvulsants
4. Evaluation and ongoing monitoring
a. Airway patency
b. Level of consciousness changes
c. Hemodynamic status
d. Breath sounds and pulse oximetry
e. Cardiac rate and rhythm
f. Intake and output

K. TRAUMATIC SUBARACHNOID HEMORRHAGE

Traumatic subarachnoid hemorrhage (tSAH) is a diffuse collection of blood between the arachnoid mater and the pia mater caused by disruption of subarachnoid blood vessels. This collection of blood then spreads throughout the cerebral spinal fluid. tSAH has been identified on

CT scans of approximately 40% of all patients with major head injuries and is present consistently with serious brain injuries caused by brain surface contusions. tSAHs have less debilitating symptoms than SAHs caused by ruptured aneurysms: nonfocal signs of headache, nausea, and meningeal irritation. tSAHs usually have an excellent prognosis but are subject to the same complications as aneurysmal SAHs: seizures, increased ICP, cerebral vasospasm, and hydrocephalus. It is important to determine whether the SAH was the result of trauma and not the cause of trauma (aneurysmal).

1. Assessment
   a. Subjective data collection
      1) History of present injury/chief complaint
         a) Mechanism of injury (see Chapter 31)
         b) Level of consciousness following the injury
         c) Trends in neurologic status
            (1) Headache
            (2) Nausea
            (3) Deteriorating level of consciousness
            (4) Nuchal rigidity
      2) Past medical history
         a) Current or preexisting diseases/illness
            (1) Neurologic disease or previous injury
            (2) Hypertension
         b) Medications
            (1) Anticoagulant or antiplatelet use
         c) Allergies
         d) Immunization status
   b. Objective data collection
      1) Physical examination
         a) General appearance
            (1) Level of consciousness, behavior, affect: disoriented to unconsciousness
            (2) Moderate to severe distress/discomfort, critically ill
         b) Inspection
            (1) Presence of surface trauma (occasional)
      2) Diagnostic procedures
         a) ABGs
         b) Head CT scan
         c) Head MRI
         d) Angiography
2. Analysis: differential nursing diagnoses/collaborative problems
   a. Ineffective tissue perfusion: cerebral
   b. Acute pain
   c. Risk for ineffective airway clearance
3. Planning and implementation/interventions
   a. Maintain airway, breathing, circulation (see Chapters 1 and 32)
   b. Provide supplemental oxygen
      1) RSI and ventilatory support in patients with airway compromise; hyperventilation is controversial because it constricts cerebral arteries and thereby decreases cerebral blood flow
      2) High-flow oxygen
   c. Establish IV access for administration of crystalloid fluids/medications/blood
   d. Prepare for/assist with medical interventions
      1) Advanced airway management
         a) Nasal or oral intubation
         b) Supraglottic airway (e.g., King, Combitube, laryngeal mask airway)
         c) Surgical airway (e.g., cricothyrotomy)
      2) Assist with medical decompression of cranial vault to decrease the ICP
         a) Increase venous outflow through elevation of head of bed, midline head and neck positioning, and avoidance of extreme hip flexion
      3) Decrease metabolic demands of the brain by
         a) Maintaining normothermia
         b) Preventing seizures
      4) Institute cardiac and pulse oximetry monitoring
      5) Maintain quiet environment
      6) Prevent use of Valsalva maneuvers
      7) Insert gastric tube and attach to suction
      8) Insert indwelling urinary catheter
      9) Assist with hospital admission
   e. Administer pharmacologic therapy as ordered
      1) RSI medications: sedatives, analgesics, neuromuscular blocking agents
      2) Osmotic diuretics (e.g., Mannitol [Osmitrol]) to decrease the water content of brain if increased ICP
      3) Analgesics: nonnarcotic agents are preferred to prevent masking a neurologic change
4. Evaluation and ongoing monitoring
   a. Airway patency
   b. Level of consciousness
   c. Hemodynamic status
   d. Breath sounds and pulse oximetry
   e. Cardiac rate and rhythm
   f. Intake and output
   g. Pain relief

Bibliography

Blackwell T, Moreira M: Prehospital care of the adult trauma patient, 2015. UpToDate. Wolters Kluwer. http://www.uptodate.com.

Decker JE, Hergenroeder AC: Overview of the musculosketetal neck injuries in the child or adolescent, 2015. UpToDate. Wolters Kluwer. http://www.uptodate.com.

Harmon KG, et al.: American Medical Society for Sports Medicine Position Statement: concussion in sport, *Clinical Journal of Sport Medicine* 23(1):1–18, 2013.

Heegaard WG, Biros M: Skull fractures in adults, 2015. UpTo-Date. Wolters Kluwer. http://www.uptodate.com.

Hemphill JC, Phan N: Traumatic brain injury: epidemiology, classification and pathophysiology, 2015. UpToDate. Wolters Kluwer. http://www.uptodate.com.

Meehan WP, O'Brien MJ: Concussion in children and adolescents: management, 2015. UpToDate. Wolters Kluwer. http://www.uptodate.com.

Raja A, Zane RD: Initial management of trauma in adults, 2015. UpToDate. Wolters Kluwer. http://www.uptodate.com.

Sidhu GS, et al.: Civilian gunshot injuries of the spinal cord: a systematic review of the current literature, *Clinical Orthopaedics and Related Research* 471:3945–3955, 2013.

Smith ER, Amin-Hanjani S: Evaluation and management of elevated intracranial pressure in adults, 2015. UpToDate. Wolters Kluwer. http://www.uptodate.com.

Stephenson RO, et al.: Autonomic dysreflexia in spinal cord injury: overview, pathophysiology, causes of autonomic dysreflexia, 2015. Medscape. http://www.medscape.com.

CHAPTER 36

Ocular and Maxillofacial Trauma

Jeff Solheim, MSN, RN, CEN, CFRN, FAEN

MAJOR TOPICS

General Strategy

Assessment

Analysis: Differential Nursing Diagnoses/Collaborative
  Problems

Planning and Implementation/Interventions

Evaluation and Ongoing Monitoring

Documentation of Interventions and Patient Response

Age-Related Considerations

Specific Traumatic Ocular Injuries

Chemical Burns

Corneal Abrasion

Extraocular Foreign Bodies

Eyelid Laceration

Globe Rupture

Hyphema

Orbital Fracture

Retinal Detachment

Specific Traumatic Maxillofacial Injuries

Facial Lacerations and Soft Tissue Injuries

Fractured Larynx

Fractured Tooth

Mandibular Fractures

Maxillary Fractures

Nasal Fracture

Subluxed/Avulsed Teeth

Temporomandibular Joint Dislocation

Zygomatic Fractures

I. General Strategy

A. ASSESSMENT

1. Primary and secondary assessment/resuscitation (see
   Chapters 1 and 32)
2. Focused assessment
   a. Subjective data collection
      1) History of present injury/chief complaint
         a) Mechanism of injury (see Chapter 31)
            (1) Blunt or penetrating forces
            (2) Chemical exposure
         b) Pain (see Chapter 8)
         c) Time of injury
         d) Airbag deployment if motor vehicle crash
         e) Treatment prior to arrival
         f) Changes in clinical status
         g) Corrective (including contact) lens/safety
            glasses use
         h) Visual acuity changes; decreased acuity,
            decreased visual fields, blurred vision,
            diplopia, tearing, eye pain
         i) Efforts to relieve symptoms
            (1) Home remedies
            (2) Alternative therapies
            (3) Medications
               (a) Prescription
               (b) OTC/herbal

2) Past medical history
   a) Current or preexisting diseases/illness
      (1) Diabetes
      (2) Cardiovascular disease
      (3) Hypertension
   b) Ocular
      (1) Corrective (including contact) or protec-
         tive lens use
      (2) Chronic eye problems; previous eye injuries
   c) Maxillofacial
      (1) Previous ear, nose, and throat (ENT) prob-
         lems, facial trauma, or surgical procedures
   d) Substance and/or alcohol use/abuse
   e) Last normal menstrual period: female
      patients of childbearing age
   f) Current medications
      (1) Prescription
      (2) OTC/herbal
   g) Allergies
   h) Immunization status
3) Psychological/social/environmental factors
   a) Behavior appropriate for age and
      developmental stage
      (1) Young male patients at higher risk for
         serious injury
      (2) Contact lens wearers at greater risk for
         corneal abrasion

b) Occupation or profession
(1) Exposure to arc welding: symptoms develop 4–8 hours after exposure
(2) Construction work involving grinding metal or use of machinery has potential for embedded foreign bodies or globe penetration
(3) Mechanics and cleaning personnel have potential for acid and/or alkali burns to eye
c) Hobbies, avocation, recreational activities
(1) Injuries involving soil and organic material have increased potential for infection
(2) Home crafts and woodworking activities increase potential for eye injuries if safety precautions not taken
(3) Ball sports increase potential for eye injuries, as do contact sports in which no protective eyewear is worn
(4) BB guns and fireworks are frequent causes of eye trauma in children
d) Possible/actual assault, abuse, intimate partner violence situations (see Chapters 3 and 40)
(1) Victims of violence often sustain ocular and/or maxillofacial injuries
(2) Victims of child maltreatment often present with findings of intraocular and/or retinal hemorrhage related to direct trauma or shaking of child
b. Objective data collection
1) General appearance
a) Level of consciousness, behavior, affect
b) Vital signs
c) Odors
d) Gait
e) Hygiene
f) Level of distress/discomfort
2) Inspection
a) Eyelids and periorbital area for soft tissue swelling and ecchymosis
b) Eye surface for foreign body, penetrating wounds, tearing, and leakage of intraocular fluid
c) Pupillary size and function, extraocular muscle movements, visual fields
d) Conjunctiva and sclera for hemorrhage
e) Blood in anterior chamber
f) Opaque, gray-white cornea
g) Facial asymmetry, wounds, bleeding
h) Soft tissue swelling, ecchymosis, obvious deformity
i) Malocclusion or trismus, intraoral trauma, tooth avulsion, missing or fragmented teeth
j) Evidence of head or neck injury
3) Palpation/percussion

a) Facial bones and periorbital structures for stability, crepitus, movement, bony step-off or deformity, tenderness
b) Head and neck for tenderness or deformity
c) Facial sensation and muscle function
3. Diagnostic procedures
a. Laboratory studies
1) Complete blood count (CBC) with differential
2) Culture of wounds, discharge
3) Arterial blood gas (ABG)
b. Imaging studies
1) Facial radiographs
a) Waters' view
b) Mandibular panoramic radiograph (Panorex)
c) Cervical spine
2) Facial, orbit, head, neck computed tomography (CT) scan or magnetic resonance imaging (MRI)
c. Other
1) Visual acuity
2) Direct ophthalmoscope examination
3) Fluorescein staining
4) Slit-lamp examination
5) Tonometry: intraocular pressure measurement

B. ANALYSIS: DIFFERENTIAL NURSING DIAGNOSES/COLLABORATIVE PROBLEMS

1. Ineffective airway clearance
2. Acute pain
3. Anxiety/fear
4. Impaired skin integrity
5. Disturbed sensory perception: visual
6. Deficient knowledge

C. PLANNING AND IMPLEMENTATION/INTERVENTIONS

1. Determine priorities of care
a. Maintain airway, breathing, circulation (see Chapters 1 and 32)
b. Provide supplemental oxygen as indicated
c. Establish IV access for administration of crystalloid fluid/blood products/medications as needed
d. Obtain and set up equipment and supplies
e. Prepare for/assist with medical interventions
f. Administer pharmacologic therapy as ordered
2. Relieve anxiety/apprehension
3. Allow significant others to remain with patient if supportive
4. Educate patient/significant others

D. EVALUATION AND ONGOING MONITORING

1. Continuously monitor and treat as indicated
2. Monitor patient response/outcomes, and modify nursing care plan as appropriate
3. If positive patient outcomes are not demonstrated, reevaluate assessment and/or plan of care

E. DOCUMENTATION OF INTERVENTIONS AND PATIENT RESPONSE

F. AGE-RELATED CONSIDERATIONS

1. Pediatrics
   a. Growth or development related
      1) Infants and small children may need to be restrained in a blanket to facilitate thorough examination
      2) Children can fixate on objects by 4 months of age
      3) Facial bone fractures in pediatric patients tend to be less severe; most common are comminuted and nondisplaced fractures because facial bones in children are softer and more pliable than in adults
      4) The tissue in the mouth and upper airway is larger in the pediatric patient than the adult patient, decreasing available space for blood, vomitus, or other foreign objects. Children are more prone to upper airway obstructions than adults
   b. "Pearls"
      1) Various alternatives to the standard Snellen chart exist to test visual acuity in the child who is not literate including the tumbling E chart, or the Lea or Allen figures eye chart. In infants, visual acuity may be tested by determining if the child's eyes will follow a brightly colored object
      2) 20/40 vision is considered normal at 3 years of age, 20/30 vision is normal by age 4, and by age 5 or 6, children should have 20/20 vision[1]
2. Geriatrics
   a. Aging related
      1) Vision diminishes gradually until approximately 70 years and then more rapidly thereafter
      2) Decreased accuracy of results from visual acuity testing
      3) Ability of eye to accommodate, or adjust, to distances decreases with age
      4) Chronic illness may cause visual changes
   b. "Pearls"
      1) Increased incidence of detached retina
      2) Maxillofacial trauma more likely associated with head and neck injuries

II. Specific Traumatic Ocular Injuries

A. CHEMICAL BURNS

Ocular injury is second only to cataracts as the leading cause of visual impairment in the United States.[2] One cause of ocular injury is chemical burns. Chemical injuries to the eye range from mildly irritating to irreversible visual impairment. Chemicals can be defined as either alkali, if the pH is >7.0 or acidic if the pH is <7.0. Acidic substances tend to denature body proteins causing a coagulative necrosis resulting in an eschar that may actually create a barrier to further penetration. Alkali substances, on the other hand, interact with fatty acids, causing tissue breakdown, allowing for deeper and more serious burns. There are two exceptions to this. Hydrofluoric acid (used by glass etchers and in certain cleaning agents) and sulfuric acid (found in car batteries) do not produce a protective eschar and these acids can cause deep ocular injuries similar to an alkali substance. The emergent treatment for a chemical exposure to the eye is neutralization of the chemical with copious irrigation. The sooner irrigation is initiated, the better the outcome for the patient. Therefore, chemical burns should result in the highest triage priority for ocular emergencies. Long-term treatment after irrigation ranges from antibiotic ointment for mild burns to surgical intervention with poor prognosis for visual acuity in severe burns.

1. Assessment
   a. Subjective data collection
      1) History of present injury/chief complaint
         a) Pain (see Chapter 8)
         b) Variable degrees of visual loss
         c) Chemical exposure
         d) Occupational hazards
      2) Past medical history
         a) Current or preexisting diseases/illness
         b) Previous eye problems
         c) Medications
         d) Allergies
         e) Immunization status
   b. Objective data collection
      1) Physical examination
         a) General appearance
            (1) Moderate to severe distress/discomfort
         b) Inspection
            (1) Burns of varying degrees
            (2) Visual acuity: decreased
            (3) Conjunctival injection
            (4) Chemosis (edema of bulbar conjunctiva)
            (5) Corneal clouding: inability to define specific eye structures
      2) Diagnostic procedures
         a) Funduscopy
         b) Fluorescein stain
         c) Slit-lamp examination
2. Analysis: differential nursing diagnoses/collaborative problems
   a. Disturbed sensory perception: visual
   b. Acute pain
   c. Fear/anxiety
   d. Deficient knowledge
   e. Risk for infection

3. Planning and implementation/interventions
   a. Maintain airway, breathing, circulation (see Chapters 1 and 32)
   b. Provide supplemental oxygen as indicated
   c. Establish IV access for administration of crystalloid fluid/medications as needed
   d. Prepare for/assist with medical interventions
      1) Immediate eye irrigation: including eversion of upper lid
         a) Irrigation should begin as soon after the injury as possible. Tap water may be used initially until other solutions are available. Lactated Ringer or normal saline may be used but irrigation should not be delayed preparing these solutions
         b) Continuous copious irrigation should be undertaken until the pH of the eye is near neutral (the pH of tears is normally 7.4, so irrigation to a pH of 7.0–8.0 is the target)[3]
         c) Wait 5 minutes after completing irrigation to check pH of the eye to ensure that pH of the irrigant is not being tested[2]
         d) Eyelid retractors or a Morgan lens may be used to facilitate thorough irrigation
      2) Possible eye patch
   e. Administer pharmacologic therapy as ordered
      1) Topical ophthalmic anesthesia
      2) Nonnarcotic analgesics
      3) Narcotics
      4) Cycloplegic agent: reduces pain related to ciliary spasm
      5) Topical ophthalmic antibiotics
      6) Tetanus immunization
4. Evaluation and ongoing monitoring
   a. Hemodynamic status
   b. Visual acuity including pH of ocular fluid
   c. Pain relief

B. CORNEAL ABRASION

Most corneal abrasions are defects of the epithelial layer of the cornea, although severe injuries may involve the deeper stromal layers of the cornea. Corneal abrasions are surprisingly common, accounting for about 10% of all ocular complaints presenting to the emergency department.[4] They are especially common in individuals who wear contacts. Corneal abrasions associated with contact lens use have a higher rate of *Pseudomonas* infection. The treatment for corneal abrasions has changed dramatically over the years. Traditional treatments such as patching of the eye, topical anesthetics, and routine use of topical antibiotics have not been found to be beneficial. Eye patches cause monocular vision, which may increase the risk of patient injury after discharge and the warm moist environment under the eye patch may encourage bacterial growth. Studies indicate that the use of eye patches does not speed healing or reduce pain. Topical anesthetics may be used to facilitate an eye exam but should not be encouraged after discharge as they may cause further injury through loss of protective reflexes and drying of the eye. Additionally, topical anesthetics have been shown to delay wound healing. There is little evidence to suggest that the routine use of antibiotics in the treatment of corneal abrasions reduces infection although they are often prescribed for abrasions associated with contact lens use. Treatment focuses mainly on pain relief through either topical or systemic nonsteroidal antiinflammatory drugs. Cycloplegic agents provide relief from photophobia and blepharospasms in patients with extensive corneal abrasions (assure that the patient does not have narrow angle glaucoma).

1. Assessment
   a. Subjective data collection
      1) History of present injury/chief complaint
         a) Ocular injury, contact lens use
         b) Pain (see Chapter 8): ranging from mild to severe, often described as a "foreign body sensation"
         c) Redness
         d) Tearing and blinking
         e) Sensitivity to light
         f) Use of corrective (including contact) or protective lenses
      2) Past medical history
         a) Current or preexisting diseases/illness
         b) Previous eye injuries or problems
         c) Medications
         d) Allergies
         e) Immunization status
   b. Objective data collection
      1) Physical examination
         a) General appearance
            (1) Mild to severe distress/discomfort
         b) Inspection
            (1) Irritated conjunctiva
            (2) Tearing, blinking
            (3) Foreign body: evert upper eyelid
            (4) Corneal ulceration
            (5) Erythema or swelling of lids and surrounding tissue
      2) Diagnostic procedures
         a) Visual acuity: usually normal unless corneal abrasion is large or located over the visual axis (line of vision)
         b) Fluorescein stain: uptake of dye if epithelial cells damaged
         c) Slit-lamp examination
2. Analysis: differential nursing diagnoses/collaborative problems
   a. Acute pain
   b. Anxiety/fear
   c. Deficient knowledge
   d. Risk for infection
3. Planning and implementation/interventions

a. Prepare for/assist with medical interventions
b. Administer pharmacologic therapy as ordered
  1) Nonsteroidal antiinflammatory topical or systemic agent
  2) Cycloplegic agent: reduces pain related to ciliary spasm in patients with extensive corneal abrasions (assure that patient does not have narrow-angle glaucoma)
  3) Topical ophthalmic antibiotics may be used in patients with a history of contact lens use
  4) Tetanus immunization may be considered in "dirty" wounds
c. Educate patient/significant others
  1) Rest eye for 12–24 hours: sunglasses, darkened room
  2) Importance of follow-up care; recheck in 24 hours if injury is the result of contact lens use
  3) Do not wear contact lenses during healing period
4. Evaluation and ongoing monitoring
  a. Pain relief

C. EXTRAOCULAR FOREIGN BODIES

Foreign bodies can enter the eye as a result of hammering, grinding, working under cars, or working above the head. Patients usually describe the sensation of "something going into the eye." Foreign bodies can range from metal to sawdust to dust particles. Foreign bodies with a metallic component are of specific concern because these objects may form a rust ring in the cornea. If the rust ring is not removed, it may continue to invade the cornea and interfere with vision. Ocular penetration with single or multiple foreign bodies must be considered with corneal injuries. This type of injury is usually related to occupation or avocation.

1. Assessment
  a. Subjective data collection
    1) History of present injury/chief complaint
      a) Mechanism of injury (see Chapter 31)
      b) Pain (see Chapter 8) often described as a foreign body sensation or photophobia
      c) Possible visual acuity changes
      d) Tearing
      e) Redness
      f) Use of protective lenses
    2) Past medical history
      a) Current or preexisting diseases/illness
      b) Previous eye injuries or problems
      c) Medications
      d) Allergies
      e) Immunization status
  b. Objective data collection
    1) Physical examination
      a) General appearance
        (1) Mild to severe distress/discomfort
      b) Inspection
        (1) Tearing, blinking

        (2) Mild to moderate conjunctival irritation
        (3) Possible visible foreign body: evert lid to inspect adequately
        (4) Visible rust ring if the object is metallic (reaction may start in as little as 2–4 hours)
    2) Diagnostic procedures
      a) Visual acuity: normal to slightly abnormal
      b) Fluorescein stain: abnormal; enhances corneal abrasion, foreign body, or rust ring if it is present
      c) Slit-lamp examination
      d) Possible orbital CT scan (especially if an extraocular foreign object is suspected but cannot be visualized; a CT scan helps identify a penetrating foreign object)
      e) MRI is contraindicated if there is the potential that the object may be metallic
2. Analysis: differential nursing diagnoses/collaborative problems
  a. Acute pain
  b. Anxiety
  c. Deficient knowledge
3. Planning and implementation/interventions
  a. Prepare for/assist with medical interventions
    1) Possible gentle eye irrigation with normal saline
    2) Foreign body removal with moistened cotton swab, 25-gauge needle, or foreign body spud
    3) Rust ring removal with ophthalmic drill
    4) Consultation with ophthalmologist if high-velocity injury suspected
  b. Administer pharmacologic therapy as ordered
    1) Topical ophthalmic anesthetic
    2) Nonnarcotic analgesics
    3) Narcotics
    4) Tetanus immunization
4. Evaluation and ongoing monitoring
  a. Pain relief
  b. Visual acuity

D. EYELID LACERATION

Lacerations of the eyelid may result from multiple types of injuries and can range from a simple laceration of the eyelid to a complex laceration involving essential structures such as the lacrimal drainage apparatus, extraocular muscles, or eyelid margins. Preservation of eyelid function, proper eyelid margin alignment, and acceptable cosmetic outcomes are the goals of emergency department management of eyelid lacerations. Complications that should be considered include injuries to the globe itself as well as disruption of the lacrimal apparatus, especially when the injury involves the inner third of the eyelid.[5]

1. Assessment
  a. Subjective data collection
    1) History of present injury/chief complaint
      a) Mechanism of injury (see Chapter 31)
      b) Any visual disturbance

2) Past medical history
   a) Current or preexisting diseases/illness
   b) Medications
   c) Allergies
   d) Immunization status
b. Objective data collection
   1) Physical examination
      a) General appearance
         (1) Mild to moderate distress/discomfort
      b) Inspection
         (1) Laceration of lid
         (2) Protrusion of orbital fat
         (3) Injury to levator muscle (resulting in ptosis) or superior rectus muscle
         (4) Observe for associated ocular injuries (e.g., globe disruption, foreign bodies, hyphema, corneal abrasion or laceration)
      c) Palpation
         (1) Periorbital soft tissue or bony injury
   2) Diagnostic procedures
      a) Facial and eye muscle function testing
      b) Funduscopy
      c) Fluorescein stain
      d) Slit-lamp examination
2. Analysis: differential nursing diagnoses/collaborative problems
   a. Impaired skin integrity
   b. Acute pain
   c. Anxiety
   d. Deficient knowledge
   e. Disturbed sensory perception: visual
   f. Risk for infection
3. Planning and implementation/interventions
   a. Prepare for/assist with medical interventions
      1) Stop bleeding: avoid direct pressure on orbit
      2) Assist with surgical repair: wound approximation and closure
      3) Refer to ophthalmologist or plastic surgeon for injury with extensive tissue loss or lacrimal duct involvement
   b. Administer pharmacologic therapy as ordered
      1) Topical ophthalmic anesthesia
      2) Nonnarcotic analgesics
      3) Narcotics
      4) Possible antibiotics
      5) Tetanus prophylaxis as indicated
4. Evaluation and ongoing monitoring
   a. Pain relief

E. GLOBE RUPTURE

This condition is a major ocular emergency and may require immediate surgical intervention. Globe rupture may be caused by blunt or penetrating forces. Forceful compression of the globe causes an increase in intraocular pressure that can result in a scleral tear. The most common site of rupture is at the limbic margin or at the insertion of the extraocular muscles where the sclera is thinnest. Penetrating injuries usually involve projectiles from pounding metal, steel-grinding wheels, or an impaled object. Globe rupture may either be easily visualized or occult; therefore, a meticulous history and physical examination are essential.

1. Assessment
   a. Subjective data collection
      1) History of present injury/chief complaint
         a) Time and mechanism of injury (see Chapter 31)
         b) Use of protective or corrective eyewear
         c) Visual changes or loss of vision
         d) Pain (see Chapter 8): minimal to severe
      2) Past medical history
         a) Current or preexisting diseases/illness
         b) Previous eye injury or problem
         c) Medications
         d) Allergies
         e) Immunization status
   b. Objective data collection
      1) Physical examination
         a) General appearance
            (1) Possible penetrating object extruding from eye
            (2) Moderate to severe distress/discomfort
         b) Inspection
            (1) Asymmetry of globes
            (2) Extrusion of aqueous or vitreous humor
            (3) Possible enophthalmos
            (4) Possible visible foreign body if located in anterior chamber
            (5) Peaked or teardrop-shaped pupil
            (6) Shallow anterior chamber: associated with poor prognosis
         c) Palpation
            (1) Periorbital soft tissue swelling and/or bony deformity
      2) Diagnostic procedures
         a) Visual acuity: decreased
         b) Orbital CT scan: to rule out occult rupture, foreign body
         c) Orbital and sinus radiographs: for foreign body or fracture
         d) Possible orbital MRI: to identify soft tissue injury to globe
         e) Slit-lamp examination
2. Analysis: differential nursing diagnoses/collaborative problems
   a. Disturbed sensory perception: visual
   b. Acute pain
   c. Anxiety
   d. Deficient knowledge
   e. Risk for infection
3. Planning and implementation/interventions
   a. Establish IV access for administration of crystalloid fluid/medications

b. Prepare for/assist with medical interventions
   1) Secure any extruding object in place
   2) Avoid all pressure around globe; if suspicion of globe rupture, do not open eye
   3) Patch lightly or shield injured eye and patch other eye as well to minimize consensual movement
   4) Keep patient at rest in semi-Fowler position
   5) Assist with obtaining ophthalmologic consultation
   6) Assist with hospital admission
c. Administer pharmacologic therapy as ordered
   1) Nonnarcotic analgesics
   2) Narcotics
   3) Parenteral antibiotics to prevent endophthalmitis
   4) Parenteral antiemetics as needed
   5) Tetanus immunization
   6) Important note: Topical medications should be avoided if a ruptured globe is suspected.
4. Evaluation and ongoing monitoring
   a. Hemodynamic status
   b. Visual acuity
   c. Pain relief

F. HYPHEMA

Disruption of blood vessels in the iris or ciliary body may cause blood to accumulate in the anterior chamber of the eye also known as a hyphema. Sometimes, the amount of blood is so minimal that it can only be seen with a slit lamp. At other times, the entire anterior chamber may fill with blood (known as an 8-ball hyphema). Hyphemas are frequently related to trauma but certain medical conditions like sickle cell disease may also be the cause. Treatment for a hyphema is largely dependent on the amount of blood and the resultant intraocular pressure. Patients with minimal elevations in intraocular pressure may be discharged and encouraged to decrease activity until the hyphema reabsorbs. Patients with hyphemas >50%, with decreased vision or significant increases in intraocular pressure, are more likely to be admitted and may be surgically treated.

1. Assessment
   a. Subjective data collection
      1) History of present injury/chief complaint
         a) Mechanism of injury (see Chapter 31)
         b) Blurred vision
         c) Blood tinged vision
         d) Pain (see Chapter 8)
         e) Use of corrective or protective eyewear
      2) Past medical history
         a) Current or preexisting diseases/illness
            (1) Sickle cell disease
            (2) Cardiovascular disease
         b) Previous eye injury or problem
         c) Medications
            (1) Antihypertensives
            (2) Anticoagulants
            (3) Nonsteroidal antiinflammatory medications (NSAIDs)
            d) Allergies
   b. Objective data collection
      1) Physical examination
         a) General appearance
            (1) Moderate distress/discomfort
         b) Inspection
            (1) Pupils: possible relative afferent pupillary defect
            (2) EOMs
            (3) Blood in the anterior chamber may be visualized
            (4) Obvious associated injuries
      2) Diagnostic procedures
         a) Visual acuity: decreased
         b) Selected radiographs and/or CT scan to determine bony injury
         c) Tonometry: may be elevated or decreased if globe rupture present
         d) Slit-lamp examination
2. Analysis: differential nursing diagnoses/collaborative problems
   a. Disturbed sensory perception: visual
   b. Anxiety/fear
   c. Deficient knowledge
   d. Self-care deficit
3. Planning and implementation/interventions
   a. Prepare for/assist with medical interventions
      1) Shield affected eye for protection and promotion of rest
      2) Place patient at bed rest with head of bed elevated 30–45 degrees to decrease intraocular pressure and pool blood inferiorly[6]
      3) Assist with obtaining ophthalmology consultation
   b. Administer pharmacologic therapy as ordered
      1) Analgesics: avoid aspirin, NSAIDs, or medications with antiplatelet effects that may contribute to recurrent bleeding
      2) Antifibrinolytic agent: topical ophthalmic, oral, or IV aminocaproic acid (Amicar)
      3) Possible topical ophthalmic atropine (1%) for large hyphemas
      4) Steroids
4. Evaluation and ongoing monitoring
   a. Visual acuity
   b. Pain relief

G. ORBITAL FRACTURE

Although any wall of the bony orbit may be fractured, the most common site of fracture is the orbital floor. The mechanism of injury is frequently a fisted blow or a ball striking the globe. The bony fragments from the fracture may sag into the underlying maxillary sinus and the inferior rectus muscle may become entrapped in the fracture line, minimizing the patient's ability to look upward. This is referred to as ocular entrapment and will usually result in visual defects such as diplopia. If the infraorbital nerve, which is located on the floor of the orbit, is affected, anesthesia over the cheek and upper lip may be noted. Other areas of the orbit may also be affected. Fractures of the medial wall are frequently associated with nasal injuries or midface fractures. The superior area of the orbit may also be fractured and in rare cases, parts of the eye may herniate into the fracture. Multiple areas of the orbit may sustain fractures. Surgical repair of these fractures is frequently indicated, but if the orbit itself is not affected, surgery may be delayed to allow for resolution of surrounding edema.[7]

1. Assessment
   a. Subjective data collection
      1) History of present injury/chief complaint
         a) Mechanism of injury (see Chapter 31)
         b) Blurred vision
         c) Diplopia: especially on lateral or upward gaze
         d) Facial numbness, especially the anteromedial cheek and upper lip if the infraorbital nerve is impacted
         e) Pain (see Chapter 8) with eye movement
      2) Past medical history
         a) Current or preexisting diseases/illness
         b) Previous facial nerve injury
         c) Medications
         d) Allergies
         e) Immunization status
   b. Objective data collection
      1) Physical examination
         a) General appearance
            (1) Level of consciousness, behavior, affect: possibly altered if associated with head injury
            (2) Moderate to severe distress/discomfort
         b) Inspection
            (1) Obvious facial trauma
            (2) Periorbital soft tissue swelling, hematoma, ecchymosis
            (3) Facial asymmetry
            (4) Subconjunctival hemorrhage
            (5) Enophthalmos if fractured area sags into the underlying sinus taking the eye with it
            (6) Exophthalmos if there is a retrobulbar hematoma
            (7) Pupils: equality, reaction
            (8) Extraocular movements (EOMs): painful or limited upward or lateral gaze
            (9) Possible ruptured tympanic membrane on affected side
            (10) Obvious associated ocular or other injuries
         c) Palpation
            (1) Bony crepitus or subcutaneous air at fracture site
            (2) Infraorbital paresthesia

      2) Diagnostic procedures
         a) Visual acuity
         b) Funduscopy
         c) Possible tonometry
         d) Orbital CT scan
         e) Orbital and facial radiograph including Waters' view (assess for air-fluid levels or teardrop sign indicating fractures involving sinuses)
         f) Possible cervical spine radiograph
2. Analysis: differential nursing diagnoses/collaborative problems
   a. Acute pain
   b. Anxiety
   c. Deficient knowledge
   d. Risk for infection
3. Planning and implementation/interventions
   a. Maintain airway, breathing, circulation (see Chapters 1 and 32)
   b. Provide supplemental oxygen as indicated
   c. Establish IV access for administration of crystalloid fluid/medications as needed
   d. Prepare for/assist with medical interventions
      1) Apply ice and elevate head of bed to decrease swelling
      2) Assist with surgical wound repair
      3) Consultation with ophthalmology, ENT, or maxillofacial specialist
   e. Administer pharmacologic therapy as ordered
      1) Nonnarcotic analgesics
      2) Narcotics
      3) Antibiotics: if sinus fracture involved
      4) Tetanus immunization
   f. Educate family/significant others
      1) Patient should avoid blowing the nose, performing Valsalva maneuver or other activities that may force air from the sinuses into subcutaneous tissue around the fracture line
      2) If patient has diplopia secondary to ocular entrapment, consider patching the eye and instructing patient not to drive or undertake other high-risk activities
4. Evaluation and ongoing monitoring
   a. Hemodynamic status
   b. Visual acuity
   c. Pain relief

H. RETINAL DETACHMENT

The retina is composed of two layers, the inner neuronal layer and choroid layer. If these two layers separate, the condition is known as a retinal detachment. Patients older than 45 years of age and those with myopia are at a higher risk of developing this condition, although it can also be associated with trauma at any age. Risk factors for this condition include hypertension, vasculitis, and central retinal venous occlusion. The retina lacks pain fibers, so a retinal detachment is painless and instead is recognized by visual disturbances including visualization of "flashes of light," floaters in the visual field, or the description of a "curtain" or "veil" obscuring part of the visual field. Small retinal detachments may be asymptomatic. The area of the retina that is detached is often ischemic so repair of this defect in a timely manner is recommended to reduce permanent vision loss. Repair of a retinal detachment is nearly always performed by ophthalmology and may involve the use of laser therapy, intraocular gas, or surgical intervention.[4]

1. Assessment
   a. Subjective data collection
      1) History of present injury/chief complaint
         a) Mechanism of injury (see Chapter 31)
         b) Painless unilateral alteration in vision (brilliant flashes of light, floaters, or "curtain," "veil," or "cobweb" defect in visual field)
            (1) Gradual (degenerative) or sudden (trauma) onset
      2) Past medical history
         a) Current or preexisting diseases/illness
            (1) Diabetes
            (2) Vasculitis
            (3) Sickle cell disease
            (4) Eclampsia
            (5) Hypertension
         b) Head or facial trauma
         c) Past eye surgery
         d) Medications, especially antihypertensives
         e) Allergies
         f) Family history of condition
   b. Objective data collection
      1) Physical examination
         a) General appearance
            (1) Condition is painless, patient may present with anxiety related to visual disturbances
         b) Inspection
            (1) Pupil reaction usually normal; may have a relative afferent pupillary defect (unequal constriction and dilation of the pupil when examined with both direct and consensual light)
            (2) Possible evidence of head or facial trauma
            (3) Possible visual field deficit
      2) Diagnostic procedures
         a) Visual acuity: diminished
         b) Funduscopy: indirect ophthalmoscopy by consultant for definitive diagnosis
         c) Slit-lamp examination
         d) Tonometry to measure intraocular pressure: may be decreased in affected eye
2. Analysis: differential nursing diagnoses/collaborative problems
   a. Disturbed sensory perception: visual
   b. Anxiety/fear

c. Deficient knowledge
d. Self-care deficit
3. Planning and implementation/interventions
   a. Prepare for/assist with medical interventions
      1) Shield both eyes to reduce eye movement and in cases of globe penetration
      2) Maintain patient at bed rest and avoid movement
      3) Assist with emergent ophthalmology consultation
      4) Assist with hospital admission: surgical repair
4. Evaluation and ongoing monitoring
   a. Visual acuity

III. Specific Traumatic Maxillofacial Injuries

A. FACIAL LACERATIONS AND SOFT TISSUE INJURIES

There are multiple causes of facial lacerations and soft tissue injuries; the most common are vehicular crashes, interpersonal altercations, violent crimes, and animal and human bites. Common types of soft tissue injuries include lacerations, abrasions, puncture wounds, contusions, and avulsion injuries. Presentations may range from simple isolated facial lacerations to those accompanied by airway obstruction, edema, hemorrhage, massive facial trauma, fractures, and multisystem injuries. As a result, it is imperative that a complete review of systems and physical assessment be done for all individuals with facial trauma. See Box 36.1 for information on lacerations to specific areas of the face.

1. Assessment
   a. Subjective data collection
      1) History of present injury/chief complaint
         a) Time/date of occurrence
         b) Mechanism of injury (see Chapter 31)
         c) Facial wounds: bleeding, swelling, asymmetry
         d) Pain (see Chapter 8)
         e) Motor/sensory deficits
         f) Presence of foreign bodies
         g) Symptoms suggestive of extensive facial injuries, central nervous system (CNS) injury, or multisystem injuries
      2) Past medical history
         a) Current or preexisting diseases/illness
         b) Medications
         c) Allergies
         d) Immunization status
   b. Objective data collection
      1) Physical examination
         a) General appearance
            (1) Mild to moderate distress/discomfort
         b) Inspection
            (1) Facial, intraoral, ocular wounds
            (2) Facial asymmetry/swelling
            (3) Bleeding

Box 36.1

Special Considerations for Facial Lacerations

Location of Laceration	Special Considerations
Lip	Improper closure may leave an uneven lip edge (vermilion border). Closure by a specialist may be considered.
Cheek	Look for either clear fluid in blood from the wound or blood in the saliva, either of which may indicate disruption of the ducts leading from the salivary glands to the mouth. If this is the case, closure by a facial specialist to maintain patency of the ducts is recommended. Lacerations in the area anterior to the tragus carry the risk of injury to the facial nerve. Careful neurological assessment is indicated.
Tongue	The tongue is vascular and heals well. Small lacerations do not require closure. Gaping lacerations, avulsions, or those prone to collection of food may require closure. Patients need to be taught to swish and spit regularly with mild antiseptic after discharge to reduce the incidence of infection.
Ears	Blunt trauma to the ear can cause blood to collect in the subperichondrial space, which, without drainage via aspiration, can result in a deformity known as "cauliflower ear." A compression dressing may be applied to the ear after drainage to prevent recurrence. Because of poor circulation to the cartilage of the ear, closure of wounds is necessary.

Table based on information obtained from: Mayersak, R. J. (2014). Facial trauma. In J. A. Marx, R. S. Hockberger, & R. M. Walls, *Rosen's emergency medicine* (pp. 368–381). Philadelphia, PA: Saunders.

c) Palpation
   (1) Motor deficits (e.g., facial muscle movement)
   (2) Sensory deficits (e.g., gustatory changes of anterior two-thirds of tongue) and other sensory deficits (e.g., loss of sensation or movement to areas of the face)
   (3) Functional changes (e.g., excessive salivation or bleeding at parotid duct opening or excessive lacrimation)
   (4) Tenderness of area
   (5) Other: close examination to determine presence of more extensive facial injuries, CNS injury, or multisystem injuries
   2) Diagnostic procedures
      a) Aerobic and/or anaerobic wound cultures
      b) Facial radiographs
      c) CT scan
2. Analysis: differential nursing diagnoses/collaborative problems
   a. Impaired skin integrity
   b. Risk for infection
   c. Acute pain
   d. Deficient knowledge
3. Planning and implementation/interventions
   a. Establish IV access for administration of crystalloid fluid/medications as needed
   b. Prepare for/assist with medical interventions
      1) Control bleeding: elevate head and apply ice to decrease bleeding and swelling
      2) Wound irrigation with normal saline

   3) Wrap any avulsed part in sterile gauze moistened with normal saline, place in plastic bag, and then place in basin with normal saline and ice
   4) Wound closure: sutures, skin adhesive; consider procedural sedation in children
      a) Patient positioning: pediatric papoose board or other restraint
      b) Never shave eyebrows or hairline
      c) Staples can be used on the scalp but should not be used on the face
   c. Administer pharmacologic therapy as ordered
      1) Anesthetics
         a) Topical
         b) Local
            (1) Lidocaine with epinephrine: provides vasoconstriction to decrease bleeding
            (2) Do not use lidocaine with epinephrine on tip of nose and ears: blood flow to area compromised by vasoconstriction from epinephrine
      2) Procedural sedation medications
      3) Nitrous oxide
      4) Nonnarcotic analgesics
      5) Narcotics
      6) Tetanus immunization
4. Evaluation and ongoing monitoring
   a. Pain relief

B. FRACTURED LARYNX

Injuries to the trachea and larynx are rare, accounting for <1% of all traumatic injuries.[8] Because the cricoid cartilage is the only solid ring in the larynx, fractures of this structure may lead to death. Common causes associated with larynx fracture include motor vehicle crashes, strangulation (both self-inflicted and accidental), and physical trauma associated with sport activities. Because of the danger of spinal cord injury, trauma to the neck must be carefully evaluated to rule out cervical spine injury. Efforts to maintain adequate airway, ventilation, and perfusion are essential because they are frequently compromised with this injury. Cricothyrotomy and tracheotomy may be necessary for airway management if the extent of trauma prevents nasal or endotracheal intubation.

1. Assessment
   a. Subjective data collection
      1) History of present injury/chief complaint
         a) Mechanism of injury (see Chapter 31)
         b) Dysphonia, aphonia, or hoarseness
         c) Pain (see Chapter 8): odynophagia (pain on swallowing)
         d) Cough, stridor, or dyspnea
         e) Hemoptysis
      2) Past medical history
         a) Current or preexisting diseases/illness
         b) Recent surgery in neck area
         c) Medications
         d) Allergies
         e) Immunization status
   b. Objective data collection
      1) Physical examination
         a) General appearance
            (1) Tachypnea
            (2) Inspiratory stridor
            (3) Severe distress/discomfort, critically ill
         b) Inspection
            (1) Ecchymosis, abrasions, soft tissue swelling of neck
            (2) Loss of normal prominence of thyroid cartilage
            (3) Suprasternal or intercostal retractions
            (4) A visible neck wound (bubbling or air leakage from the neck wound is strongly suggestive of a laryngeal injury)
         c) Palpation
            (1) Subcutaneous emphysema
            (2) Tenderness/deformity/laryngeal crepitus
      2) Diagnostic procedures
         a) CBC with differential
         b) ABGs
         c) Fiberoptic laryngoscopy: presence of edema and hematomas indicate need for tracheotomy
         d) Indirect laryngoscopy
         e) Radiographs of chest and neck soft tissues
         f) Neck CT scan: assess for fractures, hematomas, and dislocations
2. Analysis: differential nursing diagnoses/collaborative problems
   a. Ineffective airway clearance
   b. Ineffective gas exchange
   c. Ineffective breathing pattern
   d. Anxiety/fear
3. Planning and implementation/interventions
   a. Maintain airway, breathing, circulation (see Chapters 1 and 32)
   b. Provide supplemental oxygen
      1) Rapid sequence intubation (RSI) and ventilatory support
      2) High-flow oxygen
   c. Establish IV access for administration of crystalloid fluids/medications
   d. Prepare for/assist with medical interventions
      1) Advanced airway management
         a) Nasal or oral intubation: fiberoptic
         b) Supraglottic airway (e.g., King, Combitube, laryngeal mask airway)
         c) Surgical airway (e.g., cricothyrotomy)
      2) Institute cardiac and pulse oximetry monitoring
      3) Insert gastric tube and attach to suction as indicated
      4) Assist with hospital admission
   e. Administer pharmacologic therapy as ordered
      1) RSI premedications: sedatives, analgesics, neuromuscular blocking agents
      2) Nonnarcotic analgesics
      3) Narcotics
      4) Tetanus immunization
4. Evaluation and ongoing monitoring
   a. Airway patency
   b. Hemodynamic status
   c. Breath sounds and pulse oximetry
   d. Cardiac rate and rhythm
   e. Intake and output

C. FRACTURED TOOTH

Dentoalveolar trauma can cause fractures or injury to the teeth and supporting structures. Traumatic injuries are associated with falls, motor vehicle crashes, physical abuse, sports-related activities, and foreign objects that strike the oral structures. Seizures may also be responsible for intraoral injury. Tooth fractures may involve the crown, the root, or both, with or without exposure of the pulp. The Ellis classification system is commonly used to describe the fracture anatomy of teeth (Box 36.2).[9]

1. Assessment
   a. Subjective data collection
      1) History of present injury/chief complaint
         a) Mechanism of injury (see Chapter 31)
         b) Pain (see Chapter 8): affected tooth (dentin or pulp injury)
         c) Headache
         d) Nausea or vomiting
         e) Loss of consciousness or amnesia: assess for concomitant head injury (see Chapter 35)
         f) Treatment since injury

Box 36.2

Classification of Tooth Fractures

Fracture Classification	Area of Injury	Symptoms	Care Implications
Ellis I	Fractures through the enamel of the teeth	May have no visible color change or appear "chalky white." Rough edges may be palpated Nontender	Nonemergent dental referral for repair
Ellis II	Fractures extending through the enamel and into the underlying dentin	Fractured area may appear yellowish from exposed dentin Tooth is tender to touch and exposure to air	Dental referral for repair Calcium hydroxide or zinc oxide may be applied to the area to reduce sensitivity
Ellis III	Fractures through the enamel and dentin and into the underlying pulp	Visible areas of pink, red, or even blood may be present; the tooth will be tender	Urgent dental referral to reduce the risk of pulpitis and secondary infections Calcium hydroxide or zinc oxide should be applied to the area to reduce sensitivity and protect the underlying pulp

Table based on information obtained from: Thomas, J. J. (2014). Fractured teeth. Medscape. Retrieved from http://emedicine.medscape.com/article/82755-overview.

2) Past medical history
   a) Current or preexisting diseases/illness
   b) Previous dental injury, disease, surgery, or cosmetic repair (e.g., crowns)
   c) Medications
   d) Allergies
   e) Immunization status
   b. Objective data collection
   1) Physical examination
      a) General appearance
         (1) Moderate distress/discomfort
      b) Inspection
         (1) Primary or permanent teeth: number involved
         (2) Involvement of enamel, dentin, pulp, or root
         (3) Malocclusion
         (4) Intraoral or extraoral soft tissue swelling, bleeding
      c) Palpation/percussion
         (1) Tenderness of tooth
   2) Diagnostic procedures
      a) Dental radiograph: panoramic radiograph (Panorex)
      b) Facial radiographs
2. Analysis: differential nursing diagnoses/collaborative problems
   a. Acute pain
   b. Anxiety/fear
   c. Risk for infection

3. Planning and implementation/interventions
   a. Maintain airway, breathing, circulation (see Chapters 1 and 32)
   b. Establish IV access for administration of crystalloid fluid/medications as needed
   c. Prepare for/assist with medical interventions
      1) Gently suction oral cavity
      2) Fracture involving enamel and dentin
         a) Apply calcium hydroxide or zinc oxide (if available) to protect tooth from further injury or contamination from exposure to saliva and air, which may lead to pulpitis
         b) Explore soft tissues for possible tooth fragments
         c) Provide timely dental referral for definitive treatment
      3) Fracture involving pulp
         a) Apply calcium hydroxide or zinc oxide to exposed crown surface
         b) Explore soft tissues for possible tooth fragments
   d. Administer pharmacologic therapy as ordered
      1) Nonnarcotic analgesics
      2) Narcotics
      3) Antibiotics
   e. Educate patient/significant others
      1) Provide dental referral
      2) Avoid eating solid foods for 24 hours
4. Evaluation and ongoing monitoring
   a. Pain relief

Part 3

D. MANDIBULAR FRACTURES

The types of situations most likely to cause mandibular fractures are direct blows to the mandible, such as with fists or clubs, or falling forward on the chin and catapulting forward, as a driver would in a motor vehicle crash.

The mandible's facial prominence makes it a frequently injured facial bone. Its location and U shape also make it prone to multiple fractures when force from one site is transmitted to another area distant from the impact site. Common fracture sites are the body of the mandible, the angle adjacent to the wisdom tooth, and mandibular condyle. TMJ dislocation may accompany mandibular fractures.

1. Assessment
    a. Subjective data collection
        1) History of present injury/chief complaint
            a) Mechanism of injury (see Chapter 31)
            b) Pain (see Chapter 8)
            c) Malocclusion
            d) Facial asymmetry
            e) Bleeding around mouth
            f) Paresthesia/numbness of lower lip due to involvement of the inferior alveolar nerve
            g) Trismus: inability to open mouth
            h) Soft tissue swelling or hematoma formation
            i) Ruptured tympanic membrane
        2) Past medical history
            a) Current or preexisting diseases/illness
            b) Previous dental, ENT, and/or facial trauma, fractures, or surgical procedures
            c) Medications
            d) Allergies
            e) Immunization status
    b. Objective data collection
        1) Physical examination
            a) General appearance
                (1) Level of consciousness, behavior, affect: anxiety, agitation
                (2) Possible drooling
                (3) Moderate to severe distress/discomfort
            b) Inspection
                (1) Facial wounds, swelling, asymmetry
                (2) Intraoral/sublingual soft tissue swelling, bleeding, ecchymosis
                (3) Malocclusion or lateral crossbite
                (4) Bleeding at gingival margin, broken or loose teeth
                (5) Trismus: inability to open mouth
                (6) Possible ruptured tympanic membrane or hemotympanum on the side of the injury
            c) Palpation
                (1) Point tenderness at fracture site
                (2) Bony defects palpable at fracture sites
                (3) Mobility of fracture fragments
                (4) Decreased or altered sensation on affected side

        2) Diagnostic procedures
            a) Panoramic radiograph (Panorex)
            b) Facial, skull radiographs: posteroanterior, lateral, and lateral oblique views
            c) Face, head CT scan
2. Analysis: differential nursing diagnoses/collaborative problems
    a. Risk for ineffective airway
    b. Acute pain
    c. Risk for infection
    d. Deficient knowledge
3. Planning and implementation/interventions
    a. Maintain airway, breathing, circulation (see Chapters 1 and 32)
    b. Provide supplemental oxygen
    c. Establish IV access for administration of crystalloid fluid/medications
    d. Prepare for/assist with medical interventions
        1) Position patient in high Fowler position if not contraindicated
        2) Suction frequently to prevent aspiration of secretions or blood
        3) Apply ice to minimize swelling and bleeding
        4) Assist with possible admission for operative intervention; displaced symptomatic fractures require reduction and fixation with intermaxillary or direct wiring
    e. Administer pharmacologic therapy as ordered
        1) Nonnarcotic analgesics
        2) Narcotics
        3) Antibiotics
        4) Tetanus immunization
    f. Educate patient/significant others
        1) Mechanical soft diet
        2) Immobilization orders
        3) Medication instructions
        4) Follow-up care
4. Evaluation and ongoing monitoring
    a. Airway patency
    b. Hemodynamic status
    c. Amount of swelling and bleeding
    d. Pain relief

E. MAXILLARY FRACTURES

The types of situations most likely to cause maxillary fractures are sustained direct blows to the maxilla with objects such as fists or clubs and rapid deceleration from motor vehicle crashes. Maxillary fractures are less common than mandibular fractures; they are considered to reflect significant facial trauma and are frequently associated with multisystem injuries. Maxillary fractures may involve the maxilla alone; however, they frequently occur in conjunction with fractures of other bones of the midface. These fractures are categorized as follows: (1) LeFort I (transverse fracture), maxillary fracture causing transverse detachment of the entire maxilla above the teeth at the level of the nasal floor; (2) LeFort II (pyramidal fracture), fracture of the midface that involves a triangular segment of the midportion of the face and the nasal bones; and (3) LeFort III (craniofacial disjunction), complete separation of the cranial attachments from the facial bones (Fig. 36.1). Maxillary fractures are not always clearly defined, and frequently they may occur in complete or partial combination with one another, such as left LeFort II and right LeFort III fractures. Many patients with maxillary fractures require airway management and resuscitation.

1. Assessment
   a. Subjective data collection
      1) History of present injury/chief complaint
         a) Mechanism of injury (see Chapter 31)
         b) Pain (see Chapter 8): face, cervical spine
         c) Bleeding, ecchymosis
         d) Swelling/asymmetry of face
         e) Infraorbital mobility and/or paresthesia
         f) Epistaxis
         g) Malocclusion
         h) Visual disturbances
         i) Cerebrospinal rhinorrhea: with LeFort II and III fractures
      2) Past medical history
         a) Current or preexisting diseases/illness
         b) Previous dental, ENT, and/or facial trauma, fractures, or surgical procedures
         c) Medications
         d) Allergies
         e) Immunization status
   b. Objective data collection
      1) Physical examination
         a) General appearance
            (1) Moderate to severe distress/discomfort, critically ill
         b) Inspection
            (1) Facial wounds, swelling, soft tissue injury
            (2) Facial asymmetry/distortion (elongation or flattening of midface)
            (3) Malocclusion or anterior open bite
            (4) Intraoral ecchymosis
            (5) Periorbital edema, ecchymosis, bony deformity
            (6) Subconjunctival hemorrhage
            (7) Epistaxis
            (8) Cerebrospinal rhinorrhea (LeFort II and III fractures)
            (9) Evidence of intracranial and/or spinal injuries (see Chapter 35)
            (10) Evidence of multisystem injuries
         c) Palpation
            (1) Midface maxillary mobility
            (2) Infraorbital paresthesia
      2) Diagnostic procedures
         a) Facial radiographs with Waters' view
         b) Individual facial bones radiographs: mandible, zygomas, nose, orbits
         c) Face, head CT scans
2. Analysis: differential nursing diagnoses/collaborative problems
   a. Risk for ineffective airway clearance
   b. Acute pain
3. Planning and implementation/interventions
   a. Maintain airway, breathing, circulation (see Chapters 1 and 32)
   b. Provide supplemental oxygen
      1) RSI and ventilatory support for obtunded patient or if airway compromise present
      2) High-flow oxygen
   c. Establish IV access for administration of crystalloid fluid/blood products/medications
   d. Prepare for/assist with medical interventions
      1) Advanced airway management
         a) Nasal or oral intubation
         b) Supraglottic airway (e.g., King, Combitube, laryngeal mask airway)
         c) Surgical airway (e.g., cricothyrotomy)

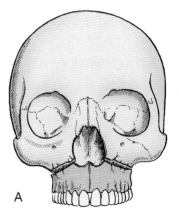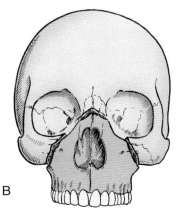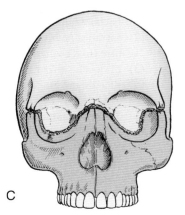

FIG. 36.1 LeFort classification of maxillary fractures: A, transverse fracture; B, pyramidal fracture; and C, craniofacial disjunction. *(From Dandy, DJ and Edwards, DJ. (2009). Essential orthopaedics and trauma (5th ed.). St. Louis, MO: Elsevier/Churchill Livingstone.)*

2) Position patient for optimal airway clearance and comfort (e.g., high Fowler position if no concurrent spine injury)
3) Gently suction oral cavity
4) Institute cardiac and pulse oximetry monitoring
5) Insert gastric tube and attach to suction as indicated
6) Assist with hospital admission for definitive treatment of fractures
   a) Open reduction
   b) Internal wiring for stabilization
   e. Administer pharmacologic therapy as ordered
1) RSI premedications: sedatives, analgesics, neuromuscular blocking agents
2) Nonnarcotic analgesics
3) Narcotics
4) Antibiotics
5) Tetanus immunization
4. Evaluation and ongoing monitoring
   a. Airway patency
   b. Hemodynamic status
   c. Breath sounds and pulse oximetry
   d. Cardiac rate and rhythm
   e. Pain relief
   f. Intake and output

F. NASAL FRACTURE

The thinness of the nasal bones, coupled with their prominent location on the face, makes them a frequent site of fracture.[7] Nasal fractures resulting from direct trauma to the nose can cause epistaxis, soft tissue swelling, nasal/septal hematoma, periorbital ecchymosis, and subconjunctival hemorrhage. Signs of deformity, asymmetry, and inflammation may be present, and crepitus may be noted on palpation of the nose. Radiologic assessment of suspected nasal fractures may be obtained to determine the extent of injury. Treatment measures include maintaining airway patency, reducing fractures, minimizing swelling, and controlling bleeding and pain. Applying ice and providing analgesic medications reduce pain and swelling. Intranasal examination is performed to rule out septal hematoma, which will appear as a large purple mass extending from the septum. When this exists, efforts to evacuate the clot immediately are undertaken to avoid secondary complications associated with septal necrosis and nasal deformity. Antibiotics may be administered to prevent infection. Cosmetic repair of nasal deformities is often delayed to allow reduction of edema.

1. Assessment
   a. Subjective data collection
      1) History of present injury/chief complaint
         a) Trauma: blunt or penetrating forces (see Chapter 31)
         b) Pain (see Chapter 8)
         c) Visual deformity of nasal bone or cartilage
         d) Swelling
         e) Nasal bleeding
         f) Nasal obstruction
         g) Loss of consciousness
      2) Past medical history
         a) Current or preexisting diseases/illness
         b) Nasal surgery or defects
         c) Medications
         d) Allergies
         e) Immunization status: if open wounds are present
   b. Objective data collection
      1) Physical examination
         a) General appearance
            (1) Level of consciousness, behavior, affect: confusion, lethargy
            (2) Moderate distress/discomfort
         b) Inspection
            (1) Nasal deformity, asymmetry, or depression
            (2) Epistaxis
            (3) Obstruction of nasal cavity on fractured side
            (4) Nasal and periorbital ecchymosis with possible subconjunctival hemorrhage
            (5) Septal fracture, hematoma, or submucosal hemorrhage
         c) Palpation
            (1) Crepitus or false motion of nasal bone
            (2) Pain or tenderness of nose
      2) Diagnostic procedures
         a) Facial/nasal radiograph: frequently not performed
         b) Facial CT scan more useful
2. Analysis: differential nursing diagnoses/collaborative problems
   a. Acute pain
   b. Anxiety/fear
3. Planning and implementation/interventions
   a. Maintain airway, breathing, circulation (see Chapters 1 and 32)
   b. Provide supplemental oxygen as indicated
   c. Establish IV access for administration of crystalloid fluids/medications as needed
   d. Prepare for/assist with medical interventions
      1) Hemorrhage control and evacuation of clot in septum as indicated
         a) Apply direct pressure to nose
         b) Assist with anterior or posterior nasal packing if necessary
   e. Administer pharmacologic therapy as ordered
      1) Anesthetics
      2) Decongestants
      3) Vasoconstrictors
      4) Nonnarcotic analgesics
      5) Narcotics
      6) Antibiotics

7) Tetanus immunization
f. Educate patient/significant others
  1) Return to emergency department if uncontrolled bleeding reoccurs
  2) Provide follow-up instructions for packing removal
  3) Fracture reduction may be performed 7–10 days after swelling subsides
4. Evaluation and ongoing monitoring
  a. Hemodynamic status
  b. Bleeding control
  c. Pain relief

G. SUBLUXED/AVULSED TEETH

Forces similar to those that result in fractured teeth are also responsible for causing subluxed (loose) or avulsed (no longer in the socket) teeth. Up to 10% of emergency department visits are due to dental trauma with subluxations accounting for 50% of tooth injuries and as many as 5 million dental avulsions occurring annually in the United States alone.[10] Examining the gingival crevice of the tooth may identify subluxation. Blood is usually visualized. Gentle finger pressure applied to the affected tooth reveals varying degrees of mobility within the socket. Minimal mobility usually heals within 2 weeks, so patients are placed on a soft diet. Referral to a dentist or oral surgeon is indicated when the pulp is exposed and the tooth is grossly mobile. When applicable, partially avulsed teeth should be repositioned for stability. Complete tooth avulsion is a dental emergency, and measures should be taken to preserve the tooth for successful replantation. Permanent retention of avulsed teeth should occur within 30 minutes to optimize successful replantation although with proper handling, the tooth may be implanted hours later. Minimal handling of avulsed teeth is encouraged, and only the crown should be handled. If debris is present, the tooth should be gently cleansed or immersed only in normal saline solution, and debris should not be scrubbed from the root surface. The tooth should be immediately placed in the tooth socket to preserve and increase viability. If replantation is delayed, the tooth should be placed in a pH-balanced transport medium, such as Hank solution (Save-A-Tooth) or milk, or inside the buccal sulcus during transport for definitive treatment. Primary deciduous, or baby teeth, should not be replanted because they heal by fusing to the bone. This may cause difficulty with the eruption of permanent teeth and could lead to cosmetic deformities.

1. Assessment
  a. Subjective data collection
    1) History of present injury/chief complaint
      a) Injury resulting in displacement of tooth from alveolar socket
      b) Pain (see Chapter 8)
      c) Blood at site of avulsion
      d) Loss of consciousness
      e) Other injuries
    2) Past medical history
      a) Current or preexisting diseases/illness
      b) Dental injuries or disease
      c) Medications
      d) Allergies
      e) Immunization status
  b. Objective data collection
    1) Physical examination
      a) General appearance
        (1) Level of consciousness: anxiety
        (2) Mild to moderate distress/discomfort
      b) Inspection
        (1) Primary or permanent teeth involved
        (2) Number of teeth involved
        (3) Oral cavity for presence of foreign objects, blood, and other injuries
        (4) Extraoral wounds
      c) Auscultation
        (1) Breath sounds: possible wheezes if aspiration occurred
    2) Diagnostic procedures
      a) Dental radiograph: panoramic radiograph (Panorex)
      b) Chest radiograph: to rule out aspiration if tooth cannot be located
2. Analysis: differential nursing diagnoses/collaborative problems
  a. Acute pain
  b. Anxiety/fear
  c. Risk for infection
  d. Risk for ineffective airway clearance
3. Planning and implementation/interventions
  a. Maintain airway, breathing, circulation (see Chapters 1 and 32)
  b. Provide supplemental oxygen as indicated
  c. Establish IV access for administration of crystalloid fluid/medication as needed
  d. Prepare for/assist with medical interventions
    1) Gently suction oral cavity
    2) Assist with replantation of avulsed tooth
      a) Clean by rinsing with normal saline or cold water (do not scrub tooth, do not handle the root of the tooth)
      b) Suction blood from socket
    3) Replant within 30 minutes of injury for best results or up to 6 hours maximum
  e. Administer pharmacologic therapy as ordered
    1) Local anesthesia
    2) Antibiotics
  f. Educate patient/significant others
    1) Instruct patient not to bite into anything with affected tooth
    2) Avoid hot and cold substances
    3) Refer to dentist or oral surgeon for further treatment and follow-up care

4. Evaluation and ongoing monitoring
   a. Airway patency
   b. Hemodynamic status
   c. Replanted tooth stability
   d. Pain relief

H. TEMPOROMANDIBULAR JOINT DISLOCATION

Temporomandibular joint (TMJ) dislocation is a displacement of the mandibular condyle outside of its function position causing spasms and muscle contractions of the jaw muscles preventing the condyles from returning to their normal position. TMJ dislocation may be unilateral or bilateral, and it may result from trauma or simply from opening one's mouth too widely, such as during yawning or when undergoing dental work.[11] TMJ dislocations may accompany mandibular fractures. Associated risk factors include malocclusion, poorly fitted dentures, grinding or clenching of the teeth (bruxism), and emotional stress, which may alter muscular balance.

1. Assessment
   a. Subjective data collection
      1) History of present injury/chief complaint
         a) Mechanism of injury (see Chapter 31)
         b) Wide and/or prolonged opening of mouth just before dislocation
         c) Inability to close mouth
         d) Malocclusion
         e) Headache
         f) Earache
         g) Pain (see Chapter 8)
            (1) Usually worsens with jaw movement ("pop, click, or snap" sensation)
            (2) Neck pain
      2) Past medical history
         a) Current or preexisting diseases/illness
            (1) Arthritis
         b) Medications
         c) Allergies
   b. Objective data collection
      1) Physical examination
         a) General appearance
            (1) Drooling
            (2) Speech difficulty
            (3) Moderate distress/discomfort
         b) Inspection
            (1) Malocclusion
            (2) Open mouth with inability to close
            (3) Limited range of motion
         c) Palpation
            (1) Pain on palpation over TMJ: a depression just below the zygomatic arch, 1–2 cm anterior to the tragus
            (2) Tenderness or spasm of masseter muscle
      2) Diagnostic procedures
         a) Open and closed mouth radiographs of TMJ; postreduction views if reduced
         b) MRI: study of choice for traumatic TMJ injury
2. Analysis: differential nursing diagnoses/collaborative problems
   a. Acute pain
   b. Deficient knowledge
   c. Anxiety/fear
   d. Risk for ineffective airway clearance
3. Planning and implementation/interventions
   a. Establish IV access for administration of crystalloid fluids/medications as needed
   b. Prepare for/assist with medical interventions
      1) Gently suction oral cavity
      2) Assist with manual reduction of jaw: consider procedural sedation (see Chapter 8)
      3) Assist with hospital admission if severe pain or spasm after reduction (rare)
   c. Administer pharmacologic therapy as ordered
      1) Nonnarcotic analgesics
      2) Narcotics
      3) Procedural sedation medications to facilitate reduction, as needed (see Chapter 8)
   d. Educate patient/significant others
      1) Soft diet for 3–4 days to reduce chewing
      2) Avoidance of stress on TMJ
      3) Medication instructions (e.g., analgesics and muscle relaxants as needed)
      4) Awareness of any habits of teeth clenching or grinding and relaxing the jaw
      5) Avoidance of wide, uncontrolled mouth opening (e.g., yawning)
4. Evaluation and ongoing monitoring
   a. Airway patency
   b. Jaw movement after relocation
   c. Pain relief

I. ZYGOMATIC FRACTURES

Motor vehicle crashes, interpersonal altercations, and other types of trauma are the most common causes of zygomatic fractures. The types of situations most likely to result in zygomatic fractures are direct blows to the prominence of the zygoma or malar eminence (e.g., with fists or clubs) and falling on the side of the face. Some zygomatic fractures are called *tripod fractures* and involve all the zygomatic suture lines. Fractures of the zygoma are frequently associated with orbital floor fractures. These are called blow-out fractures.

1. Assessment
   a. Subjective data collection
      1) History of present injury/chief complaint
         a) Mechanism of injury (see Chapter 31)
         b) Pain (see Chapter 8)
         c) Bleeding
         d) Swelling

Part 3

e) Pain with jaw movement
f) Visual disturbances
2) Past medical history
  a) Current or preexisting diseases/illness
  b) Previous dental, ENT, and/or facial trauma, fractures, or surgical procedures
  c) Medications
  d) Allergies
  e) Immunization status
b. Objective data collection
  1) Physical examination
    a) General appearance
      (1) Moderate distress/discomfort
    b) Inspection
      (1) Facial wounds
      (2) Periorbital ecchymosis (most common)
      (3) Local bleeding, soft tissue swelling, edema, ecchymosis
      (4) Facial asymmetry
        (a) Flattened cheek on affected side or bony deformity over malar eminence
        (b) Depression of infraorbital rim with downward displacement of globe of eye on affected side
      (5) Epistaxis: usually unilateral
      (6) Binocular diplopia
      (7) Subconjunctival hemorrhage
      (8) Limited movement of lower jaw
    c) Palpation
      (1) Point tenderness along zygomatic arch and lateral and infraorbital rim
      (2) Bony defect over zygomatic arch
      (3) Paresthesia of cheek, nose, and upper lip of affected side
      (4) Subcutaneous emphysema of face may indicate that fracture extends to paranasal sinuses
  2) Diagnostic procedures
    a) Facial CT scan: diagnostic imaging of choice
    b) Zygomatic radiograph: Caldwell projection provides evaluation of the zygomatic process; submental vertex view provides detail of the zygomatic arches
    c) Facial radiographs and Waters' views are less helpful
2. Analysis: differential nursing diagnoses/collaborative problems
  a. Acute pain
3. Planning and implementation/interventions
  a. Maintain airway, breathing, circulation (see Chapters 1 and 32)
  b. Provide supplemental oxygen as indicated

c. Establish IV access for administration of crystalloid fluid/medications as needed
d. Prepare for/assist with medical interventions
  1) Position patient for comfort and elevate head (if spinal injury is ruled out)
  2) Apply ice to fracture site
  3) Prepare for admission for definitive treatment of fracture by physician
    a) Open reduction
    b) Internal wire fixation
e. Administer pharmacologic therapy as ordered
  1) Nonnarcotic analgesics
  2) Narcotics
  3) Antibiotics if open fractures
  4) Tetanus immunization
4. Evaluation and ongoing monitoring
  a. Pain relief

References

1. Olitsky SE, Hug D, Plummer LS, Stahl ED, Ariss MM, Lindquist TP: Examination of the eye. In Kliegman RM, Stanton BF, St Geme JW, Schor NF, editors: *Nelson textbook of pediatrics*, ed 20, Philadelphia, PA, 2016, Mosby-Elsevier, pp 3016–3019.
2. Pargament JM, Armenia J, Nerad JA: Physical and chemical injuries to eyes and eyelids, *Clinics in Dermatology* 33(2):234–237, 2015.
3. Knoop KJ, Dennis WR, Hedges JR: Ophthalmologic procedures. In Roberts JR, Hedges JR, editors: *Roberts & Hedges' clinical procedures in emergency medicine*, ed 3, Philadelphia, PA, 2014, Saunders (chap. 62, pp. 1257–1259).
4. Bhatia K, Sharma R: Eye emergencies. In Adams JG, editor: *Emergency medicine*, Philadelphia, PA, 2013, Saunders, pp 209–225.
5. Ing E: Eyelid laceration. Medscape. Retrieved from http://emedicine.medscape.com/article/1212531-overview, 2015.
6. Sharma R, Brunette DD: Ophthalmology. In Marx JA, Hockberger RS, Walls RM, editors: *Rosen's emergency medicine*, ed 8, Philadelphia, PA, 2014, Saunders, pp 909–930.
7. Mayersak RJ: Facial trauma. In Marx JA, Hockberger RS, Walls RM, editors: *Rosen's emergency medicine*, Philadelphia, PA, 2014, Saunders, pp 368–381.
8. Newton K, Claudius I: Neck. In Marx JA, Hockberger RS, Walls RM, editors: *Rosen's emergency medicine*, ed 8, Philadelphia, PA, 2014, Saunders, pp 4210–4230.
9. Thomas JJ: Fractured teeth. Medscape. Retrieved from http://emedicine.medscape.com/article/82755-overview, 2014.
10. Fowler GC: Management of dental emergencies and reimplantation of an avulsed tooth. In Pfenninger JL, Fowler GC, editors: *Pfenninger and Fowler's procedures for primary care*, ed 3, Philadelphia, PA, 2011, Mosby-Elsevier, pp 511–515.
11. Liddell A, Perez DE: Temporomandibular joint dislocation, *Oral and Maxillofacial Surgery Clinics* 27(1):125–136, 2015.

Part 3

CHAPTER 37

Trauma in Pregnancy

Rebecca A. Steinmann, MS, APN, CPEN, CEN, TCRN, CCRN, CCNS, FAEN

Trauma is the leading nonobstetrical cause of maternal death and disability during pregnancy impacting 6–7% of all gestations. The most common type of injury in pregnant women is blunt force trauma resulting from motor vehicle crashes, which account for approximately 60% of all major injuries. Other mechanisms include intimate partner violence, falls, burns and inhalation injury, firearm, and stab wound injuries. Head injury and hemorrhagic shock account for the majority of maternal deaths. Although being pregnant does not increase the morbidity and mortality due to trauma, the presence of a gravid uterus does alter pattern injury. The most common cause of fetal death in major trauma is maternal death. Placental abruption and preterm delivery are the leading cause of fetal mortality and morbidity secondary to minor trauma. Resuscitation priorities for the injured pregnant patient are identical to those of her nonpregnant counterparts, using the "ABCDE" approach (see Chapters 1 and 32). Assessment of the fetus occurs within the secondary survey. Maternal anatomic and physiologic adaptations designed to nourish the fetus can alter the signs and symptoms of injury (Table 37.1). Pregnancy does not limit or restrict any resuscitative, diagnostic, or pharmacologic treatment. Optimal resuscitation of the mother affords the best fetal outcome. Obstetric expertise should be accessed early in the resuscitation process as the trauma team simultaneously manages two patients—the mother and the fetus.

I. General Strategy

A. ASSESSMENT

1. Primary and secondary assessment/resuscitation (see Chapters 1 and 32)

a. Every female of reproductive age with significant injuries should be considered pregnant until proven otherwise by a definitive pregnancy test or ultrasound scan[1]
b. Differences during pregnancy
  1) Primary survey: airway: greater risk for airway problems including difficult intubation; therefore, early intubation should be considered whenever airway problems are anticipated
    a) Decreased functional residual capacity
    b) Reduced respiratory system compliance
    c) Increased airway resistance
    d) Increased oxygen requirements
    e) Increased mucosal edema: consider a smaller size ETT
  2) Injured pregnant women with an unsecured airway are at increased risk for aspiration of gastric contents. Gastric emptying is delayed in pregnancy and pregnant women should be considered to have a full stomach for up to 24 hours after their last meal[1]
2. Focused assessment
a. Subjective data collection
  1) History of present injury/chief complaint
    a) Mechanism of injury (see Chapter 31)
      (1) Motor vehicle crash (MVC)
        (a) Seat belt use and placement: major risk factor for adverse outcomes during MVC is improper seat belt use
        (b) Position in the vehicle
      (2) Falls: height of fall
      (3) Other cause of blunt force or penetrating trauma

Table 37.1

Anatomic and Physiologic Changes in Pregnancy

System	Alteration	Effect
Cardiovascular	Increased total blood volume	Improved tolerance to hemorrhage
	Increased cardiac output	Increased heart rate 15–20 beats/min
	Decreased peripheral vascular	Decreased systolic (0–15 mm Hg) and diastolic resistance (10–20 mm Hg) blood pressure
	Aortocaval compression	Supine hypotensive syndrome
	Selective uterine vasoconstriction in response to hemorrhage	Fetal hypoxia
Hematologic	Increased plasma volume	Dilutional anemia (hematocrit 32–34%)
	Leukocytosis	WBC up to 20,000/mm³
	Hypercoagulability	Increased risk of disseminated intravascular coagulation with thromboplastin release
Respiratory	Increased minute ventilation	Decreased PCO_2 (30–34 mm Hg)
	Increased tidal volume	Decreased serum bicarbonate (18–22 mEq/L)
		Partially compensated respiratory alkalosis
	Elevation of diaphragm	Decreased functional residual capacity
		Decreased tolerance to hypoxia
	Increased oxygen consumption	Increased risk of maternal and fetal hypoxia
Gastrointestinal	Decreased motility and emptying	Increased risk of vomiting and aspiration
	Compartmentalization of the small intestine into the upper abdomen	Increased risk of injury
	Stretched and relaxed abdominal wall	Masked intraabdominal injury
Urinary	Elevation and compression of bladder	Increased risk of injury

PCO_2, Partial pressure of carbon dioxide; *WBC*, white blood cell.

b) Loss of consciousness: eclampsia may mimic head injury
c) Pain (see Chapter 8)
d) Vaginal bleeding or fluid leak
e) Uterine contractions/abdominal pain
f) Fetal movement prior to and since injury
g) Efforts to relieve symptoms
  (1) Home remedies
  (2) Alternative therapies
  (3) Medications
    (a) Prescription
    (b) OTC/herbal
2) Past medical history
a) Current or preexisting diseases/illness
b) Last normal menstrual period, expected date of confinement
c) Reproductive history
d) Prenatal care
e) Previous surgical procedures
f) Smoking history
g) Substance and/or alcohol use/abuse
h) Current medications
  (1) Prescription
  (2) OTC/herbal
i) Allergies
j) Immunization status

3) Psychological/social/environmental factors related to trauma in pregnancy
a) Support network
  (1) Family
  (2) Friends
  (3) Clergy or religious support
b) Stress factors
  (1) Lifestyle
  (2) Coping patterns
  (3) Precipitating event
  (4) Possible/actual assault, abuse, or intimate partner violence situations (see Chapters 3 and 40)
c) Psychological illnesses
b. Objective data collection
1) General appearance
a) Level of consciousness, behavior, affect
b) Vital signs (see Table 37.1)
c) Odors
d) Gait
e) Hygiene
f) Level of distress/discomfort
2) Inspection
a) Abdominal girth, uterine size (Fig. 37.1)
b) Abdominal ecchymosis
c) Uterine contractions

7) Kleihauer-Betke test: detects fetal red blood cells in the maternal circulation indicating fetomaternal hemorrhage
8) Serum and urine toxicology screen, blood alcohol level
9) Arterial blood gas (ABG) determination: carbon dioxide ($PaCO_2$) of 35–45 may indicate impending respiratory failure (PCO_2 levels are normally lower during pregnancy secondary to increased minute ventilation)
10) pH of vaginal secretions/fluid or bedside point-of-care test (pH of vaginal secretions is 5.0; pH of amniotic fluid is 7.5)
b. Imaging studies
1) Diagnostic imaging examinations should not be deferred because of pregnancy, but fetal exposure to radiation should be limited as much as possible. Radiologic examinations must be interpreted in the context of pregnancy-related changes
2) Transabdominal sonography/Focused Assessment Sonography for Trauma (FAST)
3) Abdominal, pelvic, or transvaginal sonography
4) Maternal radiographic procedures as indicated based on assessment findings and mechanism of injury
5) Computed tomography (CT) scan
   a) Head and chest CT if indicated
   b) Abdominal CT should be avoided in early pregnancy if possible; if CT is necessary, contrast media should be administered
c. Other
1) Cardiotocography: monitoring fetal heart rate and uterine contractions in pregnancy >20 weeks' gestation
2) 12- to 15-lead electrocardiogram (ECG): ectopic beats may increase during pregnancy
3) Possible diagnostic peritoneal lavage (DPL)

B. ANALYSIS: DIFFERENTIAL NURSING DIAGNOSES/COLLABORATIVE PROBLEMS

1. Risk for ineffective airway clearance
2. Risk for ineffective breathing patterns
3. Impaired gas exchange
4. Risk for decreased cardiac output
5. Ineffective tissue perfusion
6. Deficient fluid volume
7. Impaired skin integrity
8. Risk for infection
9. Pain
10. Anxiety/fear
11. Anticipatory grieving (potential fetal loss)
12. Risk for ineffective coping
13. Risk for other-directed violence
14. Deficient knowledge

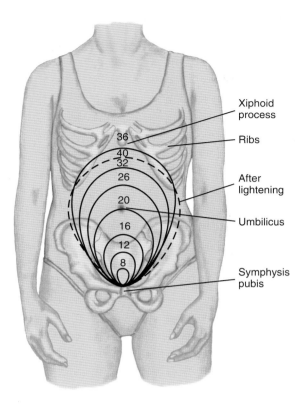

FIG. 37.1 Uterine Growth Patterns During Pregnancy (*From Murray, S. S., & McKinney, E. S. [2014]. Foundations of maternal-newborn nursing [6th ed.]. St. Louis, MO: Elsevier Saunders.*)

d) Vaginal lacerations
e) Vaginal bleeding/discharge/fluid leak
f) Crowning/presenting fetal parts
3) Auscultation
   a) Fetal heart tones (detectable by Doppler at 10–12 weeks' gestation; normal heart rate 120–160 beats/minute)
   b) Bowel sounds
4) Palpation
   a) Abdominal tenderness
   b) Fundal height (Fig. 37.2)
   c) Palpable fetal parts
   d) Contractions
3. Diagnostic procedures
a. Laboratory studies
1) Complete blood count (CBC) with differential
2) Serum chemistries including glucose, BUN, creatinine
3) Coagulation profile: prothrombin time (PT), partial thromboplastin time (PTT), fibrinogen, fibrin split products, D-dimer
4) Blood type, Rh determination, crossmatch
5) Urinalysis, pregnancy test
6) Serial hemoglobin and hematocrit

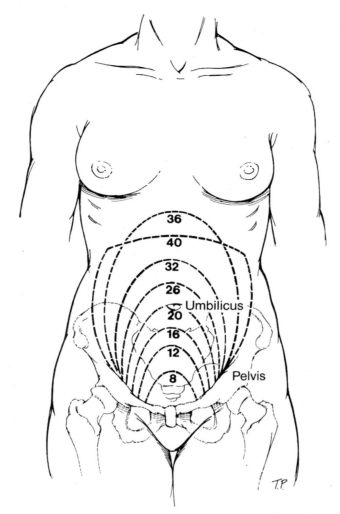

FIG. 37.2 Uterine Size and Location Reflecting Gestational Age *(From Mattson, S. & Smith, J. E. [2016]. Core Curriculum for Maternal-Newborn Nursing [5th ed.]. St. Louis, MO: Saunders/Elsevier.)*

C. PLANNING AND IMPLEMENTATION/ INTERVENTIONS

1. Determine priorities of care
   a. Maintain airway, breathing, circulation (see Chapters 1 and 32)
   b. Provide supplemental oxygen as indicated, to maintain maternal oxygen saturation >95% to ensure adequate fetal oxygenation
   c. Establish IV access for administration of crystalloid fluid/blood products/medications as needed
   d. Maintain patient in lateral decubitus position or if patient is immobilized on spinal board, tilt board 15 degrees, or manually displace gravid uterus to the left (in patients >20 weeks' gestation, compression of the inferior vena cava from the gravid uterus can decrease cardiac output as much as 30% because of decreased venous return from the lower extremities)
   e. Obtain and set up equipment and supplies

   f. Prepare for/assist with medical interventions
      1) If needed, a thoracostomy tube should be inserted in an injured pregnant woman one or two intercostal spaces higher than usual
   g. Administer pharmacologic therapy as indicated
      1) Because of their adverse effect on uteroplacental perfusion, vasopressors in pregnant women should be used only for intractable hypotension that is unresponsive to fluid resuscitation
   h. A nasogastric tube should be inserted in a semiconscious or unconscious injured pregnant woman to prevent aspiration of acidic gastric content
   i. Consider admission or transfer to a maternity facility for higher level of care and fetal monitoring
2. Relieve anxiety/apprehension
3. Allow significant others to remain with patient if supportive
4. Educate patient/significant others

D. EVALUATION AND ONGOING MONITORING

1. Continuously monitor and treat as indicated
2. Monitor patient response/outcomes, and modify nursing care plan as appropriate
3. If positive patient outcomes are not demonstrated, reevaluate assessment and/or plan of care

E. DOCUMENTATION OF INTERVENTIONS AND PATIENT RESPONSE

F. AGE-RELATED CONSIDERATIONS

1. Pediatric
   a. Growth or development related
      1) Approximately 10% of females between ages 15 and 19 years become pregnant each year
      2) Preterm labor more common in adolescent patients
   b. "Pearls"
      1) Prenatal care is frequently lacking
      2) Many adolescent mothers are from disadvantaged backgrounds
2. Geriatric/midlife pregnancies
   a. Aging related
      1) Women may become pregnant in later years through hormone replacement and either egg donation or in vitro fertilization
      2) Increased risk of fetal chromosomal abnormalities with menopausal or postmenopausal pregnancy
      3) Increased risk of osteoporosis developing during menopausal or postmenopausal pregnancy
   b. "Pearls"
      1) Other preexisting medical conditions may complicate pregnancies in older women

II. Specific Injuries of the Pregnant Trauma Patient

A. MATERNAL CARDIOPULMONARY ARREST

Viable neonates have been successfully delivered in cases of maternal cardiopulmonary arrest associated with traumatic injury. An emergent cesarean section must be performed within 20 minutes of maternal death and ideally should start within 4 minutes of maternal cardiopulmonary arrest. Hypoxia, injury to vital organs and structures, severe head injury, and extreme blood loss are all potential causes of maternal arrest. The fetus must be at least 23–24 weeks' gestation, and a team capable of neonatal resuscitation must be present with appropriate equipment. Improvement in maternal cardiopulmonary status and maternal survival after delivery has been reported in rare cases (maternal

cardiac filling is improved, thereby improving the success of cardiopulmonary resuscitation and resuscitative efforts).

1. Assessment
   a. Subjective data collection
      1) History of present injury/chief complaint
         a) Mechanism of injury (see Chapter 31)
         b) Time of arrest
         c) Gestational age of fetus
   b. Objective data collection
      1) Physical examination
         a) General appearance
            (1) Level of consciousness, behavior, affect: comatose
            (2) No maternal signs of life
            (3) Severe distress/discomfort, critically ill
         b) Inspection
            (1) Gravid uterus
         c) Auscultation
            (1) Presence/absence of fetal heart tones
      2) Diagnostic procedures
         a) Abdominal, pelvic/transvaginal sonography
2. Analysis: differential nursing diagnoses/collaborative problems
   a. Ineffective airway clearance
   b. Ineffective breathing pattern
   c. Impaired gas exchange
   d. Decreased cardiac output
   e. Deficient fluid volume
   f. Ineffective tissue perfusion
3. Planning and implementation/interventions
   a. Maintain airway, breathing, circulation (see Chapters 1 and 32)
      1) Initiate or continue Basic Life Support (BLS) and Advanced Life Support (ALS) per protocols
         a) Perform closed-chest compressions higher on the sternum, slightly above the center of the sternum
            (1) Manually displace uterus to the left for fundal height at or above the level of the umbilicus
         b) Open-chest cardiac massage may be more effective in patients with a large gravid uterus
         c) Remove fetal or uterine monitors before delivering electrical shocks for ventricular dysrhythmias
   b. Provide supplemental oxygen
      1) Intubation with ventilatory support
   c. Establish IV access for administration of crystalloid fluid/blood products/medications
   d. Prepare for/assist with medical interventions
      1) Advanced airway management
         a) Intubation
         b) Supraglottic airway (e.g., King, Combitube, laryngeal mask airway)
         c) Surgical airway (e.g., cricothyrotomy)

Part 3

2) Institute cardiac and pulse oximetry monitoring
3) Assist with collection and maintenance of physical and forensic evidence as indicated (see Chapter 44)
4) Assist with emergent cesarean delivery
5) Neonatal resuscitation as needed
   e. Administer pharmacologic therapy as ordered
      1) ALS medications per protocols
      2) Vasopressors
      3) Possible sodium bicarbonate to correct maternal acidosis
4. Evaluation and ongoing monitoring
   a. Maternal hemodynamic status following delivery
   b. Neonatal hemodynamic status

B. PLACENTAL ABRUPTION

Placental abruption (also known as abruptio placentae) is the most common cause of fetal demise following trauma where there is maternal survival. Premature separation of a portion of the placenta from the uterine wall disrupts maternal-fetal circulation. Of pregnant patients, 30–60% with major trauma, and as many as 5% with minor injuries, may experience an abruption. Placental abruption may be associated with use of lap belt restraints without shoulder restraint, which allows forward flexion of the torso and compression of the uterus. The extent to which the fetus is compromised is related to the amount of functional placenta that remains. Placental abruption may be associated with disseminated intravascular coagulation, which may develop as late as 48 hours after the initial trauma.

1. Assessment
   a. Subjective data collection
      1) History of present injury/chief complaint
         a) Mechanism of injury (see Chapter 31)
         b) Uterine tenderness
         c) Uterine contractions
         d) Pain (see Chapter 8): abdominal pain, cramping, back pain
      2) Past medical history
         a) Current or preexisting diseases/illness
            (1) Diabetes, hypertension
         b) Previous pregnancy complications
         c) Prenatal care
         d) Last normal menstrual period
         e) Medications
         f) Allergies
   b. Objective data collection
      1) Physical examination
         a) General appearance
            (1) Level of consciousness, behavior, affect: anxiety
            (2) Hypotension, tachycardia
            (3) Severe distress/discomfort, critically ill
         b) Inspection
            (1) Vaginal bleeding (may be present or absent)
            (2) Increasing fundal height or uterus that appears to be larger than normal for gestational age
            (3) Port wine–colored amniotic fluid
         c) Auscultation
            (1) Fetal heart tones: distress
               (a) Decreased fetal heart rate
               (b) Fetal heart rate decelerations
         d) Palpation
            (1) Uterine tetany, hypertonus, rigidity, irritability, or hypotonia
            (2) Preterm labor: contractions greater than six per hour
            (3) Increased or decreased fetal activity
      2) Diagnostic procedures
         a) CBC with differential
         b) Coagulation profile: PT, PTT, fibrinogen level, fibrin-split products
         c) Type and crossmatch
         d) Kleihauer-Betke test
         e) Serum chemistries
         f) Transabdominal sonography
            (1) Sonography has <50% sensitivity in the diagnosis of placental abruption
            (2) Negative initial examination should not be used as conclusive evidence to rule out placental abruption
         g) Cardiotocography for a minimum of 4 hours
2. Analysis: differential nursing diagnoses/collaborative problems
   a. Deficient fluid volume
   b. Ineffective tissue perfusion
   c. Acute pain
   d. Anticipatory grieving
3. Planning and implementation/interventions
   a. Maintain airway, breathing, circulation (see Chapters 1 and 32)
   b. Provide supplemental oxygen as indicated
   c. Establish IV access for administration of crystalloid fluid/blood products/medications as needed
   d. Maintain patient in left lateral decubitus position
   e. Prepare for/assist with medical interventions
      1) Institute cardiac and pulse oximetry monitoring
      2) Assist with collection and maintenance of physical and forensic evidence as indicated (see Chapter 44)
      3) Immediate cesarean delivery of infant
      4) Transport to labor and delivery unit when hemodynamically stable
      5) Neonatal resuscitation as needed
   f. Administer pharmacologic therapy as ordered
      1) Rh immune globulin (RhoGAM or Rhophylac) in all Rh-negative women

4. Evaluation and ongoing monitoring
   a. Maternal hemodynamic status
   b. Breath sounds and pulse oximetry
   c. Cardiac rate and rhythm
   d. Pain relief
   e. Cardiotocography
   f. Neonatal hemodynamic status

C. POSTTRAUMATIC PRETERM LABOR

Preterm labor is the most common obstetric complication in the pregnant trauma patient. Prostaglandins released after injury may cause uterine contractions. Preterm labor places the fetus at risk of premature birth and may indicate undiagnosed maternal injury. Continued contractions or uterine cramping may also be associated with placental abruption.

1. Assessment
   a. Subjective data collection
      1) History of present injury/chief complaint
         a) Mechanism of injury (see Chapter 31)
         b) Pain (see Chapter 8): abdominal pain/cramping/contractions/back pain
         c) Sudden gushes of vaginal fluid or feeling of having urinated
         d) Pelvic pressure
         e) Expected date of confinement
      2) Past medical history
         a) Current or preexisting diseases/illness
         b) Previous preterm labor or delivery
         c) Reproductive history: gravida/para
         d) Previous delivery complications
         e) Last normal menstrual period
         f) Medications
         g) Allergies
   b. Objective data collection
      1) Physical examination
         a) General appearance
            (1) Level of consciousness, behavior, affect: anxiety
            (2) Moderate distress/discomfort
         b) Inspection
            (1) Vaginal discharge
            (2) Possible presenting fetal part
         c) Auscultation
            (1) Fetal heart tones, rate: increased or decreased
         d) Palpation
            (1) Uterine contractions: greater than six per hour or occurring at least every 10 minutes
            (2) Fundal height
            (3) Cervical dilation or effacement
      2) Diagnostic procedures
         a) Cardiotocography
         b) pH of vaginal secretions

2. Analysis: differential nursing diagnoses/collaborative problems
   a. Pain
   b. Anxiety/fear
   c. Anticipatory grieving
3. Planning and implementation/interventions
   a. Provide supplemental oxygen as indicated
   b. Establish IV access for administration of crystalloid fluid/medications as needed
   c. Position mother in a lateral tilt position
   d. Prepare for/assist with medical interventions
      1) Emergency delivery if childbirth is imminent
      2) Assist with hospital admission to labor and delivery or obstetric unit
   e. Administer pharmacologic therapy as ordered
      1) Uterine contraction inhibitors if no placental abruption is present in the hemodynamically stable patient
4. Evaluation and ongoing monitoring
   a. Maternal hemodynamic status
   b. Cardiotocography for a minimum of 4 hours

D. UTERINE RUPTURE

Uterine rupture is rare, occurring in <1% of pregnant patients who have sustained major trauma, and is associated with a fetal mortality rate of almost 100%. Maternal mortality is usually associated with other injuries. Injury involving sudden deceleration, severe abdominal compression, or direct force to the abdomen can result in uterine rupture. Uterine rupture is more likely to occur in patients who have previously had a cesarean section and may also be associated with bladder rupture indicated by blood or meconium in the urine.

1. Assessment
   a. Subjective data collection
      1) History of present injury/chief complaint
         a) Mechanism of injury (see Chapter 31)
         b) Pain (see Chapter 8): abdominal pain; may be acute and severe, then decreases
         c) Uterine tenderness
      2) Past medical history
         a) Current or preexisting diseases/illness
         b) Previous pregnancy complications
         c) Prenatal care
         d) Last normal menstrual period
         e) Medications
         f) Allergies
   b. Objective data collection
      1) Physical examination
         a) General appearance
            (1) Level of consciousness, behavior; anxiety
            (2) Tachycardia, hypotension
            (3) Severe distress/discomfort, critically ill
         b) Inspection
            (1) Fundal height difficult to identify
            (2) Change or loss of contour of the uterus

(3) Vaginal bleeding: may be concealed
(4) Abnormal fetal position: extended extremities, oblique or transverse lie
   c) Auscultation
     (1) Fetal heart tones: distress or demise
       (a) Increased or decreased heart rate or no heart tones
   d) Palpation
     (1) Palpable mass or fetal parts outside the uterus
     (2) Abdominal guarding/rebound tenderness
     (3) Abdominal rigidity
     (4) Increased, decreased, or no fetal activity
  2) Diagnostic procedures
   a) Abdominal, pelvic/transvaginal sonography, FAST
   b) Abdominal CT scan
   c) Possible DPL
   d) Cardiotocography
2. Analysis: differential nursing diagnoses/collaborative problems
  a. Deficient fluid volume
  b. Ineffective tissue perfusion
  c. Acute pain
  d. Anticipatory grieving
3. Planning and implementation/interventions
  a. Maintain airway, breathing, circulation (see Chapters 1 and 32)
  b. Provide supplemental oxygen
  c. Establish IV access for administration of crystalloid fluids/blood products/medication as needed
  d. Maintain patient in left lateral decubitus position
  e. Prepare for/assist with medical interventions
   1) Institute cardiac and pulse oximetry monitoring
   2) Assist with collection and maintenance of physical and forensic evidence as indicated (see Chapter 44)
   3) Immediate cesarean delivery of infant
   4) Transport to labor and delivery unit when hemodynamically stable
   5) Neonatal resuscitation as needed
  f. Administer pharmacologic therapy as ordered
   1) Rh immune globulin (RhoGAM or Rhophylac) in all Rh-negative women
4. Evaluation and ongoing monitoring
  a. Maternal hemodynamic status
  b. Breath sounds and pulse oximetry
  c. Cardiac rate and rhythm

d. Abdomen to detect subtle changes
e. Pain relief
f. Neonatal hemodynamic status

References

1. Jain V, et al.: Guidelines for the management of pregnant trauma patient, *Journal of Obstetrics and Gynaecology Canada* 37(6):553–571, 2015.

Bibliography

American College of Surgeons: *Advanced trauma life support student course manual*, 9th ed., Chicago, IL, 2012, American College of Surgeons.

Barraco R, Chiu W, Clancy T, Como J, Ebert J, Hess L, Hoff W, Holevar M, Quirk J, Simon F, Weiss P: Practice management guidelines for the diagnosis and management of injury in the pregnant patient: The EAST Practice Management Guideline Work Group, *Journal of Trauma* 69(1):211–214, 2010.

ECC Committee, Subcommittees and Task Forces of the American Heart Association: 2015 American Heart Association for Cardiopulmonary Resuscitation and Emergency Cardiovascular Care. Part 10.1: Cardiac arrest associated with trauma, *Circulation* 132(18):S501–S518, 2015.

Emergency Nurses Association: Special populations: The pregnant trauma patient. In *Trauma nursing core course provider manual*, 7th ed., Des Plaines, IL, 2014, Emergency Nurses Association.

Kilpatrick SJ. *Trauma in pregnancy*, UpToDate, 2014. Retrieved from http://www.uptodate.com/contents/trauma-in-pregnancy.

Mendez-Figueroa H, Dahlke JD, Vrees RA, Rouse DJ: Trauma in pregnancy: an updated systematic review, *American Journal of Obstetrics & Gynecology* 209(1):1–10, 2013.

Murphy NJ, Quinlan JD: Trauma in pregnancy: Assessment, management, and prevention, *American Family Physician* 90(10):717–722, 2014.

Raja AS, Zabbo CP: Trauma in pregnancy, *Emerency Medical Clinics of North America* 30:937–948, 2013.

Repasky TM: Obstetric trauma. In Howard PK, Steinmann RA, editors: *Sheehy's emergency nursing principles and practice*, 6th ed., St. Louis, MO, 2010, Mosby/Elsevier, pp 382–392.

Trivedi N, Ylagan M, Moore TR, Bansal V, Wolfson T, Fortlage BA, Kelly T: Predicting adverse outcomes following trauma in pregnancy, *Journal of Reproductive Medicine* 57(1-2):3–8, 2012.

Wyant AR, Collett D: Trauma in pregnancy: Diagnosis and management of two patients in one, *Journal of the American Academy of Physician Assistants* 26(5):24–29, 2013.

CHAPTER 38

Orthopedic Trauma

Mary Jo Cerepani, DNP, FNP-BC, CEN

I. General Strategy

The aim in caring for the patient with an orthopedic emergency is to restore and preserve function.

A. ASSESSMENT

1. Primary and secondary assessment/resuscitation (see Chapters 1 and 32)
2. Focused assessment
   a. Subjective data collection
      1) History of present injury/chief complaint
         a) Trauma
            (1) Mechanism of injury (see Chapter 31)
               (a) Onset of symptoms
               (b) Duration of symptoms
               (c) Blunt or penetrating injury forces
               (d) Motor vehicle crash
               (e) Falls
               (f) Power tool injury
            (2) Precipitating factors: preexisting injuries, associated symptoms, medical problems
            (3) Aggravating factors
         b) Pain: PQRST (see Chapter 8)
         c) Associated symptoms
            (1) Changes in neurovascular function
            (2) Ability to bear weight
            (3) Range of motion
            (4) Weakness versus pain as presenting symptom
         d) Swollen areas
            (1) Onset
            (2) Size
            (3) Location
            (4) Symptoms: pain, tenderness, numbness, weakness
         e) Effort to relieve symptoms
            (1) Home remedies
            (2) Alternative therapies
            (3) Medications
               (a) Prescription
               (b) OTC/herbal
      2) Past medical history
         a) Current or preexisting diseases/illness
            (1) Anemia, bleeding, coagulation disorder
            (2) Cardiovascular disease (indication of peripheral vascular disease)
            (3) Diabetes mellitus (associated with peripheral neuropathy, decreased microcirculation)
            (4) Arthritis: degenerative or rheumatoid
            (5) Acute inflammatory diseases
            (6) Paget disease: localized areas of bone destruction followed by replacement

with overdeveloped, light, soft, porous bone and associated with deformities such as thickening of portions of the skull and bending of weight-bearing bones; cause unknown
- (7) Use of medications that predispose to fractures (e.g., phenytoin sodium and corticosteroids)
- (8) Disorders associated with peripheral nerve injury (Box 38.1)
- (9) Prior injury or surgery of affected extremity
- (10) Preexisting disabilities, metabolic disorders
- (11) Osteopenia or osteoporosis
- (12) Infections: septic arthritis or osteomyelitis in children
    - (a) Streptococcal infections
    - (b) Urinary tract infections
    - (c) Upper respiratory tract infections
    - (d) Ear infections
    - (e) Other infectious disorders
- b) Recent injury or problem with affected extremity
- c) Pregnancy: swelling precipitates overuse syndromes; prone to falls with pelvic ligament laxity
- d) Smoking history
- e) Substance and/or alcohol use/abuse
- f) Last normal menstrual period: female patients of childbearing age
- g) Vitamin deficiency
- h) Current medications
    - (1) Prescription
    - (2) OTC/herbal
- i) Allergies
- j) Immunization status
3) Psychological/social/environmental factors
- a) Stress factors
    - (1) Lifestyle
    - (2) Precipitating events
    - (3) Possible/actual assault, abuse, or intimate partner violence situations (see Chapters 3 and 40)

Box 38.1

Disorders Associated with Peripheral Nerve Injury

Alcoholism
Sudden significant weight loss
Carcinomatous neuropathy
Diabetic peripheral neuropathy
Previous trauma
Acute extremity compression

- b) Ability to perform activities of daily living
- c) Household or domicile residence factors
    - (1) Single, living alone
    - (2) Stairs
b. Objective data collection
1) General appearance
- a) Level of consciousness, behavior, affect
- b) Vital signs
- c) Gait
- d) Hygiene
- e) Odors
- f) Level of distress/discomfort
2) Inspection
- a) Comparison: examine both sides of body to visualize symmetry, contour, size, alignment
    - (1) Valgus: deformity of distal portion of joint that is angulated away from midline of body (e.g., knock-knees, hallux valgus)
    - (2) Varus: deformity of distal portion of joint that is angulated toward midline of body (e.g., bowleg and pigeon-toe)
- b) Skin and soft tissue
    - (1) Color changes and hair loss associated with peripheral vascular disease
    - (2) Soft tissue swelling or ecchymosis
    - (3) Gross deformities: associated with arthritis, tumors, swelling
    - (4) Muscle mass: hypertrophy and atrophy
    - (5) Scars indicative of previous injury, surgery, invasive procedures, intravenous (IV) drug abuse
- c) Joints
    - (1) Deformity (e.g., nodules in fingers, toes, knees)
    - (2) Swelling (e.g., inflammation, infection, trauma)
    - (3) Redness (e.g., inflammation associated with infection, cellulitis, and gouty arthritis)
    - (4) Range of motion (passive and active)
    - (5) Rotation: position of joint, extremity, ability to rotate internally or externally
- d) Peripheral vasculature
    - (1) Peripheral nerve assessment
    - (2) Skin for acute pallor; chronic cyanosis, pigmentation, circulatory changes
    - (3) Amount and distribution of hair
    - (4) Skin ulcers
    - (5) Veins for distention: unilateral versus bilateral
3) Palpation/percussion
- a) Skin and soft tissue
    - (1) Temperature and texture
    - (2) Swelling and pitting edema
- b) Quality of arterial pulses: brachial, radial, ulnar (overlying tissue may obscure, patency

determined by Allen test); femoral, popliteal, posterior tibial, and dorsalis pedis (may be congenitally absent or may branch higher in ankle); presence of pulse does not rule out arterial injury

    c) Grading of pulse quality (Table 38.1)
    d) Capillary refill test (Box 38.2)
    e) Muscle tone (Box 38.3)
    f) Muscle strength (Box 38.4)
    g) Deep tendon reflexes (Table 38.2)
    h) Joints
      (1) Temperature
      (2) Pain or tenderness with palpation
      (3) Crepitation with movement
      (4) Passive range of motion (done by examiner)
      (5) Joint laxity and stability (varies with each joint)
    i) Bones
      (1) Tenderness along length
      (2) Resistance to deforming force
      (3) Deformity, crepitus, tenderness

3. Diagnostic procedures
  a. Laboratory studies (Table 38.3)
    1) Complete blood count (CBC) with differential
    2) Erythrocyte sedimentation rate (ESR)
    3) Arterial blood gases (ABGs)
    4) Blood cultures
    5) Urinalysis; pregnancy test in female patients of childbearing age
  b. Imaging studies
    1) Radiographic films provide data on bone and joint changes; useful for diagnosing open joint injuries (air visible in joint space); standard imaging studies for acute fractures and

---

Table 38.1

Grading of Pulse Quality

Grade	Description
0	No pulse
1	Weak and easily obliterated with pressure
2	Difficult to palpate but easy to feel once located
3	Easily palpated and considered normal
4	Strong and bounding

Box 38.2

Capillary Refill Test

Used when unable to palpate pulses because of casts, splints, dressings

Is nonspecific measure of tissue perfusion, which can be affected by multiple factors

Normal time for color to return after blanching is 2 seconds or less

---

Box 38.3

Muscle Tone

Decreased as a result of musculoskeletal, neurologic, metabolic, or infectious disorders and/or fatigue

Increased as a result of spasms, injury, cramps, tremors (associated with electrolyte disorders, neurologic conditions, and infections such as tetanus)

Box 38.4

Muscle Strength

Assess range of motion before muscle strength, because muscular contraction may produce enough pain to inhibit further examination.

1. Ask patient to resist movement or move against resistance
2. Strength is subjectively graded by examiner on scale 1–5
3. All findings are recorded and used as a baseline
4. Grading of muscle strength
   0: Paralysis, no muscular contraction detected
   1: Only slight contractility and no joint motion
   2: Active movement, full range of motion with gravity eliminated
   3: Active movement, full range of motion against gravity
   4: Active movement, full range of motion against gravity and some resistance
   5: Active movement, full range of motion against full resistance

---

Table 38.2

Deep Tendon Reflexes*

Grading of Reflexes	
Grade	**Description**
0	No reflex
+1	Less than normal
+2	Average
+3	Stronger than average
+4	Intense (clonus)

*Assess major reflexes: biceps, brachioradialis, triceps, patellar knee jerk, Achilles tendon.

Table 38.3

Laboratory Studies to Aid Diagnosis of Orthopedic Conditions

Test	Examples
Alkaline phosphatase level	Increased with healing fractures, metabolic bone disease, osteoporosis, and metastatic tumors of bone
Calcium level	Increased with metastatic bone cancer, dehydration, Paget disease Decreased with hypoparathyroidism, advanced osteomalacia, and rickets
Creatine kinase level	Increased in dehydration, hyperthyroidism, renal failure, and rhabdomyolysis
Phosphorus level	Increased in bone metastases and hypoparathyroidism
Alanine aminotransferase	Increased in myositis (ALT), aspartate aminotransferase (AST)
Uric acid level	Increased in gout, multiple myeloma, and acute tissue destruction as a result of starvation or excessive exercise
C-reactive protein	Increased in acute inflammatory changes and rheumatoid arthritis
Antinuclear antibodies	Positive in rheumatoid arthritis, systemic lupus erythematosus, and polymyositis
Serum rheumatoid factor	Positive in rheumatoid arthritis and some chronic inflammatory diseases

dislocations; do not show soft tissue disorders except swelling
  2) Computed tomography (CT) used for diagnosis
    a) Fractures involving articular surfaces (e.g., tibial plateau, calcaneus, talus)
    b) Fracture/dislocations that are difficult to visualize or too dangerous to manipulate (e.g., pelvis for complex fractures, sacrum, acetabulum)
    c) Fracture of scapula, carpal bones, tarsal bones; dislocations of humeral and femoral heads, radioulnar or sternoclavicular joints
    d) Stress fractures
    e) Bony changes, metastatic processes
  3) Angiography: used to diagnose and treat vascular injuries, prevent hemorrhage, and relieve ischemia; useful for recognizing and selectively embolizing major bleeding vessels through an arterial catheter and injuries of extremities with suspected vascular involvement (e.g., knee dislocations or penetrating wounds)
  4) Magnetic resonance imaging (MRI): indicated for soft tissue disorders such as ligamentous injury, meniscal damage, tendon ruptures, muscle tears, tumors and hematomas, spinal structures, infection, degenerative disorders

  5) Bone scans: helpful in the identification of occult fractures and metastatic disease
  6) Arthroscopy: used to evaluate injury to joint structures
  7) Doppler sonography: assessment of arterial flow
 c. Other studies
  1) 12- to 15-lead electrocardiogram (ECG)

B. ANALYSIS: DIFFERENTIAL NURSING DIAGNOSES/COLLABORATIVE PROBLEMS

1. Acute pain
2. Activity intolerance
3. Risk for falls/injury
4. Anxiety/fear
5. Impaired skin integrity
6. Ineffective tissue perfusion
7. Risk for infection
8. Deficient knowledge

C. PLANNING AND IMPLEMENTATION/INTERVENTIONS

1. Determine priorities of care
  a. Maintain airway, breathing, circulation (see Chapters 1 and 32)
  b. Provide supplemental oxygen as indicated
  c. Establish IV access for administration of crystalloid fluids/blood products/medications as needed
  d. Obtain and set up equipment and supplies
  e. Prepare for/assist with medical interventions
  f. Administer pharmacologic therapy as ordered
2. Relieve anxiety/apprehension
3. Allow significant others to remain with patient if supportive
4. Educate patient/significant others

D. EVALUATION AND ONGOING MONITORING

1. Continuously monitor and treat as indicated
2. Monitor patient response/outcomes and modify nursing care plan as appropriate
3. If positive patient outcomes are not demonstrated, reevaluate assessment and/or plan of care

E. DOCUMENTATION OF INTERVENTIONS AND PATIENT RESPONSE

F. AGE-RELATED CONSIDERATIONS

1. Pediatric
  a. Growth or development related
    1) Child's bone structure different from adult's; children considered skeletally immature
    2) Skeleton of infant and young child is largely cartilaginous
      a) Bones narrow and flexible

3) Periosteum is thicker and resists disruption
   a) Provides circulation and nutrients to bone
   b) Allows bone to be more elastic and resists fracture
      (1) Greenstick: shaft of bone (diaphysis) fractured on one side, but cortex intact on other side
      (2) Torus: compression fracture of bone at the junction of the metaphysis and diaphysis causing "buckling"; patient often presents with pain but no deformity
4) Children have open epiphyses (growth plate) until after adolescence; this area is more susceptible to trauma; fractures to the epiphysis constitute one third of all fractures and are described according to Salter-Harris classification system (Fig. 38.1)
5) Child's ligaments are more resistant than epiphyses to trauma
   a) Dislocations rare
   b) Fractures often accompany dislocation
   c) Sprains (ligamental tears) unusual in young children but do occur in adolescents
6) General appearance
   a) Observe legs while child is walking
      (1) Infants have bowlegged (genu varum) appearance from birth to 2–3 years
      (2) Infants tend to evert feet and walk on inner aspects of feet
      (3) Between 18 and 36 months, child may appear knock-kneed (genu valgum)
      (4) Normal leg configuration should be present at approximately 6–7 years
   b) Feet appear flatfooted
      (1) Medial longitudinal arch normally obscured by fat pads until approximately 2 years
      (2) Arch better visualized when child not weight bearing (e.g., when seated or on tiptoes)
   c) Child may normally walk with in-toeing (pigeon-toed)
      (1) Rotational alignment of legs changes as skeleton matures, producing spontaneous correction
      (2) Pathologic changes may be produced by disorders of feet, lower legs, and hips
   b. "Pearls"
      1) Fractures result from significant force: history should be appropriate for pattern of injury
      2) Warning flags to consider child maltreatment: fracture in infant younger than 1 year, spiral

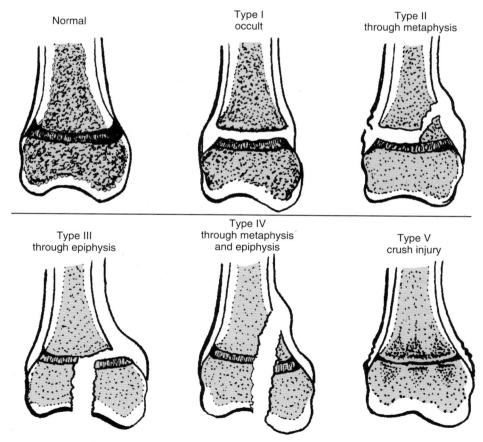

FIG. 38.1 Salter-Harris classification of pediatric fractures. *(From Simon, R. R., & Koenigsknecht, S. J. [2001]. Emergency orthopedics [4th ed.]. New York, NY: McGraw-Hill.)*

fracture, unwitnessed or unexplained injury, fractures in various healing stages, history of other fractures, fracture that does not fit mechanism of injury stated

3) Approximately 25% of fractures in children younger than 3 years caused by nonaccidental trauma

4) Torus/buckle fractures unique to children

5) Pulling injury to arm can result in "nursemaid's elbow" (subluxation of the radial head) in child commonly seen between 2 and 3 years of age

6) Limping: uncommon in children; suspect hip disorder if found

7) Unwillingness to bear weight requires further investigation

2. Geriatric
a. Aging related
1) Loss of bone minerals and mass
a) Regeneration prolonged
b) Bones become more brittle
c) Loss of vertebral body height results from compression that occurs with normal aging and leads to kyphosis
2) Muscles lose ability to regenerate new fibers to replace ones lost because of age (atrophy)
a) Decreased muscular strength and endurance, shuffling gait
b) Longer contraction time and tendency to fatigue more easily, which may cause muscle tremors, even at rest
b. "Pearls"
1) Joint stiffness and degenerative changes contribute to decreased mobility
2) Posture affected by age-related changes
3) Gait affected by posture, balance, strength, and flexibility
4) Changes in feet common
a) Foot size decreases because of loss of subcutaneous fat
b) Skin is drier; corns and calluses form at pressure points; epidermis thins and loses natural moisture
c) Decreased circulation from peripheral vascular disease may delay healing; venous stasis or arterial occlusion produces ulceration
d) Toenails thicken, affecting shoe fit
e) Bunion and toe overlapping or underriding may occur
5) Osteoporosis promotes fractures, especially in vertebral bodies, ribs, proximal femur
6) Osteoarthritis (degeneration of movable joints) affects mostly weight-bearing joints of knees, vertebrae, small joints of hand and feet
7) Rheumatoid arthritis (e.g., systemic disease of connective tissue resulting in joint inflammation) produces swelling, stiffness, ankylosis, redness, warmth of joints

8) Pathologic fracture may be caused by other chronic diseases
9) Paget disease
a) Metabolic disease that causes excessive bone resorption and deposits
b) Middle-aged and elderly men primarily affected
c) Affected bones tend to fracture easily

II. Specific Soft Tissue Injuries

The soft tissue of the extremities includes the skin, muscles, tendons, ligaments, nerves, and blood vessels. Injuries may occur with or without a bony injury, and in some cases it is difficult to determine the diagnosis. A careful clinical examination, along with radiologic studies to rule out skeletal trauma, is necessary to identify the problem. Certain disorders may result from chronic overuse and may not have an acute history of injury.

A. CONTUSIONS/HEMATOMAS

A contusion is a closed wound in which a ruptured blood vessel has hemorrhaged into the surrounding tissues. The blood may form a hematoma if bleeding is sufficient and has been contained. This can result from blunt external forces or exertional stresses. Symptoms may include swelling, discoloration, and tenderness. Populations at risk are those involved in physical activities, sports, or abusive relationships and patients who are taking anticoagulant therapy or who have a history of clotting disorders.

1. Assessment
a. Subjective data collection
1) History of present injury/chief complaint
a) Direct blow to affected area
b) Object of contact
c) Onset of swelling, discoloration
d) Therapies initiated to relieve symptoms
2) Past medical history
a) Current or preexisting diseases/illness
(1) Peripheral vascular disease
(2) Clotting factor deficiencies
b) Medications (e.g., anticoagulants, antiplatelet agents)
c) Allergies
d) Immunization status
b. Objective data collection
1) Physical examination
a) General appearance
(1) Mild to moderate distress/discomfort
b) Inspection
(1) Skin discoloration reflecting age of contusion (Box 38.5)
(2) Size
(3) Location
(a) Extension of ecchymosis to dependent areas over time (e.g., lower leg ecchymosis spreads to foot)

Box 38.5

Skin Discoloration Reflecting Age of Contusion

24–48 hours after injury: Area tender and swollen; ecchymosis may not appear; reddish blue or purple color may take up to several days to appear, depending on location of injury, distance of injured blood vessels from skin surface, and amount of bleeding

5–7 days: Color begins changing on periphery, proceeding toward center; takes on greenish tint

7–10 days: Yellow tint

10–14 days or longer: Brown

2–4 weeks: Clears

Box 38.6

Degree of Sprains/Strains

First degree: Minor tear in the fibers; minimal swelling, minor discomfort, absent or minor ecchymosis

Second degree: Partial tear; joint intact; more severe swelling, visible ecchymosis

Third degree: Complete disruption of ligament; joint may be open; minimal to severe swelling; resultant separation of muscle from muscle, muscle from tendon, or tendon from bone

      c) Palpation
        (1) Area tenderness
    2) Diagnostic procedures
      a) CBC with platelet count to rule out significant blood loss and thrombocytopenia as possible cause of bleeding
      b) Coagulation profile (prothrombin time [PT], partial thromboplastin time [PTT], international normalized ratio [INR]) to rule out coagulopathy
      c) Radiographs to rule out associated fractures
2. Analysis: differential nursing diagnoses/collaborative problems
    a. Acute pain
    b. Activity intolerance
    c. Impaired skin integrity
    d. Risk for infection
    e. Deficient knowledge
3. Planning and implementation/interventions
    a. Prepare for/assist with medical interventions
      1) Splint extremity to protect from further injury or iatrogenic injury and for pain reduction
      2) Apply pressure dressing to decrease hemorrhage and swelling
    b. Administer pharmacologic therapy as ordered
      1) Nonnarcotic analgesics
      2) Narcotics
    c. Educate patient/significant others
      1) Rest and elevate affected extremity to minimize bleeding and edema formation
      2) Apply cold packs to stimulate vasoconstriction
        a) Use for 20 minutes at a time, four times per day, for the first 2–3 days
        b) Wrap cold pack to protect skin from cold and further injury
      3) Apply and remove compressive dressing
      4) Use physical assistive devices (e.g., cane, crutches, walker)
4. Evaluation and ongoing monitoring
    a. Pain relief

B. STRAINS AND SPRAINS

Injuries to the structures around a joint are usually caused by excessive stretch or sudden force. This results in pulling on the structures, which causes tears in muscle and/or tendon. A sprain is the stretching, separation, or tear of a supporting ligament, and a strain is the separation or tear of a musculotendinous unit from a bone. Injury may result in pain, inability to weight bear fully, and swelling of the affected area. Sprains and strains are rare in small children, whose epiphyseal plates are still open and more vulnerable to forces. Athletes and obese patients resuming physical fitness are at risk for these types of injuries. Both strains and sprains are classified based on the amount of damage (Box 38.6).

1. Assessment
    a. Subjective data collection
      1) History of present injury/chief complaint
        a) Sudden stretching, twisting, or excessive force to joint (e.g., popping sound may be heard or felt)
        b) Pain (see Chapter 8): in joint (i.e., ranges from localized to severe and disabling; may be aggravated by movement, muscle tension, weight bearing)
      2) Past medical history
        a) Current or preexisting diseases/illness
          (1) Rheumatoid arthritis predisposes to tendon rupture because of associated deformity changes
          (2) Steroid injections are associated with tendon rupture; may result from injection itself or excessive volume within tendon sheath
        b) Injury, surgery, or problems with joint
        c) Medications
        d) Allergies
        e) Immunization status
    b. Objective data collection
      1) Physical examination
        a) General appearance
          (1) Gait: possible alteration
          (2) Mild to moderate distress/discomfort
        b) Inspection

(1) Swelling, deformity of affected area
(2) Ecchymosis
  c) Palpation
    (1) Tenderness over affected area
    (2) Swelling
    (3) Ottawa rules to determine if radiograph warranted
      (a) Ottawa knee rules (Box 38.7)
      (b) Ottawa ankle rules (Box 38.8)
      (c) Ottawa foot rules (Box 38.9)
    (4) Loss of motor function, ranging from minor to severe
    (5) Alteration in sensation
  2) Diagnostic procedures
    a) Radiographs of joint to rule out associated fracture or dislocation
    b) Stress view of joint may aid in detecting ligamentous injury
2. Analysis: differential nursing diagnoses/collaborative problems
  a. Acute pain
  b. Activity intolerance
  c. Risk for falls/injury
  d. Anxiety/fear
  e. Risk for ineffective tissue perfusion
  f. Deficient knowledge
3. Planning and implementation/interventions
  a. Prepare for/assist with medical interventions

Box 38.7

Ottawa Rules for Knee Radiographs*

Indications for knee radiographs
Age 55 years or older
Tenderness at head of fibula
Isolated tenderness of patella
Inability to flex knee to 90 degrees
Inability to bear weight (four steps) immediately after injury and in emergency department

---

Box 38.8

Ottawa Rules for Ankle Radiographs*

Indications for ankle radiographs in patients with acute ankle pain include pain in the ankle region plus one of the following:

Bony tenderness at the posterior edge or tip of the medial malleolus
Bony tenderness at the posterior edge or tip of the lateral malleolus
Inability to bear weight both immediately after injury and in the emergency department

---

1) Ice, elevation of extremity
2) Apply splint, immobilization devices, cast
  b. Administer pharmacologic therapy as ordered
    1) Nonnarcotic analgesics
    2) Narcotics
    3) Nonsteroidal antiinflammatory drugs (NSAIDs)
  c. Educate patient/significant others
    1) Mnemonic RICE: Rest, Ice, Compression, Elevation
      a) Rest affected joint
        (1) Non weight bearing with crutches
        (2) Protect from stress: avoid use
      b) Ice
        (1) Apply for 20 minutes at a time: perform range of motion four times per day as early as possible
        (2) Repeat regimen four times a day for the first 24 hours
        (3) Application of ice promotes vasoconstriction and reduces swelling
      c) Compression: use elastic bandage to provide support and help reduce swelling
        (1) Rewrap elastic bandage twice a day and remove at night
      d) Elevation: raise injured part to above level of heart during the first 24 hours after injury to reduce swelling
4. Evaluation and ongoing monitoring
  a. Pain relief

Box 38.9

Ottawa Rules for Foot Radiographs*

Rules for foot radiography include pain in the midfoot region plus one of the following:

Bony tenderness at the base of the fifth metatarsal
Bony tenderness over the navicular or cuboid
Inability to bear weight both immediately after injury and in the emergency department
Plain-film radiography

Ottawa foot rules predict significant midfoot fractures. If any of the following are present, a radiograph is required:

Point tenderness over the base of fifth metatarsal
Point tenderness over the navicular bone
Inability to take four steps, both immediately after injury and in the emergency department

* Clinical judgment should always take precedence over Ottawa's rules, particularly in the following circumstances:
Patient younger than 18 years
Multisystem trauma
Altered mental status
Presence of substance use/abuse
Underlying neurologic deficit affecting lower limb(s)
Communication difficulties due to language or other barriers

III. Specific Injuries of Bony Skeleton

Certain fractures and virtually all dislocations constitute an emergency in the sense that they may be a threat to the patient's life or limb.

A. DISLOCATIONS

A dislocation occurs when the articular surfaces of bones forming a joint are no longer in contact and lose their anatomic position. Bone ends may move because of congenital weakness, diseases that affect the articular and periarticular structures, and associated trauma. Dislocations are considered an emergency because of the danger of injury to adjacent nerves and blood vessels in the form of compression, stretching, or ischemia. Dislocations are described in terms of the distal segment in relation to the proximal segment (e.g., anterior, posterior, lateral, medial dislocations). Joint subluxations occur when part of the articular surface contact remains but is not complete. A person with a suspected or known orthopedic injury should be carefully assessed for both fracture and dislocation. If either one is suspected, the limb should be splinted, a neurovascular examination performed, radiographic examination completed for confirmation of diagnosis, and then the injury should be reduced as soon as possible. Table 38.4 discusses specific findings and treatment of various dislocations.

1. Assessment
   a. Subjective data collection
      1) History of present injury/chief complaint
         a) Report of significant force corresponding to type of dislocation observed
            (1) If absent, suspect preexisting condition
            (2) If caused by trauma, assess for additional injuries
         b) Symptoms since dislocation
            (1) Intense pain
            (2) Neurovascular compromise: paresthesia, hypesthesia, numbness, inability to move because of paralysis or patient's resistance to use
         c) Initial treatment
            (1) Immobilization techniques
            (2) Attempts to reduce affected joint
            (3) Use of ice or compressive dressing
            (4) Medications used

Table 38.4			
Common Dislocations			
Body Area	**Typical Mechanism of Injury**	**Clinical Findings**	**Treatment**
Phalanges			
Dorsal dislocations	Hyperextension of the joint (e.g., ball handling)	Deformity of phalanx at the proximal or distal interphalangeal joint	Radiographs with a lateral view, reduction, and splint
Thumb dislocation (e.g., gamekeeper's or ski pole thumb)	Radial stress on the ulnar collateral ligament	Painful swollen metacarpophalangeal joint of the thumb, tenderness ligament	Splint in a thumb spica and orthopedic referral over ulnar collateral
Shoulder			
Anterior	Fall on outstretched arm or direct impact on shoulder	Arm abducted, cannot bring elbow down to chest or touch opposite ear with hand	Splint in position of comfort; reduce as soon as possible
Posterior	Rare; strong blow in front of shoulder; with violent convulsions or seizures	Arm held at side, unable to rotate externally	As above
Elbow			
Radius and ulna	Fall on outstretched hand with elbow in extension	Loss of arm length, painful motion, and rapid swelling; nerve lesions may occur	As above Surgical repair if dislocation is associated with fracture to radial head or olecranon
Radius			
Head (children)	Pulled, or nursemaid's, elbow caused by sudden pull, jerk, or lift on child's wrist or hand	Pain, refusal to use arm; limited supination; can flex and extend at elbow; may have no deformity	Reduce, may place in sling; advise parents that this may recur until age 5 years
Hip			
Usually posterior	Blow to knee while hip is flexed and adducted (sitting with crossed knees); common in passengers seated in front seat	Hip flexed, adducted, internally rotated, and shortened; may have associated fracture of femur; sciatic nerve injury (lies posterior)	Splint in position of comfort; reduce as soon as possible
Patella			
	May be spontaneous	Knee flexed; can palpate patella lateral to femoral condyle	Reduce (may occur spontaneously), immobilize with cast or splint

Continued

Table 38.4

Common Dislocations—cont'd

Body Area	Typical Mechanism of Injury	Clinical Findings	Treatment
	Associated with other trauma	Excessive swelling, tenderness, and palpable soft tissue defect	Surgical repair of soft tissue injury or fractures
Knee (rare)	Direct severe blow to upper leg or forced hyperextension of knee	Ligamentous instability (requires disruption of structures); inability to straighten leg; peroneal nerve and popliteal artery injury common; must assess distal neurovascular function	Immediate neurovascular assessment; reduce
Ankle	Ankle is complex joint, with multiple ligaments providing stability; dislocation is usually associated with other injury such as fracture and soft tissue trauma	Swelling, tenderness, and loss of alignment and function	Splint; usually necessitates open reduction, because this joint has complex motion and must have accurate alignment

2) Past medical history
  a) Current or preexisting diseases/illness
  b) Previous injury or surgery, especially joint replacement, in affected joint
  c) Previous dislocation of affected joint, if any
  d) Medications
  e) Allergies
  f) Immunization status
b. Objective data collection
  1) Physical examination
    a) General appearance
      (1) Obvious deformity in affected joint
      (2) Possible altered gait or inability to ambulate
      (3) Moderate to severe distress/discomfort
    b) Inspection
      (1) Extremity length discrepancy
      (2) Abnormal position: rotation (internal or external) or alignment (angulated)
      (3) Swelling and discoloration
      (4) Open wounds
      (5) Loss of mobility as a result of
        (a) Dislocated bones
        (b) Paralysis
    c) Palpation
      (1) Tenderness
      (2) Deformity
      (3) Arterial pulses of extremity; signs of compromise
        (a) Local pulses may be difficult to palpate because of swelling
        (b) Doppler pulses may be present
        (c) Arterial flow should return after reduction is completed; if insufficiency remains, vascular injury must be ruled out

        (d) Delayed capillary refill time (<2 seconds is normal)
        (e) Temperature of extremity distal from injury
      (4) Range of motion: active and passive testing
      (5) Motor strength testing using scale 1–5
      (6) Neurologic examination: paresthesia, numbness, paralysis
  2) Diagnostic procedures
    a) Immediate radiographs to verify dislocation and identify any associated fractures
    b) Postreduction radiograph after relocation
    c) Vascular studies, as indicated by physical examination findings and history
    d) Preoperative laboratory tests if operative relocation required
2. Analysis: differential nursing diagnoses/collaborative problems
  a. Acute pain
  b. Activity intolerance
  c. Risk for falls/injury
  d. Anxiety/fear
  e. Impaired skin integrity
  f. Ineffective tissue perfusion
  g. Risk for infection
  h. Deficient knowledge
3. Planning and implementation/interventions
  a. Maintain airway, breathing, circulation (see Chapters 1 and 32)
  b. Provide supplemental oxygen as indicated
  c. Establish IV access for administration of crystalloid fluids/medications as needed
  d. Prepare for/assist with medical interventions
    1) Maintain distal neurovascular function
      a) Immobilize joint to prevent further injury and help relieve pain

b) Elevate joint
c) Apply ice to reduce swelling
2) Institute cardiac and pulse oximetry monitoring
3) Prepare for immediate reduction: procedural sedation
   a) Obtain informed consent, as necessary
   b) Apply postreduction immobilization devices
   c) Radiographs before and after reduction
   d) Assist with possible hospital admission
e. Administer pharmacologic therapy as ordered
   1) Nonnarcotic analgesics
   2) Narcotics
   3) Procedural sedation medications
f. Educate patient/significant others
   1) Maintain immobilization for prescribed time frame
   2) Apply cold packs
   3) Perform neurovascular assessment and report changes
   4) Indications/precautions for prescribed medications
4. Evaluation and ongoing monitoring
   a. Hemodynamic status
   b. Distal neurovascular supply of extremity
   c. Pain relief

B. FRACTURES

A fracture is defined as a break in the continuity of a bone. The break may result from application of repetitive action or a significant force to the bone. Fractures may also occur as a consequence of the application of an everyday force to a bone that has been weakened by a preexisting pathologic process (i.e., pathologic fracture). Fractures are classified as closed or open and by appearance. Trauma constitutes the major cause of fractures. Mechanisms of injury include motor vehicle crashes, motor versus pedestrian collisions, motorcycle collisions, falls, and sports. Open fractures place the patient at risk for wound contamination, infection, and periosteal stripping, which may lead to devascularization of the bone. Crush injuries are of special concern because of the extensive damage to surrounding soft tissues and degree of fracture comminution. Children are at lesser risk for fractures because of the elasticity of their skeletal structure. Elderly persons are more prone to fractures because of bone structure changes associated with the natural aging process and metastatic diseases. The goal in treating fractures is to restore bone alignment and function and to reduce disability. Table 38.5 provides a description of common fractures.

A focused assessment should be performed after primary and secondary surveys to identify all injuries and implement necessary interventions. Examination of fractures or the most painful area should follow the assessment of the rest of the body because muscle spasms and pain may obscure other findings. Repeated physical assessments should be completed after fracture pain has been relieved, to ensure that complications or other injuries have not been overlooked.
1. Assessment
   a. Subjective data collection

1) History of present injury/chief complaint
   a) Mechanism of injury (see Chapter 31) and estimate of force (e.g., distance of fall, how patient fell, landing surface, body part affected)
   b) Direction in which force was applied
   c) Position in which patient was found
   d) Pain (see Chapter 8); may be referred or distal to injury
   e) Associated injuries (e.g., head, chest, abdomen)
   f) Limited range of motion of affected extremity
   g) Substance and/or alcohol use/abuse
   h) Intimate partner violence/child abuse
2) Past medical history
   a) Current or preexisting diseases/illness
      (1) Diabetes mellitus
      (2) Immunosuppressive disorders
      (3) Corticosteroid use will cause delay in healing and mask symptoms
   b) Previous injury or surgery in affected extremity
   c) Nutritional status
   d) Use of tobacco products
   e) Medications
   f) Allergies
   g) Immunization status
b. Objective data collection
   1) Physical examination
      a) General appearance
         (1) Gait: possible alteration
         (2) Moderate to severe distress/discomfort
      b) Inspection
         (1) Deformity, angulation of bony structures; compare with opposite extremity
         (2) Swelling, pallor
         (3) Muscle spasm may be felt or seen
         (4) Integrity of skin (e.g., abrasions, contusions, open wounds)
         (5) Open fractures
            (a) Obvious skin wound with or without bone fragment present
            (b) Size of wound opening
            (c) Presence of contamination
            (d) Drainage from wound
      c) Palpation
         (1) Abnormal mobility at or between joints
         (2) Crepitus (grating sensation occurring as broken bone ends rub together); should never be deliberately produced
         (3) Tenderness of area
         (4) Joints above and below painful area should be palpated because referral of pain may mislead examiner
         (5) Vascular examination: assess pulses proximal and distal to fracture and compare with opposite extremity
         (6) Neurologic examination: assess for sensation, motor strength

Table 38.5

Common Fractures

Bone	Typical Mechanism of Injury	Clinical Findings*	Treatment*
Hand			
Phalanges	Direct trauma or crush injury	Pain in digit, ligament laxity	Splint; traverse, oblique, or spiral fracture of digit may require reduction or casting
Proximal to mid-phalanx fracture	Direct blow, crush injury	Subungual hematoma: nail injury	Trephination or nail removal and repair of nail bed
Distal phalanx fracture	Sudden blow to tip of the extended finger	Flexion posture or "droop" of the distal interphalangeal joint area (mallet finger)	Finger splint
Distal phalanx fracture			Mallet splint or foam-backed aluminum extension splint applied to the dorsal surface of the finger, which includes the distal and middle phalanges, for 6–8 wk; may require surgery
Metacarpal			
Second–fifth metacarpals	Crushing force or direct blow on the distal dorsal aspect of the closed fist	Swelling, rotational deformity of fingers to palm of hand	Radial or ulnar gutter splint to the fingertips with the metacarpophalangeal joints flexed 70–90 degrees, wrist extended to 20 degrees (similar to holding a tennis ball) may need surgery.
Base of thumb (Bennet fracture)	Axial load against a flexed thumb; fist fight, fall on hyperabducted or hyperflexed thumb	Pain and swelling dorsum of thumb, limited range of motion of metacarpophalangeal joint	Thumb spica splint with wrist in 30 degrees of extension, interphalangeal joint free and orthopedic referral
Humerus			
Neck	Fall on outstretched arm (may occur with dislocated shoulder)	Ecchymosis of shoulder, upper arm, and chest wall	Immobilize with sling, may splint or internally reduce if severe
Shaft	Direct trauma, twisting of arm	Radial nerve injury often occurs with fracture of lower third of bone	Immobilize with sling; use hanging arm cast if able to be mobile
Supracondylar	Fall on extended, outstretched arm (usually occurs in children)	Rapid swelling of elbow; pain	Admit to hospital for close neurovascular observation and definitive care
Radius			
Head	Fall on outstretched arm	Swelling; pain on lateral side of elbow; decreased range of motion in elbow; may have associated wrist injury	Immobilize; treatment varies according to range of motion and association with dislocated elbow
Shaft	Usually occurs with falls, altercations, and motor vehicle crash	Pain along bone (bones are mostly subcutaneous, therefore easy to palpate)	Splint for comfort (tight muscular compartments and interosseous membrane provide stabilization against movement)
Distal	Colles fracture (angulated dorsally): fall on outstretched hand	Distal fragment is deviated dorsally ("silver fork")	Immobilize with splint; reduce if displaced, cast
	Smith fracture (angulated toward volar surface): fall onto dorsum of hand	Reverse of Colles fracture	Immobilize with splint; reduce if displaced, cast
Galeazzi fracture	Oblique fracture at junction of middle and distal thirds of radius with disruption of distal radioulnar joint: fall or blow on dorsal and lateral side of wrist and distal radius (commonly occurs in adults)	Wrist and radial shaft tenderness and shortening	Usually unstable; needs open reduction
Ulna			
Monteggia fracture	Fracture of proximal third of ulna with anterior dislocation of radial head	Pain and swelling around elbow, pain worse with attempts at rotation; radial dislocation may be missed if elbow not included in radiograph	Immobilize for comfort; closed reduction for children, open for adults

Table 38.5

Common Fractures—cont'd

Bone	Typical Mechanism of Injury	Clinical Findings*	Treatment*
Nightstick fracture	Isolated, undisplaced fracture of mid-shaft of ulna as result of sharp blow	If ulna is angulated, injury to radius is also present	Immobilize; these fractures require 8–16 wk to heal
Wrist Carpus (navicular)	Usually occurs with falls on outstretched hand or direct blow; common in young men whose strong muscles prevent injury to lower radius (navicular is longest of carpal bones)	Pain in wrist, most severe in anatomic "snuff-box"; swelling; radiographs should include oblique view	Immobilize; cast for at least 3 mo to be sure fracture has reunited
Pelvis	Low velocity: elderly people; high velocity: all age groups (motor vehicle crashes, falls, and crushing forces)	Hypovolemia: retroperitoneal space can hold 4 L of blood; associated with multisystem trauma, especially genitourinary; tenderness with ilial wing compression or palpation of symphysis; ecchymosis (late sign) in flank and peritoneal area	Splint to immobilize; begin fluid resuscitation, using caution as needed (e.g., if urinary catheter is part of routine care, must assess for further injury); admit for observation and care
Femur Head or neck (intracapsular)	Caused by fall or spontaneous break (osteoporosis)	Pain in hip or referred to knee; leg shortened and externally rotated	Splint for comfort; surgical repair
Trochanter (extracapsular)	As above	Has greater blood supply; therefore, blood loss is heavier	As above
Shaft	Associated with high force	Powerful muscle groups cause angulation and overriding to produce deformity; severe pain; blood loss into tissue and from intravascular volume	Traction splint; admit for definitive care
Tibia Plateau (extends into knee joint)	Fall on extended leg, direct blow; rotation stress on extended leg (in pedestrians)	If radiographs are questionable or normal, may aspirate joint; usually associated with soft tissue injuries	Splint for comfort, compressive dressing; refer to orthopedist for definitive care
Shaft	Direct trauma: its position at distal end of leg exposes it to more trauma (e.g., car bumper); or rotation and leverage strain (as with stepping into deep hole while running) Open fractures more common because bone is subcutaneous on its anterior and medial surfaces	Associated with fractures in rest of body (ipsilateral extremity or elsewhere); must determine whether fibula is also fractured, because it acts as splint if intact Prone to complications 1. Increased incidence of compartment syndrome (tibia borders three of four myofascial compartments of lower leg) 2. Arterial injuries common with fractures of upper third	Splint for comfort; refer to specialist for evaluation and definitive care
Fibula Proximal	Direct blow to side of leg	May have concomitant peroneal nerve injury	Splint, until diagnosis made, then crutches
Distal 2 inches	As above	Associated with ankle injuries	As above
Shaft	As above	Considered minor	As above, symptomatic care
Ankle	See discussion of ankle dislocations (Table 38.4)	Sprained ankles in children are uncommon; should be evaluated for Salter-Harris I fracture	See Table 38.4

Continued

Table 38.5

Common Fractures—cont'd

Bone	Typical Mechanism of Injury	Clinical Findings*	Treatment*
Toes Second–fifth	Stubbing injury or heavy object being dropped on toes	Pain, swelling, ecchymosis possible subungual hematoma	Buddy taping to adjacent toe, gauze padding between toes

*Clinical findings and treatments listed here are in addition to general ones.

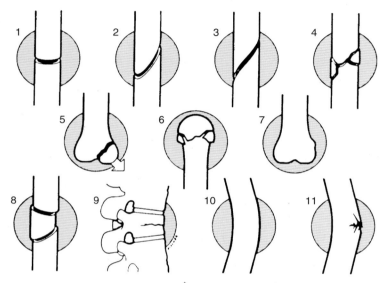

FIG. 38.2 Classification of fractures by appearance: 1, transverse; 2, oblique; 3, spiral; 4, comminuted; 5, avulsion; 6, impacted; 7, torus; 8, segmented; 9, compression; 10, bending; 11, greenstick. *(From American College of Surgeons, Committee on Trauma. [1982]. Early care of the injured patient [3rd ed., p. 283]. Philadelphia, PA: Saunders.)*

2) Diagnostic procedures
  a) Extremity radiograph
    (1) Radiographic appearance of fracture (Fig. 38.2)
      (a) Transverse
      (b) Oblique
      (c) Spiral
      (d) Comminuted: multiple splintered bone fragments
      (e) Avulsion: fragment of bone connected to ligament breaks off from rest of bone
      (f) Impacted: fracture involves bone end driven firmly into another bone end
      (g) Torus: usually seen in children; a buckling of bone surface
      (h) Compression: bone deformed by compression, usually vertebrae
      (i) Greenstick: usually seen in children; involves fracture of one side of bone
      (j) Epiphyseal fracture according to Salter-Harris classification (see Fig. 38.1)
    (2) General principles
      (a) Complete views must be done to rule out fractures
      (b) Joints above and below fracture must be seen
      (c) Children should have comparison views with opposite extremity to evaluate epiphyseal configuration (WEAK mnemonic: Wrist, Elbows, Ankles, and Knees)
      (d) Pelvis should be included if major lower limb injuries are present
      (e) Gas (air) may be evident with open fractures in soft tissue planes
      (f) Repeat films may be indicated in 7–10 days if initial films negative and continued pain-fracture may not be evident on initial films
  b) Special studies may be needed to view fracture or diagnose complication
    (1) Stress views
    (2) CT scan
    (3) Angiography

(4) MRI
(5) Nuclear bone scans
2. Analysis: differential nursing diagnoses/collaborative problems
   a. Acute pain
   b. Activity intolerance
   c. Risk for falls/injury
   d. Anxiety/fear
   e. Impaired skin integrity
   f. Ineffective tissue perfusion
   g. Risk for infection
   h. Deficient knowledge
3. Planning and implementation/interventions
   a. Maintain airway, breathing, circulation (see Chapters 1 and 32)
   b. Provide supplemental oxygen as indicated
   c. Establish IV access for administration of crystalloid fluids/blood products/medications as needed
   d. Prepare for/assist with medical interventions
      1) Elevate limb to decrease swelling
      2) Apply cold packs to decrease swelling
      3) Immobilize extremity
         a) Early use of splints, especially traction, can significantly reduce pain and swelling
         b) Immobilize joints above and below injury when possible to prevent further injury
      4) Splint fracture in position found, unless circumstances warrant movement, inability to transport patient "as is," and pulseless distal extremity
         a) Splints should be rigid and well-padded and preferably allow radiographic penetration
      5) Pneumatic antishock garment (PASG) or medical antishock trousers (MAST)
         a) May be considered for use if intraabdominal or pelvic bleeding (or both) with hypotension is present
         b) Despite the controversies that surround the use of PASG, the American College of Surgeons recommends its use to control bleeding from pelvic and lower extremity fractures; however, PASG use should not interfere with fluid resuscitation
         c) Although PASG or MAST use is controversial, when utilized, the patient must be monitored closely for circulatory compromise
      6) Assist with application of definitive cast/splint
      7) If open fracture is present, goal is to prevent infection
         a) Cover wound with sterile saline dressings
         b) Avoid use of bacteriostatic cleaning solutions in wound because they can inhibit wound healing
      8) If closed reduction is performed in emergency department

         a) Obtain informed consent as necessary
         b) Assist with regional anesthesia procedure
         c) Apply postreduction immobilization devices
      9) Assist with possible hospital admission
   e. Administer pharmacologic therapy as ordered
      1) Regional anesthesia
      2) Nonnarcotic analgesics
      3) Narcotics
      4) Antibiotics
      5) Tetanus immunization
   f. Educate patient/significant others
      1) Instructions about cast care
      2) Performing neurovascular assessment and changes to report
      3) Applying cold packs
      4) Elevating affected extremity
      5) Training with physical assistive devices (e.g., cane, crutches, walker)
      6) Using support devices (e.g., finger splints, sling, shoulder immobilizer, knee immobilizer, and fiberglass or plaster splints)
4. Evaluation and ongoing monitoring
   a. Hemodynamic status
   b. Monitor patient carefully during and after regional anesthesia procedure because patient may require large dose of medication during reduction and then become obtunded after pain is relieved
   c. If IV regional anesthesia is used, monitor tourniquet time and effectiveness every 5 minutes
   d. Evaluate immobilization devices to be sure they are properly positioned and have not caused constriction or excessive pressure
   e. Neurovascular status before and after each intervention and at regular intervals after care has been completed
   f. Pain relief

C. TRAUMATIC AMPUTATIONS

The loss of a body part presents a serious challenge to all involved in the patient's care. It is important to remain focused on the identification of life-threatening injuries and not to be distracted by limb-threatening injuries during all phases of the resuscitation.

The injury may occur alone or may be combined with other trauma as a result of tearing, crushing, or lacerating forces. The amputated part may or may not be replantable. The eventual outcome of the case depends on multiple factors. Factors decreasing the success of the outcome include excessive bacterial contamination, prolonged period of time between the injury and the institution of cooling, and severe degloving or avulsing of tissue. To avoid myonecrosis, warm ischemia time should not be >12 hours for a digit and >6 hours for parts that contain significant muscle. With cooling, major limb parts, such as those proximal to the wrist, can maintain viability for up to 12 hours, and digits may withstand up to 24 hours. Children tend to have better success with replantation than adults. Patients older than 50 years generally have more advanced vascular degenerative changes, which interfere with healing. A person's occupation is taken into account, as are the types of occupational protective devices normally used or worn during work. The amputated body part is evaluated to determine whether, after replantation, it will be functional or a hindrance to the person, especially if there will be limited motor or sensory function. Because replantation can involve lengthy hospitalization and rehabilitation, the patient's emotional status is assessed. The patient may be required to be away from work or home for long periods of time, and therefore this must be considered in the overall decision making about replantation. The patient's ability to cooperate with and tolerate a lengthy recovery and rehabilitation and the ability to withstand the pain and disability associated with the replanted part are important factors in the decision-making process.

If the patient has sustained multiple injuries, replantation may not be considered because of the potential or actual hemodynamic instability and the inability to withstand a lengthy surgical procedure. There are absolute and relative contraindications for replantation (Box 38.10). The thumb and multiple digits are carefully evaluated because they are high priority for replantation.

1. Assessment
   a. Subjective data collection
      1) History of present injury/chief complaint
         a) Mechanism of injury (see Chapter 31): object or agent causing amputation
            (1) Laceration that produces a straight-edged ("guillotine") cut has greatest potential for successful replantation
            (2) Crush injuries are associated with extensive soft tissue damage, which decreases chances for successful replantation
            (3) Avulsion injuries are associated with forceful stretching and tearing of tissue, thus making soft tissue damage more widespread, both distally and proximally
         b) Time of injury
         c) Pain (see Chapter 8)
      2) Past medical history
         a) Current or preexisting diseases/illness
            (1) Peripheral vascular disease
            (2) Bleeding disorders
         b) Smoking: nicotine is potent vasoconstrictor and decreases healing; patient is generally advised to abstain from smoking
         c) Hand dominance if hand injury involved
         d) General health and ability to withstand prolonged use of general anesthesia
         e) Medications
         f) Allergies
         g) Immunization status

   b. Objective data collection
      1) Physical examination
         a) General appearance
            (1) Moderate to severe distress/discomfort
         b) Inspection
            (1) Stump: viability of blood vessels, nerves, other tissue
            (2) Amount and type of contamination
            (3) Estimate of blood loss
            (4) Prehospital tourniquet time if used for traumatic amputation
      2) Diagnostic procedures
         a) CBC with differential
         b) Type and crossmatch
         c) CK (for crush injuries)
         d) Radiographs of stump and amputated part
2. Analysis: differential nursing diagnoses/collaborative problems
   a. Acute pain
   b. Activity intolerance
   c. Risk for falls/injury
   d. Anxiety/fear

Box 38.10

Classic Indications and Contraindications for Replantation

Indications	Contraindications
Multiple digits	Amputations in unstable patients secondary to other life-threatening injuries
Thumb	
Wrist and forearm	
Sharp amputations with minimal to moderate avulsion proximal to elbow	Multiple-level amputations
	Self-inflicted amputations
Single digits amputated between proximal and distal interphalangeal joints (distal to flexor digitorum superficialis insertion)	Single-digit amputations proximal to the flexor digitorum superficialis insertion
All pediatric amputations	Serious underlying disease such as vascular disease, complicated diabetes mellitus, congestive heart failure
Warm ischemia may be tolerated for 6–8 hours, cooling to 39.2°F (4°C) extends time to 12–24 hours with distal amputations	Extremes of age

From Antosia, R. E., & Lyn, E. (2002). General principles of orthopedic injuries. In J. A. Marx, et al. (Eds.), *Rosen's emergency medicine: Concepts and clinical practice* (5th ed., p. 477). St. Louis: Mosby.

e. Impaired skin integrity
f. Ineffective tissue perfusion
g. Risk for infection
h. Deficient knowledge
3. Planning and implementation/interventions
   a. Maintain airway, breathing, circulation (see Chapters 1 and 32)
   b. Provide supplemental oxygen as indicated
   c. Establish IV access for administration of crystalloid fluids/blood products/medications as needed
   d. Prepare for/assist with medical interventions
      1) Care of patient
         a) Control hemorrhage without causing further tissue damage
         b) Insert two large-bore IV catheters
         c) Infuse warmed normal saline solution/blood to maintain blood pressure
            (1) Apply direct pressure and pressure dressing to amputated area
            (2) Do not use tourniquet and clamps unless bleeding absolutely cannot be controlled; blood pressure cuff can be applied approximately 30 mm Hg higher than systolic pressure
         d) Splint and slightly elevate injured extremity
         e) Do not manipulate distal part if partially attached because this may potentiate injury
         f) Patient should have nothing by mouth in preparation for anticipated surgery
         g) Clean skin around stump with copious amounts of saline to remove contaminants; do not use other solutions because they may cause cellular damage
         h) Institute cardiac and pulse oximetry monitoring
         i) Assist with hospital admission, or transfer of patient to replantation center
      2) Care of amputated part
         a) Gently lift off contaminants; do not rub or clean with soap, water, or antiseptic solution
         b) Wrap in sterile gauze
         c) Moisten wrap with sterile normal saline or lactated Ringer solution: do not soak, wrap in, or use any type of water
         d) Place wrapped part in plastic bag, and seal securely to prevent entry of water from ice used during transportation
         e) Place sealed bag in ice; do not allow uncovered part to come in direct contact with ice; do not freeze, which causes further cellular damage
         f) Label plastic bag with patient's name, hospital number, and date; send with patient to operating room or replantation center
   e. Administer pharmacologic therapy as ordered
      1) Nonnarcotic analgesics
      2) Narcotics
      3) Antibiotics
      4) Tetanus immunization
      5) Medications recommended by replantation center
4. Evaluation and ongoing monitoring
   a. Hemodynamic status
   b. Neurovascular status of stump
   c. Pain relief

IV. Specific Life-Threatening Complications Associated with Orthopedic Injuries

A. COMPARTMENT SYNDROME

The extremities have multiple compartments that encase muscles, nerves, and blood vessels. They are enveloped by fascia, which is a tough and nonelastic membrane. Compartment syndrome occurs when compartmental pressures increase from an internal or an external force. Increased internal pressures result from bleeding into the compartment or internal soft tissue swelling. External forces include rigid casts, splints, air splints, and PASGs. As intracompartmental pressures rise, the vascular and neurologic structures become compressed and compromised. Initially, the low-flow microcirculation is obstructed, producing edema and further increasing the intracompartmental pressures. High-flow arteries remain patent until pressure exceeds the systolic blood pressure. Patients with decreased volume may be less prone to compartment syndrome.

Compartment syndrome tends to occur most often in the lower arm, hand, lower leg, and foot. It is rare in the upper arm and upper leg because of the larger size of the compartments, which can accommodate a greater volume. When it does occur in the upper extremity, it is usually associated with prolonged compression. These findings need to be monitored closely and documented because the patient may require an emergent fasciotomy.

1. Assessment
   a. Subjective data collection
      1) History of present injury/chief complaint
         a) Pain (see Chapter 8)
         b) Injury to extremity
            (1) Fracture, usually closed, although compartment syndrome can occur with open fractures
            (2) Crushing force
            (3) Prolonged compression
            (4) Vascular injury, especially after repair, when edema is greatest
            (5) High-pressure injections of foreign substance into deep compartment
            (6) Burns (see Chapter 34)
               (a) Circumferential or electrical
            (7) Hypothermia or frostbite (see Chapter 15)
            (8) Venomous snake or spider bites (see Chapter 15)

(9) Cannulation of artery
c) Prolonged overuse of extremity may present as chronic compartment syndrome
    (1) During forced marches
    (2) In long-distance runners
2) Past medical history
a) Current or preexisting diseases/illness
    (1) Hemophilia (increased tendency to bleed)
    (2) Nephrotic syndrome (edema resulting from increased capillary filtration)
    (3) Preexisting nerve dysfunction
b) Recent surgery on extremity
c) Use of casts, wraps, splints, circumferential tape, PASGs
d) Medications
e) Allergies
b. Objective data collection
1) Physical examination
a) General appearance
    (1) Five Ps (Box 38.11)
    (2) Severe distress/discomfort
b) Palpation
    (1) Tension over palpated compartment
    (2) Distal pulses may still be present
2) Diagnostic procedures
a) Urinalysis: myoglobinuria; pregnancy test in females of childbearing age
b) Enzyme levels: creatine kinase, lactate dehydrogenase, aspartate aminotransferase
c) Serum myoglobin
d) Serum chemistries including glucose, BUN, creatinine
e) CBC with differential
f) Coagulation profile
g) Radiograph of affected extremity: fracture pattern, soft tissue injury, occult fracture
h) CT scan: helpful in pelvic or thigh compartment syndrome
i) Doppler or arterial sonography: possible deep vein thrombosis or arterial occlusion

j) ECG
k) Compartment pressure measurement
    (1) Pressure up to 10 mm Hg considered normal
    (2) Pressure >30–40 mm Hg should be monitored for trends and clinical symptoms: may require fasciotomy
2. Analysis: differential nursing diagnoses/collaborative problems
a. Ineffective tissue perfusion
b. Acute pain
c. Anxiety/fear
d. Impaired skin integrity
e. Activity intolerance
f. Deficient knowledge
3. Planning and implementation/interventions
a. Provide supplemental oxygen as indicated
b. Establish IV access for administration of crystalloid fluids/medications
c. Prepare for/assist with medical interventions
    1) Remove all forms of external compression
    2) Avoid interventions that impede circulation
    3) Avoid application of ice because this promotes further vasoconstriction
    4) Avoid excessive elevation of limb; may impede arterial flow
    5) Prepare for and assist with fracture reduction if indicated
    6) Assist with compartment pressure measurements
    7) Institute cardiac and pulse oximetry monitoring
    8) Assist with hospital admission and possible operative fasciotomy
d. Administer pharmacologic therapy as ordered
    1) Nonnarcotic analgesics
    2) Narcotics
4. Evaluation and ongoing monitoring
a. Hemodynamic status
b. Cardiac rate and rhythm
c. Neurovascular status of involved extremity
d. Pain relief

Box 38.11

Assessment of the Five Ps

Pain that is out of proportion to injury or
  Progressive
  Intense
  Increased with palpation over compartment
  Increased with passive flexion motion of affected compartment muscles
Paresthesia (or hypothesia) along nerve that traverses affected compartment
Paralysis (or weakness) resulting from ischemia or pressure of motor fibers in affected nerve
Pallor resulting from obstructed microcirculation
Pulse usually present; pulselessness often last finding

B. FAT EMBOLISM SYNDROME

After a fracture or bone surgery, small fat globules may appear in the blood. The origin of the fat is unknown, but it is theorized to result either from the fracture site or from an alteration of lipid stability associated with the stress of trauma. The fat globules can circulate, causing occlusion of blood vessels to the brain, kidney, lungs, or other organs. Patients who have long bone fractures and pelvic fractures are at risk for fat embolism syndrome, which commonly occurs within 24–48 hours after injury. The incidence of fat emboli in long bone fractures is approximately 0.5–2%, and up to 5–10% in multiple fractures associated with pelvic injury. Fat embolism syndrome is a major cause of morbidity and mortality after musculoskeletal trauma.

1. Assessment
a. Subjective data collection

1) History of present injury/chief complaint
   a) Altered mental status (lethargy, restlessness, confusion, seizures, coma)
   b) Fracture or surgery of long bone 24–72 hours before onset of symptoms (usually lower extremity fracture and pelvis)
   c) Most common in patients with multiple injuries and those with long bone fractures
   d) Fever: 100.4–104°F (38–40°C)
   e) Rash: petechiae occur in 50–60% of patients; found over chest, axillae, and conjunctiva
   f) Episodes of syncope
2) Past medical history
   a) Current or preexisting diseases/illness
      (1) Pulmonary disease
      (2) Cardiovascular disease
   b) Medications
   c) Allergies
b. Objective data collection
   1) Physical examination
      a) General appearance
         (1) Level of consciousness, behavior, affect: restlessness, confusion
         (2) Elevated temperature: 100.4–104°F (38–40°C)
         (3) Hypotension, tachypnea
         (4) Moderate to severe distress/discomfort
      b) Inspection
         (1) Hemoptysis
         (2) Cyanosis
         (3) Hematuria
         (4) Petechiae: in buccal membranes; conjunctival sac; over chest, neck, shoulders; in anterior axillary folds
      c) Auscultation
         (1) Cough
         (2) Breath sounds: crackles
   2) Diagnostic procedures
      a) ABGs
         (1) Hypoxemia (arterial partial pressure of oxygen [PaO_2] <60 mm Hg)
         (2) Increased CO_2 retention as fat embolism syndrome develops
      b) Urinalysis: fat globules not always found
      c) CBC with differential: anemia
      d) Coagulation profile
         (1) Platelets: thrombocytopenia (platelets as low as 50,000/mm^3)
            (a) Consumed by injury and/or clotting process
            (b) Diluted with banked blood and/or IV fluids
            (c) Aggregated around fat globules
      e) ESR: elevated
      f) Chest radiograph
         (1) Initially appears normal
         (2) Serial radiographs reveal increasing bilateral diffuse haziness and interstitial edema (inflammatory response to fat microemboli) within 24–48 hours of onset of clinical findings
         (3) Changes occur late and only in approximately one third of patients with fat embolism syndrome
      g) Head CT scan without contrast: may reveal diffuse petechial hemorrhages indicating microvascular injury
      h) Ventilation-perfusion nuclear imaging of lungs: if suspicion of pulmonary embolus
      i) ECG: right-sided heart strain
2. Analysis: differential nursing diagnoses/collaborative problems
   a. Ineffective tissue perfusion
   b. Impaired gas exchange
   c. Anxiety/fear
   d. Acute pain
   e. Deficient knowledge
3. Planning and implementation/interventions
   a. Maintain airway, breathing, circulation (see Chapters 1 and 32)
   b. Provide supplemental oxygen
      1) Rapid sequence intubation (RSI) with positive end-expiratory pressure (PEEP) ventilatory support or use of continuous airway pressure if unable to maintain PaO_2 at >60 mm Hg
      2) High-flow oxygen
   c. Establish IV access for administration of crystalloid fluids/medications
   d. Prepare for/assist with medical interventions
      1) Advanced airway management
         a) Nasal or oral intubation
         b) Supraglottic airway (e.g., King, Combitube, laryngeal mask airway)
         c) Surgical airway (e.g., cricothyrotomy)
      2) Institute cardiac and pulse oximetry monitoring
      3) Insert gastric tube and attach to suction as indicated
      4) Insert indwelling urinary catheter as indicated
      5) Assist with hospital admission or transfer to higher level of care
   e. Administer pharmacologic therapy as ordered
      1) RSI premedications: sedatives, analgesics, neuromuscular blocking agents
      2) Vasopressors/inotropic support
      3) Corticosteroids
4. Evaluation and ongoing monitoring
   a. Level of consciousness
   b. Hemodynamic status
   c. Breath sounds and pulse oximetry
   d. Cardiac rate and rhythm
   e. Intake and output
   f. Pain relief

C. HEMORRHAGE FROM FRACTURES

The blood loss associated with fractures ranges from mild to severe and can be life threatening. It may be visible (e.g., in open fractures) or concealed, except for signs of soft tissue swelling, and may continue for 24–72 hours after injury. Table 38.6 lists approximate blood loss associated with the types of fracture. If the patient is already hypovolemic from other causes, or prone to bleeding because of clotting dysfunction, the magnitude of the blood loss becomes greater.

1. Assessment
   a. Subjective data collection
      1) History of present injury/chief complaint (see "Fractures" under "Specific Injuries of Bony Skeleton")
      2) Past medical history
         a) Current or preexisting diseases/illness
            (1) Bleeding disorders
            (2) Anemia
         b) Substance and/or alcohol use/abuse
         c) Medications (e.g., steroid use, anticoagulants, antiplatelet agents)
         d) Allergies
   b. Objective data collection
      1) Physical examination
         a) General appearance
            (1) Hypotension, tachycardia
            (2) Moderate to severe distress/discomfort
         b) Inspection
            (1) Length and circumference of injured extremity can be compared with uninjured side to estimate volume lost into soft tissue
         c) Palpation
            (1) Vascular examination of extremity and comparison with unaffected extremity
      2) Diagnostic procedures
         a) CBC with differential
         b) Coagulation profile
         c) Type and crossmatch
         d) Extremity/pelvis radiograph

2. Analysis: differential nursing diagnoses/collaborative problems
   a. Acute pain
   b. Ineffective tissue perfusion
   c. Anxiety/fear
   d. Impaired skin integrity
   e. Risk for infection
   f. Activity intolerance
   g. Risk for falls/injury
   h. Deficient knowledge
3. Planning and implementation/interventions
   a. Maintain airway, breathing, circulation (see Chapters 1 and 32)
   b. Provide supplemental oxygen
   c. Establish IV access for administrations of crystalloid fluids/blood products/medications
      1) Insert two large-bore IV catheters
      2) Infuse warmed normal saline solution/blood to maintain blood pressure
   d. Prepare for/assist with medical interventions
      1) Immobilize extremity/pelvis to decrease blood loss
      2) Apply and partially inflate PASG in cases of severe pelvic fractures to tamponade bleeding or provide comfort; although use of device remains controversial
      3) Traction splint for femur fracture unless contraindicated
      4) Elevate extremity to decrease blood loss
      5) Apply ice to encourage vasospasm and vasoconstriction
      6) Institute cardiac and pulse oximetry monitoring
      7) Insert gastric tube and attach to suction as indicated
      8) Insert indwelling urinary catheter as indicated
      9) Assist with hospital admission
4. Evaluation and ongoing monitoring
   a. Hemodynamic status
   b. Cardiac rate and rhythm
   c. Intake and output
   d. Extremity neurovascular status
   e. Pain relief

D. OSTEOMYELITIS

Osteomyelitis is an infection that may involve all parts of the bone. It may occur from open wounds, puncture wounds, compound fractures, or it may result from a surgical procedure that requires internal fixation. After the injury, an invasion of organisms spreads to the bone by means of exogenous or hematogenous routes. The exogenous route is the direct invasion of organisms to the bone from the outside as from a penetrating wound or fracture. The hematogenous route is the spread of organisms from another primary source such as skin abscess, otitis media, urinary tract infection, pneumonia, or abscessed teeth. The most common organisms that infect the bone are as

Table 38.6	
Blood Loss Associated with Fractures in Adults	
Bone	**Volume Loss (mL)**
Humerus	250
Elbow	500–1,500
Radius and ulna	150–250
Pelvis	1,500–3,000
Femur	1,000
Tibia and fibula	500

From Geiderman, J. M. (2002). General principles of orthopedic injuries. In J. A. Marx, et al. (Eds.), *Rosen's emergency medicine: Concepts and clinical practice* (5th ed., p. 477). St. Louis: Mosby.

follows: *S. aureus*, which is the most common, Streptococci, *Salmonella*, *Pseudomonas*, and fungal infections.

1. Assessment
   a. Subjective data collection
      1) History of present illness/injury/chief complaint
         a) Initial symptoms
            (1) Pain in the involved area
            (2) Fever
            (3) Malaise
         b) Later symptoms
            (1) Swelling, redness, and warmth over the affected area
            (2) Weakness
            (3) Irritability
            (4) Generalized signs of sepsis
      2) Past medical history
         a) Current or preexisting diseases/illness
            (1) Diabetes
            (2) Immunosuppression
            (3) Sickle cell disease
         b) Compound fracture
         c) Puncture wound, intraosseous needle insertion
         d) Surgical procedure with internal fixation
         e) IV substance abuse
         f) Medications
         g) Allergies
         h) Immunization status
   b. Objective data collection
      1) Physical examination
         a) General appearance
            (1) Possible elevated temperature
            (2) Moderate distress/discomfort
         b) Inspection
            (1) Warmth of area
            (2) Erythema
            (3) Swelling
         c) Palpation
            (1) Tenderness of area
            (2) Palpable deformity of the bone
            (3) Diminished range of motion
      2) Diagnostic procedures
         a) CBC with differential: elevated WBC count
         b) ESR: elevated
         c) C-reactive protein (CRP): elevated
         d) Blood cultures: detect bacteria in the blood; wound culture if indicated
         e) Bone scan
2. Analysis: differential nursing diagnoses/collaborative problems
   a. Acute pain
   b. Activity intolerance
   c. Risk for falls/injury
   d. Anxiety/fear
   e. Impaired skin integrity
   f. Ineffective perfusion
   g. Risk for infection
   h. Deficient knowledge
3. Planning and implementation/interventions
   a. Establish IV access for administration of crystalloid fluids/medications
   b. Prepare for/assist with medical interventions
      1) Protect other patients and personnel from infectious organism
      2) Immobilize affected extremity
      3) Assist with possible hospital admission for surgical débridement of the infected abscess or bone
   c. Administer pharmacologic therapy as ordered
      1) IV antimicrobials may be required over a 6-week period
      2) Nonnarcotic analgesics
      3) Narcotics
4. Evaluation and ongoing monitoring
   a. Pain relief

E. SEPTIC ARTHRITIS

Septic arthritis occurs when the joint has been penetrated by bacteria. There are three routes of transmission: the inoculation may be from a hematogenous event, from direct penetration injury such as a puncture wound, or by spread to the bone from an adjacent infected structure. If the condition is untreated, the destruction of the articular cartilage will be permanent and disabling. Organisms that are most common include *Staphylococcus aureus*, group B beta-hemolytic *Streptococcus*, and *Haemophilus influenzae*.

1. Assessment
   a. Subjective data collection
      1) History of present illness/injury/chief complaint
         a) High fever
         b) Pain (see Chapter 8): severe with any movement of the limb
         c) Irritability
         d) Malaise
      2) Past medical history
         a) Current or preexisting diseases/illness
            (1) Infection
            (2) Rheumatoid arthritis
            (3) Gonococcal infection
         b) Penetrating injury such as a puncture wound
         c) Medications
         d) Allergies
         e) Immunization status
   b. Objective data collection
      1) Physical examination
         a) General appearance
            (1) Possible elevated temperature
            (2) Tachycardia
            (3) Moderate distress/discomfort
         b) Inspection
            (1) Swelling of affected area
            (2) Erythema

c) Palpation
   (1) Passive motion of the joint causes severe pain
   (2) Warmth and possible effusion
2) Diagnostic procedures
   a) CBC with differential: elevated white blood cell (WBC) count
   b) ESR
   c) Blood cultures
   d) Synovial fluid analysis: Gram stain, culture, leukocyte count with differential, crystal examination
   e) Radiographs of affected joints
2. Analysis: differential nursing diagnoses/collaborative problems
   a. Acute pain
   b. Activity intolerance
   c. Risk for infection
   d. Anxiety/fear
   e. Deficient knowledge
3. Planning and implementation/interventions
   a. Establish IV access for administration of crystalloid fluids/medications as needed
   b. Prepare for/assist with medical interventions
      1) Assist with needle joint aspiration
      2) Assist with possible hospital admission for open arthrotomy if hips, shoulders, or sacroiliac joints involved
   c. Administer pharmacologic therapy as ordered
      1) Antibiotics
      2) Nonnarcotic analgesics
      3) Narcotics
4. Evaluation and ongoing monitoring
   a. Pain relief

V. Assistive Walking Devices and Splinting

A. ASSISTIVE WALKING DEVICES

1. Crutches, patient instructions (Box 38.12)
2. Cane, patient instructions (Box 38.13)
3. Walker (Box 38.14)

Box 38.12

Crutches

1. Top of crutches should reach 1–1.5 inches below axilla when standing up straight
2. Elbows should bend slightly when using hand grips
3. Use hand grips to absorb weight; patient should not lean
4. Place crutches 12 inches forward and approximately 6 inches to side
5. Body swings forward between crutches while taking normal-size steps

---

6. Clarify non-weight-bearing stance versus weight-bearing stance with patient
7. Using crutches on stairs
   a) Going up stairs
      1) Uninjured (good) leg goes up on first step
      2) Follow with injured (bad) leg and crutches
   b) Going down stairs
      1) Place crutches down one step
      2) Step down with injured leg
      3) Follow with uninjured leg

Box 38.13

Cane

1. Top of cane should reach wrist crease when standing up straight
   a. Elbow should bend slightly when holding cane
   b. Hold cane in hand opposite side of injury
   c. Cane and injured leg should swing and strike ground at the same time
   d. Using cane on stairs
      1) Going up stairs
         a) Uninjured (good) leg goes up on first step
         b) Follow with injured leg and cane
      2) Going down stairs
         a) Place cane on step
         b) Step down with bad leg
         c) Then step down with good leg
   e. General principles with crutches and cane
      1) Good leg goes up step first
      2) Bad leg goes down step first

Box 38.14

Walker

Walker should be considered in patients who cannot adapt to crutches or cane.
Walker should be considered in elderly or mentally handicapped patients.

B. SPLINTS (BOX 38.15)

Box 38.15

Splinting Principles

Splints are indicated with most fractures, dislocations, tendon injuries, or cellulitis of extremities.
Splints can reduce pain and swelling by immobilizing the extremity.

1. Assemble equipment: splinting material, elastic (Ace) bandages, padding, measuring tape, water source
2. Remove clothing and jewelry and assess area for swelling, discoloration, deformity, or open wounds

Box 38.15

Splinting Principles cont'd

3. Assess distal pulses, sensation, and capillary refill prior to and after completion of splinting
4. Dress any open wounds with sterile dressing after cleansing
5. Position patient in proper alignment using the position of function
6. Use padding to prevent pressure sores over any bony prominences or wounds
7. Measure splint to immobilize the joint above and the joint below the injured area
8. Support the limb during splinting to minimize movement, reduce pain, and ensure proper alignment
9. Splint any injured extremity when unsure of the injury

Bibliography

American College of Surgeons Committee on Trauma: Shock. In *Advanced trauma life support for doctors: Instructor course manual*, ed 7, Chicago, IL, 2004, American College of Surgeons, p 76.

Crowther CL: *Primary orthopedic care*, ed 2, St. Louis, MO, 2004, Mosby.

Griffin YL: *Essentials of musculoskeletal care*, ed 3, Rosemont, IL, 2005, American Academy of Orthopaedic Surgeons.

Hart RG, Uehara DT, Wagner MJ: *Emergency and primary care of the hand*, Dallas, TX, 2001, American College of Emergency Physicians.

Jordan KS, editors: *Emergency nursing core curriculum*, ed 5, Philadelphia, PA, 2000, Saunders and Emergency Nurses Association.

Maher-Butler A, Salmond-Warner S, Pellino TA, editors: *Orthopaedic nursing*, ed 3, Philadelphia, PA, 2001, Saunders.

Marx JA, Hockberger RS, Walls RM, editors: *Rosen's emergency medicine: Concepts and clinical practice*, ed 6, Philadelphia, PA, 2006, Elsevier Mosby.

Nettina SM: *Lippincott manual of nursing practice*, ed 7, Philadelphia, PA, 2015, Lippincott Williams & Wilkins, pp 1072–1076.

Redemann S: Modalities for immobilization. In Maher-Butler A, Salmond-Warner S, Pellino TA, editors: *Orthopaedic nursing*, ed 3, Philadelphia, PA, 2001, Saunders, pp 302–323.

Schnell ZB, Leeuwen AVM, Kranpitz TR: *Davis's comprehensive handbook of laboratory and diagnostic tests with nursing implications*, Philadelphia, PA, 2003, FA Davis.

Simon RR, Koenigsknecht SJ: *Emergency orthopedics: The extremities*, ed 4, New York, NY, 2001, McGraw-Hill.

Smith JE: Complications of orthopaedic disorders and orthopaedic surgery. In Maher-Butler A, Salmond-Warner S, Pellino TA, editors: *Orthopaedic nursing*, ed 3, Philadelphia, PA, 2001, Saunders, pp 230–266.

Thomas-Ojanen D, Bernardo LM, Herman B: *Core curriculum for pediatric emergency nursing*, Sudbury, MA, 2003, Jones and Bartlett.

Tintinalli JE, Kelen GD, Stapczynski JS, editors: *Emergency medicine: A comprehensive study guide*, ed 6, New York, NY, 2004, McGraw-Hill.

Walker J: Orthopedic emergencies. In Jordan KS, editor: *Emergency nursing core curriculum*, ed 5, Philadelphia, PA, 2000, Saunders and Emergency Nurses Association, pp 501–534.

Part 3

CHAPTER 39

Thoracic Trauma

Karen M. O'Connell, Lt Col, USAF, NC; PhD, RN, CEN, NEA-BC

MAJOR TOPICS

General Strategy
Assessment
Analysis: Differential Nursing Diagnoses/Collaborative
    Problems
Planning and Implementation/Interventions
Evaluation and Ongoing Monitoring
Documentation of Interventions and Patient Response
Age-Related Considerations

Specific Thoracic Emergencies
Aortic Injuries
Blunt Cardiac Injury
Cardiac Tamponade
Flail Chest
Hemothorax
Pneumothorax
Pulmonary Contusion
Rib and Sternal Fractures
Ruptured Diaphragm
Tension Pneumothorax
Tracheobronchial Injury

I. General Strategy

A. ASSESSMENT

1. Primary and secondary assessment/resuscitation (see Chapters 1 and 32)
2. Focused assessment
   a. Subjective data collection
      1) History of present injury/chief complaint
         a) Mechanism of injury (see Chapter 31)
         b) Pain (see Chapter 8)
         c) Level of consciousness
         d) Dyspnea
         e) Vital signs or signs of life observed prior to hospital arrival
         f) Cardiopulmonary resuscitation performed
         g) Efforts to relieve symptoms
            (1) Home remedies
            (2) Alternative therapies
            (3) Medications
               (a) Prescription
               (b) OTC/herbal
      2) Past medical history
         a) Current or preexisting diseases/illness
         b) Previous surgery
         c) Smoking history
         d) Substance and/or alcohol use/abuse
         e) Last normal menstrual period: female patients of childbearing age

      f) Current medications
         (1) Prescription
         (2) OTC/herbal
      g) Allergies
      h) Immunization status
      3) Psychological/social/environmental factors
         a) Extremes of age
         b) Possible/actual assault, abuse, or intimate partner violence situations (see Chapters 3 and 40)
   b. Objective data collection
      1) General appearance
         a) Level of consciousness, behavior, affect
         b) Posture, position of comfort
         c) Vital signs
         d) Odors
         e) Level of distress/discomfort
      2) Inspection
         a) Respiratory rate, rhythm, depth, and effort
         b) Pulse rate, cardiac rhythm, and R-wave amplitude
         c) Skin and mucosa: color
         d) Work of breathing: nasal flaring, accessory muscle use, retractions
         e) Neck veins: flat or distended
         f) Ecchymosis, abrasions, or open wounds to chest
         g) Chest wall movement with respirations: symmetric or asymmetric
         h) Paradoxical chest motion

3) Auscultation
   a) Breath sounds: present, absent
   b) Heart sounds: present, muffled, absent
   c) Bowel sounds: present, diminished, absent
4) Palpation
   a) Skin: temperature and moisture
   b) Tracheal position: midline or deviated
   c) Areas of tenderness, deformity, or bony crepitus
   d) Subcutaneous emphysema
3. Diagnostic procedures
   a. Laboratory studies
      1) Complete blood count (CBC) with differential
      2) Serial hematocrits
      3) Coagulation profile
      4) Serum chemistries including glucose, blood urea nitrogen (BUN), creatinine
      5) Cardiac enzymes
      6) Arterial blood gas (ABG)
      7) Type and screen, crossmatch
      8) Serum and urine toxicology screens
      9) Urinalysis; pregnancy test in female patients of childbearing age
   b. Imaging studies
      1) Cervical spine radiograph
      2) Chest radiograph
      3) Chest computed tomography (CT) scan
      4) Focused Assessment Sonography for Trauma (FAST)
      5) Aortography
      6) Transesophageal echocardiography (TEE)
   c. Other
      1) 12- to 15-lead electrocardiogram (ECG)
      2) Bronchoscopy or laryngoscopy
      3) Diagnostic peritoneal lavage (DPL)

B. ANALYSIS: DIFFERENTIAL NURSING DIAGNOSES/COLLABORATIVE PROBLEMS

1. Ineffective airway clearance
2. Ineffective breathing pattern
3. Impaired gas exchange
4. Decreased cardiac output
5. Fluid volume deficit
6. Acute pain
7. Anxiety/fear
8. Risk for infection
9. Knowledge deficit

C. PLANNING AND IMPLEMENTATION/ INTERVENTIONS

1. Determine priorities of care
   a. Maintain airway, breathing, circulation (see Chapters 1 and 32)
   b. Provide supplemental oxygen as indicated; maintain O₂ saturation at 94–99%

c. Establish IV access for administration of crystalloid fluids/blood products/medications
   d. Obtain and set up equipment and supplies
   e. Prepare for/assist with medical interventions
   f. Administer pharmacologic therapy as ordered
   g. Prepare for operating room, admission or transfer to higher level of care
2. Relieve anxiety/apprehension
3. Allow significant others to remain with patient if supportive
4. Educate patient/significant others

D. EVALUATION AND ONGOING MONITORING

1. Continuously monitor and treat as indicated
2. Monitor patient response/outcomes, and modify nursing care plan as appropriate
3. If positive patient outcomes are not demonstrated, reevaluate assessment and/or plan of care

E. DOCUMENTATION OF INTERVENTIONS AND PATIENT RESPONSE

F. AGE-RELATED CONSIDERATIONS

1. Pediatric
   a. Growth or development related
      1) Ribs are more compliant
      2) Mediastinum thinner, more mobile
      3) Infants are obligate nose breathers; children depend on their diaphragm for adequate chest expansion; may exhibit grunting or head bobbing with increased work of breathing (nasal flaring, accessory muscle use, and retractions)
      4) Airways are small and easily obstructed by edema or mucus
      5) Metabolic rate and oxygen consumption are much higher than those of adults. Monitor serum glucose
   b. "Pearls"
      1) Increased thoracic compliance may result in internal injury without external evidence of trauma (visual or chest radiograph findings)
      2) Airway resistance in infants is 15 times greater than in adults
      3) Less reserve muscle glycogen may affect respiratory effort—accessory muscles of inspiration tire quickly
      4) Obstructive shock and multiple varieties of dysrhythmias are unusual in pediatric patients
2. Geriatric
   a. Aging related
      1) Decreased vital capacity, forced expiratory volume, maximum midexpiratory flow
      2) Increased residual volume and functional residual capacity

3) Decreased static muscle strength and elastic lung recoil
4) Decreased diffusion capacity and arterial oxygenation
5) Increased ventilation-perfusion inequality, alveolar-arterial oxygen gradient

b. "Pearls"
1) Pulmonary defense mechanisms are reduced, making older adults more susceptible to infections
2) Diminished ventilatory response to hypoxic and hypercapnic challenge
3) Elderly persons report dyspnea as "breathlessness"
4) Causes of dyspnea in elderly patients may include
   a) Functional impairment of pulmonary or cardiopulmonary system
   b) Impaired ventilation secondary to supine positioning
5) ECG may be necessary because dyspnea may be associated with an acute myocardial infarction
6) Aspiration mortality rate of 40–70%; also significant cause of pulmonary morbidity
7) Concurrent use of medications may mask classic clinical signs following trauma
8) "Brittle" bones may fracture easily, causing penetrating injury to lungs, heart, and vessels

II. Specific Thoracic Emergencies

A. AORTIC INJURIES

Aortic injury can be the result of blunt or penetrating forces. Motor vehicle crashes and falls are the most common causes of aortic injury. Aortic injury may result in complete rupture, which often leads to sudden death at the scene of the accident (75–90%). When the aorta is subjected to accelerating, decelerating, horizontal, or vertical traumatic forces, it may tear, often at the ligamentum arteriosum, or it may be pinched between the spinal column and the manubrium. If the injury does not involve the adventitial (outermost) layer, the patient may survive. As a result of the intact adventitia, an aneurysm can form. Rupture may occur at any time. Specific signs and symptoms are often absent so diagnosis is suspected by chest radiograph and confirmed by arteriography, TEE, or CT scan. Surgical intervention is indicated.

1. Assessment
   a. Subjective data collection
      1) History of present injury/chief complaint
         a) Localized chest, midscapular, or back pain, generally severe and unrelenting (see Chapter 8)
         b) Dyspnea
         c) Mechanism of injury (see Chapter 31)

2) Past medical history
   a) Current or preexisting diseases/illness
   b) Prior thoracic surgery
   c) Medications
   d) Allergies
   e) Immunization status

b. Objective data collection
   1) Physical examination
      a) General appearance
         (1) Restlessness, disorientation, comatose
         (2) Possible cardiac arrest
         (3) Hypotension, tachycardia, tachypnea
         (4) Severe distress/discomfort, critically ill
      b) Inspection
         (1) Chest wall contusion or ecchymosis
         (2) Paraplegia
         (3) Pallor, cyanosis
         (4) Tracheal deviation
      c) Auscultation
         (1) Heart sounds: loud systolic murmur in parascapular region
         (2) Discrepancy in blood pressure between right and left arms, between upper and lower extremities
      d) Palpation
         (1) Decreased quality (amplitude) of lower extremity pulses as compared to upper extremity pulses
   2) Diagnostic procedures
      a) CBC with differential
      b) Serial hematocrits
      c) Coagulation profile
      d) Type and screen, type and crossmatch
      e) Urinalysis; pregnancy test in female patients of childbearing age
      f) Chest radiograph (Collective impression is more sensitive than single finding)
         (1) Widened mediastinum
         (2) Obliteration of the aortic knob
         (3) Presence of pleural cap
         (4) Pneumothorax
         (5) First or second rib or scapular fractures may be present
      g) Cervical spine radiograph
      h) Chest CT scan
      i) ECG
         (1) Sinus tachycardia
      j) Aortogram—diagnostic standard
         (1) Extravasation of dye
      k) TEE

2. Analysis: differential nursing diagnoses/collaborative problems
   a. Deficient fluid volume
   b. Decreased cardiac output
   c. Acute pain
   d. Anxiety/fear

3. Planning and implementation/interventions
   a. Maintain airway, breathing, circulation (see Chapters 1 and 32)
      1) Initiate or continue Basic Life Support (BLS) and Advanced Life Support (ALS) per protocols if cardiac arrest present
   b. Provide supplemental oxygen
      1) Intubation and ventilatory support in cardiac arrest patients
      2) High-flow oxygen
   c. Establish IV access for administration of crystalloid fluids/blood products/medications
      1) Insert two large-bore IV catheters
      2) Infuse warmed normal saline solution
      3) Infuse warmed blood products
   d. Prepare for/assist with medical interventions
      1) Advanced airway management
         a) Nasal or oral intubation
         b) Supraglottic airway (e.g., King, Combitube, laryngeal mask airway)
         c) Surgical airway (e.g., cricothyrotomy)
      2) Institute cardiac and pulse oximetry monitoring
      3) Prepare for emergency thoracotomy procedure
      4) Maintain normothermic body temperature
      5) Insert gastric tube and attach to suction
      6) Insert indwelling urinary catheter
      7) Assist with hospital admission or transfer to an institution providing a higher level of care for immediate surgical interventions
   e. Administer pharmacologic therapy as ordered
      1) Antihypertensives
      2) Beta blockers or calcium channel blockers
      3) ALS medications per protocols
4. Evaluation and ongoing monitoring
   a. Airway patency
   b. Hemodynamic status
   c. Breath sounds and pulse oximetry
   d. Cardiac rate and rhythm
   e. Intake and output
   f. Level of consciousness

B. BLUNT CARDIAC INJURY

Blunt cardiac injury, previously called myocardial contusion, is usually the result of blunt forces from vehicular, industrial, or sports injuries. The most common mechanism is the direct impact of the chest onto the steering wheel in motor vehicle crashes. The injury to the heart may range from subepicardial petechiae to full-thickness contusions with fragmentation and necrosis to actual rupture of the heart. The areas most frequently injured include the right anteroapical wall, the anterior interventricular septum, and the left anteroapical wall. The sequelae of blunt cardiac injury are rarely fatal; however, patients are at risk for hypotension, dysrhythmias, and rarely with a significant transmural injury, a ventricular aneurysm may develop. Motor vehicle crashes are the usual mechanism

of injury among children, whereas pedestrian-automobile crashes and falls are common mechanisms among elderly persons.

1. Assessment
   a. Subjective data collection
      1) History of present injury/chief complaint
         a) Patient may be asymptomatic
         b) Localized chest pain (see Chapter 8)
         c) Mechanism of injury (see Chapter 31)
      2) Past medical history
         a) Current or preexisting diseases/illness
            (1) Cardiovascular disease
         b) Medications
         c) Allergies
         d) Immunization status
   b. Objective data collection
      1) Physical examination
         a) General appearance
            (1) Possible hypotension, tachycardia, tachypnea
            (2) Moderate to severe distress/discomfort
         b) Inspection
            (1) Chest wall contusion or ecchymosis
         c) Auscultation
            (1) Breath sounds: diffuse crackles
            (2) Heart sounds: S_3 gallop
         d) Palpation
            (1) Localized tenderness to injured chest wall
      2) Diagnostic procedures
         a) CBC with differential
         b) Urinalysis; pregnancy test in female patients of childbearing age
         c) Chest radiograph
         d) ECG
            (1) Sinus tachycardia (most common)
            (2) ST-segment and T-wave changes
         e) Echocardiography
2. Analysis: differential nursing diagnoses/collaborative problems
   a. Decreased cardiac output
   b. Acute pain
   c. Anxiety/fear
3. Planning and implementation/interventions
   a. Maintain airway, breathing, circulation (see Chapters 1 and 32)
   b. Provide supplemental oxygen
   c. Establish IV access for administration of crystalloid fluids/medications
      1) Insert two large-bore IV catheters
   d. Prepare for/assist with medical interventions
      1) Institute cardiac and pulse oximetry monitoring
      2) Maintain normothermic body temperature
      3) Insert gastric tube and attach to suction as indicated
      4) Insert indwelling urinary catheter as indicated

5) Assist with collection and maintenance of physical and forensic evidence as indicated (see Chapter 44)
6) Assist with hospital admission or transfer to an institution providing a higher level of care
  e. Administer pharmacologic therapy as ordered
   1) Nonnarcotic or narcotic analgesics
   2) Antidysrhythmic medications as necessary
4. Evaluation and ongoing monitoring
  a. Hemodynamic status
  b. Breath sounds and pulse oximetry
  c. Cardiac rate and rhythm
  d. Intake and output
  e. Pain relief

C. CARDIAC TAMPONADE

Cardiac tamponade occurs when blood accumulates in the pericardial sac. This condition is more commonly seen in penetrating injuries of the thorax. The accumulation of blood causes an elevation in the intracardiac pressure, a progressive decrease in diastolic filling, and, subsequently, a reduction in stroke volume and cardiac output. Pericardial tamponade may be life threatening; however, clinical manifestations depend on the rate and amount of blood accumulation. It may take <100 mL of blood accumulation within the pericardial sac to produce significant and life-threatening symptoms. Prognosis depends on the timeliness of diagnosis and intervention.

1. Assessment
  a. Subjective data collection
   1) History of present injury/chief complaint
     a) Sense of impending doom
     b) Localized chest pain (see Chapter 8)
     c) Dyspnea
     d) Mechanism of injury (see Chapter 31)
   2) Past medical history
     a) Current or preexisting diseases/illness
       (1) Cardiovascular disease
     b) Medications
     c) Allergies
     d) Immunization status
  b. Objective data collection
   1) Physical examination
     a) General appearance
       (1) Decreasing level of consciousness; anxiety, agitation, restlessness, confusion, comatose
       (2) Hypotension, tachycardia, tachypnea, dyspnea, cyanosis
       (3) Severe distress/discomfort, critically ill
     b) Inspection
       (1) Chest wall contusion or ecchymosis
       (2) Skin mucosa: pale or dusky
       (3) Distended neck veins (may be absent if significant hemorrhage present)
     c) Auscultation
       (1) Heart sounds: muffled; may be difficult to appreciate; or absent
       (2) Breath sounds: equal unless lung injury is also present
       (3) Pulsus paradoxus: systolic blood pressure decreases 10 mm Hg or more during inspiration
     d) Palpation
       (1) Skin: cool and moist
       (2) Localized tenderness to injured chest wall
   2) Diagnostic procedures
     a) CBC with differential
     b) Type and crossmatch
     c) Cardiac enzymes
     d) Urinalysis; pregnancy test in female patients of childbearing age
     e) Chest radiograph
     f) ECG
       (1) Sinus tachycardia
       (2) Progressive decreased voltage of ECG complexes
       (3) Pulseless electrical activity (suggestive of cardiac tamponade)
     g) FAST: 96–100% sensitive for pericardial space blood
     h) Echocardiography
2. Analysis: differential nursing diagnoses/collaborative problems
  a. Decreased cardiac output
  b. Acute pain
  c. Anxiety/fear
3. Planning and implementation/interventions
  a. Maintain airway, breathing, circulation (see Chapters 1 and 32)
  b. Provide supplemental oxygen
  c. Establish IV access for administration of crystalloid fluids/blood products/medications
   1) Insert two large-bore IV catheters
   2) Infuse warmed normal saline solution
  d. Prepare for/assist with medical interventions
   1) Institute cardiac and pulse oximetry monitoring
   2) Catheter placement and monitoring of CVP (see Chapter 6)
   3) Prepare for pericardiocentesis, pericardial window, or emergency thoracotomy procedures
   4) Maintain normothermic body temperature
   5) Insert gastric tube and attach to suction as indicated
   6) Insert indwelling urinary catheter as indicated
   7) Assist with collection and maintenance of physical and forensic evidence as indicated (see Chapter 44)
   8) Assist with hospital admission or transfer to an institution providing a higher level of care

e. Administer pharmacologic therapy as ordered
  1) Nonnarcotic or narcotic analgesics
  2) Antidysrhythmic medications as necessary
4. Evaluation and ongoing monitoring
  a. Level of consciousness
  b. Hemodynamic status
  c. Breath sounds and pulse oximetry
  d. Cardiac rate and rhythm
  e. Intake and output
  f. Pain relief

D. FLAIL CHEST

Flail chest occurs when two or more adjacent ribs are fractured in two or more locations or when the sternum is detached. The result is a free-floating segment that is drawn inward with inspiration and outward with expiration, thus causing paradoxical motion during respiration. The flail segment may not be clinically evident for several hours after injury because of muscle spasms, splinting of the injured area, or patient intubation. Flail chest injuries are painful and cause impaired ventilation. Inefficient ventilation is caused by the loss of the bellows effect (less negative intrapleural pressure to expand the lung) and associated pulmonary contusion, dead space, and atelectasis. The patient has increased respiratory effort, decreased tidal volume, impaired cough, and hypoxia. Associated injuries may include underlying hemothorax, pneumothorax, pulmonary contusion, and blunt cardiac injury.

1. Assessment
  a. Subjective data collection
    1) History of present injury/chief complaint
      a) Localized chest pain (see Chapter 8)
      b) Dyspnea
      c) Mechanism of injury (see Chapter 31)
    2) Past medical history
      a) Current or preexisting diseases/illness
        (1) Osteodegenerative processes
        (2) Pulmonary disease
        (3) Cardiovascular disease
      b) Recent thoracic surgery
      c) Medications
      d) Allergies
      e) Immunization status
  b. Objective data collection
    1) Physical examination
      a) General appearance
        (1) Restlessness or confusion
        (2) Position intended to splint injured area
        (3) Hypotension, tachycardia, tachypnea
        (4) Severe distress/discomfort
      b) Inspection
        (1) Chest wall contusion or ecchymosis
        (2) Paradoxical chest motion (may not be seen)
        (3) Hyperventilation: rapid, shallow breathing
        (4) Increased work of breathing: nasal flaring, accessory muscle use, retractions
      c) Auscultation
        (1) Breath sounds: diminished or absent on injured side
        (2) Heart sounds: distinct
      d) Palpation
        (1) Localized point tenderness
        (2) Paradoxical chest motion
        (3) Bony deformity or crepitus
        (4) Subcutaneous emphysema if underlying pneumothorax or tracheal injury
    2) Diagnostic procedures
      a) ABGs
      b) CBC with differential
      c) Type and crossmatch
      d) Coagulation studies
      e) Cardiac enzymes
      f) Urinalysis; pregnancy test in female patients of childbearing age
      g) Chest radiograph
      h) Cervical spine radiograph
      i) ECG
2. Analysis: differential nursing diagnoses/collaborative problems
  a. Impaired gas exchange
  b. Ineffective breathing pattern
  c. Acute pain
  d. Anxiety/fear
3. Planning and implementation/interventions
  a. Maintain airway, breathing, circulation (see Chapters 1 and 32)
  b. Provide supplemental oxygen; maintain O_2 saturation at 94–99%
    1) Rapid-sequence intubation (RSI) and ventilatory support in patients with respiratory compromise
    2) High-flow humidified oxygen
  c. Establish IV access for administration of crystalloid fluids/blood products/medications
    1) Infuse warmed normal saline solution judiciously
  d. Prepare for/assist with medical interventions
    1) Advanced airway management
      a) Nasal or oral intubation
      b) Supraglottic airway (e.g., King, Combitube, laryngeal mask airway)
      c) Surgical airway (e.g., cricothyrotomy)
    2) Stabilize injured chest wall: place patient on injured side in semi-Fowler position, or position of comfort, to facilitate ventilation
    3) Institute cardiac and pulse oximetry monitoring
    4) Maintain normothermic body temperature
    5) Insert gastric tube and attach to suction
    6) Insert indwelling urinary catheter
    7) Assist with collection and maintenance of physical and forensic evidence if indicated (see Chapter 44)

8) Assist with hospital admission or transfer to an institution providing a higher level of care

e. Administer pharmacologic therapy as ordered

   1) RSI premedication: sedatives, analgesics, neuromuscular blocking agents

   2) Nonnarcotic or narcotic analgesics

   3) Tetanus immunization

4. Evaluation and ongoing monitoring

   a. Airway patency

   b. Hemodynamic status

   c. Breath sounds and pulse oximetry

   d. Cardiac rate and rhythm

   e. Intake and output

   f. Pain relief

E. HEMOTHORAX

Bleeding and accumulation of blood in the pleural space may result from injury to the chest wall, great vessels, or lungs from penetrating, blunt, or blast trauma. Accumulation of blood in the pleural space may cause the mediastinal contents to shift, resulting in impairment of venous return or lung compression with a significant blood loss (which may exceed 2,500 mL). Hypotension or shock may develop. Emergency thoracotomy may be necessary to identify and repair the bleeding source if the patient's physiological status warrants, there is at least 1,000 mL of blood drained from the chest initially or drainage >200 mL/hour for 3–4 hours.

1. Assessment

   a. Subjective data collection

      1) History of present injury/chief complaint

         a) Patient may be asymptomatic, especially if hemothorax is small

         b) Localized chest pain (see Chapter 8)

         c) Dyspnea

         d) Mechanism of injury (see Chapter 31)

      2) Past medical history

         a) Current or preexisting diseases/illness

            (1) Pulmonary disease

         b) Medications

         c) Allergies

         d) Immunization status

   b. Objective data collection

      1) Physical examination

         a) General appearance

            (1) Confusion, anxiety, restlessness

            (2) Position intended to facilitate respiration

            (3) Possible hypotension, tachycardia, tachypnea

            (4) Moderate to severe distress/discomfort, possibly critically ill

         b) Inspection

            (1) Chest wall contusion, ecchymosis, or open wound

            (2) Increased work of breathing: nasal flaring, accessory muscle use, retractions

            (3) Cyanosis, diaphoresis

         c) Auscultation

            (1) Breath sounds: decreased or absent on injured side

            (2) Bowel sounds: normal to decreased

         d) Palpation/percussion

            (1) Localized point tenderness to injured chest wall

            (2) Tracheal deviation toward uninjured side (with significant hemothorax)

            (3) Bony deformity or crepitus

            (4) Subcutaneous emphysema

            (5) Dullness on side of injury

      2) Diagnostic procedures

         a) ABGs

         b) CBC with differential: decreased hemoglobin/hematocrit if significant hemothorax

         c) Serial hematocrits

         d) Cardiac enzymes

         e) Coagulation profile

         f) Type and crossmatch

         g) Urinalysis; pregnancy test in female patients of childbearing age

         h) Chest radiograph (upright if possible)

         i) Cervical spine radiograph

         j) ECG

2. Analysis: differential nursing diagnoses/collaborative problems

   a. Impaired gas exchange

   b. Decreased cardiac output

   c. Fluid volume deficit

   d. Anxiety/fear

3. Planning and implementation/interventions

   a. Maintain airway, breathing, circulation (see Chapters 1 and 32)

   b. Provide supplemental oxygen; maintain O_2 saturation at 94–99%

   c. Establish IV access for administration of crystalloid fluids/blood products/medications

      1) Insert two large-bore IV catheters

      2) Infuse warmed normal saline solution

      3) Infuse warmed blood products

   d. Prepare for/assist with medical interventions

      1) Place in high Fowler position, unless contraindicated

      2) Assist with chest tube insertion and closed chest drainage

         a) Consider procedural sedation (see Chapter 8)

         b) 32–36 French chest tube placed in fifth intercostal space, just anterior to midaxillary line

         c) Apply dressing per facility protocol after chest tube is inserted and sutured in place

      3) Anticipate the need for autotransfusion and/or emergency thoracotomy

    4) Maintain normothermic body temperature
    5) Institute cardiac and pulse oximetry monitoring
    6) Insert gastric tube and attach to suction as indicated
    7) Insert indwelling urinary catheter as indicated
    8) Assist with collection and maintenance of physical and forensic evidence as indicated (see Chapter 44)
    9) Assist with hospital admission or transfer to an institution providing a higher level of care
  e. Administer pharmacologic therapy as ordered
    1) Nonnarcotic or narcotic analgesics
    2) Procedural sedation medications
    3) Tetanus immunization
4. Evaluation and ongoing monitoring
  a. Level of consciousness
  b. Hemodynamic status
  c. Breath sounds and pulse oximetry
  d. Cardiac rate and rhythm
  e. Intake and output
  f. Pain relief

F. PNEUMOTHORAX

Pneumothorax results when air enters the pleural space. It causes a loss of negative intrapleural pressure and subsequent partial or total collapse of the lung on the affected side. Pneumothorax may occur following either penetrating or blunt thoracic injury: a laceration occurs from either a fractured rib or penetrating object, or increased intrathoracic pressure produces a ruptured bleb. In addition, mechanical ventilation or iatrogenic procedures in the trauma patient may cause pneumothorax. Pneumothorax may be simple (no external opening) or open (sucking chest wound).

1. Assessment
  a. Subjective data collection
    1) History of present injury/chief complaint
      a) Patient may be asymptomatic, especially if small pneumothorax
      b) Localized chest pain (see Chapter 8)
      c) Dyspnea
      d) Mechanism of injury (see Chapter 31)
    2) Past medical history
      a) Current or preexisting diseases/illness
        (1) Pulmonary disease
      b) Medications
      c) Allergies
      d) Immunization status
  b. Objective data collection
    1) Physical examination
      a) General appearance
        (1) Position intended to facilitate respiration
        (2) Tachypnea, tachycardia, hypotension
        (3) Moderate to severe distress/discomfort
      b) Inspection
        (1) Chest wall contusion, ecchymosis, or open wound
        (2) Bubbles/froth from open chest wound
        (3) Hemoptysis if open wound
      c) Auscultation
        (1) Breath sounds: decreased or absent on injured side
        (2) Sucking sound or "hiss" from chest if open pneumothorax
      d) Palpation/percussion
        (1) Localized point tenderness to injured chest wall
        (2) Bony deformity or crepitus
        (3) Subcutaneous emphysema
        (4) Hyperresonance on injured side
    2) Diagnostic procedures
      a) ABGs
      b) CBC with differential
      c) Chest radiograph
      d) ECG
2. Analysis: differential nursing diagnoses/collaborative problems
  a. Impaired gas exchange
  b. Ineffective breathing pattern
  c. Anxiety/fear
3. Planning and implementation/interventions
  a. Maintain airway, breathing, circulation (see Chapters 1 and 32)
  b. Provide supplemental oxygen; maintain O_2 saturation at 94–99%
  c. Establish IV access for administration of crystalloid fluids/medications
  d. Prepare for/assist with medical interventions
    1) Cover any open chest wounds with a three-sided occlusive dressing; remove dressing if patient develops signs of tension pneumothorax
    2) Place in high Fowler position, or position of comfort, to facilitate ventilation
    3) Institute cardiac and pulse oximetry monitoring
    4) Assist with chest tube insertion and closed chest drainage
      a) Consider procedural sedation (see Chapter 8)
      b) 32–36 French chest tube placed in fifth intercostal space, just anterior to midaxillary line
      c) Apply dressing per facility protocol after chest tube is inserted and sutured in place
    5) Insert indwelling urinary catheter as indicated
    6) Assist with collection and maintenance of physical or forensic evidence as indicated (see Chapter 44)
    7) Assist with possible hospital admission or transfer to an institution providing a higher level of care
  e. Administer pharmacologic therapy as ordered
    1) Nonnarcotic or narcotic analgesics

2) Procedural sedation medications
3) Tetanus immunization
4. Evaluation and ongoing monitoring
   a. Hemodynamic status
   b. Breath sounds and pulse oximetry
   c. Cardiac rate and rhythm
   d. Pain relief

G. PULMONARY CONTUSION

Pulmonary contusion is a lung injury that may develop following high-velocity dissipation of energy to the chest. It may be localized or generalized and is usually associated with other chest injuries, such as rib fractures and flail chest. In pulmonary contusion, blood extravasates into the lung parenchyma, causing alveolar and interstitial edema and leading to tissue anoxia and a change in tissue permeability. This is followed by decreased pulmonary compliance, increased pulmonary vascular resistance, and decreased pulmonary blood flow. The signs and symptoms may not be immediately apparent; therefore, diagnosis is often made by suspecting the condition and monitoring for hypoxia. Symptoms may be delayed for 12–48 hours. Treatment may include using a specialized bed that provides continuous lateral rotation, thereby mobilizing pulmonary secretions and shifting perfusion to different regions of the lung. Unconventional modes of ventilation (e.g., pressure control combined with inverse ratio ventilation or high-frequency jet ventilation) may also be used. Pulmonary contusion occurs in almost 75% of patients with blunt chest trauma and has a 40% mortality.

1. Assessment
   a. Subjective data collection
      1) History of present injury/chief complaint
         a) Localized chest pain (see Chapter 8)
         b) Onset of nonproductive, ineffective coughing
         c) Dyspnea
         d) Mechanism of injury (see Chapter 31)
      2) Past medical history
         a) Current or preexisting diseases/illness
            (1) Pulmonary disease
         b) Medications
         c) Allergies
         d) Immunization status
   b. Objective data collection
      1) Physical examination
         a) General appearance
            (1) Increasing restlessness
            (2) Tachycardia, tachypnea, hypoxia
            (3) Moderate to severe distress/discomfort
         b) Inspection
            (1) Chest wall contusion or ecchymosis
            (2) Increased work of breathing: nasal flaring, accessory muscle use, retractions
            (3) Hemoptysis

c) Auscultation
   (1) Breath sounds: local or diffuse crackles or wheezes
d) Palpation
   (1) Localized chest point tenderness
   (2) Bony deformity or crepitus
   (3) Subcutaneous emphysema if underlying pneumothorax or tracheal injury
2) Diagnostic procedures
   a) ABGs
   b) CBC with differential
   c) Urinalysis; pregnancy test in female patients of childbearing age
   d) Chest radiograph: contusion often does not "blossom" for 6–8 hours after injury
   e) ECG
2. Analysis: differential nursing diagnoses/collaborative problems
   a. Ineffective breathing pattern
   b. Impaired gas exchange
   c. Acute pain
3. Planning and implementation/interventions
   a. Maintain airway, breathing, circulation (see Chapters 1 and 32)
   b. Provide supplemental oxygen
      1) RSI and positive-pressure ventilatory support in patients with respiratory compromise
      2) High-flow oxygen; maintain O_2 saturation at 94–99%
   c. Establish IV access for administration of crystalloid fluids/medications
      1) Restrict fluid administration if no signs of shock to prevent pulmonary overload
   d. Prepare for/assist with medical interventions
      1) Position to facilitate ventilation (usually injured side up)
      2) Advanced airway management
         a) Nasal or oral intubation
         b) Supraglottic airway (e.g., King, Combitube, laryngeal mask airway)
         c) Surgical airway (e.g., cricothyrotomy)
      3) Chest physiotherapy
      4) Institute cardiac and pulse oximetry monitoring
      5) Maintain normothermic body temperature
      6) Insert gastric tube and attach to suction as indicated
      7) Insert indwelling urinary catheter as indicated
      8) Assist with hospital admission or transfer to an institution providing a higher level of care
   e. Administer pharmacologic therapy as ordered
      1) RSI premedication: sedatives, analgesics, neuromuscular blocking agents
      2) Nonnarcotic or narcotic analgesics
      3) Diuretics
4. Evaluation and ongoing monitoring
   a. Airway patency
   b. Level of consciousness

c. Hemodynamic status
d. Breath sounds and pulse oximetry
e. Cardiac rate and rhythm
f. Intake and output
g. Pain relief

H. RIB AND STERNAL FRACTURES

Rib fractures commonly result from blunt force or crush injuries during motor vehicle crashes. Falls are also a mechanism of injury, especially in the elderly. Rib fractures are not by themselves life threatening; however, they may be associated with underlying lung injury. Fractures of the sternum, first, and second ribs rarely occur; however, they are associated with significant force that produces injury to the lungs, aortic arch, or vertebral column. First rib fractures have a 40% mortality rate because of frequently associated lacerations of the subclavian artery or vein. Left lower rib fractures are associated with splenic injury in 20% of patients. Right lower rib fractures are associated with hepatic injury in 10% of patients. Sternal fractures are associated with an increased incidence of blunt cardiac injury. Children's ribs and sternum are very flexible, making rib fractures less common in children; however, significant underlying lung or cardiac injury may be present without rib fractures. The treatment for all age groups with rib fractures is very similar.

1. Assessment
   a. Subjective data collection
      1) History of present injury/chief complaint
         a) Localized pain, aggravated by chest wall movement, palpation, or inspiration (see Chapter 8)
         b) Onset may be associated with severe coughing
         c) Dyspnea
         d) Mechanism of injury (see Chapter 31)
      2) Past medical history
         a) Current or preexisting diseases/illness
            (1) Pulmonary disease
            (2) Osteodegenerative processes
         b) Medications
         c) Allergies
         d) Immunization status
   b. Objective data collection
      1) Physical examination
         a) General appearance
            (1) Position intended to splint injured area
            (2) Facial expression of pain on movement
            (3) Moderate distress/discomfort
         b) Inspection
            (1) Chest wall contusion or ecchymosis
            (2) Hypoventilation
         c) Auscultation
            (1) Breath sounds: diminished
         d) Palpation
            (1) Localized point tenderness

            (2) Bony deformity or crepitus
            (3) Subcutaneous emphysema if underlying pneumothorax or tracheal injury
      2) Diagnostic procedures
         a) ABGs
         b) Chest radiograph (only 70% sensitive for rib fractures)
            (1) Consider CT of chest if high index of suspicion
         c) ECG
2. Analysis: differential nursing diagnoses/collaborative problems
   a. Ineffective breathing pattern
   b. Acute pain
   c. Activity intolerance
3. Planning and implementation/interventions
   a. Maintain airway, breathing, circulation (see Chapters 1 and 32)
   b. Provide supplemental oxygen as indicated; maintain O$_2$ saturation at 94–99%
   c. Establish IV access for administration of crystalloid fluids/medications as needed
   d. Prepare for/assist with medical interventions
      1) Place in high Fowler position, or position of comfort, to facilitate ventilation
      2) Institute cardiac and pulse oximetry monitoring
      3) Incentive spirometry to help prevent atelectasis during recovery
      4) Assist with collection and maintenance of physical and forensic evidence as indicated (see Chapter 44)
      5) Assist with possible hospitalization if
         a) Fractures of more than three adjacent ribs
         b) Fracture of first or second rib
         c) Suspected underlying visceral injury; sternal fracture or hypoxia
   e. Administer pharmacologic therapy as ordered
      1) Nonnarcotic or narcotic analgesics
      2) Intercostal nerve block
      3) Tetanus immunization
   f. Educate patient/significant others
      1) Importance of analgesia
      2) Appropriate splinting techniques
      3) Hydration and deep breathing exercises, including importance of incentive spirometry
      4) Do not use sandbags, strapping, or rib belts
4. Evaluation and ongoing monitoring
   a. Hemodynamic status
   b. Breath sounds and pulse oximetry
   c. Cardiac rate and rhythm
   d. Pain relief

I. RUPTURED DIAPHRAGM

A ruptured diaphragm may result from penetrating injuries to the thorax or abdomen or from high-speed deceleration forces common in motor vehicle crashes. Left diaphragmatic rupture is more common than right, possibly due to the position of the liver. Diaphragmatic rupture rarely occurs alone; other life-threatening injuries (blunt injury to the liver or spleen, or pelvic/long bone fractures) are common. There are no specific signs or symptoms so the injury is often missed. A high index of suspicion should be maintained with these other injuries. A rupture or tear to the diaphragm may allow abdominal contents to herniate into the chest cavity and cause compression of the lungs and mediastinum; a potentially life-threatening injury.

1. Assessment
   a. Subjective data collection
      1) History of present injury/chief complaint
         a) Initially patient may be asymptomatic
         b) Chest or abdominal pain radiating to left shoulder (Kehr sign)
         c) Dyspnea
         d) Mechanism of injury (see Chapter 31)
      2) Past medical history
         a) Current or preexisting diseases/illness
            (1) Gastrointestinal disease
            (2) Pulmonary disease
         b) Medications
         c) Allergies
         d) Immunization status
   b. Objective data collection
      1) Physical examination
         a) General appearance
            (1) Position intended to facilitate respiration
            (2) Hypotension, tachycardia, tachypnea, orthopnea, dysphagia
            (3) Severe distress/discomfort
         b) Inspection
            (1) Chest and/or abdominal wall contusion, ecchymosis, or open wound
            (2) Increased work of breathing: nasal flaring, accessory muscle use, retractions
            (3) Dysphagia
         c) Auscultation
            (1) Breath sounds: decreased or absent on injured side
            (2) Bowel sounds: present in lower to middle chest
            (3) Heart sounds: possible shifting to opposite side of rupture
         d) Palpation
            (1) Localized tenderness to injured chest or abdomen
            (2) Bony deformity or crepitus
      2) Diagnostic procedures
         a) ABGs
         b) CBC with differential
         c) Urinalysis; pregnancy test in female patients of childbearing age
         d) Chest radiograph
            (1) Abnormalities seen only 25% of time
            (2) Possible unilateral elevated hemidiaphragm
            (3) Possible hollow or solid mass above diaphragm
            (4) Possible mediastinal shift away from affected side
            (5) Naso/orogastric tube located in chest cavity
         e) Possible DPL
         f) FAST
         g) Minimally invasive endoscopy (laparoscopy, thorascopy)
2. Analysis: differential nursing diagnoses/collaborative problems
   a. Impaired gas exchange
   b. Ineffective breathing pattern
   c. Acute pain
   d. Anxiety/fear
   e. Risk of infection
3. Planning and implementation/interventions
   a. Maintain airway, breathing, circulation (see Chapters 1 and 32)
   b. Provide supplemental oxygen
      1) RSI and positive-pressure ventilatory support in patients with respiratory compromise
      2) High-flow oxygen
   c. Establish IV access for administration of crystalloid fluids/blood products/medications
      1) Insert two large-bore IV catheters
      2) Infuse warmed normal saline solution
   d. Prepare for/assist with medical interventions
      1) Advanced airway management
         a) Nasal or oral intubation
         b) Supraglottic airway (e.g., King, Combitube, laryngeal mask airway)
         c) Surgical airway (e.g., cricothyrotomy)
      2) Cover any open chest wounds with occlusive dressing; remove dressing if patient develops signs of tension pneumothorax
      3) Position to facilitate ventilation
      4) Prepare for possible chest tube insertion
         a) Consider procedural sedation (see Chapter 8)
         b) 32–36 French chest tube placed in fifth intercostal space, just anterior to midaxillary line
         c) Apply dressing per facility protocol after chest tube is inserted and sutured in place
      5) Institute cardiac and pulse oximetry monitoring
      6) Maintain normothermic body temperature
      7) Insert gastric tube and attach to suction
      8) Insert indwelling urinary catheter
      9) Assist with collection and maintenance of physical and forensic evidence as indicated (see Chapter 44)
      10) Assist with hospital admission or transfer to an institution providing a higher level of care

e. Administer pharmacologic therapy as ordered
  1) RSI premedications: sedatives, analgesics, neuromuscular blocking agents
  2) Procedural sedation medications
  3) Nonnarcotic or narcotic analgesics
  4) Tetanus immunization
4. Evaluation and ongoing monitoring
  a. Airway patency
  b. Hemodynamic status
  c. Breath sounds and pulse oximetry
  d. Cardiac rate and rhythm
  e. Intake and output
  f. Pain relief

J. TENSION PNEUMOTHORAX

Tension pneumothorax is a life-threatening traumatic injury. It occurs when an injury to the chest allows air to enter the pleural space on inspiration but does not allow air to escape on expiration. Trapped air causes a mediastinal shift and collapses the affected lung; compresses the heart, great vessels, and trachea; and significantly impedes venous return. If left untreated, hypotension, shock, decreased cardiac output, and vascular collapse will follow.

1. Assessment
  a. Subjective data collection
    1) History of present injury/chief complaint
      a) Sense of impending doom
      b) Localized severe chest pain (see Chapter 8)
      c) Severe dyspnea
      d) Mechanism of injury (see Chapter 31)
    2) Past medical history
      a) Current or preexisting diseases/illness
        (1) Pulmonary disease
      b) Medications
      c) Allergies
      d) Immunization status
  b. Objective data collection
    1) Physical examination
      a) General appearance
        (1) Anxiety, disorientation, confusion
        (2) Hypotension, tachycardia, tachypnea
        (3) Severe distress/discomfort, air hunger, critically ill
      b) Inspection
        (1) Chest wall contusion, ecchymosis, or open wound
        (2) Skin and mucosa: dusky color
        (3) Increased work of breathing: nasal flaring, accessory muscle use, retractions
        (4) Distended neck veins (may be absent if significant hemorrhage present)
        (5) Tracheal deviation toward uninjured side (late sign)
        (6) Cyanosis (late sign)
      c) Auscultation
        (1) Breath sounds: markedly decreased or absent on injured side
        (2) Heart tones: distinct
        (3) Bowel sounds: normal to diminished
      d) Palpation/percussion
        (1) Skin: cool temperature, and moist
        (2) Localized point tenderness to injured chest wall
        (3) Subcutaneous emphysema
        (4) Hyperresonance on injured side
    2) Diagnostic procedures
      a) ABGs
      b) CBC with differential
      c) Type and crossmatch
      d) Cardiac enzymes
      e) Urinalysis; pregnancy test in female patients of childbearing age
      f) Chest radiograph (not usually required to identify condition)
      g) Cervical spine radiograph
      h) ECG
2. Analysis: differential nursing diagnoses/collaborative problems
  a. Impaired gas exchange
  b. Decreased cardiac output
  c. Anxiety/fear
3. Planning and implementation/interventions
  a. Maintain airway, breathing, circulation (see Chapters 1 and 32)
  b. Provide supplemental oxygen; maintain O_2 saturation at 94–99%
  c. Establish IV access for administration of crystalloid fluids/medications
    1) Insert two large-bore IV catheters
    2) Infuse warmed normal saline solution
  d. Prepare for/assist with medical interventions as ordered
    1) Assist with emergent needle thoracentesis
      a) 14- to 16-gauge needle placed in second intercostal space, midclavicular line above rib
      b) Anticipate need for chest tube insertion and closed chest drainage
        (1) Consider procedural sedation (see Chapter 8)
        (2) 32–36 French chest tube placed in fifth intercostal space, just anterior to midaxillary line
        (3) Apply dressing per facility protocol after chest tube is inserted and sutured in place
    2) Place in high Fowler position, or position of comfort, to facilitate ventilation
    3) Institute cardiac and pulse oximetry monitoring
    4) Catheter placement and monitoring of central venous pressure (CVP) (see Chapter 6)
    5) Maintain normothermic body temperature
    6) Insert gastric tube and attach to suction as indicated

7) Insert indwelling urinary catheter as indicated
8) Assist with collection and maintenance of physical and forensic evidence as indicated (see Chapter 44)
9) Assist with hospital admission or transfer to an institution providing a higher level of care
   e. Administer pharmacologic therapy as ordered
      1) Nonnarcotic or narcotic analgesics
      2) Procedural sedation medications
      3) Tetanus immunization
4. Evaluation and ongoing monitoring
   a. Hemodynamic status
   b. Breath sounds and pulse oximetry
   c. Cardiac rate and rhythm
   d. Intake and output
   e. Pain relief

K. TRACHEOBRONCHIAL INJURY

Tracheobronchial injuries most commonly occur at the proximal trachea or within 1 inch of the carina, and most patients die on scene. High mortality is seen in those who arrive at a trauma center due to associated injuries that may mask this injury. Most are caused by penetrating injuries; however, severe blunt forces causing compressive shear can also be the cause. The severity of clinical signs and symptoms depends on the size of the wound, injury level, degree of injury to the lung, and resulting airflow changes. Airway continuity may be maintained by the fascia that surrounds the trachea and bronchi. Symptoms may be immediate or delayed for 3–4 days. Patients with serious injuries require urgent surgical intervention.

1. Assessment
   a. Subjective data collection
      1) History of present injury/chief complaint
         a) Localized chest pain (see Chapter 8)
         b) Dyspnea
         c) Mechanism of injury (see Chapter 31)
      2) Past medical history
         a) Current or preexisting disease/illness
            (1) Pulmonary disease
         b) Medications
         c) Allergies
         d) Immunization status
   b. Objective data collection
      1) Physical examination
         a) General appearance
            (1) Restlessness, combative
            (2) Position intended to facilitate respiration
            (3) Tachypnea or apnea (if complete obstruction), tachycardia
            (4) Hoarseness/stridor
            (5) Noisy breathing
            (6) Severe distress/discomfort, critically ill
            (7) Signs of tension pneumothorax
         b) Inspection
            (1) Possible airway obstruction

(2) Chest wall contusion, ecchymosis, or open wound
(3) Increased work of breathing: nasal flaring, accessory muscle use, retractions
(4) Hemoptysis
(5) Intercostal retractions
         c) Auscultation
            (1) Breath sounds: decreased or absent on injured side
         d) Palpation
            (1) Localized point tenderness to injured chest wall
            (2) Bony deformity or crepitus
            (3) Subcutaneous emphysema in chest that may spread to neck, face, and suprasternal area
      2) Diagnostic procedures
         a) CBC with differential
         b) ABGs
         c) Urinalysis; pregnancy test in female patients of childbearing age
         d) Chest radiograph: may reveal pneumomediastinum
         e) ECG
         f) Bronchoscopy, fiberoptic endoscopy; will confirm diagnosis
2. Analysis: differential nursing diagnoses/collaborative problems
   a. Ineffective airway clearance
   b. Impaired gas exchange
   c. Ineffective breathing pattern
   d. Anxiety/fear
   e. Acute pain
3. Planning and implementation/interventions
   a. Maintain airway, breathing, circulation (see Chapters 1 and 32)
   b. Provide supplemental oxygen
      1) Establishment of surgical airway, cricothyrotomy, and ventilatory support may be required
      2) RSI and ventilatory support if rupture is distal to end of intubation tube
   c. Establish IV access for administration of crystalloid fluids/blood products/medications
      1) Insert two large-bore IV catheters
      2) Infuse warmed normal saline solution
   d. Prepare for/assist with medical interventions
      1) Advanced airway management
         a) Nasal or oral intubation
         b) Supraglottic airway (e.g., King, Combitube, laryngeal mask airway)
         c) Surgical airway (e.g., cricothyrotomy)
      2) Cover any open chest wounds with three-sided occlusive dressing; remove dressing if patient develops signs of tension pneumothorax
      3) Place in semi-Fowler position, or position of comfort, to facilitate ventilation

4) Institute cardiac and pulse oximetry monitoring
5) Assist with chest tube insertion and closed chest drainage, as needed
   a) Consider procedural sedation (see Chapter 8)
   b) 32–36 French chest tube placed in fifth intercostal space, just anterior to midaxillary line
   c) Apply dressing per facility protocol after chest tube is inserted and sutured in place
6) Maintain normothermic body temperature
7) Insert gastric tube and attach to suction
8) Insert indwelling urinary catheter
9) Assist with collection and maintenance of physical and forensic evidence as indicated (see Chapter 44)
10) Assist with hospital admission or transfer to an institution providing a higher level of care
   e. Administer pharmacologic therapy as ordered
      1) RSI premedications: sedatives, analgesics, neuromuscular blocking agents
      2) Nonnarcotic or narcotic analgesics
      3) Local anesthesia or procedural sedation
      4) Tetanus immunization
4. Evaluation and ongoing monitoring
   a. Airway patency
   b. Level of consciousness
   c. Hemodynamic status
   d. Breath sounds and pulse oximetry
   e. Cardiac rate and rhythm
   f. Intake and output
   g. Pain relief

Bibliography

American College of Surgeons, Committee on Trauma: Thoracic trauma. In *Advanced trauma life support: Provider course manual*, ed 9, Chicago, IL, 2012, American College of Surgeons.

Bethel J: Tension pneumothorax, *Emergency Nurse*, 16(4):26–29, 2008.

Cook CC, Gleason TG: Great vessel and cardiac trauma, *Surgery Clinics of North America*, 89:797–820, 2009.

Day MW: Thoracic and neck trauma. In *Trauma nursing core course*, ed 7, Des Plaines, IL, 2014, Emergency Nurses Association.

Denlee NJ: Thoracic trauma. In Howard P, Steinmann R, editors: *Sheehy's emergency nursing principles and practice*, 6th ed., St. Louis, MO, 2010, Elselvier.

DuBose JA, O'Connor JV, Scalea TM: Lung, trachea, and esophagus. In Mattox KL, Moore EE, Feliciano DV, editors: *Trauma*, ed 7, New York, NY, 2013, McGraw-Hill.

Galketiya KP, Kerr JN, Davis IP: Blunt diaphragmatic rupture—A rare injury in blunt thoracoabdominal trauma, *Journal of Gastrointestinal Surgery*, 16:1805–1806, 2012.

Glazer ES, Meyerson SL: Delayed presentation and treatment of tracheobronchial injuries due to blunt trauma, *Journal of Surgical Education*, 65(4):302–308, 2008.

Mowery NT, Gunter OL, Collier BR, Dias JJ, Haut E, Hildreth A, Streib E: Practice management guidelines for management of hemothorax and occult pneumothorax, *Journal of Trauma, Injury, Infection and Critical Care*, 70(2):510–518, 2011.

Schuster KM, Davis KA: Diaphragm. In Mattox KL, Moore EE, Feliciano DV, editors: *Trauma*, ed 7, New York, NY, 2013, McGraw Hill.

Wall Jr MJ, Tsai P, Mattox KL: Heart and thoracic vascular injuries. In Mattox KL, Moore EE, Feliciano DV, editors: *Trauma*, ed 7, New York, NY, 2013, McGraw Hill.

CHAPTER 40

Sexual Assault

Joyce Foresman-Capuzzi, MSN, APRN, RN-BC, CCNS, CEN, CPN, CTRN, CCRN, CPEN, SANE-A, AFN-BC, EMT-P, FAEN

I. Definitions

A. SEXUAL VIOLENCE

1. Defined as a sexual act committed against someone without that person's freely given consent.
2. Sexual violence is divided into types
   a. Completed or attempted forced penetration of a victim
   b. Completed or attempted alcohol/drug-facilitated penetration of a victim
   c. Completed or attempted forced acts in which a victim is made to penetrate a perpetrator or someone else
   d. Completed or attempted alcohol/drug-facilitated acts in which a victim is made to penetrate a perpetrator or someone else
   e. Nonphysically forced penetration that occurs after a person is pressured verbally or through intimidation or misuse of authority to consent or acquiesce
   f. Unwanted sexual contact
   g. Noncontact unwanted sexual experiences[1]

B. SEXUAL ASSAULT

1. The act of forcing another person into sexual activity against his or her will and includes forced sexual intercourse, oral or anal sexual acts, incest, fondling, voyeurism, sexual harassment/threats[2]

C. RAPE

1. A legal term that denotes unlawful sexual intercourse[3]

D. EVIDENCE

1. Data presented to a jury to prove or disprove a claim
2. It can be physical or informational
3. Physical is real and tangible and can be measured, visualized or analyzed
   a. It can also be trace physical evidence, only seen microscopically
4. Informational evidence is history, excited utterances, or something observed, such as odor or appearance[4]

E. LOCARD PRINCIPLE

1. An exchange or transference of evidence when two items come in contact with each other. This transference of physical evidence is valuable to law enforcement to link a suspect or location to a victim and vice versa, because every contact leaves some type of evidence[4]

F. CHAIN OF CUSTODY

1. A paper trail necessary to ensure that no tampering of evidence occurs; this paper trail is created by documenting the possession of the evidence from the moment of collection until the moment it is introduced in court and everywhere in between[4]

II. General Strategy

Sexual assault can be defined as any type of sexual activity in which one person does not agree to engage but is forced to comply. Both psychological coercion and physical force can be parts of sexual assault. Sexual assault is not a crime of passion. In sexual assault, another person dictates the most intimate of personal choices. Girls and women and boys and men of all ages have been victims of sexual assault.

Patients who have been sexually assaulted may present to emergency departments with a myriad of complaints. Not all patients will readily admit to being sexually assaulted; therefore, the nurse has a responsibility to assess the patient and ask sensitive questions to determine whether the patient has been sexually assaulted. It is important to remember that not all sexual assaults result in physical injury; and, just as conversely, consensual sexual intercourse can result in injury. Thus, the presence or absence of physical injury neither proves nor disproves an assault occurred. While patients may present to the ED requesting a forensic nursing exam to determine if they were "raped," it is important for the ED nurse to know that it is not the role of the RN or the medical team to determine if a sexual assault occurred, but instead treat any injuries and address any emotional, psychological, and other issues. It is important to remember that "rape" is a legal term and even the presence or absence of semen or live sperm does not provide the full picture. The entire forensic team caring for the patient includes the Sexual Assault Nurse Examiner (SANE), the provider, victim advocate, local law enforcement, the legal system, and the crime laboratory.

The entire emergency team must communicate with the patient in a nonjudgmental manner. Very often guilt, fear, lack of knowledge or trust in "the system," or coercion prevents a patient from seeking timely care, or care at all. The positive hospital experience can have an important impact on the patient's physical and psychological recovery from the assault. Every sexual assault victim requires a complete and in-depth physical examination and the opportunity to consent to a sexual assault forensic examination.

Many hospitals and counties have developed Sexual Assault Response Teams (SARTs). A SART consists of a victim advocate, a police officer, and most often a Sexual Assault Nurse Examiner/Sexual Assault Forensic Examiner (SANE/SAFE). SART programs provide one-on-one comprehensive and compassionate medical care. Obtaining an appropriate forensic examination and ensuring the team meets the patient's medical, psychological, and nursing needs are the goals of the SART examination.

The SANE is a registered nurse with specialized forensic nursing training who demonstrates competency in forensic evidence collection and applies the nursing process when caring for this population. Law enforcement should be present at the hospital because, as part of the team, their presence allows for ease of information sharing and maintenance of the chain of custody. Examinations are private and usually done by the SANE or the physician—no law enforcement is to be present. The victim advocate supports the patient's emotional needs, and the patient may be given the choice to have the advocate in the examination room or not. These specialized teams have demonstrated improved care delivery to victims of sexual assault.

Although the patient may choose not to speak with law enforcement, it is important to alert the patient of the mandated reporting laws that may exist in cases of sexual assault or intimate partner violence. Requirements for the forensic examination of minors must also be determined, which can vary from state to state.

A. CLINICAL FORENSIC ISSUES

1. Evidence collection and preservation is an ED nursing competency
2. Sexual assault patient can be male, female, or gender neutral
3. Patient may not know he or she has been assaulted, but there is an index of suspicion
   a. Nonverbal child
   b. Patient with cognitive deficit
   c. Unconscious patient
4. Specific consent for the forensic exam must be obtained, as well as any photographs
   a. Foreknowledge of department-specific policy is a must
5. Purpose of sexual assault exam
   a. Medical
      1) Identify and treat injuries, assess risk of pregnancy and STI, and treat prophylactically
   b. Social
      1) Respond to emotional needs and concerns, assess patient safety, provide coping strategies and referrals
   c. Forensic and legal
      1) Collect evidence, preserve chain of custody, gather unbiased testimony
   d. Referral
      1) For medical care, advocacy and counselling
6. Use of standardized and approved sexual assault kit and documentation paperwork not necessary but helpful
   a. Sexual assault kit contains necessary items to conduct thorough forensic nursing exam with collection of physical evidence
      1) Paper bags, envelopes, glass slides, nail clippers, comb, drape, sheet, cotton-tipped applicators and boxes, tamper tape, etc.
      2) Documentation for informational evidence
         a) Blank body diagrams, consent, evidence collection logs, narrative, etc.
7. "Care of Sexual Assault and Rape Victims in the Emergency Department" is a position statement of the Emergency Nurses Association[5]
8. Care of any sexual assault patient always involves the nursing process in addition to any sexual assault nursing competencies
   a. Assessment, planning, implementation, evaluation

9. Culture, language, religion, race, values, sexual orientation, gender, immigration status, and beliefs should be assessed to provide culturally competent care[3]
10. Emergency nursing responsibilities
    a. Priority is directed toward lifesaving interventions as physical injuries can be severe and must be immediately addressed
    b. Lifesaving interventions should never be delayed or compromised in order to collect or preserve forensic evidence
    c. A safe environment must be provided for patient and personnel
    d. The nature of sexual assault cases and patients lends itself to being on high alert for workplace violence
    e. Working knowledge of legalities, reporting mandates, and patient information dissemination for jurisdiction of practice (see Chapter 45)
    f. Collection and preservation of evidence according to local, state, and federal requirements is a component of emergency nursing practice
    g. Identification of need for evidence collection and preservation
    h. Initiation and maintenance of legal records and documentation such as photographs
        1) Assessment
11. Primary and secondary assessment/resuscitation (see Chapters 1 and 32)
    a. Triage
        1) Categorized as Emergency Severity Index (ESI) 2 (see Chapter 2)
        2) Move to private area as soon as possible due to distress and for evidence preservation
            a) Medical stabilization always paramount over evidence collection
                (1) Triage for significant illness, injury, or psychiatric emergency and treat if necessary
            b) Registration
                (1) Have hospital registration occur privately
                (2) Check with local protocols for victim compensation options
    b. Focused assessment
        1) Assessment
            a) Subjective data collection and informational evidence
                (1) History of present assault/injury/chief complaint
    c. Maintain questioning demeanor
    d. Questions and documentation
        1) Documentation must be thorough and meticulous
            a) Patient's statements can be admissible in court
            b) Document what is said and what is observed
                (1) What needs to be collected as evidence is often determined by a good history of the event

                (2) Informational evidence collection
                (3) Do not analyze or judge, but simply record
            c) Patient's reflection as to what occurred during the commission of the crime
            d) Record statements in patient's own words using quotation marks
            e) Statements are not interpreted, medicalized, or sanitized
        2) If patient uses a vulgar term or slang, place correct medical term in parenthesis
            a) Answers to questions help to drive the collection of evidence, based on how patient answers
                (1) "He came (ejaculated) on my stomach" would lead the RN to collect specimens from abdominal area
        3) Date and time of assault
            a) Evidence collection and interpretation of results may need accommodations depending on elapsed time
                (1) Collection of physical evidence may be supported at 72–96 hours post assault
        4) Location of assault
            a) Known location, landmarks, in or outside, home, public place
        5) Assailant information
            a) Gender
            b) Known or unknown
            c) Number of assailants
            d) Specific information
                (1) Clothing, facial hair, markings, physical characteristics, speech, hair color and length, tattoos
        6) Nature of force used
            a) Use of penetrating foreign objects, coercion, threats, or weapons in assault
            b) Grabbing, pinching, choking, strangling, punching, slapping, etc.
        7) Physical facts of assault
            a) Area of body contacted, orifices penetrated, use of condom, etc.
        8) Consensual sexual activity within last 5 days (vaginal, oral, rectal)
            a) Findings may not be associated with crime and partner DNA will need to be ruled out
        9) Activity post assault
            a) Quality of evidence may be affected by activities post assault
                (1) Bathing, showering, douching, brushing teeth, eating, inserting tampon or using sanitary napkin, drinking, smoking, vomiting, changing clothes
                    (a) If clothes have been changed, what is the location of the clothes worn at time of assault

10) The information can be provided to local law enforcement

   a) Strangulation

     (1) Observe for ligature marks around neck or patterned injury (such as fingertips)

     (2) Observe for petechiae on face, lower lip, hairline, sclera, and conjunctiva

     (3) Patient complains of dyspnea, sore throat, hoarseness and difficulty swallowing, weakness in arms or legs

     (4) Assess for loss of consciousness, incontinence, and mental status changes

   b) Loss of memory/consciousness

     (1) What does patient last remember?

       (a) What was patient eating, drinking, or doing?

     (2) What was patient wearing during the attack?

       (a) Is that different now?

         (i) Example: wore underwear when leaving, but not on now or on inside out, shoes on wrong feet

   c) Consider drug-facilitated sexual assault (DFSA)

     (1) Voluntary substance or alcohol use and time

       (a) Involuntary drug use

         (i) Patient may describe sensation as if watching what took place, but not able to speak or move

         (ii) DFSA drugs such as flunitrazepam (Rohypnol), ketamine, and gamma-hydroxybutyric acid (GHB): follow local protocols for drug testing

         (iii) Obtain specimen early if suspected as these drugs have short half-life

         (iv) If patient vomits, collect and preserve sample

   d) Injuries that patient may have inflicted on perpetrator

   e) Contraceptive/lubricant use by perpetrator

   f) Penetration of genitalia, anus, or oral contact, no matter how slight

   g) Nongenital acts

     (1) Sucking, kissing, licking, biting

   h) Did ejaculation occur and, if so, where?

12. Past medical history

  a. Current or preexisting comorbidities

  b. Recent gynecologic/obstetric/urologic illness/injury

  c. Last normal menstrual period: female patients or transgender male (with remaining ovaries and uterus) of childbearing age

  d. Current medications

    1) Prescription, including contraceptives

    2) OTC/herbal

  e. Allergies

  f. Immunization status including tetanus

  g. Previous history of abuse/neglect

  h. Substance and/or alcohol use/abuse and if positive, last time used

13. Objective data collection

  a. Physical examination (see Chapters 1, 32, and 44)

    1) General appearance

    2) Level of consciousness, behavior, affect: alert to comatose, crying, fearful, laughing, calm, giddy

    3) Level of pain/distress/discomfort: emotional, physical, spiritual

    4) Vital signs with trending; cardiac, blood pressure, respiratory, pulse ox, and/or ET CO_2 monitoring as necessary; POCT including glucose as necessary

    5) Odors (and document)

      a) Petroleum, burning wood, chemical, alcohol, drug, vomit/urine, etc.

      b) Hazardous material odor such as bitter almonds (cyanide) or new mown hay (phosgene)

    6) Gait

    7) Hygiene

    8) Appearance

    9) Orientation of clothing, missing, or shoes on the wrong feet

      a) Could indicate that someone else dressed patient

    10) Inspection of entire unclothed body while standing on sheet on floor (see Chapter 44)

      a) Soft tissue injuries: ecchymotic areas or obvious injury/deformity with intervention as needed

      b) Burns

      c) Patterned injuries

      d) Defensive wounds

      e) "Wounds" (e.g., laceration, abrasion, avulsion, bite marks, scratches)

      f) Genital/perineal injuries

        (1) Women

          (a) Best performed in dorsal lithotomy position

            (i) Examine inner thighs, labia majora and minora, mons pubis

          (b) May use speculum

            (i) Only moistened with water, no lubricant

            (ii) Colposcope may be used to enhance visualization of potential injury and to take pictures for documentation; illuminates and magnifies view of cervix and vaginal structures

(c) TEARS mnemonic when visualizing internal and external genitalia: tears, ecchymosis, abrasion, redness, swelling

(2) Men

  (a) Some men have physical injuries after assault, but not all

  (b) Best examined prone, knee chest or bending over stretcher

  (c) Injuries tend to be soft tissue in perianal and anal areas

    (i) Separate folds

  (d) Examine inner thighs, buttocks, foreskin, urethral meatus, shaft, scrotum, perineum, glans, testes

  (e) Obtain swab, using two cotton-tipped applicators, of meatus, glans, foreskin, if present

  (f) Men can be victimized by either male or female assailants

  (g) Provide reassurance that assault is not patient's fault, as men may experience embarrassment, public disclosure, how to tell family members, inability to fight off assailant

  (h) Men may question "true" sexuality since they may have been aroused, including having an erection

    (i) Provide reassurance that this may be an involuntary response to fear, anxiety, etc.[3]

g) Buttocks injuries

  (1) Examine carefully

  (2) Document rectal vs perianal

  (3) For male or female rectal penetration, use of anoscope may be helpful

  (4) Document tears, presence of vegetation, dirt, hair, discoloration, bleeding, etc.

b. Auscultation

  1) Breath sounds

  2) Heart sounds

  3) Bowel sounds

  4) Fetal heart tones, if pregnant

c. Palpation/percussion

  1) Skin temperature, moisture

  2) Areas of tenderness, pain or deformity with evidence collection, diagnostics, and interventions as necessary

d. Diagnostic procedures

  1) Laboratory studies

    a) CBC with differential, if medically necessary

    b) Serum chemistries including glucose, BUN, creatinine, if medically necessary

    c) Serum and urine toxicology screens including testing for DFSA

    d) Type and crossmatch if necessary

    e) Urinalysis; pregnancy test in female patients and transgender male patients (with remaining ovaries and uterus) of childbearing age

    f) Baseline human immunodeficiency virus (HIV), and hepatitis B and C

    g) Rapid plasma reagin (RPR)

    h) Evidence collection swabs (e.g., anogenital [rectal, perianal, penile, cervix, vaginal] and oral areas)

      (1) Will likely go to crime laboratory after being given to police (not hospital laboratory) following chain of custody

      (2) Forensic testing: DNA, ABO blood groups

    i) Other studies as indicated by policy

  2) It is important to note that many sexual assault protocols do not include collection cultures for sexually transmitted infection (STI) at time of exam, but instead treat empirically with antibiotics and suggest follow-up with provider or clinic. Know accepted protocol

  3) Imaging studies

    a) Radiograph of injured/tender area

    b) Head, thoracic, or abdominal CT scan, as indicated by injuries

    c) 12- or 15-lead ECG if necessary

B. ANALYSIS: DIFFERENTIAL NURSING DIAGNOSES/COLLABORATIVE PROBLEMS

1. Risk for injury
2. Risk for ineffective coping
3. Risk for impaired skin integrity
4. Anxiety/fear
5. Pain
6. Risk for self-directed violence
7. Rape-trauma syndrome

C. PLANNING AND IMPLEMENTATION/ INTERVENTIONS

1. Determine priorities of care

  a. Maintain airway, breathing, circulation (see Chapters 1 and 32)

  b. Provide supplemental oxygen as indicated

  c. Establish intravenous (IV) or intraosseous (IO) access for administration of crystalloid fluids/blood products/medications

  d. Obtain and set up equipment and supplies

  e. Prepare for/assist with medical interventions

  f. Administer pharmacologic therapy as ordered

2. Relieve anxiety/apprehension
3. Allow significant others to remain with patient if supportive
4. Educate patient and significant others
5. Provide follow-up counselling
6. Provide referral for follow-up care or clinic

D. EVALUATION AND ONGOING MONITORING

1. Continuously monitor and treat as indicated
2. Monitor patient response/outcomes, and modify nursing care plan as appropriate
3. If positive patient outcomes are not demonstrated, re-evaluate assessment and/or plan of care

E. DOCUMENTATION OF INTERVENTIONS AND PATIENT RESPONSE

F. AGE AND DEVELOPMENT RELATED CONSIDERATIONS

1. Pediatrics
   a. Child abuse is reportable
      1) "Engaging of a child in sexual activities that the child cannot comprehend, for which the child is developmentally unprepared and cannot give informed consent and that violate the social taboos of society"[6]
   b. Growth or development related
      1) Children are often coerced, so maintain a high level of suspicion
         a) Presenting symptom may be general and nonspecific including regression of developmental milestones
      2) May be brought in by parent, social service, law enforcement
      3) Assess for age-appropriate behaviors
      4) Physical exam alone is not often diagnostic
      5) Dependent on caregiver to meet physical and emotional needs
      6) If an experienced pediatric examiner is not available and the assault is not acute (within 96 hours), the examination may be postponed until a time when an examiner is available. If assault is acute, consider transferring patient and caregivers to a facility that can perform a pediatric sexual assault exam
         a) Having an experienced pediatric SANE benefits the team, patient, and family
         b) Do not refer to kit as a "rape kit"
      7) Determine state law regarding consent when preparing to examine an adolescent. Patient may not want his or her parents contacted. Determine whether parental consent is required
      8) Determine adolescent's knowledge base of sexual function and terminology
   c. "Pearls"
      1) Uncooperative pediatric patient should not be restrained in order to complete an examination, to avoid further traumatization

2) Best position for examination for prepubescent children
   a) Female is knee-chest or supine in frog-leg position
      (1) Do not use digits or speculum for exam
      (2) May need specialized technique such as use of indwelling catheter balloon to visualize hymen
   b) Male is standing
3) Presence of STI is hallmark of sexual abuse in child
4) Consider differential diagnosis
   a) Foreign body
   b) Bleeding disorder
   c) Poor hygiene
   d) Urinary tract infection
5) Risk factors for abuse
   a) Infant separation at birth as a result of prematurity or illness
   b) Congenital anomalies or chronic medical conditions
   c) Behavior problems, fussy infants
   d) Developmental disabilities
   e) Nonparental male living in household
      (1) Assess for possibility of long-term molestation in the pediatric age group

2. Geriatrics
   a. Aging related
      1) Elder sexual abuse is reportable to law enforcement
      2) A pilot study of elder sexual abuse showed that 11 of 20 elderly victims died within 12 months of assault[3]
      3) May have cognitive impairment and thus cannot consent to sex, which can delay report of sexual assault
      4) Are fearful of location where sexual assault occurred and have symptoms of traumatic stress
      5) Consider consulting with geriatric nursing specialist and collaborate on assessment and care
      6) Assess for emotional trauma including regression
      7) Assess victim's sense of hearing, seeing, etc.
      8) Determine patient's degree of comfort when discussing sexual function and terminology
      9) Increased incidence of soft tissue injury resulting from force
      10) Soft tissue is more friable and may lead to increased bleeding
      11) Consider patient comfort when performing pelvic examination
      12) Dependent on caregivers to meet physical and emotional needs
      13) Examination

a) Female patients may be difficult because they cannot be placed in dorsal lithotomy position for pelvic exam due to contractures, arthritis, etc.
  (1) Supine with legs supported by assistants may be beneficial
  (2) Use small narrow speculum
  (3) Inspect both external and internal genitalia
    (a) Colposcope will be beneficial
14) Presence of STI is not conclusive for sexual assault
  a) May be preexisting
  b) Must be well documented, tested, treated, and investigated along with patient's ability to provide consent
15) Assess thoroughly for safety prior to discharge regardless of patient returning to home, assisted living, or nursing home
  b. Patients with disabilities[3]
  1) Abuse against patients with disabilities is reportable to police
  2) People with developmental disabilities are 4 to 10 times more likely to be victims of crime than other people[3]
    a) Patients with Alzheimer disease
      (1) Approach from front
      (2) Talk in low pitch and quiet tone
      (3) Explain in simple term and ask simple closed-end questions
    b) Patients with mental illness
      (1) Allow patient to become calm before intervening
      (2) Avoid touching and direct continuous eye contact
      (3) Keep conversation brief and free from distractions
    c) Patients with developmental disabilities
      (1) Treat as adults, not children
      (2) Take break every 15 minutes
      (3) Match your tempo of speech to theirs
      (4) Wait patiently for response
    d) Patients who are blind or visually impaired
      (1) Introduce yourself immediately
      (2) If you are writing and not speaking, advise patient of that
      (3) Do not pet or talk to guide dogs
      (4) Offer your arm instead of holding theirs to help them move about
    e) Patients who are deaf or hearing impaired
      (1) Obtain translator per legal requirement and policy
      (2) Determine how they want to communicate
      (3) Face patients so they see your mouth and face
      (4) Make questions short and simple[3]

G. PHYSICAL EVIDENCE COLLECTION (SEE CHAPTER 44 FOR SPECIFIC DETAILS)

1. Explain procedure to patient
  a. Advise patient that exam can take several hours and that all informational and physical evidence collected must be turned over to law enforcement, regardless if patient wants to press charges or speak with police
2. Can be modified to specific needs and comfort of patient
  a. May also be stopped at any time at patient's request
    1) Check with local law enforcement as evidence collected, regardless of how much, may be turned over to them
3. Have patient undress on clean bed sheet to collect any trace physical evidence that may come off during disrobing
  a. Fold sheet in such a way as to contain any debris and place in paper bag, then label and seal
  b. With gloved hands, place each piece of clothing in a separate paper bag, then label and seal
  c. Patient's clothing: place in paper bags, not plastic
4. Swabs/slides, during an oral, vaginal (pelvic), penile, and/or rectal examination
5. Photography (see Chapter 44)
6. Prepare for/assist with medical interventions
  a. Provide privacy for patients promptly on arrival and during all aspects of care
  b. Assist with treatment of injuries associated with assault
  c. Assist with forensic examination (see Chapter 44)
7. Evidence collected according to local or state policies. All evidence collected is placed in appropriate bag, envelope, or box, then sealed, signed, and labeled with
  a. Patient's name
  b. Medical record number
  c. Date, time
  d. Sample source
  e. Registered nurse's initials
8. Local or state policy may dictate that all swabs and slides must be air dried prior to packaging. Swab boxes, slide carriers, and envelopes should be used to house the evidence. All evidence is kept in the custody of the nurse until it is passed to the law enforcement officer
9. Obtain photographs per local policy
10. Fingernail scrapings evidence
  a. Use a cotton-tipped applicator, clean toothpick, or manicure stick to collect material under each fingernail. Place used applicator and material from each hand into a different envelope
11. Oral evidence
  a. Examine for injury, especially frenulums
    1) Swab gumlines for evidence, place on glass slide and dry swab

2) Per local policy, collect swabs for seminal fluid if patient was made to orally copulate the perpetrator. Prepare dry mount slides using swabs and label to indicate which swab was used to make which slide (see Chapter 44)

b. Buccal swabs may also be taken for a reference sample to separate DNA from that of suspect

    1) Patient must rinse mouth first with water then swab inner cheeks with gentle pressure, per directions in kit

12. Pubic hair evidence

    a. Place a paper sheet under the buttock. Using a comb or a soft brush, comb downward to remove foreign hairs/material. Evidence tape may be used if mons pubis has been previously shaved or moisten wet cotton-tipped applicators and swab mons pubis, then dry and label. Fold paper sheet, comb or brush, and collected hairs and place in envelope

13. Pelvic examination evidence

    a. Collect any foreign material or matted hairs

    b. Vaginal swabs including cervix, per local policy; swabs may be used to make dry mount slides

14. Anal/rectal examination evidence

    a. Collect any foreign material or matted hairs

        1) Cleanse perianal area after vaginal or penile specimens have been taken and foreign material has been collected

    b. Anal swabs: prepare slides as indicated by local policy

15. Administer pharmacologic therapy as ordered

    a. Antibiotics: STI prophylaxis per Centers for Disease Control and Prevention guidelines[7]

    b. HIV postexposure prophylaxis (PEP)

        1) Provider will assess level of risk and discuss option for PEP with patient

        2) Administer to patient if ordered and per policy

    c. Pregnancy-prevention medication such as levonorgestrel (Plan B) within 72 hours of the assault

        1) Must have a documented negative pregnancy test at the time of the examination before pregnancy-prevention medication can be administered

16. Ensure chain of custody

    a. Accurate documentation of the handling of evidence will establish and safeguard the integrity and competence of evidence from time of collection until it is introduced at trial

    b. Place label on outside of package and/or document the following information

        1) Patient's name or use patient's demographic hospital label

        2) Item description of what is in package

        3) Name of agency taking item

        4) Name of person sealing item with date and time

        5) Name of person releasing item with date and time

        6) Name of person receiving item with date and time

        7) Limit the number of people in the chain of custody

    c. Document in medical record

        1) Make copy for medical record

        2) Item(s) released to law enforcement

        3) Name and badge number of law enforcement officer accepting evidence

17. Educate patient/significant others

    a. Address patient safety during exam and follow policy

    b. Support patient recovery

    c. Dispel myths and misconceptions

        1) No one has the right to violate another person

        2) Patient did not cause the attack

        3) Patient did not ask for the assault by his or her actions

        4) Patient is not to blame for wearing a certain type of clothing or for drinking alcohol

    d. Follow up with primary health care provider in 1–2 weeks

    e. Offer information regarding testing for HIV and hepatitis

    f. Telephone follow-up with victim advocate

18. Evaluation and ongoing monitoring

    a. Patient safety at time of discharge or admission

    b. Continuously monitor and treat as indicated

    c. Monitor patient response/outcomes, and modify nursing care plan as appropriate

    d. If positive patient outcomes are not demonstrated, reevaluate assessment and/or plan of care

    e. Pain assessment and intervention

References

1. CDC: *Injury prevention & control: Division of Violence Prevention*, Centers for Disease Control and Prevention, 2015. Retrieved from http://www.cdc.gov/ViolencePrevention/sexualviolence/definitions.html.

2. National Center for Victims of Crime: About sexual assault, 2012. Retrieved from http://www.victimsofcrime.org/our-programs/dna-resource-center/untested-sexual-assault-kits/about-sexual-assault.

3. Brown KA: *Quick reference to adult and older adult forensics*, New York, NY, 2010, Springer.

4. Foresman-Capuzzi J: CSI and U: Evidence collection and preservation in the emergency department, *Journal of Emergency Nursing*, 229–236, 2014.

5. ENA: *Care of sexual assault and rape victims in the emergency department*, Emergency Nurses Association, 2010. Retrieved from https://www.ena.org/practice-research/Practice/Position/Pages/SexualAssaultRapeVictims.aspx.

6. Brown KA: *Quick reference to child and adolescent forensics*, New York, NY, 2010, Springer.

7. CDC: *2015 sexually transmitted disease treatment guidelines*, Centers for Disease Control and Prevention, 2015. Retrieved from http://www.cdc.gov/std/tg2015/default.htm.

Part 3

Bibliography

Brown KM, Muscari ME: *Quick reference to adult and older adult forensics*, New York, NY, 2010, Springer.

Darnell C, Michel C: *Forensic notes*, Philadelphia, PA, 2012, F.A. Davis Company.

Easter C, Muro G: An ED forensic kit, *Journal of Emergency Nursing*, 21:440–444, 1995.

Emergency Nurses Association: Position statement on forensic evidence collection. Retrieved from http://www.ena.org/Site CollectionDocuments/Position%20Statements/Forensic%20E vidence, 2010.

Foresman-Capuzzi J: CSI and U: Evidence collection and preservation in the emergency department, *Journal of Emergency Nursing*, 40(3):229–236, 2014.

Hammer R, Moynihan B, Pigliaro E: *Forensic nursing: A handbook for practice*, Burlington, MA, 2013, Jones and Bartlett.

Howard PK, Steinmann R: *Sheehy's emergency nursing: Principles and practice*, ed 6, St Louis, MO, 2010, Mosby.

International Association of Forensic Nurses: Role of the forensic nurse. Retrieved from http://iafn.org/displaycommon.cfm?an=1&subarticlenbr=137, 2006.

Lynch V: *Forensic nursing science*, ed 2, St Louis, MO, 2011, Mosby.

Pinckard JK, Wetli C, Graham MA: Release of organs and tissues for transplantation, *American Journal of Forensic Medicine and Pathology*, 28(3):202–207, 2007.

Pyrek K: *Forensic nursing*, Boca Raton, FL, 2006, CRC Press.

U.S. Department of Justice: *A national protocol for sexual assault medical examinations*, National Criminal Justice Reference Service, 2013. Retrieved from https://www.ncjrs.gov/pdffiles1/ovw/241903.pdf.

CHAPTER 41

Disaster Preparedness and Response

Sue Anne Bell, PhD, FNP-BC

Disasters are wide and varied in their scope, from natural disasters such as hurricanes, tsunamis, and earthquakes, to disease outbreaks, to chemical and radiological accidents, to terrorism including use of weapons of mass destruction, to the health-related effects of climate change. Disasters can occur as anticipated events or be sudden onset. They can also be unintentional (accidental) or human-caused intentional events. Definitions for disaster vary, including a "calamitous event that effects a large population and generally results in injury, death, and destruction of property."[1] Since 1990, the United States has experienced an average of 53 major disasters each year, with approximately 11 disasters annually warranting federal assistance under the Robert T. Stafford Disaster Relief and Emergency Assistance Act.[2] Federal disaster response is directed under the Department of Health and Human Services, where two branches have responsibility: the Federal Emergency Management Agency (FEMA) and the Assistant Secretary for Preparedness and Response (ASPR). The primary purpose of FEMA is to coordinate the response to U.S. disasters that overwhelm the resources of state and local authorities. The governor of the state in which the disaster occurs must declare a state of emergency along with a formal request from the president that FEMA and the federal government respond to the disaster. The secretary of HHS delegates to ASPR the leadership role for all health and medical services support functions in a health emergency or public health event. The National Response Framework is the governmental guide to how the nation responds to all types of disasters and emergencies. Emergency preparedness and response is best understood within the context of the emergency management cycle (Fig. 41.1), which is an ongoing process. The Incident Command System (ICS) is a method of organizing and directing emergency response, and can be applied in small or large emergency situations (Fig. 41.2).

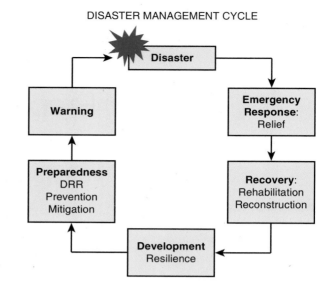

FIG. 41.1 Disaster Management Cycle. *(From Rushford, N., Thomas, K., Scherrer, V., & Pattison, M. Disaster and development, 1st ed. [2015]. St. Louis, MO: Elsevier.)*

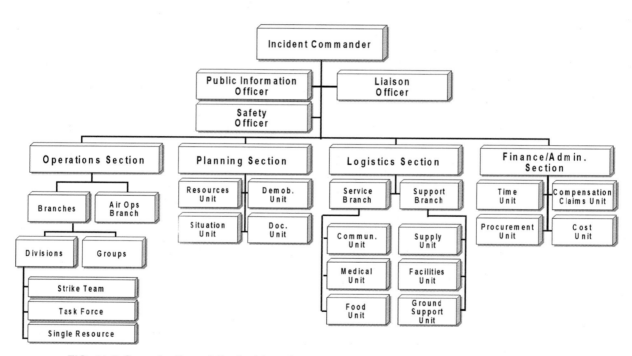

FIG. 41.2 Organization of the Incident Command System. *(From Federal Emergency Management Agency [FEMA]. [2008].* Incident Command System Training. *Available at* https://training.fema.gov /emiweb/is/icsresource/assets/reviewmaterials.pdf.*)*

I. Disasters

A. DISASTER DEFINITION

1. A disaster is a sudden, calamitous event that seriously disrupts the functioning of a community or society and causes human, material, and economic or environmental losses that exceed the community's or society's ability to cope using its own resources. Though often caused by nature, disasters can have human origins[3]

2. Any destructive event that disrupts the normal functioning of a community

B. TYPES OF DISASTER

1. Natural disaster
   a. A major adverse event that results from natural processes
      1) Examples: geological natural hazards such as earthquakes, tsunamis, landslides, sinkholes;

meteorological hazards[4] such as extreme heat or cold, tornadoes, hurricanes, or tropical storms, storm surges, floods, damaging winds, thunderstorms (lightning), hail, blizzards, ice storms, wildfires, drought, dam inundation, and volcanoes; infectious diseases and pandemics; space weather such as geomagnetic storms, solar radiation storms, radio blackouts

2. Technological disaster (formerly called "man-made" disasters)
   a. An event caused by humans that occurs in or close to cities or populated areas
      1) Examples: environmental degradation, pollution and accidents, complex emergencies/conflicts, famine, displaced populations, industrial accidents, hazardous materials exposure, and multimodal transportation accidents (air, rail, highway, marine)[5]

3. Aggravating factors
   a. Factors such as climate change, unplanned urbanization, underdevelopment, poverty and threat of pandemics can result in increased frequency, severity, and complexity of disasters

4. Intentional threats
   a. Human-caused threats and hazards including malicious cyber actors, violent actors (including active shooters and suicide bombers, domestic terrorists and homegrown violent extremists, transnational terrorists), criminal activities, and civil disturbances

II. Disaster Phases

A. WARNING

1. Definition
   a. The probability of impending danger
2. Actions
   a. Evaluate potential scope of impact
   b. Refer to all-hazards disaster plan and operate in an Incident Management System (IMS)
   c. Consider activating the hospital emergency operations center (EOC)
   d. Brief management and staff on course of actions
   e. Prepare for a potential 3- to 5-day period of self-sustaining activity
   f. Evaluate and review evacuation plans, supplies, staffing, recovery, and contingency plans to include redundant communications and critical functions

B. IMPACT

1. Definition
   a. Damage occurs in the event
2. Actions
   a. Operate using an ICS
   b. Liaison with local emergency management agencies
   c. Assess what damage or problems might occur from the event
   d. Preserve essential functions
   e. Follow the institution's emergency operations plan (EOP)

C. ISOLATION

1. Definition
   a. The period of time from impact and damage, until outside help arrives
2. Actions
   a. Assess damage
   b. Follow the institution's EOP
   c. Protect essential functions
   d. Prepare for staffing, logistics, and contingency needs, which are specific to the event and impact
   e. If needed, request assistance through established emergency management channels
   f. Prepare to function autonomously

D. RESCUE

1. Definition
   a. Assistance becomes available from external sources
2. Actions
   a. Operate with the common language of Incident Command
   b. Relay damage and needs assessment information
   c. Assign a liaison to represent the hospital at the community-based, emergency management agency's EOC (the Unified Command post)
   d. Continue to assess status of essential functions
   e. Prioritize needs for assistance

E. RESTORATION

1. Definition
   a. Emergency operations diminish, and normal functions are resuming
2. Actions
   a. Scale down emergency functions
   b. Continue to operate in Incident Command mode
   c. ICS may be scaled down as emergency operations become less complex
   d. Reconstitute nonessential functions

F. NORMAL OPERATIONS

1. Definition
   a. All functions return to baseline or a "new normal"
2. Actions
   a. Evaluate response
   b. Utilize response assessment to refine response plan

III. General Strategy

Because of the ongoing, credible threat of weapons of mass destruction (WMD) attacks, emergency nurses must be able to care for victims of WMD. Emergency personnel will have a direct, frontline role in the detection and treatment of this threat and therefore must be prepared to deal with possible patient contamination, infection, or injures from terrorist activities. Preparation for an all-hazards disaster event, such as an industrial accident or a natural hazard such as a hurricane, will assist emergency personnel in preparing for a WMD event, but a WMD event has certain characteristics that require special preparation. Preparedness includes an understanding of the location's credible threat, the facility's disaster plan, emergency personnel's role, the plan of care of the contaminated patient and the infectious patient, methods of screening for a suspicious event, forensic evidence awareness and preservation, and specific knowledge of chemical, biologic, nuclear, radiologic, and explosive event injury patterns and treatments. Additionally, a WMD event immediately elevates the local event to one of national significance, and emergency personnel must become familiar with their role in recognizing and reporting a suspicious event. First "receivers," or facility-based medical personnel, may be the initial detectors of a suspicious event such as a rapidly emerging infectious disease from a bioterrorist release. Emergency personnel need to plan, train, and exercise frequently with their colleagues and with those from other agencies such as public safety, emergency medical services, public health, hazardous materials, public information, and emergency management. An integrated, practiced response is key to a community's ability to be resilient in the face of a WMD event.

A. NATIONAL PREPAREDNESS

1. The National Response Framework—in the case of an event of national significance, such as a WMD event, the National Response Framework (NRF) will provide support and guidance to local and state response agencies
   a. Strategic National Stockpile (SNS)
      1) Managed by the Centers for Disease Control and Prevention (CDC), supported by Department of Health and Human Services
      2) Strategically located around the United States
      3) Provides large supplies of antibiotics, chemical antidotes, and medical supplies
      4) 12-hour push pack: cache of medicines and medical supplies can be delivered anywhere in the United States in 12 hours[6,7]
      5) Access through local to state emergency management or public health agencies
      6) States and high-risk jurisdictions often have additional local or state stockpiles
      7) Prior to requesting stockpile assets
         a) Identify immediately available supplies
         b) Calculate number of patients needing medications and treatment
         c) Estimate projected needs, overtime requirements
         d) Integrate preplanning with local public health
      8) Facility must be prepared for autonomous services for up to 5 days
      9) Facility recommendations include stockpiling prophylactic medications or treatment for personnel and immediate family members
2. Surveillance and notification programs
   a. Global Outbreak Alert and Response Network (GOARN) run by the World Health Organization (WHO), Program for Monitoring Emerging Diseases (ProMed), CDC Health Alert Network (HAN), and many other health intelligence networks, which collect and communicate medical surveillance data
   b. The United States has multiple, integrated surveillance systems that include public health epidemiologists, medical practitioners, electronic records, ambulance call volumes, pharmaceutical sales patterns, presenting diagnoses and illness patterns, school surveillance, and laboratory culture reports
   c. Emergency nursing role in surveillance
      1) Recognize and report suspicious symptoms
      2) Know where to find the correct treatment and diagnostic protocols
   d. Health care facilities have a role in active surveillance to detect a WMD event
      1) Ensuring educated personnel in WMD awareness and syndromic surveillance
      2) Promptly reporting suspicious illnesses to public health authorities
      3) Rapidly identifying and initiating appropriate medical screening, diagnostic tools, and agent-specific medical interventions
3. Contact resources
   a. CDC: http://www.cdc.gov
   b. WHO: http://www.who.com
   c. Local public health and/or emergency management offices serve as request and education conduits in some states. Some states also maintain caches of PPE, MCI supplies, and antidotes in strategic locations

B. REGIONAL AND LOCAL PREPAREDNESS

1. Minimize risk of contamination
2. Recognize signs and symptoms of agent
   a. Suspicion of possible initial exposure
      1) Increased death rate in hospitalized patients within 72 hours of admission
      2) Small or large outbreak of disease
      3) Clusters of patients from a single location
      4) Single case of highly unusual disease
      5) Atypical presentation of an endemic disease
      6) Rapidly increasing incidence of illness

7) Unusual increase of patients with complaints of fever, gastrointestinal (GI) symptoms, or respiratory complaints

8) Childhood disease in adults

9) Appearance of a disease off-season (e.g., flulike signs and symptoms during non-flu season)

10) Unexpected mortality rates of flulike illnesses

11) Multiple epidemics of differing illnesses

12) Unexplained blood disorders

13) Patients from a suspicious explosive event; consider contamination

14) Clusters of patients with rapidly progressing respiratory distress

15) Signs of chemical exposure

16) Commonalities of patients (e.g., in a similar area during a similar time frame)

17) Patients with presenting signs and symptoms from a CDC HAN alert

b. Second wave of infectious illnesses corresponding to incubation periods

3. Provide personnel protection

a. Use personal protective equipment (PPE)

b. Provide antidotes, prophylaxis, and vaccination when indicated

c. Provide available alternate personnel to assume duties at end of individual rotations

d. Effective equipment maintenance program

e. Differentiate between contaminated and infected patients

1) Contaminated patients have had a hazardous materials exposure, and wearing decontamination-specific PPE is indicated

a) U.S. regulatory agencies mandate the use of appropriate levels of PPE (Table 41.1)

b) PPE for receiving a contaminated patient is a minimum of level C

c) If the contaminant is not immediately known, the facility must follow the broadest PPE standards required by their annual hazards vulnerability analysis (HVA) data

d) Personnel donning PPE and providing care of the contaminated patient and/or performing decontamination must be[8]

(1) Monitored for safety issues

(2) Provided with necessary rehabilitation

(3) Medically monitored

(4) Fit tested if a fitted mask is chosen as part of the PPE ensemble

(5) Adequately trained and practiced in use of the PPE

(6) Provided with alternate personnel to assume duties at the end of their rotation

---

Table 41.1

Personal Protective Equipment

Level A PPE: Not Indicated for Use in a Health Care Facility Receiving Patients	Level B PPE: Not Indicated for Use in a Health Care Facility Receiving Patients	Level C PPE: OSHA Recommended Level of Protection for First Receivers in a Health Care Facility
1. Required for hot zone entry or hazardous environments with unknown contaminants, confined space entry, or an environment requiring the highest level of protection for skin, eyes, and the respiratory system	1. Worn when the highest level of respiratory protection is required, but less skin protection is needed, as determined by the identified contaminant or absence of aerosol or an oxygen percentage of <19.5, which is less than breathable air contains	1. Recommended by OSHA as the minimum standard PPE for first receivers; used when a hazard is present that may be absorbed through exposed skin and where the filters would remove the contaminant
2. Ensembles include fully encapsulated, liquid and vapor protective ensemble, positive pressure, full face piece, SCBA or positive pressure supplied air respirator with escape SCBA, gas tight, NIOSH-approved totally encapsulated chemical-protective suit with the highest level of permeation resistance, chemical-resistant double gloves and boots	2. Ensembles include liquid splash-resistant ensemble with the highest level of respiratory protection, positive pressure, full face piece, SCBA or positive pressure supplied air respirator with escape SCBA, gas tight, NIOSH-approved hooded, chemical-resistant clothing, chemical-resistant double gloves and boots	2. Ensemble includes liquid splash-resistant ensemble with the same level of skin protection as level B, hooded, chemical-resistant clothing, full face mask, positive air-purifying respirator with filters appropriate to the contaminant, chemical-resistant double gloves and boots
3. Difficult to wear longer than 30 minutes; hot and cumbersome, dependent on the air supply and user level of activity	3. Difficult to wear; dependent on the air supply and user level of activity	3. Requires medical monitoring and safety program, competency-based training, equipment maintenance
	4. Required for hospital-based personnel, only if a risk is indicated in the facility that would require the highest level of respiratory protection	4. PAPR batteries may run for 8 or more hours, but personnel would require monitored rotations and rehabilitation

NIOSH, National Institute for Occupational Safety and Health; *OSHA*, Occupational Safety and Health Administration; *PAPR*, powered air-purifying respirator; *PPE*, personal protective equipment; *SCBA*, self-contained breathing apparatus.

2) Infected patients usually do not require decontamination, and a minimum of standard precautions should be followed
   a) Airborne risk requires a fitted mask (e.g., N-95 respiratory mask or higher level of respiratory protection, gloves, and impervious gown)
   b) Droplet precautions include face shield, gloves, and gown
   c) Contact precautions include gloves and gown
   d) Additional infection control considerations include
      (1) Patient isolation
      (2) Cohorting patients with similar illnesses
      (3) Filtered air vents
      (4) Dedicated or decontaminated patient care equipment
      (5) Negative airflow rooms
      (6) Limited patient transportation to diminish exposure
   e) Highly infectious diseases may require
      (1) Additional PPE (e.g., powered air-purifying respirator [PAPR]), as indicated by suspicion of exposure, based on symptoms
      (2) Evaluation by infection control professionals and/or by facility policy, with recommendations available from the CDC
f. Until identification of the substance is made and it is deemed nontoxic, responders should wear their PPE
g. Levels of PPE (see Table 41.1)
4. Patient decontamination
   a. Physical process of removing contaminants from persons, equipment, and the environment
   b. Residual contaminants from exposed persons are a source of ongoing exposure and pose a risk of secondary exposure to first responders and emergency care personnel
   c. Immediate decontamination is a major treatment priority for those with exposure
      1) Initial gross field decontamination involves removal of patients from the contaminated environment followed by copious irrigation of the patient with water
      2) Patient decontamination is a medical procedure
      3) Hospitals receiving contaminated persons with or without initial field decontamination should consider the person contaminated and should provide definitive/detailed decontamination prior to entry into the facility
      4) Lifesaving interventions (e.g., assessment, airway establishment, respiratory support, bleeding stabilization, circulatory support, and fracture stabilization) should not be delayed for decontamination

5) Definitive/detailed decontamination is complete and thorough patient decontamination, not the initial gross field decontamination where only gross contaminants may be removed
6) Hospitals receiving contaminated persons should
   a) Establish an area outside the emergency department in which to perform decontamination before people and equipment are allowed to enter
   b) Minimally provide portable decontamination equipment with showers and runoff water collection systems
   c) Consider construction of external fixed "turnkey" decontamination facilities
   d) Pediatric decontamination: communication, family-centered care planning, age-related considerations
d. Decontamination preplanning
   1) OSHA guidelines state hospitals must have an EMP in place that determines numbers of patients the hospital is able to decontaminate
   2) Hospitals must be able to decontaminate patient more than one patient at time and both ambulatory and nonambulatory
   3) Health Resources and Services Administration (HRSA) indicates that hospitals should plan to be able to decontaminate all patients and providers within 3 hours from the onset of the event
   4) The Department of Homeland Security's (DHS) State Homeland Security Assessment Strategies (SHSAS) suggest that much higher numbers of presenting patients will appear commensurate with the local credible threat (e.g., mass gatherings, public event venues, and public transportation sites)
   5) Hospitals are required by The Joint Commission to conduct an annual HVA to assist in determining the likely number of patients requiring detailed/technical decontamination and the hourly throughput needed for the facility
   6) Hospitals should provide detailed/definitive decontamination procedures for presenting patients including
      a) Complete removal of clothing and jewelry
      b) Securing belongings
      c) Gender-segregated, environmentally sheltered, warm water decontamination for both ambulatory and nonambulatory patients
      d) Trained decontamination personnel with medical oversight in appropriate PPE, rehabilitation rotations, and adequate personnel to process all presenting patients rapidly
      e) Runoff collection
      f) Ability to provide lifesaving medical interventions before and during

decontamination, including the use of appropriate antidotes

    g) Gender-segregated, environmentally sheltered redress and subsequent medical screening and stabilization

  7) Community planning for a mass casualty event

  8) Rapid access to detection monitors, with trained users for radiologic, biologic, and chemical agents is recommended

  9) Hospitals should consider retrofitting or constructing the facility as a defensible facility because hospitals, as critical infrastructures in the community, may be primary and secondary terrorist targets. This involves

    a) Excluding direct line of vision access to critical areas (e.g., the emergency department and the operating room)

    b) Ability to compartmentalize the facility to offset security and contaminated patient breeches

    c) Ability to minimize damage from a direct attack (e.g., barriers for unscreened access areas to the facility by vehicles or persons)

5. Quarantine and isolation

  a. With the threat of rapidly emerging, highly infectious diseases, whether naturally occurring or from deliberate release, hospitals must have a plan to address large numbers of infected and exposed persons

  b. The plan should be integrated with local, regional, and state public health and emergency management plans because a mass casualty event is a public health emergency, not just a hospital emergency

  c. Health care facilities must be prepared to function autonomously with supplies and limited personnel for at least 5–7 days in an incident of national significance (e.g., a pandemic event)

  d. Health care facilities must be aware of state laws governing quarantine, because these laws affect their patients, visitors, and personnel

  e. Quarantine declarations are usually the domain of the lead public health official and are intended to limit spread of infectious disease; quarantine on a large scale may be voluntary, may require health care facilities to provide epidemiologic data, and may affect staffing, travel, and supplies

  f. Isolation is the medical procedure to remove an infected, contagious person from the general population

  g. Medical isolation focuses on containment of the disease

  h. Health care facilities must have plans to

    1) Rapidly increase isolation capability (e.g., by cohorting patients)

    2) Use portable isolation/filtration machines and procedures

  3) Dedicate equipment and personnel with appropriate PPE

  4) Decontaminate patients without delaying lifesaving assessment and medical treatment

  i. Community plans for a large-scale infectious disease event may include use of alternate facilities for infected patients; health care facilities should be aware of their role in the community isolation plan (e.g., staffing, supplies, referrals, transportation, and/or space)

6. Antidotes, mass prophylaxis, and vaccination

  a. Several chemical and radiologic agents have available specialized antidotes

  b. Facility responsibilities

    1) Have rapid access to the antidotes or countermeasures for agents posing a credible threat to their community

    2) Have an amount immediately available to minimally treat affected personnel and a first wave of presenting patients before requiring resupply from local or regional specialized pharmaceutical caches

    3) Have rapid access to pharmaceuticals for personnel, families, and a first wave of presenting patients, and have plans for community-based resupply

    4) Have a dispensing plan for personnel and families, and know their role in the local, regional, and state mass-dispensing plan

    5) Preserve the critical medical infrastructure for ill patients

    6) Have autonomous plans for supplies, medications, and staffing for at least 7 days, for an event of national significance

    7) Immunization plan

7. Facility evacuation

  a. Evacuation plans are mandatory

  b. In the event of a WMD event such as contamination, structural damage, or a natural disaster, plans should include autonomous offsite evacuation

  c. Evacuation plans should be integrated with local emergency management, with additional resources such as private company transportation contracts, for redundancy in the event these resources are contracted to other facilities

  d. Exercises and personnel training of the evacuation plan must occur

IV. Specific Weapons of Mass Destruction

A. BIOLOGIC AGENTS

***BACILLUS ANTHRACIS* (ANTHRAX).** Anthrax is a gram-positive, spore-forming bacterium that affects both humans and animals. The spores are hardy and can survive for decades in soil. Because of the virulence of this pathogen as a spore, many experts in biologic warfare consider anthrax to be the perfect biologic weapon. In humans, anthrax can present in three forms: inhalation, cutaneous, and GI. Anthrax is not transmissible from human to human. Inhaled anthrax is the most lethal form and results from inhaling spores, and is extremely rare. A prodromal stage of GI symptoms lasts from hours to days. Next may be a period in which improvement occurs, followed by the fulminant stage. Death may occur within 24–36 hours. Cutaneous anthrax is the most common form and is responsible for 95% of all cases. It is a local infection, usually resulting from direct contact with livestock. The incubation period is approximately 2 weeks after exposure. GI anthrax occurs from eating contaminated meat products, and the onset of symptoms is usually within 2–5 days of ingestion. It is difficult to diagnose.

1. Assessment
   a. Subjective data collection
      1) History of present illness/injury/chief complaint
         a) Inhaled anthrax
            (1) Nonspecific flulike symptoms
            (2) Fever
            (3) Myalgia
            (4) Shortness of breath
            (5) Pain (see Chapter 8)
            (6) Nonproductive cough
            (7) Vomiting
            (8) Absence of rhinorrhea or sore throat: distinguished from influenza
            (9) Diaphoresis: fulminant stage
            (10) Cyanosis: fulminant stage
            (11) Shock: fulminant stage
         b) Cutaneous anthrax
            (1) Painless, papular lesions within 1 week of exposure
            (2) 2- to 3-mm vesicle around papular lesion within 2 days
            (3) Satellite vesicles
            (4) Edematous site
            (5) Ruptured and necrotic lesions
            (6) Black eschar over ulcer
            (7) Bleeding: late stage
            (8) Fever: late stage
         c) GI anthrax
            (1) Oral ulcers
            (2) Nausea/vomiting
            (3) Malaise
            (4) Bloody diarrhea
            (5) Abdominal pain
      2) Past medical history
         a) Current or preexisting diseases/illness
         b) Medications
         c) Allergies
         d) Immunization status
   b. Objective data collection
      1) Physical examination
         a) General appearance
            (1) Level of consciousness, behavior, affect: alert, agitation, unconscious
            (2) Elevated temperature
            (3) Possible hypotension, tachycardia: advanced stages
            (4) Tachypnea: inhaled
            (5) Mild to severe distress/discomfort
         b) Inspection
            (1) Serous/serosanguineous fluid-filled vesicles: cutaneous anthrax
            (2) Necrotic lesions with black eschar: cutaneous anthrax
            (3) Oral ulceration: GI anthrax
         c) Auscultation
            (1) Breath sounds: diminished (inhaled anthrax)
            (2) Bowel sounds: diminished (GI anthrax)
         d) Palpation
            (1) Abdominal tenderness: GI anthrax
      2) Diagnostic procedures
         a) Complete blood count (CBC) with differential
         b) Serum chemistries including glucose, blood urea nitrogen (BUN), creatinine
            (1) Hypocalcemia: late finding in inhaled anthrax
            (2) Hyperkalemia: late finding in inhaled anthrax
            (3) Hyperglycemia: late finding in inhaled anthrax
         c) Blood cultures: positive
         d) Chest radiograph
         e) Chest computed tomography (CT) scan
            (1) Enlarged mediastinal and hilar lymph nodes: inhaled anthrax
            (2) Diffuse mediastinal fat edema: inhaled anthrax
            (3) Peribronchial thickening: inhaled anthrax
            (4) Pleural effusion: inhaled anthrax
2. Analysis: differential nursing diagnoses/collaborative problems
   a. Ineffective breathing pattern
   b. Deficient fluid volume
   c. Anxiety/fear
   d. Deficient knowledge
   e. Acute pain
   f. Risk for ineffective airway patency
   g. Risk for impaired skin integrity
3. Planning and implementation/interventions
   a. Maintain airway, breathing, circulation (see Chapters 1 and 32)
   b. Provide supplemental oxygen as indicated

1) Rapid sequence intubations (RSI) and ventilatory support in patients with respiratory compromise: inhaled anthrax
  c. Establish IV access for administration of crystalloid fluids/blood products/medications as needed
  d. Prepare for/assist with medical interventions
    1) Patient decontamination and personnel protection
    2) Advanced airway management: inhaled anthrax
      a) Nasal or oral intubation
      b) Supraglottic airway (e.g., King, Combitube, laryngeal mask airway)
      c) Surgical airway (e.g., cricothyrotomy)
    3) Institute cardiac and pulse oximetry monitoring
    4) Insert gastric tube and attach to suction as indicated
    5) Insert indwelling urinary catheter as indicated
    6) Assist with hospital admission (inhaled anthrax)
    7) Notification of CDC
  e. Administer pharmacologic therapy as ordered
    1) RSI premedications: sedatives, analgesics, neuromuscular blocking agents
    2) Antibiotic treatment as soon as diagnosis is suspected
      a) Ciprofloxacin (Cipro)
      b) Doxycycline (Dynapen), or antibiotic based on laboratory confirmed susceptibility
  f. Educate patient/significant others
    1) For confirmed cases, treatment should be continued for 60 days
4. Evaluation and ongoing monitoring
  a. Airway patency
  b. Level of consciousness
  c. Hemodynamic status
  d. Cardiac rate and rhythm
  e. Breath sounds and pulse oximetry
  f. Intake and output
  g. Pain relief

CLOSTRIDIUM BOTULINUM (BOTULISM).

Clostridium botulinum is the only toxin that is listed as one of the six category A biologic agents by the CDC because of its widespread availability and potency. The four forms of botulism are foodborne, wound, intestinal, and inhalation (inhalation is from the weaponization of botulism). Historically, the improper preparation and canning of foods caused deaths associated with botulism. Foodborne botulism is the most frequently occurring form of botulism as a result of the ingestion of food contaminated with *C. botulinum*. The onset of symptoms occurs within 12–36 hours after exposure.
1. Assessment
  a. Subjective data collection
    1) History of present illness/injury/chief complaint
      a) Nausea
      b) Vomiting

      c) Cramping
      d) Diarrhea
    2) Past medical history
      a) Current or preexisting diseases/illness
      b) Medications
      c) Allergies
      d) Immunization status
  b. Objective data collection
    1) Physical examination
      a) General appearance
        (1) Increased respiratory distress: late stage
        (2) Moderate to severe distress/discomfort
      b) Inspection
        (1) Cranial nerve palsies, especially eyes and oropharynx
          (a) Difficulty seeing: early stage
          (b) Difficulty speaking: early stage
          (c) Difficulty swallowing: early stage
          (d) Loss of gag reflex: late stage
        (2) Pupil dilation: late stage
      c) Palpation/percussion
        (1) Skeletal muscle weakness: early stage
        (2) Diminished deep tendon reflexes: early stage
        (3) Flaccid paralysis: early stage
          (a) Symmetric
          (b) Descending
          (c) Progressive
    2) Diagnostic procedures
      a) Serum chemistries including glucose, BUN, creatinine
      b) CBC with differential
      c) Lumbar puncture: cerebrospinal fluid (CSF) normal
      d) Mouse bioassay: gold standard
2. Analysis: differential nursing diagnoses/collaborative problems
  a. Ineffective airway clearance
  b. Ineffective breathing pattern
  c. Deficient fluid volume
  d. Anxiety/fear
  e. Deficient knowledge
  f. Pain
3. Planning and implementation/interventions
  a. Maintain airway, breathing, circulation (see Chapters 1 and 32)
  b. Provide supplemental oxygen as indicated
    1) RSI and ventilatory support in patients with respiratory compromise
    2) High-flow oxygen
  c. Establish IV access for administration of crystalloid fluids/blood products/medications as needed
  d. Prepare for/assist with medical interventions
    1) Advanced airway management
      a) Nasal or oral intubation

b) Supraglottic airway (e.g., King, Combitube, laryngeal mask airway)
c) Surgical airway (e.g., cricothyrotomy)
2) Institute cardiac and pulse oximetry monitoring
3) Prepare gastric tube and attach to suction
4) Assist with hospital admission
5) Notification of CDC
e. Administer pharmacologic therapy as ordered
1) RSI premedications: sedatives, analgesics, neuromuscular blocking agents
2) Rapid administration of antitoxin
a) Trivalent equine antitoxin if illness in progressive stage; must contact CDC for antitoxin release
b) Skin testing must be performed to avoid serum sickness or anaphylaxis
4. Evaluation and ongoing monitoring
a. Airway patency
b. Level of consciousness
c. Hemodynamic status
d. Breath sounds and pulse oximetry
e. Cardiac rate and rhythm
f. Intake and output
g. Pain relief

YERSINIA PESTIS (BUBONIC, SEPTICEMIC, AND PNEUMONIC PLAGUE). *Yersinia pestis* is infamous for killing millions of people in pandemic outbreaks, which occurred around the world throughout recent centuries. Plague still occurs naturally; therefore, a baseline knowledge of the occurrence of plague is needed. If human cases are diagnosed in nonendemic areas, in persons without risk factors, or in the absence of confirmed rodent cases, intentional release should be suspected. The three forms of plague are pneumonic, bubonic, and septicemic. Pneumonic plague is contagious through droplets, whereas bubonic and septicemic plagues are bloodborne. Septicemic plague may induce disseminated intravascular coagulopathy (DIC). The incubation period of *Yersinia pestis* is 2–3 days.
1. Assessment
a. Subjective data collection
1) History of present illness/injury/chief complaint
a) Bite by infected flea: bubonic
b) Sudden onset of fever, headache, chills, malaise: bubonic and septicemic
c) Painful and swollen grain lymph nodes (bubo): bubonic
d) Nausea/vomiting/diarrhea: septicemic
e) Pain (see Chapter 8): chest: pneumonic
f) Dyspnea: pneumonic
g) Cough: pneumonic
h) Hemoptysis: pneumonic
2) Past medical history
a) Current or preexisting diseases/illness
b) Recent travel to endemic area

c) Medications
d) Allergies
e) Immunization status
b. Objective data collection
1) Physical examination
a) General appearance
(1) Elevated temperature: bubonic, septicemic
(2) Hypotension, tachycardia: septicemic
(3) Severe distress/discomfort, critically ill
b) Inspection
(1) Erythematous bubo: bubonic
(2) Black necrotic fingertips and toes: septicemic
(3) Body rigors: septicemic
(4) External oozing of blood: septicemic
(5) Bloody sputum: pneumonic
c) Auscultation
(1) Breath sounds: wheezes, rhonchi: pneumonic
d) Palpation
(1) Painful, warm bubo: bubonic
(2) Lymphadenopathy: bubonic
2) Diagnostic procedures
a) Chest radiograph
2. Analysis: differential nursing diagnoses/collaborative problems
a. Ineffective breathing pattern
b. Deficient fluid volume
c. Deficient knowledge
d. Anxiety/fear
e. Pain
3. Planning and implementation/interventions
a. Maintain airway, breathing, circulation (see Chapters 1 and 32)
b. Provide supplemental oxygen as indicated
1) RSI with ventilatory support in patients with respiratory failure
c. Establish IV access for administration of crystalloid fluids/blood products/medications as needed
d. Prepare for/assist with medical interventions
1) Patient decontamination and personnel protection; use droplet precautions with pneumonic plague
2) Advanced airway management
a) Nasal or oral intubation
b) Supraglottic airway (e.g., King, Combitube, laryngeal mask airway)
c) Surgical airway (e.g., cricothyrotomy)
3) Institute cardiac and pulse oximetry monitoring
4) Insert gastric tube and attach to suction as indicated
5) Insert indwelling urinary catheter as indicated
6) Assist with hospital admission
7) Notification of CDC
e. Administer pharmacologic therapy as ordered

1) RSI premedications: sedatives, analgesics, neuromuscular blocking agents
2) Antibiotics: streptomycin, gentamicin (Garamycin), chloramphenicol (Chloromycetin), or doxycycline (Dynapen)
3) Prophylactic doxycycline (Dynapen) for exposed individuals
4. Evaluation and ongoing monitoring
   a. Airway patency
   b. Level of consciousness
   c. Hemodynamic status
   d. Breath sounds and pulse oximetry
   e. Cardiac rate and rhythm
   f. Intake and output
   g. Pain relief

FRANCISELLA TULARENSIS (TULAREMIA).

Francisella tularensis is a highly infectious organism that does not form spores; however, it can persist for several weeks in water, soil, vegetation, and animal products. Tularemia most commonly occurs in rural areas in all U.S. states except Hawaii. If cases are identified in nonendemic areas or in people without risk factors, a biologic weapon incident needs to be suspected. Tularemia is not transmissible from human to human, but it can be transmitted from a tick bite, by inhalation, or by ingestion of contaminated animal products. The incubation period is usually 3–5 days, but it may be as long as 20 days. Tularemia is associated with six forms: (1) ulceroglandular (most common), (2) glandular, (3) typhoidal, (4) pneumonic, (5) oropharyngeal, and (6) oculoglandular. The pneumonic form has a high mortality rate, and the typhoidal form can lead to rhabdomyolysis and renal failure, sepsis, DIC, and pneumonia.

1. Assessment
   a. Subjective data collection
      1) History of present illness/injury/chief complaint
         a) Fever/chills
         b) Rhinorrhea
         c) Myalgias
         d) Dry cough
         e) Headache
         f) Pain (see Chapter 8): pleuritic chest
         g) Dyspnea
         h) Hemoptysis
         i) Anorexia, weight loss
         j) Skin lesion
         k) Unilateral ocular pain
      2) Past medical history
         a) Current or preexisting diseases/illness
         b) Recent travel to endemic area
         c) Medications
         d) Allergies
         e) Immunization status
   b. Objective data collection
      1) Physical examination
         a) General appearance
            (1) Elevated temperature
            (2) Hypotension, tachycardia: typhoidal
            (3) Moderate to severe distress/discomfort
         b) Inspection
            (1) Single necrotic lesion with possible eschar: ulceroglandular
            (2) Exudative pharyngitis: oropharyngeal
            (3) Purulent eye discharge: oculoglandular
            (4) Ulcerative conjunctivitis: oculoglandular
         c) Auscultation
            (1) Breath sounds: wheezes, rhonchi (pneumonic)
         d) Palpation
            (1) Lesion tenderness: ulceroglandular
            (2) Lymphadenopathy: ulceroglandular, glandular, oropharyngeal
      2) Diagnostic procedures
         a) CBC with differential
         b) Serum chemistries
         c) Urinalysis: check myoglobin with typhoidal
         d) Chest radiograph: patchy infiltrates with pneumonic
2. Analysis: differential nursing diagnoses/collaborative problems
   a. Risk for ineffective breathing
   b. Risk for deficient fluid volume
   c. Anxiety/fear
   d. Deficient knowledge
   e. Acute pain
3. Planning and implementation/interventions
   a. Maintain airway, breathing, circulation (see Chapters 1 and 32)
   b. Provide supplemental oxygen as indicated
      1) RSI and ventilatory support in patients with respiratory compromise
      2) High-flow oxygen
   c. Establish IV access for administration of crystalloid fluids/blood products/medications as needed
   d. Prepare for/assist with medical interventions
      1) Institute cardiac and pulse oximetry monitoring
      2) Insert gastric tube and attach to suction as indicated
      3) Insert indwelling urinary catheter as indicated
      4) Assist with possible hospital admission
      5) Notification of CDC
   e. Administer pharmacologic therapy as ordered
      1) RSI premedications: sedatives, analgesics, neuromuscular blocking agents
      2) Antibiotics: streptomycin, gentamicin (Garamycin), or doxycycline (Dynapen)
      3) Nonnarcotic analgesics
      4) Narcotic analgesics
4. Evaluation and ongoing monitoring
   a. Airway patency
   b. Level of consciousness
   c. Hemodynamic status

d. Breath sounds and pulse oximetry
e. Cardiac rate and rhythm
f. Intake and output
g. Pain relief

SMALLPOX. Smallpox was eradicated in an aggressive campaign by the WHO in the 1970s. Today, a single case would become a global health concern and suspected as an act of terrorism. The appearance of smallpox would be considered a probable deliberate release. It is one of the most feared biologic warfare agents for the following reasons: (1) It spreads easily from person to person through aerosols, droplets, and fomites; (2) in 1972, civilian smallpox vaccination was discontinued; (3) loss of clinical familiarity with smallpox will most likely cause a delay in recognition and diagnosis; (4) the world's population is much more mobile than in the 1970s; and (5) new diseases and advances in medical treatment have made more individuals immunosuppressed. The incubation period is 12–14 days; the characteristic rash appears 2–3 days later. Secondary bacterial pneumonia may develop, resulting in a 50% mortality rate.

1. Assessment
   a. Subjective data collection
      1) History of present illness/injury/chief complaint
         a) Skin lesions similar in appearance but different from chickenpox
            (1) Begin in mouth and throat
            (2) Spread to face and extremities
            (3) Concentrated centrifugally on face, arms, and legs
            (4) Appear on palms and soles
            (5) Uniform and in same stage of development
         b) Fever/chills
         c) Malaise
         d) Vomiting
         e) Headache
      2) Past medical history
         a) Current or preexisting diseases/illness
         b) Medications
         c) Allergies
         d) Immunization status
   b. Objective data collection
      1) Physical examination
         a) General appearance
            (1) Level of consciousness, behavior, affect: alert to lethargy
            (2) Elevated temperature: >101°F (>38.4°C)
            (3) Severe distress/discomfort
         b) Inspection
            (1) Papular, vesicular lesions
         c) Auscultation
            (1) Breath sounds: wheezes, rhonchi with pneumonia
      2) Diagnostic procedures
         a) Vesicle fluid collection
            (1) Collection performed by a previously vaccinated person in PPE
            (2) Specimen should be sent to CDC or U.S. Army Medical Research Institute for Infectious Disease (USAMRIID)
         b) Direct fluorescent antibody (DFA) test, polymerase chain reaction (PCR), or electron microscopy to detect varicella-zoster virus
         c) Chest radiograph
2. Analysis: differential nursing diagnoses/collaborative problems
   a. Risk for ineffective breathing pattern
   b. Anxiety/fear
   c. Deficient knowledge
   d. Acute pain
3. Planning and implementation/interventions
   a. Personnel protection: airborne precautions at a minimum with immediate patient isolation and exposed persons quarantined
   b. Maintain airway, breathing, circulation (see Chapters 1 and 32)
   c. Provide supplemental oxygen as indicated
   d. Establish IV access for administration of crystalloid fluids/blood products/medications as needed
   e. Prepare for/assist with medical interventions
      1) Institute cardiac and pulse oximetry monitoring
      2) Assist with hospital admission
      3) Notification of CDC
   f. Administer pharmacologic therapy as ordered
      1) Immediate personnel vaccinations
      2) Immediate regional/national/international vaccinations
      3) Antivirals, which may not be effective: cidofovir (Vistide), adefovir, or ribavirin (Virazole)
4. Evaluation and ongoing monitoring
   a. Level of consciousness
   b. Hemodynamic status
   c. Breath sounds and pulse oximetry
   d. Cardiac rate and rhythm
   e. Intake and output
   f. Pain relief

FILOVIRUS, ARENAVIRUS (HEMORRHAGIC FEVERS). These fevers include Ebola, Marburg, Rift Valley, yellow, dengue, and Lassa fevers. People are not the natural reservoir for viral hemorrhagic fever (VHF) viruses, but accidental exposure can occur through contact with infected animals. The incubation period is approximately 2–21 days, with a flulike prodromal illness occurring less than 1 week after exposure. Patients with severe cases may demonstrate bleeding from orifices or under the skin. Internal organs may also bleed, leading to shock and multisystem failure. No documented use of a VHF virus as a bioweapon has occurred yet; however, it is commonly accepted that the United States, Russia, and other governments have successfully developed weaponized versions of VHFs.

1. Assessment
   a. Subjective data collection
      1) History of present illness/injury/chief complaint
         a) High fever
         b) Headache
         c) Malaise
         d) Myalgias
         e) Nausea
         f) Bloody diarrhea
      2) Past medical history
         a) Current or preexisting diseases/illness
         b) Medications
         c) Allergies
         d) Immunization status
   b. Objective data collection
      1) Physical examination
         a) General appearance
            (1) Level of consciousness, behavior, affect: lethargy to comatose
            (2) Hypotension, tachycardia
            (3) Severe distress/discomfort, critically ill
         b) Inspection
            (1) Frank blood from orifices
            (2) Petechial rash
      2) Diagnostic procedures
         a) Dependent on specific serology or virologic testing techniques
         b) EVD: initial diagnosis: antigen-capture enzyme-linked immunosorbent assay (ELISA) testing, IgM ELISA, polymerase chain reaction (PCR) and/or virus isolation, later in disease course: IgM and IgG antibodies
2. Analysis: differential nursing diagnoses/collaborative problems
   a. Deficient fluid volume
   b. Ineffective tissue perfusion
   c. Acute pain
   d. Deficient knowledge
3. Planning and implementation/interventions
   a. Strict adherence to infection control precautions and PPE use is essential: airborne, droplet, and contact precautions with patient isolation
   b. Maintain airway, breathing, circulation (see Chapters 1 and 32)
   c. Provide supplemental oxygen as indicated
      1) Intubation and ventilatory support in obtunded patients
      2) High-flow oxygen
   d. Establish IV access for administration of crystalloid fluids/blood products/medications as needed
      1) Insert large-bore IV catheters
      2) Infuse warmed normal saline solutions
      3) Infuse warmed blood products
   e. Prepare for/assist with medical interventions

1) Advanced airway management
   a) Nasal or oral intubation
   b) Supraglottic airway (e.g., King, Combitube, laryngeal mask airway)
   c) Surgical airway (e.g., cricothyrotomy)
2) Institute cardiac and pulse oximetry monitoring
3) Insert gastric tube and attach to suction
4) Insert indwelling urinary catheter
5) Assist with hospital admission
6) Notification of CDC
   f. Administer pharmacologic therapy as ordered
      1) Although a vaccine for EVD is under development, none is currently available except for yellow fever vaccine
4. Evaluation and ongoing monitoring
   a. Airway patency
   b. Level of consciousness
   c. Hemodynamic status
   d. Breath sounds and pulse oximetry
   e. Cardiac rate and rhythm
   f. Intake and output

RICIN. Ricin is widely available and easily produced. Made from the beans of the castor plant, this biological agent is largely in its own category. Delivery is via inhalation, injection, or ingestion. Liquid or crystalline ricin can potentially be delivered through contaminating food or water. Aerosolization is possible but requires more sophisticated technology to develop, which makes a mass terror event less likely. Ricin has been used more for small-scale or individual attacks. Symptoms of inhaled ricin occur 4–8 hours after exposure, but could occur up to 24 hours. Ingestion of ricin causes symptoms to appear within 10 hours. If concerns about exposure exist, move to fresh air right away by leaving the area where the ricin was released. Clothing should be removed immediately and any areas of exposed skin should be washed with copious amounts of water and soap. If ingested, do not induce vomiting or give fluids to drink.

1. Assessment
   a. Subjective data collection
      1) History of present illness/injury/chief complaint
         a) Clinical manifestations dependent on dose and route of exposure
         b) Fever
         c) Cough
         d) Ingested ricin: stomach irritation, gastroenteritis, bloody diarrhea, vomiting
         e) Inhaled ricin: respiratory distress, fever, cough, nausea, chest tightness, sweating, pulmonary edema
         f) Later symptoms: seizures and central nervous system depression
         g) Death can occur within 36–72 hours of exposure, depending on route and dose
      2) Past medical history
         a) Current or preexisting diseases/illness

b) Medications
c) Allergies
d) Immunization status
    b. Objective data collection
        1) Physical examination
            a) General appearance
                (1) Level of consciousness, behavior, affect: lethargy to comatose
                (2) Hypotension, tachycardia
                (3) Severe distress/discomfort, critically ill
            b) Inspection
        2) Diagnostic procedures
            a) Urine test for ricin at CDC-approved laboratory response centers
2. Analysis: differential nursing diagnoses/collaborative problems
    a. Risk for ineffective breathing pattern
    b. Anxiety/fear
    c. Deficient knowledge
3. Planning and implementation/interventions
    a. Universal precautions. Ricin is not contagious.
    b. Maintain airway, breathing, circulation (see Chapters 1 and 32)
    c. Provide supplemental oxygen as indicated
        1) Intubation and ventilatory support in obtunded patients
        2) High-flow oxygen
    d. Establish IV access for administration of crystalloid fluids/blood products/medications as needed
        1) Insert large-bore IV catheters
        2) Infuse warmed normal saline solutions
        3) Infuse warmed blood products
    e. Prepare for/assist with medical interventions
        1) Advanced airway management
            a) Nasal or oral intubation
            b) Supraglottic airway (e.g., King, Combitube, laryngeal mask airway)
            c) Surgical airway (e.g., cricothyrotomy)
        2) Institute cardiac and pulse oximetry monitoring
        3) Insert gastric tube and attach to suction
        4) Insert indwelling urinary catheter
        5) Assist with hospital admission
        6) Notification of CDC
    f. Administer pharmacologic therapy as ordered
        1) None available
4. Evaluation and ongoing monitoring
    a. Airway patency
    b. Level of consciousness
    c. Hemodynamic status
    d. Breath sounds and pulse oximetry
    e. Cardiac rate and rhythm
    f. Intake and output

B. CHEMICAL WEAPONS

There is risk of exposure to chemical agents from industrial accidents, terrorist attacks, and proximity military stockpiling. Industrial accidents continue to be a significant potential source of exposure to chemical weapons agents (CWAs). Although some international treaties have banned the development, production, and stockpiles of CWAs, these agents reportedly continue to be produced or stockpiled in several countries. Several characteristics of CWAs lend themselves to terrorist use. Chemical substrates used in CWAs are widely available, and recipes for CWA production may be found on the Internet. CWAs are easily transported and may be delivered by a variety of routes. Chemical agents often are difficult to protect against and quickly incapacitate the intended targets. Most civilian medical communities are inadequately prepared to deal with a large-scale chemical terrorist attack. Hospitals should also consider a more likely potential of exposures to chemicals from industrial accidents and should be prepared by reviewing local emergency planning committee (LEPC) data and material safety data sheets (MSDS), and having the appropriate PPE for the toxic industrial chemicals in their community.

NERVE AGENTS. Nerve agents are the best known, and most toxic, type of chemical agent; however, they are the most difficult to acquire or manufacture. These agents produce muscarinic, nicotinic, and direct central nervous system toxicity along with effects on the respiratory tract, cardiovascular system, GI tract, muscles, and eyes. The onset and severity of the clinical effects vary because numerous variables determine the predominant effects.

Liquid agents easily penetrate both skin and clothing, and the onset of symptoms generally occurs between 30 minutes and 18 hours after exposure. The effect may be local or systemic.

Vapor inhalation produces clinical toxicity within seconds to several minutes after exposure. The effects may involve local or systemic reactions.
1. Assessment
    a. Subjective data collection
        1) History of present illness/injury/chief complaint
            a) Mild cases
                (1) Muscle twitching
                (2) Miosis
                (3) Headache
                (4) Rhinorrhea
                (5) Salivation
                (6) Dyspnea
            b) Severe exposure
                (1) All foregoing symptoms
                (2) Severe difficulty of breathing
                (3) Generalized muscle twitching
                (4) Weakness or paralysis
                (5) Seizures
                (6) Loss of bladder and bowel control
                (7) Loss of consciousness
                (8) SLUDGE (salivation, lacrimation, urination, defecation, GI pain, and emesis) is a classic acronym for this exposure

(9) Low-level, survivable exposures may result in lacrimation only

2) Past medical history
  a) Current or preexisting diseases/illness
  b) Medications
  c) Allergies
  d) Immunization status

b. Objective data collection
  1) Physical examination
    a) General appearance
      (1) Level of consciousness, behavior, affect: alert to comatose, seizures
      (2) Hypotension, tachycardia
      (3) Severe distress/discomfort
    b) Inspection
      (1) Incontinence
      (2) Increased respiratory effort
  2) Diagnostic procedures
    a) Serum acetylcholinesterase levels
    b) Detection and monitoring using chemical monitors operated by a trained user

2. Analysis: differential nursing diagnoses/collaborative problems
  a. Deficient fluid volume
  b. Anxiety/fear
  c. Deficient knowledge
  d. Risk of inefficient airway clearance

3. Planning and implementation/interventions
  a. Patient decontamination and personnel protection, including copious lavage of eyes
  b. Maintain airway, breathing, circulation (see Chapters 1 and 32)
  c. Provide supplemental oxygen as indicated
    1) RSI and ventilatory support in patients with respiratory compromise
    2) High-flow oxygen
  d. Establish IV access for administration of crystalloid fluids/blood products/medications
  e. Prepare for/assist with medical interventions
    1) Institute cardiac and pulse oximetry monitoring
    2) Insert gastric tube and attach to suction as indicated
    3) Insert indwelling urinary catheter as indicated
    4) Assist with hospital admission
    5) Notification of CDC
  f. Administer pharmacologic therapy as ordered
    1) RSI premedications: sedatives, analgesics, neuromuscular blocking agents
    2) Atropine to manage secretory symptoms; large exposure requires high doses and longer term IV atropine maintenance until recovery
    3) 2-Pralidoxine chloride (2-PAM), preferably within 15 minutes and within 1 hour after exposure for effectiveness
    4) Benzodiazepines for seizure activity
    5) Homatropine ophthalmic solution for miosis

4. Evaluation and ongoing monitoring

a. Airway patency
b. Level of consciousness
c. Hemodynamic status
d. Breath sounds and pulse oximetry
e. Cardiac rate and rhythm
f. Intake and output
g. Pupil size and reactivity
h. Secretory status

VESICANTS. Vesicants often result in skin blistering, hence the military's nomenclature of blister agent. Examples are mustard gas (sulfur mustard, H, HD), lewisite (L), and phosgene oxime (CX) agents. Vesicants are more strategic as warfare agents because they injure instead of kill. They can cause blistering to whatever part of the body is exposed (external or internal) and can easily penetrate most fabrics and reach the skin. With exposure, 10% binds with the skin, whereas 90% is absorbed into the body. Mustard exposure can cause almost immediate cellular and bone marrow injury, whereas lewisite and phosgene oxime cause immediate symptoms but less long-term systemic injury. Immediate removal of the exposed person from the source and immediate decontamination must occur.

1. Assessment
  a. Subjective data collection
    1) History of present illness/injury/chief complaint
      a) Signs and symptoms can begin 2–48 hours after exposure (mustard)
        (1) Erythema
        (2) Blisters
        (3) Visual complaints
          (a) Irritation
          (b) Conjunctivitis
        (4) Mild upper respiratory
        (5) Nausea/vomiting
      b) Generally, symptoms are delayed, with no immediate pain on exposure, except with lewisite and phosgene oxime
    2) Past medical history
      a) Current or preexisting diseases/illness
      b) Medications
      c) Allergies
      d) Immunization status
  b. Objective data collection
    1) Physical examination
      a) General appearance
        (1) Level of consciousness, behavior, affect: alert to lethargy
        (2) Mild to severe distress/discomfort
      b) Inspection
        (1) Skin blistering
        (2) Corneal opacity
    2) Diagnostic procedures
      a) Use of chemical detectors by a trained operator

2. Analysis: differential nursing diagnoses/collaborative problems
   a. Anxiety/fear
   b. Deficient fluid volume
   c. Deficient knowledge
   d. Acute pain
   e. Risk of inefficient airway clearance
3. Planning and implementation/interventions
   a. Patient decontamination and personnel protection
      1) Decontamination is critical
      2) Wash with 0.5% bleach or baby shampoo; a surfactant is needed to remove the agent because it is oily, and water alone will not rinse the agent
      3) Avoid harsh scrubbing because it will assist in absorption
   b. Maintain airway, breathing, circulation (see Chapters 1 and 32)
   c. Provide supplemental oxygen as indicated
   d. Establish IV access for administration of crystalloid fluids/blood products/medications as needed
   e. Prepare for/assist with medical interventions
      1) Institute cardiac and pulse oximetry monitoring
      2) Assist with possible hospital admission
      3) Notification of CDC
   f. Administer pharmacologic therapy as ordered
      1) Chelating agents may be utilized
4. Evaluation and ongoing monitoring
   a. Level of consciousness
   b. Hemodynamic status
   c. Breath sounds and pulse oximetry
   d. Cardiac rate and rhythm
   e. Intake and output
   f. Pain relief

CYANIDE. Named a "blood agent" by the military because of its physiologic target of oxygen-carrying capacity on a cellular level, cyanide is a naturally occurring chemical present in a variety of food sources, soil, and water. Industrial exposures occur through many avenues including printing, agriculture, photography, and paper and plastic manufacturing. It is also a combustion product of burning synthetic materials such as carpet, furniture, and upholstery. Rail cars with 30,000-gallon tanks of cyanide can be an attractive target for terrorist threats.

1. Assessment
   a. Subjective data collection
      1) History of present illness/injury/chief complaint
         a) Symptoms depend on
            (1) Total dose of poison
            (2) Route of poison
            (3) Exposure time
         b) Occupation
      2) Past medical history
         a) Current or preexisting diseases/illness
         b) Medications
         c) Allergies
         d) Immunization status
   b. Objective data collection
      1) Physical examination
         a) General appearance
            (1) Level of consciousness, behavior, affect: unconscious
            (2) Cardiac/respiratory arrest
            (3) Severe distress/discomfort, critically ill
      2) Diagnostic procedures
         a) Serum cyanide level
2. Analysis: differential nursing diagnoses/collaborative problems
   a. Ineffective airway clearance
   b. Ineffective breathing pattern
   c. Ineffective tissue perfusion
3. Planning and implementation/interventions
   a. Removal of patient from source to fresh air
   b. Patient decontamination if clothing is wet
   c. Maintain airway, breathing, circulation (see Chapters 1 and 32)
      1) Initiate or continue Basic Life Support (BLS) and Advanced Life Support (ALS) per protocols if cardiac arrest is present
   d. Provide supplemental oxygen as indicated
      1) RSI and ventilatory support in patients with respiratory compromise
   e. Establish IV access for administration of crystalloid fluids/blood products/medications as needed
   f. Prepare for/assist with medical interventions
      1) Advanced airway management
         a) Nasal or oral intubation
         b) Supraglottic airway (e.g., King, Combitube, laryngeal mask airway)
         c) Surgical airway (e.g., cricothyrotomy)
      2) Institute cardiac and pulse oximetry monitoring
      3) Insert gastric tube and attach to suction
      4) Insert indwelling urinary catheter
      5) Assist with hospital admission if patient survives
      6) Notification of CDC
   g. Administer pharmacologic therapy as ordered
      1) Hydroxocobalamin injection: initial adult dose of 5 g IV with a possible repeat dose of 5 g IV for continued symptoms for a maximum dose of 10 g OR
      2) Cyanide antidote
         a) Amyl nitrite perles: inhaled; use until an IV is established; break onto gauze pad and hold under patient's nose, over the bag-mask ventilation intake, or place under lip of face mask; replace perle every 3 minutes
         b) Sodium nitrite: IV over 5 minutes and monitor for hypotension
         c) Sodium thiosulfate: IV after sodium nitrite and infused over 10–20 minutes; may repeat half original dose in 30 minutes if inadequate response

3) RSI premedications: sedatives, analgesics, neuromuscular blocking agents
4. Evaluation and ongoing monitoring
   a. Airway patency
   b. Level of consciousness
   c. Hemodynamic status
   d. Breath sounds and pulse oximetry
   e. Cardiac rate and rhythm
   f. Intake and output
   g. Pain relief

PULMONARY AGENTS: PHOSGENE, CHLORINE, ANHYDROUS AMMONIA. These are the most feared chemical agents for first responders because (1) they are easy to obtain and (2) no alterations are needed to use them as a weapon. They primarily attack the lungs and lung tissue after inhalation and cause irritation of the upper and lower respiratory tracts.

1. Assessment
   a. Subjective data collection
      1) History of present illness/injury/chief complaint
         a) Conjunctival irritation and lacrimation
         b) Mild coughing
         c) Pain (see Chapter 8): chest tightness
         d) Shortness of breath
         e) Skin irritation
         f) Laryngospasm: severe exposure
         g) Pulmonary edema: severe exposure
      2) Past medical history
         a) Current or preexisting diseases/illness
         b) Medications
         c) Allergies
         d) Immunization status
   b. Objective data collection
      1) Physical examination
         a) General appearance
            (1) Tachypnea, tachycardia
            (2) Severe distress/discomfort
         b) Auscultation
            (1) Breath sounds: crackles
      2) Diagnostic procedures
         a) Chest radiograph
2. Analysis: differential nursing diagnoses/collaborative problems
   a. Ineffective breathing pattern
   b. Anxiety/fear
   c. Deficient knowledge
   d. Risk for ineffective airway clearance
3. Planning and implementation/interventions
   a. Patient decontamination and personnel protection
   b. Maintain airway, breathing, circulation (see Chapters 1 and 32)
   c. Provide supplemental oxygen as indicated
      1) RSI and ventilatory support in patients with respiratory compromise or laryngospasms
      2) High-flow oxygen
   d. Establish IV access for administration of crystalloid fluids/blood products/medications as needed
   e. Prepare for/assist with medical interventions
      1) Advanced airway management
         a) Nasal or oral intubation
         b) Supraglottic airway (e.g., King, Combitube, laryngeal mask airway)
         c) Surgical airway (e.g., cricothyrotomy)
      2) Institute cardiac and pulse oximetry monitoring
      3) Insert gastric tube and attach to suction
      4) Insert indwelling urinary catheter
      5) Assist with hospital admission
      6) Notification of CDC
   f. Administer pharmacologic therapy as ordered
      1) RSI premedications: sedatives, analgesics, neuromuscular blocking agents
4. Evaluation and ongoing monitoring
   a. Airway patency
   b. Level of consciousness
   c. Hemodynamic status
   d. Breath sounds and pulse oximetry
   e. Cardiac rate and rhythm

C. NUCLEAR AND RADIOLOGIC WEAPONS

Nuclear materials in any form are understood to be a potential threat to health. Nuclear events include the concurrent presence of an explosive incident with a potential distinctive mushroom-shaped cloud (above ground or airburst detonation) and the release of gamma and neutron rays that penetrate bodies and structures. Included in nuclear detonations are the concurrent release of alpha and beta particles, which are weaker and can be stopped by clothing, skin, and barriers. Incorporation of alpha and beta particles may cause long-term health damage, depending on the amount of exposure. Gamma exposure is not a contaminant, but radioactive alpha and beta particles are. Radiation exposures require decontamination and monitoring of radiation levels, with no delay in lifesaving measures. Radiation is the transference of energy through space as electromagnetic waves or particulate matter. The energy is inversely proportional to the wavelength. Higher frequency wavelengths have higher energy and are more destructive. Threats exist in the form of radioactive dispersion devices (RDD), improvised nuclear devices (IND), or other accidental or deliberate releases of ionizing radiation.

The severity of injuries or potential injuries from nuclear exposure is based on the amount of time exposed, the distance from the nuclear source, and the levels of shielding. Persons immediately symptomatic after nuclear exposure should be considered critical, whereas long-term medical monitoring is indicated for asymptomatic but exposed persons. Any suspicious explosive event should be considered a potential hazardous materials contamination event, such as with an RDD, until monitoring proves otherwise.

Personnel should follow the facility's hazardous materials/radiation plan, to include donning of PPE, the most critical of which is respiratory protection against particulate incorporation. Persons should be removed from the source of exposure, and secondary contamination should be avoided with detailed decontamination.

1. Assessment
   a. Subjective data collection
      1) History of present illness/injury/chief complaint
         a) Acute radiation syndrome (ARS): multiorgan injury resulting from exposure to ionizing radiation; symptoms may occur minutes to hours after exposure and last several days
            (1) Nausea
            (2) Vomiting: possibly bloody
            (3) Diarrhea
            (4) Malaise
            (5) Anorexia
         b) Illness stage
            (1) Same symptoms as in prodrome
            (2) Bleeding
            (3) Bruising
            (4) Fevers
            (5) Immunodeficiency
            (6) Thrombocytopenia
            (7) Sloughing of GI epithelial cells causing
               (a) Malabsorption
               (b) Hemorrhage
               (c) Ulceration
               (d) Hypersecretion of fluid
            (8) Fluid loss
      2) Past medical history
         a) Current or preexisting diseases/illness
         b) Medications
         c) Allergies
         d) Immunization status
   b. Objective data collection
      1) Physical examination
         a) General appearance
            (1) Level of consciousness, behavior, affect: possible delirium
            (2) Possible elevated temperature
            (3) Possible hypotension, tachycardia
            (4) Moderate to severe distress/discomfort
         b) Inspection
            (1) Obvious injury
            (2) Possible bleeding
      2) Diagnostic procedures
         a) CBC with differential
         b) Serum chemistries
         c) Urinalysis
         d) Monitoring of levels of radiation contaminant using radiation detection equipment by a trained operator
2. Analysis: differential nursing diagnoses/collaborative problems

   a. Anxiety/fear
   b. Risk for deficient fluid volume
   c. Acute pain
   d. Deficient knowledge
3. Planning and implementation/interventions
   a. Immediate patient decontamination
      1) Be aware that decontamination may need to take second place to lifesaving care of the patient
      2) Decontaminate as quickly as possible
      3) Decontamination should be done outside if at all possible
   b. Maintain airway, breathing, circulation (see Chapters 1 and 32)
   c. Provide supplemental oxygen as indicated
   d. Establish IV access for administration of crystalloid fluids/blood products/medications as needed
   e. Prepare for/assist with medical interventions
      1) Institute cardiac and pulse oximetry monitoring
      2) Insert gastric tube and attach to suction as indicated
      3) Insert indwelling urinary catheter as indicated
      4) Assist with possible hospital admission
      5) Notification of CDC
   f. Administer pharmacologic therapy as ordered
      1) Chelating agents
      2) Medications to both manage symptoms and provide palliative treatments
4. Evaluation and ongoing monitoring
   a. Level of consciousness
   b. Hemodynamic status
   c. Breath sounds and pulse oximetry
   d. Cardiac rate and rhythm
   e. Intake and output
   f. Pain relief

V. Four Stages of Disaster Management

A. PREPAREDNESS

1. The goal of preparedness is to plan how to respond to, mitigate damage from, and recover from a disaster
2. Actions can include
   a. EOP (Emergency Operation Plan)
   b. An EOP should address all hazards, instead of one plan per problem, have clear organization, and be flexible enough to deal with any contingency
   c. Elements of an EOP
      1) List of potential hazards and institution vulnerabilities to these hazards
      2) Integration with community responders
      3) Critical resources needed for 5 days of autonomous functioning
      4) List of planning priorities (e.g., mitigating damage, preserving essential functions, life safety, rapid recovery)

5) Facility approach to a graduated response (e.g., scalable IMS)
6) Operational functions to include surge capacity
7) Legal basis for response to include quarantine order impact
8) Regulatory compliance
   a) Emergency Medical Treatment and Active Labor Act (EMTALA)
   b) Accreditation Emergency Management Standards (such as The Joint Commission)
   c) Occupational Safety and Health Administration (OSHA)
   d) Health Insurance and Portability Accountability Act (HIPAA)
9) Mutual aid agreements
10) Contracts for emergency support
    a) Supplies and equipment—medical (trauma, surgical, orthopaedic, biomedical, pharmaceutical, oxygen and oxygen delivery equipment, patient care support, PPE, patient movement and evacuation equipment), nonmedical (food, water, linen, fuel, environmental)
    b) Transportation
    c) Critical services
    d) Patient transfers
    e) Assessment of contract exclusivity in the event of multiple agency demands on the same resources
11) Mental/behavioral health support
12) Mass casualty ethics to include a plan to address issues of scarce lifesaving resources
13) Mass casualty triage and plan for distribution of limited resources
14) Shelter-in-place plan
15) Medical surge plan
    a) Supplies and equipment needs
    b) Space for triage, treatment, bed availability, alternate care sites
    c) Augmentation staffing plan
       (1) Integration of plan with health care coalition and community surge plan
       (2) Staff lodging, meals, off-duty but onsite activities, and other needs
       (3) Staff transportation
       (4) Plan to provide or encourage staff to have a plan for child, pet, and elder care
16) Emergency credentialing plan integrated with community emergency credentialing plans
17) Hazardous materials plan
    a) Detection capabilities for chemical and radiological agents
    b) Ongoing monitoring
    c) Decontamination (both individual and mass decontamination)
    d) Personal protective equipment
    e) Environmental remediation
    f) Lockdown procedures to protect core functions from contamination
    g) Radiation detection, response, and remediation
18) Infectious disease plan
    a) Increased surveillance
    b) Recommendations for infection control levels of personal protective equipment
    c) Plans for isolation, cohorting of patients as well as quarantine
19) Hospital as a primary or secondary target plan
20) Command and control
    a) Establish lines of authority during an emergency, utilizing the common language of a national IMS (NIMS)
    b) Contingencies should include a line of succession plan and delegations of authority in an emergency event
    c) The hospital command and control structure should be linked to the community emergency management system
    d) During an event, an EOC is established away from the front line
    e) All functions are staffed using an IMS
    f) Alternate sites should be established for the EOC and for any hospital essential functions (e.g., emergency services) in the event the primary site is rendered inoperable
21) Communications
    a) Redundant, interoperable communications should exist to cover the possibility that main channels of communication may fail during an event
    b) Should include a contingency plan for the loss of landlines, cellular phones, power, radios, and electronic communications; possible use of amateur (e.g., ham, citizen band) radios, satellite phones, and other methods of communications
    c) Need to address how response decisions are communicated to management, staff, patients, family, visitors, vendors, and the community
    d) Alert, notification, and implementation process
22) Evacuation
    a) Phased evacuation plan should include the ability to interface with potentially needed community assets
    b) Contracts or memorandums of understanding should be formalized for necessary outside assistance in the event of a facility-wide evacuation

c) Evacuation plan should be practiced with community responders and emergency management as much as possible without decreasing essential functions

d) Utilize a patient tracking system

e) Alternative preestablished care locations outside of identified risk areas

f) Address electronic medical and medication records

23) Public information

a) A risk and crisis communications plan should be developed to include the following

(1) Staff, patient, family, and community concerns

(2) Alternate languages

(3) Special populations

(4) Preformatted and prescripted messages for a variety of all-hazards events

(5) Designated public information officers for official transmission of facility messages, based at the facility and at the community joint information center (JIC)

24) Essential functions

a) In the event not all services can be sustained during an emergency, the priority essential functions should be determined in advance

b) List the logistics, staffing, and other minimum needs necessary to maintain essential functions

c) Prioritized essential functions in operation should be communicated to the staff and the community including the EOC and emergency medical services (EMSs) and dispatch

25) Security

a) Plans for facility lockdown, restricted access, or controlled ingress and egress, that can be rapidly implemented

b) Campus control of both vehicular and pedestrian access

c) Contingency planning to maintain the security plan and addressing short staffing, lack of outside law enforcement or security assistance, and locking mechanism failures

d) Cybersecurity plan for surety of electronic information

26) Mass fatality management

a) Plan for storage, identification, and decontamination of mass fatalities that is integrated with the medical examiner

3. Training

a. Didactic

1) Targeted for awareness level and clinical symptoms of specific events

a) Awareness level is for all personnel to understand their roles in an emergency event, on initial orientation, and annually

2) Protective actions should be covered for all hazards

3) Family emergency planning should be covered

b. Clinical or "hands on"

1) Targeted for specific skills

a) Donning and doffing personal protective equipment

b) Decontamination

c) Vaccination

d) Triage

c. Core nursing disaster competencies

1) International Council of Nursing (ICN) Disaster Nursing Competencies[9]

a) Risk Reduction, Disease Prevention and Health Promotion

b) Policy Development and Planning

c) Ethical Practice, Legal Practice, and Accountability

d) Communication and Information Sharing

e) Education and Preparedness

f) Care of Communities

g) Care of Individuals and Families

h) Psychological Care

i) Care of Vulnerable Populations (Special Needs Populations)

j) Long-term Care Needs

2) FEMA Emergency Management Institute

a) Established to support the Department of Homeland Security and FEMA. Purpose is to improve the knowledge and capabilities of those who have emergency management responsibilities and the general public

b) FEMA Independent Study courses

(1) Courses located online at https://training.fema.gov/is/

4. Exercises

a. Discussion based

1) Seminars

a) Increase knowledge of topics, new plans, organizational response

2) Workshops

a) Increase knowledge and skill building for specific objectives

3) Tabletop exercises (TTX)

a) Tests system reactions to a specific scenario

4) Games

a) Tests simulated operations and decision making on a hypothetical scenario using competition

b. Operations based

1) Drills

a) Supervised activities testing a specific operation or capability of a disaster response.

Examples can include decontamination drill, evacuation scenario
2) Functional exercises (FEs)
   a) Testing of multiple functions with a live response to a simulated disaster scenario. Can evaluate hospital capabilities alone or with community partners testing communications, Incident Command functions, responding to bed availability requests, and use of plans, policies, and procedures
3) Full-scale exercises
   a) Realistic scenarios with hospital incident command activation and rapid problem solving, mobilization of staff, staging area, and the need for resources. Tests major portions of an operations plan
5. Evaluation
   a. After-action reviews (including "hot washes" and reports)
   b. Use results as opportunities for improvement in corrective action improvement plans to refine plans, training, and exercises

B. MITIGATION

1. The goal of mitigation is to reduce vulnerability and diminish the effects of a disaster
2. Possible actions
   a. Hazards vulnerability analysis completed in coordination with local, regional, and state jurisdictions
   b. Assess the following
      1) Possible threats and risks (e.g., hurricanes, demonstrations, floods, terrorist events)
      2) Rate each risk on a Likert scale, with the highest number being the most severe impact and requiring the most resources
      3) Total highest numbers equal vulnerabilities most in need of preparation in the EOP
         a) Probability of occurrence
         b) Human impact
         c) Property impact
         d) Level of current preparedness and available resources
   c. Rank the hazardous events to guide EOP development and resource allocation
   d. Modifying building construction
   e. Staff and public education campaign

C. RESPONSE

1. Incident management
   a. Respond to an event utilizing an IMS to ensure common communication and clear organization (see Fig. 41.2)
2. Procedural checklists/job action sheets
   a. Lists of actions to be accomplished by designated roles in the ICS

b. Prioritized, sequential actions to take that are applicable to the specific all-hazards emergency
1) Hospital Incident Management Team key roles
   a) Command center roles
      (1) Incident commander
         (a) Provides overall direction for hospital operations and the hospital command center, has authority to make decisions for the organization
      (2) Safety officer
         (a) Organizes and enforces scene and facility protection, traffic security, and safe practices for response personnel
      (3) Liaison officer
         (a) Functions as the contact for the local, county, or regional Emergency Operations Center (EOC), other hospitals, emergency response partners, public health
      (4) Public information officer
         (a) Coordinates information sharing internally within the organization for staff messaging and hotline updates, and externally to media consistent with the EOC Joint Information Center
      (5) Scribe
         (a) Documents all activities and communications, updates status board
      (6) Medical-technical specialists
         (a) Subject matter experts for incidents involving infectious disease, hazmat exposure (biological, chemical, radiological), risk management, legal and ethical issues, pediatrics, hospital administration, clinic administration
   b) Section chiefs
      (1) Operations chief
         (a) Directs the operations section including the Staging Manager, Medical Care Branch, Infrastructure Branch, Security Branch, Hazmat Branch, Unit Leaders, Business Continuity Branch, and Patient Family Assistance Branch
      (2) Planning chief
         (a) Directs all aspects of planning by compiling information from all section chiefs. Effects long-range planning through distribution of an action plan. Responsible for the Resources Unit leader, Situation Unit leader, Documentation Unit leader, and Demobilization Unit leader
      (3) Logistics chief
         (a) Directs operations associated with the maintenance of the physical envi-

ronment and adequate levels of food, water, shelter, and supplies to support the medical objectives. Responsible for the Service Branch director and the Support Branch director

  (4) Finance chief

    (a) Monitors the utilization of financial assets necessary to carry out the hospital's medical mission by overseeing the acquisition of supplies and services, and supervising the documentation of relevant expenditures. Responsible for the Time Unit leader, Procurement Unit leader, Compensation Claims Unit leader, and Cost Unit leader

2) Incident Command forms

  a) Staffing logs

  b) Incident action plans

  c) Briefing sheets

  d) Situation reports

  e) Patient tracking logs

  f) After-action reports

  g) Decontamination team member health status tracking

3) Community integration

  a) Planning with the local/regional health care coalition, which includes emergency management, public health, other hospitals and health care agencies, law enforcement, fire-rescue, and other disaster support organizations, increases the ability of the hospital to understand community threats and resources and to conduct joint planning and exercises

  b) Planning partners

    (1) Health care coalitions: a framework to build capabilities to prepare and respond to large-scale disasters needs the support of the entire local health care system and the community infrastructure. The Office of the Assistant Secretary for Preparedness and Response (ASPR) has established a goal that 100% of communities will have local or regional coalitions representing them

    (2) Health care coalition members

      (a) Acute care hospitals, rehabilitation centers, specialty facilities (e.g., pediatric, psychiatric, long-term ventilator care), long-term care facilities

      (b) Emergency management from the local EOC

      (c) Emergency medical services

      (d) Public health

      (e) Law enforcement

      (f) Medical reserve corps

      (g) Private sector, nongovernmental organizations (e.g., Red Cross, blood centers, dialysis, Volunteer Organizations in Disasters [VOAD]), and businesses

      (h) Other partners include universities, medical examiner offices, veterinary partners, faith community representatives

    (3) Local emergency planning committees (LEPCs): mandated under the Emergency Planning and Community Right-to-Know Act to address community-based industrial hazards[10]

    (4) Partners include an overlap of the above partners and

      (a) Metropolitan medical response systems (if available locally)

      (b) Local and regional terrorism task forces

3. Mass casualty triage

  a. Utilize a system of rapid triage to sort patients into treatment priority categories

  b. Treatment priorities may vary depending on available resources and type of illness or injury (e.g., a contaminated patient receiving a known lethal dose of contaminant may warrant a different triage category than the initial appearance would normally dictate)

  c. Affix a triage tag with vital information visibly on each patient, or review patient triage tags as patients arrive by EMS and retriage patient presentations

  d. Start MCI triage[11]

    1) Simple triage and rapid treatment

    2) Goal is to assign a triage category to each patient within 30 seconds

    3) Five parameters

      a) Ability to walk

      b) Presence or absence of spontaneous respirations

      c) Respiratory rate

      d) Assessment of perfusion

      e) Ability to obey commands

  e. IDME triage colors

    1) Immediate (red tag)

      a) Priority treatment category: patients with injuries or illness that could result in loss of life or limb without immediate treatment

    2) Delayed (yellow tag)

      a) Patients that can wait for treatment until after the immediate-category patients are treated

    3) Minor (green tag)

a) Advanced medical care can wait several hours without causing further injury; patients in the minor category can wait until after patients in the immediate and delayed categories have received care
4) Expectant (black tag)
  a) Patient that has sustained injuries that overwhelm current medical resources and is not expected to survive
  b) Provide comfort care
5) Deceased (black tag)
  a) Impending death or lifeless, not salvageable with current resources
6) Contaminated (no color)
  a) Special category that can accompany any other triage category and likely to escalate patient's level of triage
  b) Patients who are potentially contaminated and need to be decontaminated
f. SALT mass casualty triage
  1) **S**ort
  2) **A**ssess
  3) **L**ifesaving interventions (hemorrhage control, open airway, needle decompression, autoinjector antidotes)
  4) **T**reatment/transport

D. RECOVERY

1. Execute a phased reconstitution of normal operations
2. Preserve continuity of operations
   a. Preserve critical business continuity of the facility by addressing key issues
   1) Plans for safety, well-being, benefits, and scheduling of personnel
   2) Access to vital records
   3) Establish lines of successions (minimum of three)
   4) Clarify delegations of authority
   5) Plan for reconstitution of essential services
   6) Prioritize essential functions

VI. United States Federal Disaster Response

A. GOVERNMENTAL PREPAREDNESS AND RESPONSE

1. Federal government supports state and local response after a formal request
2. State governments formally request federal assistance
3. Request is made by state governor, and when granted, is declared a Presidentially Declared Disaster, which allows the release of federal funding
4. Plan for autonomous response for at least 5 days

B. NATIONAL RESPONSE FRAMEWORK

1. The Department of Homeland Security developed the National Response Framework (NRF) as a guide for all response agencies at every level in the United States, including hospitals, so that they have common training, language, and responses as part of an all-hazards approach to disasters[12]
2. The NRF has 15 emergency support functions (ESFs) that summarize key federal agency roles and responsibilities
3. Framework focuses on five areas: prevention, protection, mitigation, response, and recovery[12]
4. Emergency support functions
   a. ESF 1: Transportation
   b. ESF 2: Communications
   c. ESF 3: Public Works and Engineering
   d. ESF 4: Firefighting
   e. ESF 5: Information and Planning
   f. ESF 6: Mass Care, Emergency Assistance, Temporary Housing, and Human Services
   g. ESF 7: Logistics
   h. ESF 8: Public Health and Medical Services
   i. ESF 9: Search and Rescue
   j. ESF 10: Oil and Hazardous Materials Response
   k. ESF 11: Agriculture and Natural Resources
   l. ESF 12: Energy
   m. ESF 13: Public Safety and Security
   n. ESF 14: Superseded by National Disaster Recovery Framework
   o. ESF 15: External Affairs
   p. NRP Support Annexes
   1) Mechanisms by which support is organized among private sector, NGO, and federal partners
     a) Critical Infrastructure
       (1) Financial Management
       (2) International Coordination
       (3) Private Sector Coordination
       (4) Tribal Coordination
       (5) Volunteer and Donations Management
       (6) Worker Safety and Health
   q. Incident Annexes
   1) Coordinating structures, in addition to the ESFs, that may be used to deliver core capabilities and support response missions that are unique to a specific type of incident
     a) Biological Incident
       (1) Catastrophic Incident
       (2) Cyber Incident
       (3) Food and Agriculture Incident
       (4) Mass Evacuation Incident
       (5) Nuclear/Radiological Incident
       (6) Terrorism Incident Law Enforcement and Investigation

C. NATIONAL INCIDENT MANAGEMENT SYSTEM

1. National Incident Management System (NIMS) provides the incident management basis for the NRF and defines standard command and management structures
2. NIMS is required in all federally funded jurisdictions and should be included in disaster training, exercises, and EOPs
3. NIMS training is also required for all responders that may receive federal funding; training information can be found online at the Federal Emergency Management Agency's Emergency Management Institute (https://training.fema.gov/is/)

D. NATIONAL TERRORISM ADVISORY SYSTEM

1. Replaces the color-coded Homeland Security Advisory System
2. U.S. Department of Homeland Security assesses credible terrorist threats and posts national warnings as alerts or bulletins
3. Communicates information about terrorist threats to the public[13]
4. Facilities should adjust procedures of security and increase readiness as the threat levels change
5. Threat levels
   a. Imminent Threat Alert
      1) Warns of a credible, specific, and impending terrorist threat against the United States
   b. Elevated Threat Alert
      1) Warns of a credible terrorist threat against the United States
   c. Sunset Provision
      1) Individual threat alert issued for a specific time period, which automatically expires. May be extended if new information becomes available or the threat evolves[13]

E. DISASTER RESILIENCE[14]

1. The ability of individuals, communities, organizations, and states to adapt to and recover from hazards, shocks, or stresses without compromising long-term prospects for development
2. Takes a community health focus

F. DISASTER RISK REDUCTION[15,16]

1. A systematic approach to identifying, assessing, and reducing risks of disaster
2. The concept and practice of reducing disaster risks through systematic efforts to analyze and reduce the causal factors of disasters
3. Aims to reduce socioeconomic vulnerabilities to disaster while addressing the environmental factors and other hazards that trigger disasters
4. Deaths, injuries, diseases, disabilities, psychosocial problems, and other health impacts can be avoided or reduced by disaster risk management measures involving health and other sectors

VII. Special Topics

A. WOMEN'S HEALTH

1. Pregnant women, newborns, and infants may be disproportionately harmed by natural disasters
2. Encourage patients to develop an evacuation plan in the event of a disaster
3. Inform pregnant patients on the signs of preterm labor and other obstetric emergencies
4. With work public health officials to identify facilities that can provide prenatal and obstetric services during a disaster
5. Encourage patients to develop an emergency birth kit
6. Promote lactation and relactation during a disaster
7. Encourage local and state governments to provide facilities that are safe and secure for women and children
8. Inform patients and be aware of the signs of mental distress. Promote prompt attention to mental health needs[17]

B. VULNERABLE POPULATIONS

1. Considerations include different cultures, LGBT, the disabled, very young, elderly, homeless, and people who speak limited or no English[18]

References

1. International Federation of the Red Cross and Red Crescent Societies: What is a disaster? Retrieved from http://www.ifrc.org/en/what-we-do/disaster-management/about-disasters/what-is-a-disaster/, 2015.
2. Federal Emergency Management Agency: Disaster declarations by year. Retrieved from http://www.fema.gov/disasters/grid/year, 2015.
3. ICRC 2015.
4. National Centers for Environmental Information: Billion-dollar weather and climate disasters: Overview. Retrieved from http://www.ncdc.noaa.gov/billions/, 2016.
5. International Federation of the Red Cross and Red Crescent Societies: Types of disasters: Definition of hazard. Retrieved from http://www.ifrc.org/en/what-we-do/disaster-management/about-disasters/definition-of-hazard/, 2015.
6. Centers for Disease Control and Prevention: Office of public health preparedness and response: Strategic National Stockpile (SNS). Retrieved from http://www.cdc.gov/phpr/stockpile/stockpile.htm, 2016.
7. Association of State and Territorial Health Officials: Emergency use authorization toolkit: Strategic National Stockpile. Retrieved from http://www.astho.org/Programs/Preparedness/Public-Health-Emergency-Law/Emergency-Use-Authorization-Toolkit/Strategic-National-Stockpile-Fact-Sheet/, 2016.

8. Centers for Disease Control and Prevention: Guidance on emergency responder, personal protective equipment (PPE) for response to CBRN terrorism incidents. Retrieved from http://www.cdc.gov/niosh/docs/2008-132/pdfs/2008-132.pdf, 2008.
9. World Health Organization: ICN framework of disaster nursing competencies. Retrieved from http://www.wpro.who.int/hrh/documents/icn_framework.pdf?ua=1, 2009.
10. U.S. Environmental Protection Agency: Local emergency planning committees. Retrieved from http://www2.epa.gov/epcra/local-emergency-planning-committees, 2016.
11. Veneema T: *Disaster nursing and emergency preparedness*, 3rd ed., New York, NY, 2012, Springer Publishing Company.
12. Federal Emergency Management Agency (FEMA): National Response Framework. Retrieved from http://www.fema.gov/national-response-framework, 2016.
13. Department of Homeland Security: National Terrorism Advisory System public guide. Retrieved from http://www.dhs.gov/sites/default/files/publications/ntas-public-guide_0.pdf, 2012.
14. Governance and Social Development Resource Centre (GSDRC): What is disaster resilience? Retrieved from http://www.gsdrc.org/topic-guides/disaster-resilience/concepts/what-is-disaster-resilience/, 2016.
15. The United Nations Office for Disaster Risk Reduction: What is disaster risk reduction? Retrieved from http://www.unisdr.org/who-we-are/what-is-drr, 2016.
16. World Health Organization: Disaster risk management for health fact sheets. Retrieved from http://www.who.int/hac/techguidance/preparedness/factsheets/en/, 2016.
17. The American Congress of Obstetricians and Gynecologists: Preparing for disasters: Perspectives on women. Retrieved from http://www.acog.org/Resources-And-Publications/Committee-Opinions/Committee-on-Health-Care-for-Underserved-Women/Preparing-for-Disasters-Perspectives-on-Women, 2010.
18. Emergency Management: How to include diverse, vulnerable populations in emergency preparedness. Retrieved from http://www.emergencymgmt.com/disaster/Diverse-Vulnerable-Populations-Preparedness-041111.html, 2011.

Bibliography

Adelman D, Legg T: *Disaster nursing: A handbook for practice*, Burlington, MA, 2008, Jones & Bartlett Learning.
Anderson PD: Emergency management of chemical weapons injuries, *Journal of Pharmacy Practice* 25(1):61–68, 2012, http://dx.doi.org/10.1177/0897190011420677.
Baack S, Alfred D: Nurses' preparedness and perceived competence in managing disasters, *Journal of Nursing Scholarship* 45(3):281–287, 2013, http://dx.doi.org/10.1111/jnu.12029.
Centers for Disease Control: *Response to a ricin incident: Guidelines for federal, state, and local public health and medical officials*, Washington, DC, 2006, CDC. http://emergency.cdc.gov/agent/ricin/pdf/ricin_protocol.pdf.
Centers for Disease Control: Ebola virus disease. Retrieved from http://www.cdc.gov/vhf/ebola/diagnosis, 2015.
Centers for Disease Control: Preparation and planning for bioterrorism emergencies. Retrieved from http://emergency.cdc.gov/bioterrorism/prep.asp, 2015.

Coule PL, Schwartz RB: The national disaster life support programs: A model for competency-based standardized and locally relevant training, *Journal of Public Health Management and Practice* 15(2):S25–S30, 2009, http://dx.doi.org/10.1097/01.PHH.0000345982.34551.99.
Emergency Nurses Association: *Position statement: Disaster and emergency preparedness for all hazards*, Des Plaines, IL, 2014, ENA.
Federal Emergency Management Agency: Robert T. Stafford Disaster Relief and Emergency Assistance Act (Public Law 93-288). Retrieved from http://www.fema.gov/robert-t-stafford-disaster-relief-and-emergency-assistance-act-public-law-93-288-amended, 2014.
Federal Emergency Management Agency: Disaster declarations by year. Retrieved from http://www.fema.gov/disasters/grid/year, 2015.
Federal Emergency Management Agency: National Response Framework. Retrieved from http://www.fema.gov/national-response-framework, 2015.
Foresman-Capuzzi J, Eckenrode P: When Mr Yuck meets Mr Bubble: A primer on pediatric decontamination, *Journal of Emergency Nursing* 38(5):490–492, 2012, http://dx.doi.org/10.1016/j.jen.2012.05.023.
Grey MR, Spaeth KR: *The bioterrorism sourcebook*, Columbus, OH, 2006, McGraw-Hill.
International Federation of the Red Cross/RedCrescent: What is a disaster? Retrieved from http://www.ifrc.org/en/what-we-do/disaster-management/about-disasters/what-is-a-disaster/, 2015.
Joint Commission: *Emergency management standards*, 2003. Retrieved from https://www.jointcommission.org/emergency_management.aspx.
Joint Commission: New and revised requirements address emergency management oversight. Retrieved from http://www.jointcommission.org/assets/1/18/JCP0713_Emergency_Mgmt_Oversigh.pdf, 2014.
Khoshnevis MA, Panahi Y, Ghanei M, Borna H, Sahebkar A, Aslani J: A triage model for chemical warfare casualties, *Trauma Monthly* 20(3):e16211, 2015, http://dx.doi.org/10.5812/traumamon.16211.
Leary AD, Schwartz MD, Kirk MA, Ignacio JS, Wencil EB, Cibulsky SM: Evidence-based patient decontamination: An integral component of mass exposure chemical incident planning and response, *Disaster Medicine and Public Health Preparedness* 8(3):260–266, 2014, http://dx.doi.org/10.1017/dmp.2014.41.
Mitchell CJ, Kernohan WG, Higginson R: Are emergency care nurses prepared for chemical, biological, radiological, nuclear or explosive incidents? *International Emergency Nursing* 20(3):151–161, 2012, http://dx.doi.org/10.1016/j.ienj.2011.10.001.
Occcupational Safety and Health Administration.n.d.: Best practices for hospital-based first receivers of victims from mass casualty incidents involving the release of hazardous substances. Retrieved from https://www.osha.gov/dts/osta/bestpractices/html/hospital_firstreceivers.html.
Powers R, Dailey E: *International disaster nursing*, New York, NY, 2010, Cambridge.
Ramesh AC, Kumar S: Triage, monitoring, and treatment of mass casualty events involving chemical, biological, radiological, or nuclear agents, *Journal of Pharmaceutical Bioallied Science* 2(3):239–247, 2010, http://dx.doi.org/10.4103/0975-7406.68506.

Steinfeld NI: Federal emergency and disaster requests for tribal lands. In *ISCRAM 2012 Conference Proceedings – 9th International Conference on Information Systems for Crisis Response and Management*, Madison, WI, 2012, University of Wisconsin-Madison. Retrieved from http://www.scopus.com/inward/record.url?eid=2-s2.0-84905587560&partnerID=40&md5=9707a05fb9cfc6986b50984d211dcda6.

Treat KN, Williams JM, Furbee PM, Manley WG, Russell FK, Stamper CD: Hospital preparedness for weapons of mass destruction incidents: An initial assessment, *Annuals of Emergency Medicine* 38(5):562–565, 2001, http://dx.doi.org/10.1067/mem.2001.118009.

United States Army: 21st century textbooks of military medicine – Medical aspects of biological warfare – Anthrax, ricin, smallpox, viral fevers, plague, biosafety, biosecurity. In *Emergency War Surgery Series*, Washington, DC, 2011, Progressive Management.

U.S. Department of Health and Human Services Health Resources and Services Administration: *National Bioterrorism Hospital Preparedness Program*, Washington, DC, 2005, USDHHS.

Veneema T: *Disaster nursing and emergency preparedness for chemical, biological, and radiological terrorism and other hazards*, 3rd ed., New York, NY, 2012, Springer Publishing Company.

Walsh L, Subbarao I, Gebbie K, et al.: Core competencies for disaster medicine and public health, *Disaster Medicine and Public Health Preparedness* 6(1):44–52, 2012, http://dx.doi.org/10.1001/dmp.2012.4.

Worrall J: Are emergency care staff prepared for disaster? *Emergency Nurse* 19(9):31–37, 2012, http://dx.doi.org/10.7748/en2012.02.19.9.31.c8943.

CHAPTER 42

Education: Professional, Patient, and Community

Kristine Kenney Powell, MSN, RN, CEN, NEA-BC, FAEN,
Joni Hentzen Daniels, MSN, RN, CEN, CCRN, CNS

The Emergency Nurses Association (ENA) *Emergency Nursing Scope and Standards of Practice* recognizes education as a standard of professional performance in emergency nursing. ENA is a primary resource for emergency nursing education. The ENA provides emergency nurses with opportunities to meet the educational needs of self, patients, and the community through continuing education programs, targeted topic courses, conferences, professional journals, newsletters, and other resources on current issues affecting emergency nurses, patient care, and community health and education. An understanding of learning theory, educational principles, and available resources can assist the emergency nurse with developing a framework for addressing educational needs.

I. Educational Principles

A. THEORETICAL FOUNDATIONS IN KNOWLEDGE AND LEARNING

1. Carper's Ways of Knowing: theory developed by Barbara A. Carper in 1978 that describes four patterns of knowing, which include empirical (scientific fact), ethical (morality), personal (self-awareness), and aesthetic (empathy)

2. Benner's Novice to Expert: model developed by Patricia E. Benner in 1978. The model is based on the Dreyfus Model of Skill Acquisition and describes the five stages of clinical competence in nursing (novice, advanced beginner, competent, proficient, and expert). The progression through each stage occurs as the nurse acquires knowledge through education and experience and is able to progress from concrete rules to pattern recognition to an intuitive sense of the situation as a whole. This model can be applied to any new role such as direct care nurse, triage nurse, educator, charge nurse, or nurse manager

3. Learning theory: multiple learning theories exist that attempt to explain different facets of learning. Some common categories of learning theories are listed
   a. Behaviorism: learning as defined by an observable change in behavior
   b. Cognitive theory: learning as a function of thought processes and neuroscience
   c. Constructivism: learning as the development of new ideas based on knowledge and experience
   d. Humanism: learning as a function of motivation, resilience, and need

B. ADULT LEARNING CONCEPTS

1. Basic assumptions
   a. Adult learners are independent and self-directed

b. Adult learners appreciate rationale for the existence of learning experience

c. Adult learners have past experiences that enable adaptation to new information

d. Adult learners expect and appreciate learning that is immediately applicable to the present situation

e. Adults learn best from education that is problem centered

f. Adults have extrinsic and intrinsic motivators for learning

2. Ideal conditions for adult learning

a. Climate conducive to learning is helpful, comfortable, and respectful

b. Learner has innate desire to learn

c. Clear objectives help learner recognize the experience as one that is applicable to practice

d. If possible, learner should help plan and implement the content

e. Learning program should appeal creatively to different learning styles

f. Learner's past experiences are taken into account

g. Learner has sense of personal progress toward meeting objectives

II. Professional Education

Emergency nurses deliver care to diverse patient populations in an environment that requires a broad range of knowledge and skills in a rapidly changing environment. An effective professional education program will address knowledge and skills that allow the nurse to practice safely and effectively in this type of setting.

A. EMERGENCY NURSING KNOWLEDGE AND SKILLS

1. Unique aspects of emergency nursing

a. Broad range of medical issues in diverse populations across the entire lifespan

b. Initial management of care based on chief complaint or condition rather than diagnosis

c. Need for continuous prioritization and intervention as more information becomes available, including knowledge of available internal and external resources

d. Integration of episodic outpatient and inpatient care

e. Multiple practice settings (e.g., hospital/freestanding, prehospital, transport, industrial, and recreational)

2. Knowledge and skills for clinical patient care

a. Essential clinical nursing knowledge and skills

1) Composite of clinical knowledge, population groups, and flow of patient care (Table 42.1)

2) Procedures and skills relevant to specific emergencies (e.g., airway management, wound care, medication administration)

3) Documentation of care in the patient health record

b. Communication and collaboration

1) Proficiency in public relations and customer service techniques

2) Effective communication with prehospital care providers (e.g., emergency medical technicians [EMTs], paramedics, firefighters, and law enforcement officers)

3) Effective communication and collaboration with peers and other care disciplines (e.g., physicians, laboratory, radiology, social work, and other essential care services)

Table 42.1

Emergency Nursing Knowledge Composite

Clinical Knowledge	Population Groups	Flow of Patient Care
Range of systems – maxillofacial, ocular, neurologic, circulatory, respiratory, gastrointestinal, genitourinary, musculoskeletal, medical, infectious disease, psychiatric Condition-specific – airway, obstetric, bariatric, oncology, shock, trauma, environmental, forensic, abuse/neglect, toxicology/exposures, chronic medical conditions, pain, palliative care, advanced directives, end-of-life care, medication management	Age: Newborns, neonates Infants, toddlers School-aged children Adolescents Adults Older adults Generational: 1. Traditionalist 2. Baby Boomer 3. Generation X 4. Millennial 5. Generation Z Other: Culture and ethnicity Religion Special needs and disabilities Sexual orientation	Initial patient triage Initiation of lifesaving interventions Diagnostic testing Continual interventions and patient evaluation Patient discharge and teaching Patient admission, transfer, and transport

4) Conflict management and crisis intervention
5) Safe handoffs in care transition
6) Patient and family teaching
7) Peer and student teaching
8) Varied communication styles, approaches, and devices

c. Other professional issues
1) Time management and prioritization
2) Activation and implementation of hospital and community emergency management plans including mass/multiple casualty incidents and active shooter events
3) Critical incident stress management
4) Nursing jurisprudence
5) Reading and interpreting research and evidence-based literature
6) Self-care (e.g., physical, mental, emotional)
7) Wellness, safety, and prevention

3. Work environment conditions
a. High-stress area with rapid throughput needs
b. Unexpected workload increases/decreases
c. Teamwork approach
d. Ability to transition rapidly between primary and team nursing
e. Requires mastery of emergency technology and equipment use
f. Patients represent a microcosm of general population at large
g. Risk for workplace violence
h. Incorporates utilization of telecommunication skills

B. LEARNING FACILITATOR ROLES AND RESPONSIBILITIES

1. Clinical Nurse Specialist (CNS)/Advanced Practice Nurse (APN)
a. Educator
1) Serves as resource to staff, nursing students, and other health care personnel in the acquisition of knowledge and skills related to nursing practice
b. Clinical expert
1) Models excellence in emergency nursing practice through use of assessment, planning, implementation, and evaluation
2) Assists and provides direction to nursing personnel in clinical decision making, priority setting, stabilization, and resuscitation
c. Consultant
1) Collaborates with clinical nurses, patient, family, and other members of the health care team to resolve complex clinical situations
d. Researcher
1) Critically analyzes current nursing research and disseminates relevant findings to improve patient care and patient outcomes
2) Facilitates and/or conducts nursing research

3) Teaches personnel how to evaluate nursing research
4) Implements evidence-based practice model in the emergency department

2. Nurse educator
a. Organizes and implements orientation and competency-based educational programs
b. Assesses educational needs of personnel
c. Develops, executes, and evaluates educational programs for nursing personnel
d. Serves as clinical resource
e. Utilizes evidence-based resources in the development of education programs (e.g., ENA Clinical Practice Guidelines and Translation into Practice documents)
f. Informs nurse administrator/manager of resource needs for education
g. Coordinates meetings with new staff, preceptor, and nurse administrator/manager to evaluate critical thinking, knowledge and technical skills, and readiness for independent practice on the unit

3. Nurse preceptor
a. Experienced nurse with training in orientation and precepting new personnel
b. Assignment usually for a fixed or limited time
c. Focuses on unit-specific orientation to policies, procedures, and protocols
d. Facilitates socialization into department
e. Acts as role model and clinical resource
f. Participates in development of teaching plan and evaluates learner response
g. Deploys a variety of teaching strategies (e.g., clinical inquiry and questioning, positive reinforcement, reflective practice, debriefing)
h. Able to adjust teaching style and plan to accommodate workload, patient events, learner needs, and efficient use of teachable moments

4. Nurse administrator/manager
a. Develops and nurtures ongoing learning culture and environment within the department
b. Supports and encourages involvement of personnel in education process within the department
c. Organizes committees and projects that support education
d. Holds personnel accountable for complying with educational requirements of department
e. Provides appropriate resources for departmental education programs
f. Aligns education processes with needs identified in quality improvement activities
g. Recognizes and rewards individuals and unit for achieving educational milestones and goals

5. Nurse peers
a. Involved in selection, development, delivery, and evaluation of education programs

b. Participate in unit- and hospital-based committees and workgroups to address education needs

C. DEPARTMENT ORIENTATION

1. Purpose
   a. Preparation of new employee for competent clinical practice in the targeted unit
   b. Social integration of new employee to emergency care setting
2. Program requirements and components
   a. Program requirements
      1) Active involvement of nurse manager, educator, preceptor, peers, and new employee is needed for successful completion of department orientation
      2) Orientation/teaching plan is individualized and competency based
      3) Orientation/teaching plan involves a variety of teaching/learning activities which incorporate adult learning principles with needed knowledge and skills training (e.g., simulation of clinical case studies and technical skills, preceptor-facilitated hands-on skill training, e-learning and other self-paced education modules, debriefing, reflective practice)
      4) Specific goals and objectives should be outlined in the orientation plan, and ongoing reviews of the new employee performance and competencies are documented in the employee file
      5) Specific roles in the emergency care settings require additional orientation and training (e.g., triage, flow nurse, charge nurse, preceptor)
      6) New employees should have an opportunity to provide feedback on preceptors and the orientation process
      7) Additional standardized coursework may be required by the institution
   b. Program components
      1) Review of specific unit and institutional policies, procedures, and standards of care
      2) Competency-based assessment of knowledge and skills (Table 42.2; Fig. 42.1)
      3) Orientation goals, objectives, and plan for knowledge and skills competencies
      4) Evaluation of ongoing performance and successful completion of department orientation
      5) Evaluation of orientation process by new employee

D. EMERGENCY NURSING CREDENTIALS

1. Certification
   a. Certified Emergency Nurse (CEN)
   b. Certified Pediatric Emergency Nurse (CPEN)
   c. Trauma Certified Registered Nurse (TCRN)
   d. Certified Flight Registered Nurse (CFRN)
   e. Certified Transport Registered Nurse (CTRN)
2. Verification
   a. Advanced Cardiac Life Support (ACLS)
   b. Trauma Nursing Core Course (TNCC)
   c. Emergency Nursing Pediatric Course (ENPC)
   d. Pediatric Advanced Life Support (PALS)
   e. Basic/Advanced Disaster Life Support (BDLS/ADLS)
   f. Crisis intervention, deescalation, and personal/team safety strategies
   g. Institution specific (e.g., triage, procedural sedation)

E. EDUCATIONAL APPROACHES

1. Teaching strategies
   a. Departmental in-service presentations
      1) Department- and hospital-specific issues
      2) Topical information
         a) Pain management
         b) Advance directives
         c) Updates on emerging technology, patient care
      3) Bedside teaching, dialogue, nursing rounds
      4) Equipment, pharmacology update
      5) Problem-based presentations: case studies

Table 42.2

Competency Assessment Program

Specific Program Purpose	Essential Competences	Program Components	Department Competencies	Validation Methods
1. Assess orientee's ability to perform proficiencies, tasks, skills required for baseline job performance	1. Provided to orientee on arrival to department 2. At completion of orientation, orientee must understand, complete, and demonstrate successful achievement of competencies	1. Incorporate interpersonal and technical skills with critical thinking 2. Competence standards behavioral objectives based on performance outcomes 3. Critical behaviorscriterion referenced behaviors that denote ability to perform procedures safely	1. High-volume procedures 2. High-risk, time-sensitive procedures 3. Unusual or rare procedures	1. Written test 2. Return demonstration 3. Observation of daily work 4. Exemplar 5. Case study 6. Peer review 7. Self-assessment 8. Discussion group 9. Mock events 10. Quality case reviews/audits 11. Presentation

Name:_____ Dept:__Emergency Department_____ Date:_____

ENA Regional Medical Center
Registered Nurse Competencies
2014

This form is to be completed by the employee. For each of the competency statements listed below, select which methods of validation you would like to use for validation of his or her your skill in that area. See the validation methods for details. When this form is complete, submit it to the department/unit supervisor or manager.

Competency Documentation due to Unit Manager no later than December 15, 2014.

Verification Methods	Age Specific Legend	Level of Performance
1. Written Test 2. Return Demonstration 3. Observation of daily work 4. Case studies 5. Exemplar / Reflective practice 6. Discussion / Debriefing 7. Mock Events 8. Presentations 9. Q. I. Monitors	**I** = Infant **T** = Toddler **P** = Preschool **S** = School Age **A** = Adolescent **Ad** = Adult **G** = Geriatric **All** = All Age Groups	**0** = Development Plan Required **1** = Needs Assistance **2** = Performs Independently **3** = Resourceful, able to teach others

Competency	Validation Methods	Age Specific	How Met (Method)	Level of Performance	Verified by Signature and Date
ESI Triage competency **For triage nurses only	***ESI Triage competency*** *(at least 2 of 3 demonstrated and submit evidence to unit manager)* 1. *Attend triage class and successfully complete triage test.* 2. *Submit 10 triage cases for review (at least 1 pediatric case 0-12 yrs old)* 3. *Develop 5 triage case studies and present one at a staff meeting.*	*All*	*1* *3* *4, 8*		
Code Blue *Demonstrates the ability to perform appropriate role during a code blue.*	***Mock Code*** *– At least of 5 demonstrated and submit evidence to unit manager.* 1. Participated in a Mock Code and submit completed copy of the Mock Code Evaluation Form. 2. Participated in an actual Code Blue, obtained a copy of the Interdisciplinary Code Evaluation, and has written an Exemplar (describing your role in the code and what lessons were learned). 3. Attend an initial or renewal ACLS class this year (FY2010) 4. Attend an initial or renewal PALS class this year (FY2010). 5. Attend an initial or renewal TNCC or ENPC class this year (FY2010).	*Ages that apply* *All* *All* *A, Ad, G* *I, T, P, S, A* *All*	 *7* *2,3,5,6* *1,2,4,7* *1,2,4,7* *1,2,4,7*		

Fig. 42.1 Example of Competency Validation Tool. (Courtesy of Baylor Scott & White Health)

b. Departmental/institutional resources
  1) Self-study instructional modules (e.g., assessment skills for pediatric patients)
  2) Mock scenarios (e.g., pediatric cardiac arrest, disaster drills)
  3) Simulation lab (e.g., emergent conditions such as stroke and trauma resuscitation)
  4) Demonstration/skill review (e.g., new chest tube setup, skills laboratory)
  5) Games (e.g., equipment "scavenger hunt" for new personnel)
  6) Posters (e.g., special equipment assembly, such as pediatric arterial catheter)
  7) Committee work (e.g., education committee, customer service committee)
  8) Fact sheets, newsletter
  9) Brainstorming (e.g., tackling staffing problems)

10) Learning resource center (e.g., books, journals, tapes, videos)
11) Portable education cart
12) Video or closed-circuit television
13) Computer literacy (e.g., teaching basic skills needed for computer use)
14) Computer-assisted instruction (e.g., learning modules)
15) Interactive video: screen-displayed accounts of clinical situations in which interactive process enables validation or correction of nurse's treatment plan
16) Journal clubs

c. Formalized classes, lectures
d. Seminars, conferences, workshops, symposia
e. Panel discussions, debates
f. Role modeling
g. Questioning
1) Lecture
2) Clinical practice
3) Discussion

2. Potential obstacles
a. Staffing patterns not conducive to education programs
b. Inadequate institutional funding for education and educators
c. Personnel's attitudes toward learning
d. Personnel with multiple commitments (e.g., family constraints, other employment)
e. Personnel fatigue
f. Burnout
g. Philosophic differences
h. Patient overload
i. Inappropriate needs assessment
j. Department morale
k. Lack of appropriate learning space, supplies, or facilities
l. Ineffective teaching methods for content

F. CONTINUING EDUCATION

1. Purpose
a. Promote working knowledge, competence, and skills above basic knowledge and skill expectations
b. Improve patient care and outcomes

c. Foster personal and professional development as well as career goals
2. Beneficiaries (Table 42.3)
a. Nurse
b. Patient
c. Employer
d. Nursing profession
3. Means of obtaining continuing education
a. Self-regulated learning/self-study
b. Home study/correspondence courses
c. Professional organization-sponsored continuing education (e.g., ACLS, TNCC)
d. Attendance or presentation at workshops, seminars
e. Organizational meetings (local, state, and national ENA meetings)
f. Professional journals (e.g., *Journal of Emergency Nursing*)
g. Degree advancement
h. Computer-assisted instruction (webinars, e-learning)

III. Patient Education

Patient education is an ongoing process that occurs throughout the person's emergency department visit. The information that is provided should effect changes in the patient's knowledge, attitudes, and skills in relation to his or her health or illness.

A. ESSENTIAL ELEMENTS

1. Patient teaching encompasses all disciplines of medicine
2. Patient teaching information has to be customized to patient's age, educational and developmental levels
3. Families and significant others are included in teaching
4. Teaching should be adapted to patient's culture and ethnicity
5. Effective teaching may depend on resolving language barriers
6. Patient education is a "teaching in the moment" opportunity
a. Must be short and concise
b. Must be immediately understandable and applicable
c. Focus on key items rather than comprehensive overview

Table 42.3

Beneficiaries of Professional Continuing Education

Nurse	Patient	Employer	Profession
Increases knowledge and competence	Improves patient experience of care and clinical outcomes	Increases competence of personnel	Promotes adherence to practice standards
Increases confidence and job satisfaction		Improves performance on quality measures	Promotes evidence-based practice
Enhances potential for career advancement		Decreases liability	Strengthens nursing image
		Enhances recruitment and retention of personnel	
		Enhances facility standing in the community	

d. Must be adapted to patient condition and health literacy, as well as care environment

7. Nurse must have teaching information readily available or committed to memory
   a. Teaching begins at triage
   b. Teaching is required before and during treatment
   c. Teaching is required before and after medication administration
   d. Teaching opportunities generally end at time of discharge
   e. If time and opportunity permit, teaching may encompass health and safety issues not related to patient visit (e.g., home and motor vehicle safety reminders, immunization reminders)
8. Discharge telephone calls at 24–72 hours may offer additional opportunities for assessment and enhancement of patient understanding of discharge teaching

B. LEGAL CONSIDERATIONS

1. Nurse practice acts include health guidance and health education as a responsibility of the licensed nurse
2. Patients have the right to be educated about their disease process or injury
3. Nurse must ensure that teaching has taken place before procedures and medications as patient condition permits
4. Nurse is legally responsible for teaching content and is therefore open to potential litigation

C. PROCESS

1. Data gathering
   a. Observations of patient during entire visit
   b. Prior medical records (previous hospital visits)
   c. Patient's support systems (family and friends)
   d. Interview, discussions with patient throughout visit
2. Sort data informally
3. Determine what patient wants to know
4. Identify and resolve potential barriers and obstacles to teaching/learning (Table 42.4)
5. Ascertain what will enhance patient's ability and motivation to learn
6. Devise and tailor teaching plan, keeping in mind that approach to learning is determined by past experiences, lifestyle, and personality
7. Impaired patients (physical state, drug or alcohol use, medications)
   a. Include family and significant others in teaching process
   b. Teaching may be delayed until patient is clear minded
8. Teaching is reinforced with written discharge instructions as mandated by regulatory agencies

a. Patient may be too nervous, stressed, or distracted to absorb information
b. Allows for later reference
c. Part of medicolegal record

D. TEACHING METHODS

1. Demonstration and return demonstration (e.g., crutch-walk training)
2. One-on-one discussion between nurse and patient
3. Use of preprinted information sheets for patient
4. Reiteration of physician's instructions
5. Questioning with repeat of key learning points
6. Final written instructions
7. Consultation with specialty educator (e.g., diabetes educator for use of insulin pump)
8. Educational information located in lobby or hallways
   a. Displays on bulletin boards: drawings, photographs
   b. Signs and posters
   c. Educational coloring books for children
   d. Video or educational television in lobby
   e. Pamphlets in lobby and examination rooms on various health topics
9. Referrals to community and reliable web-based resources (e.g., American Heart Association, state health departments)

E. TEACHING EFFECTIVENESS

Patient education should result in positive behavior and attitude changes in relation to health and well-being.
1. Ask patient to restate (in own words) what has been taught
2. Ask patient a question about what has been taught to test understanding of learning

Table 42.4
Potential Obstacles and Barriers to Teaching/ Learning in Patient Education
1. Lack of privacy
2. Time constraints (patient or nurse)
3. Multiple distractions
4. Ineffective nurse-patient rapport
5. Nurse's knowledge deficit or lack of teaching finesse
6. Deficiency in involvement of family of impaired patient
7. Inability to establish continuity and follow-up for reinforcement and evaluation

8. Patient barriers to learning
  a. Physiologic barrier (e.g., pain, age, critical illness, medications, cognition, sight or hearing deficits)
  b. Psychological barriers (e.g., lack of trust, anxiety, denial, depression, psychosis)
  c. Environmental barriers (e.g., lack of privacy, separation from family, noise levels)
  d. Sociocultural barrier (e.g., language barrier, ethnic background, lack of education, illiteracy)
  e. Motivation: Patient's awareness of health needs and level of desire to take responsibility for health care

3. Learning will be increased if teaching is related to something with which the patient is familiar
4. Return demonstration by patient will indicate need for correction and feedback
5. Follow-up telephone call can help nurse determine effectiveness of patient teaching
6. Follow-up questionnaire with specific questions helps nurse assess teaching effectiveness
7. Guidelines for relating information and providing feedback
   a. Be specific rather than general (e.g., instead of saying "Watch for signs of infection," state specific signs of infection)
   b. Focus on behavior, not on the person (e.g., maintain respect for patient as a person and give corrective advice in a positive manner)
   c. Avoid use of absolute words such as "always" and "never"
   d. Direct feedback toward behavior or situation that learner has the ability to change (e.g., encourage condom use for "safe sex" as opposed to advising abstinence)
   e. Do not overload patient or learner with information
   f. Do not argue with patient
   g. First give positive feedback and then discuss weaknesses
8. Patient compliance
   a. Patient has right to choose whether to follow nurse's advice
   b. Compliance with teaching depends on
      1) Recall ability
      2) Comprehension
      3) Desire to comply
      4) Ability to perform
      5) Health care literacy
9. Reinforcement of discharge instructions
   a. Provide written discharge instructions; avoid use of medical abbreviations
   b. Review discharge instructions with patient and caregivers
   c. Answer questions
   d. Clarify unclear items
   e. Explain medical terms and directions
   f. Request that physician return to clarify patient education or information needs
   g. Involve family and significant others in interaction
   h. Explain rationale for prescribed medication (e.g., drug actions, side effects)
   i. Offer specific instruction with medication (e.g., "Do not drive while taking this medication")
   j. Refer to specific community resources (e.g., American Stroke Association)
10. Arrangements for follow-up after discharge
    a. Follow-up appointment with primary care provider or specialist (e.g., orthopaedic surgeon, obstetrician, diabetic nurse educator)

b. Clinic appointment
c. Return visit to the emergency department or hospital
d. Home health care/visiting nurse/community paramedicine program
e. Social service or case management referral
f. Psychiatric facility or outpatient psychiatric program
g. Substance abuse/alcohol detoxification centers
h. Condition-specific patient and caregiver support groups

IV. Community Education

Emergency nurses are involved in community education programs directed toward promoting consumer health or reducing risk and impact of injuries. The ENA Community Injury Prevention Toolkit provides a comprehensive approach and resources to assist in community health promotion and injury prevention activities.

A. GENERAL APPROACH TO COMMUNITY HEALTH EDUCATION

1. Define the issue and target audience through needs assessments (Table 42.5)
   a. Statistical reports (e.g., trauma or cardiac registry database, state health department immunization statistics, violence and abuse statistics)
   b. Child fatality reviews
   c. Community surveys
   d. Observation studies (e.g., observing seat belt use at busy local intersection, observation of play patterns and parent supervision at local playground)
   e. Response to high-profile local, state, or national news events (e.g., bus crashes, gun crime)
2. Identify risk factors and protective factors
   a. Environmental factors
   b. Vector factors
   c. Human factors
3. Develop action plan and strategies to address the issue
   a. Primary, secondary, tertiary prevention: identifies interventions that may occur prior to, during, or after an injury event
   b. Haddon's matrix: integrates risk and protective factors with primary, secondary, tertiary interventions
   c. The five Es of prevention
      1) Education (e.g., awareness programs on risks of drinking and driving, health fairs with wellness information, educational pamphlets and public safety announcements)
      2) Enactment/enforcement (e.g., legislation and enforcement of speed limit laws)

Table 42.5

Suggested Topics for Community Health Programs

a. Traffic injuries
  1) Motor vehicle occupants
  2) Pedestrians
  3) Motorcyclists
  4) Bicyclists
b. Residential injuries
  1) Falls
  2) Fire and burns
  3) Poisoning
  4) Suffocation
c. Recreational injuries
  1) Swimming/drowning
  2) Aquatic spinal cord injuries
  3) Boating
  4) Playground
  5) Fireworks
  6) Amateur competitive sports
d. Occupational injuries
e. Violence, assault, battery
f. Intimate partner violence
g. Rape and sexual assault
h. Firearm injuries
i. Child/elder maltreatment, neglect
j. Suicide awareness, prevention, and resources
k. Alcohol, substance abuse
l. General health and wellness

3) Engineering (e.g., improved safety designs of motor vehicles, helmets, seat belts, child safety seats)
4) Economics (e.g., financial penalties for speeding tickets, Good Driver programs with lower insurance premiums)
5) Environmental (e.g., signage, changing cultural norms for acceptable behaviors)
d. Levels of intervention
  1) Individual
  2) Interpersonal
  3) Organizational
  4) Community
  5) Population
e. Venues for programs and interventions
  1) Hospital based
  2) Community based
  3) Media based (e.g., television, radio, Internet)
4. Implement action plan and evaluate program effectiveness
  a. Involvement of program facilitators and participants
  b. Acquire needed resources
  c. Evaluate process and outcome measures
5. Disseminate and share results
  a. Newsletters and other publications
  b. Websites and social media
  c. Institutions, organizations, and agencies
  d. Newspaper, radio, and other media venues

B. OTHER COMMUNITY OPPORTUNITIES

1. Careers in emergency nursing
  a. Hospital tours and information for students
  b. Junior high, high school classroom visits (e.g., career day participation)
  c. High school students' health career experiences
  d. Joint partnership with local colleges/universities
2. Paramedic/EMT or nursing school instructor or preceptor
  a. Serve as instructor in classroom settings
  b. Serve as preceptor in clinical setting
3. Legislative advocate for health care issues
4. First aid or cardiopulmonary resuscitation (CPR) instructor
  a. Schools
  b. Workplace
  c. Civic groups
  d. Community organizations
5. Volunteer activities
  a. Assisting with local health care events: health fairs
  b. Disaster work (Red Cross)
6. Emergency and disaster management
  a. Serve as member of regional disaster team
  b. Stimulate, organize, or act as resource for teaching programs for hospital disaster team
  c. Organize or participate in critical incident stress debriefing after incident
7. Serve on community boards, taskforces, and workgroups

Bibliography

American Organization of Nurse Executives: *AONE guiding principles for the newly licensed nurse transition into practice*, Chicago, IL, 2011, American Organization of Nurse Executives. Retrieved from http://www.aone.org/resources/PDFs/AONE_GP_Newly_Licensed_Nurses.pdf.

American Organization of Nurse Executives: *AONE guiding principles for mitigating violence in the workplace*, Chicago, IL, 2015, American Organization of Nurse Executives. Retrieved from http://www.aone.org/resources/PDFs/Mitigating_Violence_GP_final.pdf.

Auger RD: The "ED Mini": a novel approach to clinical education, *Journal of Emergency Nursing* 37(4):401–403, 2011.

Carnago L, Mast M: Using ways of knowing to guide emergency nursing practice, *Journal of Emergency Nursing* 41(5):387–390, 2015.

Crisis Prevention Institute: *Nonviolent crisis intervention instructor manual*, Milwaukee, WI, 2013, Crisis Prevention Institute.

Emergency Nurses Association: *Emergency nursing: Scope and standards of practice*, Des Plaines, IL, 2011, Emergency Nurses Association.

Emergency Nurses Association: *Position statement: Specialty certifications in emergency nursing*, Des Plaines, IL, 2011, Emergency Nurses Association.

Emergency Nurses Association: *Position statement: Triage qualifications*, Des Plaines, IL, 2011, Emergency Nurses Association.

Emergency Nurses Association: *Position statement: Firearm safety and injury prevention*, Des Plaines, IL, 2013, Emergency Nurses Association.

Emergency Nurses Association: *Position statement: Palliative and end-of-life care in the emergency setting*, Des Plaines, IL, 2013, Emergency Nurses Association.

Emergency Nurses Association: *Position statement: Patient handoff/transfer*, Des Plaines, IL, 2013, Emergency Nurses Association.

Emergency Nurses Association: *Position statement: Safe discharge from the emergency care setting*, Des Plaines, IL, 2013, Emergency Nurses Association.

Emergency Nurses Association: *Position statement: Prevention, wellness and disease management*, Des Plaines, IL, 2014, Emergency Nurses Association.

Emergency Nurses Association: *Community injury prevention toolkit*, Des Plaines, IL, 2015, Institute Emergency Nurses Association.

Emergency Nurses Association: *Position statement: Emergency nurse orientation*, Des Plaines, IL, 2015, Emergency Nurses Association.

Emergency Nurses Association: *Position statement: Trauma nurse education*, Des Plaines, IL, 2015, Emergency Nurses Association.

Emergency Nurses Association and International Nurses Society on Addictions: *Joint position statement: Expanded roles and responsibilities for nurses in screening, brief intervention, and referral to treatment (SBIRT) for alcohol use*, Des Plaines, IL, 2012, Emergency Nurses Association.

Gurm B: Multiple ways of knowing in teaching and learning, *International Journal for the Scholarship of Teaching and Learning* 7(1), 2013. Retrieved from http://digitalcommons.georgiasouthern.edu/ij-sotl/vol7/iss1/4.

Harding AD, Walker-Cillio GE, Duke A, Campos GJ, Stapleton SJ: A framework for creating and evaluating competencies for emergency nurses, *Journal of Emergency Nursing* 39(3):252–264, 2013.

Keller R, Frank-Bader M, Beltran K, Ascalon M, Bowar-Ferres SL: Peer education: an innovative approach for integrating standards into practice, *Journal of Nursing Care Quality* 26(2):120–127, 2011. Retrieved from http://www.researchgate.net/publication/46273798_Peer_education_an_innovative_approach_for_integrating_standards_into_practice.

Klein G, Hintze N, Saab D: *Thinking inside the box: The shadowbox method for cognitive skill development*, Marseille, France, 2013, International Conference on Naturalistic Decision Making. Retrieved from http://arpege-recherche.org/ndm11/papers/ndm11-121.pdf.

Knowles MS: *The modern practice of adult education*, New York, NY, 1970, Association Press.

Ulrich B: *Mastering precepting: A nurse's handbook for success*, Indianapolis, IN, 2012, International Honor Society of Nursing, Sigma Theta Tau International.

Wright D: *The ultimate guide to competency assessment in health care*, ed 3, Minneapolis, MN, 2005, Creative Health Care Management.

CHAPTER 43

Emergency Patient Transfer and Transport

Michael De Laby, MSN, RN, CCRN, CFRN, TCRN, NRP

I. Emergency Medical Services System

A. COMPONENTS

1. A comprehensive emergency medical services (EMS) system consists of multiple elements (Fig. 43.1)

B. SELECTED DEFINITIONS

1. EMS system
   a. Consolidated system of essential components
   b. Designed to provide a coordinated, timely, and effective response to medical emergencies
2. Medical oversight
   a. Medical authority and responsibility
      1) For all medical care provided by the service
      2) Active role in function and management of the service as it relates to patient care activities; several terms refer to the activities involved in medical oversight (Table 43.1)
3. Transfer
   a. Comprehensive infrastructure and process
   b. Involved before, during, and after moving patient from one location to another
4. Transport
   a. Physical process of moving patient from one location to another

C. PREHOSPITAL TRIAGE DECISION SCHEME

This is the scheme used to assess the severity of the patient's condition and to determine the available regional resources to treat the patient.

1. Trauma categories: *Resources for Optimal Care of the Injured Patient:* American College of Surgeons Committee on Trauma
   a. Physiologic parameters
   b. Anatomic parameters
   c. Mechanism of injury
   d. Special patient or system considerations
2. Nontrauma categories: based on a match among
   a. Patient's care requirements
   b. Facility's ability to provide care
   c. Local/regional or state protocols
   d. May include psychiatric, pediatric, geriatric, neurologic, cardiac, neonatal, spinal cord, burn cases, obstetric, or others in which patients require specialized care centers

II. Interfacility Transport

A. SELECTED DEFINITIONS

1. Critical care transport
   a. Level of transport care provided to patients with an immediate life-threatening illness or injuries associated with single or multiple organ system failure

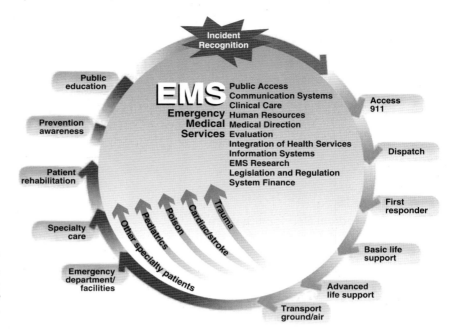

Fig. 43.1 Elements of the emergency medical services (EMS) system. *(Courtesy of the U.S. Department of Transportation, National Highway Traffic Safety Administration, Office of Emergency Medical Services [2006].)*

Table 43.1

Terminology Used in Medical Oversight

Current Terminology	Historical Reference	Historical Reference	Example
Prospective	Off-line	Indirect	Protocol development
Concurrent	On-line/On-scene	Direct	Giving orders by radio
Retrospective	Off-line	Indirect	Quality management

  b. Requirements
    1) Expert level of provider knowledge and skills
    2) Setting providing necessary equipment
    3) Ability to handle added challenge of transport
    4) High level of medical direction and sophistication of care because of patient's complex medical problems
2. Facility
  a. Licensed health care entity (e.g., hospital, clinic, rehabilitation, nursing home)
3. Interfacility transfer (IFT)
  a. Any transfer, after initial assessment and stabilization, from and to a health care facility
4. Levels of patient acuity
  a. Provider capabilities must match patient's current and potential needs
  b. Sending facility needs to determine appropriate personnel based on patient care needs, local or institutional protocols, and regulated scope of practice for all provider levels
  c. Levels: examples are provided of the types of needs the patient may have and the level of care likely to be required at each level as recommended by the National Highway Traffic Safety Administration

  1) Stable with no risk for deterioration
    a) Oxygen
    b) Monitoring of vital signs
    c) Maintenance of a saline lock (basic emergency medical care)
  2) Stable with low risk of deterioration
    a) Intravenous IV fluid line
    b) Some IV medications including pain medications
    c) Pulse oximetry monitoring/end tidal CO_2 monitoring
    d) Increased need for assessment and interpretation skills (advanced care)
  3) Stable with medium risk of deterioration
    a) Electrocardiogram (ECG) monitoring
    b) Basic cardiac medications (e.g., heparin or nitroglycerin) (advanced care plus)
  4) Stable with high risk of deterioration
    a) Requiring advanced airway management but secured, intubated, on ventilator
    b) Multiple vasoactive medication infusions (advanced care plus)
    c) Condition has been initially stabilized, but has likelihood of deterioration based

on assessment or knowledge of provider regarding specific illness/injury

5) Unstable
   a) Patient cannot be stabilized at the transferring facility
   b) Deteriorating or likely to deteriorate (e.g., patients who require invasive monitoring, intraaortic balloon pump)
   c) Postresuscitation status
   d) Sustained multiple trauma (critical care or available crew with time considerations)

5. Specialty care transport (SCT): defined by Centers for Medicare and Medicaid Services
   a. The IFT of a critically injured or ill beneficiary by a ground ambulance vehicle including the provision of medically necessary supplies and services, at a level of service beyond the scope of the EMT (Emergency Medical Technician) paramedic
   b. Necessary when a beneficiary's condition requires ongoing care that must be furnished by one or more health professionals in an appropriate specialty area (e.g., emergency or critical care nursing, emergency medicine, respiratory care, cardiovascular care, or a paramedic with additional training; i.e., critical care paramedic)

B. EMERGENCY MEDICAL TREATMENT AND ACTIVE LABOR ACT (EMTALA) (SEE CHAPTER 45)

Transfers must be carried out by qualified personnel and transportation equipment, as required by the patient condition, including the use of necessary and medically appropriate life support measures during the transfer. The physician at the transferring hospital, not the receiving facility, has the responsibility to determine appropriate mode, equipment, and medical personnel for transfer. The sending hospital is responsible to ensure that medications, equipment, and personnel are available to support anticipated patient care needs during transfer. This may include the need to assign hospital personnel to accompany the patient during transport. Receiving facilities have an obligation to accept patients based on adequate capacity and capability. This should not be decided in isolation by the medical staff but in coordination with administrative representatives who can ensure that equipment, facilities, and staffing will, in fact, be able to meet the needs of the patient.

1. Mode of transportation: ground versus air ambulance. The following recommendations are adapted from the National Association of EMS Physicians guidelines for air medical dispatch
   a. General
      1) Patients requiring critical interventions should be provided those interventions in the most expeditious manner possible

2) Patients who are stable should be transported in a manner that best addresses the needs of the patient and the system
3) Patients with critical injuries or illnesses resulting in unstable vital signs require transport by the fastest available modality, and with a transport team that has the appropriate level of care capabilities, to a center capable of providing definitive care
4) Patients with critical injuries or illnesses should be transported by a team that can provide intratransport critical care services
5) Patients who require high-level care during transport, but who do not have time-critical illnesses or injuries, may be candidates for ground critical care transport (i.e., by a specialized ground critical care transport vehicle with level of care exceeding that of local EMS) if such service is available and logistically feasible
   b. Logistical
      1) Access
      2) Time/distance factors
      3) Specialized care needed in transport
      4) Specialized equipment needed in transport
      5) Weather
      6) Terrain/road conditions between facilities
      7) Local ground resources

2. Level of service: patient condition and treatment needs en route must determine the level of service
   a. Scope of practice for each level of service varies among states, regions, and counties within the states
   b. Basic Life Support (BLS): the provision of BLS services by the EMT-Basic
      1) Oxygen
      2) Monitoring of vital signs
      3) Maintenance of a saline lock
      4) Patient administered/monitored indwelling devices
      5) Basic emergency medical care
   c. Advanced Life Support (ALS): the provision of an assessment by an ALS provider and/or the provision of one or more ALS interventions
      1) A procedure beyond the scope of an EMT-Basic
      2) May include
         a) Manual defibrillation/cardioversion
         b) Endotracheal intubation/supraglottic airway
         c) Central venous line
         d) Cardiac pacing
         e) Chest decompression
         f) Surgical airway
         g) Intraosseous line
         h) Medication administration
   d. Other common levels of providers include Intermediate Life Support (ILS) and those with additional privileges and responsibilities
   e. SCT

1) Required when patient's condition requires ongoing care that must be furnished by one or more health professionals in an appropriate specialty area
2) Invasive monitoring, balloon pump, left ventricular assist device, transvenous pacing, specialized patient populations

3. Transport team personnel: crew members should possess skills and knowledge appropriate to the level of care that patient requires during transport
   a. Must be qualified to continue advanced level of assessment and intervention initiated at referring facility
   b. Must be qualified to perform additional advanced interventions as needed during transport
   c. Team member options
      1) Physician
      2) Emergency nurse
      3) Flight nurse
      4) Adult/pediatric/neonatal intensive care/obstetrics nurse
      5) Respiratory therapist
      6) Paramedic (critical care paramedic)
      7) EMT
      8) Others to assist, as needed
4. Equipment
   a. Anticipate necessary supplies, including medications, to address the need of patients during transport
   b. Generally, ALS ambulance will have adequate airway equipment, medications, and dressings
   c. Specialized equipment and medications (beyond the basics used to provide routine EMS) must be provided by the sending facility
5. Documentation
   a. Elements of transfer form
      1) Patient condition
         a) Risks of transfer are outweighed by the anticipated benefits of transfer
         b) Record of vital signs at the time of departure
      2) Reason for transfer
         a) Medical necessity: sending facility does not have the capacity and/or capability to provide necessary treatment
         b) Patient requested
      3) Hospital acceptance
         a) Name of destination facility
         b) Name of person at receiving facility authorizing transfer
         c) Name of accepting physician
      4) Transfer risks
      5) Transfer benefits
      6) Transport mode
      7) Patient consent
   b. Elements of transfer checklist
      1) Certification of transfer completed

2) Patient identification: arm band
3) Prehospital care record
4) Initial facility record
5) Radiographs and other studies
6) Valuables: location and list of items
7) Transfer records
   a) Patient demographic data, including next of kin
   b) History of illness/mechanism of injury
   c) Patient condition on admission
   d) Diagnostic impressions
   e) Results of diagnostic studies
      (1) Include original or copies of diagnostic radiographs; if possible (do not delay transport if films are not readily available)
   f) Treatments rendered, including medications administered
   g) Status of patient at time of transfer
   h) Transfer orders
   i) Name and telephone number of referring physician
   j) Receiving physician and facility
c. Elements of the transfer record
   1) National Emergency Medical Services Information System (NEMSIS), National Highway Traffic Safety Administration (NHTSA) most current dataset version for EMS
   2) Facility based
      a) Patient demographics
      b) Vital signs
      c) Care provided
         (1) Treatment
         (2) Response
      d) Pertinent observations during transport
      e) Name/title/signature of personnel
      f) Patient status
         (1) On departure from sending facility
         (2) On arrival receiving facility

C. ADMINISTRATIVE CONSIDERATIONS

1. Certificate of Medical Necessity (for ambulance transfer)
   a. Does not pertain to emergency transfers as long as patients meet transfer criteria under 42 CFR § 1395dd (EMTALA): "Examination and treatment for emergency medical conditions and women in labor"
   b. Reason for transfer must be medically necessary and reasonable (e.g., the sending hospital does not have the capacity and/or capability necessary to care for the patient)
   c. Air ambulance services may be provided by either a fixed wing (airplane) or rotary wing (helicopter) aircraft only when patient's medical

condition requires immediate and rapid ambulance transportation that cannot be provided by ground ambulance

2. Transfer agreements
   a. Formalized between referring and receiving facilities
   b. Developed cooperatively
   c. Include transport service

3. Useful transfer policies and procedures to consider
   a. Patients to be transferred
   b. Medical and administrative authority regarding transfers (i.e., who decides) should be addressed by sending and receiving facilities
   c. Most appropriate facility for specific needs: not closest facility
   d. How to determine appropriate mode of transport
   e. How to determine personnel and equipment to accompany patient
   f. Protocols or standing orders for transport personnel
   g. How to arrange transfer and transportation
   h. How family and friends are to be included in transfer
   i. Forms used before, during, and after transfer
   j. Records to be sent with patient
   k. Documentation during transport
   l. Special circumstances: vehicle breakdown, long detours, patient deterioration, death

D. CLINICAL CONSIDERATIONS

1. Stabilization and preparation for transport within capabilities of staff and facilities
   a. Patent airway support with simultaneous cervical spine (C-spine) protection
      1) Positioning
      2) Artificial/advanced airway management
         a) Oropharyngeal-nasopharyngeal
         b) Endotracheal tube (ETT)
         c) Supraglottic airway (e.g., King, Combitube, laryngeal mask airway)
      3) Suction
      4) Stomach decompression with nasogastric or orogastric tube, unless contraindicated
   b. Breathing support and pressure support
      1) Positioning
      2) Bag-mask ventilation, as needed
      3) Supplemental oxygen
      4) Mechanical ventilation, as needed
      5) Decompression of pneumothorax or hemothorax
         a) Needle thoracostomy
         b) Chest tube insertion (Heimlich valve may be used to prevent reexpansion of pneumothorax with inadvertent disconnection of water-seal drainage set)
   c. Circulatory support
      1) Control external bleeding
      2) IV access, two sites preferred
         a) Large-caliber catheters to support volume replacement needs
      3) Fluid replacement with crystalloid fluids and/or blood products
         a) Pack blood products in ice for transport, and monitor time outside of blood bank (recommend use of blood within 1 hour)
      4) Monitor cardiac rhythm
      5) Indwelling catheter to monitor urinary output: drain urinary collection bag before transport
   d. Ongoing clinical management
      1) Maintenance of clinical care for specific patient conditions (i.e., stroke, myocardial infarction, sepsis)
      2) Maintenance of interventions/treatments (i.e., hypothermia protocols)
      3) Maintenance of pharmacologic regimens (i.e., hemodynamic support, antiarrhythmics, neuromuscular blocking agents, sedation, antibiotics)
   e. Spine precautions
      1) Long backboard with straps
      2) Special immobilization of head and neck
         a) C-spine immobilization/motion restriction device
         b) Towel rolls and tape or lateral immobilization/motion restriction device
         c) Cervical traction devices
            (1) Use with caution: acceleration and deceleration forces during transport tend to swing free-hanging weights, thus altering tension of traction and possibly injuring occupants in vehicle; locking pulley systems are preferred
            (2) Rotational stability of neck should be controlled even if long traction is applied; may be done by placing towel rolls or stabilization devices along each side of head and neck and securing to stretcher with tape
   f. Splinting of injured extremities
      1) Flexible, vacuum, padded board splints
      2) Plaster: casts should not be circumferential unless bivalved before fixed-wing transport
      3) Traction: devices may be large and bulky; anticipate problems in transport vehicles with limited working space
      4) Preserve access to distal pulse for monitoring
      5) Use air splints with caution; contraindicated for air transport secondary to gas expansion
   g. Wound care
      1) Critical life-threatening problems have priority for care
      2) Control bleeding (patient transfer should not be delayed for suturing unless hemostasis is essential)

3) Limited initial cleansing
4) Sterile dressing
5) Tetanus prophylaxis and antibiotics, when indicated
6) Burn wounds
   a) No topical ointment or ice applied before transfer
   b) Follow local burn center protocols
   c) Prevent hypothermia: cover patient with warm blankets, apply heat packs and warming lights as needed
h. Psychosocial responses of patient
   1) Fear, anxiety, anger, grief
   2) Continuously provide patient (and family) with information
      a) What happened: details of accident or illness
      b) What is currently happening: step-by-step description of events
      c) What to expect next: plans for treatment and procedures
   3) Interpret sounds, voices, and procedures for patient as needed
   4) Allow patient to see family and significant others
i. Baseline diagnostic studies
   1) Imaging studies
      a) Chest: repeat chest radiograph for ETT placement, if indicated
      b) C-spine: ensure visualization of seven cervical vertebrae before transport
      c) Pelvis
      d) Suspicious extremities
      e) CT scans
      f) Other, as indicated
   2) Laboratory studies
      a) Hemoglobin (Hgb)
      b) Hematocrit (Hct)
      c) Serum chemistries
      d) Arterial blood gases (ABGs)
      e) Urinalysis (UA)
      f) Urine (UCG), or serum chorionic gonadotropin as indicated
      g) Serum, breath, or saliva ethanol (ETOH) levels
      h) Serum and urine toxicology screen
   3) ECG
2. Protocols for treatment and transport
   a. Unless standardized regional or transport service protocols are in place, written orders must be provided by the transferring physician (consultation with receiving physician is recommended for specialized care)
   b. EMS providers should not be expected to accept patient transfers who require care exceeding their scope of practice, education, experience, and certification/licensure, although patient's needs may be satisfied by using accompanying personnel from the transferring facility to maintain a comparable level of care during transfer
   c. Each treatment and skill provided by any practitioner must be within the practitioner's scope of practice and should include the following, at a minimum
      1) Medication names, concentrations, and rates of administration
         a) Analgesia, sedation, neuromuscular blockade
            (1) Orders should contain a dosage range with a fixed time interval
            (2) Open-ended orders (e.g., "titrate for ____") are not recommended
         b) Vasoactive
            (1) Pressors
            (2) Rate and/or rhythm maintenance
         c) Other
      2) Respiratory/ventilation mode (as applicable)
         a) Oxygen settings
         b) Rate settings
         c) Volume settings
         d) Pressure settings
            (1) Positive end-expiratory pressure (PEEP)
            (2) Continuous positive airway pressure (CPAP)
            (3) Bilevel positive airway pressure (BiPAP)
      3) Circulatory
         a) Crystalloid fluids
            (1) Solution
            (2) Rate
            (3) Replacement of fluid losses (gastric, urinary, blood, burn wounds)
         b) Blood products
         c) Volume expanders
      4) Monitoring
      5) Immobilization
      6) Restraints
      7) Drains/tubes
         a) Device
            (1) Gravity
            (2) Suction/pressure
      8) Special patient care needs (if applicable)
3. Communications
   a. Before transport
      1) Referring physician to receiving physician
         a) Patient identification
         b) History of incident
         c) Initial findings, procedures, treatments
         d) Estimated time of departure and arrival
      2) Primary nurse to receiving charge or primary nurse
      3) Referring facility administrator to receiving facility administrator, as needed
      4) Referring and/or receiving physician to transferring personnel
         a) Airway and ventilatory maintenance

b) Volume replacement and management
c) Special procedures
d) Transfer orders
b. During transport
1) Contact from vehicle or aircraft to sending and/or receiving facility
2) Third-party relay contact if direct contact is not possible
3) Standing/transfer orders for treatment/interventions during transport
c. After transport
1) Follow-up report from transport team to referring physician
2) Follow-up report from receiving physician, nurse, facility to referring facility
3) Combined medical audits to identify deficits in care
4) Educational resources to remove deficits in care
5) Interfacility-interdisciplinary conference to redesign system or problem solve
6) Ongoing monitoring process to evaluate effectiveness of system
4. Nursing care required during transport
a. Age and developmental differences may require varying assessment and intervention skills
1) Pediatric population
a) Security comes from parents: allow parents to stay with patient when possible
b) If parents not allowed to ride in transport vehicle, allow them to explain their travel arrangements and plans to patient
c) Allow child to carry a toy during transport
d) Speak clearly and slowly: children may become anxious and fearful from loud and excited movements and voices
e) Be honest in providing explanations of care; explain every procedure step by step
f) Reassure child that you are there to help, not hurt
g) Respect feelings of modesty, especially with school-aged children and adolescents
2) Older adult population
a) Consider deterioration of senses: vision, hearing, touch, and thermoregulation
(1) Provide direct eye contact in clear line of vision
(2) Speak loudly, clearly, and slowly; phrase questions simply, avoid medical jargon
(3) Touch patient gently but firmly to reinforce verbal communication
(4) Older adults experience poor tolerance to cold; prevent hypothermia
b) Information and sensory overload, short-term memory losses, and delay in information processing may contribute to acute confusion

c) Underlying medical problems may affect responses to treatment
b. Assessment
1) Noise and vibration levels require extensive use of sight and touch
2) Airway and breathing: observe and feel quality and symmetry of chest wall expansion, use portable pulse oximeter to monitor oxygen saturation and end-tidal carbon dioxide to monitor ventilation and perfusion of lungs
3) Circulation: palpate pulses, determine blood pressure, observe skin moisture, observe color, use Doppler techniques to assess pulse quality and blood pressure
4) Portable electronic monitoring of heart rate and rhythm
5) Direct observation of urine output: volume and color
6) Stimulation of patient and observation of response in relation to level of consciousness
c. Interventions
1) Provide for safety of transport crew members, patient, and riders by securing transport equipment, using safety straps, and hearing protection
2) Maintain airway and ventilatory support with supplemental oxygen, bag-mask, or mechanical ventilation
3) Maintain cardiac output with volume replacement
4) Administer medications or procedures as indicated by established protocols or as ordered by referring physician
5) Maintain normothermic body temperature with warm environment, blankets, and warmed fluids
6) Maintain control in coordinating movement of patient into and out of facilities and transport vehicle
7) Institute measures to prevent problems in transport
d. Evaluation
1) Monitor patient responses for signs of improvement or deterioration
e. Documentation
1) Maintain accurate records of transport events; document responses to transport stressors
5. Arrival at receiving facility
a. Accompany patient into facility and provide interventions as needed
b. Provide receiving team with verbal report and documentation listed previously
c. Maintain close interactions with patient
d. Speak to family or friends if they have arrived
e. Notify referring facility and patient's family (as appropriate) of safe arrival of patient at receiving facility

Part 4

f. Collect equipment used for transport

g. Close interactions with receiving facility staff

6. Family members and friends

a. Crisis intervention: involve chaplain, social worker, and psychiatric personnel in care when possible

b. Need explanation of condition and reason for transfer

c. Obtain consent for transfer as necessary

d. Not responsible for arranging emergency transfer

e. Remain at sending facility until patient leaves

f. Need opportunity for brief interaction with patient before departure

g. Maps and written directions to receiving facility and parking area are helpful, reminding them not to follow the ambulance too closely

h. Explain the use of lights and sirens used during transport if necessary. Explain that it does not mean that their loved one is decompensating during transport

i. Family members who accompany patient in transport must be oriented to transport vehicle, safety procedures, and so forth; family members must be instructed as to what they can and cannot do during transport in regard to patient management

j. For safety reasons, family members who accompany patient in transport should be seated in the passenger seat at the front of the ambulance next to the driver unless their presence in the patient care area is needed to facilitate care (e.g., language interpretation, child comfort care)

E. INTERFACILITY TRIAGE CRITERIA

1. Trauma categories

a. *Resources for Optimal Care of the Injured Patient*: American College of Surgeons Committee on Trauma

1) Physiologic considerations

a) Glasgow coma scale ≤13

b) Systolic blood pressure <90 mm Hg

c) Respiratory rate <10 or >29 breaths per minute or need for ventilator support (<20 in infant younger than 1 year)

2) Anatomy of injury

a) All penetrating injuries to head, neck, torso, and extremities proximal to elbow or knee

b) Chest wall instability or deformity (i.e., flail chest)

c) Two or more proximal long bone fractures

d) Crushed, degloved, mangled, or pulseless extremity

e) Amputation proximal to wrist or ankle

f) Pelvic fractures

g) Open or depressed skull fracture

h) Paralysis

3) Mechanism of injury

a) Falls

(1) Adults >20 feet (one story is equal to 20 feet)

(2) Children >10 feet or two or three times the height of the child

b) High-risk auto crash

(1) Intrusion, including roof: >12 inches occupant site; >18 inches any site

(2) Ejection (partial or complete) from automobile

(3) Death in same passenger compartment

(4) Vehicle with telemetry data consistent with a high-risk injury

c) Auto vs. pedestrian/bicyclist thrown, run over, or with significant (>20 mph) impact

d) Motorcycle crash >20 mph

4) Special patient or system considerations

a) Older adults

(1) Risk of injury/death increases after age 55 years

(2) SBP <110 may represent shock after age 65

(3) Low impact mechanism (i.e., ground level falls) may result in severe injury

b) Children

(1) Should be triaged preferentially to pediatric capable trauma centers

c) Anticoagulants and bleeding disorders

(1) Patients with head injury are at high risk for rapid deterioration

d) Burns

(1) Without trauma mechanism: triage to burn facility

(2) With trauma mechanism: triage to trauma center

e) Pregnancy >20 weeks

f) EMS provider judgement

2. Nontrauma categories: based on a match between

a. Patient's care requirements

b. Facility's ability to provide care

c. Local/regional or state protocols

d. May include psychiatric, pediatric, geriatric, neurologic, cardiac, neonatal, spinal cord, burn cases, obstetric, or others in which patients require specialized care centers

III. National Standards Related to Transport

A. NATIONAL EMERGENCY MEDICAL SERVICES EDUCATION AGENDA

The National EMS Education Agenda is a vision for the future of EMS education and a proposal for an improved structured system to educate the next generation of EMS professionals. The Education Agenda builds on broad concepts from the 1996 EMS Agenda for the Future to create a vision for an education system, similar to those of other health professions that will result in improved efficiency for the national EMS education process. The proposed system maximizes consistency of instruction quality and student competence by prescribing a high degree of structure, coordination, and interdependence among the five components. Under the auspices of the National Highway Traffic Safety Administration, the EMS Education Agenda will serve to define the qualities, skills, and knowledge among EMS professionals that will inevitably be critical in the realm of patient transport for years to come.

1. National EMS Core Content
   a. Identifies complete domain of knowledge and skills: comprehensive list of knowledge and skills needed for out-of-hospital emergency care
2. National EMS Scope of Practice
   a. Divides content into levels of practice
      1) Defines minimum knowledge and skills for each level of EMS provider
      2) Replaces the National EMS Education and Practice Blueprint
      3) Serve as a model for levels of state EMS licensing
3. National EMS Education Standards
   a. Establishes learning objectives
      1) Specifies minimum terminal learning objectives for each level of EMS practice
      2) Replaces preexisting National Standard Curricula
      3) Has minimum learning objectives for each EMS provider level
4. National EMS Training Accreditation
   a. Full coverage and universal utilization by training institutes
   b. Uses educational standards appropriate for each level
   c. Curriculum must meet national standards
   d. Program accreditation includes all nationally recognized levels of EMS instruction
   e. Enhances consistency of quality of instruction and educational outcomes at all levels of EMS education
   f. Educational institutions and other EMS instruction providers deliver instructional programming that is consistent with the National EMS education standards
5. National EMS certification
   a. Universal utilization by all levels of EMS practitioners in all states
   b. To be certified, or eligible for national EMS certification, individuals must graduate from nationally accredited programs
   c. National EMS certification is available for all levels of EMS providers
   d. National certification enhances the consistency of the quality of educational programs and thereby enhances the quality of the EMS care delivered by nationally certified graduates of accredited institutions

B. NATIONAL TRANSPORT CERTIFICATION

1. Board of Certification for Emergency Nursing
   a. Certified Flight Registered Nurse (CFRN)
   b. Certified Transport Registered Nurse (CTRN)
2. Board for Critical Care Transport Paramedic Certification
   a. Certified Flight Paramedic (FP-C)
   b. Certified Critical Care Paramedic (CCP-C)

C. ACCREDITATION AND SAFETY STANDARDS FOR AMBULANCE COMPANIES

1. Ground
   a. Commission on Accreditation of Ambulance Services
   b. Commission on Accreditation of Medical Transport Services
2. Air
   a. Commission on Accreditation of Medical Transport Services

Bibliography

Air and Surface Transport Nurses Association: *Air and surface patient transport principles and practice*, ed 4, St. Louis, MO, 2009, Mosby.

American Academy of Pediatrics: *Guidelines for air and ground transport of neonatal and pediatric patients*, ed 4, Elk Grove Village, IL, 2015, American Academy of Pediatrics.

American College of Surgeons, Committee on Trauma: *Resources for optimal care of the injured patient*, Chicago, IL, 2014, American College of Surgeons.

Commission on Accreditation of Ambulance Services: *Accreditation standards (v3.0)*, Glenview, IL, 2009, Commission on Accreditation of Ambulance Services.

Commission on Accreditation of Medical Transport Services: Accreditation standards. Retrieved from http://www.camts.org, 2006.

Department of Health and Human Services Centers for Medicare and Medicaid Services: Medicare ambulance services. Retrieved from https://www.cms.gov/Outreach-and-Education/Medicare-Learning-Network-MLN/MLNProducts/downloads/Medicare_Ambulance_Services_ICN903194.pdf, 2011.

Emergency Nurses Association: *Standards of emergency nursing practice*, ed 4, St. Louis, MO, 1999, Mosby-Year Book.

Emergency Nurses Association: *Sheehy's manual of emergency care*, ed 7, St. Louis, MO, 2012, Mosby.

National Association of EMS Physicians: Position paper: Guidelines for air medical dispatch. Retrieved from http://www.naemsp.org/Position%20Papers/AirMedical Dispatch.pdf, 2003.

National Highway Traffic Safety Administration: National EMS education agenda. Retrieved from http://www.nhtsa.dot.gov/people/injury/ems/EdAgenda/final, 2000.

National Highway Traffic Safety Administration: National EMS core content. Retrieved from http://www.nhtsa.dot.gov/people/injury/ems/EMSCoreContent/index.htm, 2005.

National Highway Traffic Safety Administration: *Guide for interfacility patient transfer*, Washington, DC, 2006, National Highway Traffic Safety Administration.

National Highway Traffic Safety Administration: *National EMS scope of practice*. Washington, DC, 2007, National Highway Traffic Safety Administration.

Newberry, LN, editor: *Sheehy's emergency nursing principles and practice*. ed 5, St. Louis, MO,, 2013, Mosby Elsevier and Emergency Nurses Association.

Society for Critical Care Medicine: Guidelines for the inter- and intra-hospital transport of critically ill patients. Retrieved from http://www.learnicu.org/Docs/Guidelines/Inter-IntrahospitalTransport.pdf, 2004.

CHAPTER 44

Forensic Aspects of Emergency Nursing

Joyce Foresman-Capuzzi, MSN, APRN, RN-BC, CCNS, CEN,
CPN, CTRN, CCRN, CPEN, AFN-BC, SANE-A, EMT-P, FAEN

The term *forensic* confers a relationship with the legal system; it is derived from the Latin word *forensis*, meaning "public." The nurse who will work in the emergency department (ED) takes care of patients who fall into the "FORENSIC" category, sometimes on a daily basis. With the rise in incidence of trauma and violence, ED nurses are in the special position to identify, evaluate, and treat such patients; and at the same time collect and preserve evidence. Forensic evidence collection is a core competency of the ED nurse, which is supported by a position statement on Forensic Evidence Collection. It remains incumbent on ED nurses to remember that even though they are an integral member of the multidisciplinary team that may include law enforcement agencies and the court system, the nursing process of assessment, planning, intervention, and evaluation continues to be priority. Having an unbiased approach as an advocate for truth and justice, all the while providing holistic care to the patient, is foundational. The nurse is ethically bound to advocate for any patient, regardless of whether the patient is a victim or an offender.[1]

I. General Overview

A. DEFINITIONS

1. Evidence
   a. Data presented to a jury to prove or disprove a claim
   b. It can be physical or informational
      1) Physical is real and tangible and can be measured, visualized, or analyzed
      2) It can also be trace physical evidence, only seen microscopically
      3) Informational evidence is history, excited utterances, or something observed such as odor or appearance[1]
2. Locard principle
   a. An exchange or transference of evidence when two items come in contact with each other
   b. This transference of physical evidence is valuable to law enforcement to link a suspect or location to a victim and vice versa, because every contact leaves some type of evidence[1]
3. Chain of custody

a. A paper trail necessary to ensure that no tampering of evidence occurs; this paper trail is created by documenting the possession of the evidence from the moment of collection until the moment it is introduced in court and everywhere in between[1]

B. CLINICAL FORENSIC ISSUES

1. Evidence collection and preservation is an ED nursing competency
2. Care of the forensic patient always involves the nursing process in addition to any forensic nursing competencies
3. Early identification of a forensic patient is necessary
4. All trauma patients should also be categorized as forensic patients
5. Trauma and violence spans a multitude of presentations in adult and pediatric patients
   a. Include but are not limited to motor vehicle collisions (MVC), accidents, falls, assault or crimes, unidentified patients, VIPs, faulty equipment, bioterrorist acts, mass disasters, motor vehicle crashes, missile injuries, burns, workplace violence, elder abuse, child maltreatment, self-directed violence, sexual assault, pediatric patients, and domestic or intimate partner violence (IPV)
6. Resultant patient outcomes range from emotional devastation to morbidity and mortality
7. Culture, language, religion, race, values, sexual orientation, gender, immigration status, and beliefs should be assessed to provide culturally competent care[2]

C. EMERGENCY NURSING RESPONSIBILITIES

1. First is to ensure a safe environment for the patient and personnel
   a. The nature of forensic cases and patients lends itself to being on high alert for violence to extend into the work/care setting
   b. An injured nurse cannot provide care
   c. Follow institutional polices
      1) Use fictitious name for patient, if necessary
      2) Notify or involve police/security
2. Once safety is ensured, next priority is directed toward lifesaving interventions
   a. Lifesaving interventions should never be delayed or compromised in order to collect or preserve forensic evidence
3. Working knowledge of legalities, reporting mandates, and patient information dissemination for jurisdiction of practice must be understood (see Chapter 45)
4. Identify the need for forensic evidence collection and preservation
5. Initiate and maintain legal records and documentation
6. Collect and preserve forensic evidence according to local, state, and federal requirements as part of emergency nursing practice

II. Assessment

A. DOCUMENTATION

1. Record statements in patient's own words, using quotation marks
2. Patient's statements can be admissible in court
3. Do NOT analyze or judge, but simply record facts and statements
4. Statements are NOT interpreted, medicalized, or sanitized

B. COMPREHENSIVE ASSESSMENT (SEE CHAPTERS 1 AND 32)

C. FOCUSED ASSESSMENT

1. Subjective data collection
   a. Chief complaint
      1) Quote the patient's own words
   b. History of present injury (HPI)
      1) Complete, clear, and concise accounting of the event including mechanism of injury and time of injury
      2) Patient's reflection as to what occurred during the commission of the crime
      3) Be alert for what is both said and unsaid
      4) What needs to be collected as evidence is often determined by a good history of the event
   c. Past medical history
      1) Current or preexisting comorbidities including medical and psychiatric
      2) Surgical history
      3) Substance and/or alcohol use/abuse and if positive, last time used
      4) Last normal menstrual period: female patients or transgender male (with remaining ovaries and uterus) of childbearing age
      5) Current medications
         a) Prescription
         b) OTC
         c) Herbals
         d) Birth control (if applicable)
      6) Allergies to medications and foods include reaction
      7) Immunization status including tetanus
2. Objective data collection
   a. Overall general appearance
      1) Nonjudgmental
      2) Include only accurate statements
      3) Orientation of clothing, missing clothing, or shoes on the wrong feet
         a) Could indicate that someone else dressed the patient
         b) Consider drug-facilitated assault
         c) Can help determine speed of car if patient was struck
            (1) Shoes can be knocked off a patient struck by a car going 35 mph

(2) Where injury occurred on the body such as lower leg, upper leg, or pelvis

b. Level of consciousness
1) Range from alert to comatose
2) Orientation to person, place, time, and event

c. Behavioral
1) Such as aggressive, scared, crying, fearful, laughing, calm, giddy, nervous, pacing
2) Preoccupation with a particular item, person, or situation
   a) Repeatedly asks questions about item, person(s), or situation

d. Vital signs with trending
1) Cardiac monitoring
2) Blood pressure
3) Respiratory
4) Pulse oximetry and/or ET CO_2 monitoring (if necessary)
5) Point of care testing, including glucose (if necessary)

e. Odors
1) Petroleum, burning wood, chemical, alcohol, drug, vomit/urine, etc.
2) Hazardous materials' odor such as bitter almonds (cyanide) or new mown hay (phosgene)

f. Gait

g. Pain level

h. Inspection
1) Obvious injury/deformity with interventions as needed
2) Skin color

i. Palpation
1) Skin temperature
2) Areas of tenderness/deformity, percussion

j. Auscultation
1) Breath sounds
2) Heart sounds
3) Bowel sounds

D. PLANNING AND IMPLEMENTATION/ INTERVENTIONS

1. Maintain airway, breathing, circulation (see Chapters 1 and 32)
2. Provide supplemental oxygen as indicated
3. Establish intravenous (IV) or intraosseous (IO) access for administration of crystalloid fluids/blood products/medications
4. Obtain and set up equipment and supplies
5. Prepare for/assist with medical interventions
6. Administer pharmacologic therapy as ordered or per protocol

E. EVALUATION AND ONGOING MONITORING

1. Patient safety
2. Continuously monitor and treat as indicated

3. Monitor patient response/outcomes, and modify nursing care plan as appropriate
4. If positive patient outcomes are not demonstrated, reevaluate assessment and/or plan of care
5. Pain assessment and intervention

F. ANALYSIS (DIFFERENTIAL NURSING DIAGNOSES/COLLABORATIVE PROBLEMS)

1. Risk for injury
2. Risk for ineffective coping
3. Risk for impaired skin integrity
4. Anxiety/fear
5. Pain
6. Risk for bleeding
7. Risk for ineffective respiratory pattern
8. Risk for shock/ineffective tissue perfusion

III. Physical Forensic Evidence

A. NECESSITY OF COLLECTION AND PRESERVATION

A combination of the importance and value of physical evidence in criminal and civil investigations and the continuing advance of the applications of science and technology has caused the role of physical evidence to grow to unprecedented levels within the legal arena. Collecting and maintaining uncontaminated forensic evidence is of paramount importance. Although most crime laboratories follow the Federal Bureau of Investigations (FBI) crime laboratory standards of evidence collection, labeling, and/or packaging, there may be some local or state differences. Consult institution protocols, as well as law enforcement officers, who can provide specific regional and local policies. The use of an evidence collection kit will aid the nurse in the collection and preservation of physical evidence, and may be easily moved to other departments, such as the operating room (OR), should the patient need to be relocated (Table 44.1).

B. BASICS OF GENERAL PHYSICAL EVIDENCE COLLECTION

1. Place patient into clean room to limit cross-contamination from previous patient
2. Collect and preserve all evidence separately and individually
3. Maintain running inventory list of items collected
4. Use personal protective equipment (PPE)
   a. Handle all evidence with gloved hands (preferably powder free) and change after each piece of evidence is collected
   b. Wear protective gown and hair covering to avoid contamination of evidence
5. Collect items in only paper bags to limit static electricity and mold growth of biologic material

Table 44.1

Evidence Collection Kit

Part One: Supplies
- Plastic box with lid
- Plain white 8.5 × 11 inch paper
- Roll of newsprint (ends of rolls often can be obtained free of charge from newspaper publishers)
- Brown paper bags (large, medium, and lunchsize)
- Coin envelopes
- Envelopes of various sizes
- Sealed specimen containers
- Sterile cotton-tip applicator swabs
- Styrofoam cups
- Glass slides and blood tubes
- Labels, labels, and more labels
- Adhesive tape
- Tamper tape
- Permanent black marker
- Small bottles of sterile water
- Cardboard boxes of various sizes (optional)
- Empty dry sterile water bottle (optional)
- Red biohazard bag (all paper bags are placed in this bag for transport during handoff)
- Rubber-tipped tweezers and forceps

Part Two: Notebook
- Hospital policy and procedure on evidence collection
- Phone numbers
  - Local and state law enforcement
  - Multidisciplinary agencies (e.g., district attorney, FBI, child abuse, domestic abuse, services for aging, flight programs, ground transport, fire departments, poison control, game and wildlife, emergency preparedness resource, hazardous materials team, fire departments, animal control, and emergency dispatch)
  - Hospital resources (e.g., pagers and direct numbers for the department director, supervisor, medical director, radiation officer, emergency preparedness officer, security, and sexual assault nurse examiner, if applicable)
  - Hotline numbers for advocate groups
  - Organ procurement organizations
- Forms and resources
  - Photography consents
  - Chain of custody forms
  - Blank body diagrams
- Hints and reminders on evidence collection and for postmortem care

a. Only place one item of evidence into individual bags
b. Label as described and seal with evidence tamper tape

6. All pieces of physical evidence collected separately and should be placed individually into bag, envelope, or container, then sealed and labeled
   a. Have plenty of patient demographic labels on hand to assist in this process
   b. Patient name and ID
   c. Name of collector
   d. Date and time collected
   e. Site of collection

f. Seal items used to preserve evidence with the above information, using label and evidence tamper-proof tape
g. Collector's signature should be written across seal
h. Never lick envelope adhesive or use staples to seal

7. Collect and preserve bedsheet from EMS stretcher and label and document as such
8. Do not toss clothing or other items from patient onto floor
   a. If unable to immediately bag items, place on counter on which a sheet has been placed
   b. Place sheet between each clothing item to prevent cross-contamination
   c. Do not shake out, wash off, or ball up clothing, to avoid losing trace evidence or distorting any blood or body fluid pattern
9. Do not throw anything away (receipts, stickers, soil, leaves, insects, etc.)
   a. Label all items, and if item is unknown, label as "debris" on inventory list
10. Do not have patient use or delete any information on cell phone
11. Attempt to dry all collected items per policy and if not feasible, let law enforcement know that items may be wet
12. Refrain if possible from IV insertion in hand(s) of suspected shooter
13. Draw extra blood tubes before medication, blood, or IV fluid is administered
14. Do not give any personal items to friends or family without checking with law enforcement
15. Do not cut through any holes, stains, blood spatter, or other defects in patient's clothing
16. Look for small evidence collected onto paper
    a. Make a paper bindle (Fig. 44.1)

C. PATIENT CLOTHING AND ITEMS (BOX 44.1)

1. Collect and preserve shoes from patient as soon as possible
   a. Package each separately
   b. Material collects in grooves and linked to scene
   c. Footwear patterns or prints
2. Package each clothing item separately
3. Avoid excessive handling of clothing
4. Do not shake out or ball up clothing
5. Change gloves after each item is collected
6. Collect and preserve jewelry, especially rings as they can contain DNA from perpetrator

D. BULLETS/GUNSHOT WOUNDS

1. Cover victim's hands with paper bags for anyone involved in a shooting
2. Minimize handling of bullet to prevent loss of evidence on bullet
3. Avoid using metal forceps, if possible, to remove bullet

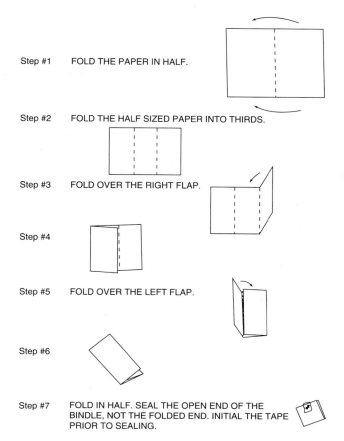

Step #1   FOLD THE PAPER IN HALF.

Step #2   FOLD THE HALF SIZED PAPER INTO THIRDS.

Step #3   FOLD OVER THE RIGHT FLAP.

Step #4

Step #5   FOLD OVER THE LEFT FLAP.

Step #6

Step #7   FOLD IN HALF. SEAL THE OPEN END OF THE
           BINDLE, NOT THE FOLDED END. INITIAL THE TAPE
           PRIOR TO SEALING.

FIG. 44.1 Make a paper bindle. (*From Lynch, VA, Duval JB.* Forensic nursing science, *ed 2, 2011. St. Louis, MO: Elsevier/Mosby.*)

Box 44.1

Clothing Preservation for Forensic Evidence

Place clean sheet or table paper on floor to act as a barrier (out of traffic flow).

Place a second sheet or layer of table paper on top of the barrier.

Place each clothing item at a separate location on the sheet/paper.

Do not put clothing items in a pile.

Maintain and package any prehospital linen used for patient.

When Patient Stabilization Permits

Label each clothing item, with patient name and collector's initials, and carefully avoid any rip, stain, or affected area.

Place each clothing item in an individual clean paper bag.

Fold and place the top sheet/table paper in a separate paper bag.

Double-fold edge of paper bag.

Apply tape from one end of the fold all the way across to the other end to provide a complete seal (never use staples).

Write collector's initials across tape onto bag to provide tamper-resistant seal.

Complete and attach chain of custody label.

Special Situations

If stains are present, place clean paper over the stains prior to folding, to avoid cross-contamination

If any items are wet, leave the paper bag open to continue to air dry until given to law enforcement

Identify paper bag as wet and notify law enforcement of situation

---

  a. Forceps teeth may damage bullet exterior
  b. If metal forceps must be used, use rubber tipped
4. Place bullet inside cup or envelope lined with gauze
  a. Only one bullet per container
  b. Fragments of same bullet may be placed in single container
  c. Seal as previously discussed, identifying where bullet was located and place signature across seal

5. Make no markings on retrieved bullet
6. Surrounding gunpowder or bullet wipe
  a. If asked by law enforcement and prior to placing paper bags around the hands of patient, obtain photographs of wound and surrounding gunpowder
7. Gunpowder may be removed with tape; place tape on glass slide, label it and place the slide into an envelope and label the envelope

8. Do not refer, document, or label wound as an "entrance" or "exit" wound
   a. For example, describe as "2 mm and oval"

E. BASIC COLLECTION RANDOM HAIR, DEBRIS AND FIBERS BY PICKING, LIFTING, SCRAPING, COMBING, OR CLIPPING

1. Do not discount anything as too small or unimportant
2. Collect hair, paint, glass, plastic, dirt, vegetation, rug or clothing fibers, fingernails, dirt, insects, or unknown "debris," with rubber-tipped forceps and place in bindle. Label and seal as previously described (see Fig. 44.1)
3. A lint roller, piece of tape, or edge of a "sticky note" can also be used to collect and preserve this material; then label and seal

F. BODY FLUIDS/SKIN CELLS OR DEBRIS

1. Any wet items, large or small, should be air dried prior to preserving
2. Air dry prior to placing in envelope
   a. Air drying of cotton-tipped applicators can be done by inverting a Styrofoam cup and push applicator(s) through bottom or top
   b. If drying more than one applicator, label each with location from where retrieved to avoid confusion
3. Examine victim's skin using high-intensity lamp or Wood's lamp
   a. Body fluids may fluoresce, leading to area for evidence collection
4. If area is wet, use cotton-tipped applicator to remove fluid
5. If area is dry, obtain evidence by moistening cotton-tipped applicator or gauze with sterile water and swab over area
6. Scrape or swab under each fingernail with orange-type stick
   a. Allow evidence to fall onto clean paper separately labeled "right hand" and "left hand"
   b. Make paper bindle
   c. Clip broken fingernails and place on separate piece of paper
7. If poisoning is suspected, consider how toxin could have entered body
   a. If patient vomits, collect and preserve vomitus
   b. An empty sterile water bottle works as a good container for this
   c. Seal and label as described

G. BITES

1. Human bites often oval or circular; animal may be oblong with deep wounds
2. If dressing exists on wound, collect and label as such, for DNA of biter may be present
3. If possible, do not clean until a swab of the wound has been collected and preserved using a cotton-tipped swab

4. If wound is wet, dry cotton-tipped applicator before preserving
5. If wound is dry, moisten cotton-tipped applicator with sterile water and swab over area; then allow to air dry

H. PATTERN INJURIES

1. Blunt objects leave a pattern of causative agent on patient's body
2. Shows features of object that produced it
   a. Example: stitching of baseball, finger marks, belt buckle, tire imprint
3. Document what is seen, but do not make definitive statement as to source
   a. Instead document "baseball-like" or "tire-like"

I. BRUISES/CONTUSIONS/ ECCHYMOSIS

1. From blunt force trauma
2. Use care labeling the wound as such when documenting
   a. Can be called into question in court
3. Describe distribution of bruises
4. Do not stage bruise by color
5. Photographs are extremely helpful

J. SHARP EDGED WEAPONS (KNIFE, ICE PICK, AXE, NEEDLE, ETC.)

1. Deeper than long
2. If remaining in patient, remove in such a way so as not to destroy fingerprints
3. Do not wash or wipe off weapon after it has been removed
4. Place in rigid container and label as previously described
5. Place needle in empty glass tube, such as blood tube
6. Pattern injury may be present so document in writing, on blank body diagram and with photographs
7. Inspect posterior surfaces of forearms, palms of hands, and back of thighs for defensive injuries

K. STRANGULATION

1. Observe for ligature marks around neck or patterned injury (such as fingertips)
2. Observe for petechiae on face, lower lip, hairline, sclera, and conjunctiva
3. Patient complaints of dyspnea, sore throat, hoarseness and difficulty swallowing, weakness in arms or legs
4. Assess for loss of consciousness, incontinence, and mental status changes

L. SEXUAL ASSAULT (SEE CHAPTER 40)

M. POSTMORTEM

1. A forensic case does not negate the option for organ procurement, so check with your local or regional agency

2. Minimize handling of the body, including typical cleaning or preparation of body
3. IV/IO lines, catheters, tubes, etc. should be left in body
4. Circle venepuncture or resuscitation wounds with a permanent marker and document resuscitation wounds can be dressed
5. Leave preexisting wounds undressed
6. Check with law enforcement before allowing anyone in to view the body and never leave the body alone, even with family members
7. Give no personal items to family members without checking with law enforcement

IV. Informational Forensic Evidence

A. BASIC WRITTEN RECORD DOCUMENTATION REQUIREMENTS

1. Use same clock or watch to avoid discrepancies
2. Use institution's standard documentation for patient assessment
3. Document all injuries, including areas of pain, discoloration, minor wounds, point tenderness, redness
4. Must be accurate and precise
5. Be as descriptive as possible to give the reader the most accurate reflection of what occurred
6. Provides nurse ability to recall events years later if case goes to court
7. Seemingly random details may prove important when law enforcement looks at the big picture
8. Use quotation marks and document what patient has said verbatim and not sanitized or medicalized, even if term is slang or vulgar
9. Correct medical terminology can be placed in parenthesis
10. Do not make a summary of what was said, even if it takes extra time
11. Excited utterances
    a. Made by someone very upset during or soon after an event, and often when the person thinks he or she is about to die
    b. Use quotation marks and document time carefully
12. Do not use the term "alleged"
    a. Infers that the nurse does not believe the patient
    b. Instead use "reported" or "suspected"
13. Laboratory technicians, as well as law enforcement, will be referring to this patient record
14. Reflect size (standard measurement, millimeters, centimeters)
15. Identify specific location on the body
16. Use recognized anatomic landmarks (e.g., sternum, external ear canal)
17. Describe the injury as a "wound"
    a. Laceration is not a cut

b. Ecchymosis is not bruise/contusion
c. Strangulation is not choking
d. NEVER make assumptions such as classifying gunshot wounds by caliber or entrance or exit wounds

B. BLANK BODY DIAGRAM

1. Can be male, female, or nongender
2. Creates a visual record of an injury or from whence evidence was collected to convey location of injuries or physical evidence
3. Documentation should reflect location, size, and description of findings
4. Never depend on photographs to reconstruct diagram information

C. PHOTOGRAPHS

1. Crucial component of evidence collection
2. Considered a true and accurate representation of what was seen and treatment provided on a particular date
3. Supplemental and does not replace blank body diagram
4. Department policy to be referenced for
   a. Separate patient photograph consent
   b. Releasing photos to law enforcement using chain of custody
5. Confer with local law enforcement or district attorney regarding their preferred format (digital vs. film/prints)
   a. If printing photos, they must be high quality and a duplicate set kept for medical records
   b. If downloading digital photos, place them onto appropriate requested format, keeping a copy for the medical record
6. Obtain user-friendly camera
7. If not using digital format, do not write directly on the picture
8. Identify the photograph or digital format with the patient's name, photographer's name, and date and time photo taken
   a. A patient demographic label can be placed on the back of the picture to aid in this
9. Keep a photograph log of all photos taken
10. Standard forensic photography is three views
    a. Full picture of patient, moving in by one third toward the injury, and then the last a close-up of the injury
11. Identify body location of photograph; ruler, standardized measurement such as a coin or a colorimetric chart may be added to aid in identifying size and type of injury, but not covering wound

D. CHAIN OF CUSTODY

1. Place label on outside of each package and/or item and document the following information
   a. Patient's name or use patient's demographic hospital label
   b. Item description of what is in package

c. Name of agency taking item
d. Name of person sealing item with date and time
e. Name of person releasing item with date and time
f. Name of person receiving item with date and time

E. DOCUMENTATION IN MEDICAL RECORD

1. Make copy of chain of custody for medical record
2. List all item(s) released to law enforcement
3. Provide the name and badge number of law enforcement officer accepting evidence

References

1. Foresman-Capuzzi J: CSI and U: evidence collection and preservation in the emergency department, *Journal of Emergency Nursing* 229–236, 2014.
2. Brown KM, Muscari ME: *Quick reference to adult and older adult forensics*, New York, NY, 2010, Springer.

Bibliography

Darnell C, Michel C: *Forensic notes*, Philadelphia, PA, 2012, F.A. Davis Company.
Easter C, Muro G: An ED forensic kit, *Journal of Emergency Nursing* 21:440–444, 1995.

Emergency Nurses Association: Forensic evidence collection. Retrieved from https://www.ena.org/practice-research/Practice/Position/Pages/ForensicEvidence.aspx, 2010.
Emergency Nurses Association: Position statement on forensic evidence collection. Retrieved from http://www.ena.org/SiteCollectionDocuments/Position%20Statements/Forensic%20Evidence.pdf, 2010.
Foresman-Capuzzi J: CSI and U: evidence collection and preservation in the emergency department, *Journal of Emergency Nursing* 40(3):229–236, 2014.
Hammer R, Moynihan B, Pigliaro E: *Forensic nursing: a handbook for practice*, Burlington, MA, 2013, Jones and Bartlett.
Howard PK, Steinmann R, editors: *Sheehy's emergency nursing: Principles and practice*, ed 6, St. Louis, MO, 2010, Mosby.
International Association of Forensic Nurses: Role of the forensic nurse. Retrieved from http://iafn.org/displaycommon.cfm?an=1&subarticlenbr=137, 2006.
Lynch V: *Forensic nursing science*, ed 2, St. Louis, MO, 2011, Mosby.
Pinckard JK, Wetli C, Graham MA: Release of organs and tissues for transplantation, *American Journal of Forensic Medicine Pathology* 28(3):202–207, 2007.
Pyrek K: *Forensic nursing*, Boca Raton, FL, 2006, CRC Press.

Part 4

CHAPTER 45
Legal and Regulatory Issues

Tamara C. McConnell, RN, MSN, LNC, PHN

When determining whether general principles of law and regulatory standards have been modified for a particular state, it is necessary to refer to the applicable state law or case law for the state in question. Federal law should be consulted for federal facilities.

Published standards of regulatory agencies, established professional references, and position papers of the national Emergency Nurses Association are available to assist in the formulation of emergency department (ED) policies. Additionally, hospital legal counsel is a resource when seeking advice on the development of policies and procedures to address medical-legal issues.

I. General Overview

The health care industry is one of the most highly regulated sectors in the United States as evidenced by the vast array of laws and regulations related to health access, quality, licensing, safety, cost, and the like. Health care regulations are developed and enforced by all levels of government: federal, state, and local and also by private organizations. Each state has its own regulatory structure reflective of various public-private partnerships comprised of working professionals with technical expertise and governmental oversight agencies. Several layers of law have blended to form rules, statutes, regulations, case law, codes, and opinions that vary between states and other jurisdictions. It is incumbent upon all health care providers to understand the general principles of law related to the industry; recognize professional standards of care; and have the ability to access appropriate state or federal laws applicable to their practice setting.

A. SOURCES OF LAW

1. Constitutional law
   a. Constitutional law is derived from the United States and state constitutions and encompasses laws, principles, and amendments intended to guarantee individuals certain rights, such as privacy, speech, and equal protection
2. Statutory law
   a. Statutory law is enacted by federal, state, and local legislative bodies
   b. Health-care-related stch681atutes include the reporting of elder and child abuse and communicable diseases

3. Administrative law
   a. Administrative law is derived from administrative agencies that are under the arm of the executive branch of government and include state health departments and boards of nursing
   b. Administrative agencies promulgate rules and regulations, conduct investigations, and ensure enforcement of the practice acts
   c. In California and several other states, for example, grounds for disciplinary action against a certified or licensed nurse include:
      1) Unprofessional conduct, which includes, but is not limited to the following
         a) Incompetence or gross negligence in carrying out usual certified or licensed nursing function
      2) Procuring his or her certificate or license by fraud, misrepresentation, or mistake
      3) Conviction of a felony or any offense substantially related to the qualifications, functions, and duties of a registered nurse, in which event the record of the conviction shall be conclusive evidence thereof
      4) Impersonating another certified or licensed practitioner, or permitting or allowing another person to use his or her certificate or license for the purpose of nursing the sick or afflicted
4. Common law
   a. Common law is a body of law based on custom and general principles embodied in case law, which serves as precedent and is applied to situations not covered by statute
   b. It applies only to civil cases and is generally uncodified, meaning that there is no comprehensive compilation of legal rules and statutes
   c. The precedents, or judicial decisions, made during civil cases are found through court records and applied in decisions of new cases

B. TYPES OF LAW

1. Civil law
   a. Civil law applies to the rights of individuals or entities
   b. In general, plaintiffs pursue remedies such as money to make them *whole* again
      1) The remedies or damages may be determined by a jury following a trial
2. Criminal law
   a. Criminal law is defined as a body of rules and statutes that defines conduct prohibited by the government because it threatens and harms public safety and welfare
   b. It defines crimes and may establish punishments
   c. Health-care-related crimes committed by nurses include drug diversion, patient abuse, and sexual misconduct

3. Contract law
   a. Contract law comprises agreements between parties, individuals, and entities
   b. Three requirements for a contract include offer, acceptance, and consideration
   c. Depending upon the subject matter and reason for contract, they can be in oral or written form
   d. Health-care-related contracts include those between employee/employer and contracts with health maintenance organizations, suppliers, and facilities
4. Tort law
   a. Tort law is an area of civil law that involves three categories dependent upon the defendant's conduct: intentional torts, negligence, and strict liability
   b. A tort is a wrongful act that is committed by someone and causes injury to another's person or property
   c. Simply defined, a tort is a *wrong; injury; opposite of right*
      1) An *intentional tort* requires that the person committing the tort have the intent to commit the wrongful act
      2) Examples in the health care setting
         a) Assault: intention to cause harm to an individual without touching but with present ability to commit injury
         b) Battery: nonconsensual, physical violence, constraint, or offensive touching
         c) False imprisonment
         d) Invasion of privacy: public disclosure of person's privacy right
            (1) Strict liability most often applies to hazardous activities or product-liability cases. Liability is not dependent on actual negligence or intent to harm, rather it is based on the breach of an absolute duty to make something safe

C. NEGLIGENCE

1. Negligence is a failure to act as an ordinary prudent person or "reasonable person" under similar circumstances
2. In the context of a nurse-patient relationship, a medical malpractice claim must prove four elements of negligence
   a. A *duty* must be owed to the patient. The duty usually occurs when the nurse accepts responsibility for the care and treatment of that patient
      1) *Wilmington General Hospital v. Manlove*, 194 A.2d 135 (Del. 1961): court decision held that if a hospital has an ED, it has the duty to provide emergency care; internal hospital policies cannot be used to negate the duty owed to the community at large

2) The Hospital Survey and Construction Act, also known as the "Hill-Burton Act," Title 42, Part 124, (1946): federal law required hospitals receiving federal funds under this act to provide care to patients regardless of ability to pay

3) *Lunsford v. the Board of Nurse Examiners*, 648 SW 2d 391 (Tex. App. 3 Dist., 1983): court held that nurses have a duty to patients just as physicians owe a duty, and that duty stems from the privilege granted by the state in nurse licensure

b. There is a *breach* of duty or standard of care by the nurse. The standard of care for the nursing specialty and treatment must be established to determine if there has been an act of omission or commission that has caused damage to the patient

1) Standard of care: degree of care that a reasonable, prudent professional would exercise in the same or similar circumstances

2) Standard of care is presented in court through the use of expert witnesses and documents (e.g., the State Nurse Practice Act), institutional policies and procedures, professional standards of practice, professional position statements, statutes, regulations, and authoritative textbooks

3) Example: an IV infusion set requires a special filter to be used to prevent an air embolism, but if the nurse fails to set up the system properly by omitting the filter, a breach has occurred

c. A *proximate cause* or casual connection must be evident between the breach of duty and the harm or *damages* that occurred to the patient/plaintiff

d. *Damages* or injuries suffered by the patient/plaintiff. Damages may include but are not limited to pain and suffering; past, present, and future medical expenses; disfigurement; premature death; loss of life

3. Jury instructions are intended to provide jurors with a plain-English explanation of the law

a. An example of this is found in the Judicial Council of California Civil Injury Instructions: 504. Standard of Care for Nurses

A Registered Nurse is negligent is she fails to use the level of skill, knowledge, and care in diagnosis and treatment that other reasonably careful Registered Nurses would use in the same or similar circumstances. This level of skill, knowledge, and are is sometimes referred to as "the standard of care." You must determine the level of skill, knowledge, and care that other reasonably careful Registered Nurses would use in the same or similar circumstances, based on the testimony of the expert witness including the defendant who have testified in this case.

4. Examples of professional negligence due to breaches of duty include failure to

a. Detect signs and symptoms of bleeding, resulting in hemorrhage and death

b. Properly position the patient during procedures, resulting in a paralyzed limb

c. Check properly and administer the correct medication, resulting in death

d. Properly monitor restrained patients, resulting in asphyxia, brain damage, or death

5. All four elements of negligence were proven in *Gordon v. Wills Knighton Medical Center*, 661 So.2d 991, La (1995)

a. The court awarded $350,000 for wrongful death damages and $60,000 for the patient's pain and suffering upon finding that the patient's myocardial infarct was caused by lack of oxygen to the heart attributable to the following breaches in care

1) Upon arrival to the ED, the patient should have been classified as an "urgent cardiac patient"

2) The patient should have been immediately evaluated by a nurse and physician within 15 minutes

3) The patient should have been given oxygen. Upon transfer from EMS to hospital, the ED nurses removed the oxygen that had been placed on the patient by paramedics

6. Categories of negligence resulting in malpractice lawsuits

a. Failure to follow standards of care including failure to

1) Perform complete admission assessment

2) Adhere to standardized protocols or policies and procedures

3) Follow written or verbal physician order

b. Failure to use equipment in a responsible manner including failure to

1) Follow manufacturer's recommendations for operating equipment

2) Perform safety check of equipment prior to use

c. Failure to communicate, including failure to

1) Notify a physician in a timely manner when warranted

2) Listen to a patient's complaint and act

3) Communicate effectively with a patient

4) Seek higher medical authorization for treatment

d. Failure to document including failure to note within the medical record

1) Patient condition, progress, and response to treatment

2) Pertinent nursing assessment information such as drug allergies

3) Medical orders

4) Telephone conversations with physicians including time, content of communication, and actions taken

Part 4

5) Transfer of care to another health care professional

6) Inconsistent timing of entries and chronology of events

e. Failure to assess and monitor, including failure to
   1) Complete a shift assessment
   2) Implement a plan of care
   3) Observe a patient's ongoing progress
   4) Interpret patient signs and symptoms

f. Failure to act as a patient advocate, including failure to
   1) Question inappropriate discharge orders
   2) Question illegible or incomplete medical
   3) Provide a safe environment (i.e., patient falls)

g. Medication errors related to the rights of medication administration: Wrong patient; Wrong medication; Wrong dose; Wrong route, Wrong time; Wrong documentation; Wrong reason; Wrong response

D. OTHER LEGAL CONCEPTS

1. "But for" test
   a. Used in malpractice and negligence cases to determine whether there would have been injury or damages "but for" the defendant's actions

2. Due process
   a. Legal process that protects rights of both sides for a fair trial by an impartial judge or jury due them by constitutional right

3. Duty to follow physician's orders
   a. Negligence may be attributed to physician if nurse is following physician orders
   b. Nurse may also be held liable for following improper orders

4. Liability
   a. Lawful accountability and obligations required
   b. Defendants judged and decisions based on the issues in question

5. Res ipsa loquitor
   a. The action speaks for itself
   b. A rule of evidence where negligence may be inferred because an accident occurred (e.g., incorrect body part amputated)

6. Respondeat superior
   a. Employers have vicarious liability for negligent actions of their employees acting within the scope of their employment
   b. Hospital employer is legally liable for the acts of its staff members while they are performing work duties

7. Good Samaritan laws
   a. Enacted to encourage rendering of assistance in emergency situations outside the hospital setting without fear of liability
   b. Laws vary among states
   c. May not apply if health care professional was grossly negligent or received compensation for services provide

8. Indemnification
   a. An employer may be required to pay settlement for an employee found liable for professional negligence
   b. If so, the employer may require the employee to repay the employer for money lost (indemnification)

9. Malpractice insurance
   a. Hospitals insure nurses for malpractice within the scope of the nurse's employment for benefit of the hospital
   b. Privately available and recommended for nurses to cover costs associated with litigation of professional negligence cases and expenses of settlement or verdict in the event that hospital insurance doesn't cover actions contrary to employer policies and procedures; out-of-hospital events; other licensure representation

II. Consent

A. TYPES OF CONSENT

1. Expressed consent
   a. Voluntary consent of individual seeking medical treatment
   b. Predicated on patient's mental competency
   c. Does not waive patient's ability to sue for presumed negligence

2. Implied consent
   a. Individual in a life- or limb-threatening situation and unable to provide expressed consent
   b. Law assumes implied consent is present
   c. Attempts should be made to obtain expressed consent from family or patient

3. Involuntary consent
   a. Incompetent individual refuses to consent to needed medical treatment
   b. Often utilized by physicians, psychiatrists, or police to ensure mentally incompetent individual receives treatment
   c. If medical care required in excess of 48 hours, most states require a hearing before a judge
   d. Documentation must include psychiatric evaluation to assess mental capacity

4. Informed consent
   a. Essential components
      1) Description of procedure to be performed
      2) Alternatives available to procedure explained
      3) Risks and benefits of procedures explained
      4) Patient's understanding of risks, benefits, and alternatives
   b. Most states mandate that physicians present consent information

B. CONSENT ISSUES

1. Minors
   a. Age of consent varies among state statutes

b. Emancipated (e.g., economically independent, married) minor may be allowed to provide consent regardless of age

c. Minors are frequently able to consent to treatment in specific areas (e.g., birth control counseling, sexually transmitted disease treatment, substance abuse or alcohol rehabilitation, and female patients seeking care for pregnancy-related issues)

2. Religious conviction

a. Competent adults may refuse lifesaving care: decision should be based on complete knowledge of risks of refusal

b. Social policy may override patient's decision if decision would leave minor child without a parent

c. Courts have held that parents cannot make religious martyrs of their children

d. If patient is a minor and parents refuse medical care, it may be necessary to involve hospital administration and/or legal counsel to consider obtaining a court order to treat

3. Managed care

a. Managed care plans may control decisions regarding payment for services rendered, but these plans do not have the right to consent to or refuse treatment of a patient

b. Managed care organizations should not be contacted until a medical screening examination (MSE) and stabilization have been completed

c. After completion of an MSE and stabilization, managed care organizations can provide assistance in identifying services and follow-up care covered under the plan

4. Refusal of treatment/leaving against medical advice/elopement

a. If a patient refuses medically indicated treatment, it is essential that a determination be made regarding the patient's mental competency to make such a decision

b. If a patient is found to be competent, the emergency physician must provide a comprehensive explanation of the risks involved in refusing treatment; the details of the patient conference, as well as patient's understanding, must be thoroughly documented in the medical record

c. Patients should be requested to sign a "release of responsibility" form; if a patient refuses to sign the form, document the refusal in the medical record

d. If a patient's refusal of treatment puts the patient at risk and there is a question of the patient's competency, contact the hospital administrator or designee to consider court-ordered treatment; obtain a psychiatric consultation to evaluate mental capacity

e. Patient discovered missing (elopement): hospital should have policy indicating recall attempts were made when necessary

5. Patients in custody of law enforcement

a. Consent for treatment generally remains with the individual, not with law enforcement personnel

b. Conflict may occur if a patient is in custody for suspected alcohol or drug intoxication or ingestion; state law governs whether the individual in custody can refuse consent for withdrawal of blood and other body fluid specimens for police or forensic purposes; court order may be obtained in absence of patient consent

c. Invasive surgical procedures to remove suspected ingested balloons or bags of illegal drugs generally require a court order if the patient refuses removal; the court may not order the removal because of the risk associated with the surgery; the court weighs the interests of the state and the individual in custody

   1) Exception: physician believes within a reasonable degree of medical certainly that the patient is in imminent danger, thus creating a medical emergency

d. Legal counsel should be consulted for specific direction for policy development

6. Consent regarding withholding or withdrawal of life support

a. Patient Self-Determination Act (1991)

   1) Federal law

   2) Intent to provide hospitalized patients with information regarding advance directives

      a) Patient must be asked during the admission phase whether he or she has an advance directive in place

      b) If signed copies available, must be placed in the medical record

      c) If no advance directive exists, information about advance directives must be provided

      d) Interaction must then be documented in the medical record

b. Living will

   1) An advanced care document

   2) States a person's wishes regarding medical care should he or she become terminally ill and incompetent or unable to communicate

   3) Applies to decisions made by the patient's designated person after the terminally ill patient has no reasonable chance of recovery

   4) Often used in combination with a durable power of attorney

c. Durable power of attorney for health care decisions (health care proxy)

   1) Extension of the traditional durable power of attorney concept

   2) Allows competent individuals to select someone (attorney-in-fact) to act for them in the area of health care decisions should they become unable to make their own decisions

3) Attorney-in-fact (who does not have to be an attorney-at-law) assumes responsibility to speak for the individual regarding all treatment decisions unless his or her power is specifically limited in the durable power
  d. Do-not-resuscitate (DNR) orders
   1) The majority of states have enacted legislation authorizing and prescribing guidelines for DNR orders
   2) Differs from written directives in that they are executed by a physician with the patient or their representative's consent when the physician believes that a situation requiring a resuscitation is anticipated

III. Patient Treatment and Transfer Issues

A. EMERGENCY MEDICAL TREATMENT AND ACTIVE LABOR ACT (EMTALA)

1. EMTALA
   a. The Consolidated Omnibus Budget Reconciliation Act (COBRA) is a federal mandate, enacted in 1986. A portion of the act, known as EMTALA, was designed to prevent inappropriate transfers ("patient dumping") by hospitals. EMTALA creates two basic obligations: screening and stabilization. The act requires the medical screening of individuals seeking emergency care to determine whether an emergency condition exists and, if so, stabilization of the patient, to the best of the hospital's capabilities, prior to discharge or transfer.
2. ED requirements
   a. Anyone presenting on hospital property requesting emergency medical treatment must receive an appropriate medical screening examination (MSE) to determine whether an emergency condition exists and, if so, must be stabilized prior to discharge or transfer
    1) Hospital property refers to the main campus and any area within 250 yards of the building to include parking lots, sidewalks, and driveways of the hospital or hospital departments; the hospital has the obligation to provide emergency response capabilities and to call 911
    2) MSEs
     a) Must not be delayed to obtain financial information
     b) Require the determination, with reasonable medical certainty, as to whether an emergency medical condition exists or whether a woman is in active labor
     c) Screening must be done within the facility's capabilities using available personnel, including on-call physicians

     d) Ongoing processes should continue until the patient is either stabilized or appropriately transferred
     e) The MSE must be performed by a physician or qualified medical personnel (QMP)
      (1) QMP are nonphysician personnel as defined by the hospital's medical staff bylaws and its rules and regulations
      (2) QMP must be approved by the hospital's governing board to perform the initial MSE
      (3) Nursing triage does not constitute an MSE for EMTALA purposes
     f) Screening typically occurs in the ED unless a more appropriate location is determined (e.g., screening of a pregnant woman on the inpatient obstetric unit)
      (1) Women in active labor are not considered to be stabilized until after the delivery of the placenta
      (2) Patients should not be moved to a hospital-owned, noncontiguous area unless all patients with the same medical condition are moved to that area regardless of ability to pay, there is a good reason, and a physician or QMP is available to care for them
     g) If a patient chooses to leave the ED prior to a MSE, he or she should sign a release form
   b. EMTALA includes ambulances owned and/or operated by the hospital
    1) Exception is if the ambulance is operating under community-wide EMS protocols that direct it to another hospital or is operating at the direction of a physician who is not employed or affiliated with the hospital that owns the ambulance
    2) Does not include ambulances with patients on the hospital property for the sole purpose of meeting a helicopter for transport to another destination, so long as the ambulance or helicopter does not request medical assistance
   c. EMTALA is no longer applicable when
    1) A physician or QMP decides, after an MSE, that no emergency medical condition exists
    2) A physician or QMP decides an emergency medical condition exists and an appropriate transfer occurs after stabilization
    3) A physician or QMP decides an emergency medical condition exists and the patient is admitted to the hospital for further stabilizing treatment
   d. All Medicare-participating EDs must have signs posted prominently in the waiting, admission, and triage areas
    1) Specifies the patient's rights with respect to examination and treatment for emergency medical conditions

2) Should be written in the languages of the most frequent visitors
3. Emergency medical condition
   a. Definition: a medical condition manifesting itself by acute symptoms of sufficient severity such that the absence of immediate medical attention could reasonably be expected to result in increased morbidity or mortality
      1) A condition that is a danger to health and safety of a patient or fetus
      2) May result in a risk of impairment or dysfunction of any bodily organ or body part
   b. Examples
      1) Undiagnosed, acute pain sufficient to impair normal function
      2) Pregnancy with contractions present
      3) Symptoms of substance abuse
      4) Psychiatric disturbances
4. Dedicated ED (DED)
   a. Licensed by the state as an emergency room or ED
   b. Holds itself out to the public as providing emergency care on an urgent basis without requiring a scheduled appointment
   c. During the preceding calendar year, must have provided at least one third of its outpatient visits for the treatment of emergency medical conditions without requiring a scheduled appointment
   d. If a patient presents in a hospital department off the hospital's main campus other than a DED, EMTALA would not apply
5. On-call physician coverage
   a. Should be prearranged and a schedule available for those medical specialties generally engaged in the delivery of care necessary to serve the community needs under Medicare Conditions of Participation
   b. Backup plan for coverage should also be prearranged, and on-call lists must be kept for 5 years
   c. On-call physicians can provide coverage at more than one hospital at a time and may schedule elective surgical cases while on call
   d. On-call physicians must respond in a timely manner and provide stabilizing care
   e. On-call physicians may not act independently on behalf of the hospital to refuse or accept patient transfers for evaluation in a DED
6. Documentation requirements
   a. Documentation
      1) Log entry of patient visit with patient name, date, time of arrival, complaint/diagnosis, disposition, and time of disposition
      2) Triage record with notations including complaint duration and level of distress
      3) Ongoing vital signs
      4) Oral history
      5) Physician examination: affected systems, potentially affected systems, and known chronic conditions
      6) Diagnostic testing necessary to rule out presence of legally defined emergency medical conditions
      7) Monitoring and interventions
      8) Use of on-call personnel and physicians
      9) Resolution of abnormal findings or diagnostic test results
      10) Intake and discharge/transfer vital signs
7. Patient transfers (see Chapter 43)
   a. Patients should be transferred to another facility only for services or care not available at facility or on patient request
   b. Receiving hospital must accept all transfers of patients needing specialty services not available at the transferring hospital if services and capacity are available at the receiving hospital; advance acceptance and documentation of the transfer should be obtained
   c. Receiving hospital must have an accepting physician, whose name must be documented
   d. Transfer documents must also include patient's consent or refusal for transfer and physician certification that the risks of transfer are outweighed by the benefits; medical records, reports, and consultation records should accompany the patient
   e. Medically appropriate transportation: life support equipment and personnel appropriate for the patient's condition should be used to transport the patient to the receiving hospital
8. EMTALA violations
   a. Any suspected violations of EMTALA by another facility that result in a facility's improperly receiving a patient without EMTALA compliance or another facility's refusal to accept transfer patients from a hospital to an appropriate destination hospital with specialized services not available at the facility must be reported
   b. Suspected EMTALA violations are investigated by the Office of Inspector General (OIG) and the state's Attorney General
   c. If violation is found to have occurred, imposed fines are up to $50,000 per violation for hospitals of 100 beds or more, $25,000 per violation for hospitals of 99 beds or less, and $50,000 per violation per physician
   d. If Centers for Medicare and Medicaid Services (CMS) determines that Conditions of Participation have been violated, the hospital may face termination from Medicare and state Medicaid programs

B. PATIENT CONFIDENTIALITY

1. Health Insurance Portability and Accountability Act and the Privacy Rule
   a. Shortly following the enactment of HIPAA, the U.S. Department of Health and Human Services issued the Privacy Rule standards. These standards address the use and disclosure of individuals' health information ("protected health information") by organizations ("covered entities") subject to the Privacy Rule as well as standards for individuals' privacy rights to understand and control how their health information is used. The Rule balances permitted uses of information while protecting the privacy of people who seek care
   b. Protected health information (PHI) may be used without consent of the patient by the medical provider only for treatment, payment, and health care operations activities
      1) Treatment is defined as the provision, coordination, or management of health care and related services
      2) Includes consultation between providers regarding a patient and referral of a patient by one provider to another
   c. Patient's personal information must be protected in all public and uncontrolled settings
   d. Communications should be with the patient or authorized representative
      1) Information can be provided to family members or close friends only on patient consent
   e. Release of information to law enforcement
      1) In civil litigation, medical records are released to attorneys on receipt of a HIPAA-compliant authorization
      2) HIPAA allows covered entities, including hospitals, to disclose protected health information to law enforcement officials for certain limited purposes without patient authorization, although state limitation may be more stringent
         a) Court-ordered subpoenas, warrants, or summonses
         b) Grand jury subpoenas
         c) Administrative requests, subpoenas, or summonses by a federal or state agency or law enforcement agency
         d) In situations regarding identification and location of a suspect, fugitive, material witness, or missing person the following may be released
            (1) Name and address
            (2) Date and place of birth
            (3) Social Security number
            (4) ABO blood type
            (5) Type of injury
            (6) Date and time of treatment
            (7) Date and time of death (if applicable)
            (8) Description of any distinguishing physical characteristics
         e) Victims of a crime
         f) Custodial situations where a correctional institution needs the information to ensure the health and safety of the patient, inmate, or officers
         g) Hospital reporting required by law
         h) Death caused by criminal conduct
         i) Criminal conduct on hospital premises
         j) Criminal conduct offsite
         k) To avert a serious threat to health or safety (e.g., a patient believed to have escaped from a correctional facility or a patient making a statement admitting participation in a violent crime)

IV. Reportable Situations

A. REQUIREMENTS

1. Individual states have legally defined certain situations that require health care professionals to breach patient confidentiality and report the situation to a specified agency or individual
2. Because of variances by state, each ED needs to obtain copies of its particular state laws related to mandatory reporting requirements
3. Examples of mandatory reporting include homicide or suicide attempts, child maltreatment, elder abuse, rape, communicable diseases, and deaths within 48 hours of hospital admission

B. NURSING RESPONSIBILITY

1. If the situation requires either a physician or a nurse to report the incident, nurses should not assume that the physician will be the person responsible; the nurse shares equally in this legal responsibility
2. If the nurse believes in good faith that the incident meets the statutory reporting requirements but the physician disagrees, it remains the nurse's responsibility to report to the designated authority or document that social services have assumed responsibility for the case

V. Documentation

A. MEDICAL RECORD REQUIREMENTS

1. Must be initiated and maintained on every individual who seeks emergency care
2. Serves a variety of functions
   a. Communication system for health care professionals providing patient care

b. Chronicle of the patient's progress

c. Medical-legal record of all care provided

d. Justification for billing

3. Requirements for what must be included in medical record documentation vary on an institutional basis

4. Accredited hospitals are required to have certain information on the medical record

5. Trauma centers are often required to track specific information on the medical records of injured patients

6. State law may dictate the minimum requirements of what is included in medical records

B. EMERGENCY DEPARTMENT CONSIDERATIONS

1. Should reflect that past medical records were ordered, received, or not available

2. When rapid interventions are occurring, it is optimal to have someone making contemporaneous and chronologic documentation

3. Critically ill or injured patients should have documented evidence that intensive nursing care, through the frequent recording of vital signs or interventions, was being performed; care in the ED must be consistent with what would be provided in the intensive care unit (ICU)

4. Unusual occurrences or events that are not part of routine care or operations and result in, or have the potential to result in, harm to patient should be documented

a. Document a description of the event, in objective, factual terms, in the medical record

b. If pertinent, provide a description of the environment (e.g., "side rails up and locked" or "water on floor")

c. Do not document in the medical record that the unusual occurrence form was completed

5. If a problem is found (e.g., esophageal intubation), resolution should also be documented (e.g., endotracheal tube replaced into trachea with equal breath sounds present)

6. All communication with or attempted communication with physicians, supervisors, or administrators regarding the patient's status should be documented; failure to follow the chain of command to benefit the patient is the focus in many lawsuits

7. Documentation must reflect compliance with state laws (e.g., evidence of organ request in the case of death and documentation of the patient's decision regarding life support for the patient admitted from the ED)

8. All appropriate forms and consents must be included in the medical record

9. Discharge instructions

a. Every discharged patient should receive written and verbal discharge instructions

b. Copy of discharge instructions must be a permanent part of the medical record

c. Documented evidence that written instructions were discussed with patient and the patient indicated understanding

d. Language of discharge instructions should not be more complex than sixth-grade reading level

e. Discharge instructions should be available in the predominant languages of the area population

f. Claims of inadequate discharge instructions are frequent issues in ED lawsuits

VI. Trauma Center Legalities

A. APPLICATION TO EMERGENCY DEPARTMENTS

1. A "designated trauma center" is a facility that has met the requirements of government or other authorized entities. Most states have their own evaluation process to determine designation, which may include "verification" by the American College of Surgeons Committee on Trauma of the presence of trauma resources

a. If the ED is designated or verified trauma center, it is legally responsible to provide nationally described resources based on its designation level

b. Required to accept appropriate transfers of injured patients if capacity is present to provide care

2. Undesignated hospitals are not required to have all the resources available as the designated centers

a. They are expected to provide rapid intervention or transfer of the patient, after stabilization, to a hospital that can provide the care

3. Hospitals claiming to be a trauma center are held legally accountable to the standards of a trauma center

4. Accountable to state trauma system regulations

VII. Affordable Care Act

A. THE PATIENT PROTECTION AND AFFORDABLE CARE ACT (PPACA) OR AFFORDABLE CARE ACT (ACA)

1. Was signed into law to reform the health care industry by President Barack Obama on March 23, 2010, and upheld by the Supreme Court on June 28, 2012

2. The ACA expands the affordability, quality, and availability of private and public health insurance through consumer protections, regulations, subsidies, taxes, insurance exchanges, and other reforms and went into effect January 1, 2014

3. Its enactment and implementation have not been without controversy as each of America's 50 states decided to either create a state-run health insurance exchange or follow a federally operated exchange

VIII. Hospital Accreditation Organizations

A. PRIMARY REASONS FOR SEEKING ACCREDITATION

1. Each of the private accreditation organizations develop sets of standards to help hospitals demonstrate they have voluntarily gone beyond minimum federal standards related quality, health, and safety
2. For teaching hospitals, accreditation is mandatory for practicing interns
3. Helps hospital meet the necessary reimbursement criteria under the Centers for Medicare & Medicaid Services (CMS) Conditions of Participation (CoPs)

B. ACCREDITING ORGANIZATIONS

1. For over 40 years, there were two federally approved programs; however, following the enactment of the Medicare Improvements for Patients and Providers Act (MIPPA) of 2008, oversight shifted
2. Today, the accrediting organizations maintain oversight for participating hospitals and CMS maintains oversight for them
3. Currently there are four hospital programs with deeming authority to determine compliance with corresponding CMS regulations
   a. The Joint Commission
   b. Health Care Facilities Accreditation Program (HFAP)
   c. Det Norske Veritas (DNV GL) National Integrated Accreditation for Healthcare Organizations
   d. Center for Improvement in Healthcare Quality (CIHQ)

Bibliography

American Association of Nurse Attorneys. (2015). Available at http://www.taana.org.

American College of Emergency. (2015). EMTALA main points. Retrieved from http://www.acep.org/News-Media-top-banner/EMTALA/.

American College of Legal Medicine: *Legal medicine*, ed 7, St. Louis, MO, 2007, Mosby.

American Hospital Association, National Association of Police Organizations: *Guidelines for releasing patient information to law enforcement*, Chicago, IL, 2005, American Hospital Association.

American Society for Healthcare Engineering: Advocacy report. Retrieved from http://www.ashe.org/resources/pdfs/ashe_advocacy_report_2014.pdf, 2014.

Black's law dictionary online Retrieved from http://thelawdictionary.org/, 2015.

Brent NJ: *Nurses and the law: a guide to principles and applications*, ed 2, Chicago, IL, 2000, W.B. Saunders.

California Judicial Branch: Judicial Council of California civil jury instructions. Retrieved from http://www.courts.ca.gov/partners/317.htm, 2015.

California Nurse Practice Act Retrieved from http://www.rn.ca.gov/regulations/bpc, 2015.

Centers for Medicare and Medicaid Services: Emergency medical treatment and labor act. Retrieved from https://www.cms.gov/Regulations-and-Guidance/Legislation/EMTALA/index.html, 2015.

Cipriano J: The importance of professional liability insurance in managing risk: American Nurses Association. Retrieved from http://ana.nursingworld.org/mods/archive/mod312/cerm301.htm, 2001.

Croke E: Nurses, negligence, and malpractice, *American Journal of Nursing* 103(9):54–63, 2003.

Emergency Nurses Association: Position statement on telephone triage. Retrieved from http://www.ena.org, 2010.

Emergency Nurses Association: *Standards of emergency nursing practice*, ed 6, St. Louis, MO, 2010, Mosby.

Emergency Nurses Association: Position statement on professional liability and risk management. Retrieved from http://www.ena.org, 2012.

Field RI: Why is health care regulation so complex? *Pharmacy and Therapeutics* 33(10):607–608, 2008. Retrieved from http://www.ncbi.nlm.nih.gov/pmc/articles/PMC2730786/.

Gordon v: Wills Knighton Medical Center, 661 So.2d 991, La 1995.

Lee NG: *Legal concepts and issues in emergency care*, Philadelphia, PA, 2001, Saunders.

Lunsford v: Board of Nurse Examiners, 648 SW 2d 391 (Tex. App. 3 Dist.), 1983.

Meisel A: *The right to die*, 2nd ed., New York, NY, 1995, Wiley.

National Council on Aging: Medicare Improvements for Patients and Providers Act (MIPPA). Retrieved from https://www.ncoa.org/centerforbenefits/mippa/, 2015.

Patient Self-Determination Act (PSDA), Title 42, U.S.C.A. section 1395 1995(Suppl 1995).

Peterson AM, Kopishke L, editors: *Legal nurse consulting principles*, ed 3, Boca Raton, FL, 2010, American Association of Legal Nurse Consultants.

Prosser WL: *Handbook on the law of torts*, ed 4, St. Paul, MN, 1971, West.

Refolo MA: The Patient Self-Determination Act of 1990: Health care's own Miranda, *Journal of Contemporary Health Law & Policy* 8(1):26, 1992. Retrieved from http://scholarship.law.edu/chlp/vol8/iss1/26,http://scholarship.law.edu/jchlp/vol8/iss1/26/?utm_source=scholarship.law.edu%2Fjchlp%2Fvol8%2Fiss1%2F26&utm_medium=PDF&utm_campaign=PDFCoverPages.

Roach Jr WH, Aspen Health Law Center: *Medical records and the law*, ed 4, Gaithersburg, MD, 2006, American Health Information Management Association.

Rosenbaum S: The enduring role of the emergency medical treatment and active labor act, *Health Affairs* 32(12):2075–2081, 2013. Retrieved from http://hsrc.himmelfarb.gwu.edu/sphhs_policy_facpubs/165/.

Rothenberg MA: *Emergency medicine malpractice*, 2nd ed., New York, NY, 1994, Wiley (suppl. published 1997).

Rotundo MF, Cribari C, Smith RS, editors: *Resources for optimal care of the injured patient*, ed 6, Chicago, IL, 2014, American College of Surgeons.

Rozovsky FA: *Consent to treatment: A practical guide*, 2nd ed., Boston, 1990, Little, Brown.

Rozovsky FA: *Consent to treatment: A practical guide*, 2nd ed., suppl., Boston, 1995, Little, Brown.

The Joint Commission. (n.d.). Retrieved from http://www.jointcommission.org/accreditation/hospitals.aspx.

United States Department of Health and Human Services: Affordable Care Act. Retrieved from http://www.hhs.gov/regulations/index.html, 2015.

United States Department of Health and Human Services: Summary of the HIPAA Privacy Rule. Retrieved from http://www.hhs.gov/ocr/privacy/hipaa/understanding/summary/index.html, 2015.

United States Department of Health & Human Services, Centers for Medicare & Medicaid Services: Transmittal 60: Revisions to Appendix V–Interpretive Guidelines–responsibilities of Medicare Participating Hospitals in Emergency Care. Retrieved from https://www.google.com/url?sa=t&rct=j&q=&esrc=s&frm=1&source=web&cd=1&ved=0ahUKEwjAztqdz6fJAhUGOIgKHdB0AfAQFggdMAA&url=https%3A%2F%2Fwww.cms.gov%2FRegulations-and-Guidance%2FGuidance%2FTransmittals%2Fdownloads%2FR60SOMA.pdf&usg=AFQjCNGNwtXM2CpTU898o9_jN_lX3ZOLWA&bvm=bv.108194040,d.cGU, 2010.

Wartenber D, Thompson WD: Privacy versus public health: The impact of current confidentiality rules, *Health Policy and Ethics* 100(3):407–412, 2010.

Wilmington General Hospital v. Manlove 194 A.2d 135 (State Court, Del.), 1961.

Part 4

CHAPTER 46

Professionalism and Leadership

Denise Bayer, MSN, RN, CEN, FAEN, Nancy M. Bonalumi, DNP, RN, CEN, FAEN,
Vicki Sweet, MSN, RN, MICN, CEN, FAEN

I. Professionalism

A. COMPONENTS OF PROFESSIONALISM[1]

1. Profession: a type of occupation that meets certain criteria that rise to a level above that of an occupation
2. Professional: a person who belongs to and practices a profession
3. Professionalism: the demonstration of high-level personal, ethical, and skill characteristics of a member of a profession
4. Traits that define a profession
   a. High intellectual level
   b. High level of individual responsibility and accountability
   c. Specialized body of knowledge
   d. Relatively high degree of autonomy and independence of practice
   e. Need for a well-organized and strong organization representing the members of the profession and controlling the quality of practice
   f. Code of ethics that guides the members of the profession in their practice
   g. Demonstration of professional competency and possession of a legally recognized license

B. RESPONSIBLE USE OF SOCIAL MEDIA[2,3]

1. Social media sites

a. May promote professional connections and collaboration

b. May enhance networking opportunities

c. May be used to share educational content

2. Social media platforms must be used with caution

   a. Posted activities and messages may

      1) Violate others' privacy

      2) Be viewed by national boards of nursing as potentially unprofessional or unethical

   b. Emergency nurses should understand federal, state, and agency regulations and policies governing use of social media in the workplace setting

3. Know professional resources related to use of social media

   a. Example: ENA Position Statement: Social Networking by Emergency Nurses

II. Scope and Standards of Emergency Nursing[4]

A *standard* is an acknowledged measure or quantitative or qualitative value and is designed to set forth a combination of skills, education, and performance that a nurse should strive to achieve. It is not a legal model to determine competence. The standards of emergency nursing practice are authoritative statements of the duties for emergency nurses. They may be utilized as evidence of the standard of care.

Competent level identifies sound clinical judgment in autonomous practice. *Excellent* practice surpasses the competent level and contributes to the growth of emergency nursing practice. *Excellent* practice can reflect the role of the Advanced Practice RN (APRN).

A. APPLICATION OF STANDARDS

1. Criteria-based job descriptions
2. Criteria-based performance evaluations
3. Department policies and procedures
4. Interviewing/hiring practices
5. Orientation, in-service, and continuing education programs
6. Creation/revision of emergency care forms
7. Quality improvement programs and activities

B. CLINICAL STANDARDS (TABLE 46.1)

C. PROFESSIONAL STANDARDS (TABLE 46.2)

III. Career Development

A. CONCEPTS AND BEHAVIORS (BOX 46.1)

B. PROFESSIONAL DEVELOPMENT

Nurses today can expect a career that will stretch over 40 years. While many may choose a hospital-based

Table 46.1

Standards of Practice

Assessment	Collect comprehensive data pertinent to the health consumer's need or situation. a. Each patient is triaged using age, developmentally appropriate, and culturally sensitive practices to prioritize and optimize patient flow
Diagnosis	Analyze collected data to determine diagnosis or issues
Outcomes Identification	Identify expected outcomes for each individual patient
Planning	Develop a plan of care with strategies to attain expected outcomes
Implementation	Implement the plan of care by: a. Coordinating care delivery b. Utilizing teaching strategies to promote health and a safe practice environment c. Consulting with the health care team to influence the plan of care and effect change d. Using prescriptive authority, procedures, referrals, treatments, and therapies within applicable laws and regulations (APRN only)
Evaluation	Evaluate progress toward attainment of outcomes

Table 46.2

Standards of Professional Performance

Standard	Behavior
Ethics	Practices nursing using ethical principles
Education	Attains knowledge and competence that reflects current nursing practice
Evidence-Based Practice and Research	Integrates evidence and research findings into practice
Quality of Practice	Contributes to quality nursing practice
Communication	Communicates effectively in a variety of formats in all areas of practice
Leadership	Demonstrates leadership in the professional practice setting and the profession
Collaboration	Collaborates with health care consumers, families, and others in the conduct of nursing practice
Professional Practice Evaluation	Evaluates self in relation to professional practice standards and guidelines, relevant statutes, rules, and regulations
Resource Utilization	Uses appropriate resources to plan and provide nursing services that are safe, effective, and financially responsible
Environmental Health	Practices in an environmentally safe and healthy manner

Part 4

Part 4

BOX 46.1

Career Development Concepts and Behaviors

Concepts/Definitions

1. Career development includes a commitment to further one's education through mentors, professional organizations, academia, and employers
2. Career mapping is a strategic plan for one's career and provides direction for formal education, experience, continuing education, professional associations, and networking
3. Emergency nursing practice is dynamic, fluid, and continually evolving; therefore, continuing education is essential to remaining current with emergency nursing practice
4. Certification promotes professionalism and assures the public and other professionals that the professional registered nurse has attained a level of knowledge and clinical judgment necessary to provide high-quality care

Behaviors (Educational)

1. The registered nurse attains knowledge and competency that reflect current nursing practice through academia, continuing education, and certification
2. Attains certification in emergency nursing
3. Attains other knowledge specific to emergency nursing (e.g., Trauma Nursing Core Course, Emergency Nursing Pediatric Course, and Course in Advanced Trauma Nursing)
4. May choose to pursue an advanced nursing degree at the master's level with a focus on Clinical Nurse Specialist, Nurse Practitioner, Nurse Educator, or Nurse Administrator
5. Demonstrates a commitment to continuous, lifelong learning for self and others

Behaviors (Professional Associations)

1. Networks with peers at the local, state, and/or national levels
2. Maintains membership in professional nursing organizations (e.g., Emergency Nurses Association or American Nurses Association)
3. Participates in professional nursing organizations at the local, state, and/or national level
4. Participates in developing and presenting educational programs and activities, conferences, research, and articles for publication

Behaviors (e.g., Hospital/Department Involvement)

1. Participates in departmental/hospital committees and workgroups
2. Works to influence decision-making bodies to improve patient care, health services, and policies

---

emergency department (ED) as the place for clinical practice during their career, the environment where emergency care is needed and can be given is extremely diverse.

1. Other practice environments for emergency nurses
   a. Freestanding EDs
   b. Urgent care centers
   c. Poison control centers
   d. Cruise ships
   e. Sports arenas
   f. Telephone triage programs
   g. EMS/prehospital environment including ambulances, helicopters, airplanes
2. Emergency nursing role specialization
   a. Informatics
   b. Quality and patient safety
   c. Population health
   d. Health care policy
   e. Management and leadership
   f. Education[5]

Some, but not all, of these specializations will require certifications or an advanced degree to attain the required skills and competencies needed for these roles.

3. Certifications available for emergency nurses
   a. Certification in Emergency Nursing (CEN®)[6]
   b. Certification in Pediatric Emergency Nursing (CPEN®)[6]
   c. Certified Transport Registered Nurse (CTRN®)[6]
   d. Trauma Certified Registered Nurse (TCRN®)[6]
   e. Certified Flight Registered Nurse (CFRN®)
4. Other courses to attain competency
   a. Trauma Nurse Core Curriculum (TNCC™)[7]
   b. Emergency Nursing Pediatric Course (ENPC™)[7]
   c. Course in Advanced Trauma Nursing (CATN™)[6]
   Continuing education promotes career development. Most states require a minimum number of continuing education hours to maintain nursing licensure. Local, state, and national ENA meetings offer opportunities to be updated on the latest in emergency nursing practice, earn continuing education credit hours, and network with other emergency nurses.

C. CAREER GOALS

Developing career goals is one of the most important activities that an individual can do to enhance professional development and ensure upward mobility in the nursing profession. It's important to consider these points when developing goals:

1. Identify your passions and interests
2. Develop a broad career goal based on your education, skills, abilities, and life experiences
3. Develop short-term goals. These goals will allow you to pursue your career aspirations gradually without becoming overwhelmed with the long-term goal
4. Don't be discouraged if life situations get in the way of attaining your goals. Take a break and then get back on the career ladder as soon as possible
5. Stay current on what's happening in the nursing profession
6. Surround yourself with people who are positive influences in your life
7. Present yourself as a professional role model for nursing who puts people first
8. Develop a résumé that showcases your talents[8]

D. ACADEMIC CAREER PROGRESSION

There are many levels of education within the nursing profession. Entry to practice can be through a diploma or associate or baccalaureate degree. Advanced degrees may be required for certain roles within emergency nursing. Table 46.3 summarizes the various academic levels in nursing. A comparison of research (PhD) and practice (DNP) doctorates is found in Table 46.4.

Table 46.3

Comparison of Academic Nursing Education Levels

Diploma	2–3 years to complete Usually is hospital based Least common entry-to-practice program and being phased out in the United States
Associate Degree in Nursing (ADN)	2 years to complete Community college or vocational/trade school based
Bachelor of Science in Nursing (BSN)	4 years to complete (1–2 years if applicant has ADN) University based Coursework offered on campus or online
Masters of Science in Nursing	1.5–2 years to complete (may be longer if applicant does not have a BSN) University-based program Coursework offered on campus or online Specialties include: • Nurse Practitioner (NP) • Certified Nurse Midwife (CNM) • Clinical Nurse Specialist (CNS) • Certified Nurse Anesthetist (CRNA) • Clinical Nurse Leader (CNL) • Nurse Educator • School Nursing
Doctor of Nursing (DNP/PhD/DNSc)	3–6 years to complete University based Coursework offered on campus or online

(Adapted from Wilson, A. [2011]. http://nursejournal.org/articles/types-of-nursing-degrees.)

IV. Advanced Practice Roles in the Emergency Care System

A. EMERGENCY NURSES ASSOCIATION POSITION STATEMENT ON ADVANCED PRACTICE ROLES IN EMERGENCY NURSING[9]

1. Advanced Practice Registered Nurses (APRNs) are highly qualified clinicians who are positioned to serve an integral role in emergency health care systems
2. APRN is a regulatory title, and four advanced practice roles have been delineated by the American Nurses Association in The Consensus Model for the Advanced Practice Registered Nurse
3. These roles are
   a. Certified Registered Nurse Anesthetist
   b. Certified Nurse Midwife
   c. Certified Nurse Practitioner
   d. Clinical Nurse Specialist
4. APRNs have a broad depth of knowledge and expertise in their specialty and can manage complex clinical and system issues

Table 46.4

Key Differences between DNP and PhD/DNS Programs

	DNP	PHD/DNS
Program of Study	*Objectives:* Prepare nurse leaders at the highest level of nursing practice to improve patient outcomes and translate research into practice *Competencies:* See AACN's *Essentials of Doctoral Education for Advanced Nursing Practice* (2006)	*Objectives:* Prepare nurses at the highest level of nursing science to conduct research to advance the science of nursing *Content:* See *The Research-Focused Doctoral Program in Nursing: Pathways to Excellence* (2010)
Students	Commitment to practice career Oriented toward improving outcomes of patient care and population health	Commitment to research career Oriented toward developing new nursing knowledge and scientific inquiry
Program Faculty	Practice or research doctorate in nursing, and expertise in area teaching Leadership experience in area of role and population practice High level of expertise in practice congruent with focus of academic program	Research doctorate in nursing or related field Leadership experience in area of sustained research funding High level of expertise in research congruent with focus of academic program
Resources	Mentors and/or preceptors in leadership positions across practice settings Access to diverse practice settings with appropriate resources for areas of practice Access to financial aid Access to information and patient-care technology resources congruent with areas of study	Mentors and/or preceptors in research settings Access to research settings with appropriate resources Access to dissertation support dollars and financial aid Access to information and research technology resources congruent with program of research
Program Assessment and Evaluation	*Program Outcome:* Health care improvements and contributions via practice, policy change, and practice scholarship Receives accreditation by nursing accreditor	*Program Outcome:* Contributes to health care improvements via the development of new knowledge and scholarly products that provide the foundation for the advancement of nursing science Oversight by the institution's authorized bodies (i.e., graduate school) and regional accreditors

(From American Association of Colleges of Nursing. [2014]. Doctor of Nursing Practice. DNP Contrast Grid. http://www.aacn.nche.edu/dnp/ContrastGrid.pdf.)

5. Nurses in advanced clinical practice provide comprehensive health assessments and demonstrate a high level of autonomy and expert skill in the diagnosis and treatment of many complex problems
6. In the emergency setting APRNs are uniquely prepared to develop and apply theory, conduct research, educate health care providers and consumers, and develop standards of practice that contribute to optimum patient outcomes
7. It is the position of the Emergency Nurses Association that:
   a. APRNs can practice effectively in an emergency environment and use their abilities, knowledge, and specialized skills to meet the needs of patients and their families or significant others at the point of crisis or need
   b. APRNs can effectively extend themselves into the communities by providing educational opportunities that assist individuals and communities in the promotion of safe practices, healthy behaviors, and prevention of injury and illness[9]

V. Networking

A. DEFINITION

1. Creating a group of acquaintances and associates and keeping it active through regular communication for mutual benefit[10]
2. A supportive system of sharing information and services among individuals and groups having a common interest[11]

B. WHERE TO NETWORK

1. Work
2. Professional association meetings/groups
3. Conferences
4. Internet/social media
5. Networking events/groups
6. Social gatherings/events
7. Community events

C. WHO TO NETWORK WITH

1. Existing connections (friends, classmates, family, work colleagues)

2. People at work who you do not directly work with (i.e., other departments)
3. Others within your industry who work for other employers
4. Individuals outside of your industry
5. Individuals in positions you aspire to obtain

D. HOW TO NETWORK

1. Be open-minded, communicative, and approachable
2. Have a networking goal
   a. To gather information
   b. To make contacts
   c. To connect with specific individuals
   d. To seek advice on a problem/situation
   e. To find solutions
   f. To expand client referrals
   g. To create mutually benefiting relationships
3. Introduce yourself
   a. Have a prepared self-introduction that sums up your professional self that can be delivered quickly
   b. Have professional-looking business cards to hand out
4. Communicate
   a. Have some prepared questions/ice-breaker questions
   b. Ask a question and then listen
   c. Ask for advice or for their opinion on a topic
   d. Ask curious and open-ended questions
   e. Share about yourself
   f. Always offer to assist the other person
5. Keep in touch
   a. When someone gives you their business card, make a notation on the back of the card to help you remember them (i.e., date and place you met, shared interests, area of expertise)
   b. Follow up after meeting someone (a simple email to say thank you, or send him or her an interesting article on a topic you discussed when you met)
   c. Do not wait until you need something to follow up with your contacts; follow up periodically just to say hello and check in with them
   d. Send your contacts referrals
   e. Congratulate your contacts on business achievements

E. HOW NOT TO NETWORK

1. Do not approach networking from a "How can I profit?" approach; instead approach it from "How can I help?"
2. Blatant self-promotion
3. Interrupting others in mid-speech; instead actively listen
4. Be cautious about personal use of social media sites

VI. Leadership Traits and Styles

A. FUNDAMENTAL TRAITS OF A LEADER

1. Challenging the process
   a. Seek and accept challenge

   b. Change the status quo
   c. Pioneers; willing to step out into the unknown
   d. Willing to take risk, innovate and experiment to find a new and better way of doing things
   e. Recognizes the good ideas of others and supports those ideas
2. Inspiring a shared vision
   a. They have visions and dreams of what could be, and they have absolute and total belief in those dreams and confidence in their ability to make extraordinary things happen
   b. Their clear image of the future pulls them forward
   c. They inspire others to commit to their vision through forging a unity of purpose and by showing others how the dream is for the common good
3. Enabling others to act
   a. Recognize it will take a team effort to accomplish the work
   b. Involve key stakeholders and those who must live with the results
   c. Empower others and make it possible for them to do good work
   d. They don't hoard power but instead give it away
   e. Build teamwork, trust, and empowerment
4. Modeling the way
   a. Understand actions are more important than words and work to ensure their words and actions are consistent
   b. They "walk the walk and talk the talk"
5. Encouraging the heart
   a. Encourages others, especially in hard times
   b. Celebrates small and large accomplishments
   c. Recognizes and rewards the efforts of others

VII. Leadership Competencies

Leadership competencies are the measurable or observable knowledge, skills, abilities, and behaviors (KSABs) critical to successful job performance. The concepts and behaviors of these competencies are identified in Table 46.5.

A. COLLABORATION

B. EMOTIONAL INTELLIGENCE

C. SYSTEMS THINKING

D. HUMAN RESOURCE MANAGEMENT

E. CHANGE

F. COMMUNICATION

G. CONFLICT MANAGEMENT

Table 46.5		
Leadership Competencies		
Competency	**Concept/Definition**	**Behavior**
Collaboration	1. To work with another person or group to achieve or do something 2. Bringing together people with different views and perspectives to discuss issues openly and supportively in an attempt to find ways of helping each other solve a larger problem or achieve broader goals	1. Places goals of the organization ahead of personal goals 2. Consistently demonstrates transparent decision making 3. Creates a shared purpose 4. Leads by example, questions own ideas, take risks, and listens to all views/ideas 5. Builds productive working relationships with coworkers, staff, and others 6. Gains the cooperation and support of others by seeking to understand what they think/need and by rapidly establishing trust and respect
Emotional Intelligence	The five domains of emotional intelligence include: 1. Self-awareness 2. Self-management 3. Self-motivation 4. Empathy; recognizing emotions in others 5. Relationship management Emotional intelligence is the single most significant predictor of performance in the workplace	1. Able to identify and manage their own emotions in any given situation 2. Able to identify and understand the emotions of others with whom they are interacting 3. Has an accurate understanding of personal strengths and weaknesses and strives to improve 4. Maintains a professional demeanor and serves as a role model for staff 5. Manages self effectively in emotionally charged situations 6. Actively listens to understand 7. Explains decisions to others 8. Builds trust with others 9. Acknowledges others' feelings 10. Provides direct and constructive feedback while being aware of the other person's feelings
Systems Thinking	Systems thinking is a management discipline that focuses on understanding a system/organization by examining the linkages and interactions between the components/departments that comprise the entirety of that defined system/organization	1. Establishes collaborative relationships throughout the organization 2. Considers the impact of actions/decisions on the entire organization/system 3. Understands the political nature of the organization and works appropriately within this culture 4. Deals effectively with contradictory requirements or inconsistencies in the organization
Human Resource Management	1. Human resource management is a process of managing staff in a structured and thorough manner 2. Human resource management requires an understanding of state and federal laws/regulations, hospital policy and procedure as well as how to inspire, motivate, and influence others 3. Effective human resource management is critical for the success of the department/organization	1. Works collaboratively to recruit, interview, and select exceptional staff 2. Addresses morale issues and establishes a healthy work environment 3. Establishes departmental performance expectations and staff competencies 4. Provides staff reward and recognition programs 5. Communicates performance expectations to staff and assesses staff competency 6. Ensures staff receive appropriate education/training/orientation to perform duties 7. Coaches and counsels staff on performance issues 8. Delegates duties to others based on their ability 9. Provides staff with growth opportunities 10. Stays current on human resources regulations, policies, and procedures

Table 46.5

Leadership Competencies—cont'd

Competency	Concept/Definition	Behavior
Change	1. The role of a change agent is multifaceted and includes the ability to effect change in themselves and to build the capacity to change in others 2. A change agent alters the organizational system and alters human capabilities by supporting and influencing others toward change 3. A change agent is one who works to bring about a change 4. Change is inevitable and necessary for growth 5. Change often produces fear and anxiety 6. Nurses at all levels in the organization are in key positions to identify and drive changes that will enhance the health care system	1. Leads and/or participates in the change process through identification, planning, implementation, and evaluation of process improvement initiatives 2. Leads change by example 3. Accepts change as positive 4. Adapts plans as necessary 5. Considers/responds to other's concerns during change 6. Involves key stakeholders in the design and implementation of change 7. Adjusts management style to changing situations
Communication	1. Communication is the complex exchange of thoughts, ideas, or information both verbally and nonverbally 2. Communication is a complex, ongoing, dynamic process in which the participants simultaneously create shared meaning in an interaction 3. Collaboration is an assertive and cooperative means of communication in which both parties try to find mutually satisfying solutions 4. Communication requires intentional knowledge sharing styles and is based on mutual respect for each other's unique perspective and contributions to the situation 5. Conflict results from differences in ideas, values, or feelings between two or more people and is manifested as internal or external discord; other sources of conflict include scarce resources and poorly defined role expectations	1. Expresses ideas cogently, fluently, and eloquently 2. Communicates important decisions, plans, and activities in a timely and proactive manner 3. Encourages direct and open discussion about important issues/topics 4. Communications with peers, colleagues, patients, and others are open, honest, and respectful 5. Facilitates and participates in two-way communication 6. Continuously strives to improve communication and interpersonal skills 7. Actively and objectively listens to others and seeks to understand 8. Utilizes assertive communication skills and avoids passive/aggressive communication styles 9. Collaborates with peers, colleagues, patients, and others regarding the patient's needs and plan of care 10. Seeks a win-win solution to conflict through collaboration, problem solving, and consensus
Conflict management	Conflict results from differences in ideas, values, or feelings between two or more people and is manifested as internal or external discord; other sources of conflict include scarce resources and poorly defined role expectations	1. Acts decisively and fairly when faced with tough decisions and managing problem employees 2. Identifies performance issues early and takes appropriate action quickly to resolve issues 3. Appropriately documents performance issues 4. Effectively deescalates highly emotional situations and individuals 5. Assists staff to manage and resolve conflict
Employee development	1. Mentoring includes sharing knowledge and experience, providing emotional support, role-modeling, and guiding 2. A mentor is a wiser and more experienced person	1. Encourages staff to share in decision making and change 2. Is visible and available to staff 3. Identifies upcoming leaders and nurtures their talents 4. Is available to establish one-on-one mentoring relationships 5. Establishes performance expectations 6. Assists staff with analyzing their performance and provides feedback on areas for improvement 7. Acts as a sounding board for ideas and encourages creative thinking and problem solving 8. Supports staff in taking on new challenges

Continued

Table 46.5

Leadership Competencies—cont'd

Competency	Concept/Definition	Behavior
Integrity	1. Ethics is the systematic study of what a person's conduct and actions should be with regard to himself or herself, other human beings, and the environment 2. Registered nurses are bound by a professional code of ethics 3. The emergency nurse provides care based on philosophical and ethical concepts; these concepts include reverence for life, respect for the dignity, worth, autonomy, and individuality of each human being; and an acknowledgment of the diversity of all people 4. Registered nurses must be principle-centered leaders and individuals	1. Acts as an advocate for the department, staff, and patients 2. Is trustworthy and produces trust in employees 3. Has credibility with the employees 4. Builds and maintains strong relationships with staff 5. Follows through on commitments and agreements 6. Demonstrates fairness when dealing with all levels of staff 7. Treats people fairly and with consistency

Critical Thinking	1. Critical thinking is a rational reasoning process that involves applying knowledge, skills, attitudes, and values for the purpose of making a decision that affects patient care
	2. Critical thinking uses clinical and professional judgment in each phase of the nursing process
	3. Critical thinking is a higher-level cognitive skill that includes creativity, problem solving, and decision-making techniques
	4. Problem solving is a process of identifying and solving a problem
	5. Decision making is a process involving selection of one of several alternatives: it is initiated when there is a perceived gap between what is actually happening and what should be happening, and it ends with action that will narrow or close that gap
		1. Applies critical thinking skills while utilizing the nursing process
		2. Critical thinking skills include:
		  a. Analyzing: separating or breaking a whole into parts to discover its nature, function, and relationships
		  b. Applying standards: judging according to established personal, professional, or social rules or criteria
		  c. Discriminating: recognizing differences and similarities among things or situations
		  d. Information seeking: searching for evidence, facts, or knowledge by identifying relevant sources and gathering objective, subjective, historical, and current data from those sources
		  e. Logical reasoning: drawing inferences or conclusions that are supported or justified by evidence
		  f. Predicting: envisioning a plan and its consequences
		  g. Transforming knowledge: changing or converting the condition, nature, form, or function of concepts among contexts
		3. Applies critical thinking, problem solving, decision making, and creative thinking skills

Financial Management	1. Financial management is critical to the success of every organization and department 2. Nurse leaders are generally responsible for the capital and noncapital budget for their department 3. The major components of the departmental budget include revenue and expenses; the two major expenses are typically labor and supplies	1. Tracks and analyzes staffing, equipment, and supply expenses through the year; responds to and adjusts operations based on variances 2. Educates staff on financial issue that impact the unit and on best uses of budget resources 3. Considers organizational profit and loss information in making budget decisions 4. Holds staff accountable for the efficient use of resources 5. Remains current on reimbursement issues and methodology as well as financial issues that impact health care systems

H. EMPLOYEE DEVELOPMENT

I. INTEGRITY

J. CRITICAL THINKING

K. FINANCIAL MANAGEMENT

VIII. Work Environment

A. HEALTHY WORK ENVIRONMENT

Workplace culture is one of the biggest factors that increase employee commitment, engagement, and job satisfaction. Healthy work environments are defined as "supportive of the whole human being, are patient-focused, and are joyful workplaces."[12] Hospitals perform better when employees are engaged with what they are doing and committed to their jobs.[13] There is a large body of evidence confirming the inextricable link between healthy work environments and optimal outcomes for patients, health care professionals, and health care organizations.[14]

It is almost universally acknowledged that EDs are stressful places to work.[13] ED nurse leaders should be aware of these stressors and implement support strategies to minimize their effect.

1. Negative stressors
   a. Lack of participation in operational decision making
   b. ED crowding
   c. Staff workload
2. Support strategies
   a. Ability of management to offer flexible working arrangements
   b. Good quality leadership
   c. Balancing patient acuity, staff skill mix, and resources
   d. Work-life balance and control of total working hours
   e. Respect for multidisciplinary expertise[15]

B. WORKPLACE VIOLENCE (SEE CHAPTER 48)

1. Workplace violence is any act or threat of physical violence, harassment, intimidation, or other threatening disruptive behavior that occurs at the worksite. It ranges from threats and verbal abuse to physical assaults and even homicide. It can affect and involve employees, clients, customers, and visitors[16]
2. Bullying, also referred to as horizontal violence, is a form of workplace violence and consists of three main elements
   a. An imbalance of power, this can be due to formal or perceived power
   b. An intent to cause harm
   c. Repetition of bullying behaviors[17]
3. Sources
   a. Patients, visitors
   b. Supervisors, peers, physicians, colleagues
4. Prevalence
   a. Workplace violence occurs in emergency departments worldwide[18]
   b. Verbal abuse is the most common form of workplace violence; however, high rates of physical abuse are reported in the emergency department setting as well
   c. There is significant underreporting of workplace violence
5. Impact
   a. The consequences of workplace violence are far reaching, it is detrimental to the work environment and the profession of nursing. In addition, it is a contributing factor to the nursing shortage.[18] Common outcomes of workplace violence include
   b. Physical and psychological
      1) Headaches
      2) Stress, irritability, anxiety
      3) Sleep disturbances
      4) Depression, fatigue, loss of concentration
      5) Excessive worry, impaired social skills
      6) Posttraumatic stress disorder
      7) Psychosomatic complaints
   c. Performance
      1) Absenteeism
      2) Medical errors
      3) Decreased moral and teamwork
      4) Decreased communication
      5) The performance of the entire team suffers, not just the performance of the victim
   d. Retention and turnover
      1) Job abandonment
      2) Increased turnover[18]
6. Leadership's responsibility[19]
   a. Often department leadership is unaware of workplace bullying
   b. Policy and procedures that support a zero tolerance
   c. Provide staff education
   d. Create a culture of respect and safety
   e. Provide for adequate staffing
   f. Council employees privately, not publicly
   g. Implementation of a code of conduct/behavior/ethics to reinforce professionalism among all staff; refer to:
      1) Emergency Nurses Association Code of Ethics
      2) American Nurses Association Position Statement on Incivility, Bullying and Workplace Violence

C. ETHICAL ISSUES IN EMERGENCY NURSING[20,21,22]

1. Emergency nurses should understand basic ethical issues in nursing. It is important for emergency nurses to understand their resources for addressing ethical situations encountered in the workplace. There are four main ethical principles
   a. Autonomy
      1) Respecting the decision of the patient
      2) Example: issues of consent or refusal of care
   b. Beneficence
      1) Toward the greater good or promotion of well-being
      2) Example: discharge teaching
   c. Nonmaleficence
      1) Avoidance of harm
      2) Example: policies aimed at reduction of medical errors
   d. Justice
      1) Fairness or equality
      2) Example: medical screening examinations for all patients presenting to the ED
   e. Many organizations have a formal code of ethics
      1) See Emergency Nurses Association Code of Ethics, available through the organization

f. Ethical dilemmas may arise in several areas of emergency nursing, including but not limited to
1) Biomedical issues affecting populations or specific patients
a) End-of-life options
2) Access to care
3) Availability of resources
a) Disaster triage
4) Patients' rights and autonomy
5) Moral distress

D. JUST CULTURE (SEE TABLE 46.6)

1. Historically, health care has punished people for making errors, with little to no regard for the system the error occurred within. This has led to a culture of fear and nonreporting of errors. The Just Culture model aims to change the culture of error reporting and management[23]
2. The Just Culture model acknowledges the interaction between the individual and the system within which they work; while individuals make choices, the system is often flawed, which contributes to the error[23]
3. In a Just Culture model the system is modified and the individual is held accountable for his or her choices in a fair and just way, to prevent future errors[23]
4. The Just Culture model is based on an algorithm to help guide leaders when holding individuals accountable for their choices[24]
5. A key premise of the Just Culture model is that choices are made with intentions and you must first understand the intention behind the choice. The model defines four levels of intent and identifies recommendations related to coaching/counseling/discipline for each level of intent[24]
6. Implementation of a Just Culture model can be a significant paradigm shift and will require[25]
a. Education of the staff and leaders within the organization
b. Trust between staff and leadership
c. A commitment to changing/improving processes and systems

IX. The Impaired Nurse

A. EMERGENCY NURSES ASSOCIATION POSITION STATEMENT

1. According to the Position Statement, Chemical Impairment of Emergency Nurses,[26] the incidence of substance abuse in the nursing community is approximately 10%, equaling that of the general population. It is estimated by the American Nurses Association that 6–8% of nurses use enough alcohol or drugs to impair nursing judgment. The basis of professional nursing licensure is to protect the patient. Nurses who are impaired due to substance abuse affect employers, coworkers, patients, families, and communities as a whole. Nurses who remain silent about suspected substance abuse are culpable since their inaction could lead to putting patient safety at risk. Chemical dependency is a treatable, medical disease. Nurse managers must understand chemical dependency so they may identify signs and symptoms and intervene accordingly based on their state board of nursing rules and regulations. Resources are available for emergency nurse leaders to guide policies and strategies for addressing the impaired nurse.

B. EMERGENCY NURSES ASSOCIATION POSITION ON CHEMICAL IMPAIRMENT OF EMERGENCY NURSES[26]

C. AMERICAN NURSES ASSOCIATION POSITION ON IMPAIRED NURSES (IMPAIRED NURSES RESOURCE CENTER)[27]

Table 46.6

Just Culture Algorithm

Human Error	At-Risk Behavior	Reckless Behavior
Inadvertent action: slip, lapse, mistake	A choice: risk not recognized or believed justified	Conscious disregard of unreasonable risk
Manage through changes in: Process Procedures Training Design	Manage through: Removing incentives for at-risk behavior Creating incentives for healthy behaviors Increasing situational awareness	Manage through: Remedial action Punitive action
CONSOLE	COACH	PUNISH

(Copyright 2016, Outcome Engenuity, LLC. All rights reserved. Available at https://www.outcome-eng.com/getting-to-know-just-culture/.)

References

1. Zerwekh J, Zerwekh Garneau A: Nursing: a developing profession. In *Nursing today: Transition and trends*, ed 8, St. Louis, MO, 2015, Elsevier.
2. Milton CL: Power with social media: a nursing perspective, *Nursing Science Quarterly* 29(2):113–115, 2016.
3. Henderson M, Dahnke MD: The ethical use of social media in nursing practice, *MedSurg Nursing* 24(1):62–64, 2015.
4. Emergency Nurses Association: *Emergency nursing scope and standards of practice*, Des Plaines, IL, 2011, Emergency Nurses Association.
5. Nurses for a Healthier Tomorrow. (n.d.). Retrieved from http://www.nursesource.org/emergency.html.
6. Get certified. (n.d.). Retrieved from http://www.bcencertifications.org/Get-Certified.aspx.
7. Emergency Nurses Association – Safe Practice, Safe Care: (n.d.). Retrieved from https://www.ena.org/education/Pages/default.aspx.
8. Nurse Journal. (n.d.). Best types of nursing degrees. Retrieved from http://nursejournal.org/articles/types-of-nursing-degrees/.
9. Emergency Nurses Association: *Position statement: Advanced practice in emergency nursing*, Des Plains, IL, 2012, Emergency Nurses Association.
10. How has this term impacted your life? (n.d.). Retrieved from http://www.businessdictionary.com/definition/networking.html#ixzz3uE7ZMK4G.
11. Dictionary.com. (n.d.). Networking. Retrieved from http://www.dictionary.com/browse/networking.
12. Morton PG: Creating and sustaining healthy work environments, *Journal of Professional Nursing* 31(3):165–167, 2015. http://dx.doi.org/10.1016/j.profnurs.2015.04.002.
13. Brunges M, Foley-Brinza C: Projects for increasing job satisfaction and creating a healthy work environment, *AORN Journal* 100(6):670–681, 2014. http://dx.doi.org/10.1016/j.aorn.2014.01.029.
14. American Association of Critical Care Nursing: *Standards for establishing and sustaining healthy work environments*, Aliso Viejo, CA, 2005, American Association of Critical Care Nursing.
15. Johnston A, Abraham L, Greenslade J, Thom O, Carlstrom E, Wallis M, Crilly J: Review article: staff perception of the emergency department working environment: Integrative review of the literature, *Emergency Medicine Australasia* 28(1):7–26, 2016. http://dx.doi.org/10.1111/1742-6723.12522.
16. United States Department of Labor. (n.d.). Retrieved from https://www.osha.gov/SLTC/workplaceviolence/.
17. Edward K, Ousey K, Warelow P, Lui S: Nursing and aggression in the workplace: a systematic review, *British Journal of Nursing* 23(12), 2014.
18. Granstra K: Nurse against nurse: horizontal bullying in the nursing profession, *Journal of Healthcare Management* 60(4), 2015.
19. Rammer F, Ball C: Perceptions of horizontal violence in staff nurses and intent to leave, *IOS Press* 15:91, 2015.
20. Epstein B, Turner M: The nursing code of ethics: its value, its history, *The Online Journal of Issues in Nursing* 20(2):4, 2015.
21. Ganz FD, Wagner N, Toren O: Nurse middle manager ethical dilemmas and moral distress, *Nursing Ethics* 22(1):43–45, 2014.
22. Wagner JM, Dahnke MD: Nursing ethics and disaster triage: applying utilitarian ethical theory, *Journal of Emergency Nursing* 41(4):300–306, 2015.
23. Boysen II PG: Just culture: a foundation for balanced accountability and patient safety, *The Ochsner Journal* 13:400–406, 2013.
24. Team, B. T. (n.d.). What does our model of accountability look like? Retrieved from https://www.outcome-eng.com/getting-to-know-just-culture.
25. Frank-Cooper M: The justice behind a just culture, *Nephrology Nursing Journal* 41(1), 2014.
26. Emergency Nurses Association: *Position statement: Chemical impairment of emergency nurses*, Des Plaines, IL, 2010, Emergency Nurses Association.
27. American Nurses Association. (n.d.). Impaired nurses resource center. Retrieved from http://nursingworld.org/impaired.

Bibliography

Peck JL: Social media in nursing education: Responsible integration for meaningful use, *Journal of Nursing Education* 53(3):164–169, 2014.
Simpson RL: Social media creates significant risks for nursing, *Nursing Administration Quarterly* 38(1):96–108, 2014.

Part 4

CHAPTER 47

Research and Evidence-Based Practice

Lisa Adams Wolf, PhD, RN, CEN, FAEN

Nursing research and evidence-based practice are an integral aspect of daily emergency nursing practice. The application of research findings is essential to ensure that the care provided will result in the best clinical outcomes possible for the patient.

Research is a process of systematic inquiry; a question exists, investigation occurs, data are analyzed, and conclusions are reached. In reviewing evidence, emergency nurses look at what is known about a specific clinical condition or circumstance, evaluate the evidence, and derive best practices from the interpretations. The use of research and evidence and their incorporation into practice is an iterative loop in which research findings inform practice, which in turn contributes to the body of evidence with regard to a clinical situation or problem.

I. Purpose

A. ESTABLISHES THE SCIENTIFIC BASIS FOR PRACTICE

B. IDENTIFIES THE SCOPE OF EMERGENCY NURSING PRACTICE

C. FACILITATES EVALUATION OF EMERGENCY NURSING PRACTICE

D. PROVIDES A BASIS FOR ACCOUNTABILITY

E. DOCUMENTS EMERGENCY NURSING CONTRIBUTIONS TO HEALTH CARE

F. ASSESSES OUTCOMES OF EMERGENCY NURSING CARE

G. VALIDATES AND REFINES EXISTING EMERGENCY NURSING KNOWLEDGE

H. GENERATES NEW KNOWLEDGE RELATED TO NURSING CARE OF EMERGENCY PATIENTS

I. DESCRIBES AND PROMOTES THE UNDERSTANDING OF HUMAN EXPERIENCES

II. Nursing Education and Research Functions

A. EDUCATION INSTITUTIONS

1. Educational institutions should incorporate research courses and opportunities into nursing programs to familiarize nurses with the research process and related responsibilities

B. NURSING RESEARCH AND EVIDENCE-BASED PRACTICE

1. Nursing research and evidence-based practice are an integral aspect of daily emergency nursing practice.
2. Every single day the use of research findings is essential to ensure that the care provided will result in the best clinical outcomes that are possible for the patient.

3. A compelling need to provide the best nursing care causes nurses to seek out evidence that supports best practice.
4. Research is a process of systematic inquiry; a question exists, investigation occurs, data are analyzed, and conclusions are reached.
5. In using evidence-based practice, emergency nurses look at what is known about a specific clinical condition or circumstance, evaluate the evidence, and derive best practices from the interpretations.
6. The use of research and evidence and their incorporation into practice is an iterative loop in which research findings inform practice, which in turn contributes to the body of evidence with regard to a clinical situation or problem.

III. Research Projects

A. RESEARCH STUDY

1. Uses formal plan to study a problem
2. Ideally should be based on theory or generate theory
3. Uses appropriate data collection and analysis methods for the question being asked
4. Is concerned with issues of reliability and validity in quantitative research and auditability, credibility, and fittingness in qualitative research
5. May suggest solutions with wide applications for quantitative research or describe and give meaning to life experiences for qualitative research

IV. Research Methodologies

A. QUANTITATIVE (TABLE 47.1)

1. Described as a formal, objective, and systemic process: deductive process
2. Uses numeric data to quantify findings
3. Used to describe variables, examine relationships among variables, and determine cause-and-effect interactions between variables
4. Is most frequently used method of research studies
5. Identification of dependent and independent variables
   a. Dependent variables: what the researcher is interested in exploring, understanding, and measuring; it is the answer or outcome response
   b. Independent variables: what the researcher believes to be the cause of or influence on dependent variables; variable manipulated by the researcher; it is factor that contributes to the outcome
      1) Example: "What effect is there on turnover among emergency nurses who work in level I trauma centers versus those who work in freestanding urgent care centers?"

Table 47.1

Comparison of Four Quantitative Research Methods

Method	Sample Research Question	Setting/Participants	Examples	Types of Results
Descriptive	Does the use of a five-level triage method increase the triage nurse's confidence when assigning triage acuities?	Urban ED/triage nurses with at least 1 year of experience	Surveys using Likert-type scales 1 = no change 2 = neutral 3 = improved confidence	Research that describes phenomena as they exist
Correlational (prospective or retrospective)	Was triage acuity predictive of length of stay in the ED?	All ED visits will be reviewed for a 30-day period	Retrospective chart review of acuity and length of stay	Variables are not manipulated; researcher uses measures of association to study their relations
Quasi-experimental	Do triage nurses assign acuity levels more accurately using a three-level or a five-level triage method?	Urban and rural EDs will be selected to participate	ED visit acuities will be reassessed by experienced triage nurses for interrater reliability	Manipulates some independent variables but cannot randomly assign subjects to control/experimental groups
Experimental	Do selected teachable-moment messages reduce repeat ED visits?	ED patients with an acuity level of 4 or 5	ED patients will be randomly assigned to either: standard care (no teachable-moment messages) versus teachable-moment messages	Strength is in random assignment (e.g., number of ED visits by group will be delineated and appropriate inferential statistics will be performed to determine statistical significance)

ED, Emergency department.

Table 47.2

Comparison of Three Qualitative Research Methods

Method	Sample Research Question	Setting/Participants	Strategies	Types of Results
Phenomenology	What is the lived experienced by those individual family members who witness an ED resuscitation?	Individual interviews are conducted at a time and location most convenient for participant, soon after the event	Expansive audiotaped conversations Analysis of data for congruent themes	Comprehensive reflective description experience of the grief present during resuscitation
Grounded theory	What is the process of being present during a resuscitation of a family member in the ED presence?	Individual interviews of participants to saturation of data	Audiotape interviews	Grounded theory development related to the process of witnessing resuscitation
Ethnography	What are the observed patterns of behavior experienced by family members present during resuscitation?	ED observation during family presence 25–50 participant interviews	Observer data	Data analysis related to observations of behavioral patterns

ED, Emergency department.

a) Dependent variable: turnover rates of emergency nurses
b) Independent variable: type of emergency setting (level I trauma or freestanding urgent care centers)

B. QUALITATIVE (TABLE 47.2)

1. Described as a systematic, interactive, and subjective approach
2. Uses words, not numbers, to give meaning to data
3. Used to describe life experiences and give them meaning
4. Is used less frequently than quantitative research, often generates rich, meaningful data
5. Inductive methods

C. MIXED METHODS

1. Provides both the description of a problem as well as explicating contextual factors and possible solutions
2. Can be employed in both quantitative and qualitative studies; can include a blending of both methodologies

3. Allows limitations of two methodologies to be overcome by comparing findings from different perspectives
4. May be used to overcome weaknesses in a specific method of data collection by using many strategies to avoid potential deficiencies of a single methodology or theory

V. Research Process Steps

A. QUESTION OR PROBLEM FORMULATION (FOR QUANTITATIVE)

1. Definition of problem
   a. Is derived from gaps in the literature
   b. Describes the setting and population for which the problem is relevant
   c. Is current and relevant to the present and future of nursing
   d. Is clear, concise, and cogent
   e. Provides direction for the research project
2. Research question
   a. Directs research
   b. Includes one topic per question
   c. Provides basis for study methodology
   d. Example: "What effect does performing a brief intervention have on the number of emergency department visits for alcohol-related injuries?"

B. PROBLEM STATEMENT

1. Definition
   a. Introduction of research topic
   b. Explanation of importance of problem
   c. What the investigator hopes to investigate
   d. Full exposure of idea that needs to be studied
   e. Logical ordering of thoughts about problem
2. Elements in formulating the problem statement
   a. Initial literature search
      1) Substantiates rationale for development and narrowing of problem
      2) Provides references that support researcher's justification for studying problem
   b. Rationale for developing research question includes
      1) Why there is a need for this particular research topic (identifying the gap in knowledge)
      2) Why an answer for this question is so important from a nursing standpoint
      3) How the findings might be applied to practice
3. Theoretical or conceptual framework
   a. Both describe framework for study
   b. Theoretical frameworks are composed of a set of concepts in which the relationships among concepts are described
   c. Conceptual frameworks are the building blocks of theoretical frameworks; they may include

multiple concepts related to a common theme (e.g., child maltreatment, anger) and tend to be more global and less testable than theoretical frameworks
   d. Not all research studies have a fully developed conceptual or theoretical framework (e.g., descriptive or exploratory research studies)

C. LITERATURE REVIEW

1. A critique or analysis of existing research that should help researcher identify and evaluate data from previous research studies; can provide or examine three types of information
   a. Findings from previous studies
   b. Theoretical or conceptual basis
   c. Sources of methodology: instruments to be used to measure variables
   d. Synthesizes similar findings and highlights discrepancies and gaps in the literature, and yields
      1) A summary of major agreements and disagreements in the literature
      2) A summary of general conclusions that are being drawn
      3) Possible ways to address your own problem
   e. Establishes need for proposed or completed study
2. Steps to use when critiquing a research study for review of literature
   a. Usefulness of study
      1) Literature reviewed can be used in research study
         a) Similar clinical problem
         b) Setting
         c) Sample population
         d) Classic source or current literature usually less than 5 years old
         e) IRB process followed
         f) Applicable to emergency nursing practice
   b. Completeness
      1) Study being reviewed follows a sequence expected of a research study
      2) Steps in the research process flow in logical order and are described in appropriate depth and scope in the reviewed study
      3) Method is consistent with and supportive of what was described in the problem statement and hypothesis

D. HYPOTHESIS FORMULATION (IF APPROPRIATE)

1. Can have a theoretical basis
2. Is a method of showing a relationship among two or more variables
3. Example: "An emergency nursing–sponsored community health program on bicycle safety and helmet use will result in a decreased number of head injuries in those who attend all six sessions"

E. DEFINITION OF TERMS

1. Operational definitions: specify what the researcher wants to study and how he or she wants to study it (e.g., an emergency nurse can be operationally defined as a registered nurse with a baccalaureate degree in nursing who works in an emergency care setting)
2. Theoretical definitions: abstract definitions that arise from theory or conceptual framework used (e.g., an emergency nurse can be theoretically defined as a person who provides nursing care to patients in an emergency care facility)

F. METHODOLOGY

1. Research approaches: the selection of a specific approach depends on research purposes. Approaches can be categorized as
   a. Quantitative
   b. Qualitative
2. Research instruments
   a. Methods used to collect, measure, and record data
   b. Types of research instruments
      1) Interviews: involve interviews with each participant in the study; interviews are recorded for further analysis
      2) Questionnaires: involve written responses of participants to open or closed questions
      3) Observational tools: entail recording observations of patients, families, or staff by the researcher for later analysis
      4) Physiologic tools: may involve noninvasive measures (e.g., electrocardiogram [ECG]) or invasive measures (e.g., serum blood samples and values)
      5) Record analysis: involves careful auditing of charts and records to obtain data for analysis
   c. Reliability and validity of instrument or tool
      1) Researcher needs to show reliability and validity of instrument that is being used
      2) Reliability of instrument or tool is support for how consistently tool measures what it is supposed to measure (e.g., internal consistency, interrater, intrarater)
      3) Validity of instrument or tool refers to extent to which tool or instrument measures what it is supposed to measure; there are several ways to measure an instrument's validity (i.e., content, criterion related, construct)
3. Sample and population
   a. The population includes all persons who fit specific characteristics the researcher wants to study; it serves as basis for sample selections
   b. Not every member of a population can be studied, so the researcher takes a sample of the population (e.g., it may be difficult to study the treatment-seeking delay patterns of every patient with acute coronary syndrome who is admitted from the emergency department; therefore, a sample of this population is used)
   c. Population needs to be carefully defined with regard to critical variables to delineate clearly the objects of research study (e.g., does researcher want to study treatment-seeking delay patterns of every patient with acute coronary syndrome who is admitted from the emergency department or only a certain age group, ethnicity, or gender?)
   d. Sample and population must be of adequate size and depend on the research design and problem to be investigated to allow for the research question or purpose to be answered with statistical meaning
   e. Sample methodology depends on financial resources, available time, and availability of subjects; there are various methods of sample selection
      1) Probability
         a) Random
         b) Stratified random
         c) Cluster
         d) Systematic
      2) Nonprobability
         a) Convenience
         b) Quota
         c) Purpose
4. Informed consent
   a. Protection of human subjects: there are key elements that should always be included when obtaining informed consent
      1) In certain emergency situations, informed consent may be waived; however, in most cases, Institutional Review Board (IRB) approval must be obtained as well as patient consent
   b. Code of Federal Regulations (2005) establishes basic elements of informed consent (applies to quantitative and qualitative research [Table 47.3])
   c. Bilingual forms are available when appropriate; it is not sufficient to have emergency department personnel translate documents; all research consents and study documents must be formally translated and back-translated and approved by the IRB prior to use
   d. Approval for research is obtained from appropriate IRB, as required, and Health Insurance Portability and Accountability Act (HIPAA) authorization
      1) Examines investigator's efforts to determine whether proposed study protects subjects' rights
      2) Returns comments and decision of support or nonsupport to investigator

Table 47.3

Elements of Informed Consent

Elements	Justification
Statement that study involves research	Purpose of the research and anticipated number of subjects Expected duration of subject's participation Description of procedures to be followed Identification of experimental procedures
Risks	Description of foreseeable subject risks or discomfort
Benefits	Description of benefits to subject or others that may be reasonably expected from the research
Alternative treatments	Disclosure of appropriate alternate treatments that could be beneficial to the subject
Confidentiality	Description of the extent to which the subject can expect confidentiality to be maintained
More than minimal risk	Explanation of compensation and whether or not medical treatment will be provided if research-related injury occurs
Rights as a research subject	How to obtain additional information, who to contact in the event of research-related injury, and who to contact to answer research-related questions
Voluntary participation	Disclosure that research participation is voluntary and that participation will not result in penalty or loss of benefits
Early study termination	Description of circumstances where the investigator and/or study sponsor may end the study without the subject's consent; description of how the subject can choose to withdraw from the study
Costs	Any additional costs that the subject may incur as a result of the research
New findings	Statement that significant new findings that may affect the subject's willingness to continue will be provided to the subject

From Code of Federal Regulations. (2005). Protection of human subjects: 21CFR50, April 1, 2005. Available at http://www.acess.gpo.gov/nara/cfr/waisidx_05/21cfr50_05.html.

G. DATA ANALYSIS

1. Summarizes all data collected from research study
2. Analysis of numeric data
   a. Descriptive analysis
      1) Provides description of data collected from sample
      2) Usually used with descriptive or exploratory research designs
      3) Describes what was seen or found in sample
      4) Example: median, mode, range, standard deviation, correlation coefficients
      5) Does not make any comparisons between groups
   b. Inferential analysis
      1) Based on analysis and derives inferences about population from sample
      2) Tests hypothesis to determine whether scientific hunch was correct
      3) Depending data type (categorical or continuous variables) and distribution, can use either parametric or nonparametric statistics
3. Analysis of nonnumeric data
   a. Used to provide a description and thematic interpretation of people, places, situations, happenings, opinions, attitudes, or behaviors
   b. Can be used to generate theory or hypothesis for future testing
   c. Data usually come from written documents or notes related to unstructured interviews, observations, medical records, open-ended responses to questions on questionnaires, and other written accounts
   d. Involves reviewing written material for categories, themes, or patterns in data
   e. Analysis of interviews with patients about care received in the emergency department may reveal the following themes: patients were satisfied with nursing care received, patients were dissatisfied with their waiting time to be seen, and nurses were viewed as being concerned about patient's condition or illness

H. FINDINGS/RESULTS, CONCLUSIONS, AND RECOMMENDATIONS

1. Should be structured according to the research question(s). Initially, a description of the results of data analysis should be presented
2. If the question is qualitative, using the example *How do nurses identify sepsis patients in triage?* there may be a description of emerging themes (commonalities in the experience), such as *eyeballing the patient, feeling that something isn't right, pressing for detail, etc…*, which describe a *process.*
3. The research question, *How accurately do emergency nurses identify sepsis in triage?* Is answered using quantitative data, and results should reflect that by reporting comparative statistical data

(t-tests, Pearson's r, Chi-square, regression analysis, ANOVA).

4. Results are stated and data may be displayed in tables or graphs
5. Based on results of data analysis, conclusions are drawn
6. Based on study's results and conclusions, recommendations are made for interventions as appropriate and future research
7. Limitations are acknowledged

I. COMMUNICATION OF FINDINGS

This is the final step of the research process, which is necessary if research findings are to be integrated into practice.

1. Professional journals (e.g., *Journal of Emergency Nursing; Nursing Research*)
2. Professional meetings (e.g., Emergency Nurses Association Annual Conference Research Presentation)

VI. Research Ethics

A. HUMAN SUBJECTS AND ETHICAL GUIDELINES

1. Developed as a result of recognition of unethical treatment of and harm to subjects in earlier research studies, such as withholding treatment to persons with syphilis to study effects of the disease
2. IRBs were developed to review all research studies to ensure that research subjects' rights and safety are maintained
3. Department of Health and Human Services instituted the following regulations in 1983
   a. Requirements for and documentation of informed consent
   b. IRB review of research proposals
   c. Procedures for expedited and exempt reviews
   d. Criteria for IRB approval of research proposals
4. Human rights to be maintained while participating in a research project
   a. Right to self-determination
   b. Right to privacy and dignity
   c. Right to anonymity and confidentiality
   d. Right to fair treatment
   e. Right to protection from discomfort and harm
5. Protection of human rights is ensured through informed consent

B. ANIMAL SUBJECTS AND ETHICAL GUIDELINES

1. Rights of animals used in research are controlled by legislation in the United States
2. Animal Care and Use Committees (ACUCs) are the equivalent of the IRB for protecting animal rights
3. Research involving animals must be approved by the ACUC

C. SCIENTIFIC FRAUD AND MISCONDUCT

1. Includes the following circumstances
   a. Inventing data for a project
   b. Falsifying or altering data
   c. Reporting another researcher's results as one's own
   d. Plagiarism
   e. Violating animal or human rights
2. Agencies exist to investigate allegations of scientific misconduct or fraud

VII. Application to Clinical Practice

Before the findings of a research study can be used in clinical practice, several questions need to be answered.

A. DO STUDY FINDINGS ADDRESS CURRENT CLINICAL PROBLEMS? IS THERE RELEVANCE TO CLINICAL PRACTICE?

B. DOES STUDY INCLUDE AN APPROPRIATE SUBJECT POPULATION?

C. WERE SUBJECTS' RIGHTS PROTECTED?

D. WAS STUDY ETHICAL, LEGAL, AND FEASIBLE?

E. WAS A CRITICAL REVIEW OF THE LITERATURE DONE?

F. IS STUDY'S SETTING SIMILAR TO OR DIFFERENT FROM INTENDED PRACTICE SETTING?

G. IS SAMPLE SIMILAR TO INTENDED POPULATION TO WHICH YOU HOPE TO APPLY FINDINGS?

H. ARE THE RESEARCH INSTRUMENTS OR TOOLS USED RELIABLE AND VALID?

I. ARE FINDINGS CONSISTENT WITH PRACTICE?

J. DO OTHER STUDIES REPORT SIMILAR OR DIFFERENT FINDINGS?

VIII. Critiquing Research

A. QUANTITATIVE RESEARCH STUDIES

1. Title
   a. Readily understood
   b. Related to content of study
2. Abstract
   a. Background information briefly described
   b. Problem or purpose, hypothesis, or questions are outlined clearly and concisely
   c. Methodology is identified and described briefly
   d. Analysis of data is succinctly described
   e. Important results/findings discussed
   f. Conclusions are clear
3. Problem statement/purposes
   a. General problem statement is narrowed to a specific statement
   b. Definite statement of problem and purposes of study
   c. Information is clear and concise
   d. Definitions of terms are complete
   e. Precise information about variables studied
   f. Background information clearly and concisely describes importance of study
4. Review of literature
   a. Literature reviews information relevant to problem and purpose of study
   b. Literature review is adequate (content saturation achieved)
   c. Literature review is taken from peer reviewed journals, books, and general scientific sources; primary sources preferred
   d. Review of literature is clear, concise, and logically organized
   e. Research used in literature review is critically analyzed, and the review concludes with synopsis of literature and its implications for this study
5. Framework: theoretical-conceptual
   a. Linkage of problem to theory or concept
   b. Selected framework makes sense and is relevant to research focus
   c. Deductions from theory or conceptual framework are clear, correct, and well defined
6. Hypothesis and questions of study
   a. Study identifies hypothesis or questions for the research proposed
   b. Each question or hypothesis shows a relationship between two or more variables
   c. Hypotheses and questions are testable
   d. Hypothesis and questions are worthy of study
7. Method
   a. Research design examples
      1) Descriptive
      2) Correlational
      3) Quasi-experimental
      4) Experimental
   b. Research procedure
      1) Method chosen for study is described in detail
      2) Contamination of groups is adequately addressed
      3) Research is conducted in proper setting
      4) Subjects are protected
   c. Subjects
      1) Sample size is appropriate to provide enough data for significant findings to be revealed
      2) Sample is representative of population studied
      3) Population is clearly defined
      4) Inclusion and exclusion criteria are appropriately described and applied to the study
      5) Subject selection is described
   d. Data collection
      1) Instruments or tools used are clearly defined and described
      2) Instruments or tools are reliable and valid for use in the study
      3) Methods used to collect the data are appropriate
      4) If new instruments or tools were developed, there is evidence that they were properly tested and described
   e. Data analysis
      1) Detailed description of how the data are analyzed
      2) Chosen statistical methods used are appropriate for the study data
      3) Confidentiality is provided for and ensured
      4) Internal consistency in data analysis is sought
   f. Results
      1) Sample is clearly described (number and characteristics)
      2) Results are reported and interpreted correctly
      3) Hypothesis and questions are answered
      4) Tables and graphs are presented clearly, correctly, and concisely
      5) Readers can understand tables and graphs and determine results
      6) Consistency is found in data interpretation and table construction
8. Discussion section
   a. Research discussed in the context of the current literature
      1) Methodologic problems are discussed
   b. Meaning of research findings discussed
   c. Limitations of project identified
9. Conclusions
   a. Clearly stated and concise
   b. Substantiated by data analysis
   c. Results are generalizable to population identified in study
10. Implications for further research
    a. Clear and applicable
    b. Based on data analysis
    c. Meaningful and realistic

Part 4

B. QUALITATIVE RESEARCH STUDIES

1. Title
   a. Readily understood
   b. Related to content of study
2. Abstract
   a. Background information briefly described
   b. Problem or purpose, or questions are clearly and concisely outlined
   c. Methodology is identified and briefly described
   d. Analysis of data is succinctly summarized
   e. Important results/findings are described and discussed
   f. Conclusions are clear
3. Problem statement/purposes/study context
   a. Research questions and purpose of study are well written and easily understood
   b. Phenomenon, idea, culture, or topic is clearly defined
   c. There is adequate description of people, places, events, and/or site of study
   d. The philosophic basis for study is described
   e. Background information clearly and concisely describes importance of study (this can include a brief review of literature which describes the gap being explored by the study)
4. Framework: theoretical-conceptual
   a. Linkage of problem to theory or concept
   b. Selected framework makes sense and is relevant to research focus
   c. Conceptual framework is well defined
5. Questions of research study
   a. Qualitative method used to collect data is identified and described in detail
   b. Method is consistent with research questions and purpose
   c. Researcher follows method consistently
   d. Sampling procedures are explained
   e. Sampling procedures are appropriate for type of qualitative method used
   f. Participants selected are able to provide data required for this project (i.e., they have they experienced the phenomenon or been a member of the culture under study)
   g. Sample size is adequate to ensure data saturation or to provide a complete picture of the culture, behavior, or events
   h. Steps used to collect data are described
   i. Data collection strategies are consistent with research method selected
   j. Data collection strategies provide the type of data required for this study
   k. Human subjects are protected
6. Method
   a. Research design examples
      1) Phenomenology
      2) Grounded theory
      3) Ethnography
   b. Research procedure
      1) Method chosen for study is described in detail
      2) Research is conducted in proper setting
      3) Participants are protected
   c. Participants
      1) Appropriate number of participants to provide adequate data
      2) Population of interest is clearly defined
      3) Inclusion and exclusion are appropriately described and applied to the study
      4) Participant selected is described
   d. Data collection
      1) Data collection procedure is clearly defined and described
      2) Data collected is trustworthy
      3) Methods used to collect the data are appropriate
   e. Data analysis
      1) Detailed description of how the data are analyzed
      2) Analysis methods are appropriate to data and study aims/purpose
      3) Confidentiality is provided for and ensured
   f. Findings
      1) Sample characteristics are clearly described
      2) Findings are reported and interpreted correctly
      3) Study purpose is addressed
      4) Tables and graphs are set up clearly, correctly, and concisely
      5) Readers can understand tables, graphs, and study findings
      6) Consistency is found in data interpretation and table construction
7. Discussion section
   a. Research discussed in the context of the current literature (this incorporates the review of literature)
      1) Methodologic problems are discussed
   b. Meaning of research findings discussed
   c. Limitations to generalizability discussed
8. Conclusions
   a. Clearly and concisely stated
   b. Substantiated by data analysis
9. Implications for further research
   a. Clear and applicable
   b. Based on data analysis
   c. Meaningful and realistic

IX. Using Evidence-Based Practice

A. COMPONENTS OF EVIDENCE-BASED PRACTICE

1. Evidence from research, evidence-based theories, leaders, and expert panels

Table 47.4

Rating System for Hierarchy of Evidence

Level	Criteria
I	Evidence from systematic review or meta-analyses of relevant randomized controlled trials or evidence-based clinical practice guidelines based on randomized clinical trials
II	Evidence from at least one well-designed randomized clinical trial
III	Evidence obtained from nonrandomized well-designed controlled trials
IV	Evidence from well-designed case-control or cohort studies
V	Evidence from systematic reviews of descriptive or qualitative studies
VI	Evidence from a single descriptive or qualitative study
VII	Evidence from opinions of content authorities or reports of expert panels

2. Evidence from clinical assessment of the patient and availability of health care resources
3. Clinical expertise
4. Information about patient preferences and values

B. ESSENTIAL STEPS OF EVIDENCE-BASED PRACTICE

1. Formulate the critical clinical question
2. Collect most relevant and best evidence
3. Critically evaluate the evidence (Table 47.4)
4. Integrate the evidence with personal clinical expertise, patient preferences, and values in determining a practice decision or change
5. Evaluate the practice decision or change

Bibliography

Code of Federal Regulations: Protection of human subjects: 21CFR50. Retrieved from http://www.acess.gpo.gov/nara/cfr/waisidx_05/21cfr50_05.html, 2005.

Code of Federal Regulations: Protection of human subjects: 45CFR46. Retrieved from http://www.acess.gpo.gov/nara/cfr/waisidx_05/45cfr46_05.html, 2005.

Crabtree B, Miller W: *Doing qualitative research*, ed 2, Thousand Oaks, CA, 1999, Sage.

Melnyk B, Fineout-Overholt E: *Evidence-based practice in nursing and healthcare*, Philadelphia, PA, 2005, Lippincott Williams & Wilkins.

Polit D, Beck C: *Nursing research principles and methods*, ed 7, Philadelphia, PA, 2004, Lippincott Williams & Wilkins.

Wood M, Ross-Kerr J: *Basic steps in planning nursing research from question to proposal*, ed 6, Sudbury, MA, 2006, Jones and Bartlett.

Part 4

CHAPTER 48

Violence in the Emergency Care Setting

Lisa Adams Wolf, PhD, RN, CEN, FAEN

Although violence in the emergency care setting has been previously documented, the precursors and sequelae of violence perpetrated against emergency nurses and other health care workers by patients and visitors are not well understood. It is known that emergency department incidents of violence cause physical and psychological damage and that emergency nurses leave the profession as a result. An understanding of the nature and types of violence that emergency nurses may encounter and strategies to recognize and mitigate violence in the emergency setting are warranted. Findings from research studies identify some of the physical and psychological long-term consequences of violence experienced by nurses while they are providing patient care. These consequences lead to lost productivity, contribute to the attrition from the emergency nursing profession, and impede nurses' ability to effectively deliver patient care. With the clear and long-lasting impact of workplace violence, it is imperative that hospitals and emergency care workers address the issue proactively through adoption of violence prevention education, zero tolerance policies, safety measures, and procedures for reporting and responding to incidents of workplace violence when they do occur.

I. Definitions

A. WORKPLACE VIOLENCE

1. Any action, incident, or behavior that departs from reasonable conduct in which a person is assaulted, threatened, harmed, injured in the course of, or as a direct result of, his or her work[1]

B. INTERNAL WORKPLACE VIOLENCE

1. That which takes place between workers, including managers and supervisors

C. EXTERNAL WORKPLACE VIOLENCE

1. That which takes place between workers (and managers and supervisors) and any other person present at the workplace

II. Bowie's Expanded Typology of Violence[2]

A. TYPE 1 - EXTERNAL/INTRUSIVE VIOLENCE

1. Criminal intent by strangers
2. Terrorist acts including sabotage and kidnappings
3. Protest violence
4. Mental illness or drug-related aggression
5. Random violence

B. TYPE 2 – CONSUMER-RELATED VIOLENCE

1. Consumer/clients/patients (and family) violence against staff
2. Vicarious trauma to staff
3. Staff violence against clients/consumers, including terrorist acts

C. TYPE 3 - STAFF-RELATED VIOLENCE

1. Staff-on-staff violence and bullying, including terrorist acts
2. Domestic violence and sexual harassment at work
3. Third-party violence

D. TYPE 4 - ORGANIZATIONAL VIOLENCE

1. Organizational violence against staff
2. Organizational violence against consumers/clients/patients
3. Organizational violence against other organizations or communities
4. Organizationally condoned or sponsored terrorist acts

III. Violence Against ED Nurses

Violence against ED nurses is common (56.7% reported violence in the previous 7 days).[3]

A. HOW NURSES FEEL

1. Workplaces are unsafe (57.6% of nurses rated the safety of their ED as a 5 or lower on a 1–10 scale)
2. There is little institutional support to protect them
3. Not confident to manage a violent patient in the ED
4. They are substantially more committed to eliminating violence against nurses than their hospital administrations
5. One third of emergency nurses surveyed had considered leaving their ED or emergency nursing because of ED violence

B. CONTRIBUTING FACTORS TO WORKPLACE VIOLENCE[3]

1. Alcohol (79%)
2. Boarding of admitted patients (43.3%)
3. Acceptance of violence as a coping method (47.9%)
4. Drug-seeking behavior (88.2%)
5. Dementia/Alzheimer patients (44.2%)
6. Crowding (78.4%)

C. ELEMENTS OF VIOLENCE MANAGEMENT PROGRAMS[4]

1. Necessary foundational behaviors
   a. What is the social environment of my institution or unit?
   b. How do nurses relate to each other?
   c. What is the hierarchical structure of a given unit? The entire institution?
   d. Is there a sense of collaboration, or are disciplines working in silos?
2. Essential elements of a zero-tolerance program
   a. A JCAHO leadership standard effective January 1, 2009, requires hospitals and other accredited organizations to adopt and implement a code of conduct that defines and manages disruptive or inappropriate behavior by physicians and administrators
   b. The development of an identification system for potential violence, response to threats or violent events, and constructive support procedures after the event will contribute to zero tolerance of violence in the workplace[5]
   c. "Zero tolerance" that the organization acknowledges the threat of violence and puts in place infrastructure to identify and mitigate its impact on staff
   d. "A comprehensive organizational violence prevention program should include a reporting and documentation system for acts of violence and a workplace violence prevention policy that includes specific strategies that can be instituted system-wide in the event of a violent incident, as well as post-event support and adequate training of personnel for pre and post-event incident management."[6,7,8]
3. Ensuring ownership and accountability
   a. Ensuring that all staff understand both the overall culture around violence in the workplace and the specific behaviors that comprise violence in its myriad forms
   b. Lateral (staff–staff)
   c. Organizational (administration–staff)
   d. External (patients/visitors–staff)
4. Proper training and education
   a. Evidence-based training in
      1) Violence recognition and mitigation
      2) Deescalation techniques
      3) Communication strategies
      4) Security strategies
5. Outcome metrics
   a. How can an institution measure outcomes?
      1) Increased reporting of violent incidents
      2) Interventions in place to reduce escalation and assault
      3) Tracking of the nature and number of incidents institution-wide
      4) Perception of safety by staff
      5) Cultural changes in the acceptance of violence of all kinds
6. Nurse-to-nurse (lateral) violence
   a. Nurse-to-nurse aggression with overtly or covertly directed dissatisfaction toward another
   b. Origins include role issues, oppression, strict hierarchy, disenfranchising work practices, low self-esteem, powerlessness perception, anger, and circuits of power.[9] Research suggests that up to 90% of nurses experience some form of lateral violence at work[10]
      1) Implications for job satisfaction, burnout, and patient safety

a) Nurses report increased anxiety, depression, and sleeplessness[11]

2) Up to 60% of new graduate nurses left their first job because of lateral violence and poor resolution of coworker conflict[12]

3) Lateral violence can become "normalized" and part of the culture of a unit if not checked

4) Interventions that improve communication strategies for nurses can help mitigate lateral violence[10]

References

1. International Labor Organization: Work-related violence and its integration into existing surveys. Retrieved from http://www.ilo.org/wcmsp5/groups/public/—dgreports/—stat/documents/meetingdocument/wcms_222231.pdf, 2003.

2. Bowie V, Fisher B, & Cooper C: *Workplace violence: Issues, trends, strategies*, London, 2011, Willan.

3. Emergency Nurses Association: Emergency department violence surveillance study. Retrieved from https://www.ena.org/practice-research/research/Documents/ENAEDVSReportNovember2011.pdf, 2011.

4. American Organization of Nurse Executives: AONE/ENA tool kit for mitigating violence in the workplace. Retrieved from http://www.aone.org/resources/final_toolkit.pdf, 2015.

5. Clements PT, et al.: Workplace violence and corporate policy for health care settings, *Nursing Economics* 23(3):119–124, 2005. Retrieved from http://www.ncbi.nlm.nih.gov/pubmed/16033140.

6. Bruser S: Workplace violence: Getting hospitals focused on prevention, *American Nurse* 30(3):11, 1998.

7. Burgess AW, Douglas JE, Burgess AG, Baker T, Suave H, Gariti K: Hospital communication threats and intervention, *Journal of Psychosocial Nursing & Mental Health Services* 35(8):42–43, 1997.

8. Williams ML, Robertson K: Workplace violence: Prevalence, prevention and first line interventions, *Critical Care Clinics of North America* 9(2):221–228, 1997.

9. Embree JL & White AH: Concept analysis: Nurse-to-nurse lateral violence, *Nursing Forum* 45(3):166–173, 2010.

10. Ceravolo DJ, Schwartz DG, Foltz-Ramos KM, Castner J: Strengthening communication to overcome lateral violence, *Journal of Nursing Management* 1–8, 2012.

11. Hutchinson M, Wilkes L, Vickers M, & Jackson D: The development and validation of a bullying inventory for the nursing workplace, *Nurse Researcher* 15(2):19–29, 2008.

12. Griffin M: Teaching cognitive rehearsal as a shield for lateral violence: An intervention for newly licensed nurses, *The Journal of Continuing Education in Nursing* 35(6):257–263, 2004.

Coma Scales

Comparison of the FOUR Score with the Glasgow Coma Scale

Glasgow Coma Scale	FOUR Score
Eye response 4 = eyes open spontaneously 3 = eye opening to verbal command 2 = eye opening to pain 1 = no eye opening	**Eye response** 4 = eyelids open or opened, tracking, or blinking to command 3 = eyelids open but not tracking 2 = eyelids closed but open to loud voice 1 = eyelids closed but open to pain 0 = eyelids remain closed with pain
Motor response 6 = obeys commands 5 = localizing pain 4 = withdrawal from pain 3 = flexion response to pain 2 = extension response to pain 1 = no motor response	**Motor response** 4 = thumbs-up, fist, or peace sign 3 = localizing to pain 2 = flexion response to pain 1 = extension response to pain 0 = no response to pain or generalized myoclonus status
Verbal response 5 = oriented 4 = confused 3 = inappropriate words 2 = incomprehensible sounds 1 = no verbal response	**Brainstem reflexes** 4 = pupil and corneal reflexes present 3 = one pupil wide and fixed 2 = pupil or corneal reflexes absent 1 = pupil and corneal reflexes absent 0 = absent pupil, corneal, and cough reflex
	Respiration 4 = not intubated, regular breathing pattern 3 = not intubated, Cheyne-Stokes breathing pattern 2 = not intubated, irregular breathing 1 = breathes above ventilator rate 0 = breathes at ventilator rate or apnea

FOUR = Full Outline of UnResponsiveness.

(From Wijdicks MD, Bamlet WR, Maramattom BV, Manno EM, & McClelland RL. [2005]. Validation of a new coma scale: The FOUR score. Annals of Neurology, 58 [4], 585-593.)

Glasgow Coma Scale

Category	Score	Response
Eye opening	4	Spontaneous: eyes open spontaneously without stimulation
	3	To speech: eyes open with verbal stimulation but not necessarily to command
	2	To pain: eyes open with noxious stimuli
	1	None: no eye opening regardless of stimulation
Verbal response	5	Oriented: accurate information about person, place, time, reason for hospitalization, and personal data
	4	Confused: answers not appropriate to question but use of language is correct
	3	Inappropriate words: disorganized, random speech, no sustained conversation
	2	Incomprehensible sounds: moans, groans, and incomprehensible mumbles
	1	None: no verbalization despite stimulation
Best motor response	6	Obeys commands: performs simple tasks on command; able to repeat performance
	5	Localizes to pain: organized attempt to localize to remove painful stimuli
	4	Withdraws from pain: withdraws extremity from source of painful stimuli
	3	Abnormal flexion: decorticate posturing spontaneously or in response to noxious stimuli
	2	Extension: decerebrate posturing spontaneously or in response to noxious stimuli
	1	None: no response to noxious stimuli; flaccid

From ENA (2013). Sheehy's manual of emergency care (7th ed.). St. Louis, MO: Elsevier/Mosby; Data from Urden, L. D., Stacy, K. M., & Lough, M. E. (2010). Critical care nursing: Diagnosis and management (6th ed.). St. Louis, MO: Mosby.

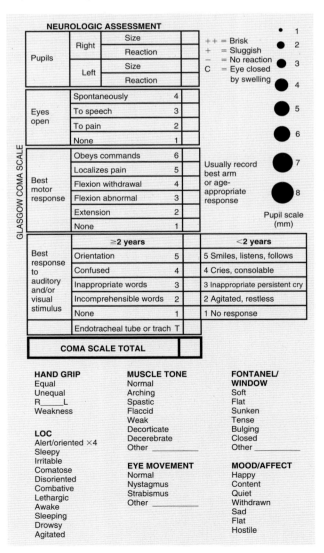

Pediatric Glasgow Coma Scale. *(From Wilson, D. and Hockenberry, M.J. (2012). Wong's clinical manual of pediatric nursing (8th ed.) St. Louis, MO: Elsevier/Mosby.).*

Age-Specific Vital Signs

Normal Vital Signs by Age

Age	Heart Rate (beats/min)	Respiratory Rate (breaths/min)	Systolic Blood Pressure (mm Hg)	Weight (kg)
Preterm	120-180	55-65	40-60	2
Term newborn	90-170	40-60	52-92	3
1 month	110-180	30-50	60-104	4
6 months	110-180	25-35	65-125	7
1 year	80-160	20-30	70-118	10
2 years	80-130	20-30	73-117	12
4 years	80-120	20-30	65-117	16
6 years	75-115	18-24	76-116	20
8 years	70-110	18-22	76-119	25
10 years	70-110	16-20	82-122	30
12 years	60-110	16-20	84-128	40
14 years	60-105	16-20	85-136	50

From ENA: Sheehy's emergency nursing: Principles and practice, ed 6, St. Louis, 2009, Mosby; Modified from Barken RM, Rosen P: Emergency pediatrics, ed 6, St. Louis, 2003, Mosby.

Infant Pain Scales

Neonatal Infant Pain Scale (NIPS)*

Variables	Scoring Range
Facial expression	0–1
Cry	0–2
Breathing patterns	0–1
Arms	0–1
Legs	0–1
State of arousal	0–1

*Scoring range: 0 = no pain; 7 = worst pain.

Pain Assessment Tool (PAT)*

Variables	Scoring Range
Posture/tone	1–2
Sleep pattern	0–2
Expression	1–2
Color	0–2
Cry	0–2
Respiration	1–2
Heart rate	1–2
Oxygen saturation	0–2
Blood pressure	0–2
Nurse's perception	0–2

*Scoring range 4 = no pain; 20 = worst pain.
Modified from Hockenberry M. J., Wilson, D., Winkelstein, M. L., & Kline, N. E. (Eds.). (2003). *Wong's nursing care of infants and children* (7th ed.). St. Louis, MO: Mosby.

FLACC (Face, Legs, Activity, Cry, and Consolability): 3 Months to 7 Years

Categories	Scoring		
	0	**1**	**2**
Face	No particular expression or smile	Occasional grimace or frown; withdrawn, disinterested	Frequent to constant frown, clenched jaw, quivering chin
Legs	Normal position or relaxed	Uneasy, restless, tense	Kicking or legs drawn up
Activity	Lying quietly, normal position, moves easily	Squirming, shifting back and forth, tense	Arched, rigid, or jerking
Cry	No cry (awake or asleep)	Moans or whimpers, occasional complaint	Crying steadily, screams, or sobs; frequent complaints
Consolability	Content, relaxed	Reassured by occasional touching, hugging, or being talked to; distractable	Difficult to console or comfort

Each of the 5 categories is scored from 0 to 2, resulting in a total score between 0 and 10. Prior to scoring, awake children are observed for 2 minutes, asleep for 5 minutes.

From Malviya, S., Voepel-Lewis, T., Burke, C., Merkel, S., & Tait, A. R. (2006). The revised FLACC observational pain tool: improved reliability and validity for pain assessment in children with cognitive impairment. *Pediatric Anesthesia, 16*(3), 258–265.

Revised Trauma Score

Area of Measurement	Coded Value
Systolic Blood Pressure (mm Hg)	
Greater than 89	4
76–89	3
50–75	2
1–49	1
0	0
Respiratory Rate (spontaneous inspirations/minute)*	
Greater than 29	4
10–29	3
6–9	2
1–5	1
0	0
Glasgow Coma Scale Score	
13–15	4
9–12	3
6–8	2
4–5	1
3	0
Total possible points: 0–12	

*patient initiated, not artificial ventilations

From Champion, H. R., Sacco, W. J., Copes, W. S., Gann, D. S., Gennarelli, T. A., & Flanagan, M. E. (1989). A revision of the trauma score. *J Trauma,* 29, 623–629.

Page numbers followed by *f* indicate figures, *t* indicate tables, and *b* indicate boxes.